AMA
AMERICAN MEDICAL ASSOCIATION

2019

ICD-10-PCS

The Complete Official Codebook

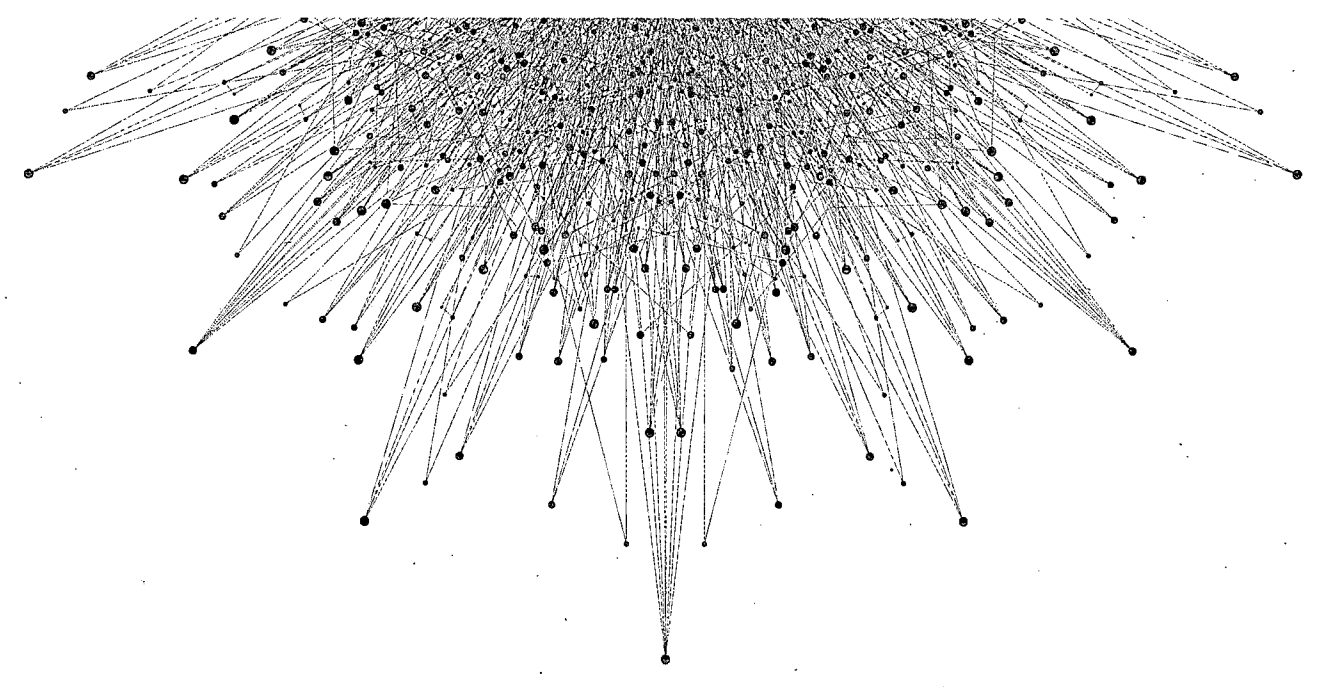

Notice

ICD-10-PCS: The Complete Official Codebook is designed to be an accurate and authoritative source regarding coding and every reasonable effort has been made to ensure accuracy and completeness of the content. However, the AMA makes no guarantee, warranty, or representation that this publication is accurate, complete, or without errors. It is understood that the AMA is not rendering any legal or other professional services or advice in this publication and that the AMA bears no liability for any results or consequences that may arise from the use of this book.

Our Commitment to Accuracy

The AMA is committed to producing accurate and reliable materials. To report corrections, please call the AMA Unified Service Center at (800) 621-8335. AMA product updates, errata, and addendum can be found at amaproductupdates.org.

To purchase additional copies, contact the American Medical Association at 800 621-8335 or visit the AMA store at amastore.com. Refer to product number OP201119.

Copyright

OP201119
BQ45: 8/18

Acknowledgments

Marianne Randall, CPC, *Product Manager*
Karen Schmidt, BSN, *Technical Director*
Anita Schmidt, BS, RHIT, AHIMA-approved ICD-10-CM/PCS Trainer, *Clinical Technical Editor*
Peggy Willard, CCS, AHIMA-approved ICD-10-CM/PCS Trainer, *Clinical Technical Editor*
Stacy Perry, *Manager, Desktop Publishing*
Tracy Betzler, *Senior Desktop Publishing Specialist*
Hope M. Dunn, *Senior Desktop Publishing Specialist*
Katie Russell, *Desktop Publishing Specialist*
Kate Holden, *Editor*

Anita Schmidt, BS, RHIT, AHIMA-approved ICD-10-CM/PCS Trainer

Ms. Schmidt has expertise in Level I adult and pediatric trauma hospital coding, specializing in ICD-9-CM, ICD-10-CM/PCS, DRG, and CPT coding. Her experience includes analysis of medical record documentation, assignment of ICD-10-CM and PCS codes, DRG validation, as well as CPT code assignments for same-day surgery cases. She has conducted coding training and auditing, including DRG validation, conducted electronic health record training, and worked with clinical documentation specialists to identify documentation needs and potential areas for physician education. Most recently she has been developing content for resource and educational products related to ICD-10-CM and ICD-10-PCS. Ms. Schmidt is an AHIMA-approved ICD-10-CM/PCS trainer, and is an active member of the American Health Information Management Association (AHIMA) and the Minnesota Health Information Management Association (MHIMA).

Peggy Willard, CCS, AHIMA-approved ICD-10-CM/PCS Trainer

Ms. Willard has 18 years of experience in the healthcare field. Her expertise is in ICD-10-CM and ICD-10-PCS, including in-depth analysis of medical record documentation, ICD-10-CM/PCS code and DRG assignment, as well as clinical documentation improvement (CDI). In recent years Ms. Willard has been responsible for the creation and development of several products for Optum360 Coding Solutions that are designed to assist with appropriate application of the ICD-10-CM and ICD-10-PCS coding systems. She has several years of prior experience in Level I adult and pediatric trauma hospital and inpatient rehabilitation facility (IRF) coding, specializing in ICD-9-CM diagnosis and procedural coding, with emphasis in conducting coding audits, and conducting coding training for coding staff and clinical documentation specialists. Ms. Willard is an AHIMA-approved ICD-10 CM/PCS trainer and is an active member of the American Health Information Management Association (AHIMA) and the Minnesota Health Information Management Association (MHIMA).

Contents

Notes

Notes

What's New for 2019

The Centers for Medicare and Medicaid Services is the agency charged with maintaining and updating ICD-10-PCS. CMS released the most current revisions, a summary of which may be found on the CMS website at: https://www.cms.gov/Medicare/Coding/ICD10/2019-ICD-10-PCS-and-GEMs.html

Due to the unique structure of ICD-10-PCS, a change in a character value may affect individual codes and several code tables.

Change Summary Table

2018 Total	New Codes	Revised Titles	Deleted Codes	2019 Total
78,705	392	8	216	78,881

ICD-10-PCS Code FY 2019 Totals, By Section

Medical and Surgical	68,639
Obstetrics	302
Placement	861
Administration	1,445
Measurement and Monitoring	414
Extracorporeal or Systemic Assistance and Performance	45
Extracorporeal or Systemic Therapies	46
Osteopathic	100
Other Procedures	60
Chiropractic	90
Imaging	2,941
Nuclear Medicine	463
Radiation Therapy	1,939
Physical Rehabilitation and Diagnostic Audiology	1,380
Mental Health	30
Substance Abuse Treatment	59
New Technology	67
Total	78,881

ICD-10-PCS Changes Highlights

- In the Medical and Surgical section, body part values revised or streamlined for clarity and usefulness as coded data
- ICD-10-PCS guidelines updated with new and revised guidelines
- Root operation Control was added to the Ear, Nose and Sinus body system for the body part of Nasal Mucosa and Soft Tissue
- Root Operation Extraction was added to the Hepatobiliary System and Pancreas body system
- The No Device value was removed from the Fusion root operation tables
- Unicondylar devices (Medial and Lateral) and Articulating Spacers were added to the Removal table and Replacement table in the Lower Joints body system
- New qualifiers were added to identify:
  - — More specificity for Bypass procedures
  - — Drug coated balloon use in Dilation procedures
  - — Stent Retriever use in Extirpation procedures
  - — Use of irreversible electroporation in Destruction procedures

New Definitions Addenda

Section 0 - Medical and Surgical

Body Part Definitions

ICD-10-PCS Value	Definition
Head and Neck Bursa and Ligament	Delete Interspinous ligament Add Interspinous ligament, cervical Add Intertransverse ligament, cervical Add Ligamentum flavum, cervical
Lower Spine Bursa and Ligament	Delete Interspinous ligament Delete Intertransverse ligament Delete Ligamentum flavum Add Interspinous ligament, lumbar Add Intertransverse ligament, lumbar Add Ligamentum flavum, lumbar
Add Mediastinum	Add Mediastinal cavity Add Mediastinal space
Retroperitoneum	Add Retroperitoneal cavity
Rib(s) Bursa and Ligament	Delete Costoxiphoid ligament Delete Sternocostal ligament
Sternum Bursa and Ligament	Delete Costotransverse ligament
Upper Spine Bursa and Ligament	Delete Interspinous ligament Delete Intertransverse ligament Delete Ligamentum flavum Add Interspinous ligament, thoracic Add Intertransverse ligament, thoracic Add Ligamentum flavum, thoracic

Section 0 - Medical and Surgical

Device Definitions

ICD-10-PCS Value	Definition
Add Articulating Spacer in Lower Joints	Add Articulating Spacer (Antibiotic) Add Spacer, Articulating (Antibiotic)
Spacer in Lower Joints	Add Spacer, Static (Antibiotic) Add Static Spacer (Antibiotic)

Section 0 - Medical and Surgical

Device Aggregation Table

Specific Device	for Operation	in Body System	General Device
Delete Synthetic Substitute, Unicondylar	Delete Replacement	Delete Lower Joints	Delete J Synthetic Substitute

Section X - New Technology

Root Operation

ICD-10-PCS Value	Definition
Add Destruction	Add Definition: Physical eradication of all or a portion of a body part by the direct use of energy, force, or a destructive agent Add Explanation: None of the body part is physically taken out Add Includes/Examples: Fulguration of rectal polyp, cautery of skin lesion

Section X - New Technology

Approach

ICD-10-PCS Value	Definition
Add Via Natural or Artificial Opening Endoscopic	Add Definition: Entry of instrumentation through a natural or artificial external opening to reach and visualize the site of the procedure

Section X - New Technology

Device / Substance / Technology

ICD-10-PCS Value	Definition
Engineered Autologous Chimeric Antigen Receptor T-cell Immunotherapy	Add KYMRIAH Add Tisagenlecleucel
Add Synthetic Human Angiotensin II	Add Angiotensin II Add GIAPREZA™ Add Human angiotensin II, synthetic

List of Updated Files

2019 Official ICD-10-PCS Coding Guidelines

- New Guideline B3.17 added in response to public comment.
- Guidelines A10, B3.7, and B6.1a revised in response to public comment and internal review.
- Downloadable PDF, file name pcs_guidelines_2019.pdf

2019 ICD-10-PCS Code Tables and Index (Zip file)

- Code tables for use beginning October 1, 2018
- Downloadable PDF, file name is pcs_2019.pdf
- Downloadable xml files for developers, file names are icd10pcs_tables_2019.xml, icd10pcs_index_2019.xml, icd10pcs_definitions_2019.xml
- Accompanying schema for developers, file names are icd10pcs_tables.xsd, icd10pcs_index.xsd, icd10pcs_definitions.xsd

2019 ICD-10-PCS Codes File (Zip file)

- ICD-10-PCS Codes file is a simple format for non-technical uses, containing the valid FY 2019 ICD-10-PCS codes and their long titles.
- File is in text file format, file name is icd10pcs_codes_2019.txt
- Accompanying documentation for codes file, file name is icd10pcsCodesFile.pdf
- Codes file addenda in text format, file name is codes_addenda_2019.txt

2019 ICD-10-PCS Order File (Long and Abbreviated Titles) (Zip file)

- ICD-10-PCS order file is for developers, provides a unique five-digit "order number" for each ICD-10-PCS table and code, as well as a long and abbreviated code title.
- ICD-10-PCS order file name is icd10pcs_order_2019.txt
- Accompanying documentation for tabular order file, file name is icd10pcsOrderFile.pdf
- Tabular order file addenda in text format, file name is order_addenda_2019.txt

2019 ICD-10-PCS Final Addenda (Zip file)

- Addenda files in downloadable PDF, file names are tables_addenda_2019.pdf, index_addenda_2019.pdf, definitions_addenda_2019.pdf
- Addenda files also in machine readable text format for developers, file names are tables_addenda_2019.txt, index_addenda_2019.txt, definitions_addenda_2019.txt

2019 ICD-10-PCS Conversion Table (Zip file)

- ICD-10-PCS code conversion table is provided to assist users in data retrieval, in downloadable Excel spreadsheet, file name is icd10pcs_conversion_table_2019.xlsx
- Conversion table also in machine readable text format for developers, file name is icd10pcs_conversion_table_2019.txt
- Accompanying documentation for code conversion table, file name is icd10pcsConversionTable.pdf

Introduction

History of ICD-10-PCS

The World Health Organization has maintained the International Classification of Diseases (ICD) for recording cause of death since 1893. It has updated the ICD periodically to reflect new discoveries in epidemiology and changes in medical understanding of disease.

The International Classification of Diseases Tenth Revision (ICD-10), published in 1992, is the latest revision of the ICD. The WHO authorized the National Center for Health Statistics (NCHS) to develop a clinical modification of ICD-10 for use in the United States. This version, called ICD-10-CM, is intended to replace the previous U.S. clinical modification, ICD-9-CM, that has been in use since 1979. ICD-9-CM contains a procedure classification; ICD-10-CM does not.

CMS, the agency responsible for maintaining the inpatient procedure code set in the United States, contracted with 3M Health Information Systems in 1993 to design and then develop a procedure classification system to replace volume 3 of ICD-9-CM.

The result, ICD-10-PCS, was initially completed in 1998. The code set has been updated annually since that time to ensure that ICD-10-PCS includes classifications for new procedures, devices, and technologies.

The development of ICD-10-PCS had as its goal the incorporation of the following major attributes:

- **Completeness:** There should be a unique code for all substantially different procedures.
- **Unique definitions:** Because ICD-10-PCS codes are constructed of individual values rather than lists of fixed codes and text descriptions, the unique, stable definition of a code in the system is retained. New values may be added to the system to represent a specific new approach or device or qualifier, but whole codes by design cannot be given new meanings and reused.
- **Expandability:** As new procedures are developed, the structure of ICD-10-PCS should allow them to be easily incorporated as unique codes.
- **Multi-axial codes:** ICD-10-PCS codes should consist of independent characters, with each individual component retaining its meaning across broad ranges of codes to the extent possible.
- **Standardized terminology:** ICD-10-PCS should include definitions of the terminology used. While the meaning of specific words varies in common usage, ICD-10-PCS should not include multiple meanings for the same term, and each term must be assigned a specific meaning. There are no eponyms or common procedure terms in ICD-10-PCS.
- **Structural integrity:** ICD-10-PCS can be easily expanded without disrupting the structure of the system. ICD-10-PCS allows unique new codes to be added to the system because values for the seven characters that make up a code can be combined as needed. The system can evolve as medical technology and clinical practice evolve, without disrupting the ICD-10-PCS structure.

In the development of ICD-10-PCS, several additional general characteristics were added:

- **Diagnostic information is not included in procedure description:** When procedures are performed for specific diseases or disorders, the disease or disorder is not contained in the procedure code. The diagnosis codes, not the procedure codes, specify the disease or disorder.
- **Explicit not otherwise specified (NOS) options are restricted:** Explicit "not otherwise specified," (NOS) options are restricted in ICD-10-PCS. A minimal level of specificity is required for each component of the procedure.
- **Limited use of not elsewhere classified (NEC) option:** Because all significant components of a procedure are specified in ICD-10-PCS, there is generally no need for a "not elsewhere classified" (NEC) code option. However, limited NEC options are incorporated into ICD-10-PCS where necessary. For example, new devices are frequently developed, and therefore it is necessary to provide an "other device" option for use until the new device can be explicitly added to the coding system.
- **Level of specificity:** All procedures currently performed can be specified in ICD-10-PCS. The frequency with which a procedure is performed was not a consideration in the development of the system. A unique code is available for variations of a procedure that can be performed.

ICD-10-PCS code structure results in qualities that optimize the performance of the system in electronic applications, and maximize the usefulness of the coded healthcare data. These qualities include:

- **Optimal search capability:** ICD-10-PCS is designed for maximum versatility in the ability to aggregate coded data. Values belonging to the same character as defined in a section or sections can be easily compared, since they occupy the same position in a code. This provides a high degree of flexibility and functionality for data mining.
- **Consistent characters and values:** Stability of characters and values across vast ranges of codes provides the maximum degree of functionality and flexibility for the collection and analysis of data. Because the character definition is consistent, and only the individual values assigned to that character differ as needed, meaningful comparisons of data over time can be conducted across a virtually infinite range of procedures.
- **Code readability:** ICD-10-PCS resembles a language in the sense that it is made up of semi-independent values combined by following the rules of the system, much the way a sentence is formed by combining words and following the rules of grammar and syntax. As with words in their context, the meaning of any single value is a combination of its position in the code and any preceding values on which it may be dependent.

ICD-10-PCS Code Structure

ICD-10-PCS has a seven-character alphanumeric code structure. Each character contains up to 34 possible values. Each value represents a specific option for the general character definition. The 10 digits Ø–9 and the 24 letters A–H, J–N, and P–Z may be used in each character. The letters O and I are not used so as to avoid confusion with the digits Ø and 1. An ICD-10-PCS code is the result of a process rather than as a single fixed set of digits or alphabetic characters. The process consists of combining semi-independent values from among a selection of values, according to the rules governing the construction of codes.

	Section	Body System	Root Operation	Body Part	Approach	Device	Qualifier
Characters:	1	2	3	4	5	6	7

A code is derived by choosing a specific value for each of the seven characters. Based on details about the procedure performed, values for each character specifying the section, body system, root operation, body part, approach, device, and qualifier are assigned. Because the definition of each character is also a function of its physical position in the code, the same letter or number placed in a different position in the code has a different meaning.

The seven characters that make up a complete code have specific meanings that vary for each of the 17 sections of the manual.

Procedures are then divided into sections that identify the general type of procedure (e.g., Medical and Surgical, Obstetrics, Imaging). The first character of the procedure code always specifies the section. The second through seventh characters have the same meaning within each section, but may mean different things in other sections. In all sections, the third character specifies the general type of procedure performed (e.g., Resection, Transfusion, Fluoroscopy), while the other characters give additional information such as the body part and approach.

In ICD-10-PCS, the term *procedure* refers to the complete specification of the seven characters.

Number of Codes in ICD-10-PCS

The table structure of ICD-10-PCS permits the specification of a large number of codes on a single page. At the time of this publication, there are 78,881 codes in the 2019 ICD-10-PCS.

ICD-10-PCS Manual

Index

Codes may be found in the index based on the general type of procedure (e.g., resection, transfusion, fluoroscopy), or a more commonly used term (e.g., appendectomy). For example, the code for percutaneous intraluminal dilation of the coronary arteries with an intraluminal device can be found in the Index under *Dilation*, or a synonym of *Dilation* (e.g., angioplasty). The Index then specifies the first three or four values of the code or directs the user to see another term.

Example:

Dilation
  Artery
    Coronary
      One Artery Ø27Ø

Based on the first three values of the code provided in the Index, the corresponding table can be located. In the example above, the first three values indicate table Ø27 is to be referenced for code completion.

The tables and characters are arranged first by number and then by letter for each character (tables for ØØ-, Ø1-, Ø2-, etc., are followed by those for ØB-, ØC-, ØD-, etc., followed by ØB1, ØB2, etc., followed by ØBB, ØBC, ØBD, etc.).

Note: The Tables section must be used to construct a complete and valid code by specifying the last three or four values.

Tables

The Tables are composed of rows that specify the valid combinations of code values. In most sections of the system, the upper portion of each table contains a description of the first three characters of the procedure code. In the Medical and Surgical section, for example, the first three characters contain the name of the section, the body system, and the root operation performed.

For instance, the values *Ø27* specify the section *Medical and Surgical* (Ø), the body system *Heart and Great Vessels* (2) and the root operation *Dilation* (7). As shown in table Ø27, the root operation (*Dilation*) is accompanied by its definition.

The lower portion of the table specifies all the valid combinations of characters 4 through 7. The four columns in the table specify the last four characters. In the Medical and Surgical section they are labeled body part, approach, device and qualifier, respectively. Each row in the table specifies the valid combination of values for characters 4 through 7.

Table 1: Row from table Ø27

Ø Medical and Surgical
2 Heart and Great Vessels
7 Dilation Definition: Expanding an orifice or the lumen of a tubular body part
Explanation: The orifice can be a natural orifice or an artificially created orifice. Accomplished by stretching a tubular body part using intraluminal pressure or by cutting part of the orifice or wall of the tubular body part.

Body Part Character 4	Approach Character 5	Device Character 6	Qualifier Character 7
Ø Coronary Artery, One Artery 1 Coronary Artery, Two Arteries 2 Coronary Artery, Three Arteries 3 Coronary Artery, Four or More Arteries	Ø Open 3 Percutaneous 4 Percutaneous Endoscopic	4 Intraluminal Device, Drug-eluting 5 Intraluminal Device, Drug-eluting, Two 6 Intraluminal Device, Drug-eluting, Three 7 Intraluminal Device, Drug-eluting, Four or More D Intraluminal Device E Intraluminal Device, Two F Intraluminal Device, Three G Intraluminal Device, Four or More T Intraluminal Device, Radioactive Z No Device	6 Bifurcation Z No Qualifier

The rows of this table can be used to construct 240 unique procedure codes. For example, code Ø27Ø3DZ specifies the procedure for dilation of one coronary artery using an intraluminal device via percutaneous approach (i.e., percutaneous transluminal coronary angioplasty with stent).

The valid codes shown in table 2 are constructed using the first body part value in table 1 (i.e., one coronary artery), combined with all the valid approaches and devices listed in the table, and the value "No Qualifier".

Table 2: Code titles for dilation of one coronary artery (Ø27Ø)

Ø27ØØ4Z	Dilation of Coronary Artery, One Artery with Drug-eluting Intraluminal Device, Open Approach
Ø27ØØ5Z	Dilation of Coronary Artery, One Artery with Two Drug-eluting Intraluminal Devices, Open Approach
Ø27ØØ6Z	Dilation of Coronary Artery, One Artery with Three Drug-eluting Intraluminal Devices, Open Approach
Ø27ØØ7Z	Dilation of Coronary Artery, One Artery with Four or More Drug-eluting Intraluminal Devices, Open Approach
Ø27ØØDZ	Dilation of Coronary Artery, One Artery with Intraluminal Device, Open Approach
Ø27ØØEZ	Dilation of Coronary Artery, One Artery with Two Intraluminal Devices, Open Approach
Ø27ØØFZ	Dilation of Coronary Artery, One Artery with Three Intraluminal Devices, Open Approach
Ø27ØØGZ	Dilation of Coronary Artery, One Artery with Four or More Intraluminal Devices, Open Approach
Ø27ØØTZ	Dilation of Coronary Artery, One Artery with Radioactive Intraluminal Device, Open Approach
Ø27ØØZZ	Dilation of Coronary Artery, One Artery, Open Approach
Ø27Ø34Z	Dilation of Coronary Artery, One Artery with Drug-eluting Intraluminal Device, Percutaneous Approach
Ø27Ø35Z	Dilation of Coronary Artery, One Artery with Two Drug-eluting Intraluminal Devices, Percutaneous Approach
Ø27Ø36Z	Dilation of Coronary Artery, One Artery with Three Drug-eluting Intraluminal Devices, Percutaneous Approach
Ø27Ø37Z	Dilation of Coronary Artery, One Artery with Four or More Drug-eluting Intraluminal Devices, Percutaneous Approach
Ø27Ø3DZ	Dilation of Coronary Artery, One Artery with Intraluminal Device, Percutaneous Approach
Ø27Ø3EZ	Dilation of Coronary Artery, One Artery with Two Intraluminal Devices, Percutaneous Approach
Ø27Ø3FZ	Dilation of Coronary Artery, One Artery with Three Intraluminal Devices, Percutaneous Approach
Ø27Ø3GZ	Dilation of Coronary Artery, One Artery with Four or More Intraluminal Devices, Percutaneous Approach
Ø27Ø3TZ	Dilation of Coronary Artery, One Artery with Radioactive Intraluminal Device, Percutaneous Approach
Ø27Ø3ZZ	Dilation of Coronary Artery, One Artery, Percutaneous Approach
Ø27Ø44Z	Dilation of Coronary Artery, One Artery with Drug-eluting Intraluminal Device, Percutaneous Endoscopic Approach
Ø27Ø45Z	Dilation of Coronary Artery, One Artery with Two Drug-eluting Intraluminal Devices, Percutaneous Endoscopic Approach
Ø27Ø46Z	Dilation of Coronary Artery, One Artery with Three Drug-eluting Intraluminal Devices, Percutaneous Endoscopic Approach
Ø27Ø47Z	Dilation of Coronary Artery, One Artery with Four or More Drug-eluting Intraluminal Devices, Percutaneous Endoscopic Approach
Ø27Ø4DZ	Dilation of Coronary Artery, One Artery with Intraluminal Device, Percutaneous Endoscopic Approach
Ø27Ø4EZ	Dilation of Coronary Artery, One Artery with Two Intraluminal Devices, Percutaneous Endoscopic Approach
Ø27Ø4FZ	Dilation of Coronary Artery, One Artery with Three Intraluminal Devices, Percutaneous Endoscopic Approach
Ø27Ø4GZ	Dilation of Coronary Artery, One Artery with Four or More Intraluminal Devices, Percutaneous Endoscopic Approach
Ø27Ø4TZ	Dilation of Coronary Artery, One Artery with Radioactive Intraluminal Device, Percutaneous Endoscopic Approach
Ø27Ø4ZZ	Dilation of Coronary Artery, One Artery, Percutaneous Endoscopic Approach

Table 3: Rows from table ØØH

Ø Medical and Surgical
Ø Central Nervous System and Cranial Nerves
H Insertion Definition: Putting in a nonbiological appliance that monitors, assists, performs, or prevents a physiological function but does not physically take the place of a body part
Explanation: None

Body Part Character 4		Approach Character 5	Device Character 6	Qualifier Character 7
Ø Brain Cerebrum Corpus callosum Encephalon		**Ø** Open	**2** Monitoring Device **3** Infusion Device **4** Radioactive Element, Cesium-131 Collagen Implant **M** Neurostimulator Lead **Y** Other Device	**Z** No Qualifier
Ø Brain Cerebrum Corpus callosum Encephalon		**3** Percutaneous **4** Percutaneous Endoscopic	**2** Monitoring Device **3** Infusion Device **M** Neurostimulator Lead **Y** Other Device	**Z** No Qualifier
6 Cerebral Ventricle Aqueduct of Sylvius Cerebral aqueduct (Sylvius) Choroid plexus Ependyma Foramen of Monro (intraventricular) Fourth ventricle Interventricular foramen (Monro) Left lateral ventricle Right lateral ventricle Third ventricle	**E** Cranial Nerve **U** Spinal Canal Epidural space, spinal Extradural space, spinal Subarachnoid space, spinal Subdural space, spinal Vertebral canal **V** Spinal Cord	**Ø** Open **3** Percutaneous **4** Percutaneous Endoscopic	**2** Monitoring Device **3** Infusion Device **M** Neurostimulator Lead **Y** Other Device	**Z** No Qualifier

Table 3, is split into three rows; values of characters must all be selected from within the same row of the table. Row 1 and 2 indicate that the body part (character 4) value Ø and Qualifier value Z may both be used in combination with device values 2, 3, M or Y. However, the approach (character 5) and device (character 6) values are not exactly the same for both rows. As shown in row 1, Body part value Brain (Ø) with Device value Radioactive Element, Cesium-131 Collagen Implant (4) can only be used with approach value Open (Ø). In other words, code ØØHØ34Z would be invalid as the approach value 3 is only applicable to row 2 and the device value 4 is only applicable to row 1. It would be inappropriate to build a code for body part Ø if all of the values are not contained in its own row.

Note: In this manual, there are instances in which some tables due to length must be continued on the next page. Each section must be used separately and value selection must be made within the same row of the table.

Character Meanings

In each section, each character has a specific meaning, and this character meaning remains constant within that section. Character meaning tables have been provided at the beginning of each section or, in the case of the Medical and Surgical section (Ø), at the beginning of each body system to help the user identify the character members available within that section. These tables have purple headers, unlike the official code tables that have green headers and **SHOULD NOT** be used to build a PCS code. Following is an excerpt of a character meaning table.

Table 4: Rows from Central Nervous System and Cranial Nerves - Character Meanings Table

Operation–Character 3	Body Part–Character 4	Approach–Character 5	Device–Character 6	Qualifier–Character 7
1 Bypass	Ø Brain	Ø Open	Ø Drainage Device	Ø Nasopharynx
2 Change	1 Cerebral Meninges	3 Percutaneous	2 Monitoring Device	1 Mastoid Sinus
5 Destruction	2 Dura Mater	4 Percutaneous Endoscopic	3 Infusion Device	2 Atrium
7 Dilation	3 Epidural Space, Intracranial	X External	4 Radioactive Element, Cesium-131 Collagen Implant	3 Blood Vessel
8 Division	4 Subdural Space, Intracranial		7 Autologous Tissue Substitute	4 Pleural Cavity
9 Drainage	5 Subarachnoid Space, Intracranial		J Synthetic Substitute	5 Intestine
B Excision	6 Cerebral Ventricle		K Nonautologous Tissue Substitute	6 Peritoneal Cavity
C Extirpation	7 Cerebral Hemisphere		M Neurostimulator Lead	7 Urinary Tract
D Extraction	8 Basal Ganglia		Y Other Device	8 Bone Marrow
F Fragmentation	9 Thalamus		Z No Device	9 Fallopian Tube
H Insertion	A Hypothalamus			B Cerebral Cisterns
J Inspection	B Pons			F Olfactory Nerve

Sections

Procedures are divided into sections that identify the general type of procedure (e.g., Medical and Surgical, Obstetrics, Imaging). The first character of the procedure code always specifies the section.

The sections are listed below:

Medical and Surgical section

Ø Medical and Surgical

Medical and Surgical-related sections

1 Obstetrics

2 Placement

3 Administration

4 Measurement and Monitoring

5 Extracorporeal or Systemic Assistance and Performance

6 Extracorporeal or Systemic Therapies

7 Osteopathic

8 Other Procedures

9 Chiropractic

Ancillary Sections

B Imaging

C Nuclear Medicine

D Radiation Therapy

F Physical Rehabilitation and Diagnostic Audiology

G Mental Health

H Substance Abuse Treatment

New Technology Section

X New Technology

Medical and Surgical Section (Ø)

Character Meaning

The seven characters for Medical and Surgical procedures have the following meaning:

Character	Meaning
1	Section
2	Body System
3	Root Operation
4	Body Part
5	Approach
6	Device
7	Qualifier

The Medical and Surgical section constitutes the vast majority of procedures reported in an inpatient setting. Medical and Surgical procedure codes all have a first character value of Ø. The second character indicates the general body system (e.g., Mouth and Throat, Gastrointestinal). The third character indicates the root operation, or specific objective, of the procedure (e.g., Excision). The fourth character indicates the specific body part on which the procedure was performed (e.g., Tonsils, Duodenum). The fifth character indicates the approach used to reach the procedure site (e.g., Open). The sixth character indicates whether a device was left in place during the procedure (e.g., Synthetic Substitute). The seventh character is qualifier, which has a specific meaning for each root operation. For example, the qualifier can be used to identify the destination site of a *Bypass*. The first through fifth characters are always assigned a specific value, but the device (sixth character) and the qualifier (seventh character) are not applicable to all procedures. The value *Z* is used for the sixth and seventh characters to indicate that a specific device or qualifier does not apply to the procedure.

Section (Character 1)

Medical and Surgical procedure codes all have a first character value of *Ø*.

Body Systems (Character 2)

Body systems for Medical and Surgical section codes are specified in the second character.

Body Systems

Ø Central Nervous System and Cranial Nerves

1 Peripheral Nervous System

2 Heart and Great Vessels

3 Upper Arteries

4 Lower Arteries

5 Upper Veins

6 Lower Veins

7 Lymphatic and Hemic Systems

8 Eye

9 Ear, Nose, Sinus

B Respiratory System

C Mouth and Throat

D Gastrointestinal System

F Hepatobiliary System and Pancreas

G Endocrine System

H Skin and Breast

J Subcutaneous Tissue and Fascia

K Muscles

L Tendons

M Bursae and Ligaments

N Head and Facial Bones

P Upper Bones

Q Lower Bones

R Upper Joints

S Lower Joints

T Urinary System

U Female Reproductive System

V Male Reproductive System

W Anatomical Regions, General

X Anatomical Regions, Upper Extremities

Y Anatomical Regions, Lower Extremities

Root Operations (Character 3)

The root operation is specified in the third character. In the Medical and Surgical section there are 31 different root operations. The root operation identifies the objective of the procedure. Each root operation has a precise definition.

- *Alteration:* Modifying the natural anatomic structure of a body part without affecting the function of the body part
- *Bypass:* Altering the route of passage of the contents of a tubular body part
- *Change:* Taking out or off a device from a body part and putting back an identical or similar device in or on the same body part without cutting or puncturing the skin or a mucous membrane
- *Control:* Stopping, or attempting to stop, postprocedural or other acute bleeding
- *Creation:* Putting in or on biological or synthetic material to form a new body part that to the extent possible replicates the anatomic structure or function of an absent body part
- *Destruction:* Physical eradication of all or a portion of a body part by the direct use of energy, force, or a destructive agent
- *Detachment:* Cutting off all or a portion of the upper or lower extremities
- *Dilation:* Expanding an orifice or the lumen of a tubular body part
- *Division:* Cutting into a body part without draining fluids and/or gases from the body part in order to separate or transect a body part
- *Drainage:* Taking or letting out fluids and/or gases from a body part
- *Excision:* Cutting out or off, without replacement, a portion of a body part
- *Extirpation:* Taking or cutting out solid matter from a body part
- *Extraction:* Pulling or stripping out or off all or a portion of a body part by the use of force
- *Fragmentation:* Breaking solid matter in a body part into pieces
- *Fusion:* Joining together portions of an articular body part rendering the articular body part immobile
- *Insertion:* Putting in a nonbiological appliance that monitors, assists, performs, or prevents a physiological function but does not physically take the place of a body part
- *Inspection:* Visually and/or manually exploring a body part
- *Map:* Locating the route of passage of electrical impulses and/or locating functional areas in a body part
- *Occlusion:* Completely closing an orifice or lumen of a tubular body part
- *Reattachment:* Putting back in or on all or a portion of a separated body part to its normal location or other suitable location
- *Release:* Freeing a body part from an abnormal physical constraint by cutting or by use of force
- *Removal:* Taking out or off a device from a body part
- *Repair:* Restoring, to the extent possible, a body part to its normal anatomic structure and function
- *Replacement:* Putting in or on biological or synthetic material that physically takes the place and/or function of all or a portion of a body part
- *Reposition:* Moving to its normal location or other suitable location all or a portion of a body part
- *Resection:* Cutting out or off, without replacement, all of a body part
- *Restriction:* Partially closing an orifice or lumen of a tubular body part
- *Revision:* Correcting, to the extent possible, a portion of a malfunctioning device or the position of a displaced device
- *Supplement:* Putting in or on biological or synthetic material that physically reinforces and/or augments the function of a portion of a body part
- *Transfer:* Moving, without taking out, all or a portion of a body part to another location to take over the function of all or a portion of a body part
- *Transplantation:* Putting in or on all or a portion of a living body part taken from another individual or animal to physically take the place and/or function of all or a portion of a similar body part

The above definitions of root operations illustrate the precision of code values defined in the system. There is a clear distinction between each root operation.

A root operation specifies the objective of the procedure. The term *anastomosis* is not a root operation, because it is a means of joining and is always an integral part of another procedure (e.g., Bypass, Resection) with a specific objective. Similarly, *incision* is not a root operation, since it is always part of the objective of another procedure (e.g., Division, Drainage). The root operation *Repair* in the Medical and Surgical section functions as a "not elsewhere classified" option. *Repair* is used when the procedure performed is not one of the other specific root operations.

Appendix B provides additional explanation and representative examples of the Medical and Surgical root operations. Appendix C groups all root operations in the Medical and Surgical section into subcategories and provides an example of each root operation.

Body Part (Character 4)

The body part is specified in the fourth character. The body part indicates the specific anatomical site of the body system on which the procedure was performed (e.g., Duodenum). Tubular body parts are defined in ICD-10-PCS as those hollow body parts that provide a route of passage for solids, liquids, or gases. They include the cardiovascular system and body parts such as those contained in the gastrointestinal tract, genitourinary tract, biliary tract, and respiratory tract.

Approach (Character 5)

The technique used to reach the site of the procedure is specified in the fifth character. There are seven different approaches:

- *Open*: Cutting through the skin or mucous membrane and any other body layers necessary to expose the site of the procedure
- *Percutaneous*: Entry, by puncture or minor incision, of instrumentation through the skin or mucous membrane and any other body layers necessary to reach the site of the procedure
- *Percutaneous Endoscopic*: Entry, by puncture or minor incision, of instrumentation through the skin or mucous membrane and any other body layers necessary to reach and visualize the site of the procedure
- *Via Natural or Artificial Opening*: Entry of instrumentation through a natural or artificial external opening to reach the site of the procedure
- *Via Natural or Artificial Opening Endoscopic*: Entry of instrumentation through a natural or artificial external opening to reach and visualize the site of the procedure

- *Via Natural or Artificial Opening with Percutaneous Endoscopic Assistance:* Entry of instrumentation through a natural or artificial external opening and entry, by puncture or minor incision, of instrumentation through the skin or mucous membrane and any other body layers necessary to aid in the performance of the procedure
- *External*: Procedures performed directly on the skin or mucous membrane and procedures performed indirectly by the application of external force through the skin or mucous membrane

The approach comprises three components: the access location, method, and type of instrumentation.

Access location: For procedures performed on an internal body part, the access location specifies the external site through which the site of the procedure is reached. There are two general types of access locations: skin or mucous membranes, and external orifices. Every approach value except external includes one of these two access locations. The skin or mucous membrane can be cut or punctured to reach the procedure site. All open and percutaneous approach values use this access location. The site of a procedure can also be reached through an external opening. External openings can be natural (e.g., mouth) or artificial (e.g., colostomy stoma).

Method: For procedures performed on an internal body part, the method specifies how the external access location is entered. An open method specifies cutting through the skin or mucous membrane and any other intervening body layers necessary to expose the site of the procedure. An instrumentation method specifies the entry of instrumentation through the access location to the internal procedure site. Instrumentation can be introduced by puncture or minor incision, or through an external opening. The puncture or minor incision does not constitute an open approach because it does not expose the site of the procedure. An approach can define multiple methods. For example, *Via Natural or Artificial Opening with Percutaneous Endoscopic Assistance* includes both the initial entry of instrumentation to reach the site of the procedure, and the placement of additional percutaneous instrumentation into the body part to visualize and assist in the performance of the procedure.

Type of instrumentation: For procedures performed on an internal body part, instrumentation means that specialized equipment is used to perform the procedure. Instrumentation is used in all internal approaches other than the basic open approach. Instrumentation may or may not include the capacity to visualize the procedure site. For example, the instrumentation used to perform a sigmoidoscopy permits the internal site of the procedure to be visualized, while the instrumentation used to perform a needle biopsy of the liver does not. The term "endoscopic" as used in approach values refers to instrumentation that permits a site to be visualized.

Procedures performed directly on the skin or mucous membrane are identified by the external approach (e.g., skin excision). Procedures performed indirectly by the application of external force are also identified by the external approach (e.g., closed reduction of fracture).

Appendix A compares the components (access location, method, and type of instrumentation) of each approach and provides an example and illustration of each approach.

Device (Character 6)

The device is specified in the sixth character and is used only to specify devices that remain after the procedure is completed. There are four general types of devices:

- Biological or synthetic material that takes the place of all or a portion of a body part (e.g, skin graft, joint prosthesis).
- Biological or synthetic material that assists or prevents a physiological function (e.g., IUD).
- Therapeutic material that is not absorbed by, eliminated by, or incorporated into a body part (e.g., radioactive implant).
- Mechanical or electronic appliances used to assist, monitor, take the place of or prevent a physiological function (e.g., cardiac pacemaker, orthopedic pin).

While all devices can be removed, some cannot be removed without putting in another nonbiological appliance or body-part substitute.

When a specific device value is used to identify the device for a root operation, such as *Insertion* and that same device value is not an option for a more broad range root operation such as *Removal*, select the general device value. For example, in the body system Heart and Great Vessels, the specific device character for Cardiac Lead, Pacemaker in root operation *Insertion* is J. For the root operation *Removal*, the general device character M Cardiac Lead would be selected for the pacemaker lead.

ICD-10-PCS contains a PCS Device Aggregation Table (see appendix F) that crosswalks the *specific* device character values that have been created for specific root operations and specific body part character values to the *general* device character value that would be used for root operations that represent a broad range of procedures and general body part character values, such as Removal and Revision.

Instruments used to visualize the procedure site are specified in the approach, not the device, value.

If the objective of the procedure is to put in the device, then the root operation is *Insertion*. If the device is put in to meet an objective other than *Insertion*, then the root operation defining the underlying objective of the procedure is used, with the device specified in the device character. For example, if a procedure to replace the hip joint is performed, the root operation *Replacement* is coded, and the prosthetic device is specified in the device character. Materials that are incidental to a procedure such as clips, ligatures, and sutures are not specified in the device character. Because new devices can be developed, the value *Other Device* is provided as a temporary option for use until a specific device value is added to the system.

Qualifier (Character 7)

The qualifier is specified in the seventh character. The qualifier contains unique values for individual procedures. For example, the qualifier can be used to identify the destination site in a *Bypass*.

Medical and Surgical Section Principles

In developing the Medical and Surgical procedure codes, several specific principles were followed:

Composite Terms Are Not Root Operations

Composite terms such as colonoscopy, sigmoidectomy, or appendectomy do not describe root operations, but they do specify multiple components of a specific root operation. In ICD-10-PCS, the components of a procedure are defined separately by the characters making up the complete code. The only component of a procedure specified in the root operation is the objective of the procedure. With each complete code the underlying objective of the procedure is specified by the root operation (third character), the precise part is specified by the body part (fourth character), and the method used to reach and visualize the procedure site is specified by the approach (fifth character). While colonoscopy, sigmoidectomy, and appendectomy are included in the Index, they do not constitute root operations in the Tables section. The objective of colonoscopy is the visualization of the colon and the root operation (character 3) is *Inspection*. Character 4 specifies the body part, which in this case is part of the colon. These composite terms, like colonoscopy or appendectomy, are included as cross-reference only. The index provides the correct root operation reference. Examples of other types of composite terms not representative of root operations are *partial* sigmoidectomy, *total* hysterectomy, and *partial* hip replacement. Always refer to the correct root operation in the Index and Tables section.

Root Operation Based on Objective of Procedure

The root operation is based on the objective of the procedure, such as *Resection* of transverse colon or *Dilation* of an artery. The assignment of the root operation is based on the procedure actually performed, which may or may not have been the intended procedure. If the intended procedure is modified or discontinued (e.g., excision instead of resection is performed), the root operation is determined by the procedure actually performed. If the desired result is not attained after completing the procedure (i.e., the artery does not remain expanded after the dilation procedure), the root operation is still determined by the procedure actually performed.

Examples:

- Dilating the urethra is coded as *Dilation* since the objective of the procedure is to dilate the urethra. If dilation of the urethra includes putting in an intraluminal stent, the root operation remains *Dilation* and not *Insertion* of the intraluminal device because the underlying objective of the procedure is dilation of the urethra. The stent is identified by the intraluminal device value in the sixth character of the dilation procedure code.
- If the objective is solely to put a radioactive element in the urethra, then the procedure is coded to the root operation *Insertion*, with the radioactive element identified in the sixth character of the code.
- If the objective of the procedure is to correct a malfunctioning or displaced device, then the procedure is coded to the root operation *Revision*. In the root operation *Revision*, the original device being revised is identified in the device character. *Revision* is typically performed on mechanical appliances (e.g., pacemaker) or materials used in replacement procedures (e.g., synthetic substitute). Typical revision procedures include adjustment of pacemaker position and correction of malfunctioning knee prosthesis.

Combination Procedures Are Coded Separately

If multiple procedures as defined by distinct objectives are performed during an operative episode, then multiple codes are used. For example, obtaining the vein graft used for coronary bypass surgery is coded as a separate procedure from the bypass itself.

Redo of Procedures

The complete or partial redo of the original procedure is coded to the root operation that identifies the procedure performed rather than *Revision*.

Example:

A complete redo of a hip replacement procedure that requires putting in a new prosthesis is coded to the root operation *Replacement* rather than *Revision*.

The correction of complications arising from the original procedure, other than device complications, is coded to the procedure performed. Correction of a malfunctioning or displaced device would be coded to the root operation *Revision*.

Example:

A procedure to control hemorrhage arising from the original procedure is coded to *Control* rather than *Revision*.

Examples of Procedures Coded in the Medical Surgical Section

The following are examples of procedures from the Medical and Surgical section, coded in ICD-10-PCS.

- Suture of skin laceration, left lower arm: ØHQEXZZ

  Medical and Surgical section (Ø), body system *Skin and Breast* (H), root operation *Repair* (Q), body part *Skin, Left Lower Arm* (E), *External* Approach (X) *No device* (Z), and *No qualifier* (Z).

- Laparoscopic appendectomy: ØDTJ4ZZ

  Medical and Surgical section (Ø), body system *Gastrointestinal* (D), root operation *Resection* (T), body part *Appendix* (J), *Percutaneous Endoscopic* approach (4), No Device (Z), and No qualifier (Z).

- Sigmoidoscopy with biopsy: ØDBN8ZX

  Medical and Surgical section (Ø), body system *Gastrointestinal* (D), root operation *Excision* (B), body part *Sigmoid Colon* (N), *Via Natural or Artificial Opening Endoscopic* approach (8), *No Device* (Z), and with qualifier *Diagnostic* (X).

- Tracheostomy with tracheostomy tube: ØB11ØF4

  Medical and Surgical section (Ø), body system *Respiratory* (B), root operation *Bypass* (1), body part *Trachea* (1), *Open* approach (Ø), with *Tracheostomy Device* (F), and qualifier *Cutaneous* (4).

Obstetrics Section (1)

Character Meanings

The seven characters in the Obstetrics section have the same meaning as in the Medical and Surgical section.

Character	Meaning
1	Section
2	Body System
3	Root Operation
4	Body Part
5	Approach
6	Device
7	Qualifier

The Obstetrics section includes procedures performed on the products of conception only. Procedures on the pregnant female are coded in the Medical and Surgical section (e.g., episiotomy). The term "products of conception" refers to all physical components of a pregnancy, including the fetus, amnion, umbilical cord, and placenta. There is no differentiation of the products of conception based on gestational age. Thus, the specification of the products of conception as a zygote, embryo or fetus, or the trimester of the pregnancy is not part of the procedure code but can be found in the diagnosis code.

Section (Character 1)

Obstetrics procedure codes have a first character value of *1*.

Body System (Character 2)

The second character value for body system is *Pregnancy*.

Root Operation (Character 3)

The root operations *Change, Drainage, Extraction, Insertion, Inspection, Removal, Repair, Reposition, Resection,* and *Transplantation* are used in the obstetrics section and have the same meaning as in the Medical and Surgical section.

The Obstetrics section also includes two additional root operations, *Abortion* and *Delivery*, defined below:

- *Abortion*: Artificially terminating a pregnancy
- *Delivery*: Assisting the passage of the products of conception from the genital canal

A cesarean section is not a separate root operation because the underlying objective is *Extraction* (i.e., pulling out all or a portion of a body part).

Body Part (Character 4)

The body part values in the obstetrics section are:

- *Products of conception*
- *Products of conception, retained*
- *Products of conception, ectopic*

Approach (Character 5)

The fifth character specifies approaches and is defined as are those in the Medical and Surgical section. In the case of an abortion procedure that uses a laminaria or an abortifacient, the approach is *Via Natural or Artificial Opening*.

Device (Character 6)

The sixth character is used for devices such as fetal monitoring electrodes.

Qualifier (Character 7)

Qualifier values are specific to the root operation and are used to specify the type of extraction (e.g., low forceps, high forceps, etc.), the type of cesarean section (e.g., classical, low cervical, etc.), or the type of fluid taken out during a drainage procedure (e.g., amniotic fluid, fetal blood, etc.).

Placement Section (2)

Character Meanings

The seven characters in the Placement section have the following meaning:

Character	Meaning
1	Section
2	Body System
3	Root Operation
4	Body Region
5	Approach
6	Device
7	Qualifier

Placement section codes represent procedures for putting a device in or on a body region for the purpose of protection, immobilization, stretching, compression, or packing.

Section (Character 1)

Placement procedure codes have a first character value of *2*.

Body System (Character 2)

The second character contains two values specifying either *Anatomical Regions* or *Anatomical Orifices*.

Root Operation (Character 3)

The root operations in the Placement section include only those procedures that are performed without making an incision or a puncture. The root operations *Change* and *Removal* are in the Placement section and have the same meaning as in the Medical and Surgical section.

The Placement section also includes five additional root operations, defined as follows:

- *Compression*: Putting pressure on a body region
- *Dressing*: Putting material on a body region for protection
- *Immobilization*: Limiting or preventing motion of an external body region
- *Packing*: Putting material in a body region or orifice
- *Traction*: Exerting a pulling force on a body region in a distal direction

Body Region (Character 4)

The fourth character values are either body regions (e.g., *Upper Leg*) or natural orifices (e.g., *Ear*).

Approach (Character 5)

Since all placement procedures are performed directly on the skin or mucous membrane, or performed indirectly by applying external force through the skin or mucous membrane, the approach value is always *External*.

Device (Character 6)

The device character is always specified (except in the case of manual traction) and indicates the device placed during the procedure (e.g., cast, splint, bandage, etc.). Except for casts for fractures and dislocations, devices in the Placement section are off the shelf and do not require any extensive design, fabrication, or fitting. Placement of devices that require extensive design, fabrication, or fitting are coded in the Rehabilitation section.

Qualifier (Character 7)
The qualifier character is not specified in the Placement section; the qualifier value is always *No Qualifier.*

Administration Section (3)

Character Meanings
The seven characters in the Administration section have the following meaning:

Character	Meaning
1	Section
2	Body System
3	Root Operation
4	Body System/Region
5	Approach
6	Substance
7	Qualifier

Administration section codes represent procedures for putting in or on a therapeutic, prophylactic, protective, diagnostic, nutritional, or physiological substance. The section includes transfusions, infusions, and injections, along with other similar services such as irrigation and tattooing.

Section (Character 1)
Administration procedure codes have a first character value of *3*.

Body System (Character 2)
The body system character contains only three values: *Indwelling Device, Physiological Systems and Anatomical Regions,* or *Circulatory System*. The *Circulatory System* is used for transfusion procedures.

Root Operation (Character 3)
There are three root operations in the Administration section.

- *Introduction*: Putting in or on a therapeutic, diagnostic, nutritional, physiological, or prophylactic substance except blood or blood products
- *Irrigation*: Putting in or on a cleansing substance
- *Transfusion*: Putting in blood or blood products

Body/System Region (Character 4)
The fourth character specifies the body system/region. The fourth character identifies the site where the substance is administered, not the site where the substance administered takes effect. Sites include *Skin and Mucous Membranes, Subcutaneous Tissue,* and *Muscle*. These differentiate intradermal, subcutaneous, and intramuscular injections, respectively. Other sites include *Eye, Respiratory Tract, Peritoneal Cavity,* and *Epidural Space.*

The body systems/regions for arteries and veins are *Peripheral Artery, Central Artery, Peripheral Vein,* and *Central Vein*. The *Peripheral Artery* or *Vein* is typically used when a substance is introduced locally into an artery or vein. For example, chemotherapy is the introduction of an antineoplastic substance into a peripheral artery or vein by a percutaneous approach. In general, the substance introduced into a peripheral artery or vein has a systemic effect.

The *Central Artery* or *Vein* is typically used when the site where the substance is introduced is distant from the point of entry into the artery or vein. For example, the introduction of a substance directly at the site of a clot within an artery or vein using a catheter is coded as an introduction of a thrombolytic substance into a central artery or vein by a percutaneous approach. In general, the substance introduced into a central artery or vein has a local effect.

Approach (Character 5)
The fifth character specifies approaches as defined in the Medical and Surgical section. The approach for intradermal, subcutaneous, and intramuscular introductions (i.e., injections) is *Percutaneous.* If a catheter is placed to introduce a substance into an internal site within the circulatory system, then the approach is also *Percutaneous.* For example, if a catheter is used to introduce contrast directly into the heart for angiography, then the procedure would be coded as a percutaneous introduction of contrast into the heart.

Substance (Character 6)
The sixth character specifies the substance being introduced. Broad categories of substances are defined, such as anesthetic, contrast, dialysate, and blood products such as platelets.

Qualifier (Character 7)
The seventh character is a qualifier and is used to indicate whether the substance is *Autologous* or *Nonautologous*, or to further specify the substance.

Measurement and Monitoring Section (4)

Character Meanings
The seven characters in the Measurement and Monitoring section have the following meaning:

Character	Meaning
1	Section
2	Body System
3	Root Operation
4	Body System
5	Approach
6	Function/Device
7	Qualifier

Measurement and Monitoring section codes represent procedures for determining the level of a physiological or physical function.

Section (Character 1)
Measurement and Monitoring procedure codes have a first character value of *4*.

Body System (Character 2)
The second character values for body system are A, *Physiological Systems* or *B, Physiological Devices.*

Root Operation (Character 3)
There are two root operations in the Measurement and Monitoring section, as defined below:

- *Measurement*: Determining the level of a physiological or physical function at a point in time

- *Monitoring*: Determining the level of a physiological or physical function repetitively over a period of time

Body System (Character 4)
The fourth character specifies the specific body system measured or monitored.

Approach (Character 5)
The fifth character specifies approaches as defined in the Medical and Surgical section.

Function/Device (Character 6)
The sixth character specifies the physiological or physical function being measured or monitored. Examples of physiological or physical functions are *Conductivity, Metabolism, Pulse, Temperature,* and *Volume.* If a device used to perform the measurement or monitoring is inserted and left in, then insertion of the device is coded as a separate Medical and Surgical procedure.

Qualifier (Character 7)
The seventh character qualifier contains specific values as needed to further specify the body part (e.g., central, portal, pulmonary) or a variation of the procedure performed (e.g., ambulatory, stress). Examples of typical procedures coded in this section are EKG, EEG, and cardiac catheterization. An EKG is the measurement of cardiac electrical activity, while an EEG is the measurement of electrical activity of the central nervous system. A cardiac catheterization performed to measure the pressure in the heart is coded as the measurement of cardiac pressure by percutaneous approach.

Extracorporeal or Systemic Assistance and Performance Section (5)

Character Meanings
The seven characters in the Extracorporeal or Systemic Assistance and Performance section have the following meaning:

Character	Meaning
1	Section
2	Body System
3	Root Operation
4	Body System
5	Duration
6	Function
7	Qualifier

In Extracorporeal or Systemic Assistance and Performance procedures, equipment outside the body is used to assist or perform a physiological function. The section includes procedures performed in a critical care setting, such as mechanical ventilation and cardioversion; it also includes other services such as hyperbaric oxygen treatment and hemodialysis.

Section (Character 1)
Extracorporeal or Systemic Assistance and Performance procedure codes have a first character value of *5*.

Body System (Character 2)
The second character value for body system is A, *Physiological Systems.*

Root Operation (Character 3)
There are three root operations in the Extracorporeal or Systemic Assistance and Performance section, as defined below.

- *Assistance*: Taking over a portion of a physiological function by extracorporeal means
- *Performance*: Completely taking over a physiological function by extracorporeal means
- *Restoration*: Returning, or attempting to return, a physiological function to its natural state by extracorporeal means

The root operation *Restoration* contains a single procedure code that identifies extracorporeal cardioversion.

Body System (Character 4)
The fourth character specifies the body system (e.g., cardiac, respiratory) to which extracorporeal or systemic assistance or performance is applied.

Duration (Character 5)
The fifth character specifies the duration of the procedure—*Single, Intermittent*, or *Continuous.* For respiratory ventilation assistance or performance, the duration is specified in hours— *< 24 Consecutive Hours, 24–96 Consecutive Hours,* or *> 96 Consecutive Hours.* For urinary procedures, duration is specified as *Intermittent, Less than 6 Hours Per Day; Prolonged Intermittent, 6-18 hours Per Day;* or *Continuous, Greater than 18 hours Per Day.* Value 6, *Multiple* identifies serial procedure treatment.

Function (Character 6)
The sixth character specifies the physiological function assisted or performed (e.g., oxygenation, ventilation) during the procedure.

Qualifier (Character 7)
The seventh character qualifier specifies the type of equipment used, if any.

Extracorporeal or Systemic Therapies Section (6)

Character Meanings
The seven characters in the Extracorporeal or Systemic Therapies section have the following meaning:

Character	Meaning
1	Section
2	Body System
3	Root Operation
4	Body System
5	Duration
6	Qualifier
7	Qualifier

In extracorporeal or systemic therapy, equipment outside the body is used for a therapeutic purpose that does not involve the assistance or performance of a physiological function.

Section (Character 1)

Extracorporeal or Systemic Therapy procedure codes have a first character value of 6.

Body System (Character 2)

The second character value for body system is *Physiological Systems*.

Root Operation (Character 3)

There are 11 root operations in the Extracorporeal or Systemic Therapy section, as defined below.

- *Atmospheric Control*: Extracorporeal control of atmospheric pressure and composition
- *Decompression*: Extracorporeal elimination of undissolved gas from body fluids

  Coding note: The root operation *Decompression* involves only one type of procedure: treatment for decompression sickness (the bends) in a hyperbaric chamber.
- *Electromagnetic Therapy*: Extracorporeal treatment by electromagnetic rays
- *Hyperthermia*: Extracorporeal raising of body temperature

  Coding note: The term hyperthermia is used to describe both a temperature imbalance treatment and also as an adjunct radiation treatment for cancer. When treating the temperature imbalance, it is coded to this section; for the cancer treatment, it is coded in section *D Radiation Therapy.*
- *Hypothermia*: Extracorporeal lowering of body temperature
- *Perfusion*: Extracorporeal treatment by diffusion of therapeutic fluid
- *Pheresis*: Extracorporeal separation of blood products

  Coding note: Pheresis may be used for two main purposes: to treat diseases when too much of a blood component is produced (e.g., leukemia) and to remove a blood product such as platelets from a donor, for transfusion into another patient.
- *Phototherapy*: Extracorporeal treatment by light rays

  Coding note: Phototherapy involves using a machine that exposes the blood to light rays outside the body, recirculates it, and then returns it to the body.
- *Shock Wave Therapy*: Extracorporeal treatment by shock waves
- *Ultrasound Therapy*: Extracorporeal treatment by ultrasound
- *Ultraviolet Light Therapy*: Extracorporeal treatment by ultraviolet light

Body System (Character 4)

The fourth character specifies the body system on which the extracorporeal or systemic therapy is performed (e.g., skin, circulatory).

Duration (Character 5)

The fifth character specifies the duration of the procedure (e.g., single or intermittent).

Qualifier (Character 6)

The sixth character for Extracorporeal or Systemic Therapies is *No Qualifier*, except for root operation Perfusion which has a sixth character qualifier of *Donor Organ*.

Qualifier (Character 7)

The seventh character qualifier is used in the root operation *Pheresis* to specify the blood component on which pheresis is performed and in the root operation *Ultrasound Therapy* to specify site of treatment.

Osteopathic Section (7)

Character Meanings

The seven characters in the Osteopathic section have the following meaning:

Character	Meaning
1	Section
2	Body System
3	Root Operation
4	Body Region
5	Approach
6	Method
7	Qualifier

Section (Character 1)

Osteopathic procedure codes have a first character value of *7*.

Body System (Character 2)

The body system character contains the value *Anatomical Regions*.

Root Operation (Character 3)

There is only one root operation in the Osteopathic section.

- *Treatment*: Manual treatment to eliminate or alleviate somatic dysfunction and related disorders

Body Region (Character 4)

The fourth character specifies the body region on which the osteopathic treatment is performed.

Approach (Character 5)

The approach for osteopathic treatment is always *External*.

Method (Character 6)

The sixth character specifies the method by which the treatment is accomplished.

Qualifier (Character 7)

The seventh character is not specified in the Osteopathic section and always has the value *None*.

Other Procedures Section (8)

Character Meanings

The seven characters in the Other Procedures section have the following meaning:

Character	Meaning
1	Section
2	Body System
3	Root Operation
4	Body Region
5	Approach
6	Method
7	Qualifier

The Other Procedures section includes acupuncture, suture removal, and in vitro fertilization.

Section (Character 1)

Other Procedure section codes have a first character value of *8*.

Body System (Character 2)

The second character values for body systems are *Physiological Systems and Anatomical Regions* and *Indwelling Device.*

Root Operation (Character 3)

The Other Procedures section has only one root operation, defined as follows:

- *Other Procedures*: Methodologies that attempt to remediate or cure a disorder or disease.

Body Region (Character 4)

The fourth character contains specified body-region values, and also the body-region value *None.*

Approach (Character 5)

The fifth character specifies approaches as defined in the Medical and Surgical section.

Method (Character 6)

The sixth character specifies the method (e.g., *Acupuncture, Therapeutic Massage*).

Qualifier (Character 7)

The seventh character is a qualifier and contains specific values as needed.

Chiropractic Section (9)

Character Meanings

The seven characters in the Chiropractic section have the following meaning:

Character	Meaning
1	Section
2	Body System
3	Root Operation
4	Body Region
5	Approach
6	Method
7	Qualifier

Section (Character 1)

Chiropractic section procedure codes have a first character value of *9.*

Body System (Character 2)

The second character value for body system is *Anatomical Regions.*

Root Operation (Character 3)

There is only one root operation in the *Chiropractic* section.

- *Manipulation:* Manual procedure that involves a directed thrust to move a joint past the physiological range of motion, without exceeding the anatomical limit.

Body Region (Character 4)

The fourth character specifies the body region on which the chiropractic manipulation is performed.

Approach (Character 5)

The approach for chiropractic manipulation is always *External.*

Method (Character 6)

The sixth character is the method by which the manipulation is accomplished.

Qualifier (Character 7)

The seventh character is not specified in the Chiropractic section and always has the value *None.*

Imaging Section (B)

Character Meanings

The seven characters in Imaging procedures have the following meaning:

Character	Meaning
1	Section
2	Body System
3	Type
4	Body Part
5	Contrast
6	Qualifier
7	Qualifier

Imaging procedures include plain radiography, fluoroscopy, CT, MRI, and ultrasound. Nuclear medicine procedures, including PET, uptakes, and scans, are in the nuclear medicine section. Therapeutic radiation procedure codes are in a separate radiation therapy section.

Section (Character 1)

Imaging procedure codes have a first character value of *B*.

Body System (Character 2)

In the Imaging section, the second character defines the body system, such as *Heart* or *Gastrointestinal System*.

Type (Character 3)

The third character defines the type of imaging procedure (e.g., MRI, ultrasound). The following list includes all types in the *Imaging* section with a definition of each type:

- *Computerized Tomography (CT Scan)*: Computer reformatted digital display of multiplanar images developed from the capture of multiple exposures of external ionizing radiation
- *Fluoroscopy*: Single plane or bi-plane real time display of an image developed from the capture of external ionizing radiation on a fluorescent screen. The image may also be stored by either digital or analog means
- *Magnetic Resonance Imaging (MRI)*: Computer reformatted digital display of multiplanar images developed from the capture of radiofrequency signals emitted by nuclei in a body site excited within a magnetic field
- *Plain Radiography*: Planar display of an image developed from the capture of external ionizing radiation on photographic or photoconductive plate
- *Ultrasonography*: Real time display of images of anatomy or flow information developed from the capture of reflected and attenuated high frequency sound waves

Body Part (Character 4)

The fourth character defines the body part with different values for each body system (character 2) value.

Contrast (Character 5)

The fifth character specifies whether the contrast material used in the imaging procedure is *High Osmolar, Low Osmolar*, or *Other Contrast* when applicable.

Qualifier (Character 6)

The sixth character qualifier provides further detail regarding the nature of the substance or technologies used, such as *Unenhanced and Enhanced (contrast), Laser, or Intravascular Optical Coherence.*

Qualifier (Character 7)

The seventh character is a qualifier that may be used to specify certain procedural circumstances, the method by which the procedure was performed, or technologies utilized, such as *Intraoperative, Intravascular, or Transesophageal.*

Nuclear Medicine Section (C)

Character Meanings

The seven characters in the Nuclear Medicine section have the following meaning:

Character	Meaning
1	Section
2	Body System
3	Type
4	Body Part
5	Radionuclide
6	Qualifier
7	Qualifier

Nuclear Medicine is the introduction of radioactive material into the body to create an image, to diagnose and treat pathologic conditions, or to assess metabolic functions. The Nuclear Medicine section does not include the introduction of encapsulated radioactive material for the treatment of cancer. These procedures are included in the Radiation Therapy section.

Section (Character 1)

Nuclear Medicine procedure codes have a first character value of *C*.

Body System (Character 2)

The second character specifies the body system on which the nuclear medicine procedure is performed.

Type (Character 3)

The third character indicates the type of nuclear medicine procedure (e.g., planar imaging or nonimaging uptake). The following list includes the types of nuclear medicine procedures with a definition of each type.

- *Nonimaging Nuclear Medicine Assay:* Introduction of radioactive materials into the body for the study of body fluids and blood elements, by the detection of radioactive emissions
- *Nonimaging Nuclear Medicine Probe:* Introduction of radioactive materials into the body for the study of distribution and fate of certain substances by the detection of radioactive emissions; or alternatively, measurement of absorption of radioactive emissions from an external source
- *Nonimaging Nuclear Medicine Uptake:* Introduction of radioactive materials into the body for measurements of organ function, from the detection of radioactive emissions
- *Planar Nuclear Medicine Imaging*: Introduction of radioactive materials into the body for single-plane display of images developed from the capture of radioactive emissions
- *Positron Emission Tomography (PET) Imaging:* Introduction of radioactive materials into the body for three dimensional display of images developed from the simultaneous capture, 180 degrees apart, of radioactive emissions
- *Systemic Nuclear Medicine Therapy:* Introduction of unsealed radioactive materials into the body for treatment
- *Tomographic (Tomo) Nuclear Medicine Imaging*: Introduction of radioactive materials into the body for three dimensional display of images developed from the capture of radioactive emissions

Body Part (Character 4)
The fourth character indicates the body part or body region studied; with regional (e.g., *lower extremity veins*) and combination (e.g., *liver and spleen*) body parts commonly used.

Radionuclide (Character 5)
The fifth character specifies the radionuclide, the radiation source. The option *Other Radionuclide* is provided in the nuclear medicine section for newly approved radionuclides until they can be added to the coding system. If more than one radiopharmaceutical is given to perform the procedure, then more than one code is used.

Qualifier (Character 6 and 7)
The sixth and seventh characters are qualifiers but are not specified in the *Nuclear Medicine* section; the value is always *None*.

Radiation Therapy Section (D)

Character Meanings
The seven characters in the Radiation Therapy section have the following meaning:

Character	Meaning
1	Section
2	Body System
3	Modality
4	Treatment Site
5	Modality Qualifier
6	Isotope
7	Qualifier

Section (Character 1)
Radiation therapy procedure codes have a first character value of *D*.

Body System (Character 2)
The second character specifies the body system (e.g., central nervous system, musculoskeletal) irradiated.

Modality (Character 3)
The third character specifies the general modality used (e.g., beam radiation).

Treatment Site (Character 4)
The fourth character specifies the body part that is the focus of the radiation therapy.

Modality Qualifier (Character 5)
The fifth character further specifies the radiation modality used (e.g., photons, electrons).

Isotope (Character 6)
The sixth character specifies the isotopes introduced into the body, if applicable.

Qualifier (Character 7)
The seventh character may specify whether the procedure was performed intraoperatively.

Physical Rehabilitation and Diagnostic Audiology Section (F)

Character Meanings
The seven characters in the Physical Rehabilitation and Diagnostic Audiology section have the following meaning:

Character	Meaning
1	Section
2	Section Qualifier
3	Type
4	Body System/Region
5	Type Qualifier
6	Equipment
7	Qualifier

Physical rehabilitation procedures include physical therapy, occupational therapy, and speech-language pathology. Osteopathic procedures and chiropractic procedures are in separate sections.

Section (Character 1)
Physical Rehabilitation and Diagnostic Audiology procedure codes have a first character value of *F*.

Section Qualifier (Character 2)
The section qualifier *Rehabilitation* or *Diagnostic Audiology* is specified in the second character.

Type (Character 3)
The third character specifies the type. There are 14 different values, which can be classified into four basic types of rehabilitation and diagnostic audiology procedures, defined as follows:

Assessment: Includes a determination of the patient's diagnosis when appropriate, need for treatment, planning for treatment, periodic assessment, and documentation related to these activities

Assessments are further classified into more than 100 different tests or methods. The majority of these focus on the faculties of hearing and speech, but others focus on various aspects of body function, and on the patient's quality of life, such as muscle performance, neuromotor development, and reintegration skills.

- *Speech Assessment*: Measurement of speech and related functions
- *Motor and/or Nerve Function Assessment*: Measurement of motor, nerve, and related functions
- *Activities of Daily Living Assessment*: Measurement of functional level for activities of daily living
- *Hearing Assessment*: Measurement of hearing and related functions
- *Hearing Aid Assessment*: Measurement of the appropriateness and/or effectiveness of a hearing device
- *Vestibular Assessment*: Measurement of the vestibular system and related functions

Caregiver Training: Educating caregiver with the skills and knowledge used to interact with and assist the patient

Caregiver Training is divided into 18 different broad subjects taught to help a caregiver provide proper patient care.

- *Caregiver Training*: Training in activities to support patient's optimal level of function

Fitting(s): Design, fabrication, modification, selection, and/or application of splint, orthosis, prosthesis, hearing aids, and/or other rehabilitation device

The fifth character used in *Device Fitting* procedures describes the device being fitted rather than the method used to fit the device. Definitions of devices, when provided, are located in the definitions portion of the ICD-10-PCS tables and index, under section F, character 5.

- *Device Fitting*: Fitting of a device designed to facilitate or support achievement of a higher level of function

Treatment: Use of specific activities or methods to develop, improve, and/or restore the performance of necessary functions, compensate for dysfunction and/or minimize debilitation

Treatment procedures include swallowing dysfunction exercises, bathing and showering techniques, wound management, gait training, and a host of activities typically associated with rehabilitation.

- *Speech Treatment*: Application of techniques to improve, augment, or compensate for speech and related functional impairment
- *Motor Treatment*: Exercise or activities to increase or facilitate motor function
- *Activities of Daily Living Treatment*: Exercise or activities to facilitate functional competence for activities of daily living
- *Hearing Treatment*: Application of techniques to improve, augment, or compensate for hearing and related functional impairment
- *Cochlear Implant Treatment*: Application of techniques to improve the communication abilities of individuals with cochlear implant
- *Vestibular Treatment*: Application of techniques to improve, augment, or compensate for vestibular and related functional impairment

The type of treatment includes training as well as activities that restore function.

Body System/Region (Character 4)

The fourth character specifies the body region and/or system on which the procedure is performed.

Type Qualifier (Character 5)

The fifth character is a type qualifier that further specifies the procedure performed. Examples include therapy to improve the range of motion and training for bathing techniques. Refer to appendix I for definitions of these types of procedures.

Equipment (Character 6)

The sixth character specifies the equipment used. Specific equipment is not defined in the equipment value. Instead, broad categories of equipment are specified (e.g., aerobic endurance and conditioning, assistive/adaptive/supportive, etc.)

Qualifier (Character 7)

The seventh character is not specified in the Physical Rehabilitation and Diagnostic Audiology section and always has the value *None*.

Mental Health Section (G)

Character Meanings

The seven characters in the Mental Health section have the following meaning:

Character	Meaning
1	Section
2	Body System
3	Type
4	Qualifier
5	Qualifier
6	Qualifier
7	Qualifier

Section (Character 1)

Mental health procedure codes have a first character value of *G*.

Body System (Character 2)

The second character is used to identify the body system elsewhere in ICD-10-PCS. In this section it always has the value *None*.

Type (Character 3)

The third character specifies the procedure type, such as crisis intervention or counseling. There are 12 types of mental health procedures.

- *Psychological Tests:* The administration and interpretation of standardized psychological tests and measurement instruments for the assessment of psychological function
- *Crisis Intervention:* Treatment of a traumatized, acutely disturbed, or distressed individual for the purpose of short-term stabilization
- *Medication Management:* Monitoring and adjusting the use of medications for the treatment of a mental health disorder
- *Individual Psychotherapy:* Treatment of an individual with a mental health disorder by behavioral, cognitive, psychoanalytic, psychodynamic, or psychophysiological means to improve functioning or well-being
- *Counseling:* The application of psychological methods to treat an individual with normal developmental issues and psychological problems in order to increase function, improve well-being, alleviate distress, maladjustment, or resolve crises
- *Family Psychotherapy:* Treatment that includes one or more family members of an individual with a mental health disorder by behavioral, cognitive, psychoanalytic, psychodynamic, or psychophysiological means to improve functioning or well-being
- *Electroconvulsive Therapy:* The application of controlled electrical voltages to treat a mental health disorder
- *Biofeedback:* Provision of information from the monitoring and regulating of physiological processes in conjunction with cognitive-behavioral techniques to improve patient functioning or well-being

- *Hypnosis:* Induction of a state of heightened suggestibility by auditory, visual, and tactile techniques to elicit an emotional or behavioral response
- *Narcosynthesis:* Administration of intravenous barbiturates in order to release suppressed or repressed thoughts
- *Group Psychotherapy:* Treatment of two or more individuals with a mental health disorder by behavioral, cognitive, psychoanalytic, psychodynamic, or psychophysiological means to improve functioning or well-being
- *Light Therapy:* Application of specialized light treatments to improve functioning or well-being

Qualifier (Character 4)

The fourth character is a qualifier to indicate that counseling was educational or vocational or to indicate type of test or method of therapy.

Qualifier (Character 5, 6 and 7)

The fifth, sixth, and seventh characters are not specified and always have the value *None.*

Substance Abuse Treatment Section (H)

Character Meanings

The seven characters in the Substance Abuse Treatment section have the following meaning:

Character	Meaning
1	Section
2	Body System
3	Type
4	Qualifier
5	Qualifier
6	Qualifier
7	Qualifier

Section (Character 1)

Substance Abuse Treatment codes have a first character value of *H.*

Body System (Character 2)

The second character is used to identify the body system elsewhere in ICD-10-PCS. In this section, it always has the value *None.*

Type (Character 3)

The third character specifies the type of procedure. There are seven values classified in this section, as listed below:

- *Detoxification Services:* Detoxification from alcohol and/or drugs
- *Individual Counseling:* The application of psychological methods to treat an individual with addictive behavior
- *Group Counseling:* The application of psychological methods to treat two or more individuals with addictive behavior
- *Individual Psychotherapy:* Treatment of an individual with addictive behavior by behavioral, cognitive, psychoanalytic, psychodynamic, or psychophysiological means
- *Family Counseling:* The application of psychological methods that includes one or more family members to treat an individual with addictive behavior
- *Medication Management:* Monitoring and adjusting the use of replacement medications for the treatment of addiction
- *Pharmacotherapy:* The use of replacement medications for the treatment of addiction

Qualifier (Character 4)

The fourth character further specifies the procedure type. These qualifier values vary dependent upon the Root Type procedure (Character 3). Root type 2, *Detoxification Services* contains only the value Z, *None* and Root type 6, *Family Counseling* contains only the value 3; *Other Family Counseling,* whereas the remainder Root Type procedures include multiple possible values.

Qualifier (Character 5, 6 and 7)

The fifth through seventh characters are designated as qualifiers but are never specified, so they always have the value *None.*

New Technology Section (X)

General Information

Section X New Technology is a section added to ICD-10-PCS beginning October 1, 2015. The new section provides a place for codes that uniquely identify procedures requested via the New Technology Application Process or that capture other new technologies not currently classified in ICD-10-PCS.

Section X does not introduce any new coding concepts or unusual guidelines for correct coding. In fact, Section X codes maintain continuity with the other sections in ICD-10-PCS by using the same root operation and body part values as their closest counterparts in other sections of ICD-10-PCS. For example, the codes for the infusion of ceftazidime-avibactam, use the same root operation (Introduction) and body part values (Central Vein and Peripheral Vein) in section X as the infusion codes in section 3 Administration, which are their closest counterparts in the other sections of ICD-10-PCS.

Character Meanings

The seven characters in the new technology section have the following meaning:

Character	Meaning
1	Section
2	Body System
3	Root Operation
4	Body Part
5	Approach
6	Device/Substance/Technology
7	Qualifier

Section (Character 1)

New technology procedure codes have a first character value of *X.*

Body System (Character 2)

The second character values for body system combine the uses of body system, body region, and physiological system as specified in other sections in ICD-10-PCS.

Root Operation (Character 3)

The third character utilizes the same root operation values as their counterparts in other sections of ICD-10-PCS.

Body Part (Character 4)

The fourth character specifies the same body part values as their closest counterparts in other sections of ICD-10-PCS.

Approach (Character 5)

The fifth character specifies approaches as defined in the Medical and Surgical section.

Device/Substance/Technology (Character 6)

The sixth character specifies the key feature of the new technology procedure. It may be specified as a new device, a new substance, or other new technology. Examples of sixth character values are *blinatumomab antineoplastic immunotherapy, orbital atherectomy technology,* and *intraoperative knee replacement sensor.*

Qualifier (Character 7)

The seventh character qualifier is used exclusively to specify the new technology group, a number or letter that changes each year that new technology codes are added to the system. For example, Section X codes added for the first year have the seventh character value 1, *New Technology Group 1*, and the next year that Section X codes are added have the seventh character value 2, *New Technology Group 2*, and so on. Changing the seventh character value to a unique letter or number every year that there are new codes in the new technology section allows the ICD-10-PCS to "recycle" the values in the third, fourth, and sixth characters as needed.

New Technology Coding Instruction

Section X codes are standalone codes. They are not supplemental codes. Section X codes fully represent the specific procedure described in the code title, and do not require any additional codes from other sections of ICD-10-PCS. When section X contains a code title which describes a specific new technology procedure, only that X code is reported for the procedure. There is no need to report a broader, non-specific code in another section of ICD-10-PCS.

For example, code XWØ4321 Introduction of Ceftazidime-Avibactam Anti-infective into Central Vein, Percutaneous Approach, New Technology Group 1, would be reported to indicate that Ceftazidime-Avibactam Anti-infective was administered via central vein. A separate code from table 3EØ in the Administration section of ICD-10-PCS would not be reported in addition to this code. The X section code fully identifies the administration of the ceftazidime-avibactam antibiotic, and no additional code is needed.

The New Technology section codes are easily found by looking in the ICD-10-PCS Index or the Tables. In the Index, the name of the new technology device, substance or technology for a section X code is included as a main term. In addition, all codes in section X are listed under the main term New Technology. The new technology code index entry for ceftazidime-avibactam is shown below.

Ceftazidime-Avibactam Anti-infective XWØ

New Technology
  Ceftazidime-Avibactam Anti-infective XWØ

Appendixes

The resources described below have been included as appendixes for *ICD-10-PCS The Complete Official Code Set.* These resources further instruct the coder on the appropriate application of the ICD-10-PCS code set.

Appendix A: Components of the Medical and Surgical Approach Definitions

This resource further defines the approach characters used in the Medical and Surgical (Ø) section. Complementing the detailed definition of the approach, additional information includes whether or not instrumentation is a part of the approach, the typical access location, the method used to initiate the approach, related procedural examples, and illustrations all of which will help the user determine the appropriate approach value.

Appendix B: Root Operation Definitions

This resource is a compilation of all root operations found in the Medical and Surgical-related sections (Ø-9) of this PCS manual. It provides a definition and in some cases a more detailed explanation of the root operation, to better reflect the purpose or objective. Examples of related procedure(s) may also be provided.

Appendix C: Comparison of Medical and Surgical Root Operations

The Medical and Surgical root operations are divided into groups that share similar attributes. These groups, and the root operations in each group, are listed in this resource along with information identifying the target of the root operation, the action used to perform the root operation, any clarification or further explanation on the objective of the root operation, and procedure examples.

Appendix D: Body Part Key

When an anatomical term or description is provided in the documentation but does not have a specific body part character within a table, the user can reference this resource to search for the anatomical description or site noted in the documentation to determine if there is a specific PCS body part character (character 4) to which the anatomical description or site could be coded.

Appendix E: Body Part Definitions

This resource is the reverse look-up of the Body Part Key. Each table in the Medical and Surgical section (Ø) of the PCS manual contains anatomical terms linked to a body part character or value, for example, in Table ØBB the Body Part (character 4) of 1 is Trachea. The body part Trachea may have anatomical structures or descriptions that may be used in procedure documentation instead of the term trachea. The Body Part Definitions list other anatomical structures or synonyms that are included in specific ICD-10-PCS body part values. According to the body part definitions, in the example above, cricoid cartilage is included in the Trachea (character 1) body part.

Appendix F: Device Key and Aggregation Table

The Device Key relates specific devices used in the medical profession, such as stents or bovine pericardial valves, with the appropriate device character (character 6).

The Aggregation Table crosswalks specific device character value definitions for specific root operations in a specific body system to the more general device character value to be used when the root operation covers a wide range of body parts and the device character represents an entire family of devices.

Appendix G: Device Definitions

This resource is a reverse look-up to the Device Key. The user may reference this resource to see all the specific devices that may be grouped to a particular device character (character 6).

Appendix H: Substance Key/Substance Definitions

The Substance Key lists substances by trade name or synonym and relates them to a PCS character in the Administration (3) or New Technology (X) section in the sixth character Substance or seventh character Qualifier column.

The Substance Definitions table is the reverse look-up of the substance key, relating all substance categories, the sixth- or seventh character values, to all trade name or synonyms that may be classified to that particular character.

Appendix I: Sections B-H Character Definitions

In each ancillary section (B-H) the characters in a particular column may have different meanings depending on which ancillary section the user is working from. This resource provides the values for the characters in that particular ancillary section as well as a definition of the character value.

Appendix J: Hospital Acquired Conditions

This comprehensive table displays codes identifying conditions that are considered reasonably preventable when occurring during the hospital admission and may prevent the case from grouping to a higher-paying MS-DRG. Many of these HACs are conditional and are based on reporting of a specific ICD-10-CM diagnosis code in combination with certain ICD-10-PCS procedure codes, all of which are noted in this table.

Appendix K: Coding Exercises with Answers

This resource provides the coding exercises with answers, and in some cases a brief explanation as to the reason that particular code was used.

Appendix L: Procedure Combination Tables

The procedure combination tables provided in this resource illustrate certain procedure combinations that must occur in order to assign a specific MS-DRG.

Sources

All material contained in this manual is derived from the ICD-10-PCS Coding System files, revised and distributed by the Centers for Medicare and Medicaid Services, FY 2019.

ICD-10-PCS Index and Tabular Format

The *ICD-10-PCS: The Complete Official Code Set* is based on the official version of the International Classification of Diseases, 10th Revision, Procedure Classification System, issued by the U.S. Department of Health and Human Services, Centers for Medicare and Medicaid Services. This book is consistent with the content of the government's version of ICD-10-PCS and follows their official format.

Index

The Alphabetic Index can be used to locate the appropriate table containing all the information necessary to construct a procedure code, however, the PCS tables should always be consulted to find the most appropriate valid code. Users may choose a valid code directly from the tables—he or she need not consult the index before proceeding to the tables to complete the code.

Main Terms

The Alphabetic Index reflects the structure of the tables. Therefore, the index is organized as an alphabetic listing. The index:

- Is based on the value of the third character
- Contains common procedure terms
- Lists anatomic sites
- Uses device terms

The main terms in the Alphabetic Index are root operations, root procedure types, or common procedure names. In addition, anatomic sites from the Body Part Key and device terms from the Device Key have been added for ease of use.

Examples:

Resection (root operation)

Fluoroscopy (root type)

Prostatectomy (common procedure name)

Brachial artery (body part)

Bard® Dulex™ mesh (device)

The index provides at least the first three or four values of the code, and some entries may provide complete valid codes. However, the user should always consult the appropriate table to verify that the most appropriate valid code has been selected.

Root Operation and Procedure Type Main Terms

For the *Medical and Surgical* and related sections, the root operation values are used as main terms in the index. The subterms under the root operation main terms are body parts. For the Ancillary section of the tables, the main terms in the index are the general type of procedure performed.

Examples:

Biofeedback GZC9ZZZ
Destruction
  Acetabulum
    Left ØQ55
    Right ØQ54
  Adenoids ØC5Q
  Ampulla of Vater ØF5C
Planar Nuclear Medicine Imaging
  Abdomen CW1Ø

See Reference

The second type of term in the index uses common procedure names, such as "appendectomy" or "fundoplication." These common terms are listed as main terms with a "see" reference noting the PCS root operations that are possible valid code tables based on the objective of the procedure.

Examples:

Tendonectomy
  see Excision, Tendons ØLB
  see Resection, Tendons ØLT

Use Reference

The index also lists anatomic sites from the Body Part Key and device terms from the Device Key. These terms are listed with a "use" reference. The purpose of these references is to act as an additional reference to the terms located in the Appendix Keys. The term provided is the Body Part value or Device value to be selected when constructing a procedure code using the code tables. This type of index reference is not intended to direct the user to another term in the index, but to provide guidance regarding character value selection. Therefore, "use" references generally do not refer to specific valid code tables.

Examples:

CoAxia NeuroFlo catheter
  use Intraluminal Device
Epitrochlear lymph node
  use Lymphatic, Right Upper Extremity
  use Lymphatic, Left Upper Extremity
SynCardia Total Artificial Heart
  use Synthetic Substitute

Code Tables

ICD-10-PCS contains 17 sections of Code Tables organized by general type of procedure. The first three characters of a procedure code define each table. The tables consist of columns providing the possible last four characters of codes and rows providing valid values for each character. Within a PCS table, valid codes include all combinations of choices in characters 4 through 7 contained in the same row of the table. All seven characters must be specified to form a valid code.

There are three main sections of tables:

- Medical and Surgical section:
  - *Medical and Surgical* (Ø)
- Medical and Surgical-related sections:
  - *Obstetrics* (1)
  - *Placement* (2)
  - *Administration* (3)
  - *Measurement and Monitoring* (4)
  - *Extracorporeal or Systemic Assistance and Performance* (5)
  - *Extracorporeal or Systemic Therapies* (6)
  - *Osteopathic* (7)
  - *Other Procedures* (8)
  - *Chiropractic* (9)

- Ancillary sections:
  - — *Imaging* (B)
  - — *Nuclear Medicine* (C)
  - — *Radiation Therapy* (D)
  - — *Physical Rehabilitation and Diagnostic Audiology* (F)
  - — *Mental Health* (G)
  - — *Substance Abuse Treatment* (H)
- New Technology section:
  - — *New Technology* (X)

The first three character values define each table. The root operation or root type designated for each table is accompanied by its official definition.

Example:
Table ØØF provides codes for procedures on the central nervous system that involve breaking up of solid matter into pieces:

Character 1, Section	Ø: Medical and Surgical
Character 2, Body System	Ø: Central Nervous System and Cranial Nerves
Character 3, Root Operation	F: Fragmentation: Breaking solid matter in a body part into pieces

Tables are arranged numerically, then alphabetically.

When reviewing tables, the user should keep in mind that:

- Some tables may cover multiple pages in the code book—to ensure maximum clarity about character choices, valid entries do not split rows between pages. For instance, the entire table of valid characters completing a code beginning with 4A1 is split between two pages, but the split is between, not within, rows. This means that all the valid sixth and seventh characters for, say, body system *Arterial* (3) and approach *External* (X) are contained on one page.
- Individual entries may be listed in several horizontal "selection" lines.
- When a table is continued onto another page, a note to this effect has been added in red.

Body Part Definitions:
An exclusive feature in the tables is the incorporation of the body part definitions provided in appendix E into the Medical and Surgical section (Ø) tables under their appropriate body part characters in the fourth column (character 4). This provides the user a direct reference to all anatomical descriptions, terms, and sites that could be coded to that particular body part value.

Paired body parts typically have values for the right and left side and in some cases a value for bilateral. These paired body parts often have the same list of inclusive body part definitions. When there are paired body parts with the same body part definitions, the first listed body part (usually the right side) contains the list of body part definitions while the second listed body part (usually the left side) contains a ***See*** instruction. This ***See*** instruction references the body part value that contains the body part definitions. In the table below, body part value P – Upper Eyelid, Left is followed by a ***See*** instruction that states ***See*** *N Upper Eyelid, Right.* All body part descriptions under value N also apply to body part value P.

Example:

Ø Medical and Surgical
8 Eye
M Reattachment Definition: Putting back in or on all or a portion of a separated body part to its normal location or other suitable location
Explanation: Vascular circulation and nervous pathways may or may not be reestablished

Body Part Character 4	Approach Character 5	Device Character 6	Qualifier Character 7
N Upper Eyelid, Right Lateral canthus Levator palpebrae superioris muscle Orbicularis oculi muscle Superior tarsal plate **P** Upper Eyelid, Left *See N Upper Eyelid, Right* **Q** Lower Eyelid, Right Inferior tarsal plate Medial canthus **R** Lower Eyelid, Left *See Q Lower Eyelid, Right*	**X** External	**Z** No Device	**Z** No Qualifier

ICD-10-PCS Additional Features

Use of Official Sources

The *ICD-10-PCS: The Complete Official Code Set* contains the official U.S. Department of Health and Human Services, Tenth Revision, Procedure Classification System, effective for the current year.

Color-coding, symbol, and other annotations in this manual that identify coding and reimbursement issues are derived from various official federal government sources, including Medicare Code Editor (MCE), version 35, ICD-10 MS-DRG Definitions Manual Files, version 35, and the *Federal Register*, volume 83, number 88, May 7, 2018 ("Hospital Inpatient Prospective Payment Systems for Acute Care Hospitals and the Long Term Care Hospital Prospective Payment System and Proposed Policy Changes and Fiscal Year 2019 Rates; Proposed Rule"). For the most current files related to IPPS, please refer to the following:

https://www.cms.gov/Medicare/Medicare-Fee-for-Service-Payment/AcuteInpatientPPS/IPPS-Regulations-and-Notices.html.

Table Notations

Many tables in ICD-10-PCS contain color or symbol annotations that may aid in code selection, provide clinical or coding information, or alert the coder to reimbursement issues affected by the PCS code assignment. These annotations are most often displayed on or next to a character 4 value. Some character 4 values may have more than one annotation.

Refer to the color/symbol legend at the bottom of each page in the tables section for an abridged description of each color and symbol.

Annotation Box

An annotation box has been appended to all tables that contain color-coding or symbol annotations. The color bar or symbol attached to a character 4 value is provided in the box, as well as a list of the valid PCS code(s) to which that edit applies. The box may also list conditional criteria that must be met to satisfy the edit.

For example, see Table ØØF. Four character 4 body part values have a gray color bar. In the annotation box below the table, the gray color bar is defined as "Non-OR," or a nonoperating room procedure edit. Following the Non-OR annotation are the PCS codes that are considered nonoperating room procedures from that row of Table ØØF.

Bracketed Code Notation

The use of bracketed codes is an efficient convention to provide all valid character value alternatives for a specific set of circumstances. The character values in the brackets correspond to the valid values for the character in the position the bracket appears.

Examples:

In the annotation box for Table ØØF the Noncovered Procedure edit (NC) applies to codes represented in the bracketed code ØØF[3,4,5,6]XZZ.

ØØF[3,4,5,6]XZZ Fragmentation in (Central Nervous System and Cranial Nerves), External Approach

The valid fourth character values (Body Part) that may be selected for this specific circumstance are as follows:

3 Epidural Space, Intracranial

4 Subdural Space, Intracranial

5 Subarachnoid Space, Intracranial

6 Cerebral Ventricle

The fragmentation of matter in the spinal canal, Body Part value U, is not included in the noncovered procedure code edits.

Color-Coding/Symbols

New and Revised Text

To highlight changes to the PCS tables for the current year, the new and revised text is provided in green font.

Medicare Code Edits

Medicare administrative contractors (MACs) and many payers use Medicare code edits to check the coding accuracy on claims. The coding edits in this manual are only those directly related to ICD-10-PCS codes and are used for acute care hospital inpatient admissions.

The PCS related Medicare code edits are listed below:

- Invalid procedure code
- *Sex conflict
- *Noncovered procedure
- *Limited coverage procedure

Starred edits above that are related to PCS issues are identified in this manual by symbols as described below.

Sex Edit Symbols

The sex edit symbols below address MCE and are used to detect inconsistencies between the patient's sex and the procedure. The symbols below most often appear to the right of a character 4 value but may also be found to the right of a character 7 value:

♂ Male procedure only

♀ Female procedure only

NC Noncovered Procedure

Medicare does not cover all procedures. However, some noncovered procedures, due to the presence of certain diagnoses, are reimbursed.

LC Limited Coverage

For certain procedures whose medical complexity and serious nature incur extraordinary associated costs, Medicare limits coverage to a portion of the cost. The limited coverage edit indicates the type of limited coverage.

ICD-10 MS-DRG Definitions Manual Edits

An MS-DRG is assigned based on specific patient attributes, such as principal diagnosis, secondary diagnoses, procedures, and discharge status. The attributes (edits) provided in this manual are only those directly related to ICD-10-PCS codes and are used for acute care hospital inpatient admissions.

Non-Operating Room Procedures Not Affecting MS-DRG Assignment

In the Medical and Surgical section (ØØ1-ØYW) and the Obstetric section (1Ø2-1ØY) tables **only,** ICD-10-PCS procedures codes that DO NOT affect MS-DRG assignment are identified by a **gray color bar** over the character 4 value and are considered non-operating room (non-OR) procedures.

NOTE: The majority of the ICD-10-PCS codes in the Medical and Surgical-Related, Ancillary and New Technology section tables are non-operating room procedures that do not typically affect MS-DRG assignment. Only the Valid Operating Room and DRG Non-Operating Room procedures are highlighted in these sections, *see* Non-Operating Room Procedures Affecting MS-DRG Assignment and Valid OR Procedure description below.

Non-Operating Room Procedures Affecting MS-DRG Assignment

Some ICD-10-PCS procedure codes, although considered non-operating room procedures, may still affect MS-DRG assignment. In all sections of the ICD-10-PCS book, these procedures are identified by a **purple color bar** over the character 4 value.

Valid OR Procedure

In the Medical and Surgical-Related (2WØ-9WB), Ancillary (BØØ-HZ9) and New Technology (X2A-XYØ) section tables **only,** any codes that are considered a valid operating room procedure are identified with a **blue color bar** over the character 4 value and will affect MS-DRG assignment. All codes without a color bar (blue or purple) are considered non-operating room procedures.

Hospital-Acquired Condition Related Procedures

Procedures associated with hospital-acquired conditions (HAC) are identified with the **yellow color bar** over the body part value.

Combination Only

Some ICD-10-PCS procedure codes are considered "noncovered procedures" except when reported in combination with certain other procedure codes. Such codes are designated by a **red color bar** over the character 4 value.

⊞ **Combination Member**

A combination member is an ICD-10-PCS procedure code that can influence MS-DRG assignment either on its own or in combination with other specific ICD-10-PCS procedure codes. Combination member codes are designated by a plus sign (⊞) to the right of the body part value.

See Appendix L for Procedure Combinations

Under certain circumstances, more than one procedure code is needed in order to group to a specific MS-DRG. When codes within a table have been identified as a Combination Only (**red color bar**) or Combination Member (⊞) code, there is also a footnote instructing the coder to *see Appendix L*. Appendix L contains tables that identify the other procedure codes needed in the combination and the title and number of the MS-DRG to which the combination will group.

Other Table Notations

AHA Coding Clinic:

Official citations from AHA's *Coding Clinic for ICD-10-CM/PCS* have been provided at the beginning of each section, when applicable. Each specific citation is listed below a header identifying the table to which that particular *Coding Clinic* citation applies. The citations appear in purple type with the year, quarter, and page of the reference as well as the title of the question as it appears in that *Coding Clinic's* table of contents. *Coding Clinic* citations included in this edition have been updated through first quarter 2018.

Index Notations

▽ Subterms under main terms may continue to the next column or page. This warning statement is a reminder to always check for additional subterms and information that may continue onto the next page or column before making a final selection.

ICD-10-PCS Official Guidelines for Coding and Reporting 2019

Narrative changes appear in **bold** text.

The Centers for Medicare and Medicaid Services (CMS) and the National Center for Health Statistics (NCHS), two departments within the U.S. Federal Government's Department of Health and Human Services (DHHS) provide the following guidelines for coding and reporting using the International Classification of Diseases, 10th Revision, Procedure Coding System (ICD-10-PCS). These guidelines should be used as a companion document to the official version of the ICD-10-PCS as published on the CMS website. The ICD-10-PCS is a procedure classification published by the United States for classifying procedures performed in hospital inpatient health care settings.

These guidelines have been approved by the four organizations that make up the Cooperating Parties for the ICD-10-PCS: the American Hospital Association (AHA), the American Health Information Management Association (AHIMA), CMS, and NCHS.

These guidelines are a set of rules that have been developed to accompany and complement the official conventions and instructions provided within the ICD-10-PCS itself. The instructions and conventions of the classification take precedence over guidelines. These guidelines are based on the coding and sequencing instructions in the Tables, Index and Definitions of ICD-10-PCS, but provide additional instruction. Adherence to these guidelines when assigning ICD-10-PCS procedure codes is required under the Health Insurance Portability and Accountability Act (HIPAA). The procedure codes have been adopted under HIPAA for hospital inpatient healthcare settings. A joint effort between the healthcare provider and the coder is essential to achieve complete and accurate documentation, code assignment, and reporting of diagnoses and procedures. These guidelines have been developed to assist both the healthcare provider and the coder in identifying those procedures that are to be reported. The importance of consistent, complete documentation in the medical record cannot be overemphasized. Without such documentation accurate coding cannot be achieved.

Conventions

A1. ICD-10-PCS codes are composed of seven characters. Each character is an axis of classification that specifies information about the procedure performed. Within a defined code range, a character specifies the same type of information in that axis of classification.

Example: The fifth axis of classification specifies the approach in sections Ø through 4 and 7 through 9 of the system.

A2. One of 34 possible values can be assigned to each axis of classification in the seven-character code: they are the numbers Ø through 9 and the alphabet (except I and O because they are easily confused with the numbers 1 and Ø). The number of unique values used in an axis of classification differs as needed.

Example: Where the fifth axis of classification specifies the approach, seven different approach values are currently used to specify the approach.

A3. The valid values for an axis of classification can be added to as needed.

Example: If a significantly distinct type of device is used in a new procedure, a new device value can be added to the system.

A4. As with words in their context, the meaning of any single value is a combination of its axis of classification and any preceding values on which it may be dependent.

Example: The meaning of a body part value in the Medical and Surgical section is always dependent on the body system value. The body part value Ø in the Central Nervous body system specifies Brain and the body part value Ø in the Peripheral Nervous body system specifies Cervical Plexus.

A5. As the system is expanded to become increasingly detailed, over time more values will depend on preceding values for their meaning.

Example: In the Lower Joints body system, the device value 3 in the root operation Insertion specifies Infusion Device and the device value 3 in the root operation Replacement specifies Ceramic Synthetic Substitute.

A6. The purpose of the alphabetic index is to locate the appropriate table that contains all information necessary to construct a procedure code. The PCS Tables should always be consulted to find the most appropriate valid code.

A7. It is not required to consult the index first before proceeding to the tables to complete the code. A valid code may be chosen directly from the tables.

A8. All seven characters must be specified to be a valid code. If the documentation is incomplete for coding purposes, the physician should be queried for the necessary information.

A9. Within a PCS table, valid codes include all combinations of choices in characters 4 through 7 contained in the same row of the table. In the example below, ØJHT3VZ is a valid code, and ØJHW3VZ is *not* a valid code.

Section: Ø **Medical and Surgical**
Body System: J **Subcutaneous Tissue and Fascia**
Operation: H **Insertion** Putting in a nonbiological appliance that monitors, assists, performs, or prevents a physiological function but does not physically take the place of a body part

Body Part	Approach	Device	Qualifier
S Subcutaneous Tissue and Fascia, Head and Neck **V** Subcutaneous Tissue and Fascia, Upper Extremity **W** Subcutaneous Tissue and Fascia, Lower Extremity	**Ø** Open **3** Percutaneous	**1** Radioactive Element **3** Infusion Device	**Z** No Qualifier
T Subcutaneous Tissue and Fascia, Trunk	**Ø** Open **3** Percutaneous	**1** Radioactive Element **3** Infusion Device **V** Infusion Pump	**Z** No Qualifier

A10. "And," when used in a code description, means "and/or," **except when used to describe a combination of multiple body parts for which separate values exist for each body part (e.g., Skin and Subcutaneous Tissue used as a qualifier, where there are separate body part values for "Skin" and "Subcutaneous Tissue").**

Example: Lower Arm and Wrist Muscle means lower arm and/or wrist muscle.

A11. Many of the terms used to construct PCS codes are defined within the system. It is the coder's responsibility to determine what the documentation in the medical record equates to in the PCS definitions. The physician is not expected to use the terms used in PCS code descriptions, nor is the coder required to query the physician when the correlation between the documentation and the defined PCS terms is clear.

Example: When the physician documents "partial resection" the coder can independently correlate "partial resection" to the root operation Excision without querying the physician for clarification.

Medical and Surgical Section Guidelines (section Ø)

B2. Body System

General guidelines

B2.1a. The procedure codes in the general anatomical regions body systems can be used when the procedure is performed on an anatomical region rather than a specific body part (e.g., root operations Control and Detachment, Drainage of a body cavity) or on the rare occasion when no information is available to support assignment of a code to a specific body part.

Examples: Control of postoperative hemorrhage is coded to the root operation Control found in the general anatomical regions body systems.

Chest tube drainage of the pleural cavity is coded to the root operation Drainage found in the general anatomical regions body systems. Suture repair of the abdominal wall is coded to the root operation Repair in the general anatomical regions body system.

B2.1b. Where the general body part values "upper" and "lower" are provided as an option in the Upper Arteries, Lower Arteries, Upper Veins, Lower Veins, Muscles and Tendons body systems, "upper" or "lower "specifies body parts located above or below the diaphragm respectively.

Example: Vein body parts above the diaphragm are found in the Upper Veins body system; vein body parts below the diaphragm are found in the Lower Veins body system.

B3. Root Operation

General guidelines

B3.1a. In order to determine the appropriate root operation, the full definition of the root operation as contained in the PCS Tables must be applied.

B3.1b. Components of a procedure specified in the root operation definition and explanation are not coded separately. Procedural steps necessary to reach the operative site and close the operative site, including anastomosis of a tubular body part, are also not coded separately.

Examples: Resection of a joint as part of a joint replacement procedure is included in the root operation definition of Replacement and is not coded separately.

Laparotomy performed to reach the site of an open liver biopsy is not coded separately. In a resection of sigmoid colon with anastomosis of descending colon to rectum, the anastomosis is not coded separately.

Multiple procedures

B3.2. During the same operative episode, multiple procedures are coded if:

a. The same root operation is performed on different body parts as defined by distinct values of the body part character.

   Examples: Diagnostic excision of liver and pancreas are coded separately.

   Excision of lesion in the ascending colon and excision of lesion in the transverse colon are coded separately.

b. The same root operation is repeated in multiple body parts, and those body parts are separate and distinct body parts classified to a single ICD-10-PCS body part value.

   Examples: Excision of the sartorius muscle and excision of the gracilis muscle are both included in the upper leg muscle body part value, and multiple procedures are coded.

   Extraction of multiple toenails are coded separately.

c. Multiple root operations with distinct objectives are performed on the same body part.

   Example: Destruction of sigmoid lesion and bypass of sigmoid colon are coded separately.

d. The intended root operation is attempted using one approach, but is converted to a different approach.

   Example: Laparoscopic cholecystectomy converted to an open cholecystectomy is coded as percutaneous endoscopic Inspection and open Resection.

Discontinued or incomplete procedures

B3.3. If the intended procedure is discontinued or otherwise not completed, code the procedure to the root operation performed. If a procedure is discontinued before any other root operation is performed, code the root operation Inspection of the body part or anatomical region inspected.

Example: A planned aortic valve replacement procedure is discontinued after the initial thoracotomy and before any incision is made in the heart muscle, when the patient becomes hemodynamically unstable. This procedure is coded as an open Inspection of the mediastinum.

Biopsy procedures

B3.4a. Biopsy procedures are coded using the root operations Excision, Extraction, or Drainage and the qualifier Diagnostic.

Examples: Fine needle aspiration biopsy of fluid in the lung is coded to the root operation Drainage with the qualifier Diagnostic.

Biopsy of bone marrow is coded to the root operation Extraction with the qualifier Diagnostic.

Lymph node sampling for biopsy is coded to the root operation Excision with the qualifier Diagnostic.

Biopsy followed by more definitive treatment

B3.4b. If a diagnostic Excision, Extraction, or Drainage procedure (biopsy) is followed by a more definitive procedure, such as Destruction, Excision or Resection at the same procedure site, both the biopsy and the more definitive treatment are coded.

Example: Biopsy of breast followed by partial mastectomy at the same procedure site, both the biopsy and the partial mastectomy procedure are coded.

Overlapping body layers

B3.5. If the root operations Excision, Repair or Inspection are performed on overlapping layers of the musculoskeletal system, the body part specifying the deepest layer is coded.

Example: Excisional debridement that includes skin and subcutaneous tissue and muscle is coded to the muscle body part.

Bypass procedures

B3.6a. Bypass procedures are coded by identifying the body part bypassed "from" and the body part bypassed "to." The fourth character body part specifies the body part bypassed from, and the qualifier specifies the body part bypassed to.

Example: Bypass from stomach to jejunum, stomach is the body part and jejunum is the qualifier.

B3.6b. Coronary artery bypass procedures are coded differently than other bypass procedures as described in the previous guideline. Rather than identifying the body part bypassed from, the body part identifies the number of coronary arteries bypassed to, and the qualifier specifies the vessel bypassed from.

Example: Aortocoronary artery bypass of the left anterior descending coronary artery and the obtuse marginal coronary artery is classified in the body part axis of classification as two coronary arteries, and the qualifier specifies the aorta as the body part bypassed from.

B3.6c. If multiple coronary arteries are bypassed, a separate procedure is coded for each coronary artery that uses a different device and/or qualifier.

Example: Aortocoronary artery bypass and internal mammary coronary artery bypass are coded separately.

Control vs. more definitive root operations

B3.7. The root operation Control is defined as, "Stopping, or attempting to stop, postprocedural or other acute bleeding." If an attempt to stop postprocedural or other acute bleeding is ~~initially~~ unsuccessful, and to stop the bleeding requires performing a more definitive root operation, such as Bypass, Detachment, Excision, Extraction, Reposition, Replacement, or Resection, then the more definitive root operation is coded instead of Control.

Example: Resection of spleen to stop bleeding is coded to Resection instead of Control.

Excision vs. Resection

B3.8. PCS contains specific body parts for anatomical subdivisions of a body part, such as lobes of the lungs or liver and regions of the intestine. Resection of the specific body part is coded whenever all of the body part is cut out or off, rather than coding Excision of a less specific body part.

Example: Left upper lung lobectomy is coded to Resection of Upper Lung Lobe, Left rather than Excision of Lung, Left.

Excision for graft

B3.9. If an autograft is obtained from a different procedure site in order to complete the objective of the procedure, a separate procedure is coded.

Example: Coronary bypass with excision of saphenous vein graft, excision of saphenous vein is coded separately.

Fusion procedures of the spine

B3.10a. The body part coded for a spinal vertebral joint(s) rendered immobile by a spinal fusion procedure is classified by the level of the spine (e.g. thoracic). There are distinct body part values for a single vertebral joint and for multiple vertebral joints at each spinal level.

Example: Body part values specify Lumbar Vertebral Joint, Lumbar Vertebral Joints, 2 or More and Lumbosacral Vertebral Joint.

B3.10b. If multiple vertebral joints are fused, a separate procedure is coded for each vertebral joint that uses a different device and/or qualifier.

Example: Fusion of lumbar vertebral joint, posterior approach, anterior column and fusion of lumbar vertebral joint, posterior approach, posterior column are coded separately.

B3.10c. Combinations of devices and materials are often used on a vertebral joint to render the joint immobile. When combinations of devices are used on the same vertebral joint, the device value coded for the procedure is as follows:

- If an interbody fusion device is used to render the joint immobile (alone or containing other material like bone graft), the procedure is coded with the device value Interbody Fusion Device
- If bone graft is the *only* device used to render the joint immobile, the procedure is coded with the device value Nonautologous Tissue Substitute or Autologous Tissue Substitute
- If a mixture of autologous and nonautologous bone graft (with or without biological or synthetic extenders or binders) is used to render the joint immobile, code the procedure with the device value Autologous Tissue Substitute

Examples: Fusion of a vertebral joint using a cage style interbody fusion device containing morsellized bone graft is coded to the device Interbody Fusion Device.

Fusion of a vertebral joint using a bone dowel interbody fusion device made of cadaver bone and packed with a mixture of local morsellized bone and demineralized bone matrix is coded to the device Interbody Fusion Device.

Fusion of a vertebral joint using both autologous bone graft and bone bank bone graft is coded to the device Autologous Tissue Substitute.

Inspection procedures

B3.11a. Inspection of a body part(s) performed in order to achieve the objective of a procedure is not coded separately.

Example: Fiberoptic bronchoscopy performed for irrigation of bronchus, only the irrigation procedure is coded.

B3.11b. If multiple tubular body parts are inspected, the most distal body part (the body part furthest from the starting point of the inspection) is coded. If multiple non-tubular body parts in a region are inspected, the body part that specifies the entire area inspected is coded.

Examples: Cystoureteroscopy with inspection of bladder and ureters is coded to the ureter body part value.

Exploratory laparotomy with general inspection of abdominal contents is coded to the peritoneal cavity body part value.

B3.11c. When both an Inspection procedure and another procedure are performed on the same body part during the same episode, if the Inspection procedure is performed using a different approach than the other procedure, the Inspection procedure is coded separately.

Example: Endoscopic Inspection of the duodenum is coded separately when open Excision of the duodenum is performed during the same procedural episode.

Occlusion vs. Restriction for vessel embolization procedures

B3.12. If the objective of an embolization procedure is to completely close a vessel, the root operation Occlusion is coded. If the objective of an embolization procedure is to narrow the lumen of a vessel, the root operation Restriction is coded.

Examples: Tumor embolization is coded to the root operation Occlusion, because the objective of the procedure is to cut off the blood supply to the vessel.

Embolization of a cerebral aneurysm is coded to the root operation Restriction, because the objective of the procedure is not to close off the vessel entirely, but to narrow the lumen of the vessel at the site of the aneurysm where it is abnormally wide.

Release procedures

B3.13. In the root operation Release, the body part value coded is the body part being freed and not the tissue being manipulated or cut to free the body part.

Example: Lysis of intestinal adhesions is coded to the specific intestine body part value.

Release vs. Division

B3.14. If the sole objective of the procedure is freeing a body part without cutting the body part, the root operation is Release. If the sole objective of the procedure is separating or transecting a body part, the root operation is Division.

Examples: Freeing a nerve root from surrounding scar tissue to relieve pain is coded to the root operation Release.

Severing a nerve root to relieve pain is coded to the root operation Division.

Reposition for fracture treatment

B3.15. Reduction of a displaced fracture is coded to the root operation Reposition and the application of a cast or splint in conjunction with the Reposition procedure is not coded separately. Treatment of a nondisplaced fracture is coded to the procedure performed.

Examples: Casting of a nondisplaced fracture is coded to the root operation Immobilization in the Placement section.

Putting a pin in a nondisplaced fracture is coded to the root operation Insertion.

Transplantation vs. Administration

B3.16. Putting in a mature and functioning living body part taken from another individual or animal is coded to the root operation Transplantation. Putting in autologous or nonautologous cells is coded to the Administration section.

Example: Putting in autologous or nonautologous bone marrow, pancreatic islet cells or stem cells is coded to the Administration section.

Transfer procedures using multiple tissue layers

B3.17. The root operation Transfer contains qualifiers that can be used to specify when a transfer flap is composed of more than one tissue layer, such as a musculocutaneous flap. For procedures involving transfer of multiple tissue layers including skin, subcutaneous tissue, fascia or muscle, the procedure is coded to the body part value that describes the deepest tissue layer in the flap, and the qualifier can be used to describe the other tissue layer(s) in the transfer flap.

***Example:* A musculocutaneous flap transfer is coded to the appropriate body part value in the body system Muscles, and the qualifier is used to describe the additional tissue layer(s) in the transfer flap.**

B4. Body Part

General guidelines

B4.1a. If a procedure is performed on a portion of a body part that does not have a separate body part value, code the body part value corresponding to the whole body part.

Example: A procedure performed on the alveolar process of the mandible is coded to the mandible body part.

B4.1b. If the prefix "peri" is combined with a body part to identify the site of the procedure, and the site of the procedure is not further specified, then the procedure is coded to the body part named. This guideline applies only when a more specific body part value is not available.

Examples: A procedure site identified as perirenal is coded to the kidney body part when the site of the procedure is not further specified.

A procedure site described in the documentation as peri-urethral, and the documentation also indicates that it is the vulvar tissue and not the urethral tissue that is the site of the procedure, then the procedure is coded to the vulva body part.

B4.1c. If a procedure is performed on a continuous section of a tubular body part, code the body part value corresponding to the furthest anatomical site from the point of entry.

Example: A procedure performed on a continuous section of artery from the femoral artery to the external iliac artery with the point of entry at the femoral artery is coded to the external iliac body part.

Branches of body parts

B4.2. Where a specific branch of a body part does not have its own body part value in PCS, the body part is typically coded to the closest proximal branch that has a specific body part value. In the cardiovascular body systems, if a general body part is available in the correct root operation table, and coding to a proximal branch would require assigning a code in a different body system, the procedure is coded using the general body part value.

Examples: A procedure performed on the mandibular branch of the trigeminal nerve is coded to the trigeminal nerve body part value.

Occlusion of the bronchial artery is coded to the body part value Upper Artery in the body system Upper Arteries, and not to the body part value Thoracic Aorta, Descending in the body system Heart and Great Vessels.

Bilateral body part values

B4.3. Bilateral body part values are available for a limited number of body parts. If the identical procedure is performed on contralateral body parts, and a bilateral body part value exists for that body part, a single procedure is coded using the bilateral body part value. If no bilateral body part value exists, each procedure is coded separately using the appropriate body part value.

Examples: The identical procedure performed on both fallopian tubes is coded once using the body part value Fallopian Tube, Bilateral.

The identical procedure performed on both knee joints is coded twice using the body part values Knee Joint, Right and Knee Joint, Left.

Coronary arteries

B4.4. The coronary arteries are classified as a single body part that is further specified by number of arteries treated. One procedure code specifying multiple arteries is used when the same procedure is performed, including the same device and qualifier values.

Examples: Angioplasty of two distinct coronary arteries with placement of two stents is coded as Dilation of Coronary Artery, Two Arteries with Two Intraluminal Devices.

Angioplasty of two distinct coronary arteries, one with stent placed and one without, is coded separately as Dilation of Coronary Artery, One Artery with Intraluminal Device, and Dilation of Coronary Artery, One Artery with no device.

Tendons, ligaments, bursae and fascia near a joint

B4.5. Procedures performed on tendons, ligaments, bursae and fascia supporting a joint are coded to the body part in the respective body system that is the focus of the procedure. Procedures performed on joint structures themselves are coded to the body part in the joint body systems.

Examples: Repair of the anterior cruciate ligament of the knee is coded to the knee bursa and ligament body part in the bursae and ligaments body system.

Knee arthroscopy with shaving of articular cartilage is coded to the knee joint body part in the Lower Joints body system.

Skin, subcutaneous tissue and fascia overlying a joint

B4.6. If a procedure is performed on the skin, subcutaneous tissue or fascia overlying a joint, the procedure is coded to the following body part:

- Shoulder is coded to Upper Arm
- Elbow is coded to Lower Arm
- Wrist is coded to Lower Arm
- Hip is coded to Upper Leg
- Knee is coded to Lower Leg
- Ankle is coded to Foot

Fingers and toes

B4.7. If a body system does not contain a separate body part value for fingers, procedures performed on the fingers are coded to the body part value for the hand. If a body system does not contain a separate body part value for toes, procedures performed on the toes are coded to the body part value for the foot.

Example: Excision of finger muscle is coded to one of the hand muscle body part values in the Muscles body system.

Upper and lower intestinal tract

B4.8. In the Gastrointestinal body system, the general body part values Upper Intestinal Tract and Lower Intestinal Tract are provided as an option for the root operations Change, Inspection, Removal and Revision. Upper Intestinal Tract includes the portion of the gastrointestinal tract from the esophagus down to and including the duodenum, and Lower Intestinal Tract includes the portion of the gastrointestinal tract from the jejunum down to and including the rectum and anus.

Example: In the root operation Change table, change of a device in the jejunum is coded using the body part Lower Intestinal Tract.

B5. Approach

Open approach with percutaneous endoscopic assistance

B5.2. Procedures performed using the open approach with percutaneous endoscopic assistance are coded to the approach Open.

Example: Laparoscopic-assisted sigmoidectomy is coded to the approach Open.

External approach

B5.3a. Procedures performed within an orifice on structures that are visible without the aid of any instrumentation are coded to the approach External.

Example: Resection of tonsils is coded to the approach External.

B5.3b. Procedures performed indirectly by the application of external force through the intervening body layers are coded to the approach External.

Example: Closed reduction of fracture is coded to the approach External.

Percutaneous procedure via device

B5.4. Procedures performed percutaneously via a device placed for the procedure are coded to the approach Percutaneous.

Example: Fragmentation of kidney stone performed via percutaneous nephrostomy is coded to the approach Percutaneous.

B6. Device

General guidelines

B6.1a. A device is coded only if a device remains after the procedure is completed. If no device remains, the device value No Device is coded. In limited root operations, the classification provides the qualifier values Temporary and Intraoperative, for specific procedures involving clinically significant devices, where the purpose of the device is to be utilized for a brief duration during the procedure or current inpatient stay. **If a device that is intended to remain after the procedure is completed requires removal before the end of the operative episode in which it was inserted (for example, the device size is**

inadequate or a complication occurs), both the insertion and removal of the device should be coded.

B6.1b. Materials such as sutures, ligatures, radiological markers and temporary post-operative wound drains are considered integral to the performance of a procedure and are not coded as devices.

B6.1c. Procedures performed on a device only and not on a body part are specified in the root operations Change, Irrigation, Removal and Revision, and are coded to the procedure performed.

Example: Irrigation of percutaneous nephrostomy tube is coded to the root operation Irrigation of indwelling device in the Administration section.

Drainage device

B6.2. A separate procedure to put in a drainage device is coded to the root operation Drainage with the device value Drainage Device.

Obstetric Section Guidelines (section 1)

C. Obstetrics Section

Products of conception

C1. Procedures performed on the products of conception are coded to the Obstetrics section. Procedures performed on the pregnant female other than the products of conception are coded to the appropriate root operation in the Medical and Surgical section.

Example: Amniocentesis is coded to the products of conception body part in the Obstetrics section. Repair of obstetric urethral laceration is coded to the urethra body part in the Medical and Surgical section.

Procedures following delivery or abortion

C2. Procedures performed following a delivery or abortion for curettage of the endometrium or evacuation of retained products of conception are all coded in the Obstetrics section, to the root operation Extraction and the body part Products of Conception, Retained.

Diagnostic or therapeutic dilation and curettage performed during times other than the postpartum or post-abortion period are all coded in the Medical and Surgical section, to the root operation Extraction and the body part Endometrium.

New Technology Section Guidelines (section X)

D. New Technology Section

General guidelines

D1. Section X codes are standalone codes. They are not supplemental codes. Section X codes fully represent the specific procedure described in the code title, and do not require any additional codes from other sections of ICD-10-PCS. When section X contains a code title which describes a specific new technology procedure, only that X code is reported for the procedure. There is no need to report a broader, non-specific code in another section of ICD-10-PCS.

Example: XWØ4321 Introduction of Ceftazidime-Avibactam Anti-infective into Central Vein, Percutaneous Approach, New Technology Group 1, can be coded to indicate that Ceftazidime-Avibactam Anti-infective was administered via a central vein. A separate code from table 3EØ in the Administration section of ICD-10-PCS is not coded in addition to this code.

Selection of Principal Procedure

The following instructions should be applied in the selection of principal procedure and clarification on the importance of the relation to the principal diagnosis when more than one procedure is performed:

1. Procedure performed for definitive treatment of both principal diagnosis and secondary diagnosis
   a. Sequence procedure performed for definitive treatment most related to principal diagnosis as principal procedure.
2. Procedure performed for definitive treatment and diagnostic procedures performed for both principal diagnosis and secondary diagnosis.
   a. Sequence procedure performed for definitive treatment most related to principal diagnosis as principal procedure
3. A diagnostic procedure was performed for the principal diagnosis and a procedure is performed for definitive treatment of a secondary diagnosis.
   a. Sequence diagnostic procedure as principal procedure, since the procedure most related to the principal diagnosis takes precedence.
4. No procedures performed that are related to principal diagnosis; procedures performed for definitive treatment and diagnostic procedures were performed for secondary diagnosis
   a. Sequence procedure performed for definitive treatment of secondary diagnosis as principal procedure, since there are no procedures (definitive or nondefinitive treatment) related to principal diagnosis.

Arytenoid cartilage *use* Larynx
Arytenoid muscle
 use Neck Muscle, Left
 use Neck Muscle, Right
Arytenoidectomy *see* Excision, Larynx, ØCBS
Arytenoidopexy *see* Repair, Larynx, ØCQS
Ascenda Intrathecal Catheter *use* Infusion Device
Ascending aorta *use* Thoracic Aorta, Ascending/Arch
Ascending palatine artery *use* Face Artery
Ascending pharyngeal artery
 use External Carotid Artery, Left
 use External Carotid Artery, Right
Aspiration, fine needle
 Fluid or gas *see* Drainage
 Tissue biopsy
 see Excision
 see Extraction
Assessment
 Activities of daily living *see* Activities of Daily Living
 Assessment, Rehabilitation, FØ2
 Hearing *see* Hearing Assessment, Diagnostic Audiol-
 ogy, F13
 Hearing aid *see* Hearing Aid Assessment, Diagnostic
 Audiology, F14
 Intravascular perfusion, using indocyanine green (ICG)
 dye *see* Monitoring, Physiological Systems, 4A1
 Motor function *see* Motor Function Assessment, Re-
 habilitation, FØ1
 Nerve function *see* Motor Function Assessment, Re-
 habilitation, FØ1
 Speech *see* Speech Assessment, Rehabilitation, FØØ
 Vestibular *see* Vestibular Assessment, Diagnostic
 Audiology, F15
 Vocational *see* Activities of Daily Living Treatment,
 Rehabilitation, FØ8
Assistance
 Cardiac
 Continuous
 Balloon Pump, 5AØ221Ø
 Impeller Pump, 5AØ221D
 Other Pump, 5AØ2216
 Pulsatile Compression, 5AØ2215
 Intermittent
 Balloon Pump, 5AØ211Ø
 Impeller Pump, 5AØ211D
 Other Pump, 5AØ2116
 Pulsatile Compression, 5AØ2115
 Circulatory
 Continuous
 Hyperbaric, 5AØ5221
 Supersaturated, 5AØ522C
 Intermittent
 Hyperbaric, 5AØ5121
 Supersaturated, 5AØ512C
 Respiratory
 24-96 Consecutive Hours
 Continuous Negative Airway Pressure,
 5AØ9459
 Continuous Positive Airway Pressure,
 5AØ9457
 Intermittent Negative Airway Pressure,
 5AØ945B
 Intermittent Positive Airway Pressure,
 5AØ9458
 No Qualifier, 5AØ945Z
 Continuous, Filtration, 5AØ92ØZ
 Greater than 96 Consecutive Hours
 Continuous Negative Airway Pressure,
 5AØ9559
 Continuous Positive Airway Pressure,
 5AØ9557
 Intermittent Negative Airway Pressure,
 5AØ955B
 Intermittent Positive Airway Pressure,
 5AØ9558
 No Qualifier, 5AØ955Z
 Less than 24 Consecutive Hours
 Continuous Negative Airway Pressure,
 5AØ9359
 Continuous Positive Airway Pressure,
 5AØ9357
 Intermittent Negative Airway Pressure,
 5AØ935B
 Intermittent Positive Airway Pressure,
 5AØ9358
 No Qualifier, 5AØ935Z
Assurant (Cobalt) stent *use* Intraluminal Device

Atherectomy
 see Extirpation, Heart and Great Vessels, Ø2C
 see Extirpation, Lower Arteries, Ø4C
 see Extirpation, Upper Arteries, Ø3C
Atlantoaxial joint *use* Cervical Vertebral Joint
Atmospheric Control, 6AØZ
AtriClip LAA Exclusion System *use* Extraluminal Device
Atrioseptoplasty
 see Repair, Heart and Great Vessels, Ø2Q
 see Replacement, Heart and Great Vessels, Ø2R
 see Supplement, Heart and Great Vessels, Ø2U
Atrioventricular node *use* Conduction Mechanism
Atrium dextrum cordis *use* Atrium, Right
Atrium pulmonale *use* Atrium, Left
Attain Ability® lead, Ø2H
 use Cardiac Lead, Defibrillator in, Ø2H
 use Cardiac Lead, Pacemaker in, Ø2H
Attain Starfix® (OTW) lead
 use Cardiac Lead, Defibrillator in, Ø2H
 use Cardiac Lead, Pacemaker in, Ø2H
Audiology, diagnostic
 see Hearing Aid Assessment, Diagnostic Audiology,
 F14
 see Hearing Assessment, Diagnostic Audiology, F13
 see Vestibular Assessment, Diagnostic Audiology, F15
Audiometry *see* Hearing Assessment, Diagnostic Audiology, F13
Auditory tube
 use Eustachian Tube, Left
 use Eustachian Tube, Right
Auerbach's (myenteric) plexus *use* Abdominal Sympathetic Nerve
Auricle
 use External Ear, Bilateral
 use External Ear, Left
 use External Ear, Right
Auricularis muscle *use* Head Muscle
Autograft *use* Autologous Tissue Substitute
Autologous artery graft
 use Autologous Arterial Tissue in Heart and Great
 Vessels
 use Autologous Arterial Tissue in Lower Arteries
 use Autologous Arterial Tissue in Lower Veins
 use Autologous Arterial Tissue in Upper Arteries
 use Autologous Arterial Tissue in Upper Veins
Autologous vein graft
 use Autologous Venous Tissue in Heart and Great
 Vessels
 use Autologous Venous Tissue in Lower Arteries
 use Autologous Venous Tissue in Lower Veins
 use Autologous Venous Tissue in Upper Arteries
 use Autologous Venous Tissue in Upper Veins
Autotransfusion *see* Transfusion
Autotransplant
 Adrenal tissue *see* Reposition, Endocrine System, ØGS
 Kidney *see* Reposition, Urinary System, ØTS
 Pancreatic tissue *see* Reposition, Pancreas, ØFSG
 Parathyroid tissue *see* Reposition, Endocrine System,
 ØGS
 Thyroid tissue *see* Reposition, Endocrine System, ØGS
 Tooth *see* Reattachment, Mouth and Throat, ØCM
Avulsion *see* Extraction
Axial Lumbar Interbody Fusion System *use* Interbody
 Fusion Device in Lower Joints
AxiaLIF® System *use* Interbody Fusion Device in Lower
 Joints
Axicabtagene Ciloeucel *use* Engineered Autologous
 Chimeric Antigen Receptor T-cell Immunotherapy
Axillary fascia
 use Subcutaneous Tissue and Fascia, Left Upper Arm
 use Subcutaneous Tissue and Fascia, Right Upper Arm
Axillary nerve *use* Brachial Plexus

B

BAK/C® Interbody Cervical Fusion System *use* Inter-
 body Fusion Device in Upper Joints
BAL (bronchial alveolar lavage), diagnostic *see*
 Drainage, Respiratory System, ØB9
Balanoplasty
 see Repair, Penis, ØVQS
 see Supplement, Penis, ØVUS
Balloon atrial septostomy (BAS), Ø2163Z7
Balloon Pump
 Continuous, Output, 5AØ221Ø
 Intermittent, Output, 5AØ211Ø

Bandage, Elastic *see* Compression
Banding
 see Occlusion
 see Restriction
Banding, esophageal varices *see* Occlusion, Vein,
 Esophageal, Ø6L3
Banding, laparoscopic (adjustable) gastric
 Initial procedure, ØDV64CZ
 Surgical correction *see* Revision of device in, Stomach,
 ØDW6
Bard® Composix® Kugel® patch *use* Synthetic Substitute
Bard® Composix® (E/X) (LP) mesh *use* Synthetic Substi-
 tute
Bard® Dulex™ mesh *use* Synthetic Substitute
Bard® Ventralex™ Hernia Patch *use* Synthetic Substitute
Barium swallow *see* Fluoroscopy, Gastrointestinal System,
 BD1
Baroreflex Activation Therapy® (BAT®)
 use Stimulator Generator in Subcutaneous Tissue and
 Fascia
 use Stimulator Lead in Upper Arteries
Bartholin's (greater vestibular) gland *use* Vestibular
 Gland
Basal (internal) cerebral vein *use* Intracranial Vein
Basal metabolic rate (BMR) *see* Measurement, Physio-
 logical Systems, 4AØZ
Basal nuclei *use* Basal Ganglia
Base of Tongue *use* Pharynx
Basilar artery *use* Intracranial Artery
Basis pontis *use* Pons
Beam Radiation
 Abdomen, DWØ3
 Intraoperative, DWØ33ZØ
 Adrenal Gland, DGØ2
 Intraoperative, DGØ23ZØ
 Bile Ducts, DFØ2
 Intraoperative, DFØ23ZØ
 Bladder, DTØ2
 Intraoperative, DTØ23ZØ
 Bone
 Intraoperative, DPØC3ZØ
 Other, DPØC
 Bone Marrow, D7ØØ
 Intraoperative, D7ØØ3ZØ
 Brain, DØØØ
 Intraoperative, DØØØ3ZØ
 Brain Stem, DØØ1
 Intraoperative, DØØ13ZØ
 Breast
 Left, DMØØ
 Intraoperative, DMØØ3ZØ
 Right, DMØ1
 Intraoperative, DMØ13ZØ
 Bronchus, DBØ1
 Intraoperative, DBØ13ZØ
 Cervix, DUØ1
 Intraoperative, DUØ13ZØ
 Chest, DWØ2
 Intraoperative, DWØ23ZØ
 Chest Wall, DBØ7
 Intraoperative, DBØ73ZØ
 Colon, DDØ5
 Intraoperative, DDØ53ZØ
 Diaphragm, DBØ8
 Intraoperative, DBØ83ZØ
 Duodenum, DDØ2
 Intraoperative, DDØ23ZØ
 Ear, D9ØØ
 Intraoperative, D9ØØ3ZØ
 Esophagus, DDØØ
 Intraoperative, DDØØ3ZØ
 Eye, D8ØØ
 Intraoperative, D8ØØ3ZØ
 Femur, DPØ9
 Intraoperative, DPØ93ZØ
 Fibula, DPØB
 Intraoperative, DPØB3ZØ
 Gallbladder, DFØ1
 Intraoperative, DFØ13ZØ
 Gland
 Adrenal, DGØ2
 Intraoperative, DGØ23ZØ
 Parathyroid, DGØ4
 Intraoperative, DGØ43ZØ
 Pituitary, DGØØ
 Intraoperative, DGØØ3ZØ
 Thyroid, DGØ5
 Intraoperative, DGØ53ZØ

Beam Radiation — *continued*
Glands
Intraoperative, D9063Z0
Salivary, D906
Head and Neck, DW01
Intraoperative, DW013Z0
Hemibody, DW04
Intraoperative, DW043Z0
Humerus, DP06
Intraoperative, DP063Z0
Hypopharynx, D903
Intraoperative, D9033Z0
Ileum, DD04
Intraoperative, DD043Z0
Jejunum, DD03
Intraoperative, DD033Z0
Kidney, DT00
Intraoperative, DT003Z0
Larynx, D90B
Intraoperative, D90B3Z0
Liver, DF00
Intraoperative, DF003Z0
Lung, DB02
Intraoperative, DB023Z0
Lymphatics
Abdomen, D706
Intraoperative, D7063Z0
Axillary, D704
Intraoperative, D7043Z0
Inguinal, D708
Intraoperative, D7083Z0
Neck, D703
Intraoperative, D7033Z0
Pelvis, D707
Intraoperative, D7073Z0
Thorax, D705
Intraoperative, D7053Z0
Mandible, DP03
Intraoperative, DP033Z0
Maxilla, DP02
Intraoperative, DP023Z0
Mediastinum, DB06
Intraoperative, DB063Z0
Mouth, D904
Intraoperative, D9043Z0
Nasopharynx, D90D
Intraoperative, D90D3Z0
Neck and Head, DW01
Intraoperative, DW013Z0
Nerve
Intraoperative, D0073Z0
Peripheral, D007
Nose, D901
Intraoperative, D9013Z0
Oropharynx, D90F
Intraoperative, D90F3Z0
Ovary, DU00
Intraoperative, DU003Z0
Palate
Hard, D908
Intraoperative, D9083Z0
Soft, D909
Intraoperative, D9093Z0
Pancreas, DF03
Intraoperative, DF033Z0
Parathyroid Gland, DG04
Intraoperative, DG043Z0
Pelvic Bones, DP08
Intraoperative, DP083Z0
Pelvic Region, DW06
Intraoperative, DW063Z0
Pineal Body, DG01
Intraoperative, DG013Z0
Pituitary Gland, DG00
Intraoperative, DG003Z0
Pleura, DB05
Intraoperative, DB053Z0
Prostate, DV00
Intraoperative, DV003Z0
Radius, DP07
Intraoperative, DP073Z0
Rectum, DD07
Intraoperative, DD073Z0
Rib, DP05
Intraoperative, DP053Z0
Sinuses, D907
Intraoperative, D9073Z0
Skin
Abdomen, DH08

Beam Radiation — *continued*
Skin — *continued*
Abdomen — *continued*
Intraoperative, DH083Z0
Arm, DH04
Intraoperative, DH043Z0
Back, DH07
Intraoperative, DH073Z0
Buttock, DH09
Intraoperative, DH093Z0
Chest, DH06
Intraoperative, DH063Z0
Face, DH02
Intraoperative, DH023Z0
Leg, DH0B
Intraoperative, DH0B3Z0
Neck, DH03
Intraoperative, DH033Z0
Skull, DP00
Intraoperative, DP003Z0
Spinal Cord, D006
Intraoperative, D0063Z0
Spleen, D702
Intraoperative, D7023Z0
Sternum, DP04
Intraoperative, DP043Z0
Stomach, DD01
Intraoperative, DD013Z0
Testis, DV01
Intraoperative, DV013Z0
Thymus, D701
Intraoperative, D7013Z0
Thyroid Gland, DG05
Intraoperative, DG053Z0
Tibia, DP0B
Intraoperative, DP0B3Z0
Tongue, D905
Intraoperative, D9053Z0
Trachea, DB00
Intraoperative, DB003Z0
Ulna, DP07
Intraoperative, DP073Z0
Ureter, DT01
Intraoperative, DT013Z0
Urethra, DT03
Intraoperative, DT033Z0
Uterus, DU02
Intraoperative, DU023Z0
Whole Body, DW05
Intraoperative, DW053Z0
Bedside swallow, F00ZJWZ
Berlin Heart Ventricular Assist Device *use* Implantable Heart Assist System in Heart and Great Vessels
Bezlotoxumab Monoclonal Antibody, XW0
Biceps brachii muscle
use Upper Arm Muscle, Left
use Upper Arm Muscle, Right
Biceps femoris muscle
use Upper Leg Muscle, Left
use Upper Leg Muscle, Right
Bicipital aponeurosis
use Subcutaneous Tissue and Fascia, Left Lower Arm
use Subcutaneous Tissue and Fascia, Right Lower Arm
Bicuspid valve *use* Mitral Valve
Bili light therapy *see* Phototherapy, Skin, 6A60
Bioactive embolization coil(s) *use* Intraluminal Device, Bioactive in Upper Arteries
Biofeedback, GZC9ZZZ
Biopsy
see Drainage with qualifier Diagnostic
see Excision with qualifier Diagnostic
see Extraction with qualifier Diagnostic
BiPAP *see* Assistance, Respiratory, 5A09
Bisection *see* Division
Biventricular external heart assist system *use* Short-term External Heart Assist System in Heart and Great Vessels
Blepharectomy
see Excision, Eye, 08B
see Resection, Eye, 08T
Blepharoplasty
see Repair, Eye, 08Q
see Replacement, Eye, 08R
see Reposition, Eye, 08S
see Supplement, Eye, 08U
Blepharorrhaphy *see* Repair, Eye, 08Q
Blepharotomy *see* Drainage, Eye, 089
Blinatumomab Antineoplastic Immunotherapy, XW0

Block, Nerve, anesthetic injection
Blood glucose monitoring system *use* Monitoring Device
Blood pressure *see* Measurement, Arterial, 4A03
BMR (basal metabolic rate) *see* Measurement, Physiological Systems, 4A0Z
Body of femur
use Femoral Shaft, Left
use Femoral Shaft, Right
Body of fibula
use Fibula, Left
use Fibula, Right
Bone anchored hearing device
use Hearing Device, Bone Conduction in, 09H
use Hearing Device in Head and Facial Bones
Bone bank bone graft *use* Nonautologous Tissue Substitute
Bone Growth Stimulator
Insertion of device in
Bone
Facial, 0NHW
Lower, 0QHY
Nasal, 0NHB
Upper, 0PHY
Skull, 0NH0
Removal of device from
Bone
Facial, 0NPW
Lower, 0QPY
Nasal, 0NPB
Upper, 0PPY
Skull, 0NP0
Revision of device in
Bone
Facial, 0NWW
Lower, 0QWY
Nasal, 0NWB
Upper, 0PWY
Skull, 0NW0
Bone marrow transplant *see* Transfusion, Circulatory, 302
Bone morphogenetic protein 2 (BMP 2) *use* Recombinant Bone Morphogenetic Protein
Bone screw (interlocking) (lag) (pedicle) (recessed)
use Internal Fixation Device in Head and Facial Bones
use Internal Fixation Device in Lower Bones
use Internal Fixation Device in Upper Bones
Bony labyrinth
use Inner Ear, Left
use Inner Ear, Right
Bony orbit
use Orbit, Left
use Orbit, Right
Bony vestibule
use Inner Ear, Left
use Inner Ear, Right
Botallo's duct *use* Pulmonary Artery, Left
Bovine pericardial valve *use* Zooplastic Tissue in Heart and Great Vessels
Bovine pericardium graft *use* Zooplastic Tissue in Heart and Great Vessels
BP (blood pressure) *see* Measurement, Arterial, 4A03
Brachial (lateral) lymph node
use Lymphatic, Left Axillary
use Lymphatic, Right Axillary
Brachialis muscle
use Upper Arm Muscle, Left
use Upper Arm Muscle, Right
Brachiocephalic artery *use* Innominate Artery
Brachiocephalic trunk *use* Innominate Artery
Brachiocephalic vein
use Innominate Vein, Left
use Innominate Vein, Right
Brachioradialis muscle
use Lower Arm and Wrist Muscle, Left
use Lower Arm and Wrist Muscle, Right
Brachytherapy
Abdomen, DW13
Adrenal Gland, DG12
Bile Ducts, DF12
Bladder, DT12
Bone Marrow, D710
Brain, D010
Brain Stem, D011
Breast
Left, DM10
Right, DM11

Brachytherapy — *continued*
Bronchus, DB11
Cervix, DU11
Chest, DW12
Chest Wall, DB17
Colon, DD15
Diaphragm, DB18
Duodenum, DD12
Ear, D910
Esophagus, DD10
Eye, D810
Gallbladder, DF11
Gland
Adrenal, DG12
Parathyroid, DG14
Pituitary, DG10
Thyroid, DG15
Glands, Salivary, D916
Head and Neck, DW11
Hypopharynx, D913
Ileum, DD14
Jejunum, DD13
Kidney, DT10
Larynx, D91B
Liver, DF10
Lung, DB12
Lymphatics
Abdomen, D716
Axillary, D714
Inguinal, D718
Neck, D713
Pelvis, D717
Thorax, D715
Mediastinum, DB16
Mouth, D914
Nasopharynx, D91D
Neck and Head, DW11
Nerve, Peripheral, D017
Nose, D911
Oropharynx, D91F
Ovary, DU10
Palate
Hard, D918
Soft, D919
Pancreas, DF13
Parathyroid Gland, DG14
Pelvic Region, DW16
Pineal Body, DG11
Pituitary Gland, DG10
Pleura, DB15
Prostate, DV10
Rectum, DD17
Sinuses, D917
Spinal Cord, D016
Spleen, D712
Stomach, DD11
Testis, DV11
Thymus, D711
Thyroid Gland, DG15
Tongue, D915
Trachea, DB10
Ureter, DT11
Urethra, DT13
Uterus, DU12
Brachytherapy seeds *use* Radioactive Element
Broad ligament *use* Uterine Supporting Structure
Bronchial artery *use* Upper Artery
Bronchography
see Fluoroscopy, Respiratory System, BB1
see Plain Radiography, Respiratory System, BB0
Bronchoplasty
see Repair, Respiratory System, 0BQ
see Supplement, Respiratory System, 0BU
Bronchorrhaphy *see* Repair, Respiratory System, 0BQ
Bronchoscopy, 0BJ08ZZ
Bronchotomy *see* Drainage, Respiratory System, 0B9
Bronchus Intermedius *use* Main Bronchus, Right
BRYAN® Cervical Disc System *use* Synthetic Substitute
Buccal gland *use* Buccal Mucosa
Buccinator lymph node *use* Lymphatic, Head
Buccinator muscle *use* Facial Muscle
Buckling, scleral with implant *see* Supplement, Eye, 08U
Bulbospongiosus muscle *use* Perineum Muscle
Bulbourethral (Cowper's) gland *use* Urethra
Bundle of His *use* Conduction Mechanism
Bundle of Kent *use* Conduction Mechanism
Bunionectomy *see* Excision, Lower Bones, 0QB

Bursectomy
see Excision, Bursae and Ligaments, 0MB
see Resection, Bursae and Ligaments, 0MT
Bursocentesis *see* Drainage, Bursae and Ligaments, 0M9
Bursography
see Plain Radiography, Non-Axial Lower Bones, BQ0
see Plain Radiography, Non-Axial Upper Bones, BP0
Bursotomy
see Division, Bursae and Ligaments, 0M8
see Drainage, Bursae and Ligaments, 0M9
BVS 5000 Ventricular Assist Device *use* Short-term External Heart Assist System in Heart and Great Vessels
Bypass
Anterior Chamber
Left, 08133
Right, 08123
Aorta
Abdominal, 0410
Thoracic
Ascending/Arch, 021X
Descending, 021W
Artery
Anterior Tibial
Left, 041Q
Right, 041P
Axillary
Left, 03160
Right, 03150
Brachial
Left, 03180
Right, 03170
Common Carotid
Left, 031J0
Right, 031H0
Common Iliac
Left, 041D
Right, 041C
Coronary
Four or More Arteries, 0213
One Artery, 0210
Three Arteries, 0212
Two Arteries, 0211
External Carotid
Left, 031N0
Right, 031M0
External Iliac
Left, 041J
Right, 041H
Femoral
Left, 041L
Right, 041K
Foot
Left, 041W
Right, 041V
Hepatic, 0413
Innominate, 03120
Internal Carotid
Left, 031L0
Right, 031K0
Internal Iliac
Left, 041F
Right, 041E
Intracranial, 031G0
Peroneal
Left, 041U
Right, 041T
Popliteal
Left, 041N
Right, 041M
Posterior Tibial
Left, 041S
Right, 041R
Pulmonary
Left, 021R
Right, 021Q
Pulmonary Trunk, 021P
Radial
Left, 031C0
Right, 031B0
Splenic, 0414
Subclavian
Left, 03140
Right, 03130
Temporal
Left, 031T0
Right, 031S0
Ulnar
Left, 031A0

Bypass — *continued*
Artery — *continued*
Ulnar — *continued*
Right, 03190
Atrium
Left, 0217
Right, 0216
Bladder, 0T1B
Cavity, Cranial, 0W110J
Cecum, 0D1H
Cerebral Ventricle, 0016
Colon
Ascending, 0D1K
Descending, 0D1M
Sigmoid, 0D1N
Transverse, 0D1L
Duct
Common Bile, 0F19
Cystic, 0F18
Hepatic
Common, 0F17
Left, 0F16
Right, 0F15
Lacrimal
Left, 081Y
Right, 081X
Pancreatic, 0F1D
Accessory, 0F1F
Duodenum, 0D19
Ear
Left, 091E0
Right, 091D0
Esophagus, 0D15
Lower, 0D13
Middle, 0D12
Upper, 0D11
Fallopian Tube
Left, 0U16
Right, 0U15
Gallbladder, 0F14
Ileum, 0D1B
Jejunum, 0D1A
Kidney Pelvis
Left, 0T14
Right, 0T13
Pancreas, 0F1G
Pelvic Cavity, 0W1J
Peritoneal Cavity, 0W1G
Pleural Cavity
Left, 0W1B
Right, 0W19
Spinal Canal, 001U
Stomach, 0D16
Trachea, 0B11
Ureter
Left, 0T17
Right, 0T16
Ureters, Bilateral, 0T18
Vas Deferens
Bilateral, 0V1Q
Left, 0V1P
Right, 0V1N
Vein
Axillary
Left, 0518
Right, 0517
Azygos, 0510
Basilic
Left, 051C
Right, 051B
Brachial
Left, 051A
Right, 0519
Cephalic
Left, 051F
Right, 051D
Colic, 0617
Common Iliac
Left, 061D
Right, 061C
Esophageal, 0613
External Iliac
Left, 061G
Right, 061F
External Jugular
Left, 051Q
Right, 051P
Face
Left, 051V

Bypass — *continued*
 Vein — *continued*
 Face — *continued*
 Right, 051T
 Femoral
 Left, 061N
 Right, 061M
 Foot
 Left, 061V
 Right, 061T
 Gastric, 0612
 Hand
 Left, 051H
 Right, 051G
 Hemiazygos, 0511
 Hepatic, 0614
 Hypogastric
 Left, 061J
 Right, 061H
 Inferior Mesenteric, 0616
 Innominate
 Left, 0514
 Right, 0513
 Internal Jugular
 Left, 051N
 Right, 051M
 Intracranial, 051L
 Portal, 0618
 Renal
 Left, 061B
 Right, 0619
 Saphenous
 Left, 061Q
 Right, 061P
 Splenic, 0611
 Subclavian
 Left, 0516
 Right, 0515
 Superior Mesenteric, 0615
 Vertebral
 Left, 051S
 Right, 051R
 Vena Cava
 Inferior, 0610
 Superior, 021V
 Ventricle
 Left, 021L
 Right, 021K
Bypass, cardiopulmonary, 5A1221Z

C

Caesarean section *see* Extraction, Products of Conception, 10D0
Calcaneocuboid joint
 use Tarsal Joint, Left
 use Tarsal Joint, Right
Calcaneocuboid ligament
 use Foot Bursa and Ligament, Left
 use Foot Bursa and Ligament, Right
Calcaneofibular ligament
 use Ankle Bursa and Ligament, Left
 use Ankle Bursa and Ligament, Right
Calcaneus
 use Tarsal, Left
 use Tarsal, Right
Cannulation
 see Bypass
 see Dilation
 see Drainage
 see Irrigation
Canthorrhaphy *see* Repair, Eye, 08Q
Canthotomy *see* Release, Eye, 08N
Capitate bone
 use Carpal, Left
 use Carpal, Right
Capsulectomy, lens *see* Excision, Eye, 08B
Capsulorrhaphy, joint
 see Repair, Lower Joints, 0SQ
 see Repair, Upper Joints, 0RQ
Cardia *use* Esophagogastric Junction
Cardiac contractility modulation lead *use* Cardiac Lead in Heart and Great Vessels
Cardiac event recorder *use* Monitoring Device

Cardiac Lead
 Defibrillator
 Atrium
 Left, 02H7
 Right, 02H6
 Pericardium, 02HN
 Vein, Coronary, 02H4
 Ventricle
 Left, 02HL
 Right, 02HK
 Insertion of device in
 Atrium
 Left, 02H7
 Right, 02H6
 Pericardium, 02HN
 Vein, Coronary, 02H4
 Ventricle
 Left, 02HL
 Right, 02HK
 Pacemaker
 Atrium
 Left, 02H7
 Right, 02H6
 Pericardium, 02HN
 Vein, Coronary, 02H4
 Ventricle
 Left, 02HL
 Right, 02HK
 Removal of device from, Heart, 02PA
 Revision of device in, Heart, 02WA
Cardiac plexus *use* Thoracic Sympathetic Nerve
Cardiac Resynchronization Defibrillator Pulse Generator
 Abdomen, 0JH8
 Chest, 0JH6
Cardiac Resynchronization Pacemaker Pulse Generator
 Abdomen, 0JH8
 Chest, 0JH6
Cardiac resynchronization therapy (CRT) lead
 use Cardiac Lead, Defibrillator in, 02H
 use Cardiac Lead, Pacemaker in, 02H
Cardiac Rhythm Related Device
 Insertion of device in
 Abdomen, 0JH8
 Chest, 0JH6
 Removal of device from, Subcutaneous Tissue and Fascia, Trunk, 0JPT
 Revision of device in, Subcutaneous Tissue and Fascia, Trunk, 0JWT
Cardiocentesis *see* Drainage, Pericardial Cavity, 0W9D
Cardioesophageal junction *use* Esophagogastric Junction
Cardiolysis *see* Release, Heart and Great Vessels, 02N
CardioMEMS® pressure sensor *use* Monitoring Device, Pressure Sensor in, 02H
Cardiomyotomy *see* Division, Esophagogastric Junction, 0D84
Cardioplegia *see* Introduction of substance in or on, Heart, 3E08
Cardiorrhaphy *see* Repair, Heart and Great Vessels, 02Q
Cardioversion, 5A2204Z
Caregiver Training, F0FZ
Caroticotympanic artery
 use Internal Carotid Artery, Left
 use Internal Carotid Artery, Right
Carotid glomus
 use Carotid Bodies, Bilateral
 use Carotid Body, Left
 use Carotid Body, Right
Carotid sinus
 use Internal Carotid Artery, Left
 use Internal Carotid Artery, Right
Carotid (artery) sinus (baroreceptor) lead *use* Stimulator Lead in Upper Arteries
Carotid sinus nerve *use* Glossopharyngeal Nerve
Carotid WALLSTENT® Monorail® Endoprosthesis *use* Intraluminal Device
Carpectomy
 see Excision, Upper Bones, 0PB
 see Resection, Upper Bones, 0PT
Carpometacarpal ligament
 use Hand Bursa and Ligament, Left
 use Hand Bursa and Ligament, Right
Casting *see* Immobilization
CAT scan *see* Computerized Tomography (CT Scan)

Catheterization
 see Dilation
 see Drainage
 see Insertion of device in
 see Irrigation
 Heart *see* Measurement, Cardiac, 4A02
 Umbilical vein, for infusion, 06H033T
Cauda equina *use* Lumbar Spinal Cord
Cauterization
 see Destruction
 see Repair
Cavernous plexus *use* Head and Neck Sympathetic Nerve
CBMA (Concentrated Bone Marrow Aspirate) *use* Concentrated Bone Marrow Aspirate
CBMA (Concentrated Bone Marrow Aspirate) injection, intramuscular, XK02303
Cecectomy
 see Excision, Cecum, 0DBH
 see Resection, Cecum, 0DTH
Cecocolostomy
 see Bypass, Gastrointestinal System, 0D1
 see Drainage, Gastrointestinal System, 0D9
Cecopexy
 see Repair, Cecum, 0DQH
 see Reposition, Cecum, 0DSH
Cecoplication *see* Restriction, Cecum, 0DVH
Cecorrhaphy *see* Repair, Cecum, 0DQH
Cecostomy
 see Bypass, Cecum, 0D1H
 see Drainage, Cecum, 0D9H
Cecotomy *see* Drainage, Cecum, 0D9H
Ceftazidime-Avibactam Anti-infective, XW0
Celiac ganglion *use* Abdominal Sympathetic Nerve
Celiac lymph node *use* Lymphatic, Aortic
Celiac (solar) plexus *use* Abdominal Sympathetic Nerve
Celiac trunk *use* Celiac Artery
Central axillary lymph node
 use Lymphatic, Left Axillary
 use Lymphatic, Right Axillary
Central venous pressure *see* Measurement, Venous, 4A04
Centrimag® Blood Pump *use* Short-term External Heart Assist System in Heart and Great Vessels
Cephalogram, BN00ZZZ
Ceramic on ceramic bearing surface *use* Synthetic Substitute, Ceramic in, 0SR
Cerclage *see* Restriction
Cerebral aqueduct (Sylvius) *use* Cerebral Ventricle
Cerebral Embolic Filtration, Dual Filter, X2A5312
Cerebrum *use* Brain
Cervical esophagus *use* Esophagus, Upper
Cervical facet joint
 use Cervical Vertebral Joint
 use Cervical Vertebral Joint, 2 or more
Cervical ganglion *use* Head and Neck Sympathetic Nerve
Cervical interspinous ligament *use* Head and Neck Bursa and Ligament
Cervical intertransverse ligament *use* Head and Neck Bursa and Ligament
Cervical ligamentum flavum *use* Head and Neck Bursa and Ligament
Cervical lymph node
 use Lymphatic, Left Neck
 use Lymphatic, Right Neck
Cervicectomy
 see Excision, Cervix, 0UBC
 see Resection, Cervix, 0UTC
Cervicothoracic facet joint *use* Cervicothoracic Vertebral Joint
Cesarean section *see* Extraction, Products of Conception, 10D0
Cesium-131 Collagen Implant *use* Radioactive Element, Cesium-131 Collagen Implant in 00H
Change device in
 Abdominal Wall, 0W2FX
 Back
 Lower, 0W2LX
 Upper, 0W2KX
 Bladder, 0T2BX
 Bone
 Facial, 0N2WX
 Lower, 0Q2YX
 Nasal, 0N2BX
 Upper, 0P2YX
 Bone Marrow, 072TX
 Brain, 0020X

Closure — *continued*
- *see* Repair

Clysis *see* Introduction of substance in or on
Coagulation *see* Destruction
COALESCE® radiolucent interbody fusion device *use* Interbody Fusion Device, Radiolucent Porous in New Technology
CoAxia NeuroFlo catheter *use* Intraluminal Device
Cobalt/chromium head and polyethylene socket *use* Synthetic Substitute, Metal on Polyethylene in, ØSR
Cobalt/chromium head and socket *use* Synthetic Substitute, Metal in, ØSR
Coccygeal body *use* Coccygeal Glomus
Coccygeus muscle
- *use* Trunk Muscle, Left
- *use* Trunk Muscle, Right

Cochlea
- *use* Inner Ear, Left
- *use* Inner Ear, Right

Cochlear implant (CI), multiple channel (electrode)
- *use* Hearing Device, Multiple Channel Cochlear Prosthesis in, Ø9H

Cochlear implant (CI), single channel (electrode) *use* Hearing Device, Single Channel Cochlear Prosthesis in, Ø9H
Cochlear Implant Treatment, FØBZØ
Cochlear nerve *use* Acoustic Nerve
COGNIS® CRT-D *use* Cardiac Resynchronization Defibrillator Pulse Generator in, ØJH
COHERE® radiolucent interbody fusion device *use* Interbody Fusion Device, Radiolucent Porous in New Technology
Colectomy
- *see* Excision, Gastrointestinal System, ØDB
- *see* Resection, Gastrointestinal System, ØDT

Collapse *see* Occlusion
Collection from
- Breast, Breast Milk, 8EØHX62
- Indwelling Device
  - Circulatory System
    - Blood, 8CØ2X6K
    - Other Fluid, 8CØ2X6L
  - Nervous System
    - Cerebrospinal Fluid, 8CØ1X6J
    - Other Fluid, 8CØ1X6L
- Integumentary System, Breast Milk, 8EØHX62
- Reproductive System, Male, Sperm, 8EØVX63

Colocentesis *see* Drainage, Gastrointestinal System, ØD9
Colofixation
- *see* Repair, Gastrointestinal System, ØDQ
- *see* Reposition, Gastrointestinal System, ØDS

Cololysis *see* Release, Gastrointestinal System, ØDN
Colonic Z-Stent® *use* Intraluminal Device
Colonoscopy, ØDJD8ZZ
Colopexy
- *see* Repair, Gastrointestinal System, ØDQ
- *see* Reposition, Gastrointestinal System, ØDS

Coloplication *see* Restriction, Gastrointestinal System, ØDV
Coloproctectomy
- *see* Excision, Gastrointestinal System, ØDB
- *see* Resection, Gastrointestinal System, ØDT

Coloproctostomy
- *see* Bypass, Gastrointestinal System, ØD1
- *see* Drainage, Gastrointestinal System, ØD9

Colopuncture *see* Drainage, Gastrointestinal System, ØD9
Colorrhaphy *see* Repair, Gastrointestinal System, ØDQ
Colostomy
- *see* Bypass, Gastrointestinal System, ØD1
- *see* Drainage, Gastrointestinal System, ØD9

Colpectomy
- *see* Excision, Vagina, ØUBG
- *see* Resection, Vagina, ØUTG

Colpocentesis *see* Drainage, Vagina, ØU9G
Colpopexy
- *see* Repair, Vagina, ØUQG
- *see* Reposition, Vagina, ØUSG

Colpoplasty
- *see* Repair, Vagina, ØUQG
- *see* Supplement, Vagina, ØUUG

Colporrhaphy *see* Repair, Vagina, ØUQG
Colposcopy, ØUJH8ZZ
Columella *use* Nasal Mucosa and Soft Tissue
Common digital vein
- *use* Foot Vein, Left
- *use* Foot Vein, Right

Common facial vein
- *use* Face Vein, Left
- *use* Face Vein, Right

Common fibular nerve *use* Peroneal Nerve
Common hepatic artery *use* Hepatic Artery
Common iliac (subaortic) lymph node *use* Lymphatic, Pelvis
Common interosseous artery
- *use* Ulnar Artery, Left
- *use* Ulnar Artery, Right

Common peroneal nerve *use* Peroneal Nerve
Complete (SE) stent *use* Intraluminal Device
Compression
- *see* Restriction
- Abdominal Wall, 2W13X
- Arm
  - Lower
    - Left, 2W1DX
    - Right, 2W1CX
  - Upper
    - Left, 2W1BX
    - Right, 2W1AX
- Back, 2W15X
- Chest Wall, 2W14X
- Extremity
  - Lower
    - Left, 2W1MX
    - Right, 2W1LX
  - Upper
    - Left, 2W19X
    - Right, 2W18X
- Face, 2W11X
- Finger
  - Left, 2W1KX
  - Right, 2W1JX
- Foot
  - Left, 2W1TX
  - Right, 2W1SX
- Hand
  - Left, 2W1FX
  - Right, 2W1EX
- Head, 2W1ØX
- Inguinal Region
  - Left, 2W17X
  - Right, 2W16X
- Leg
  - Lower
    - Left, 2W1RX
    - Right, 2W1QX
  - Upper
    - Left, 2W1PX
    - Right, 2W1NX
- Neck, 2W12X
- Thumb
  - Left, 2W1HX
  - Right, 2W1GX
- Toe
  - Left, 2W1VX
  - Right, 2W1UX

Computer Assisted Procedure
- Extremity
  - Lower
    - With Computerized Tomography, 8EØYXBG
    - With Fluoroscopy, 8EØYXBF
    - With Magnetic Resonance Imaging, 8EØYXBH
    - No Qualifier, 8EØYXBZ
  - Upper
    - With Computerized Tomography, 8EØXXBG
    - With Fluoroscopy, 8EØXXBF
    - With Magnetic Resonance Imaging, 8EØXXBH
    - No Qualifier, 8EØXXBZ
- Head and Neck Region
  - With Computerized Tomography, 8EØ9XBG
  - With Fluoroscopy, 8EØ9XBF
  - With Magnetic Resonance Imaging, 8EØ9XBH
  - No Qualifier, 8EØ9XBZ
- Trunk Region
  - With Computerized Tomography, 8EØWXBG
  - With Fluoroscopy, 8EØWXBF
  - With Magnetic Resonance Imaging, 8EØWXBH
  - No Qualifier, 8EØWXBZ

Computerized Tomography (CT Scan)
- Abdomen, BW2Ø
  - Chest and Pelvis, BW25

Computerized Tomography (CT Scan) — *continued*
- Abdomen and Chest, BW24
- Abdomen and Pelvis, BW21
- Airway, Trachea, BB2F
- Ankle
  - Left, BQ2H
  - Right, BQ2G
- Aorta
  - Abdominal, B42Ø
    - Intravascular Optical Coherence, B42ØZ2Z
  - Thoracic, B32Ø
    - Intravascular Optical Coherence, B32ØZ2Z
- Arm
  - Left, BP2F
  - Right, BP2E
- Artery
  - Celiac, B421
    - Intravascular Optical Coherence, B421Z2Z
  - Common Carotid
    - Bilateral, B325
    - Intravascular Optical Coherence, B325Z2Z
  - Coronary
    - Bypass Graft
      - Intravascular Optical Coherence, B223Z2Z
      - Multiple, B223
    - Multiple, B221
      - Intravascular Optical Coherence, B221Z2Z
  - Internal Carotid
    - Bilateral, B328
    - Intravascular Optical Coherence, B328Z2Z
  - Intracranial, B32R
    - Intravascular Optical Coherence, B32RZ2Z
  - Lower Extremity
    - Bilateral, B42H
      - Intravascular Optical Coherence, B42HZ2Z
    - Left, B42G
      - Intravascular Optical Coherence, B42GZ2Z
    - Right, B42F
      - Intravascular Optical Coherence, B42FZ2Z
  - Pelvic, B42C
    - Intravascular Optical Coherence, B42CZ2Z
  - Pulmonary
    - Left, B32T
      - Intravascular Optical Coherence, B32TZ2Z
    - Right, B32S
      - Intravascular Optical Coherence, B32SZ2Z
  - Renal
    - Bilateral, B428
      - Intravascular Optical Coherence, B428Z2Z
    - Transplant, B42M
      - Intravascular Optical Coherence, B42MZ2Z
  - Superior Mesenteric, B424
    - Intravascular Optical Coherence, B424Z2Z
  - Vertebral
    - Bilateral, B32G
    - Intravascular Optical Coherence, B32GZ2Z
- Bladder, BT2Ø
- Bone
  - Facial, BN25
  - Temporal, BN2F
- Brain, BØ2Ø
- Calcaneus
  - Left, BQ2K
  - Right, BQ2J
- Cerebral Ventricle, BØ28
- Chest, Abdomen and Pelvis, BW25
- Chest and Abdomen, BW24
- Cisterna, BØ27
- Clavicle
  - Left, BP25
  - Right, BP24
- Coccyx, BR2F
- Colon, BD24
- Ear, B92Ø
- Elbow
  - Left, BP2H
  - Right, BP2G
- Extremity
  - Lower
    - Left, BQ2S

38

Subterms under main terms may continue to next column or page

Closure — Computerized Tomography (CT Scan) Index

Index Computerized Tomography (CT Scan) — Contact Radiation

D

Densitometry — *continued*
Plain Radiography — *continued*
Hip
Left, BQØ1ZZ1
Right, BQØØZZ1
Spine
Cervical, BRØØZZ1
Lumbar, BRØ9ZZ1
Thoracic, BRØ7ZZ1
Whole, BRØGZZ1
Ultrasonography
Elbow
Left, BP4HZZ1
Right, BP4GZZ1
Hand
Left, BP4PZZ1
Right, BP4NZZ1
Shoulder
Left, BP49ZZ1
Right, BP48ZZ1
Wrist
Left, BP4MZZ1
Right, BP4LZZ1
Denticulate (dentate) ligament *use* Spinal Meninges
Depressor anguli oris muscle *use* Facial Muscle
Depressor labii inferioris muscle *use* Facial Muscle
Depressor septi nasi muscle *use* Facial Muscle
Depressor supercilii muscle *use* Facial Muscle
Dermabrasion *see* Extraction, Skin and Breast, ØHD
Dermis *use* Skin
Descending genicular artery
use Femoral Artery, Left
use Femoral Artery, Right
Destruction
Acetabulum
Left, ØQ55
Right, ØQ54
Adenoids, ØC5Q
Ampulla of Vater, ØF5C
Anal Sphincter, ØD5R
Anterior Chamber
Left, Ø8533ZZ
Right, Ø8523ZZ
Anus, ØD5Q
Aorta
Abdominal
Thoracic
Ascending/Arch, Ø25X
Descending, Ø25W
Aortic Body, ØG5D
Appendix, ØD5J
Artery
Anterior Tibial
Left, Ø45Q
Right, Ø45P
Axillary
Left, Ø356
Right, Ø355
Brachial
Left, Ø358
Right, Ø357
Celiac, Ø451
Colic
Left, Ø457
Middle, Ø458
Right, Ø456
Common Carotid
Left, Ø35J
Right, Ø35H
Common Iliac
Left, Ø45D
Right, Ø45C
External Carotid
Left, Ø35N
Right, Ø35M
External Iliac
Left, Ø45J
Right, Ø45H
Face, Ø35R
Femoral
Left, Ø45L
Right, Ø45K
Foot
Left, Ø45W
Right, Ø45V
Gastric, Ø452
Hand
Left, Ø35F

Destruction — *continued*
Artery — *continued*
Hand — *continued*
Right, Ø35D
Hepatic, Ø453
Inferior Mesenteric, Ø45B
Innominate, Ø352
Internal Carotid
Left, Ø35L
Right, Ø35K
Internal Iliac
Left, Ø45F
Right, Ø45E
Internal Mammary
Left, Ø351
Right, Ø35Ø
Intracranial, Ø35G
Lower, Ø45Y
Peroneal
Left, Ø45U
Right, Ø45T
Popliteal
Left, Ø45N
Right, Ø45M
Posterior Tibial
Left, Ø45S
Right, Ø45R
Pulmonary
Left, Ø25R
Right, Ø25Q
Pulmonary Trunk, Ø25P
Radial
Left, Ø35C
Right, Ø35B
Renal
Left, Ø45A
Right, Ø459
Splenic, Ø454
Subclavian
Left, Ø354
Right, Ø353
Superior Mesenteric, Ø455
Temporal
Left, Ø35T
Right, Ø35S
Thyroid
Left, Ø35V
Right, Ø35U
Ulnar
Left, Ø35A
Right, Ø359
Upper, Ø35Y
Vertebral
Left, Ø35Q
Right, Ø35P
Atrium
Left, Ø257
Right, Ø256
Auditory Ossicle
Left, Ø95A
Right, Ø959
Basal Ganglia, ØØ58
Bladder, ØT5B
Bladder Neck, ØT5C
Bone
Ethmoid
Left, ØN5G
Right, ØN5F
Frontal, ØN51
Hyoid, ØN5X
Lacrimal
Left, ØN5J
Right, ØN5H
Nasal, ØN5B
Occipital, ØN57
Palatine
Left, ØN5L
Right, ØN5K
Parietal
Left, ØN54
Right, ØN53
Pelvic
Left, ØQ53
Right, ØQ52
Sphenoid, ØN5C
Temporal
Left, ØN56
Right, ØN55

Destruction — *continued*
Bone — *continued*
Zygomatic
Left, ØN5N
Right, ØN5M
Brain, ØØ5Ø
Breast
Bilateral, ØH5V
Left, ØH5U
Right, ØH5T
Bronchus
Lingula, ØB59
Lower Lobe
Left, ØB5B
Right, ØB56
Main
Left, ØB57
Right, ØB53
Middle Lobe, Right, ØB55
Upper Lobe
Left, ØB58
Right, ØB54
Buccal Mucosa, ØC54
Bursa and Ligament
Abdomen
Left, ØM5J
Right, ØM5H
Ankle
Left, ØM5R
Right, ØM5Q
Elbow
Left, ØM54
Right, ØM53
Foot
Left, ØM5T
Right, ØM5S
Hand
Left, ØM58
Right, ØM57
Head and Neck, ØM5Ø
Hip
Left, ØM5M
Right, ØM5L
Knee
Left, ØM5P
Right, ØM5N
Lower Extremity
Left, ØM5W
Right, ØM5V
Perineum, ØM5K
Rib(s), ØM5G
Shoulder
Left, ØM52
Right, ØM51
Spine
Lower, ØM5D
Upper, ØM5C
Sternum, ØM5F
Upper Extremity
Left, ØM5B
Right, ØM59
Wrist
Left, ØM56
Right, ØM55
Carina, ØB52
Carotid Bodies, Bilateral, ØG58
Carotid Body
Left, ØG56
Right, ØG57
Carpal
Left, ØP5N
Right, ØP5M
Cecum, ØD5H
Cerebellum, ØØ5C
Cerebral Hemisphere, ØØ57
Cerebral Meninges, ØØ51
Cerebral Ventricle, ØØ56
Cervix, ØU5C
Chordae Tendineae, Ø259
Choroid
Left, Ø85B
Right, Ø85A
Cisterna Chyli, Ø75L
Clavicle
Left, ØP5B
Right, ØP59
Clitoris, ØU5J
Coccygeal Glomus, ØG5B
Coccyx, ØQ5S

Destruction — *continued*

Colon
- Ascending, 0D5K
- Descending, 0D5M
- Sigmoid, 0D5N
- Transverse, 0D5L

Conduction Mechanism, 0258

Conjunctiva
- Left, 085TXZZ
- Right, 085SXZZ

Cord
- Bilateral, 0V5H
- Left, 0V5G
- Right, 0V5F

Cornea
- Left, 0859XZZ
- Right, 0858XZZ

Cul-de-sac, 0U5F

Diaphragm, 0B5T

Disc
- Cervical Vertebral, 0R53
- Cervicothoracic Vertebral, 0R55
- Lumbar Vertebral, 0S52
- Lumbosacral, 0S54
- Thoracic Vertebral, 0R59
- Thoracolumbar Vertebral, 0R5B

Duct
- Common Bile, 0F59
- Cystic, 0F58
- Hepatic
 - Common, 0F57
 - Left, 0F56
 - Right, 0F55
- Lacrimal
 - Left, 085Y
 - Right, 085X
- Pancreatic, 0F5D
 - Accessory, 0F5F
- Parotid
 - Left, 0C5C
 - Right, 0C5B

Duodenum, 0D59

Dura Mater, 0052

Ear
- External
 - Left, 0951
 - Right, 0950
- External Auditory Canal
 - Left, 0954
 - Right, 0953
- Inner
 - Left, 095E
 - Right, 095D
- Middle
 - Left, 0956
 - Right, 0955

Endometrium, 0U5B

Epididymis
- Bilateral, 0V5L
- Left, 0V5K
- Right, 0V5J

Epiglottis, 0C5R

Esophagogastric Junction, 0D54

Esophagus, 0D55
- Lower, 0D53
- Middle, 0D52
- Upper, 0D51

Eustachian Tube
- Left, 095G
- Right, 095F

Eye
- Left, 0851XZZ
- Right, 0850XZZ

Eyelid
- Lower
 - Left, 085R
 - Right, 085Q
- Upper
 - Left, 085P
 - Right, 085N

Fallopian Tube
- Left, 0U56
- Right, 0U55

Fallopian Tubes, Bilateral, 0U57

Femoral Shaft
- Left, 0Q59
- Right, 0Q58

Destruction — *continued*

Femur
- Lower
 - Left, 0Q5C
 - Right, 0Q5B
- Upper
 - Left, 0Q57
 - Right, 0Q56

Fibula
- Left, 0Q5K
- Right, 0Q5J

Finger Nail, 0H5QXZZ

Gallbladder, 0F54

Gingiva
- Lower, 0C56
- Upper, 0C55

Gland
- Adrenal
 - Bilateral, 0G54
 - Left, 0G52
 - Right, 0G53
- Lacrimal
 - Left, 085W
 - Right, 085V
- Minor Salivary, 0C5J
- Parotid
 - Left, 0C59
 - Right, 0C58
- Pituitary, 0G50
- Sublingual
 - Left, 0C5F
 - Right, 0C5D
- Submaxillary
 - Left, 0C5H
 - Right, 0C5G
- Vestibular, 0U5L

Glenoid Cavity
- Left, 0P58
- Right, 0P57

Glomus Jugulare, 0G5C

Humeral Head
- Left, 0P5D
- Right, 0P5C

Humeral Shaft
- Left, 0P5G
- Right, 0P5F

Hymen, 0U5K

Hypothalamus, 005A

Ileocecal Valve, 0D5C

Ileum, 0D5B

Intestine
- Large, 0D5E
 - Left, 0D5G
 - Right, 0D5F
- Small, 0D58

Iris
- Left, 085D3ZZ
- Right, 085C3ZZ

Jejunum, 0D5A

Joint
- Acromioclavicular
 - Left, 0R5H
 - Right, 0R5G
- Ankle
 - Left, 0S5G
 - Right, 0S5F
- Carpal
 - Left, 0R5R
 - Right, 0R5Q
- Carpometacarpal
 - Left, 0R5T
 - Right, 0R5S
- Cervical Vertebral, 0R51
- Cervicothoracic Vertebral, 0R54
- Coccygeal, 0S56
- Elbow
 - Left, 0R5M
 - Right, 0R5L
- Finger Phalangeal
 - Left, 0R5X
 - Right, 0R5W
- Hip
 - Left, 0S5B
 - Right, 0S59
- Knee
 - Left, 0S5D
 - Right, 0S5C
- Lumbar Vertebral, 0S50
- Lumbosacral, 0S53

Destruction — *continued*

Joint — *continued*
- Metacarpophalangeal
 - Left, 0R5V
 - Right, 0R5U
- Metatarsal-Phalangeal
 - Left, 0S5N
 - Right, 0S5M
- Occipital-cervical, 0R50
- Sacrococcygeal, 0S55
- Sacroiliac
 - Left, 0S58
 - Right, 0S57
- Shoulder
 - Left, 0R5K
 - Right, 0R5J
- Sternoclavicular
 - Left, 0R5F
 - Right, 0R5E
- Tarsal
 - Left, 0S5J
 - Right, 0S5H
- Tarsometatarsal
 - Left, 0S5L
 - Right, 0S5K
- Temporomandibular
 - Left, 0R5D
 - Right, 0R5C
- Thoracic Vertebral, 0R56
- Thoracolumbar Vertebral, 0R5A
- Toe Phalangeal
 - Left, 0S5Q
 - Right, 0S5P
- Wrist
 - Left, 0R5P
 - Right, 0R5N

Kidney
- Left, 0T51
- Right, 0T50

Kidney Pelvis
- Left, 0T54
- Right, 0T53

Larynx, 0C5S

Lens
- Left, 085K3ZZ
- Right, 085J3ZZ

Lip
- Lower, 0C51
- Upper, 0C50

Liver, 0F50
- Left Lobe, 0F52
- Right Lobe, 0F51

Lung
- Bilateral, 0B5M
- Left, 0B5L
- Lower Lobe
 - Left, 0B5J
 - Right, 0B5F
- Middle Lobe, Right, 0B5D
- Right, 0B5K
- Upper Lobe
 - Left, 0B5G
 - Right, 0B5C

Lung Lingula, 0B5H

Lymphatic
- Aortic, 075D
- Axillary
 - Left, 0756
 - Right, 0755
- Head, 0750
- Inguinal
 - Left, 075J
 - Right, 075H
- Internal Mammary
 - Left, 0759
 - Right, 0758
- Lower Extremity
 - Left, 075G
 - Right, 075F
- Mesenteric, 075B
- Neck
 - Left, 0752
 - Right, 0751
- Pelvis, 075C
- Thoracic Duct, 075K
- Thorax, 0757
- Upper Extremity
 - Left, 0754
 - Right, 0753

Destruction — *continued*
　Mandible
　　Left, ØN5V
　　Right, ØN5T
　Maxilla, ØN5R
　Medulla Oblongata, ØØ5D
　Mesentery, ØD5V
　Metacarpal
　　Left, ØP5Q
　　Right, ØP5P
　Metatarsal
　　Left, ØQ5P
　　Right, ØQ5N
　Muscle
　　Abdomen
　　　Left, ØK5L
　　　Right, ØK5K
　　Extraocular
　　　Left, Ø85M
　　　Right, Ø85L
　　Facial, ØK51
　　Foot
　　　Left, ØK5W
　　　Right, ØK5V
　　Hand
　　　Left, ØK5D
　　　Right, ØK5C
　　Head, ØK50
　　Hip
　　　Left, ØK5P
　　　Right, ØK5N
　　Lower Arm and Wrist
　　　Left, ØK5B
　　　Right, ØK59
　　Lower Leg
　　　Left, ØK5T
　　　Right, ØK5S
　　Neck
　　　Left, ØK53
　　　Right, ØK52
　　Papillary, Ø25D
　　Perineum, ØK5M
　　Shoulder
　　　Left, ØK56
　　　Right, ØK55
　　Thorax
　　　Left, ØK5J
　　　Right, ØK5H
　　Tongue, Palate, Pharynx, ØK54
　　Trunk
　　　Left, ØK5G
　　　Right, ØK5F
　　Upper Arm
　　　Left, ØK58
　　　Right, ØK57
　　Upper Leg
　　　Left, ØK5R
　　　Right, ØK5Q
　Nasal Mucosa and Soft Tissue, Ø95K
　Nasopharynx, Ø95N
　Nerve
　　Abdominal Sympathetic, Ø15M
　　Abducens, ØØ5L
　　Accessory, ØØ5R
　　Acoustic, ØØ5N
　　Brachial Plexus, Ø153
　　Cervical, Ø151
　　Cervical Plexus, Ø15Ø
　　Facial, ØØ5M
　　Femoral, Ø15D
　　Glossopharyngeal, ØØ5P
　　Head and Neck Sympathetic, Ø15K
　　Hypoglossal, ØØ5S
　　Lumbar, Ø15B
　　Lumbar Plexus, Ø159
　　Lumbar Sympathetic, Ø15N
　　Lumbosacral Plexus, Ø15A
　　Median, Ø155
　　Oculomotor, ØØ5H
　　Olfactory, ØØ5F
　　Optic, ØØ5G
　　Peroneal, Ø15H
　　Phrenic, Ø152
　　Pudendal, Ø15C
　　Radial, Ø156
　　Sacral, Ø15R
　　Sacral Plexus, Ø15Q
　　Sacral Sympathetic, Ø15P
　　Sciatic, Ø15F

Destruction — *continued*
　Nerve — *continued*
　　Thoracic, Ø158
　　Thoracic Sympathetic, Ø15L
　　Tibial, Ø15G
　　Trigeminal, ØØ5K
　　Trochlear, ØØ5J
　　Ulnar, Ø154
　　Vagus, ØØ5Q
　Nipple
　　Left, ØH5X
　　Right, ØH5W
　Omentum, ØD5U
　Orbit
　　Left, ØN5Q
　　Right, ØN5P
　Ovary
　　Bilateral, ØU52
　　Left, ØU51
　　Right, ØU50
　Palate
　　Hard, ØC52
　　Soft, ØC53
　Pancreas, ØF5G
　Para-aortic Body, ØG59
　Paraganglion Extremity, ØG5F
　Parathyroid Gland, ØG5R
　　Inferior
　　　Left, ØG5P
　　　Right, ØG5N
　　Multiple, ØG5Q
　　Superior
　　　Left, ØG5M
　　　Right, ØG5L
　Patella
　　Left, ØQ5F
　　Right, ØQ5D
　Penis, ØV5S
　Pericardium, Ø25N
　Peritoneum, ØD5W
　Phalanx
　　Finger
　　　Left, ØP5V
　　　Right, ØP5T
　　Thumb
　　　Left, ØP5S
　　　Right, ØP5R
　　Toe
　　　Left, ØQ5R
　　　Right, ØQ5Q
　Pharynx, ØC5M
　Pineal Body, ØG51
　Pleura
　　Left, ØB5P
　　Right, ØB5N
　Pons, ØØ5B
　Prepuce, ØV5T
　Prostate, ØV50
　　Robotic Waterjet Ablation, XV5Ø8A4
　Radius
　　Left, ØP5J
　　Right, ØP5H
　Rectum, ØD5P
　Retina
　　Left, Ø85F3ZZ
　　Right, Ø85E3ZZ
　Retinal Vessel
　　Left, Ø85H3ZZ
　　Right, Ø85G3ZZ
　Ribs
　　1 to 2, ØP51
　　3 or More, ØP52
　Sacrum, ØQ51
　Scapula
　　Left, ØP56
　　Right, ØP55
　Sclera
　　Left, Ø857XZZ
　　Right, Ø856XZZ
　Scrotum, ØV55
　Septum
　　Atrial, Ø255
　　Nasal, Ø95M
　　Ventricular, Ø25M
　Sinus
　　Accessory, Ø95P
　　Ethmoid
　　　Left, Ø95V
　　　Right, Ø95U

Destruction — *continued*
　Sinus — *continued*
　　Frontal
　　　Left, Ø95T
　　　Right, Ø95S
　　Mastoid
　　　Left, Ø95C
　　　Right, Ø95B
　　Maxillary
　　　Left, Ø95R
　　　Right, Ø95Q
　　Sphenoid
　　　Left, Ø95X
　　　Right, Ø95W
　Skin
　　Abdomen, ØH57XZ
　　Back, ØH56XZ
　　Buttock, ØH58XZ
　　Chest, ØH55XZ
　　Ear
　　　Left, ØH53XZ
　　　Right, ØH52XZ
　　Face, ØH51XZ
　　Foot
　　　Left, ØH5NXZ
　　　Right, ØH5MXZ
　　Hand
　　　Left, ØH5GXZ
　　　Right, ØH5FXZ
　　Inguinal, ØH5AXZ
　　Lower Arm
　　　Left, ØH5EXZ
　　　Right, ØH5DXZ
　　Lower Leg
　　　Left, ØH5LXZ
　　　Right, ØH5KXZ
　　Neck, ØH54XZ
　　Perineum, ØH59XZ
　　Scalp, ØH5ØXZ
　　Upper Arm
　　　Left, ØH5CXZ
　　　Right, ØH5BXZ
　　Upper Leg
　　　Left, ØH5JXZ
　　　Right, ØH5HXZ
　Skull, ØN50
　Spinal Cord
　　Cervical, ØØ5W
　　Lumbar, ØØ5Y
　　Thoracic, ØØ5X
　Spinal Meninges, ØØ5T
　Spleen, Ø75P
　Sternum, ØP5Ø
　Stomach, ØD56
　　Pylorus, ØD57
　Subcutaneous Tissue and Fascia
　　Abdomen, ØJ58
　　Back, ØJ57
　　Buttock, ØJ59
　　Chest, ØJ56
　　Face, ØJ51
　　Foot
　　　Left, ØJ5R
　　　Right, ØJ5Q
　　Hand
　　　Left, ØJ5K
　　　Right, ØJ5J
　　Lower Arm
　　　Left, ØJ5H
　　　Right, ØJ5G
　　Lower Leg
　　　Left, ØJ5P
　　　Right, ØJ5N
　　Neck
　　　Left, ØJ55
　　　Right, ØJ54
　　Pelvic Region, ØJ5C
　　Perineum, ØJ5B
　　Scalp, ØJ50
　　Upper Arm
　　　Left, ØJ5F
　　　Right, ØJ5D
　　Upper Leg
　　　Left, ØJ5M
　　　Right, ØJ5L
　Tarsal
　　Left, ØQ5M
　　Right, ØQ5L

Destruction — *continued*
Tendon
 Abdomen
 Left, 0L5G
 Right, 0L5F
 Ankle
 Left, 0L5T
 Right, 0L5S
 Foot
 Left, 0L5W
 Right, 0L5V
 Hand
 Left, 0L58
 Right, 0L57
 Head and Neck, 0L50
 Hip
 Left, 0L5K
 Right, 0L5J
 Knee
 Left, 0L5R
 Right, 0L5Q
 Lower Arm and Wrist
 Left, 0L56
 Right, 0L55
 Lower Leg
 Left, 0L5P
 Right, 0L5N
 Perineum, 0L5H
 Shoulder
 Left, 0L52
 Right, 0L51
 Thorax
 Left, 0L5D
 Right, 0L5C
 Trunk
 Left, 0L5B
 Right, 0L59
 Upper Arm
 Left, 0L54
 Right, 0L53
 Upper Leg
 Left, 0L5M
 Right, 0L5L
Testis
 Bilateral, 0V5C
 Left, 0V5B
 Right, 0V59
Thalamus, 0059
Thymus, 075M
Thyroid Gland, 0G5K
 Left Lobe, 0G5G
 Right Lobe, 0G5H
Tibia
 Left, 0Q5H
 Right, 0Q5G
Toe Nail, 0H5RXZZ
Tongue, 0C57
Tonsils, 0C5P
Tooth
 Lower, 0C5X
 Upper, 0C5W
Trachea, 0B51
Tunica Vaginalis
 Left, 0V57
 Right, 0V56
Turbinate, Nasal, 095L
Tympanic Membrane
 Left, 0958
 Right, 0957
Ulna
 Left, 0P5L
 Right, 0P5K
Ureter
 Left, 0T57
 Right, 0T56
Urethra, 0T5D
Uterine Supporting Structure, 0U54
Uterus, 0U59
Uvula, 0C5N
Vagina, 0U5G
Valve
 Aortic, 025F
 Mitral, 025G
 Pulmonary, 025H
 Tricuspid, 025J
Vas Deferens
 Bilateral, 0V5Q
 Left, 0V5P
 Right, 0V5N

Destruction — *continued*
Vein
 Axillary
 Left, 0558
 Right, 0557
 Azygos, 0550
 Basilic
 Left, 055C
 Right, 055B
 Brachial
 Left, 055A
 Right, 0559
 Cephalic
 Left, 055F
 Right, 055D
 Colic, 0657
 Common Iliac
 Left, 065D
 Right, 065C
 Coronary, 0254
 Esophageal, 0653
 External Iliac
 Left, 065G
 Right, 065F
 External Jugular
 Left, 055Q
 Right, 055P
 Face
 Left, 055V
 Right, 055T
 Femoral
 Left, 065N
 Right, 065M
 Foot
 Left, 065V
 Right, 065T
 Gastric, 0652
 Hand
 Left, 055H
 Right, 055G
 Hemiazygos, 0551
 Hepatic, 0654
 Hypogastric
 Left, 065J
 Right, 065H
 Inferior Mesenteric, 0656
 Innominate
 Left, 0554
 Right, 0553
 Internal Jugular
 Left, 055N
 Right, 055M
 Intracranial, 055L
 Lower, 065Y
 Portal, 0658
 Pulmonary
 Left, 025T
 Right, 025S
 Renal
 Left, 065B
 Right, 0659
 Saphenous
 Left, 065Q
 Right, 065P
 Splenic, 0651
 Subclavian
 Left, 0556
 Right, 0555
 Superior Mesenteric, 0655
 Upper, 055Y
 Vertebral
 Left, 055S
 Right, 055R
Vena Cava
 Inferior, 0650
 Superior, 025V
Ventricle
 Left, 025L
 Right, 025K
Vertebra
 Cervical, 0P53
 Lumbar, 0Q50
 Thoracic, 0P54
Vesicle
 Bilateral, 0V53
 Left, 0V52
 Right, 0V51
Vitreous
 Left, 08553ZZ

Destruction — *continued*
Vitreous — *continued*
 Right, 08543ZZ
Vocal Cord
 Left, 0C5V
 Right, 0C5T
Vulva, 0U5M
Detachment
Arm
 Lower
 Left, 0X6F0Z
 Right, 0X6D0Z
 Upper
 Left, 0X690Z
 Right, 0X680Z
Elbow Region
 Left, 0X6C0ZZ
 Right, 0X6B0ZZ
Femoral Region
 Left, 0Y680ZZ
 Right, 0Y670ZZ
Finger
 Index
 Left, 0X6P0Z
 Right, 0X6N0Z
 Little
 Left, 0X6W0Z
 Right, 0X6V0Z
 Middle
 Left, 0X6R0Z
 Right, 0X6Q0Z
 Ring
 Left, 0X6T0Z
 Right, 0X6S0Z
Foot
 Left, 0Y6N0Z
 Right, 0Y6M0Z
Forequarter
 Left, 0X610ZZ
 Right, 0X600ZZ
Hand
 Left, 0X6K0Z
 Right, 0X6J0Z
Hindquarter
 Bilateral, 0Y640ZZ
 Left, 0Y630ZZ
 Right, 0Y620ZZ
Knee Region
 Left, 0Y6G0ZZ
 Right, 0Y6F0ZZ
Leg
 Lower
 Left, 0Y6J0Z
 Right, 0Y6H0Z
 Upper
 Left, 0Y6D0Z
 Right, 0Y6C0Z
Shoulder Region
 Left, 0X630ZZ
 Right, 0X620ZZ
Thumb
 Left, 0X6M0Z
 Right, 0X6L0Z
Toe
 1st
 Left, 0Y6Q0Z
 Right, 0Y6P0Z
 2nd
 Left, 0Y6S0Z
 Right, 0Y6R0Z
 3rd
 Left, 0Y6U0Z
 Right, 0Y6T0Z
 4th
 Left, 0Y6W0Z
 Right, 0Y6V0Z
 5th
 Left, 0Y6Y0Z
 Right, 0Y6X0Z
Determination, Mental status, GZ14ZZZ
Detorsion
 see Release
 see Reposition
Detoxification Services, for substance abuse, HZ2ZZZZ
Device Fitting, F0DZ
Diagnostic Audiology *see* Audiology, Diagnostic
Diagnostic imaging *see* Imaging, Diagnostic
Diagnostic radiology *see* Imaging, Diagnostic

Dilation — *continued*
 Vein — *continued*
 Superior Mesenteric, 0675
 Upper, 057Y
 Vertebral
 Left, 057S
 Right, 057R
 Vena Cava
 Inferior, 0670
 Superior, 027V
 Ventricle
 Left, 027L
 Right, 027K
Direct Lateral Interbody Fusion (DLIF) device *use* Interbody Fusion Device in Lower Joints
Disarticulation *see* Detachment
Discectomy, diskectomy
 see Excision, Lower Joints, 0SB
 see Excision, Upper Joints, 0RB
 see Resection, Lower Joints, 0ST
 see Resection, Upper Joints, 0RT
Discography
 see Fluoroscopy, Axial Skeleton, Except Skull and Facial Bones, BR1
 see Plain Radiography, Axial Skeleton, Except Skull and Facial Bones, BR0
Distal humerus
 use Humeral Shaft, Left
 use Humeral Shaft, Right
Distal humerus, involving joint
 use Elbow Joint, Left
 use Elbow Joint, Right
Distal radioulnar joint
 use Wrist Joint, Left
 use Wrist Joint, Right
Diversion *see* Bypass
Diverticulectomy *see* Excision, Gastrointestinal System, 0DB
Division
 Acetabulum
 Left, 0Q85
 Right, 0Q84
 Anal Sphincter, 0D8R
 Basal Ganglia, 0088
 Bladder Neck, 0T8C
 Bone
 Ethmoid
 Left, 0N8G
 Right, 0N8F
 Frontal, 0N81
 Hyoid, 0N8X
 Lacrimal
 Left, 0N8J
 Right, 0N8H
 Nasal, 0N8B
 Occipital, 0N87
 Palatine
 Left, 0N8L
 Right, 0N8K
 Parietal
 Left, 0N84
 Right, 0N83
 Pelvic
 Left, 0Q83
 Right, 0Q82
 Sphenoid, 0N8C
 Temporal
 Left, 0N86
 Right, 0N85
 Zygomatic
 Left, 0N8N
 Right, 0N8M
 Brain, 0080
 Bursa and Ligament
 Abdomen
 Left, 0M8J
 Right, 0M8H
 Ankle
 Left, 0M8R
 Right, 0M8Q
 Elbow
 Left, 0M84
 Right, 0M83
 Foot
 Left, 0M8T
 Right, 0M8S
 Hand
 Left, 0M88

Division — *continued*
 Bursa and Ligament — *continued*
 Hand — *continued*
 Right, 0M87
 Head and Neck, 0M80
 Hip
 Left, 0M8M
 Right, 0M8L
 Knee
 Left, 0M8P
 Right, 0M8N
 Lower Extremity
 Left, 0M8W
 Right, 0M8V
 Perineum, 0M8K
 Rib(s), 0M8G
 Shoulder
 Left, 0M82
 Right, 0M81
 Spine
 Lower, 0M8D
 Upper, 0M8C
 Sternum, 0M8F
 Upper Extremity
 Left, 0M8B
 Right, 0M89
 Wrist
 Left, 0M86
 Right, 0M85
 Carpal
 Left, 0P8N
 Right, 0P8M
 Cerebral Hemisphere, 0087
 Chordae Tendineae, 0289
 Clavicle
 Left, 0P8B
 Right, 0P89
 Coccyx, 0Q8S
 Conduction Mechanism, 0288
 Esophagogastric Junction, 0D84
 Femoral Shaft
 Left, 0Q89
 Right, 0Q88
 Femur
 Lower
 Left, 0Q8C
 Right, 0Q8B
 Upper
 Left, 0Q87
 Right, 0Q86
 Fibula
 Left, 0Q8K
 Right, 0Q8J
 Gland, Pituitary, 0G80
 Glenoid Cavity
 Left, 0P88
 Right, 0P87
 Humeral Head
 Left, 0P8D
 Right, 0P8C
 Humeral Shaft
 Left, 0P8G
 Right, 0P8F
 Hymen, 0U8K
 Kidneys, Bilateral, 0T82
 Mandible
 Left, 0N8V
 Right, 0N8T
 Maxilla, 0N8R
 Metacarpal
 Left, 0P8Q
 Right, 0P8P
 Metatarsal
 Left, 0Q8P
 Right, 0Q8N
 Muscle
 Abdomen
 Left, 0K8L
 Right, 0K8K
 Facial, 0K81
 Foot
 Left, 0K8W
 Right, 0K8V
 Hand
 Left, 0K8D
 Right, 0K8C
 Head, 0K80
 Hip
 Left, 0K8P

Division — *continued*
 Muscle — *continued*
 Hip — *continued*
 Right, 0K8N
 Lower Arm and Wrist
 Left, 0K8B
 Right, 0K89
 Lower Leg
 Left, 0K8T
 Right, 0K8S
 Neck
 Left, 0K83
 Right, 0K82
 Papillary, 028D
 Perineum, 0K8M
 Shoulder
 Left, 0K86
 Right, 0K85
 Thorax
 Left, 0K8J
 Right, 0K8H
 Tongue, Palate, Pharynx, 0K84
 Trunk
 Left, 0K8G
 Right, 0K8F
 Upper Arm
 Left, 0K88
 Right, 0K87
 Upper Leg
 Left, 0K8R
 Right, 0K8Q
 Nerve
 Abdominal Sympathetic, 018M
 Abducens, 008L
 Accessory, 008R
 Acoustic, 008N
 Brachial Plexus, 0183
 Cervical, 0181
 Cervical Plexus, 0180
 Facial, 008M
 Femoral, 018D
 Glossopharyngeal, 008P
 Head and Neck Sympathetic, 018K
 Hypoglossal, 008S
 Lumbar, 018B
 Lumbar Plexus, 0189
 Lumbar Sympathetic, 018N
 Lumbosacral Plexus, 018A
 Median, 0185
 Oculomotor, 008H
 Olfactory, 008F
 Optic, 008G
 Peroneal, 018H
 Phrenic, 0182
 Pudendal, 018C
 Radial, 0186
 Sacral, 018R
 Sacral Plexus, 018Q
 Sacral Sympathetic, 018P
 Sciatic, 018F
 Thoracic, 0188
 Thoracic Sympathetic, 018L
 Tibial, 018G
 Trigeminal, 008K
 Trochlear, 008J
 Ulnar, 0184
 Vagus, 008Q
 Orbit
 Left, 0N8Q
 Right, 0N8P
 Ovary
 Bilateral, 0U82
 Left, 0U81
 Right, 0U80
 Pancreas, 0F8G
 Patella
 Left, 0Q8F
 Right, 0Q8D
 Perineum, Female, 0W8NXZZ
 Phalanx
 Finger
 Left, 0P8V
 Right, 0P8T
 Thumb
 Left, 0P8S
 Right, 0P8R
 Toe
 Left, 0Q8R
 Right, 0Q8Q

Division — *continued*
Radius
 Left, 0P8J
 Right, 0P8H
Ribs
 1 to 2, 0P81
 3 or More, 0P82
Sacrum, 0Q81
Scapula
 Left, 0P86
 Right, 0P85
Skin
 Abdomen, 0H87XZZ
 Back, 0H86XZZ
 Buttock, 0H88XZZ
 Chest, 0H85XZZ
 Ear
 Left, 0H83XZZ
 Right, 0H82XZZ
 Face, 0H81XZZ
 Foot
 Left, 0H8NXZZ
 Right, 0H8MXZZ
 Hand
 Left, 0H8GXZZ
 Right, 0H8FXZZ
 Inguinal, 0H8AXZZ
 Lower Arm
 Left, 0H8EXZZ
 Right, 0H8DXZZ
 Lower Leg
 Left, 0H8LXZZ
 Right, 0H8KXZZ
 Neck, 0H84XZZ
 Perineum, 0H89XZZ
 Scalp, 0H80XZZ
 Upper Arm
 Left, 0H8CXZZ
 Right, 0H8BXZZ
 Upper Leg
 Left, 0H8JXZZ
 Right, 0H8HXZZ
Skull, 0N80
Spinal Cord
 Cervical, 008W
 Lumbar, 008Y
 Thoracic, 008X
Sternum, 0P80
Stomach, Pylorus, 0D87
Subcutaneous Tissue and Fascia
 Abdomen, 0J88
 Back, 0J87
 Buttock, 0J89
 Chest, 0J86
 Face, 0J81
 Foot
 Left, 0J8R
 Right, 0J8Q
 Hand
 Left, 0J8K
 Right, 0J8J
 Head and Neck, 0J8S
 Lower Arm
 Left, 0J8H
 Right, 0J8G
 Lower Extremity, 0J8W
 Lower Leg
 Left, 0J8P
 Right, 0J8N
 Neck
 Left, 0J85
 Right, 0J84
 Pelvic Region, 0J8C
 Perineum, 0J8B
 Scalp, 0J80
 Trunk, 0J8T
 Upper Arm
 Left, 0J8F
 Right, 0J8D
 Upper Extremity, 0J8V
 Upper Leg
 Left, 0J8M
 Right, 0J8L
Tarsal
 Left, 0Q8M
 Right, 0Q8L
Tendon
 Abdomen
 Left, 0L8G

Division — *continued*
Tendon — *continued*
 Abdomen — *continued*
 Right, 0L8F
 Ankle
 Left, 0L8T
 Right, 0L8S
 Foot
 Left, 0L8W
 Right, 0L8V
 Hand
 Left, 0L88
 Right, 0L87
 Head and Neck, 0L80
 Hip
 Left, 0L8K
 Right, 0L8J
 Knee
 Left, 0L8R
 Right, 0L8Q
 Lower Arm and Wrist
 Left, 0L86
 Right, 0L85
 Lower Leg
 Left, 0L8P
 Right, 0L8N
 Perineum, 0L8H
 Shoulder
 Left, 0L82
 Right, 0L81
 Thorax
 Left, 0L8D
 Right, 0L8C
 Trunk
 Left, 0L8B
 Right, 0L89
 Upper Arm
 Left, 0L84
 Right, 0L83
 Upper Leg
 Left, 0L8M
 Right, 0L8L
Thyroid Gland Isthmus, 0G8J
Tibia
 Left, 0Q8H
 Right, 0Q8G
Turbinate, Nasal, 098L
Ulna
 Left, 0P8L
 Right, 0P8K
Uterine Supporting Structure, 0U84
Vertebra
 Cervical, 0P83
 Lumbar, 0Q80
 Thoracic, 0P84
Doppler study *see* Ultrasonography
Dorsal digital nerve *use* Radial Nerve
Dorsal metacarpal vein
 use Hand Vein, Left
 use Hand Vein, Right
Dorsal metatarsal artery
 use Foot Artery, Left
 use Foot Artery, Right
Dorsal metatarsal vein
 use Foot Vein, Left
 use Foot Vein, Right
Dorsal scapular artery
 use Subclavian Artery, Left
 use Subclavian Artery, Right
Dorsal scapular nerve *use* Brachial Plexus
Dorsal venous arch
 use Foot Vein, Left
 use Foot Vein, Right
Dorsalis pedis artery
 use Anterior Tibial Artery, Left
 use Anterior Tibial Artery, Right
DownStream® System, 5A0512C, 5A0522C
Drainage
 Abdominal Wall, 0W9F
 Acetabulum
 Left, 0Q95
 Right, 0Q94
 Adenoids, 0C9Q
 Ampulla of Vater, 0F9C
 Anal Sphincter, 0D9R
 Ankle Region
 Left, 0Y9L
 Right, 0Y9K

Drainage — *continued*
Anterior Chamber
 Left, 0893
 Right, 0892
Anus, 0D9Q
Aorta, Abdominal, 0490
Aortic Body, 0G9D
Appendix, 0D9J
Arm
 Lower
 Left, 0X9F
 Right, 0X9D
 Upper
 Left, 0X99
 Right, 0X98
Artery
 Anterior Tibial
 Left, 049Q
 Right, 049P
 Axillary
 Left, 0396
 Right, 0395
 Brachial
 Left, 0398
 Right, 0397
 Celiac, 0491
 Colic
 Left, 0497
 Middle, 0498
 Right, 0496
 Common Carotid
 Left, 039J
 Right, 039H
 Common Iliac
 Left, 049D
 Right, 049C
 External Carotid
 Left, 039N
 Right, 039M
 External Iliac
 Left, 049J
 Right, 049H
 Face, 039R
 Femoral
 Left, 049L
 Right, 049K
 Foot
 Left, 049W
 Right, 049V
 Gastric, 0492
 Hand
 Left, 039F
 Right, 039D
 Hepatic, 0493
 Inferior Mesenteric, 049B
 Innominate, 0392
 Internal Carotid
 Left, 039L
 Right, 039K
 Internal Iliac
 Left, 049F
 Right, 049E
 Internal Mammary
 Left, 0391
 Right, 0390
 Intracranial, 039G
 Lower, 049Y
 Peroneal
 Left, 049U
 Right, 049T
 Popliteal
 Left, 049N
 Right, 049M
 Posterior Tibial
 Left, 049S
 Right, 049R
 Radial
 Left, 039C
 Right, 039B
 Renal
 Left, 049A
 Right, 0499
 Splenic, 0494
 Subclavian
 Left, 0394
 Right, 0393
 Superior Mesenteric, 0495
 Temporal
 Left, 039T

Drainage — continued
 Nerve — continued
 Radial, 0196
 Sacral, 019R
 Sacral Plexus, 019Q
 Sacral Sympathetic, 019P
 Sciatic, 019F
 Thoracic, 0198
 Thoracic Sympathetic, 019L
 Tibial, 019G
 Trigeminal, 009K
 Trochlear, 009J
 Ulnar, 0194
 Vagus, 009Q
 Nipple
 Left, 0H9X
 Right, 0H9W
 Omentum, 0D9U
 Oral Cavity and Throat, 0W93
 Orbit
 Left, 0N9Q
 Right, 0N9P
 Ovary
 Bilateral, 0U92
 Left, 0U91
 Right, 0U90
 Palate
 Hard, 0C92
 Soft, 0C93
 Pancreas, 0F9G
 Para-aortic Body, 0G99
 Paraganglion Extremity, 0G9F
 Parathyroid Gland, 0G9R
 Inferior
 Left, 0G9P
 Right, 0G9N
 Multiple, 0G9Q
 Superior
 Left, 0G9M
 Right, 0G9L
 Patella
 Left, 0Q9F
 Right, 0Q9D
 Pelvic Cavity, 0W9J
 Penis, 0V9S
 Pericardial Cavity, 0W9D
 Perineum
 Female, 0W9N
 Male, 0W9M
 Peritoneal Cavity, 0W9G
 Peritoneum, 0D9W
 Phalanx
 Finger
 Left, 0P9V
 Right, 0P9T
 Thumb
 Left, 0P9S
 Right, 0P9R
 Toe
 Left, 0Q9R
 Right, 0Q9Q
 Pharynx, 0C9M
 Pineal Body, 0G91
 Pleura
 Left, 0B9P
 Right, 0B9N
 Pleural Cavity
 Left, 0W9B
 Right, 0W99
 Pons, 009B
 Prepuce, 0V9T
 Products of Conception
 Amniotic Fluid
 Diagnostic, 1090
 Therapeutic, 1090
 Fetal Blood, 1090
 Fetal Cerebrospinal Fluid, 1090
 Fetal Fluid, Other, 1090
 Fluid, Other, 1090
 Prostate, 0V90
 Radius
 Left, 0P9J
 Right, 0P9H
 Rectum, 0D9P
 Retina
 Left, 089F
 Right, 089E
 Retinal Vessel
 Left, 089H

Drainage — continued
 Retinal Vessel — continued
 Right, 089G
 Retroperitoneum, 0W9H
 Ribs
 1 to 2, 0P91
 3 or More, 0P92
 Sacrum, 0Q91
 Scapula
 Left, 0P96
 Right, 0P95
 Sclera
 Left, 0897
 Right, 0896
 Scrotum, 0V95
 Septum, Nasal, 099M
 Shoulder Region
 Left, 0X93
 Right, 0X92
 Sinus
 Accessory, 099P
 Ethmoid
 Left, 099V
 Right, 099U
 Frontal
 Left, 099T
 Right, 099S
 Mastoid
 Left, 099C
 Right, 099B
 Maxillary
 Left, 099R
 Right, 099Q
 Sphenoid
 Left, 099X
 Right, 099W
 Skin
 Abdomen, 0H97
 Back, 0H96
 Buttock, 0H98
 Chest, 0H95
 Ear
 Left, 0H93
 Right, 0H92
 Face, 0H91
 Foot
 Left, 0H9N
 Right, 0H9M
 Hand
 Left, 0H9G
 Right, 0H9F
 Inguinal, 0H9A
 Lower Arm
 Left, 0H9E
 Right, 0H9D
 Lower Leg
 Left, 0H9L
 Right, 0H9K
 Neck, 0H94
 Perineum, 0H99
 Scalp, 0H90
 Upper Arm
 Left, 0H9C
 Right, 0H9B
 Upper Leg
 Left, 0H9J
 Right, 0H9H
 Skull, 0N90
 Spinal Canal, 009U
 Spinal Cord
 Cervical, 009W
 Lumbar, 009Y
 Thoracic, 009X
 Spinal Meninges, 009T
 Spleen, 079P
 Sternum, 0P90
 Stomach, 0D96
 Pylorus, 0D97
 Subarachnoid Space, Intracranial, 0095
 Subcutaneous Tissue and Fascia
 Abdomen, 0J98
 Back, 0J97
 Buttock, 0J99
 Chest, 0J96
 Face, 0J91
 Foot
 Left, 0J9R
 Right, 0J9Q

Drainage — continued
 Subcutaneous Tissue and Fascia — continued
 Hand
 Left, 0J9K
 Right, 0J9J
 Lower Arm
 Left, 0J9H
 Right, 0J9G
 Lower Leg
 Left, 0J9P
 Right, 0J9N
 Neck
 Left, 0J95
 Right, 0J94
 Pelvic Region, 0J9C
 Perineum, 0J9B
 Scalp, 0J90
 Upper Arm
 Left, 0J9F
 Right, 0J9D
 Upper Leg
 Left, 0J9M
 Right, 0J9L
 Subdural Space, Intracranial, 0094
 Tarsal
 Left, 0Q9M
 Right, 0Q9L
 Tendon
 Abdomen
 Left, 0L9G
 Right, 0L9F
 Ankle
 Left, 0L9T
 Right, 0L9S
 Foot
 Left, 0L9W
 Right, 0L9V
 Hand
 Left, 0L98
 Right, 0L97
 Head and Neck, 0L90
 Hip
 Left, 0L9K
 Right, 0L9J
 Knee
 Left, 0L9R
 Right, 0L9Q
 Lower Arm and Wrist
 Left, 0L96
 Right, 0L95
 Lower Leg
 Left, 0L9P
 Right, 0L9N
 Perineum, 0L9H
 Shoulder
 Left, 0L92
 Right, 0L91
 Thorax
 Left, 0L9D
 Right, 0L9C
 Trunk
 Left, 0L9B
 Right, 0L99
 Upper Arm
 Left, 0L94
 Right, 0L93
 Upper Leg
 Left, 0L9M
 Right, 0L9L
 Testis
 Bilateral, 0V9C
 Left, 0V9B
 Right, 0V99
 Thalamus, 0099
 Thymus, 079M
 Thyroid Gland, 0G9K
 Left Lobe, 0G9G
 Right Lobe, 0G9H
 Tibia
 Left, 0Q9H
 Right, 0Q9G
 Toe Nail, 0H9R
 Tongue, 0C97
 Tonsils, 0C9P
 Tooth
 Lower, 0C9X
 Upper, 0C9W
 Trachea, 0B91

Drainage — *continued*
- Tunica Vaginalis
  - Left, ØV97
  - Right, ØV96
- Turbinate, Nasal, Ø99L
- Tympanic Membrane
  - Left, Ø998
  - Right, Ø997
- Ulna
  - Left, ØP9L
  - Right, ØP9K
- Ureter
  - Left, ØT97
  - Right, ØT96
- Ureters, Bilateral, ØT98
- Urethra, ØT9D
- Uterine Supporting Structure, ØU94
- Uterus, ØU99
- Uvula, ØC9N
- Vagina, ØU9G
- Vas Deferens
  - Bilateral, ØV9Q
  - Left, ØV9P
  - Right, ØV9N
- Vein
  - Axillary
    - Left, Ø598
    - Right, Ø597
  - Azygos, Ø59Ø
  - Basilic
    - Left, Ø59C
    - Right, Ø59B
  - Brachial
    - Left, Ø59A
    - Right, Ø599
  - Cephalic
    - Left, Ø59F
    - Right, Ø59D
  - Colic, Ø697
  - Common Iliac
    - Left, Ø69D
    - Right, Ø69C
  - Esophageal, Ø693
  - External Iliac
    - Left, Ø69G
    - Right, Ø69F
  - External Jugular
    - Left, Ø59Q
    - Right, Ø59P
  - Face
    - Left, Ø59V
    - Right, Ø59T
  - Femoral
    - Left, Ø69N
    - Right, Ø69M
  - Foot
    - Left, Ø69V
    - Right, Ø69T
  - Gastric, Ø692
  - Hand
    - Left, Ø59H
    - Right, Ø59G
  - Hemiazygos, Ø591
  - Hepatic, Ø694
  - Hypogastric
    - Left, Ø69J
    - Right, Ø69H
  - Inferior Mesenteric, Ø696
  - Innominate
    - Left, Ø594
    - Right, Ø593
  - Internal Jugular
    - Left, Ø59N
    - Right, Ø59M
  - Intracranial, Ø59L
  - Lower, Ø69Y
  - Portal, Ø698
  - Renal
    - Left, Ø69B
    - Right, Ø699
  - Saphenous
    - Left, Ø69Q
    - Right, Ø69P
  - Splenic, Ø691
  - Subclavian
    - Left, Ø596
    - Right, Ø595
  - Superior Mesenteric, Ø695
  - Upper, Ø59Y

Drainage — *continued*
- Vein — *continued*
  - Vertebral
    - Left, Ø59S
    - Right, Ø59R
- Vena Cava, Inferior, Ø69Ø
- Vertebra
  - Cervical, ØP93
  - Lumbar, ØQ9Ø
  - Thoracic, ØP94
- Vesicle
  - Bilateral, ØV93
  - Left, ØV92
  - Right, ØV91
- Vitreous
  - Left, Ø895
  - Right, Ø894
- Vocal Cord
  - Left, ØC9V
  - Right, ØC9T
- Vulva, ØU9M
- Wrist Region
  - Left, ØX9H
  - Right, ØX9G

Dressing
- Abdominal Wall, 2W23X4Z
- Arm
  - Lower
    - Left, 2W2DX4Z
    - Right, 2W2CX4Z
  - Upper
    - Left, 2W2BX4Z
    - Right, 2W2AX4Z
- Back, 2W25X4Z
- Chest Wall, 2W24X4Z
- Extremity
  - Lower
    - Left, 2W2MX4Z
    - Right, 2W2LX4Z
  - Upper
    - Left, 2W29X4Z
    - Right, 2W28X4Z
- Face, 2W21X4Z
- Finger
  - Left, 2W2KX4Z
  - Right, 2W2JX4Z
- Foot
  - Left, 2W2TX4Z
  - Right, 2W2SX4Z
- Hand
  - Left, 2W2FX4Z
  - Right, 2W2EX4Z
- Head, 2W2ØX4Z
- Inguinal Region
  - Left, 2W27X4Z
  - Right, 2W26X4Z
- Leg
  - Lower
    - Left, 2W2RX4Z
    - Right, 2W2QX4Z
  - Upper
    - Left, 2W2PX4Z
    - Right, 2W2NX4Z
- Neck, 2W22X4Z
- Thumb
  - Left, 2W2HX4Z
  - Right, 2W2GX4Z
- Toe
  - Left, 2W2VX4Z
  - Right, 2W2UX4Z

Driver stent (RX) (OTW) *use* Intraluminal Device

Drotrecogin alfa, infusion *see* Introduction of Recombinant Human-activated Protein C

Duct of Santorini *use* Pancreatic Duct, Accessory

Duct of Wirsung *use* Pancreatic Duct

Ductogram, mammary *see* Plain Radiography, Skin, Subcutaneous Tissue and Breast, BHØ

Ductography, mammary *see* Plain Radiography, Skin, Subcutaneous Tissue and Breast, BHØ

Ductus deferens
- *use* Vas Deferens
- *use* Vas Deferens, Bilateral
- *use* Vas Deferens, Left
- *use* Vas Deferens, Right

Duodenal ampulla *use* Ampulla of Vater

Duodenectomy
- *see* Excision, Duodenum, ØDB9
- *see* Resection, Duodenum, ØDT9

Duodenocholedochotomy *see* Drainage, Gallbladder, ØF94

Duodenocystostomy
- *see* Bypass, Gallbladder, ØF14
- *see* Drainage, Gallbladder, ØF94

Duodenoenterostomy
- *see* Bypass, Gastrointestinal System, ØD1
- *see* Drainage, Gastrointestinal System, ØD9

Duodenojejunal flexure *use* Jejunum

Duodenolysis *see* Release, Duodenum, ØDN9

Duodenorrhaphy *see* Repair, Duodenum, ØDQ9

Duodenostomy
- *see* Bypass, Duodenum, ØD19
- *see* Drainage, Duodenum, ØD99

Duodenotomy *see* Drainage, Duodenum, ØD99

Dura mater, intracranial *use* Dura Mater

Dura mater, spinal *use* Spinal Meninges

DuraGraft® Endothelial Damage Inhibitor *use* Endothelial Damage Inhibitor

DuraHeart Left Ventricular Assist System *use* Implantable Heart Assist System in Heart and Great Vessels

Dural venous sinus *use* Intracranial Vein

Durata® Defibrillation Lead *use* Cardiac Lead, Defibrillator in, Ø2H

Dynesys® Dynamic Stabilization System
- *use* Spinal Stabilization Device, Pedicle-Based in, ØRH
- *use* Spinal Stabilization Device, Pedicle-Based in, ØSH

E

Earlobe
- *use* Ear, External, Bilateral
- *use* Ear, External, Left
- *use* Ear, External, Right

ECCO2R (Extracorporeal Carbon Dioxide Removal), 5AØ92ØZ

Echocardiogram *see* Ultrasonography, Heart, B24

Echography *see* Ultrasonography

ECMO *see* Performance, Circulatory, 5A15

EDWARDS INTUITY Elite valve system *use* Zooplastic Tissue, Rapid Deployment Technique in New Technology

EEG (electroencephalogram) *see* Measurement, Central Nervous, 4AØØ

EGD (esophagogastroduodenoscopy), ØDJØ8ZZ

Eighth cranial nerve *use* Acoustic Nerve

Ejaculatory duct
- *use* Vas Deferens
- *use* Vas Deferens, Bilateral
- *use* Vas Deferens, Left
- *use* Vas Deferens, Right

EKG (electrocardiogram) *see* Measurement, Cardiac, 4AØ2

Electrical bone growth stimulator (EBGS)
- *use* Bone Growth Stimulator in Head and Facial Bones
- *use* Bone Growth Stimulator in Lower Bones
- *use* Bone Growth Stimulator in Upper Bones

Electrical muscle stimulation (EMS) lead *use* Stimulator Lead in Muscles

Electrocautery
- Destruction *see* Destruction
- Repair *see* Repair

Electroconvulsive Therapy
- Bilateral-Multiple Seizure, GZB3ZZZ
- Bilateral-Single Seizure, GZB2ZZZ
- Electroconvulsive Therapy, Other, GZB4ZZZ
- Unilateral-Multiple Seizure, GZB1ZZZ
- Unilateral-Single Seizure, GZBØZZZ

Electroencephalogram (EEG) *see* Measurement, Central Nervous, 4AØØ

Electromagnetic Therapy
- Central Nervous, 6A22
- Urinary, 6A21

Electronic muscle stimulator lead *use* Stimulator Lead in Muscles

Electrophysiologic stimulation (EPS) *see* Measurement, Cardiac, 4AØ2

Electroshock therapy *see* Electroconvulsive Therapy

Elevation, bone fragments, skull *see* Reposition, Head and Facial Bones, ØNS

Eleventh cranial nerve *use* Accessory Nerve

E-Luminexx™ (Biliary) (Vascular) Stent *use* Intraluminal Device

Embolectomy *see* Extirpation

Subterms under main terms may continue to next column or page

Embolization
 see Occlusion
 see Restriction
Embolization coil(s) *use* Intraluminal Device
EMG (electromyogram) *see* Measurement, Musculoskeletal, 4A0F
Encephalon *use* Brain
Endarterectomy
 see Extirpation, Lower Arteries, 04C
 see Extirpation, Upper Arteries, 03C
Endeavor® (III) (IV) (Sprint) Zotarolimus-eluting Coronary Stent System *use* Intraluminal Device, Drug-eluting in Heart and Great Vessels
Endologix® AFX Endovascular AAA System *use* Intraluminal Device
EndoSure® sensor *use* Monitoring Device, Pressure Sensor in, 02H
ENDOTAK RELIANCE® (G) Defibrillation Lead *use* Cardiac Lead, Defibrillator in, 02H
Endothelial damage inhibitor, applied to vein graft, XY0VX83
Endotracheal tube (cuffed) (double-lumen) *use* Intraluminal Device, Endotracheal Airway in Respiratory System
Endurant® Endovascular Stent Graft *use* Intraluminal Device
Endurant® II AAA stent graft system *use* Intraluminal Device
Engineered Autologous Chimeric Antigen Receptor T-cell Immunotherapy, XW0
Enlargement
 see Dilation
 see Repair
EnRhythm *use* Pacemaker, Dual Chamber in, 0JH
Enterorrhaphy *see* Repair, Gastrointestinal System, 0DQ
Enterra gastric neurostimulator *use* Stimulator Generator, Multiple Array in, 0JH
Enucleation
 Eyeball *see* Resection, Eye, 08T
 Eyeball with prosthetic implant *see* Replacement, Eye, 08R
Ependyma *use* Cerebral Ventricle
Epicel® cultured epidermal autograft *use* Autologous Tissue Substitute
Epic™ Stented Tissue Valve (aortic) *use* Zooplastic Tissue in Heart and Great Vessels
Epidermis *use* Skin
Epididymectomy
 see Excision, Male Reproductive System, 0VB
 see Resection, Male Reproductive System, 0VT
Epididymoplasty
 see Repair, Male Reproductive System, 0VQ
 see Supplement, Male Reproductive System, 0VU
Epididymorrhaphy *see* Repair, Male Reproductive System, 0VQ
Epididymotomy *see* Drainage, Male Reproductive System, 0V9
Epidural space, spinal *use* Spinal Canal
Epiphysiodesis
 see Insertion of device in, Lower Bones, 0QH
 see Insertion of device in, Upper Bones, 0PH
 see Repair, Lower Bones, 0QQ
 see Repair, Upper Bones, 0PQ
Epiploic foramen *use* Peritoneum
Epiretinal Visual Prosthesis
 Left, 08H105Z
 Right, 08H005Z
Episiorrhaphy *see* Repair, Perineum, Female, 0WQN
Episiotomy *see* Division, Perineum, Female, 0W8N
Epithalamus *use* Thalamus
Epitrochlear lymph node
 use Lymphatic, Left Upper Extremity
 use Lymphatic, Right Upper Extremity
EPS (electrophysiologic stimulation) *see* Measurement, Cardiac, 4A02
Eptifibatide, infusion *see* Introduction of Platelet Inhibitor
ERCP (endoscopic retrograde cholangiopancreatography) *see* Fluoroscopy, Hepatobiliary System and Pancreas, BF1
Erector spinae muscle
 use Trunk Muscle, Left
 use Trunk Muscle, Right
Esophageal artery *use* Upper Artery
Esophageal obturator airway (EOA) *use* Intraluminal Device, Airway in Gastrointestinal System
Esophageal plexus *use* Thoracic Sympathetic Nerve

Esophagectomy
 see Excision, Gastrointestinal System, 0DB
 see Resection, Gastrointestinal System, 0DT
Esophagocoloplasty
 see Repair, Gastrointestinal System, 0DQ
 see Supplement, Gastrointestinal System, 0DU
Esophagoenterostomy
 see Bypass, Gastrointestinal System, 0D1
 see Drainage, Gastrointestinal System, 0D9
Esophagoesophagostomy
 see Bypass, Gastrointestinal System, 0D1
 see Drainage, Gastrointestinal System, 0D9
Esophagogastrectomy
 see Excision, Gastrointestinal System, 0DB
 see Resection, Gastrointestinal System, 0DT
Esophagogastroduodenoscopy (EGD), 0DJ08ZZ
Esophagogastroplasty
 see Repair, Gastrointestinal System, 0DQ
 see Supplement, Gastrointestinal System, 0DU
Esophagogastroscopy, 0DJ68ZZ
Esophagogastrostomy
 see Bypass, Gastrointestinal System, 0D1
 see Drainage, Gastrointestinal System, 0D9
Esophagojejunoplasty *see* Supplement, Gastrointestinal System, 0DU
Esophagojejunostomy
 see Bypass, Gastrointestinal System, 0D1
 see Drainage, Gastrointestinal System, 0D9
Esophagomyotomy *see* Division, Esophagogastric Junction, 0D84
Esophagoplasty
 see Repair, Gastrointestinal System, 0DQ
 see Replacement, Esophagus, 0DR5
 see Supplement, Gastrointestinal System, 0DU
Esophagoplication *see* Restriction, Gastrointestinal System, 0DV
Esophagorrhaphy *see* Repair, Gastrointestinal System, 0DQ
Esophagoscopy, 0DJ08ZZ
Esophagotomy *see* Drainage, Gastrointestinal System, 0D9
Esteem® implantable hearing system *use* Hearing Device in Ear, Nose, Sinus
ESWL (extracorporeal shock wave lithotripsy) *see* Fragmentation
Ethmoidal air cell
 use Ethmoid Sinus, Left
 use Ethmoid Sinus, Right
Ethmoidectomy
 see Excision, Ear, Nose, Sinus, 09B
 see Excision, Head and Facial Bones, 0NB
 see Resection, Ear, Nose, Sinus, 09T
 see Resection, Head and Facial Bones, 0NT
Ethmoidotomy *see* Drainage, Ear, Nose, Sinus, 099
Evacuation
 Hematoma *see* Extirpation
 Other Fluid *see* Drainage
Evera (XT) (S) (DR/VR) *use* Defibrillator Generator in, 0JH
Everolimus-eluting coronary stent *use* Intraluminal Device, Drug-eluting in Heart and Great Vessels
Evisceration
 Eyeball *see* Resection, Eye, 08T
 Eyeball with prosthetic implant *see* Replacement, Eye, 08R
Examination *see* Inspection
Exchange *see* Change device in
Excision
 Abdominal Wall, 0WBF
 Acetabulum
 Left, 0QB5
 Right, 0QB4
 Adenoids, 0CBQ
 Ampulla of Vater, 0FBC
 Anal Sphincter, 0DBR
 Ankle Region
 Left, 0YBL
 Right, 0YBK
 Anus, 0DBQ
 Aorta
 Abdominal
 Thoracic
 Ascending/Arch, 02BX
 Descending, 02BW
 Aortic Body, 0GBD
 Appendix, 0DBJ

Excision — *continued*
 Arm
 Lower
 Left, 0XBF
 Right, 0XBD
 Upper
 Left, 0XB9
 Right, 0XB8
 Artery
 Anterior Tibial
 Left, 04BQ
 Right, 04BP
 Axillary
 Left, 03B6
 Right, 03B5
 Brachial
 Left, 03B8
 Right, 03B7
 Celiac, 04B1
 Colic
 Left, 04B7
 Middle, 04B8
 Right, 04B6
 Common Carotid
 Left, 03BJ
 Right, 03BH
 Common Iliac
 Left, 04BD
 Right, 04BC
 External Carotid
 Left, 03BN
 Right, 03BM
 External Iliac
 Left, 04BJ
 Right, 04BH
 Face, 03BR
 Femoral
 Left, 04BL
 Right, 04BK
 Foot
 Left, 04BW
 Right, 04BV
 Gastric, 04B2
 Hand
 Left, 03BF
 Right, 03BD
 Hepatic, 04B3
 Inferior Mesenteric, 04BB
 Innominate, 03B2
 Internal Carotid
 Left, 03BL
 Right, 03BK
 Internal Iliac
 Left, 04BF
 Right, 04BE
 Internal Mammary
 Left, 03B1
 Right, 03B0
 Intracranial, 03BG
 Lower, 04BY
 Peroneal
 Left, 04BU
 Right, 04BT
 Popliteal
 Left, 04BN
 Right, 04BM
 Posterior Tibial
 Left, 04BS
 Right, 04BR
 Pulmonary
 Left, 02BR
 Right, 02BQ
 Pulmonary Trunk, 02BP
 Radial
 Left, 03BC
 Right, 03BB
 Renal
 Left, 04BA
 Right, 04B9
 Splenic, 04B4
 Subclavian
 Left, 03B4
 Right, 03B3
 Superior Mesenteric, 04B5
 Temporal
 Left, 03BT
 Right, 03BS
 Thyroid
 Left, 03BV

Excision — *continued*
 Artery — *continued*
 Thyroid — *continued*
 Right, 03BU
 Ulnar
 Left, 03BA
 Right, 03B9
 Upper, 03BY
 Vertebral
 Left, 03BQ
 Right, 03BP
 Atrium
 Left, 02B7
 Right, 02B6
 Auditory Ossicle
 Left, 09BA
 Right, 09B9
 Axilla
 Left, 0XB5
 Right, 0XB4
 Back
 Lower, 0WBL
 Upper, 0WBK
 Basal Ganglia, 00B8
 Bladder, 0TBB
 Bladder Neck, 0TBC
 Bone
 Ethmoid
 Left, 0NBG
 Right, 0NBF
 Frontal, 0NB1
 Hyoid, 0NBX
 Lacrimal
 Left, 0NBJ
 Right, 0NBH
 Nasal, 0NBB
 Occipital, 0NB7
 Palatine
 Left, 0NBL
 Right, 0NBK
 Parietal
 Left, 0NB4
 Right, 0NB3
 Pelvic
 Left, 0QB3
 Right, 0QB2
 Sphenoid, 0NBC
 Temporal
 Left, 0NB6
 Right, 0NB5
 Zygomatic
 Left, 0NBN
 Right, 0NBM
 Brain, 00B0
 Breast
 Bilateral, 0HBV
 Left, 0HBU
 Right, 0HBT
 Supernumerary, 0HBY
 Bronchus
 Lingula, 0BB9
 Lower Lobe
 Left, 0BBB
 Right, 0BB6
 Main
 Left, 0BB7
 Right, 0BB3
 Middle Lobe, Right, 0BB5
 Upper Lobe
 Left, 0BB8
 Right, 0BB4
 Buccal Mucosa, 0CB4
 Bursa and Ligament
 Abdomen
 Left, 0MBJ
 Right, 0MBH
 Ankle
 Left, 0MBR
 Right, 0MBQ
 Elbow
 Left, 0MB4
 Right, 0MB3
 Foot
 Left, 0MBT
 Right, 0MBS
 Hand
 Left, 0MB8
 Right, 0MB7
 Head and Neck, 0MB0

Excision — *continued*
 Bursa and Ligament — *continued*
 Hip
 Left, 0MBM
 Right, 0MBL
 Knee
 Left, 0MBP
 Right, 0MBN
 Lower Extremity
 Left, 0MBW
 Right, 0MBV
 Perineum, 0MBK
 Rib(s), 0MBG
 Shoulder
 Left, 0MB2
 Right, 0MB1
 Spine
 Lower, 0MBD
 Upper, 0MBC
 Sternum, 0MBF
 Upper Extremity
 Left, 0MBB
 Right, 0MB9
 Wrist
 Left, 0MB6
 Right, 0MB5
 Buttock
 Left, 0YB1
 Right, 0YB0
 Carina, 0BB2
 Carotid Bodies, Bilateral, 0GB8
 Carotid Body
 Left, 0GB6
 Right, 0GB7
 Carpal
 Left, 0PBN
 Right, 0PBM
 Cecum, 0DBH
 Cerebellum, 00BC
 Cerebral Hemisphere, 00B7
 Cerebral Meninges, 00B1
 Cerebral Ventricle, 00B6
 Cervix, 0UBC
 Chest Wall, 0WB8
 Chordae Tendineae, 02B9
 Choroid
 Left, 08BB
 Right, 08BA
 Cisterna Chyli, 07BL
 Clavicle
 Left, 0PBB
 Right, 0PB9
 Clitoris, 0UBJ
 Coccygeal Glomus, 0GBB
 Coccyx, 0QBS
 Colon
 Ascending, 0DBK
 Descending, 0DBM
 Sigmoid, 0DBN
 Transverse, 0DBL
 Conduction Mechanism, 02B8
 Conjunctiva
 Left, 08BTXZ
 Right, 08BSXZ
 Cord
 Bilateral, 0VBH
 Left, 0VBG
 Right, 0VBF
 Cornea
 Left, 08B9XZ
 Right, 08B8XZ
 Cul-de-sac, 0UBF
 Diaphragm, 0BBT
 Disc
 Cervical Vertebral, 0RB3
 Cervicothoracic Vertebral, 0RB5
 Lumbar Vertebral, 0SB2
 Lumbosacral, 0SB4
 Thoracic Vertebral, 0RB9
 Thoracolumbar Vertebral, 0RBB
 Duct
 Common Bile, 0FB9
 Cystic, 0FB8
 Hepatic
 Common, 0FB7
 Left, 0FB6
 Right, 0FB5
 Lacrimal
 Left, 08BY

Excision — *continued*
 Duct — *continued*
 Lacrimal — *continued*
 Right, 08BX
 Pancreatic, 0FBD
 Accessory, 0FBF
 Parotid
 Left, 0CBC
 Right, 0CBB
 Duodenum, 0DB9
 Dura Mater, 00B2
 Ear
 External
 Left, 09B1
 Right, 09B0
 External Auditory Canal
 Left, 09B4
 Right, 09B3
 Inner
 Left, 09BE
 Right, 09BD
 Middle
 Left, 09B6
 Right, 09B5
 Elbow Region
 Left, 0XBC
 Right, 0XBB
 Epididymis
 Bilateral, 0VBL
 Left, 0VBK
 Right, 0VBJ
 Epiglottis, 0CBR
 Esophagogastric Junction, 0DB4
 Esophagus, 0DB5
 Lower, 0DB3
 Middle, 0DB2
 Upper, 0DB1
 Eustachian Tube
 Left, 09BG
 Right, 09BF
 Extremity
 Lower
 Left, 0YBB
 Right, 0YB9
 Upper
 Left, 0XB7
 Right, 0XB6
 Eye
 Left, 08B1
 Right, 08B0
 Eyelid
 Lower
 Left, 08BR
 Right, 08BQ
 Upper
 Left, 08BP
 Right, 08BN
 Face, 0WB2
 Fallopian Tube
 Left, 0UB6
 Right, 0UB5
 Fallopian Tubes, Bilateral, 0UB7
 Femoral Region
 Left, 0YB8
 Right, 0YB7
 Femoral Shaft
 Left, 0QB9
 Right, 0QB8
 Femur
 Lower
 Left, 0QBC
 Right, 0QBB
 Upper
 Left, 0QB7
 Right, 0QB6
 Fibula
 Left, 0QBK
 Right, 0QBJ
 Finger Nail, 0HBQXZ
 Floor of mouth *see* Excision, Oral Cavity and Throat, 0WB3
 Foot
 Left, 0YBN
 Right, 0YBM
 Gallbladder, 0FB4
 Gingiva
 Lower, 0CB6
 Upper, 0CB5

Subterms under main terms may continue to next column or page

Extirpation — *continued*
Palate
 Hard, ØCC2
 Soft, ØCC3
Pancreas, ØFCG
Para-aortic Body, ØGC9
Paraganglion Extremity, ØGCF
Parathyroid Gland, ØGCR
 Inferior
 Left, ØGCP
 Right, ØGCN
 Multiple, ØGCQ
 Superior
 Left, ØGCM
 Right, ØGCL
Patella
 Left, ØQCF
 Right, ØQCD
Pelvic Cavity, ØWCJ
Penis, ØVCS
Pericardial Cavity, ØWCD
Pericardium, Ø2CN
Peritoneal Cavity, ØWCG
Peritoneum, ØDCW
Phalanx
 Finger
 Left, ØPCV
 Right, ØPCT
 Thumb
 Left, ØPCS
 Right, ØPCR
 Toe
 Left, ØQCR
 Right, ØQCQ
Pharynx, ØCCM
Pineal Body, ØGC1
Pleura
 Left, ØBCP
 Right, ØBCN
Pleural Cavity
 Left, ØWCB
 Right, ØWC9
Pons, ØØCB
Prepuce, ØVCT
Prostate, ØVCØ
Radius
 Left, ØPCJ
 Right, ØPCH
Rectum, ØDCP
Respiratory Tract, ØWCQ
Retina
 Left, Ø8CF
 Right, Ø8CE
Retinal Vessel
 Left, Ø8CH
 Right, Ø8CG
Retroperitoneum, ØWCH
Ribs
 1 to 2, ØPC1
 3 or More, ØPC2
Sacrum, ØQC1
Scapula
 Left, ØPC6
 Right, ØPC5
Sclera
 Left, Ø8C7XZZ
 Right, Ø8C6XZZ
Scrotum, ØVC5
Septum
 Atrial, Ø2C5
 Nasal, Ø9CM
 Ventricular, Ø2CM
Sinus
 Accessory, Ø9CP
 Ethmoid
 Left, Ø9CV
 Right, Ø9CU
 Frontal
 Left, Ø9CT
 Right, Ø9CS
 Mastoid
 Left, Ø9CC
 Right, Ø9CB
 Maxillary
 Left, Ø9CR
 Right, Ø9CQ
 Sphenoid
 Left, Ø9CX
 Right, Ø9CW

Extirpation — *continued*
Skin
 Abdomen, ØHC7XZZ
 Back, ØHC6XZZ
 Buttock, ØHC8XZZ
 Chest, ØHC5XZZ
 Ear
 Left, ØHC3XZZ
 Right, ØHC2XZZ
 Face, ØHC1XZZ
 Foot
 Left, ØHCNXZZ
 Right, ØHCMXZZ
 Hand
 Left, ØHCGXZZ
 Right, ØHCFXZZ
 Inguinal, ØHCAXZZ
 Lower Arm
 Left, ØHCEXZZ
 Right, ØHCDXZZ
 Lower Leg
 Left, ØHCLXZZ
 Right, ØHCKXZZ
 Neck, ØHC4XZZ
 Perineum, ØHC9XZZ
 Scalp, ØHCØXZZ
 Upper Arm
 Left, ØHCCXZZ
 Right, ØHCBXZZ
 Upper Leg
 Left, ØHCJXZZ
 Right, ØHCHXZZ
Spinal Canal, ØØCU
Spinal Cord
 Cervical, ØØCW
 Lumbar, ØØCY
 Thoracic, ØØCX
Spinal Meninges, ØØCT
Spleen, Ø7CP
Sternum, ØPCØ
Stomach, ØDC6
 Pylorus, ØDC7
Subarachnoid Space, Intracranial, ØØC5
Subcutaneous Tissue and Fascia
 Abdomen, ØJC8
 Back, ØJC7
 Buttock, ØJC9
 Chest, ØJC6
 Face, ØJC1
 Foot
 Left, ØJCR
 Right, ØJCQ
 Hand
 Left, ØJCK
 Right, ØJCJ
 Lower Arm
 Left, ØJCH
 Right, ØJCG
 Lower Leg
 Left, ØJCP
 Right, ØJCN
 Neck
 Left, ØJC5
 Right, ØJC4
 Pelvic Region, ØJCC
 Perineum, ØJCB
 Scalp, ØJCØ
 Upper Arm
 Left, ØJCF
 Right, ØJCD
 Upper Leg
 Left, ØJCM
 Right, ØJCL
Subdural Space, Intracranial, ØØC4
Tarsal
 Left, ØQCM
 Right, ØQCL
Tendon
 Abdomen
 Left, ØLCG
 Right, ØLCF
 Ankle
 Left, ØLCT
 Right, ØLCS
 Foot
 Left, ØLCW
 Right, ØLCV
 Hand
 Left, ØLC8

Extirpation — *continued*
Tendon — *continued*
 Hand — *continued*
 Right, ØLC7
 Head and Neck, ØLCØ
 Hip
 Left, ØLCK
 Right, ØLCJ
 Knee
 Left, ØLCR
 Right, ØLCQ
 Lower Arm and Wrist
 Left, ØLC6
 Right, ØLC5
 Lower Leg
 Left, ØLCP
 Right, ØLCN
 Perineum, ØLCH
 Shoulder
 Left, ØLC2
 Right, ØLC1
 Thorax
 Left, ØLCD
 Right, ØLCC
 Trunk
 Left, ØLCB
 Right, ØLC9
 Upper Arm
 Left, ØLC4
 Right, ØLC3
 Upper Leg
 Left, ØLCM
 Right, ØLCL
Testis
 Bilateral, ØVCC
 Left, ØVCB
 Right, ØVC9
Thalamus, ØØC9
Thymus, Ø7CM
Thyroid Gland, ØGCK
 Left Lobe, ØGCG
 Right Lobe, ØGCH
Tibia
 Left, ØQCH
 Right, ØQCG
Toe Nail, ØHCRXZZ
Tongue, ØCC7
Tonsils, ØCCP
Tooth
 Lower, ØCCX
 Upper, ØCCW
Trachea, ØBC1
Tunica Vaginalis
 Left, ØVC7
 Right, ØVC6
Turbinate, Nasal, Ø9CL
Tympanic Membrane
 Left, Ø9C8
 Right, Ø9C7
Ulna
 Left, ØPCL
 Right, ØPCK
Ureter
 Left, ØTC7
 Right, ØTC6
Urethra, ØTCD
Uterine Supporting Structure, ØUC4
Uterus, ØUC9
Uvula, ØCCN
Vagina, ØUCG
Valve
 Aortic, Ø2CF
 Mitral, Ø2CG
 Pulmonary, Ø2CH
 Tricuspid, Ø2CJ
Vas Deferens
 Bilateral, ØVCQ
 Left, ØVCP
 Right, ØVCN
Vein
 Axillary
 Left, Ø5C8
 Right, Ø5C7
 Azygos, Ø5CØ
 Basilic
 Left, Ø5CC
 Right, Ø5CB
 Brachial
 Left, Ø5CA

▽ **Subterms under main terms may continue to next column or page**

Extirpation — *continued*
Vein — *continued*
 Brachial — *continued*
 Right, 05C9
 Cephalic
 Left, 05CF
 Right, 05CD
 Colic, 06C7
 Common Iliac
 Left, 06CD
 Right, 06CC
 Coronary, 02C4
 Esophageal, 06C3
 External Iliac
 Left, 06CG
 Right, 06CF
 External Jugular
 Left, 05CQ
 Right, 05CP
 Face
 Left, 05CV
 Right, 05CT
 Femoral
 Left, 06CN
 Right, 06CM
 Foot
 Left, 06CV
 Right, 06CT
 Gastric, 06C2
 Hand
 Left, 05CH
 Right, 05CG
 Hemiazygos, 05C1
 Hepatic, 06C4
 Hypogastric
 Left, 06CJ
 Right, 06CH
 Inferior Mesenteric, 06C6
 Innominate
 Left, 05C4
 Right, 05C3
 Internal Jugular
 Left, 05CN
 Right, 05CM
 Intracranial, 05CL
 Lower, 06CY
 Portal, 06C8
 Pulmonary
 Left, 02CT
 Right, 02CS
 Renal
 Left, 06CB
 Right, 06C9
 Saphenous
 Left, 06CQ
 Right, 06CP
 Splenic, 06C1
 Subclavian
 Left, 05C6
 Right, 05C5
 Superior Mesenteric, 06C5
 Upper, 05CY
 Vertebral
 Left, 05CS
 Right, 05CR
Vena Cava
 Inferior, 06C0
 Superior, 02CV
Ventricle
 Left, 02CL
 Right, 02CK
Vertebra
 Cervical, 0PC3
 Lumbar, 0QC0
 Thoracic, 0PC4
Vesicle
 Bilateral, 0VC3
 Left, 0VC2
 Right, 0VC1
Vitreous
 Left, 08C5
 Right, 08C4
Vocal Cord
 Left, 0CCV
 Right, 0CCT
Vulva, 0UCM
Extracorporeal Carbon Dioxide Removal (ECCO2R),
 5A0920Z

Extracorporeal shock wave lithotripsy *see* Fragmentation
Extracranial-intracranial bypass (EC-IC) *see* Bypass, Upper Arteries, 031
Extraction
Acetabulum
 Left, 0QD50ZZ
 Right, 0QD40ZZ
Ampulla of Vater, 0FDC
Anus, 0DDQ
Appendix, 0DDJ
Auditory Ossicle
 Left, 09DA0ZZ
 Right, 09D90ZZ
Bone
 Ethmoid
 Left, 0NDG0ZZ
 Right, 0NDF0ZZ
 Frontal, 0ND10ZZ
 Hyoid, 0NDX0ZZ
 Lacrimal
 Left, 0NDJ0ZZ
 Right, 0NDH0ZZ
 Nasal, 0NDB0ZZ
 Occipital, 0ND70ZZ
 Palatine
 Left, 0NDL0ZZ
 Right, 0NDK0ZZ
 Parietal
 Left, 0ND40ZZ
 Right, 0ND30ZZ
 Pelvic
 Left, 0QD30ZZ
 Right, 0QD20ZZ
 Sphenoid, 0NDC0ZZ
 Temporal
 Left, 0ND60ZZ
 Right, 0ND50ZZ
 Zygomatic
 Left, 0NDN0ZZ
 Right, 0NDM0ZZ
Bone Marrow
 Iliac, 07DR
 Sternum, 07DQ
 Vertebral, 07DS
Bronchus
 Lingula, 0BD9
 Lower Lobe
 Left, 0BDB
 Right, 0BD6
 Main
 Left, 0BD7
 Right, 0BD3
 Middle Lobe, Right, 0BD5
 Upper Lobe
 Left, 0BD8
 Right, 0BD4
Bursa and Ligament
 Abdomen
 Left, 0MDJ
 Right, 0MDH
 Ankle
 Left, 0MDR
 Right, 0MDQ
 Elbow
 Left, 0MD4
 Right, 0MD3
 Foot
 Left, 0MDT
 Right, 0MDS
 Hand
 Left, 0MD8
 Right, 0MD7
 Head and Neck, 0MD0
 Hip
 Left, 0MDM
 Right, 0MDL
 Knee
 Left, 0MDP
 Right, 0MDN
 Lower Extremity
 Left, 0MDW
 Right, 0MDV
 Perineum, 0MDK
 Rib(s), 0MDG
 Shoulder
 Left, 0MD2
 Right, 0MD1

Extraction — *continued*
Bursa and Ligament — *continued*
 Spine
 Lower, 0MDD
 Upper, 0MDC
 Sternum, 0MDF
 Upper Extremity
 Left, 0MDB
 Right, 0MD9
 Wrist
 Left, 0MD6
 Right, 0MD5
Carina, 0BD2
Carpal
 Left, 0PDN0ZZ
 Right, 0PDM0ZZ
Cecum, 0DDH
Cerebral Meninges, 00D1
Cisterna Chyli, 07DL
Clavicle
 Left, 0PDB0ZZ
 Right, 0PD90ZZ
Coccyx, 0QDS0ZZ
Colon
 Ascending, 0DDK
 Descending, 0DDM
 Sigmoid, 0DDN
 Transverse, 0DDL
Cornea
 Left, 08D9XZ
 Right, 08D8XZ
Duct
 Common Bile, 0FD9
 Cystic, 0FD8
 Hepatic
 Common, 0FD7
 Left, 0FD6
 Right, 0FD5
 Pancreatic, 0FDD
 Accessory, 0FDF
Duodenum, 0DD9
Dura Mater, 00D2
Endometrium, 0UDB
Esophagogastric Junction, 0DD4
Esophagus, 0DD5
 Lower, 0DD3
 Middle, 0DD2
 Upper, 0DD1
Femoral Shaft
 Left, 0QD90ZZ
 Right, 0QD80ZZ
Femur
 Lower
 Left, 0QDC0ZZ
 Right, 0QDB0ZZ
 Upper
 Left, 0QD70ZZ
 Right, 0QD60ZZ
Fibula
 Left, 0QDK0ZZ
 Right, 0QDJ0ZZ
Finger Nail, 0HDQXZZ
Gallbladder, 0FD4
Glenoid Cavity
 Left, 0PD80ZZ
 Right, 0PD70ZZ
Hair, 0HDSXZZ
Humeral Head
 Left, 0PDD0ZZ
 Right, 0PDC0ZZ
Humeral Shaft
 Left, 0PDG0ZZ
 Right, 0PDF0ZZ
Ileocecal Valve, 0DDC
Ileum, 0DDB
Intestine
 Large, 0DDE
 Left, 0DDG
 Right, 0DDF
 Small, 0DD8
Jejunum, 0DDA
Kidney
 Left, 0TD1
 Right, 0TD0
Lens
 Left, 08DK3ZZ
 Right, 08DJ3ZZ
Liver, 0FD0
 Left Lobe, 0FD2

Extraction — *continued*
Liver — *continued*
Right Lobe, 0FD1
Lung
Bilateral, 0BDM
Left, 0BDL
Lower Lobe
Left, 0BDJ
Right, 0BDF
Middle Lobe, Right, 0BDD
Right, 0BDK
Upper Lobe
Left, 0BDG
Right, 0BDC
Lung Lingula, 0BDH
Lymphatic
Aortic, 07DD
Axillary
Left, 07D6
Right, 07D5
Head, 07D0
Inguinal
Left, 07DJ
Right, 07DH
Internal Mammary
Left, 07D9
Right, 07D8
Lower Extremity
Left, 07DG
Right, 07DF
Mesenteric, 07DB
Neck
Left, 07D2
Right, 07D1
Pelvis, 07DC
Thoracic Duct, 07DK
Thorax, 07D7
Upper Extremity
Left, 07D4
Right, 07D3
Mandible
Left, 0NDV0ZZ
Right, 0NDT0ZZ
Maxilla, 0NDR0ZZ
Metacarpal
Left, 0PDQ0ZZ
Right, 0PDP0ZZ
Metatarsal
Left, 0QDP0ZZ
Right, 0QDN0ZZ
Muscle
Abdomen
Left, 0KDL0ZZ
Right, 0KDK0ZZ
Facial, 0KD10ZZ
Foot
Left, 0KDW0ZZ
Right, 0KDV0ZZ
Hand
Left, 0KDD0ZZ
Right, 0KDC0ZZ
Head, 0KD00ZZ
Hip
Left, 0KDP0ZZ
Right, 0KDN0ZZ
Lower Arm and Wrist
Left, 0KDB0ZZ
Right, 0KD90ZZ
Lower Leg
Left, 0KDT0ZZ
Right, 0KDS0ZZ
Neck
Left, 0KD30ZZ
Right, 0KD20ZZ
Perineum, 0KDM0ZZ
Shoulder
Left, 0KD60ZZ
Right, 0KD50ZZ
Thorax
Left, 0KDJ0ZZ
Right, 0KDH0ZZ
Tongue, Palate, Pharynx, 0KD40ZZ
Trunk
Left, 0KDG0ZZ
Right, 0KDF0ZZ
Upper Arm
Left, 0KD80ZZ
Right, 0KD70ZZ

Extraction — *continued*
Muscle — *continued*
Upper Leg
Left, 0KDR0ZZ
Right, 0KDQ0ZZ
Nerve
Abdominal Sympathetic, 01DM
Abducens, 00DL
Accessory, 00DR
Acoustic, 00DN
Brachial Plexus, 01D3
Cervical, 01D1
Cervical Plexus, 01D0
Facial, 00DM
Femoral, 01DD
Glossopharyngeal, 00DP
Head and Neck Sympathetic, 01DK
Hypoglossal, 00DS
Lumbar, 01DB
Lumbar Plexus, 01D9
Lumbar Sympathetic, 01DN
Lumbosacral Plexus, 01DA
Median, 01D5
Oculomotor, 00DH
Olfactory, 00DF
Optic, 00DG
Peroneal, 01DH
Phrenic, 01D2
Pudendal, 01DC
Radial, 01D6
Sacral, 01DR
Sacral Plexus, 01DQ
Sacral Sympathetic, 01DP
Sciatic, 01DF
Thoracic, 01D8
Thoracic Sympathetic, 01DL
Tibial, 01DG
Trigeminal, 00DK
Trochlear, 00DJ
Ulnar, 01D4
Vagus, 00DQ
Orbit
Left, 0NDQ0ZZ
Right, 0NDP0ZZ
Ova, 0UDN
Pancreas, 0FDG
Patella
Left, 0QDF0ZZ
Right, 0QDD0ZZ
Phalanx
Finger
Left, 0PDV0ZZ
Right, 0PDT0ZZ
Thumb
Left, 0PDS0ZZ
Right, 0PDR0ZZ
Toe
Left, 0QDR0ZZ
Right, 0QDQ0ZZ
Pleura
Left, 0BDP
Right, 0BDN
Products of Conception
Ectopic, 10D2
Extraperitoneal, 10D00Z2
High, 10D00Z0
High Forceps, 10D07Z5
Internal Version, 10D07Z7
Low, 10D00Z1
Low Forceps, 10D07Z3
Mid Forceps, 10D07Z4
Other, 10D07Z8
Retained, 10D1
Vacuum, 10D07Z6
Radius
Left, 0PDJ0ZZ
Right, 0PDH0ZZ
Rectum, 0DDP
Ribs
1 to 2, 0PD10ZZ
3 or More, 0PD20ZZ
Sacrum, 0QD10ZZ
Scapula
Left, 0PD60ZZ
Right, 0PD50ZZ
Septum, Nasal, 09DM
Sinus
Accessory, 09DP

Extraction — *continued*
Sinus — *continued*
Ethmoid
Left, 09DV
Right, 09DU
Frontal
Left, 09DT
Right, 09DS
Mastoid
Left, 09DC
Right, 09DB
Maxillary
Left, 09DR
Right, 09DQ
Sphenoid
Left, 09DX
Right, 09DW
Skin
Abdomen, 0HD7XZZ
Back, 0HD6XZZ
Buttock, 0HD8XZZ
Chest, 0HD5XZZ
Ear
Left, 0HD3XZZ
Right, 0HD2XZZ
Face, 0HD1XZZ
Foot
Left, 0HDNXZZ
Right, 0HDMXZZ
Hand
Left, 0HDGXZZ
Right, 0HDFXZZ
Inguinal, 0HDAXZZ
Lower Arm
Left, 0HDEXZZ
Right, 0HDDXZZ
Lower Leg
Left, 0HDLXZZ
Right, 0HDKXZZ
Neck, 0HD4XZZ
Perineum, 0HD9XZZ
Scalp, 0HD0XZZ
Upper Arm
Left, 0HDCXZZ
Right, 0HDBXZZ
Upper Leg
Left, 0HDJXZZ
Right, 0HDHXZZ
Skull, 0ND00ZZ
Spinal Meninges, 00DT
Spleen, 07DP
Sternum, 0PD00ZZ
Stomach, 0DD6
Pylorus, 0DD7
Subcutaneous Tissue and Fascia
Abdomen, 0JD8
Back, 0JD7
Buttock, 0JD9
Chest, 0JD6
Face, 0JD1
Foot
Left, 0JDR
Right, 0JDQ
Hand
Left, 0JDK
Right, 0JDJ
Lower Arm
Left, 0JDH
Right, 0JDG
Lower Leg
Left, 0JDP
Right, 0JDN
Neck
Left, 0JD5
Right, 0JD4
Pelvic Region, 0JDC
Perineum, 0JDB
Scalp, 0JD0
Upper Arm
Left, 0JDF
Right, 0JDD
Upper Leg
Left, 0JDM
Right, 0JDL
Tarsal
Left, 0QDM0ZZ
Right, 0QDL0ZZ

▽ Subterms under main terms may continue to next column or page

Extraction — *continued*
 Tendon
 Abdomen
 Left, ØLDGØZZ
 Right, ØLDFØZZ
 Ankle
 Left, ØLDTØZZ
 Right, ØLDSØZZ
 Foot
 Left, ØLDWØZZ
 Right, ØLDVØZZ
 Hand
 Left, ØLD8ØZZ
 Right, ØLD7ØZZ
 Head and Neck, ØLDØØZZ
 Hip
 Left, ØLDKØZZ
 Right, ØLDJØZZ
 Knee
 Left, ØLDRØZZ
 Right, ØLDQØZZ
 Lower Arm and Wrist
 Left, ØLD6ØZZ
 Right, ØLD5ØZZ
 Lower Leg
 Left, ØLDPØZZ
 Right, ØLDNØZZ
 Perineum, ØLDHØZZ
 Shoulder
 Left, ØLD2ØZZ
 Right, ØLD1ØZZ
 Thorax
 Left, ØLDDØZZ
 Right, ØLDCØZZ
 Trunk
 Left, ØLDBØZZ
 Right, ØLD9ØZZ
 Upper Arm
 Left, ØLD4ØZZ
 Right, ØLD3ØZZ
 Upper Leg
 Left, ØLDMØZZ
 Right, ØLDLØZZ
 Thymus, Ø7DM
 Tibia
 Left, ØQDHØZZ
 Right, ØQDGØZZ
 Toe Nail, ØHDRXZZ
 Tooth
 Lower, ØCDXXZ
 Upper, ØCDWXZ
 Trachea, ØBD1
 Turbinate, Nasal, Ø9DL
 Tympanic Membrane
 Left, Ø9D8
 Right, Ø9D7
 Ulna
 Left, ØPDLØZZ
 Right, ØPDKØZZ
 Vein
 Basilic
 Left, Ø5DC
 Right, Ø5DB
 Brachial
 Left, Ø5DA
 Right, Ø5D9
 Cephalic
 Left, Ø5DF
 Right, Ø5DD
 Femoral
 Left, Ø6DN
 Right, Ø6DM
 Foot
 Left, Ø6DV
 Right, Ø6DT
 Hand
 Left, Ø5DH
 Right, Ø5DG
 Lower, Ø6DY
 Saphenous
 Left, Ø6DQ
 Right, Ø6DP
 Upper, Ø5DY
 Vertebra
 Cervical, ØPD3ØZZ
 Lumbar, ØQDØØZZ
 Thoracic, ØPD4ØZZ
 Vocal Cord
 Left, ØCDV

Extraction — *continued*
 Vocal Cord — *continued*
 Right, ØCDT
Extradural space, intracranial *use* Epidural Space, Intracranial
Extradural space, spinal *use* Spinal Canal
EXtreme Lateral Interbody Fusion (XLIF) device *use* Interbody Fusion Device in Lower Joints

F

Face lift *see* Alteration, Face, ØWØ2
Facet replacement spinal stabilization device
 use Spinal Stabilization Device, Facet Replacement in, ØRH
 use Spinal Stabilization Device, Facet Replacement in, ØSH
Facial artery *use* Face Artery
Factor Xa Inhibitor Reversal Agent, Andexanet Alfa
 use Andexanet Alfa, Factor Xa Inhibitor Reversal Agent
False vocal cord *use* Larynx
Falx cerebri *use* Dura Mater
Fascia lata
 use Subcutaneous Tissue and Fascia, Left Upper Leg
 use Subcutaneous Tissue and Fascia, Right Upper Leg
Fasciaplasty, fascioplasty
 see Repair, Subcutaneous Tissue and Fascia, ØJQ
 see Replacement, Subcutaneous Tissue and Fascia, ØJR
Fasciectomy *see* Excision, Subcutaneous Tissue and Fascia, ØJB
Fasciorrhaphy *see* Repair, Subcutaneous Tissue and Fascia, ØJQ
Fasciotomy
 see Division, Subcutaneous Tissue and Fascia, ØJ8
 see Drainage, Subcutaneous Tissue and Fascia, ØJ9
 see Release
Feeding Device
 Change device in
 Lower, ØD2DXUZ
 Upper, ØD2ØXUZ
 Insertion of device in
 Duodenum, ØDH9
 Esophagus, ØDH5
 Ileum, ØDHB
 Intestine, Small, ØDH8
 Jejunum, ØDHA
 Stomach, ØDH6
 Removal of device from
 Esophagus, ØDP5
 Intestinal Tract
 Lower, ØDPD
 Upper, ØDPØ
 Stomach, ØDP6
 Revision of device in
 Intestinal Tract
 Lower, ØDWD
 Upper, ØDWØ
 Stomach, ØDW6
Femoral head
 use Upper Femur, Left
 use Upper Femur, Right
Femoral lymph node
 use Lymphatic, Left Lower Extremity
 use Lymphatic, Right Lower Extremity
Femoropatellar joint
 use Knee Joint, Left
 use Knee Joint, Left, Tibial Surface
 use Knee Joint, Right
 use Knee Joint, Right, Femoral Surface
Femorotibial joint
 use Knee Joint, Left
 use Knee Joint, Left, Tibial Surface
 use Knee Joint, Right
 use Knee Joint, Right, Tibial Surface
Fibular artery
 use Peroneal Artery, Left
 use Peroneal Artery, Right
Fibularis brevis muscle
 use Lower Leg Muscle, Left
 use Lower Leg Muscle, Right
Fibularis longus muscle
 use Lower Leg Muscle, Left
 use Lower Leg Muscle, Right
Fifth cranial nerve *use* Trigeminal Nerve

Filum terminale *use* Spinal Meninges
Fimbriectomy
 see Excision, Female Reproductive System, ØUB
 see Resection, Female Reproductive System, ØUT
Fine needle aspiration
 Fluid or gas *see* Drainage
 Tissue biopsy
 see Excision
 see Extraction
First cranial nerve *use* Olfactory Nerve
First intercostal nerve *use* Brachial Plexus
Fistulization
 see Bypass
 see Drainage
 see Repair
Fitting
 Arch bars, for fracture reduction *see* Reposition, Mouth and Throat, ØCS
 Arch bars, for immobilization *see* Immobilization, Face, 2W31
 Artificial limb *see* Device Fitting, Rehabilitation, FØD
 Hearing aid *see* Device Fitting, Rehabilitation, FØD
 Ocular prosthesis, FØDZ8UZ
 Prosthesis, limb *see* Device Fitting, Rehabilitation, FØD
 Prosthesis, ocular, FØDZ8UZ
Fixation, bone
 External, with fracture reduction *see* Reposition
 External, without fracture reduction *see* Insertion
 Internal, with fracture reduction *see* Reposition
 Internal, without fracture reduction *see* Insertion
FLAIR® Endovascular Stent Graft *use* Intraluminal Device
Flexible Composite Mesh *use* Synthetic Substitute
Flexor carpi radialis muscle
 use Lower Arm and Wrist Muscle, Left
 use Lower Arm and Wrist Muscle, Right
Flexor carpi ulnaris muscle
 use Lower Arm and Wrist Muscle, Left
 use Lower Arm and Wrist Muscle, Right
Flexor digitorum brevis muscle
 use Foot Muscle, Left
 use Foot Muscle, Right
Flexor digitorum longus muscle
 use Lower Leg Muscle, Left
 use Lower Leg Muscle, Right
Flexor hallucis brevis muscle
 use Foot Muscle, Left
 use Foot Muscle, Right
Flexor hallucis longus muscle
 use Lower Leg Muscle, Left
 use Lower Leg Muscle, Right
Flexor pollicis longus muscle
 use Lower Arm and Wrist Muscle, Left
 use Lower Arm and Wrist Muscle, Right
Fluoroscopy
 Abdomen and Pelvis, BW11
 Airway, Upper, BB1DZZZ
 Ankle
 Left, BQ1H
 Right, BQ1G
 Aorta
 Abdominal, B41Ø
 Laser, Intraoperative, B41Ø
 Thoracic, B31Ø
 Laser, Intraoperative, B31Ø
 Thoraco-Abdominal, B31P
 Laser, Intraoperative, B31P
 Aorta and Bilateral Lower Extremity Arteries, B41D
 Laser, Intraoperative, B41D
 Arm
 Left, BP1FZZZ
 Right, BP1EZZZ
 Artery
 Brachiocephalic-Subclavian
 Laser, Intraoperative, B311
 Right, B311
 Bronchial, B31L
 Laser, Intraoperative, B31L
 Bypass Graft, Other, B21F
 Cervico-Cerebral Arch, B31Q
 Laser, Intraoperative, B31Q
 Common Carotid
 Bilateral, B315
 Laser, Intraoperative, B315
 Left, B314
 Laser, Intraoperative, B314
 Right, B313

Fluoroscopy — *continued*
Ureter — *continued*
Right, BT16
Urethra, BT15
Urethra and Bladder, BT1B
Uterus, BU16
Uterus and Fallopian Tube, BU18
Vagina, BU19
Vasa Vasorum, BV18
Vein
Cerebellar, B511
Cerebral, B511
Epidural, B510
Jugular
Bilateral, B515
Left, B514
Right, B513
Lower Extremity
Bilateral, B51D
Left, B51C
Right, B51B
Other, B51V
Pelvic (Iliac)
Left, B51G
Right, B51F
Pelvic (Iliac) Bilateral, B51H
Portal, B51T
Pulmonary
Bilateral, B51S
Left, B51R
Right, B51Q
Renal
Bilateral, B51L
Left, B51K
Right, B51J
Spanchnic, B51T
Subclavian
Left, B517
Right, B516
Upper Extremity
Bilateral, B51P
Left, B51N
Right, B51M
Vena Cava
Inferior, B519
Superior, B518
Wrist
Left, BP1M
Right, BP1L
Fluoroscopy, laser intraoperative
see Fluoroscopy, Heart, B21
see Fluoroscopy, Lower Arteries, B41
see Fluoroscopy, Upper Arteries, B31
Flushing *see* Irrigation
Foley catheter *use* Drainage Device
Fontan completion procedure Stage II *see* Bypass, Vena Cava, Inferior, 0610
Foramen magnum *use* Occipital Bone
Foramen of Monro (intraventricular) *use* Cerebral Ventricle
Foreskin *use* Prepuce
Formula™ Balloon-Expandable Renal Stent System *use* Intraluminal Device
Fossa of Rosenmuller *use* Nasopharynx
Fourth cranial nerve *use* Trochlear Nerve
Fourth ventricle *use* Cerebral Ventricle
Fovea
use Retina, Left
use Retina, Right
Fragmentation
Ampulla of Vater, 0FFC
Anus, 0DFQ
Appendix, 0DFJ
Bladder, 0TFB
Bladder Neck, 0TFC
Bronchus
Lingula, 0BF9
Lower Lobe
Left, 0BFB
Right, 0BF6
Main
Left, 0BF7
Right, 0BF3
Middle Lobe, Right, 0BF5
Upper Lobe
Left, 0BF8
Right, 0BF4
Carina, 0BF2

Fragmentation — *continued*
Cavity, Cranial, 0WF1
Cecum, 0DFH
Cerebral Ventricle, 00F6
Colon
Ascending, 0DFK
Descending, 0DFM
Sigmoid, 0DFN
Transverse, 0DFL
Duct
Common Bile, 0FF9
Cystic, 0FF8
Hepatic
Common, 0FF7
Left, 0FF6
Right, 0FF5
Pancreatic, 0FFD
Accessory, 0FFF
Parotid
Left, 0CFC
Right, 0CFB
Duodenum, 0DF9
Epidural Space, Intracranial, 00F3
Esophagus, 0DF5
Fallopian Tube
Left, 0UF6
Right, 0UF5
Fallopian Tubes, Bilateral, 0UF7
Gallbladder, 0FF4
Gastrointestinal Tract, 0WFP
Genitourinary Tract, 0WFR
Ileum, 0DFB
Intestine
Large, 0DFE
Left, 0DFG
Right, 0DFF
Small, 0DF8
Jejunum, 0DFA
Kidney Pelvis
Left, 0TF4
Right, 0TF3
Mediastinum, 0WFC
Oral Cavity and Throat, 0WF3
Pelvic Cavity, 0WFJ
Pericardial Cavity, 0WFD
Pericardium, 02FN
Peritoneal Cavity, 0WFG
Pleural Cavity
Left, 0WFB
Right, 0WF9
Rectum, 0DFP
Respiratory Tract, 0WFQ
Spinal Canal, 00FU
Stomach, 0DF6
Subarachnoid Space, Intracranial, 00F5
Subdural Space, Intracranial, 00F4
Trachea, 0BF1
Ureter
Left, 0TF7
Right, 0TF6
Urethra, 0TFD
Uterus, 0UF9
Vitreous
Left, 08F5
Right, 08F4
Freestyle (Stentless) Aortic Root Bioprosthesis *use* Zooplastic Tissue in Heart and Great Vessels
Frenectomy
see Excision, Mouth and Throat, 0CB
see Resection, Mouth and Throat, 0CT
Frenoplasty, frenuloplasty
see Repair, Mouth and Throat, 0CQ
see Replacement, Mouth and Throat, 0CR
see Supplement, Mouth and Throat, 0CU
Frenotomy
see Drainage, Mouth and Throat, 0C9
see Release, Mouth and Throat, 0CN
Frenulotomy
see Drainage, Mouth and Throat, 0C9
see Release, Mouth and Throat, 0CN
Frenulum labii inferioris *use* Lower Lip
Frenulum labii superioris *use* Upper Lip
Frenulum linguae *use* Tongue
Frenulumectomy
see Excision, Mouth and Throat, 0CB
see Resection, Mouth and Throat, 0CT
Frontal lobe *use* Cerebral Hemisphere

Frontal vein
use Face Vein, Left
use Face Vein, Right
Fulguration *see* Destruction
Fundoplication, gastroesophageal *see* Restriction, Esophagogastric Junction, 0DV4
Fundus uteri *use* Uterus
Fusion
Acromioclavicular
Left, 0RGH
Right, 0RGG
Ankle
Left, 0SGG
Right, 0SGF
Carpal
Left, 0RGR
Right, 0RGQ
Carpometacarpal
Left, 0RGT
Right, 0RGS
Cervical Vertebral, 0RG1
2 or more, 0RG2
Interbody Fusion Device
Nanotextured Surface, XRG2092
Radiolucent Porous, XRG20F3
Interbody Fusion Device
Nanotextured Surface, XRG1092
Radiolucent Porous, XRG10F3
Cervicothoracic Vertebral, 0RG4
Interbody Fusion Device
Nanotextured Surface, XRG4092
Radiolucent Porous, XRG40F3
Coccygeal, 0SG6
Elbow
Left, 0RGM
Right, 0RGL
Finger Phalangeal
Left, 0RGX
Right, 0RGW
Hip
Left, 0SGB
Right, 0SG9
Knee
Left, 0SGD
Right, 0SGC
Lumbar Vertebral, 0SG0
2 or more, 0SG1
Interbody Fusion Device
Nanotextured Surface, XRGC092
Radiolucent Porous, XRGC0F3
Interbody Fusion Device
Nanotextured Surface, XRGB092
Radiolucent Porous, XRGB0F3
Lumbosacral, 0SG3
Interbody Fusion Device
Nanotextured Surface, XRGD092
Radiolucent Porous, XRGD0F3
Metacarpophalangeal
Left, 0RGV
Right, 0RGU
Metatarsal-Phalangeal
Left, 0SGN
Right, 0SGM
Occipital-cervical, 0RG0
Interbody Fusion Device
Nanotextured Surface, XRG0092
Radiolucent Porous, XRG00F3
Sacrococcygeal, 0SG5
Sacroiliac
Left, 0SG8
Right, 0SG7
Shoulder
Left, 0RGK
Right, 0RGJ
Sternoclavicular
Left, 0RGF
Right, 0RGE
Tarsal
Left, 0SGJ
Right, 0SGH
Tarsometatarsal
Left, 0SGL
Right, 0SGK
Temporomandibular
Left, 0RGD
Right, 0RGC
Thoracic Vertebral, 0RG6
2 to 7, 0RG7

Subterms under main terms may continue to next column or page

HeartMate XVE® Left Ventricular Assist Device (LVAD) *use* Implantable Heart Assist System in Heart and Great Vessels
HeartMate® implantable heart assist system *see* Insertion of device in, Heart, Ø2HA
Helix
use Ear, External, Bilateral
use Ear, External, Left
use Ear, External, Right
Hematopoietic cell transplant (HCT) *see* Transfusion, Circulatory, 3Ø2
Hemicolectomy *see* Resection, Gastrointestinal System, ØDT
Hemicystectomy *see* Excision, Urinary System, ØTB
Hemigastrectomy *see* Excision, Gastrointestinal System, ØDB
Hemiglossectomy *see* Excision, Mouth and Throat, ØCB
Hemilaminectomy
see Excision, Lower Bones, ØQB
see Excision, Upper Bones, ØPB
Hemilaminotomy
see Drainage, Lower Bones, ØQ9
see Drainage, Upper Bones, ØP9
see Excision, Lower Bones, ØQB
see Excision, Upper Bones, ØPB
see Release, Central Nervous System and Cranial Nerves, ØØN
see Release, Lower Bones, ØQN
see Release, Peripheral Nervous System, Ø1N
see Release, Upper Bones, ØPN
Hemilaryngectomy *see* Excision, Larynx, ØCBS
Hemimandibulectomy *see* Excision, Head and Facial Bones, ØNB
Hemimaxillectomy *see* Excision, Head and Facial Bones, ØNB
Hemipylorectomy *see* Excision, Gastrointestinal System, ØDB
Hemispherectomy
see Excision, Central Nervous System and Cranial Nerves, ØØB
see Resection, Central Nervous System and Cranial Nerves, ØØT
Hemithyroidectomy
see Excision, Endocrine System, ØGB
see Resection, Endocrine System, ØGT
Hemodialysis *see* Performance, Urinary, 5A1D
Hemolung® Respiratory Assist System (RAS), 5AØ92ØZ
Hepatectomy
see Excision, Hepatobiliary System and Pancreas, ØFB
see Resection, Hepatobiliary System and Pancreas, ØFT
Hepatic artery proper *use* Hepatic Artery
Hepatic flexure *use* Transverse Colon
Hepatic lymph node *use* Lymphatic, Aortic
Hepatic plexus *use* Abdominal Sympathetic Nerve
Hepatic portal vein *use* Portal Vein
Hepaticoduodenostomy
see Bypass, Hepatobiliary System and Pancreas, ØF1
see Drainage, Hepatobiliary System and Pancreas, ØF9
Hepaticotomy *see* Drainage, Hepatobiliary System and Pancreas, ØF9
Hepatocholedochostomy *see* Drainage, Duct, Common Bile, ØF99
Hepatogastric ligament *use* Omentum
Hepatopancreatic ampulla *use* Ampulla of Vater
Hepatopexy
see Repair, Hepatobiliary System and Pancreas, ØFQ
see Reposition, Hepatobiliary System and Pancreas, ØFS
Hepatorrhaphy *see* Repair, Hepatobiliary System and Pancreas, ØFQ
Hepatotomy *see* Drainage, Hepatobiliary System and Pancreas, ØF9
Herculink (RX) Elite Renal Stent System *use* Intraluminal Device
Herniorrhaphy
With synthetic substitute
see Supplement, Anatomical Regions, General, ØWU
see Supplement, Anatomical Regions, Lower Extremities, ØYU
see Repair, Anatomical Regions, General, ØWQ
see Repair, Anatomical Regions, Lower Extremities, ØYQ
Hip (joint) liner *use* Liner in Lower Joints
Holter monitoring, 4A12X45
Holter valve ventricular shunt *use* Synthetic Substitute
Human angiotensin II, synthetic *use* Synthetic Human Angiotensin II
Humeroradial joint
use Elbow Joint, Left
use Elbow Joint, Right
Humeroulnar joint
use Elbow Joint, Left
use Elbow Joint, Right
Humerus, distal
use Humeral Shaft, Left
use Humeral Shaft, Right
Hydrocelectomy *see* Excision, Male Reproductive System, ØVB
Hydrotherapy
Assisted exercise in pool *see* Motor Treatment, Rehabilitation, FØ7
Whirlpool *see* Activities of Daily Living Treatment, Rehabilitation, FØ8
Hymenectomy
see Excision, Hymen, ØUBK
see Resection, Hymen, ØUTK
Hymenoplasty
see Repair, Hymen, ØUQK
see Supplement, Hymen, ØUUK
Hymenorrhaphy *see* Repair, Hymen, ØUQK
Hymenotomy
see Division, Hymen, ØU8K
see Drainage, Hymen, ØU9K
Hyoglossus muscle *use* Tongue, Palate, Pharynx Muscle
Hyoid artery
use Thyroid Artery, Left
use Thyroid Artery, Right
Hyperalimentation *see* Introduction of substance in or on
Hyperbaric oxygenation
Decompression sickness treatment *see* Decompression, Circulatory, 6A15
Wound treatment *see* Assistance, Circulatory, 5AØ5
Hyperthermia
Radiation Therapy
Abdomen, DWY38ZZ
Adrenal Gland, DGY28ZZ
Bile Ducts, DFY28ZZ
Bladder, DTY28ZZ
Bone Marrow, D7YØ8ZZ
Bone, Other, DPYC8ZZ
Brain, DØYØ8ZZ
Brain Stem, DØY18ZZ
Breast
Left, DMYØ8ZZ
Right, DMY18ZZ
Bronchus, DBY18ZZ
Cervix, DUY18ZZ
Chest, DWY28ZZ
Chest Wall, DBY78ZZ
Colon, DDY58ZZ
Diaphragm, DBY88ZZ
Duodenum, DDY28ZZ
Ear, D9YØ8ZZ
Esophagus, DDYØ8ZZ
Eye, D8YØ8ZZ
Femur, DPY98ZZ
Fibula, DPYB8ZZ
Gallbladder, DFY18ZZ
Gland
Adrenal, DGY28ZZ
Parathyroid, DGY48ZZ
Pituitary, DGYØ8ZZ
Thyroid, DGY58ZZ
Glands, Salivary, D9Y68ZZ
Head and Neck, DWY18ZZ
Hemibody, DWY48ZZ
Humerus, DPY68ZZ
Hypopharynx, D9Y38ZZ
Ileum, DDY48ZZ
Jejunum, DDY38ZZ
Kidney, DTYØ8ZZ
Larynx, D9YB8ZZ
Liver, DFYØ8ZZ
Lung, DBY28ZZ
Lymphatics
Abdomen, D7Y68ZZ
Axillary, D7Y48ZZ
Inguinal, D7Y88ZZ
Neck, D7Y38ZZ
Pelvis, D7Y78ZZ
Thorax, D7Y58ZZ
Hyperthermia — *continued*
Radiation Therapy — *continued*
Mandible, DPY38ZZ
Maxilla, DPY28ZZ
Mediastinum, DBY68ZZ
Mouth, D9Y48ZZ
Nasopharynx, D9YD8ZZ
Neck and Head, DWY18ZZ
Nerve, Peripheral, DØY78ZZ
Nose, D9Y18ZZ
Oropharynx, D9YF8ZZ
Ovary, DUYØ8ZZ
Palate
Hard, D9Y88ZZ
Soft, D9Y98ZZ
Pancreas, DFY38ZZ
Parathyroid Gland, DGY48ZZ
Pelvic Bones, DPY88ZZ
Pelvic Region, DWY68ZZ
Pineal Body, DGY18ZZ
Pituitary Gland, DGYØ8ZZ
Pleura, DBY58ZZ
Prostate, DVYØ8ZZ
Radius, DPY78ZZ
Rectum, DDY78ZZ
Rib, DPY58ZZ
Sinuses, D9Y78ZZ
Skin
Abdomen, DHY88ZZ
Arm, DHY48ZZ
Back, DHY78ZZ
Buttock, DHY98ZZ
Chest, DHY68ZZ
Face, DHY28ZZ
Leg, DHYB8ZZ
Neck, DHY38ZZ
Skull, DPYØ8ZZ
Spinal Cord, DØY68ZZ
Spleen, D7Y28ZZ
Sternum, DPY48ZZ
Stomach, DDY18ZZ
Testis, DVY18ZZ
Thymus, D7Y18ZZ
Thyroid Gland, DGY58ZZ
Tibia, DPYB8ZZ
Tongue, D9Y58ZZ
Trachea, DBYØ8ZZ
Ulna, DPY78ZZ
Ureter, DTY18ZZ
Urethra, DTY38ZZ
Uterus, DUY28ZZ
Whole Body, DWY58ZZ
Whole Body, 6A3Z
Hypnosis, GZFZZZZ
Hypogastric artery
use Internal Iliac Artery, Left
use Internal Iliac Artery, Right
Hypopharynx *use* Pharynx
Hypophysectomy
see Excision, Gland, Pituitary, ØGBØ
see Resection, Gland, Pituitary, ØGTØ
Hypophysis *use* Pituitary Gland
Hypothalamotomy *see* Destruction, Thalamus, ØØ59
Hypothenar muscle
use Hand Muscle, Left
use Hand Muscle, Right
Hypothermia, Whole Body, 6A4Z
Hysterectomy
Supracervical *see* Resection, Uterus, ØUT9
Total *see* Resection, Uterus, ØUT9
Hysterolysis *see* Release, Uterus, ØUN9
Hysteropexy
see Repair, Uterus, ØUQ9
see Reposition, Uterus, ØUS9
Hysteroplasty *see* Repair, Uterus, ØUQ9
Hysterorrhaphy *see* Repair, Uterus, ØUQ9
Hysteroscopy, ØUJD8ZZ
Hysterotomy *see* Drainage, Uterus, ØU99
Hysterotrachelectomy
see Resection, Cervix, ØUTC
see Resection, Uterus, ØUT9
Hysterotracheloplasty *see* Repair, Uterus, ØUQ9
Hysterotrachelorrhaphy *see* Repair, Uterus, ØUQ9

I

Subterms under main terms may continue to next column or page

- **Inspection** — *continued*
  - Joint — *continued*
    - Tarsal
      - Left, ØSJJ
      - Right, ØSJH
    - Tarsometatarsal
      - Left, ØSJL
      - Right, ØSJK
    - Temporomandibular
      - Left, ØRJD
      - Right, ØRJC
    - Thoracic Vertebral, ØRJ6
    - Thoracolumbar Vertebral, ØRJA
    - Toe Phalangeal
      - Left, ØSJQ
      - Right, ØSJP
    - Wrist
      - Left, ØRJP
      - Right, ØRJN
  - Kidney, ØTJ5
  - Knee Region
    - Left, ØYJG
    - Right, ØYJF
  - Larynx, ØCJS
  - Leg
    - Lower
      - Left, ØYJJ
      - Right, ØYJH
    - Upper
      - Left, ØYJD
      - Right, ØYJC
  - Lens
    - Left, Ø8JKXZZ
    - Right, Ø8JJXZZ
  - Liver, ØFJØ
  - Lung
    - Left, ØBJL
    - Right, ØBJK
  - Lymphatic, Ø7JN
    - Thoracic Duct, Ø7JK
  - Mediastinum, ØWJC
  - Mesentery, ØDJV
  - Mouth and Throat, ØCJY
  - Muscle
    - Extraocular
      - Left, Ø8JM
      - Right, Ø8JL
    - Lower, ØKJY
    - Upper, ØKJX
  - Nasal Mucosa and Soft Tissue, Ø9JK
  - Neck, ØWJ6
  - Nerve
    - Cranial, ØØJE
    - Peripheral, Ø1JY
  - Omentum, ØDJU
  - Oral Cavity and Throat, ØWJ3
  - Ovary, ØUJ3
  - Pancreas, ØFJG
  - Parathyroid Gland, ØGJR
  - Pelvic Cavity, ØWJJ
  - Penis, ØVJS
  - Pericardial Cavity, ØWJD
  - Perineum
    - Female, ØWJN
    - Male, ØWJM
  - Peritoneal Cavity, ØWJG
  - Peritoneum, ØDJW
  - Pineal Body, ØGJ1
  - Pleura, ØBJQ
  - Pleural Cavity
    - Left, ØWJB
    - Right, ØWJ9
  - Products of Conception, 1ØJØ
    - Ectopic, 1ØJ2
    - Retained, 1ØJ1
  - Prostate and Seminal Vesicles, ØVJ4
  - Respiratory Tract, ØWJQ
  - Retroperitoneum, ØWJH
  - Scrotum and Tunica Vaginalis, ØVJ8
  - Shoulder Region
    - Left, ØXJ3
    - Right, ØXJ2
  - Sinus, Ø9JY
  - Skin, ØHJPXZZ
  - Skull, ØNJØ
  - Spinal Canal, ØØJU
  - Spinal Cord, ØØJV
  - Spleen, Ø7JP
  - Stomach, ØDJ6

- **Inspection** — *continued*
  - Subcutaneous Tissue and Fascia
    - Head and Neck, ØJJS
    - Lower Extremity, ØJJW
    - Trunk, ØJJT
    - Upper Extremity, ØJJV
  - Tendon
    - Lower, ØLJY
    - Upper, ØLJX
  - Testis, ØVJD
  - Thymus, Ø7JM
  - Thyroid Gland, ØGJK
  - Toe Nail, ØHJRXZZ
  - Trachea, ØBJ1
  - Tracheobronchial Tree, ØBJØ
  - Tympanic Membrane
    - Left, Ø9J8
    - Right, Ø9J7
  - Ureter, ØTJ9
  - Urethra, ØTJD
  - Uterus and Cervix, ØUJD
  - Vagina and Cul-de-sac, ØUJH
  - Vas Deferens, ØVJR
  - Vein
    - Lower, Ø6JY
    - Upper, Ø5JY
  - Vulva, ØUJM
  - Wrist Region
    - Left, ØXJH
    - Right, ØXJG
- **Instillation** *see* Introduction of substance in or on
- **Insufflation** *see* Introduction of substance in or on
- **Interatrial septum** *use* Atrial Septum
- **Interbody fusion (spine) cage**
  - *use* Interbody Fusion Device in Lower Joints
  - *use* Interbody Fusion Device in Upper Joints
- **Interbody Fusion Device**
  - Nanotextured Surface
    - Cervical Vertebral, XRG1Ø92
      - 2 or more, XRG2Ø92
    - Cervicothoracic Vertebral, XRG4Ø92
    - Lumbar Vertebral, XRGBØ92
      - 2 or more, XRGCØ92
    - Lumbosacral, XRGDØ92
    - Occipital-cervical, XRGØØ92
    - Thoracic Vertebral, XRG6Ø92
      - 2 to 7, XRG7Ø92
      - 8 or more, XRG8Ø92
    - Thoracolumbar Vertebral, XRGAØ92
  - Radiolucent Porous
    - Cervical Vertebral, XRG1ØF3
      - 2 or more, XRG2ØF3
    - Cervicothoracic Vertebral, XRG4ØF3
    - Lumbar Vertebral, XRGBØF3
      - 2 or more, XRGCØF3
    - Lumbosacral, XRGDØF3
    - Occipital-cervical, XRGØØF3
    - Thoracic Vertebral, XRG6ØF3
      - 2 to 7, XRG7ØF3
      - 8 or more, XRG8ØF3
    - Thoracolumbar Vertebral, XRGAØF3
- **Intercarpal joint**
  - *use* Carpal Joint, Left
  - *use* Carpal Joint, Right
- **Intercarpal ligament**
  - *use* Hand Bursa and Ligament, Left
  - *use* Hand Bursa and Ligament, Right
- **Interclavicular ligament**
  - *use* Shoulder Bursa and Ligament, Left
  - *use* Shoulder Bursa and Ligament, Right
- **Intercostal lymph node** *use* Lymphatic, Thorax
- **Intercostal muscle**
  - *use* Thorax Muscle, Left
  - *use* Thorax Muscle, Right
- **Intercostal nerve** *use* Thoracic Nerve
- **Intercostobrachial nerve** *use* Thoracic Nerve
- **Intercuneiform joint**
  - *use* Tarsal Joint, Left
  - *use* Tarsal Joint, Right
- **Intercuneiform ligament**
  - *use* Foot Bursa and Ligament, Left
  - *use* Foot Bursa and Ligament, Right
- **Intermediate bronchus** *use* Main Bronchus, Right
- **Intermediate cuneiform bone**
  - *use* Tarsal, Left
  - *use* Tarsal, Right
- **Intermittent hemodialysis (IHD)**, 5A1D7ØZ

- **Intermittent mandatory ventilation** *see* Assistance, Respiratory, 5AØ9
- **Intermittent Negative Airway Pressure**
  - 24-96 Consecutive Hours, Ventilation, 5AØ945B
  - Greater than 96 Consecutive Hours, Ventilation, 5AØ955B
  - Less than 24 Consecutive Hours, Ventilation, 5AØ935B
- **Intermittent Positive Airway Pressure**
  - 24-96 Consecutive Hours, Ventilation, 5AØ9458
  - Greater than 96 Consecutive Hours, Ventilation, 5AØ9558
  - Less than 24 Consecutive Hours, Ventilation, 5AØ9358
- **Intermittent positive pressure breathing** *see* Assistance, Respiratory, 5AØ9
- **Internal anal sphincter** *use* Anal Sphincter
- **Internal carotid artery, intracranial portion** *use* Intracranial Artery
- **Internal carotid plexus** *use* Head and Neck Sympathetic Nerve
- **Internal (basal) cerebral vein** *use* Intracranial Vein
- **Internal iliac vein**
  - *use* Hypogastric Vein, Left
  - *use* Hypogastric Vein, Right
- **Internal maxillary artery**
  - *use* External Carotid Artery, Left
  - *use* External Carotid Artery, Right
- **Internal naris** *use* Nasal Mucosa and Soft Tissue
- **Internal oblique muscle**
  - *use* Abdomen Muscle, Left
  - *use* Abdomen Muscle, Right
- **Internal pudendal artery**
  - *use* Internal Iliac Artery, Left
  - *use* Internal Iliac Artery, Right
- **Internal pudendal vein**
  - *use* Hypogastric Vein, Left
  - *use* Hypogastric Vein, Right
- **Internal thoracic artery**
  - *use* Internal Mammary Artery, Left
  - *use* Internal Mammary Artery, Right
  - *use* Subclavian Artery, Left
  - *use* Subclavian Artery, Right
- **Internal urethral sphincter** *use* Urethra
- **Interphalangeal (IP) joint**
  - *use* Finger Phalangeal Joint, Left
  - *use* Finger Phalangeal Joint, Right
  - *use* Toe Phalangeal Joint, Left
  - *use* Toe Phalangeal Joint, Right
- **Interphalangeal ligament**
  - *use* Foot Bursa and Ligament, Left
  - *use* Foot Bursa and Ligament, Right
  - *use* Hand Bursa and Ligament, Left
  - *use* Hand Bursa and Ligament, Right
- **Interrogation, cardiac rhythm related device**
  - With cardiac function testing *see* Measurement, Cardiac, 4AØ2
  - Interrogation only *see* Measurement, Cardiac, 4BØ2
- **Interruption** *see* Occlusion
- **Interspinalis muscle**
  - *use* Trunk Muscle, Left
  - *use* Trunk Muscle, Right
- **Interspinous ligament, cervical** *use* Head and Neck Bursa and Ligament
- **Interspinous ligament, lumbar** *use* Lower Spine Bursa and Ligament
- **Interspinous ligament, thoracic** *use* Upper Spine Bursa and Ligament
- **Interspinous process spinal stabilization device**
  - *use* Spinal Stabilization Device, Interspinous Process in, ØRH
  - *use* Spinal Stabilization Device, Interspinous Process in, ØSH
- **InterStim® Therapy lead** *use* Neurostimulator Lead in Peripheral Nervous System
- **InterStim® Therapy neurostimulator** *use* Stimulator Generator, Single Array in, ØJH
- **Intertransversarius muscle**
  - *use* Trunk Muscle, Left
  - *use* Trunk Muscle, Right
- **Intertransverse ligament, cervical** *use* Head and Neck Bursa and Ligament
- **Intertransverse ligament, lumbar** *use* Lower Spine Bursa and Ligament
- **Intertransverse ligament, thoracic** *use* Upper Spine Bursa and Ligament
- **Interventricular foramen (Monro)** *use* Cerebral Ventricle
- **Interventricular septum** *use* Ventricular Septum
- **Intestinal lymphatic trunk** *use* Cisterna Chyli

Introduction of substance in or on — *continued*
 Gastrointestinal Tract — *continued*
 Lower — *continued*
 Destructive Agent, 3E0H
 Diagnostic Substance, Other, 3E0H
 Electrolytic Substance, 3E0H
 Gas, 3E0H
 Hypnotics, 3E0H
 Nutritional Substance, 3E0H
 Radioactive Substance, 3E0H
 Sedatives, 3E0H
 Water Balance Substance, 3E0H
 Upper, 3E0G
 Analgesics, 3E0G
 Anesthetic Agent, 3E0G
 Anti-infective, 3E0G
 Anti-inflammatory, 3E0G
 Antineoplastic, 3E0G
 Destructive Agent, 3E0G
 Diagnostic Substance, Other, 3E0G
 Electrolytic Substance, 3E0G
 Gas, 3E0G
 Hypnotics, 3E0G
 Nutritional Substance, 3E0G
 Radioactive Substance, 3E0G
 Sedatives, 3E0G
 Water Balance Substance, 3E0G
 Genitourinary Tract, 3E0K
 Analgesics, 3E0K
 Anesthetic Agent, 3E0K
 Anti-infective, 3E0K
 Anti-inflammatory, 3E0K
 Antineoplastic, 3E0K
 Destructive Agent, 3E0K
 Diagnostic Substance, Other, 3E0K
 Electrolytic Substance, 3E0K
 Gas, 3E0K
 Hypnotics, 3E0K
 Nutritional Substance, 3E0K
 Radioactive Substance, 3E0K
 Sedatives, 3E0K
 Water Balance Substance, 3E0K
 Heart, 3E08
 Diagnostic Substance, Other, 3E08
 Platelet Inhibitor, 3E08
 Thrombolytic, 3E08
 Joint, 3E0U
 Analgesics, 3E0U3NZ
 Anesthetic Agent, 3E0U3BZ
 Anti-infective, 3E0U
 Anti-inflammatory, 3E0U33Z
 Antineoplastic, 3E0U30
 Destructive Agent, 3E0U3TZ
 Diagnostic Substance, Other, 3E0U3KZ
 Electrolytic Substance, 3E0U37Z
 Gas, 3E0U3SF
 Hypnotics, 3E0U3NZ
 Nutritional Substance, 3E0U36Z
 Radioactive Substance, 3E0U3HZ
 Sedatives, 3E0U3NZ
 Water Balance Substance, 3E0U37Z
 Lymphatic, 3E0W3GC
 Analgesics, 3E0W3NZ
 Anesthetic Agent, 3E0W3BZ
 Anti-infective, 3E0W32
 Anti-inflammatory, 3E0W33Z
 Antineoplastic, 3E0W30
 Destructive Agent, 3E0W3TZ
 Diagnostic Substance, Other, 3E0W3KZ
 Electrolytic Substance, 3E0W37Z
 Hypnotics, 3E0W3NZ
 Nutritional Substance, 3E0W36Z
 Radioactive Substance, 3E0W3HZ
 Sedatives, 3E0W3NZ
 Water Balance Substance, 3E0W37Z
 Mouth, 3E0D
 Analgesics, 3E0D
 Anesthetic Agent, 3E0D
 Antiarrhythmic, 3E0D
 Anti-infective, 3E0D
 Anti-inflammatory, 3E0D
 Antineoplastic, 3E0D
 Destructive Agent, 3E0D
 Diagnostic Substance, Other, 3E0D
 Electrolytic Substance, 3E0D
 Hypnotics, 3E0D
 Nutritional Substance, 3E0D
 Radioactive Substance, 3E0D
 Sedatives, 3E0D

Introduction of substance in or on — *continued*
 Mouth — *continued*
 Serum, 3E0D
 Toxoid, 3E0D
 Vaccine, 3E0D
 Water Balance Substance, 3E0D
 Mucous Membrane, 3E00XGC
 Analgesics, 3E00XNZ
 Anesthetic Agent, 3E00XBZ
 Anti-infective, 3E00X2
 Anti-inflammatory, 3E00X3Z
 Antineoplastic, 3E00X0
 Destructive Agent, 3E00XTZ
 Diagnostic Substance, Other, 3E00XKZ
 Hypnotics, 3E00XNZ
 Pigment, 3E00XMZ
 Sedatives, 3E00XNZ
 Serum, 3E00X4Z
 Toxoid, 3E00X4Z
 Vaccine, 3E00X4Z
 Muscle, 3E023GC
 Analgesics, 3E023NZ
 Anesthetic Agent, 3E023BZ
 Anti-infective, 3E0232
 Anti-inflammatory, 3E0233Z
 Antineoplastic, 3E0230
 Destructive Agent, 3E023TZ
 Diagnostic Substance, Other, 3E023KZ
 Electrolytic Substance, 3E0237Z
 Hypnotics, 3E023NZ
 Nutritional Substance, 3E0236Z
 Radioactive Substance, 3E023HZ
 Sedatives, 3E023NZ
 Serum, 3E0234Z
 Toxoid, 3E0234Z
 Vaccine, 3E0234Z
 Water Balance Substance, 3E0237Z
 Nerve
 Cranial, 3E0X3GC
 Anesthetic Agent, 3E0X3BZ
 Anti-inflammatory, 3E0X33Z
 Destructive Agent, 3E0X3TZ
 Peripheral, 3E0T3GC
 Anesthetic Agent, 3E0T3BZ
 Anti-inflammatory, 3E0T33Z
 Destructive Agent, 3E0T3TZ
 Plexus, 3E0T3GC
 Anesthetic Agent, 3E0T3BZ
 Anti-inflammatory, 3E0T33Z
 Destructive Agent, 3E0T3TZ
 Nose, 3E09
 Analgesics, 3E09
 Anesthetic Agent, 3E09
 Anti-infective, 3E09
 Anti-inflammatory, 3E09
 Antineoplastic, 3E09
 Destructive Agent, 3E09
 Diagnostic Substance, Other, 3E09
 Hypnotics, 3E09
 Radioactive Substance, 3E09
 Sedatives, 3E09
 Serum, 3E09
 Toxoid, 3E09
 Vaccine, 3E09
 Pancreatic Tract, 3E0J
 Analgesics, 3E0J
 Anesthetic Agent, 3E0J
 Anti-infective, 3E0J
 Anti-inflammatory, 3E0J
 Antineoplastic, 3E0J
 Destructive Agent, 3E0J
 Diagnostic Substance, Other, 3E0J
 Electrolytic Substance, 3E0J
 Gas, 3E0J
 Hypnotics, 3E0J
 Islet Cells, Pancreatic, 3E0J
 Nutritional Substance, 3E0J
 Radioactive Substance, 3E0J
 Sedatives, 3E0J
 Water Balance Substance, 3E0J
 Pericardial Cavity, 3E0Y
 Analgesics, 3E0Y3NZ
 Anesthetic Agent, 3E0Y3BZ
 Anti-infective, 3E0Y32
 Anti-inflammatory, 3E0Y33Z
 Antineoplastic, 3E0Y
 Destructive Agent, 3E0Y3TZ
 Diagnostic Substance, Other, 3E0Y3KZ
 Electrolytic Substance, 3E0Y37Z

Introduction of substance in or on — *continued*
 Pericardial Cavity — *continued*
 Gas, 3E0Y
 Hypnotics, 3E0Y3NZ
 Nutritional Substance, 3E0Y36Z
 Radioactive Substance, 3E0Y3HZ
 Sedatives, 3E0Y3NZ
 Water Balance Substance, 3E0Y37Z
 Peritoneal Cavity, 3E0M
 Adhesion Barrier, 3E0M
 Analgesics, 3E0M3NZ
 Anesthetic Agent, 3E0M3BZ
 Anti-infective, 3E0M32
 Anti-inflammatory, 3E0M33Z
 Antineoplastic, 3E0M
 Destructive Agent, 3E0M3TZ
 Diagnostic Substance, Other, 3E0M3KZ
 Electrolytic Substance, 3E0M37Z
 Gas, 3E0M
 Hypnotics, 3E0M3NZ
 Nutritional Substance, 3E0M36Z
 Radioactive Substance, 3E0M3HZ
 Sedatives, 3E0M3NZ
 Water Balance Substance, 3E0M37Z
 Pharynx, 3E0D
 Analgesics, 3E0D
 Anesthetic Agent, 3E0D
 Antiarrhythmic, 3E0D
 Anti-infective, 3E0D
 Anti-inflammatory, 3E0D
 Antineoplastic, 3E0D
 Destructive Agent, 3E0D
 Diagnostic Substance, Other, 3E0D
 Electrolytic Substance, 3E0D
 Hypnotics, 3E0D
 Nutritional Substance, 3E0D
 Radioactive Substance, 3E0D
 Sedatives, 3E0D
 Serum, 3E0D
 Toxoid, 3E0D
 Vaccine, 3E0D
 Water Balance Substance, 3E0D
 Pleural Cavity, 3E0L
 Adhesion Barrier, 3E0L
 Analgesics, 3E0L3NZ
 Anesthetic Agent, 3E0L3BZ
 Anti-infective, 3E0L32
 Anti-inflammatory, 3E0L33Z
 Antineoplastic, 3E0L
 Destructive Agent, 3E0L3TZ
 Diagnostic Substance, Other, 3E0L3KZ
 Electrolytic Substance, 3E0L37Z
 Gas, 3E0L
 Hypnotics, 3E0L3NZ
 Nutritional Substance, 3E0L36Z
 Radioactive Substance, 3E0L3HZ
 Sedatives, 3E0L3NZ
 Water Balance Substance, 3E0L37Z
 Products of Conception, 3E0E
 Analgesics, 3E0E
 Anesthetic Agent, 3E0E
 Anti-infective, 3E0E
 Anti-inflammatory, 3E0E
 Antineoplastic, 3E0E
 Destructive Agent, 3E0E
 Diagnostic Substance, Other, 3E0E
 Electrolytic Substance, 3E0E
 Gas, 3E0E
 Hypnotics, 3E0E
 Nutritional Substance, 3E0E
 Radioactive Substance, 3E0E
 Sedatives, 3E0E
 Water Balance Substance, 3E0E
 Reproductive
 Female, 3E0P
 Adhesion Barrier, 3E0P
 Analgesics, 3E0P
 Anesthetic Agent, 3E0P
 Anti-infective, 3E0P
 Anti-inflammatory, 3E0P
 Antineoplastic, 3E0P
 Destructive Agent, 3E0P
 Diagnostic Substance, Other, 3E0P
 Electrolytic Substance, 3E0P
 Gas, 3E0P
 Hormone, 3E0P
 Hypnotics, 3E0P
 Nutritional Substance, 3E0P
 Ovum, Fertilized, 3E0P

Subterms under main terms may continue to next column or page

Introduction of substance in or on — *continued*
Reproductive — *continued*
Female — *continued*
Radioactive Substance, 3EØP
Sedatives, 3EØP
Sperm, 3EØP
Water Balance Substance, 3EØP
Male, 3EØN
Analgesics, 3EØN
Anesthetic Agent, 3EØN
Anti-infective, 3EØN
Anti-inflammatory, 3EØN
Antineoplastic, 3EØN
Destructive Agent, 3EØN
Diagnostic Substance, Other, 3EØN
Electrolytic Substance, 3EØN
Gas, 3EØN
Hypnotics, 3EØN
Nutritional Substance, 3EØN
Radioactive Substance, 3EØN
Sedatives, 3EØN
Water Balance Substance, 3EØN
Respiratory Tract, 3EØF
Analgesics, 3EØF
Anesthetic Agent, 3EØF
Anti-infective, 3EØF
Anti-inflammatory, 3EØF
Antineoplastic, 3EØF
Destructive Agent, 3EØF
Diagnostic Substance, Other, 3EØF
Electrolytic Substance, 3EØF
Gas, 3EØF
Hypnotics, 3EØF
Nutritional Substance, 3EØF
Radioactive Substance, 3EØF
Sedatives, 3EØF
Water Balance Substance, 3EØF
Skin, 3EØØXGC
Analgesics, 3EØØXNZ
Anesthetic Agent, 3EØØXBZ
Anti-infective, 3EØØX2
Anti-inflammatory, 3EØØX3Z
Antineoplastic, 3EØØXØ
Destructive Agent, 3EØØXTZ
Diagnostic Substance, Other, 3EØØXKZ
Hypnotics, 3EØØXNZ
Pigment, 3EØØXMZ
Sedatives, 3EØØXNZ
Serum, 3EØØX4Z
Toxoid, 3EØØX4Z
Vaccine, 3EØØX4Z
Spinal Canal, 3EØR3GC
Analgesics, 3EØR3NZ
Anesthetic Agent, 3EØR3BZ
Anti-infective, 3EØR32
Anti-inflammatory, 3EØR33Z
Antineoplastic, 3EØR3Ø
Destructive Agent, 3EØR3TZ
Diagnostic Substance, Other, 3EØR3KZ
Electrolytic Substance, 3EØR37Z
Gas, 3EØR
Hypnotics, 3EØR3NZ
Nutritional Substance, 3EØR36Z
Radioactive Substance, 3EØR3HZ
Sedatives, 3EØR3NZ
Stem Cells
Embryonic, 3EØR
Somatic, 3EØR
Water Balance Substance, 3EØR37Z
Subcutaneous Tissue, 3EØ13GC
Analgesics, 3EØ13NZ
Anesthetic Agent, 3EØ13BZ
Anti-infective, 3EØ1
Anti-inflammatory, 3EØ133Z
Antineoplastic, 3EØ13Ø
Destructive Agent, 3EØ13TZ
Diagnostic Substance, Other, 3EØ13KZ
Electrolytic Substance, 3EØ137Z
Hormone, 3EØ13V
Hypnotics, 3EØ13NZ
Nutritional Substance, 3EØ136Z
Radioactive Substance, 3EØ13HZ
Sedatives, 3EØ13NZ
Serum, 3EØ134Z
Toxoid, 3EØ134Z
Vaccine, 3EØ134Z
Water Balance Substance, 3EØ137Z
Vein
Central, 3EØ4

Introduction of substance in or on — *continued*
Vein — *continued*
Central — *continued*
Analgesics, 3EØ4
Anesthetic, Intracirculatory, 3EØ4
Antiarrhythmic, 3EØ4
Anti-infective, 3EØ4
Anti-inflammatory, 3EØ4
Antineoplastic, 3EØ4
Destructive Agent, 3EØ4
Diagnostic Substance, Other, 3EØ4
Electrolytic Substance, 3EØ4
Hormone, 3EØ4
Hypnotics, 3EØ4
Immunotherapeutic, 3EØ4
Nutritional Substance, 3EØ4
Platelet Inhibitor, 3EØ4
Radioactive Substance, 3EØ4
Sedatives, 3EØ4
Serum, 3EØ4
Thrombolytic, 3EØ4
Toxoid, 3EØ4
Vaccine, 3EØ4
Vasopressor, 3EØ4
Water Balance Substance, 3EØ4
Peripheral, 3EØ3
Analgesics, 3EØ3
Anesthetic, Intracirculatory, 3EØ3
Antiarrhythmic, 3EØ3
Anti-infective, 3EØ3
Anti-inflammatory, 3EØ3
Antineoplastic, 3EØ3
Destructive Agent, 3EØ3
Diagnostic Substance, Other, 3EØ3
Electrolytic Substance, 3EØ3
Hormone, 3EØ3
Hypnotics, 3EØ3
Immunotherapeutic, 3EØ3
Islet Cells, Pancreatic, 3EØ3
Nutritional Substance, 3EØ3
Platelet Inhibitor, 3EØ3
Radioactive Substance, 3EØ3
Sedatives, 3EØ3
Serum, 3EØ3
Thrombolytic, 3EØ3
Toxoid, 3EØ3
Vaccine, 3EØ3
Vasopressor, 3EØ3
Water Balance Substance, 3EØ3
Intubation
Airway
see Insertion of device in, Esophagus, ØDH5
see Insertion of device in, Mouth and Throat, ØCHY
see Insertion of device in, Trachea, ØBH1
Drainage device *see* Drainage
Feeding Device *see* Insertion of device in, Gastrointestinal System, ØDH
INTUITY Elite valve system, EDWARDS *use* Zooplastic Tissue, Rapid Deployment Technique in New Technology
IPPB (intermittent positive pressure breathing) *see* Assistance, Respiratory, 5AØ9
IRE (Irreversible Electroporation) *see* Destruction, Hepatobiliary System and Pancreas, ØF5
Iridectomy
see Excision, Eye, Ø8B
see Resection, Eye, Ø8T
Iridoplasty
see Repair, Eye, Ø8Q
see Replacement, Eye, Ø8R
see Supplement, Eye, Ø8U
Iridotomy *see* Drainage, Eye, Ø89
Irreversible Electroporation (IRE) *see* Destruction, Hepatobiliary System and Pancreas, ØF5
Irrigation
Biliary Tract, Irrigating Substance, 3E1J
Brain, Irrigating Substance, 3E1Q38Z
Cranial Cavity, Irrigating Substance, 3E1Q38Z
Ear, Irrigating Substance, 3E1B
Epidural Space, Irrigating Substance, 3E1S38Z
Eye, Irrigating Substance, 3E1C
Gastrointestinal Tract
Lower, Irrigating Substance, 3E1H
Upper, Irrigating Substance, 3E1G
Genitourinary Tract, Irrigating Substance, 3E1K
Irrigating Substance, 3C1ZX8Z
Joint, Irrigating Substance, 3E1U38Z

Irrigation — *continued*
Mucous Membrane, Irrigating Substance, 3E1Ø
Nose, Irrigating Substance, 3E19
Pancreatic Tract, Irrigating Substance, 3E1J
Pericardial Cavity, Irrigating Substance, 3E1Y38Z
Peritoneal Cavity
Dialysate, 3E1M39Z
Irrigating Substance, 3E1M38Z
Pleural Cavity, Irrigating Substance, 3E1L38Z
Reproductive
Female, Irrigating Substance, 3E1P
Male, Irrigating Substance, 3E1N
Respiratory Tract, Irrigating Substance, 3E1F
Skin, Irrigating Substance, 3E1Ø
Spinal Canal, Irrigating Substance, 3E1R38Z
Isavuconazole Anti-infective, XWØ
Ischiatic nerve *use* Sciatic Nerve
Ischiocavernosus muscle *use* Perineum Muscle
Ischiofemoral ligament
use Hip Bursa and Ligament, Left
use Hip Bursa and Ligament, Right
Ischium
use Pelvic Bone, Left
use Pelvic Bone, Right
Isolation, 8EØZXY6
Isotope Administration, Whole Body, DWY5G
Itrel (3) (4) neurostimulator *use* Stimulator Generator, Single Array in, ØJH

J

Jejunal artery *use* Superior Mesenteric Artery
Jejunectomy
see Excision, Jejunum, ØDBA
see Resection, Jejunum, ØDTA
Jejunocolostomy
see Bypass, Gastrointestinal System, ØD1
see Drainage, Gastrointestinal System, ØD9
Jejunopexy
see Repair, Jejunum, ØDQA
see Reposition, Jejunum, ØDSA
Jejunostomy
see Bypass, Jejunum, ØD1A
see Drainage, Jejunum, ØD9A
Jejunotomy *see* Drainage, Jejunum, ØD9A
Joint fixation plate
use Internal Fixation Device in Lower Joints
use Internal Fixation Device in Upper Joints
Joint liner (insert) *use* Liner in Lower Joints
Joint spacer (antibiotic)
use Spacer in Lower Joints
use Spacer in Upper Joints
Jugular body *use* Glomus Jugulare
Jugular lymph node
use Lymphatic, Left Neck
use Lymphatic, Right Neck

K

Kappa *use* Pacemaker, Dual Chamber in, ØJH
Kcentra *use* 4-Factor Prothrombin Complex Concentrate
Keratectomy, kerectomy
see Excision, Eye, Ø8B
see Resection, Eye, Ø8T
Keratocentesis *see* Drainage, Eye, Ø89
Keratoplasty
see Repair, Eye, Ø8Q
see Replacement, Eye, Ø8R
see Supplement, Eye, Ø8U
Keratotomy
see Drainage, Eye, Ø89
see Repair, Eye, Ø8Q
Kirschner wire (K-wire)
use Internal Fixation Device in Head and Facial Bones
use Internal Fixation Device in Lower Bones
use Internal Fixation Device in Lower Joints
use Internal Fixation Device in Upper Bones
use Internal Fixation Device in Upper Joints
Knee (implant) insert *use* Liner in Lower Joints
KUB x-ray *see* Plain Radiography, Kidney, Ureter and Bladder, BTØ4
Kuntscher nail
use Internal Fixation Device, Intramedullary in Lower Bones

Kuntscher nail — *continued*
use Internal Fixation Device, Intramedullary in Upper Bones
KYMRIAH *use* Engineered Autologous Chimeric Antigen Receptor T-cell Immunotherapy

L

Labia majora *use* Vulva
Labia minora *use* Vulva
Labial gland
use Lower Lip
use Upper Lip
Labiectomy
see Excision, Female Reproductive System, ØUB
see Resection, Female Reproductive System, ØUT
Lacrimal canaliculus
use Lacrimal Duct, Left
use Lacrimal Duct, Right
Lacrimal punctum
use Lacrimal Duct, Left
use Lacrimal Duct, Right
Lacrimal sac
use Lacrimal Duct, Left
use Lacrimal Duct, Right
LAGB (laparoscopic adjustable gastric banding)
Initial procedure, ØDV64CZ
Surgical correction *see* Revision of device in, Stomach, ØDW6
Laminectomy
see Excision, Lower Bones, ØQB
see Excision, Upper Bones, ØPB
see Release, Central Nervous System and Cranial Nerves, ØØN
see Release, Peripheral Nervous System, Ø1N
Laminotomy
see Drainage, Lower Bones, ØQ9
see Drainage, Upper Bones, ØP9
see Excision, Lower Bones, ØQB
see Excision, Upper Bones, ØPB
see Release, Central Nervous System and Cranial Nerves, ØØN
see Release, Lower Bones, ØQN
see Release, Peripheral Nervous System, Ø1N
see Release, Upper Bones, ØPN
Laparoscopic-assisted transanal pull-through
see Excision, Gastrointestinal System, ØDB
see Resection, Gastrointestinal System, ØDT
Laparoscopy *see* Inspection
Laparotomy
Drainage *see* Drainage, Peritoneal Cavity, ØW9G
Exploratory *see* Inspection, Peritoneal Cavity, ØWJG
LAP-BAND® Adjustable Gastric Banding System *use* Extraluminal Device
Laryngectomy
see Excision, Larynx, ØCBS
see Resection, Larynx, ØCTS
Laryngocentesis *see* Drainage, Larynx, ØC9S
Laryngogram *see* Fluoroscopy, Larynx, B91J
Laryngopexy *see* Repair, Larynx, ØCQS
Laryngopharynx *use* Pharynx
Laryngoplasty
see Repair, Larynx, ØCQS
see Replacement, Larynx, ØCRS
see Supplement, Larynx, ØCUS
Laryngorrhaphy *see* Repair, Larynx, ØCQS
Laryngoscopy, ØCJS8ZZ
Laryngotomy *see* Drainage, Larynx, ØC9S
Laser Interstitial Thermal Therapy
Adrenal Gland, DGY2KZZ
Anus, DDY8KZZ
Bile Ducts, DFY2KZZ
Brain, DØYØKZZ
Brain Stem, DØY1KZZ
Breast
Left, DMYØKZZ
Right, DMY1KZZ
Bronchus, DBY1KZZ
Chest Wall, DBY7KZZ
Colon, DDY5KZZ
Diaphragm, DBY8KZZ
Duodenum, DDY2KZZ
Esophagus, DDYØKZZ
Gallbladder, DFY1KZZ
Gland
Adrenal, DGY2KZZ
Laser Interstitial Thermal Therapy — *continued*
Gland — *continued*
Parathyroid, DGY4KZZ
Pituitary, DGYØKZZ
Thyroid, DGY5KZZ
Ileum, DDY4KZZ
Jejunum, DDY3KZZ
Liver, DFYØKZZ
Lung, DBY2KZZ
Mediastinum, DBY6KZZ
Nerve, Peripheral, DØY7KZZ
Pancreas, DFY3KZZ
Parathyroid Gland, DGY4KZZ
Pineal Body, DGY1KZZ
Pituitary Gland, DGYØKZZ
Pleura, DBY5KZZ
Prostate, DVYØKZZ
Rectum, DDY7KZZ
Spinal Cord, DØY6KZZ
Stomach, DDY1KZZ
Thyroid Gland, DGY5KZZ
Trachea, DBYØKZZ
Lateral canthus
use Upper Eyelid, Left
use Upper Eyelid, Right
Lateral collateral ligament (LCL)
use Knee Bursa and Ligament, Left
use Knee Bursa and Ligament, Right
Lateral condyle of femur
use Lower Femur, Left
use Lower Femur, Right
Lateral condyle of tibia
use Tibia, Left
use Tibia, Right
Lateral cuneiform bone
use Tarsal, Left
use Tarsal, Right
Lateral epicondyle of femur
use Lower Femur, Left
use Lower Femur, Right
Lateral epicondyle of humerus
use Humeral Shaft, Left
use Humeral Shaft, Right
Lateral femoral cutaneous nerve *use* Lumbar Plexus
Lateral (brachial) lymph node
use Lymphatic, Left Axillary
use Lymphatic, Right Axillary
Lateral malleolus
use Fibula, Left
use Fibula, Right
Lateral meniscus
use Knee Joint, Left
use Knee Joint, Right
Lateral nasal cartilage *use* Nasal Mucosa and Soft Tissue
Lateral plantar artery
use Foot Artery, Left
use Foot Artery, Right
Lateral plantar nerve *use* Tibial Nerve
Lateral rectus muscle
use Extraocular Muscle, Left
use Extraocular Muscle, Right
Lateral sacral artery
use Internal Iliac Artery, Left
use Internal Iliac Artery, Right
Lateral sacral vein
use Hypogastric Vein, Left
use Hypogastric Vein, Right
Lateral sural cutaneous nerve *use* Peroneal Nerve
Lateral tarsal artery
use Foot Artery, Left
use Foot Artery, Right
Lateral temporomandibular ligament *use* Head and Neck Bursa and Ligament
Lateral thoracic artery
use Axillary Artery, Left
use Axillary Artery, Right
Latissimus dorsi muscle
use Trunk Muscle, Left
use Trunk Muscle, Right
Latissimus Dorsi Myocutaneous Flap
Replacement
Bilateral, ØHRVØ75
Left, ØHRUØ75
Right, ØHRTØ75
Transfer
Left, ØKXG
Right, ØKXF
Lavage
see Irrigation
Bronchial alveolar, diagnostic *see* Drainage, Respiratory System, ØB9
Least splanchnic nerve *use* Thoracic Sympathetic Nerve
Left ascending lumbar vein *use* Hemiazygos Vein
Left atrioventricular valve *use* Mitral Valve
Left auricular appendix *use* Atrium, Left
Left colic vein *use* Colic Vein
Left coronary sulcus *use* Heart, Left
Left gastric artery *use* Gastric Artery
Left gastroepiploic artery *use* Splenic Artery
Left gastroepiploic vein *use* Splenic Vein
Left inferior phrenic vein *use* Renal Vein, Left
Left inferior pulmonary vein *use* Pulmonary Vein, Left
Left jugular trunk *use* Thoracic Duct
Left lateral ventricle *use* Cerebral Ventricle
Left ovarian vein *use* Renal Vein, Left
Left second lumbar vein *use* Renal Vein, Left
Left subclavian trunk *use* Thoracic Duct
Left subcostal vein *use* Hemiazygos Vein
Left superior pulmonary vein *use* Pulmonary Vein, Left
Left suprarenal vein *use* Renal Vein, Left
Left testicular vein *use* Renal Vein, Left
Lengthening
Bone, with device *see* Insertion of Limb Lengthening Device
Muscle, by incision *see* Division, Muscles, ØK8
Tendon, by incision *see* Division, Tendons, ØL8
Leptomeninges, intracranial *use* Cerebral Meninges
Leptomeninges, spinal *use* Spinal Meninges
Lesser alar cartilage *use* Nasal Mucosa and Soft Tissue
Lesser occipital nerve *use* Cervical Plexus
Lesser Omentum *use* Omentum
Lesser saphenous vein
use Saphenous Vein, Left
use Saphenous Vein, Right
Lesser splanchnic nerve *use* Thoracic Sympathetic Nerve
Lesser trochanter
use Upper Femur, Left
use Upper Femur, Right
Lesser tuberosity
use Humeral Head, Left
use Humeral Head, Right
Lesser wing *use* Sphenoid Bone
Leukopheresis, therapeutic *see* Pheresis, Circulatory, 6A55
Levator anguli oris muscle *use* Facial Muscle
Levator ani muscle *use* Perineum Muscle
Levator labii superioris alaeque nasi muscle *use* Facial Muscle
Levator labii superioris muscle *use* Facial Muscle
Levator palpebrae superioris muscle
use Upper Eyelid, Left
use Upper Eyelid, Right
Levator scapulae muscle
use Neck Muscle, Left
use Neck Muscle, Right
Levator veli palatini muscle *use* Tongue, Palate, Pharynx Muscle
Levatores costarum muscle
use Thorax Muscle, Left
use Thorax Muscle, Right
LifeStent® (Flexstar) (XL) Vascular Stent System *use* Intraluminal Device
Ligament of head of fibula
use Knee Bursa and Ligament, Left
use Knee Bursa and Ligament, Right
Ligament of the lateral malleolus
use Ankle Bursa and Ligament, Left
use Ankle Bursa and Ligament, Right
Ligamentum flavum, cervical *use* Head and Neck Bursa and Ligament
Ligamentum flavum, lumbar *use* Lower Spine Bursa and Ligament
Ligamentum flavum, thoracic *use* Upper Spine Bursa and Ligament
Ligation *see* Occlusion
Ligation, hemorrhoid *see* Occlusion, Lower Veins, Hemorrhoidal Plexus
Light Therapy, GZJZZZZ
Liner
Removal of device from
Hip
Left, ØSPBØ9Z
Right, ØSP9Ø9Z

M

Magnetic Resonance Imaging (MRI) — continued
 Tendon
 Lower Extremity, BL33
 Upper Extremity, BL32
 Testicle
 Bilateral, BV37
 Left, BV36
 Right, BV35
 Toe
 Left, BQ3Q
 Right, BQ3P
 Uterus, BU36
 Pregnant, BU3B
 Uterus and Ovary, BU3C
 Vagina, BU39
 Vein
 Cerebellar, B531
 Cerebral, B531
 Jugular, Bilateral, B535
 Lower Extremity
 Bilateral, B53D
 Left, B53C
 Right, B53B
 Other, B53V
 Pelvic (Iliac) Bilateral, B53H
 Portal, B53T
 Pulmonary, Bilateral, B53S
 Renal, Bilateral, B53L
 Spanchnic, B53T
 Upper Extremity
 Bilateral, B53P
 Left, B53N
 Right, B53M
 Vena Cava
 Inferior, B539
 Superior, B538
 Wrist
 Left, BP3M
 Right, BP3L
Magnetically Controlled Growth Rod(s)
 Cervical, XNS3
 Lumbar, XNS0
 Thoracic, XNS4
Malleotomy see Drainage, Ear, Nose, Sinus, 099
Malleus
 use Auditory Ossicle, Left
 use Auditory Ossicle, Right
Mammaplasty, mammoplasty
 see Alteration, Skin and Breast, 0H0
 see Repair, Skin and Breast, 0HQ
 see Replacement, Skin and Breast, 0HR
 see Supplement, Skin and Breast, 0HU
Mammary duct
 use Breast, Bilateral
 use Breast, Left
 use Breast, Right
Mammary gland
 use Breast, Bilateral
 use Breast, Left
 use Breast, Right
Mammectomy
 see Excision, Skin and Breast, 0HB
 see Resection, Skin and Breast, 0HT
Mammillary body use Hypothalamus
Mammography see Plain Radiography, Skin, Subcutaneous Tissue and Breast, BH0
Mammotomy see Drainage, Skin and Breast, 0H9
Mandibular nerve use Trigeminal Nerve
Mandibular notch
 use Mandible, Left
 use Mandible, Right
Mandibulectomy
 see Excision, Head and Facial Bones, 0NB
 see Resection, Head and Facial Bones, 0NT
Manipulation
 Adhesions see Release
 Chiropractic see Chiropractic Manipulation
Manual removal, retained placenta see Extraction, Products of Conception, Retained, 10D1
Manubrium use Sternum
Map
 Basal Ganglia, 00K8
 Brain, 00K0
 Cerebellum, 00KC
 Cerebral Hemisphere, 00K7
 Conduction Mechanism, 02K8
 Hypothalamus, 00KA
 Medulla Oblongata, 00KD

Map — continued
 Pons, 00KB
 Thalamus, 00K9
Mapping
 Doppler ultrasound see Ultrasonography
 Electrocardiogram only see Measurement, Cardiac, 4A02
Mark IV Breathing Pacemaker System use Stimulator Generator in Subcutaneous Tissue and Fascia
Marsupialization
 see Drainage
 see Excision
Massage, cardiac
 External, 5A12012
 Open, 02QA0ZZ
Masseter muscle use Head Muscle
Masseteric fascia use Subcutaneous Tissue and Fascia, Face
Mastectomy
 see Excision, Skin and Breast, 0HB
 see Resection, Skin and Breast, 0HT
Mastoid air cells
 use Mastoid Sinus, Left
 use Mastoid Sinus, Right
Mastoid (postauricular) lymph node
 use Lymphatic, Left Neck
 use Lymphatic, Right Neck
Mastoid process
 use Temporal Bone, Left
 use Temporal Bone, Right
Mastoidectomy
 see Excision, Ear, Nose, Sinus, 09B
 see Resection, Ear, Nose, Sinus, 09T
Mastoidotomy see Drainage, Ear, Nose, Sinus, 099
Mastopexy
 see Repair, Skin and Breast, 0HQ
 see Reposition, Skin and Breast, 0HS
Mastorrhaphy see Repair, Skin and Breast, 0HQ
Mastotomy see Drainage, Skin and Breast, 0H9
Maxillary artery
 use External Carotid Artery, Left
 use External Carotid Artery, Right
Maxillary nerve use Trigeminal Nerve
Maximo II DR (VR) use Defibrillator Generator in, 0JH
Maximo II DR CRT-D use Cardiac Resynchronization Defibrillator Pulse Generator in, 0JH
Measurement
 Arterial
 Flow
 Coronary, 4A03
 Peripheral, 4A03
 Pulmonary, 4A03
 Pressure
 Coronary, 4A03
 Peripheral, 4A03
 Pulmonary, 4A03
 Thoracic, Other, 4A03
 Pulse
 Coronary, 4A03
 Peripheral, 4A03
 Pulmonary, 4A03
 Saturation, Peripheral, 4A03
 Sound, Peripheral, 4A03
 Biliary
 Flow, 4A0C
 Pressure, 4A0C
 Cardiac
 Action Currents, 4A02
 Defibrillator, 4B02XTZ
 Electrical Activity, 4A02
 Guidance, 4A02X4A
 No Qualifier, 4A02X4Z
 Output, 4A02
 Pacemaker, 4B02XSZ
 Rate, 4A02
 Rhythm, 4A02
 Sampling and Pressure
 Bilateral, 4A02
 Left Heart, 4A02
 Right Heart, 4A02
 Sound, 4A02
 Total Activity, Stress, 4A02XM4
 Central Nervous
 Conductivity, 4A00
 Electrical Activity, 4A00
 Pressure, 4A000BZ
 Intracranial, 4A00
 Saturation, Intracranial, 4A00

Measurement — continued
 Central Nervous — continued
 Stimulator, 4B00XVZ
 Temperature, Intracranial, 4A00
 Circulatory, Volume, 4A05XLZ
 Gastrointestinal
 Motility, 4A0B
 Pressure, 4A0B
 Secretion, 4A0B
 Lymphatic
 Flow, 4A06
 Pressure, 4A06
 Metabolism, 4A0Z
 Musculoskeletal
 Contractility, 4A0F
 Stimulator, 4B0FXVZ
 Olfactory, Acuity, 4A08X0Z
 Peripheral Nervous
 Conductivity
 Motor, 4A01
 Sensory, 4A01
 Electrical Activity, 4A01
 Stimulator, 4B01XVZ
 Products of Conception
 Cardiac
 Electrical Activity, 4A0H
 Rate, 4A0H
 Rhythm, 4A0H
 Sound, 4A0H
 Nervous
 Conductivity, 4A0J
 Electrical Activity, 4A0J
 Pressure, 4A0J
 Respiratory
 Capacity, 4A09
 Flow, 4A09
 Pacemaker, 4B09XSZ
 Rate, 4A09
 Resistance, 4A09
 Total Activity, 4A09
 Volume, 4A09
 Sleep, 4A0ZXQZ
 Temperature, 4A0Z
 Urinary
 Contractility, 4A0D
 Flow, 4A0D
 Pressure, 4A0D
 Resistance, 4A0D
 Volume, 4A0D
 Venous
 Flow
 Central, 4A04
 Peripheral, 4A04
 Portal, 4A04
 Pulmonary, 4A04
 Pressure
 Central, 4A04
 Peripheral, 4A04
 Portal, 4A04
 Pulmonary, 4A04
 Pulse
 Central, 4A04
 Peripheral, 4A04
 Portal, 4A04
 Pulmonary, 4A04
 Saturation, Peripheral, 4A04
 Visual
 Acuity, 4A07X0Z
 Mobility, 4A07X7Z
 Pressure, 4A07XBZ
Meatoplasty, urethra see Repair, Urethra, 0TQD
Meatotomy see Drainage, Urinary System, 0T9
Mechanical ventilation see Performance, Respiratory, 5A19
Medial canthus
 use Lower Eyelid, Left
 use Lower Eyelid, Right
Medial collateral ligament (MCL)
 use Knee Bursa and Ligament, Left
 use Knee Bursa and Ligament, Right
Medial condyle of femur
 use Lower Femur, Left
 use Lower Femur, Right
Medial condyle of tibia
 use Tibia, Left
 use Tibia, Right
Medial cuneiform bone
 use Tarsal, Left

▽ Subterms under main terms may continue to next column or page

Medial cuneiform bone — *continued*
use Tarsal, Right
Medial epicondyle of femur
use Lower Femur, Left
use Lower Femur, Right
Medial epicondyle of humerus
use Humeral Shaft, Left
use Humeral Shaft, Right
Medial malleolus
use Tibia, Left
use Tibia, Right
Medial meniscus
use Knee Joint, Left
use Knee Joint, Right
Medial plantar artery
use Foot Artery, Left
use Foot Artery, Right
Medial plantar nerve *use* Tibial Nerve
Medial popliteal nerve *use* Tibial Nerve
Medial rectus muscle
use Extraocular Muscle, Left
use Extraocular Muscle, Right
Medial sural cutaneous nerve *use* Tibial Nerve
Median antebrachial vein
use Basilic Vein, Left
use Basilic Vein, Right
Median cubital vein
use Basilic Vein, Left
use Basilic Vein, Right
Median sacral artery *use* Abdominal Aorta
Mediastinal cavity *use* Mediastinum
Mediastinal lymph node *use* Lymphatic, Thorax
Mediastinal space *use* Mediastinum
Mediastinoscopy, 0WJC4ZZ
Medication Management, GZ3ZZZZ
for substance abuse
Antabuse, HZ83ZZZ
Bupropion, HZ87ZZZ
Clonidine, HZ86ZZZ
Levo-alpha-acetyl-methadol (LAAM), HZ82ZZZ
Methadone Maintenance, HZ81ZZZ
Naloxone, HZ85ZZZ
Naltrexone, HZ84ZZZ
Nicotine Replacement, HZ80ZZZ
Other Replacement Medication, HZ89ZZZ
Psychiatric Medication, HZ88ZZZ
Meditation, 8E0ZXY5
Medtronic Endurant® II AAA stent graft system *use* Intraluminal Device
Meissner's (submucous) plexus *use* Abdominal Sympathetic Nerve
Melody® transcatheter pulmonary valve *use* Zooplastic Tissue in Heart and Great Vessels
Membranous urethra *use* Urethra
Meningeorrhaphy
see Repair, Cerebral Meninges, 00Q1
see Repair, Spinal Meninges, 00QT
Meniscectomy, knee
see Excision, Joint, Knee, Left, 0SBD
see Excision, Joint, Knee, Right, 0SBC
Mental foramen
use Mandible, Left
use Mandible, Right
Mentalis muscle *use* Facial Muscle
Mentoplasty *see* Alteration, Jaw, Lower, 0W05
Mesenterectomy *see* Excision, Mesentery, 0DBV
Mesenteriorrhaphy, mesenterorrhaphy *see* Repair, Mesentery, 0DQV
Mesenteriplication *see* Repair, Mesentery, 0DQV
Mesoappendix *use* Mesentery
Mesocolon *use* Mesentery
Metacarpal ligament
use Hand Bursa and Ligament, Left
use Hand Bursa and Ligament, Right
Metacarpophalangeal ligament
use Hand Bursa and Ligament, Left
use Hand Bursa and Ligament, Right
Metal on metal bearing surface *use* Synthetic Substitute, Metal in, 0SR
Metatarsal ligament
use Foot Bursa and Ligament, Left
use Foot Bursa and Ligament, Right
Metatarsectomy
see Excision, Lower Bones, 0QB
see Resection, Lower Bones, 0QT
Metatarsophalangeal (MTP) joint
use Metatarsal-Phalangeal Joint, Left
Metatarsophalangeal (MTP) joint — *continued*
use Metatarsal-Phalangeal Joint, Right
Metatarsophalangeal ligament
use Foot Bursa and Ligament, Left
use Foot Bursa and Ligament, Right
Metathalamus *use* Thalamus
Micro-Driver stent (RX) (OTW) *use* Intraluminal Device
MicroMed HeartAssist *use* Implantable Heart Assist System in Heart and Great Vessels
Micrus CERECYTE Microcoil *use* Intraluminal Device, Bioactive in Upper Arteries
Midcarpal joint
use Carpal Joint, Left
use Carpal Joint, Right
Middle cardiac nerve *use* Thoracic Sympathetic Nerve
Middle cerebral artery *use* Intracranial Artery
Middle cerebral vein *use* Intracranial Vein
Middle colic vein *use* Colic Vein
Middle genicular artery
use Popliteal Artery, Left
use Popliteal Artery, Right
Middle hemorrhoidal vein
use Hypogastric Vein, Left
use Hypogastric Vein, Right
Middle rectal artery
use Internal Iliac Artery, Left
use Internal Iliac Artery, Right
Middle suprarenal artery *use* Abdominal Aorta
Middle temporal artery
use Temporal Artery, Left
use Temporal Artery, Right
Middle turbinate *use* Nasal Turbinate
MIRODERM™ Biologic Wound Matrix *use* Skin Substitute, Porcine Liver Derived in New Technology
MitraClip valve repair system *use* Synthetic Substitute
Mitral annulus *use* Mitral Valve
Mitroflow® Aortic Pericardial Heart Valve *use* Zooplastic Tissue in Heart and Great Vessels
Mobilization, adhesions *see* Release
Molar gland *use* Buccal Mucosa
Monitoring
Arterial
Flow
Coronary, 4A13
Peripheral, 4A13
Pulmonary, 4A13
Pressure
Coronary, 4A13
Peripheral, 4A13
Pulmonary, 4A13
Pulse
Coronary, 4A13
Peripheral, 4A13
Pulmonary, 4A13
Saturation, Peripheral, 4A13
Sound, Peripheral, 4A13
Cardiac
Electrical Activity, 4A12
Ambulatory, 4A12X45
No Qualifier, 4A12X4Z
Output, 4A12
Rate, 4A12
Rhythm, 4A12
Sound, 4A12
Total Activity, Stress, 4A12XM4
Vascular Perfusion, Indocyanine Green Dye, 4A12XSH
Central Nervous
Conductivity, 4A10
Electrical Activity
Intraoperative, 4A10
No Qualifier, 4A10
Pressure, 4A100BZ
Intracranial, 4A10
Saturation, Intracranial, 4A10
Temperature, Intracranial, 4A10
Gastrointestinal
Motility, 4A1B
Pressure, 4A1B
Secretion, 4A1B
Vascular Perfusion, Indocyanine Green Dye, 4A1BXSH
Intraoperative Knee Replacement Sensor, XR2
Lymphatic
Flow, 4A16
Pressure, 4A16
Monitoring — *continued*
Peripheral Nervous
Conductivity
Motor, 4A11
Sensory, 4A11
Electrical Activity
Intraoperative, 4A11
No Qualifier, 4A11
Products of Conception
Cardiac
Electrical Activity, 4A1H
Rate, 4A1H
Rhythm, 4A1H
Sound, 4A1H
Nervous
Conductivity, 4A1J
Electrical Activity, 4A1J
Pressure, 4A1J
Respiratory
Capacity, 4A19
Flow, 4A19
Rate, 4A19
Resistance, 4A19
Volume, 4A19
Skin and Breast, Vascular Perfusion, Indocyanine Green Dye, 4A1GXSH
Sleep, 4A1ZXQZ
Temperature, 4A1Z
Urinary
Contractility, 4A1D
Flow, 4A1D
Pressure, 4A1D
Resistance, 4A1D
Volume, 4A1D
Venous
Flow
Central, 4A14
Peripheral, 4A14
Portal, 4A14
Pulmonary, 4A14
Pressure
Central, 4A14
Peripheral, 4A14
Portal, 4A14
Pulmonary, 4A14
Pulse
Central, 4A14
Peripheral, 4A14
Portal, 4A14
Pulmonary, 4A14
Saturation
Central, 4A14
Portal, 4A14
Pulmonary, 4A14
Monitoring Device, Hemodynamic
Abdomen, 0JH8
Chest, 0JH6
Mosaic Bioprosthesis (aortic) (mitral) valve *use* Zooplastic Tissue in Heart and Great Vessels
Motor Function Assessment, F01
Motor Treatment, F07
MR Angiography
see Magnetic Resonance Imaging (MRI), Heart, B23
see Magnetic Resonance Imaging (MRI), Lower Arteries, B43
see Magnetic Resonance Imaging (MRI), Upper Arteries, B33
MULTI-LINK (VISION) (MINI-VISION) (ULTRA) Coronary Stent System *use* Intraluminal Device
Multiple sleep latency test, 4A0ZXQZ
Musculocutaneous nerve *use* Brachial Plexus
Musculopexy
see Repair, Muscles, 0KQ
see Reposition, Muscles, 0KS
Musculophrenic artery
use Internal Mammary Artery, Left
use Internal Mammary Artery, Right
Musculoplasty
see Repair, Muscles, 0KQ
see Supplement, Muscles, 0KU
Musculorrhaphy *see* Repair, Muscles, 0KQ
Musculospiral nerve *use* Radial Nerve
Myectomy
see Excision, Muscles, 0KB
see Resection, Muscles, 0KT
Myelencephalon *use* Medulla Oblongata

N

New Technology — *continued*
- Synthetic Human Angiotensin II, XWØ
- Uridine Triacetate, XWØDX82

Ninth cranial nerve *use* Glossopharyngeal Nerve
Nitinol framed polymer mesh *use* Synthetic Substitute
Nonimaging Nuclear Medicine Assay
- Bladder, Kidneys and Ureters, CT63
- Blood, C763
- Kidneys, Ureters and Bladder, CT63
- Lymphatics and Hematologic System, C76YYZZ
- Ureters, Kidneys and Bladder, CT63
- Urinary System, CT6YYZZ

Nonimaging Nuclear Medicine Probe
- Abdomen, CW5Ø
- Abdomen and Chest, CW54
- Abdomen and Pelvis, CW51
- Brain, CØ5Ø
- Central Nervous System, CØ5YYZZ
- Chest, CW53
- Chest and Abdomen, CW54
- Chest and Neck, CW56
- Extremity
  - Lower, CP5PZZZ
  - Upper, CP5NZZZ
- Head and Neck, CW5B
- Heart, C25YYZZ
  - Right and Left, C256
- Lymphatics
  - Head, C75J
  - Head and Neck, C755
  - Lower Extremity, C75P
  - Neck, C75K
  - Pelvic, C75D
  - Trunk, C75M
  - Upper Chest, C75L
  - Upper Extremity, C75N
- Lymphatics and Hematologic System, C75YYZZ
- Musculoskeletal System, Other, CP5YYZZ
- Neck and Chest, CW56
- Neck and Head, CW5B
- Pelvic Region, CW5J
- Pelvis and Abdomen, CW51
- Spine, CP55ZZZ

Nonimaging Nuclear Medicine Uptake
- Endocrine System, CG4YYZZ
- Gland, Thyroid, CG42

Non-tunneled central venous catheter *use* Infusion Device
Nostril *use* Nasal Mucosa and Soft Tissue
Novacor Left Ventricular Assist Device *use* Implantable Heart Assist System in Heart and Great Vessels
Novation® Ceramic AHS® (Articulation Hip System) *use* Synthetic Substitute, Ceramic in, ØSR
Nuclear medicine
- *see* Nonimaging Nuclear Medicine Assay
- *see* Nonimaging Nuclear Medicine Probe
- *see* Nonimaging Nuclear Medicine Uptake
- *see* Planar Nuclear Medicine Imaging
- *see* Positron Emission Tomographic (PET) Imaging
- *see* Systemic Nuclear Medicine Therapy
- *see* Tomographic (Tomo) Nuclear Medicine Imaging

Nuclear scintigraphy *see* Nuclear Medicine
Nutrition, concentrated substances
- Enteral infusion, 3EØG36Z
- Parenteral (peripheral) infusion *see* Introduction of Nutritional Substance

O

Obliteration *see* Destruction
Obturator artery
- *use* Internal Iliac Artery, Left
- *use* Internal Iliac Artery, Right

Obturator lymph node *use* Lymphatic, Pelvis
Obturator muscle
- *use* Hip Muscle, Left
- *use* Hip Muscle, Right

Obturator nerve *use* Lumbar Plexus
Obturator vein
- *use* Hypogastric Vein, Left
- *use* Hypogastric Vein, Right

Obtuse margin *use* Heart, Left
Occipital artery
- *use* External Carotid Artery, Left
- *use* External Carotid Artery, Right

Occipital lobe *use* Cerebral Hemisphere
Occipital lymph node
- *use* Lymphatic, Left Neck
- *use* Lymphatic, Right Neck

Occipitofrontalis muscle *use* Facial Muscle
Occlusion
- Ampulla of Vater, ØFLC
- Anus, ØDLQ
- Aorta
  - Abdominal, Ø4LØ
  - Thoracic, Descending, Ø2LW3DJ
- Artery
  - Anterior Tibial
    - Left, Ø4LQ
    - Right, Ø4LP
  - Axillary
    - Left, Ø3L6
    - Right, Ø3L5
  - Brachial
    - Left, Ø3L8
    - Right, Ø3L7
  - Celiac, Ø4L1
  - Colic
    - Left, Ø4L7
    - Middle, Ø4L8
    - Right, Ø4L6
  - Common Carotid
    - Left, Ø3LJ
    - Right, Ø3LH
  - Common Iliac
    - Left, Ø4LD
    - Right, Ø4LC
  - External Carotid
    - Left, Ø3LN
    - Right, Ø3LM
  - External Iliac
    - Left, Ø4LJ
    - Right, Ø4LH
  - Face, Ø3LR
  - Femoral
    - Left, Ø4LL
    - Right, Ø4LK
  - Foot
    - Left, Ø4LW
    - Right, Ø4LV
  - Gastric, Ø4L2
  - Hand
    - Left, Ø3LF
    - Right, Ø3LD
  - Hepatic, Ø4L3
  - Inferior Mesenteric, Ø4LB
  - Innominate, Ø3L2
  - Internal Carotid
    - Left, Ø3LL
    - Right, Ø3LK
  - Internal Iliac
    - Left, Ø4LF
    - Right, Ø4LE
  - Internal Mammary
    - Left, Ø3L1
    - Right, Ø3LØ
  - Intracranial, Ø3LG
  - Lower, Ø4LY
  - Peroneal
    - Left, Ø4LU
    - Right, Ø4LT
  - Popliteal
    - Left, Ø4LN
    - Right, Ø4LM
  - Posterior Tibial
    - Left, Ø4LS
    - Right, Ø4LR
  - Pulmonary
    - Left, Ø2LR
    - Right, Ø2LQ
  - Pulmonary Trunk, Ø2LP
  - Radial
    - Left, Ø3LC
    - Right, Ø3LB
  - Renal
    - Left, Ø4LA
    - Right, Ø4L9
  - Splenic, Ø4L4
  - Subclavian
    - Left, Ø3L4
    - Right, Ø3L3
  - Superior Mesenteric, Ø4L5
  - Temporal
    - Left, Ø3LT
    - Right, Ø3LS

Occlusion — *continued*
- Artery — *continued*
  - Thyroid
    - Left, Ø3LV
    - Right, Ø3LU
  - Ulnar
    - Left, Ø3LA
    - Right, Ø3L9
  - Upper, Ø3LY
  - Vertebral
    - Left, Ø3LQ
    - Right, Ø3LP
- Atrium, Left, Ø2L7
- Bladder, ØTLB
- Bladder Neck, ØTLC
- Bronchus
  - Lingula, ØBL9
  - Lower Lobe
    - Left, ØBLB
    - Right, ØBL6
  - Main
    - Left, ØBL7
    - Right, ØBL3
  - Middle Lobe, Right, ØBL5
  - Upper Lobe
    - Left, ØBL8
    - Right, ØBL4
- Carina, ØBL2
- Cecum, ØDLH
- Cisterna Chyli, Ø7LL
- Colon
  - Ascending, ØDLK
  - Descending, ØDLM
  - Sigmoid, ØDLN
  - Transverse, ØDLL
- Cord
  - Bilateral, ØVLH
  - Left, ØVLG
  - Right, ØVLF
- Cul-de-sac, ØULF
- Duct
  - Common Bile, ØFL9
  - Cystic, ØFL8
  - Hepatic
    - Common, ØFL7
    - Left, ØFL6
    - Right, ØFL5
  - Lacrimal
    - Left, Ø8LY
    - Right, Ø8LX
  - Pancreatic, ØFLD
    - Accessory, ØFLF
  - Parotid
    - Left, ØCLC
    - Right, ØCLB
- Duodenum, ØDL9
- Esophagogastric Junction, ØDL4
- Esophagus, ØDL5
  - Lower, ØDL3
  - Middle, ØDL2
  - Upper, ØDL1
- Fallopian Tube
  - Left, ØUL6
  - Right, ØUL5
- Fallopian Tubes, Bilateral, ØUL7
- Ileocecal Valve, ØDLC
- Ileum, ØDLB
- Intestine
  - Large, ØDLE
    - Left, ØDLG
    - Right, ØDLF
  - Small, ØDL8
- Jejunum, ØDLA
- Kidney Pelvis
  - Left, ØTL4
  - Right, ØTL3
- Left atrial appendage (LAA) *see* Occlusion, Atrium, Left, Ø2L7
- Lymphatic
  - Aortic, Ø7LD
  - Axillary
    - Left, Ø7L6
    - Right, Ø7L5
  - Head, Ø7LØ
  - Inguinal
    - Left, Ø7LJ
    - Right, Ø7LH
  - Internal Mammary
    - Left, Ø7L9

Occlusion — *continued*
 Lymphatic — *continued*
 Internal Mammary — *continued*
 Right, 07L8
 Lower Extremity
 Left, 07LG
 Right, 07LF
 Mesenteric, 07LB
 Neck
 Left, 07L2
 Right, 07L1
 Pelvis, 07LC
 Thoracic Duct, 07LK
 Thorax, 07L7
 Upper Extremity
 Left, 07L4
 Right, 07L3
 Rectum, 0DLP
 Stomach, 0DL6
 Pylorus, 0DL7
 Trachea, 0BL1
 Ureter
 Left, 0TL7
 Right, 0TL6
 Urethra, 0TLD
 Vagina, 0ULG
 Valve, Pulmonary, 02LH
 Vas Deferens
 Bilateral, 0VLQ
 Left, 0VLP
 Right, 0VLN
 Vein
 Axillary
 Left, 05L8
 Right, 05L7
 Azygos, 05L0
 Basilic
 Left, 05LC
 Right, 05LB
 Brachial
 Left, 05LA
 Right, 05L9
 Cephalic
 Left, 05LF
 Right, 05LD
 Colic, 06L7
 Common Iliac
 Left, 06LD
 Right, 06LC
 Esophageal, 06L3
 External Iliac
 Left, 06LG
 Right, 06LF
 External Jugular
 Left, 05LQ
 Right, 05LP
 Face
 Left, 05LV
 Right, 05LT
 Femoral
 Left, 06LN
 Right, 06LM
 Foot
 Left, 06LV
 Right, 06LT
 Gastric, 06L2
 Hand
 Left, 05LH
 Right, 05LG
 Hemiazygos, 05L1
 Hepatic, 06L4
 Hypogastric
 Left, 06LJ
 Right, 06LH
 Inferior Mesenteric, 06L6
 Innominate
 Left, 05L4
 Right, 05L3
 Internal Jugular
 Left, 05LN
 Right, 05LM
 Intracranial, 05LL
 Lower, 06LY
 Portal, 06L8
 Pulmonary
 Left, 02LT
 Right, 02LS
 Renal
 Left, 06LB

Occlusion — *continued*
 Vein — *continued*
 Renal — *continued*
 Right, 06L9
 Saphenous
 Left, 06LQ
 Right, 06LP
 Splenic, 06L1
 Subclavian
 Left, 05L6
 Right, 05L5
 Superior Mesenteric, 06L5
 Upper, 05LY
 Vertebral
 Left, 05LS
 Right, 05LR
 Vena Cava
 Inferior, 06L0
 Superior, 02LV
Occlusion, REBOA (resuscitative endovascular balloon occlusion of the aorta)
 02LW3DJ
 04L03DJ
Occupational therapy *see* Activities of Daily Living Treatment, Rehabilitation, F08
Odentectomy
 see Excision, Mouth and Throat, 0CB
 see Resection, Mouth and Throat, 0CT
Odontoid process *use* Cervical Vertebra
Olecranon bursa
 use Elbow Bursa and Ligament, Left
 use Elbow Bursa and Ligament, Right
Olecranon process
 use Ulna, Left
 use Ulna, Right
Olfactory bulb *use* Olfactory Nerve
Omentectomy, omentumectomy
 see Excision, Gastrointestinal System, 0DB
 see Resection, Gastrointestinal System, 0DT
Omentofixation *see* Repair, Gastrointestinal System, 0DQ
Omentoplasty
 see Repair, Gastrointestinal System, 0DQ
 see Replacement, Gastrointestinal System, 0DR
 see Supplement, Gastrointestinal System, 0DU
Omentorrhaphy *see* Repair, Gastrointestinal System, 0DQ
Omentotomy *see* Drainage, Gastrointestinal System, 0D9
Omnilink Elite Vascular Balloon Expandable Stent System *use* Intraluminal Device
Onychectomy
 see Excision, Skin and Breast, 0HB
 see Resection, Skin and Breast, 0HT
Onychoplasty
 see Repair, Skin and Breast, 0HQ
 see Replacement, Skin and Breast, 0HR
Onychotomy *see* Drainage, Skin and Breast, 0H9
Oophorectomy
 see Excision, Female Reproductive System, 0UB
 see Resection, Female Reproductive System, 0UT
Oophoropexy
 see Repair, Female Reproductive System, 0UQ
 see Reposition, Female Reproductive System, 0US
Oophoroplasty
 see Repair, Female Reproductive System, 0UQ
 see Supplement, Female Reproductive System, 0UU
Oophororrhaphy *see* Repair, Female Reproductive System, 0UQ
Oophorostomy *see* Drainage, Female Reproductive System, 0U9
Oophorotomy
 see Division, Female Reproductive System, 0U8
 see Drainage, Female Reproductive System, 0U9
Oophorrhaphy *see* Repair, Female Reproductive System, 0UQ
Open Pivot Aortic Valve Graft (AVG) *use* Synthetic Substitute
Open Pivot (mechanical) Valve *use* Synthetic Substitute
Ophthalmic artery *use* Intracranial Artery
Ophthalmic nerve *use* Trigeminal Nerve
Ophthalmic vein *use* Intracranial Vein
Opponensplasty
 Tendon replacement *see* Replacement, Tendons, 0LR
 Tendon transfer *see* Transfer, Tendons, 0LX
Optic chiasma *use* Optic Nerve
Optic disc
 use Retina, Left
 use Retina, Right
Optic foramen *use* Sphenoid Bone

Optical coherence tomography, intravascular *see* Computerized Tomography (CT Scan)
Optimizer™ III implantable pulse generator *use* Contractility Modulation Device in, 0JH
Orbicularis oculi muscle
 use Upper Eyelid, Left
 use Upper Eyelid, Right
Orbicularis oris muscle *use* Facial Muscle
Orbital Atherectomy Technology, X2C
Orbital fascia *use* Subcutaneous Tissue and Fascia, Face
Orbital portion of ethmoid bone
 use Orbit, Left
 use Orbit, Right
Orbital portion of frontal bone
 use Orbit, Left
 use Orbit, Right
Orbital portion of lacrimal bone
 use Orbit, Left
 use Orbit, Right
Orbital portion of maxilla
 use Orbit, Left
 use Orbit, Right
Orbital portion of palatine bone
 use Orbit, Left
 use Orbit, Right
Orbital portion of sphenoid bone
 use Orbit, Left
 use Orbit, Right
Orbital portion of zygomatic bone
 use Orbit, Left
 use Orbit, Right
Orchectomy, orchidectomy, orchiectomy
 see Excision, Male Reproductive System, 0VB
 see Resection, Male Reproductive System, 0VT
Orchidoplasty, orchioplasty
 see Repair, Male Reproductive System, 0VQ
 see Replacement, Male Reproductive System, 0VR
 see Supplement, Male Reproductive System, 0VU
Orchidorrhaphy, orchiorrhaphy *see* Repair, Male Reproductive System, 0VQ
Orchidotomy, orchiotomy, orchotomy *see* Drainage, Male Reproductive System, 0V9
Orchiopexy
 see Repair, Male Reproductive System, 0VQ
 see Reposition, Male Reproductive System, 0VS
Oropharyngeal airway (OPA) *use* Intraluminal Device, Airway in Mouth and Throat
Oropharynx *use* Pharynx
Ossiculectomy
 see Excision, Ear, Nose, Sinus, 09B
 see Resection, Ear, Nose, Sinus, 09T
Ossiculotomy *see* Drainage, Ear, Nose, Sinus, 099
Ostectomy
 see Excision, Head and Facial Bones, 0NB
 see Excision, Lower Bones, 0QB
 see Excision, Upper Bones, 0PB
 see Resection, Head and Facial Bones, 0NT
 see Resection, Lower Bones, 0QT
 see Resection, Upper Bones, 0PT
Osteoclasis
 see Division, Head and Facial Bones, 0N8
 see Division, Lower Bones, 0Q8
 see Division, Upper Bones, 0P8
Osteolysis
 see Release, Head and Facial Bones, 0NN
 see Release, Lower Bones, 0QN
 see Release, Upper Bones, 0PN
Osteopathic Treatment
 Abdomen, 7W09X
 Cervical, 7W01X
 Extremity
 Lower, 7W06X
 Upper, 7W07X
 Head, 7W00X
 Lumbar, 7W03X
 Pelvis, 7W05X
 Rib Cage, 7W08X
 Sacrum, 7W04X
 Thoracic, 7W02X
Osteopexy
 see Repair, Head and Facial Bones, 0NQ
 see Repair, Lower Bones, 0QQ
 see Repair, Upper Bones, 0PQ
 see Reposition, Head and Facial Bones, 0NS
 see Reposition, Lower Bones, 0QS
 see Reposition, Upper Bones, 0PS

P

Plain Radiography — *continued*
 Artery — *continued*
 Common Carotid
 Bilateral, B305
 Left, B304
 Right, B303
 Coronary
 Bypass Graft
 Multiple, B203
 Single, B202
 Multiple, B201
 Single, B200
 External Carotid
 Bilateral, B30C
 Left, B30B
 Right, B309
 Hepatic, B402
 Inferior Mesenteric, B405
 Intercostal, B30L
 Internal Carotid
 Bilateral, B308
 Left, B307
 Right, B306
 Internal Mammary Bypass Graft
 Left, B208
 Right, B207
 Intra-Abdominal, Other, B40B
 Intracranial, B30R
 Lower Extremity
 Bilateral and Aorta, B40D
 Left, B40G
 Right, B40F
 Lower, Other, B40J
 Lumbar, B409
 Pelvic, B40C
 Pulmonary
 Left, B30T
 Right, B30S
 Renal
 Bilateral, B408
 Left, B407
 Right, B406
 Transplant, B40M
 Spinal, B30M
 Splenic, B403
 Subclavian, Left, B302
 Superior Mesenteric, B404
 Upper Extremity
 Bilateral, B30K
 Left, B30J
 Right, B30H
 Upper, Other, B30N
 Vertebral
 Bilateral, B30G
 Left, B30F
 Right, B30D
 Bile Duct, BF00
 Bile Duct and Gallbladder, BF03
 Bladder, BT00
 Kidney and Ureter, BT04
 Bladder and Urethra, BT0B
 Bone
 Facial, BN05ZZZ
 Nasal, BN04ZZZ
 Bones, Long, All, BW0BZZZ
 Breast
 Bilateral, BH02ZZZ
 Left, BH01ZZZ
 Right, BH00ZZZ
 Calcaneus
 Left, BQ0KZZZ
 Right, BQ0JZZZ
 Chest, BW03ZZZ
 Clavicle
 Left, BP05ZZZ
 Right, BP04ZZZ
 Coccyx, BR0FZZZ
 Corpora Cavernosa, BV00
 Dialysis Fistula, B50W
 Dialysis Shunt, B50W
 Disc
 Cervical, BR01
 Lumbar, BR03
 Thoracic, BR02
 Duct
 Lacrimal
 Bilateral, B802
 Left, B801
 Right, B800

Plain Radiography — *continued*
 Duct — *continued*
 Mammary
 Multiple
 Left, BH06
 Right, BH05
 Single
 Left, BH04
 Right, BH03
 Elbow
 Left, BP0H
 Right, BP0G
 Epididymis
 Left, BV02
 Right, BV01
 Extremity
 Lower, BW0CZZZ
 Upper, BW0JZZZ
 Eye
 Bilateral, B807ZZZ
 Left, B806ZZZ
 Right, B805ZZZ
 Facet Joint
 Cervical, BR04
 Lumbar, BR06
 Thoracic, BR05
 Fallopian Tube
 Bilateral, BU02
 Left, BU01
 Right, BU00
 Fallopian Tube and Uterus, BU08
 Femur
 Left, Densitometry, BQ04ZZ1
 Right, Densitometry, BQ03ZZ1
 Finger
 Left, BP0SZZZ
 Right, BP0RZZZ
 Foot
 Left, BQ0MZZZ
 Right, BQ0LZZZ
 Forearm
 Left, BP0KZZZ
 Right, BP0JZZZ
 Gallbladder and Bile Duct, BF03
 Gland
 Parotid
 Bilateral, B906
 Left, B905
 Right, B904
 Salivary
 Bilateral, B90D
 Left, B90C
 Right, B90B
 Submandibular
 Bilateral, B909
 Left, B908
 Right, B907
 Hand
 Left, BP0PZZZ
 Right, BP0NZZZ
 Heart
 Left, B205
 Right, B204
 Right and Left, B206
 Hepatobiliary System, All, BF0C
 Hip
 Left, BQ01
 Densitometry, BQ01ZZ1
 Right, BQ00
 Densitometry, BQ00ZZ1
 Humerus
 Left, BP0BZZZ
 Right, BP0AZZZ
 Ileal Diversion Loop, BT0C
 Intracranial Sinus, B502
 Joint
 Acromioclavicular, Bilateral, BP03ZZZ
 Finger
 Left, BP0D
 Right, BP0C
 Foot
 Left, BQ0Y
 Right, BQ0X
 Hand
 Left, BP0D
 Right, BP0C
 Lumbosacral, BR0BZZZ
 Sacroiliac, BR0D

Plain Radiography — *continued*
 Joint — *continued*
 Sternoclavicular
 Bilateral, BP02ZZZ
 Left, BP01ZZZ
 Right, BP00ZZZ
 Temporomandibular
 Bilateral, BN09
 Left, BN08
 Right, BN07
 Thoracolumbar, BR08ZZZ
 Toe
 Left, BQ0Y
 Right, BQ0X
 Kidney
 Bilateral, BT03
 Left, BT02
 Right, BT01
 Ureter and Bladder, BT04
 Knee
 Left, BQ08
 Right, BQ07
 Leg
 Left, BQ0FZZZ
 Right, BQ0DZZZ
 Lymphatic
 Head, B704
 Lower Extremity
 Bilateral, B70B
 Left, B709
 Right, B708
 Neck, B704
 Pelvic, B70C
 Upper Extremity
 Bilateral, B707
 Left, B706
 Right, B705
 Mandible, BN06ZZZ
 Mastoid, B90HZZZ
 Nasopharynx, B90FZZZ
 Optic Foramina
 Left, B804ZZZ
 Right, B803ZZZ
 Orbit
 Bilateral, BN03ZZZ
 Left, BN02ZZZ
 Right, BN01ZZZ
 Oropharynx, B90FZZZ
 Patella
 Left, BQ0WZZZ
 Right, BQ0VZZZ
 Pelvis, BR0CZZZ
 Pelvis and Abdomen, BW01ZZZ
 Prostate, BV03
 Retroperitoneal Lymphatic
 Bilateral, B701
 Unilateral, B700
 Ribs
 Left, BP0YZZZ
 Right, BP0XZZZ
 Sacrum, BR0FZZZ
 Scapula
 Left, BP07ZZZ
 Right, BP06ZZZ
 Shoulder
 Left, BP09
 Right, BP08
 Sinus
 Intracranial, B502
 Paranasal, B902ZZZ
 Skull, BN00ZZZ
 Spinal Cord, B00B
 Spine
 Cervical, Densitometry, BR00ZZ1
 Lumbar, Densitometry, BR09ZZ1
 Thoracic, Densitometry, BR07ZZ1
 Whole, Densitometry, BR0GZZ1
 Sternum, BR0HZZZ
 Teeth
 All, BN0JZZZ
 Multiple, BN0HZZZ
 Testicle
 Left, BV06
 Right, BV05
 Toe
 Left, BQ0QZZZ
 Right, BQ0PZZZ
 Tooth, Single, BN0GZZZ

▽ **Subterms under main terms may continue to next column or page**

Index

Plain Radiography

Plain Radiography — Plain Radiography

Psychotherapy — *continued*
Individual — *continued*
Mental Health Services — *continued*
Interpersonal, GZ53ZZZ
Psychoanalysis, GZ54ZZZ
Psychodynamic, GZ55ZZZ
Psychophysiological, GZ59ZZZ
Supportive, GZ56ZZZ
PTCA (percutaneous transluminal coronary angioplasty) *see* Dilation, Heart and Great Vessels, Ø27
Pterygoid muscle *use* Head Muscle
Pterygoid process *use* Sphenoid Bone
Pterygopalatine (sphenopalatine) ganglion *use* Head and Neck Sympathetic Nerve
Pubis
use Pelvic Bone, Left
use Pelvic Bone, Right
Pubofemoral ligament
use Hip Bursa and Ligament, Left
use Hip Bursa and Ligament, Right
Pudendal nerve *use* Sacral Plexus
Pull-through, laparoscopic-assisted transanal
see Excision, Gastrointestinal System, ØDB
see Resection, Gastrointestinal System, ØDT
Pull-through, rectal *see* Resection, Rectum, ØDTP
Pulmoaortic canal *use* Pulmonary Artery, Left
Pulmonary annulus *use* Pulmonary Valve
Pulmonary artery wedge monitoring *see* Monitoring, Arterial, 4A13
Pulmonary plexus
use Thoracic Sympathetic Nerve
use Vagus Nerve
Pulmonic valve *use* Pulmonary Valve
Pulpectomy *see* Excision, Mouth and Throat, ØCB
Pulverization *see* Fragmentation
Pulvinar *use* Thalamus
Pump reservoir *use* Infusion Device, Pump in Subcutaneous Tissue and Fascia
Punch biopsy *see* Excision with qualifier Diagnostic
Puncture *see* Drainage
Puncture, lumbar *see* Drainage, Spinal Canal, ØØ9U
Pyelography
see Fluoroscopy, Urinary System, BT1
see Plain Radiography, Urinary System, BTØ
Pyeloileostomy, urinary diversion *see* Bypass, Urinary System, ØT1
Pyeloplasty
see Repair, Urinary System, ØTQ
see Replacement, Urinary System, ØTR
see Supplement, Urinary System, ØTU
Pyelorrhaphy *see* Repair, Urinary System, ØTQ
Pyeloscopy, ØTJ58ZZ
Pyelostomy
see Bypass, Urinary System, ØT1
see Drainage, Urinary System, ØT9
Pyelotomy *see* Drainage, Urinary System, ØT9
Pylorectomy
see Excision, Stomach, Pylorus, ØDB7
see Resection, Stomach, Pylorus, ØDT7
Pyloric antrum *use* Stomach, Pylorus
Pyloric canal *use* Stomach, Pylorus
Pyloric sphincter *use* Stomach, Pylorus
Pylorodiosis *see* Dilation, Stomach, Pylorus, ØD77
Pylorogastrectomy
see Excision, Gastrointestinal System, ØDB
see Resection, Gastrointestinal System, ØDT
Pyloroplasty
see Repair, Stomach, Pylorus, ØDQ7
see Supplement, Stomach, Pylorus, ØDU7
Pyloroscopy, ØDJ68ZZ
Pylorotomy *see* Drainage, Stomach, Pylorus, ØD97
Pyramidalis muscle
use Abdomen Muscle, Left
use Abdomen Muscle, Right

Q

Quadrangular cartilage *use* Nasal Septum
Quadrant resection of breast *see* Excision, Skin and Breast, ØHB
Quadrate lobe *use* Liver
Quadratus femoris muscle
use Hip Muscle, Left
use Hip Muscle, Right
Quadratus lumborum muscle
use Trunk Muscle, Left
use Trunk Muscle, Right
Quadratus plantae muscle
use Foot Muscle, Left
use Foot Muscle, Right
Quadriceps (femoris)
use Upper Leg Muscle, Left
use Upper Leg Muscle, Right
Quarantine, 8EØZXY6

R

Radial collateral carpal ligament
use Wrist Bursa and Ligament, Left
use Wrist Bursa and Ligament, Right
Radial collateral ligament
use Elbow Bursa and Ligament, Left
use Elbow Bursa and Ligament, Right
Radial notch
use Ulna, Left
use Ulna, Right
Radial recurrent artery
use Radial Artery, Left
use Radial Artery, Right
Radial vein
use Brachial Vein, Left
use Brachial Vein, Right
Radialis indicis
use Hand Artery, Left
use Hand Artery, Right
Radiation Therapy
see Beam Radiation
see Brachytherapy
see Stereotactic Radiosurgery
Radiation treatment *see* Radiation Therapy
Radiocarpal joint
use Wrist Joint, Left
use Wrist Joint, Right
Radiocarpal ligament
use Wrist Bursa and Ligament, Left
use Wrist Bursa and Ligament, Right
Radiography *see* Plain Radiography
Radiology, analog *see* Plain Radiography
Radiology, diagnostic *see* Imaging, Diagnostic
Radioulnar ligament
use Wrist Bursa and Ligament, Left
use Wrist Bursa and Ligament, Right
Range of motion testing *see* Motor Function Assessment, Rehabilitation, FØ1
REALIZE® Adjustable Gastric Band *use* Extraluminal Device
Reattachment
Abdominal Wall, ØWMFØZZ
Ampulla of Vater, ØFMC
Ankle Region
Left, ØYMLØZZ
Right, ØYMKØZZ
Arm
Lower
Left, ØXMFØZZ
Right, ØXMDØZZ
Upper
Left, ØXM9ØZZ
Right, ØXM8ØZZ
Axilla
Left, ØXM5ØZZ
Right, ØXM4ØZZ
Back
Lower, ØWMLØZZ
Upper, ØWMKØZZ
Bladder, ØTMB
Bladder Neck, ØTMC
Breast
Bilateral, ØHMVXZZ
Left, ØHMUXZZ
Right, ØHMTXZZ
Bronchus
Lingula, ØBM9ØZZ
Lower Lobe
Left, ØBMBØZZ
Right, ØBM6ØZZ
Main
Left, ØBM7ØZZ
Right, ØBM3ØZZ
Middle Lobe, Right, ØBM5ØZZ
Reattachment — *continued*
Bronchus — *continued*
Upper Lobe
Left, ØBM8ØZZ
Right, ØBM4ØZZ
Bursa and Ligament
Abdomen
Left, ØMMJ
Right, ØMMH
Ankle
Left, ØMMR
Right, ØMMQ
Elbow
Left, ØMM4
Right, ØMM3
Foot
Left, ØMMT
Right, ØMMS
Hand
Left, ØMM8
Right, ØMM7
Head and Neck, ØMMØ
Hip
Left, ØMMM
Right, ØMML
Knee
Left, ØMMP
Right, ØMMN
Lower Extremity
Left, ØMMW
Right, ØMMV
Perineum, ØMMK
Rib(s), ØMMG
Shoulder
Left, ØMM2
Right, ØMM1
Spine
Lower, ØMMD
Upper, ØMMC
Sternum, ØMMF
Upper Extremity
Left, ØMMB
Right, ØMM9
Wrist
Left, ØMM6
Right, ØMM5
Buttock
Left, ØYM1ØZZ
Right, ØYMØØZZ
Carina, ØBM2ØZZ
Cecum, ØDMH
Cervix, ØUMC
Chest Wall, ØWM8ØZZ
Clitoris, ØUMJXZZ
Colon
Ascending, ØDMK
Descending, ØDMM
Sigmoid, ØDMN
Transverse, ØDML
Cord
Bilateral, ØVMH
Left, ØVMG
Right, ØVMF
Cul-de-sac, ØUMF
Diaphragm, ØBMTØZZ
Duct
Common Bile, ØFM9
Cystic, ØFM8
Hepatic
Common, ØFM7
Left, ØFM6
Right, ØFM5
Pancreatic, ØFMD
Accessory, ØFMF
Duodenum, ØDM9
Ear
Left, Ø9M1XZZ
Right, Ø9MØXZZ
Elbow Region
Left, ØXMCØZZ
Right, ØXMBØZZ
Esophagus, ØDM5
Extremity
Lower
Left, ØYMBØZZ
Right, ØYM9ØZZ
Upper
Left, ØXM7ØZZ
Right, ØXM6ØZZ

Release — continued

Joint — continued

Tarsal — continued

Right, 0SNH

Tarsometatarsal

Left, 0SNL

Right, 0SNK

Temporomandibular

Left, 0RND

Right, 0RNC

Thoracic Vertebral, 0RN6

Thoracolumbar Vertebral, 0RNA

Toe Phalangeal

Left, 0SNQ

Right, 0SNP

Wrist

Left, 0RNP

Right, 0RNN

Kidney

Left, 0TN1

Right, 0TN0

Kidney Pelvis

Left, 0TN4

Right, 0TN3

Larynx, 0CNS

Lens

Left, 08NK3ZZ

Right, 08NJ3ZZ

Lip

Lower, 0CN1

Upper, 0CN0

Liver, 0FN0

Left Lobe, 0FN2

Right Lobe, 0FN1

Lung

Bilateral, 0BNM

Left, 0BNL

Lower Lobe

Left, 0BNJ

Right, 0BNF

Middle Lobe, Right, 0BND

Right, 0BNK

Upper Lobe

Left, 0BNG

Right, 0BNC

Lung Lingula, 0BNH

Lymphatic

Aortic, 07ND

Axillary

Left, 07N6

Right, 07N5

Head, 07N0

Inguinal

Left, 07NJ

Right, 07NH

Internal Mammary

Left, 07N9

Right, 07N8

Lower Extremity

Left, 07NG

Right, 07NF

Mesenteric, 07NB

Neck

Left, 07N2

Right, 07N1

Pelvis, 07NC

Thoracic Duct, 07NK

Thorax, 07N7

Upper Extremity

Left, 07N4

Right, 07N3

Mandible

Left, 0NNV

Right, 0NNT

Maxilla, 0NNR

Medulla Oblongata, 00ND

Mesentery, 0DNV

Metacarpal

Left, 0PNQ

Right, 0PNP

Metatarsal

Left, 0QNP

Right, 0QNN

Muscle

Abdomen

Left, 0KNL

Right, 0KNK

Extraocular

Left, 08NM

Release — continued

Muscle — continued

Extraocular — continued

Right, 08NL

Facial, 0KN1

Foot

Left, 0KNW

Right, 0KNV

Hand

Left, 0KND

Right, 0KNC

Head, 0KN0

Hip

Left, 0KNP

Right, 0KNN

Lower Arm and Wrist

Left, 0KNB

Right, 0KN9

Lower Leg

Left, 0KNT

Right, 0KNS

Neck

Left, 0KN3

Right, 0KN2

Papillary, 02ND

Perineum, 0KNM

Shoulder

Left, 0KN6

Right, 0KN5

Thorax

Left, 0KNJ

Right, 0KNH

Tongue, Palate, Pharynx, 0KN4

Trunk

Left, 0KNG

Right, 0KNF

Upper Arm

Left, 0KN8

Right, 0KN7

Upper Leg

Left, 0KNR

Right, 0KNQ

Myocardial Bridge see Release, Artery, Coronary

Nasal Mucosa and Soft Tissue, 09NK

Nasopharynx, 09NN

Nerve

Abdominal Sympathetic, 01NM

Abducens, 00NL

Accessory, 00NR

Acoustic, 00NN

Brachial Plexus, 01N3

Cervical, 01N1

Cervical Plexus, 01N0

Facial, 00NM

Femoral, 01ND

Glossopharyngeal, 00NP

Head and Neck Sympathetic, 01NK

Hypoglossal, 00NS

Lumbar, 01NB

Lumbar Plexus, 01N9

Lumbar Sympathetic, 01NN

Lumbosacral Plexus, 01NA

Median, 01N5

Oculomotor, 00NH

Olfactory, 00NF

Optic, 00NG

Peroneal, 01NH

Phrenic, 01N2

Pudendal, 01NC

Radial, 01N6

Sacral, 01NR

Sacral Plexus, 01NQ

Sacral Sympathetic, 01NP

Sciatic, 01NF

Thoracic, 01N8

Thoracic Sympathetic, 01NL

Tibial, 01NG

Trigeminal, 00NK

Trochlear, 00NJ

Ulnar, 01N4

Vagus, 00NQ

Nipple

Left, 0HNX

Right, 0HNW

Omentum, 0DNU

Orbit

Left, 0NNQ

Right, 0NNP

Release — continued

Ovary

Bilateral, 0UN2

Left, 0UN1

Right, 0UN0

Palate

Hard, 0CN2

Soft, 0CN3

Pancreas, 0FNG

Para-aortic Body, 0GN9

Paraganglion Extremity, 0GNF

Parathyroid Gland, 0GNR

Inferior

Left, 0GNP

Right, 0GNN

Multiple, 0GNQ

Superior

Left, 0GNM

Right, 0GNL

Patella

Left, 0QNF

Right, 0QND

Penis, 0VNS

Pericardium, 02NN

Peritoneum, 0DNW

Phalanx

Finger

Left, 0PNV

Right, 0PNT

Thumb

Left, 0PNS

Right, 0PNR

Toe

Left, 0QNR

Right, 0QNQ

Pharynx, 0CNM

Pineal Body, 0GN1

Pleura

Left, 0BNP

Right, 0BNN

Pons, 00NB

Prepuce, 0VNT

Prostate, 0VN0

Radius

Left, 0PNJ

Right, 0PNH

Rectum, 0DNP

Retina

Left, 08NF3ZZ

Right, 08NE3ZZ

Retinal Vessel

Left, 08NH3ZZ

Right, 08NG3ZZ

Ribs

1 to 2, 0PN1

3 or More, 0PN2

Sacrum, 0QN1

Scapula

Left, 0PN6

Right, 0PN5

Sclera

Left, 08N7XZZ

Right, 08N6XZZ

Scrotum, 0VN5

Septum

Atrial, 02N5

Nasal, 09NM

Ventricular, 02NM

Sinus

Accessory, 09NP

Ethmoid

Left, 09NV

Right, 09NU

Frontal

Left, 09NT

Right, 09NS

Mastoid

Left, 09NC

Right, 09NB

Maxillary

Left, 09NR

Right, 09NQ

Sphenoid

Left, 09NX

Right, 09NW

Skin

Abdomen, 0HN7XZZ

Back, 0HN6XZZ

Buttock, 0HN8XZZ

▽ Subterms under main terms may continue to next column or page

Release — continued
 Skin — continued
 Chest, ØHN5XZZ
 Ear
 Left, ØHN3XZZ
 Right, ØHN2XZZ
 Face, ØHN1XZZ
 Foot
 Left, ØHNNXZZ
 Right, ØHNMXZZ
 Hand
 Left, ØHNGXZZ
 Right, ØHNFXZZ
 Inguinal, ØHNAXZZ
 Lower Arm
 Left, ØHNEXZZ
 Right, ØHNDXZZ
 Lower Leg
 Left, ØHNLXZZ
 Right, ØHNKXZZ
 Neck, ØHN4XZZ
 Perineum, ØHN9XZZ
 Scalp, ØHNØXZZ
 Upper Arm
 Left, ØHNCXZZ
 Right, ØHNBXZZ
 Upper Leg
 Left, ØHNJXZZ
 Right, ØHNHXZZ
 Spinal Cord
 Cervical, ØØNW
 Lumbar, ØØNY
 Thoracic, ØØNX
 Spinal Meninges, ØØNT
 Spleen, Ø7NP
 Sternum, ØPNØ
 Stomach, ØDN6
 Pylorus, ØDN7
 Subcutaneous Tissue and Fascia
 Abdomen, ØJN8
 Back, ØJN7
 Buttock, ØJN9
 Chest, ØJN6
 Face, ØJN1
 Foot
 Left, ØJNR
 Right, ØJNQ
 Hand
 Left, ØJNK
 Right, ØJNJ
 Lower Arm
 Left, ØJNH
 Right, ØJNG
 Lower Leg
 Left, ØJNP
 Right, ØJNN
 Neck
 Left, ØJN5
 Right, ØJN4
 Pelvic Region, ØJNC
 Perineum, ØJNB
 Scalp, ØJNØ
 Upper Arm
 Left, ØJNF
 Right, ØJND
 Upper Leg
 Left, ØJNM
 Right, ØJNL
 Tarsal
 Left, ØQNM
 Right, ØQNL
 Tendon
 Abdomen
 Left, ØLNG
 Right, ØLNF
 Ankle
 Left, ØLNT
 Right, ØLNS
 Foot
 Left, ØLNW
 Right, ØLNV
 Hand
 Left, ØLN8
 Right, ØLN7
 Head and Neck, ØLNØ
 Hip
 Left, ØLNK
 Right, ØLNJ

Release — continued
 Tendon — continued
 Knee
 Left, ØLNR
 Right, ØLNQ
 Lower Arm and Wrist
 Left, ØLN6
 Right, ØLN5
 Lower Leg
 Left, ØLNP
 Right, ØLNN
 Perineum, ØLNH
 Shoulder
 Left, ØLN2
 Right, ØLN1
 Thorax
 Left, ØLND
 Right, ØLNC
 Trunk
 Left, ØLNB
 Right, ØLN9
 Upper Arm
 Left, ØLN4
 Right, ØLN3
 Upper Leg
 Left, ØLNM
 Right, ØLNL
 Testis
 Bilateral, ØVNC
 Left, ØVNB
 Right, ØVN9
 Thalamus, ØØN9
 Thymus, Ø7NM
 Thyroid Gland, ØGNK
 Left Lobe, ØGNG
 Right Lobe, ØGNH
 Tibia
 Left, ØQNH
 Right, ØQNG
 Toe Nail, ØHNRXZZ
 Tongue, ØCN7
 Tonsils, ØCNP
 Tooth
 Lower, ØCNX
 Upper, ØCNW
 Trachea, ØBN1
 Tunica Vaginalis
 Left, ØVN7
 Right, ØVN6
 Turbinate, Nasal, Ø9NL
 Tympanic Membrane
 Left, Ø9N8
 Right, Ø9N7
 Ulna
 Left, ØPNL
 Right, ØPNK
 Ureter
 Left, ØTN7
 Right, ØTN6
 Urethra, ØTND
 Uterine Supporting Structure, ØUN4
 Uterus, ØUN9
 Uvula, ØCNN
 Vagina, ØUNG
 Valve
 Aortic, Ø2NF
 Mitral, Ø2NG
 Pulmonary, Ø2NH
 Tricuspid, Ø2NJ
 Vas Deferens
 Bilateral, ØVNQ
 Left, ØVNP
 Right, ØVNN
 Vein
 Axillary
 Left, Ø5N8
 Right, Ø5N7
 Azygos, Ø5NØ
 Basilic
 Left, Ø5NC
 Right, Ø5NB
 Brachial
 Left, Ø5NA
 Right, Ø5N9
 Cephalic
 Left, Ø5NF
 Right, Ø5ND
 Colic, Ø6N7

Release — continued
 Vein — continued
 Common Iliac
 Left, Ø6ND
 Right, Ø6NC
 Coronary, Ø2N4
 Esophageal, Ø6N3
 External Iliac
 Left, Ø6NG
 Right, Ø6NF
 External Jugular
 Left, Ø5NQ
 Right, Ø5NP
 Face
 Left, Ø5NV
 Right, Ø5NT
 Femoral
 Left, Ø6NN
 Right, Ø6NM
 Foot
 Left, Ø6NV
 Right, Ø6NT
 Gastric, Ø6N2
 Hand
 Left, Ø5NH
 Right, Ø5NG
 Hemiazygos, Ø5N1
 Hepatic, Ø6N4
 Hypogastric
 Left, Ø6NJ
 Right, Ø6NH
 Inferior Mesenteric, Ø6N6
 Innominate
 Left, Ø5N4
 Right, Ø5N3
 Internal Jugular
 Left, Ø5NN
 Right, Ø5NM
 Intracranial, Ø5NL
 Lower, Ø6NY
 Portal, Ø6N8
 Pulmonary
 Left, Ø2NT
 Right, Ø2NS
 Renal
 Left, Ø6NB
 Right, Ø6N9
 Saphenous
 Left, Ø6NQ
 Right, Ø6NP
 Splenic, Ø6N1
 Subclavian
 Left, Ø5N6
 Right, Ø5N5
 Superior Mesenteric, Ø6N5
 Upper, Ø5NY
 Vertebral
 Left, Ø5NS
 Right, Ø5NR
 Vena Cava
 Inferior, Ø6NØ
 Superior, Ø2NV
 Ventricle
 Left, Ø2NL
 Right, Ø2NK
 Vertebra
 Cervical, ØPN3
 Lumbar, ØQNØ
 Thoracic, ØPN4
 Vesicle
 Bilateral, ØVN3
 Left, ØVN2
 Right, ØVN1
 Vitreous
 Left, Ø8N53ZZ
 Right, Ø8N43ZZ
 Vocal Cord
 Left, ØCNV
 Right, ØCNT
 Vulva, ØUNM
Relocation see Reposition
Removal
 Abdominal Wall, 2W53X
 Anorectal, 2Y53X5Z
 Arm
 Lower
 Left, 2W5DX
 Right, 2W5CX

Removal of device from — *continued*
Omentum, ØDPU
Ovary, ØUP3
Pancreas, ØFPG
Parathyroid Gland, ØGPR
Patella
Left, ØQPF
Right, ØQPD
Pelvic Cavity, ØWPJ
Penis, ØVPS
Pericardial Cavity, ØWPD
Perineum
Female, ØWPN
Male, ØWPM
Peritoneal Cavity, ØWPG
Peritoneum, ØDPW
Phalanx
Finger
Left, ØPPV
Right, ØPPT
Thumb
Left, ØPPS
Right, ØPPR
Toe
Left, ØQPR
Right, ØQPQ
Pineal Body, ØGP1
Pleura, ØBPQ
Pleural Cavity
Left, ØWPB
Right, ØWP9
Products of Conception, 1ØPØ
Prostate and Seminal Vesicles, ØVP4
Radius
Left, ØPPJ
Right, ØPPH
Rectum, ØDPP
Respiratory Tract, ØWPQ
Retroperitoneum, ØWPH
Ribs
1 to 2, ØPP1
3 or More, ØPP2
Sacrum, ØQP1
Scapula
Left, ØPP6
Right, ØPP5
Scrotum and Tunica Vaginalis, ØVP8
Sinus, Ø9PY
Skin, ØHPPX
Skull, ØNPØ
Spinal Canal, ØØPU
Spinal Cord, ØØPV
Spleen, Ø7PP
Sternum, ØPPØ
Stomach, ØDP6
Subcutaneous Tissue and Fascia
Head and Neck, ØJPS
Lower Extremity, ØJPW
Trunk, ØJPT
Upper Extremity, ØJPV
Tarsal
Left, ØQPM
Right, ØQPL
Tendon
Lower, ØLPY
Upper, ØLPX
Testis, ØVPD
Thymus, Ø7PM
Thyroid Gland, ØGPK
Tibia
Left, ØQPH
Right, ØQPG
Toe Nail, ØHPRX
Trachea, ØBP1
Tracheobronchial Tree, ØBPØ
Tympanic Membrane
Left, Ø9P8
Right, Ø9P7
Ulna
Left, ØPPL
Right, ØPPK
Ureter, ØTP9
Urethra, ØTPD
Uterus and Cervix, ØUPD
Vagina and Cul-de-sac, ØUPH
Vas Deferens, ØVPR
Vein
Azygos, Ø5PØ

Removal of device from — *continued*
Vein — *continued*
Innominate
Left, Ø5P4
Right, Ø5P3
Lower, Ø6PY
Upper, Ø5PY
Vertebra
Cervical, ØPP3
Lumbar, ØQPØ
Thoracic, ØPP4
Vulva, ØUPM
Renal calyx
use Kidney
use Kidney, Left
use Kidney, Right
use Kidneys, Bilateral
Renal capsule
use Kidney
use Kidney, Left
use Kidney, Right
use Kidneys, Bilateral
Renal cortex
use Kidney
use Kidney, Left
use Kidney, Right
use Kidneys, Bilateral
Renal dialysis *see* Performance, Urinary, 5A1D
Renal plexus *use* Abdominal Sympathetic Nerve
Renal segment
use Kidney
use Kidney, Left
use Kidney, Right
use Kidneys, Bilateral
Renal segmental artery
use Renal Artery, Left
use Renal Artery, Right
Reopening, operative site
Control of bleeding *see* Control bleeding in
Inspection only *see* Inspection
Repair
Abdominal Wall, ØWQF
Acetabulum
Left, ØQQ5
Right, ØQQ4
Adenoids, ØCQQ
Ampulla of Vater, ØFQC
Anal Sphincter, ØDQR
Ankle Region
Left, ØYQL
Right, ØYQK
Anterior Chamber
Left, Ø8Q33ZZ
Right, Ø8Q23ZZ
Anus, ØDQQ
Aorta
Abdominal, Ø4QØ
Thoracic
Ascending/Arch, Ø2QX
Descending, Ø2QW
Aortic Body, ØGQD
Appendix, ØDQJ
Arm
Lower
Left, ØXQF
Right, ØXQD
Upper
Left, ØXQ9
Right, ØXQ8
Artery
Anterior Tibial
Left, Ø4QQ
Right, Ø4QP
Axillary
Left, Ø3Q6
Right, Ø3Q5
Brachial
Left, Ø3Q8
Right, Ø3Q7
Celiac, Ø4Q1
Colic
Left, Ø4Q7
Middle, Ø4Q8
Right, Ø4Q6
Common Carotid
Left, Ø3QJ
Right, Ø3QH

Repair — *continued*
Artery — *continued*
Common Iliac
Left, Ø4QD
Right, Ø4QC
Coronary
Four or More Arteries, Ø2Q3
One Artery, Ø2QØ
Three Arteries, Ø2Q2
Two Arteries, Ø2Q1
External Carotid
Left, Ø3QN
Right, Ø3QM
External Iliac
Left, Ø4QJ
Right, Ø4QH
Face, Ø3QR
Femoral
Left, Ø4QL
Right, Ø4QK
Foot
Left, Ø4QW
Right, Ø4QV
Gastric, Ø4Q2
Hand
Left, Ø3QF
Right, Ø3QD
Hepatic, Ø4Q3
Inferior Mesenteric, Ø4QB
Innominate, Ø3Q2
Internal Carotid
Left, Ø3QL
Right, Ø3QK
Internal Iliac
Left, Ø4QF
Right, Ø4QE
Internal Mammary
Left, Ø3Q1
Right, Ø3QØ
Intracranial, Ø3QG
Lower, Ø4QY
Peroneal
Left, Ø4QU
Right, Ø4QT
Popliteal
Left, Ø4QN
Right, Ø4QM
Posterior Tibial
Left, Ø4QS
Right, Ø4QR
Pulmonary
Left, Ø2QR
Right, Ø2QQ
Pulmonary Trunk, Ø2QP
Radial
Left, Ø3QC
Right, Ø3QB
Renal
Left, Ø4QA
Right, Ø4Q9
Splenic, Ø4Q4
Subclavian
Left, Ø3Q4
Right, Ø3Q3
Superior Mesenteric, Ø4Q5
Temporal
Left, Ø3QT
Right, Ø3QS
Thyroid
Left, Ø3QV
Right, Ø3QU
Ulnar
Left, Ø3QA
Right, Ø3Q9
Upper, Ø3QY
Vertebral
Left, Ø3QQ
Right, Ø3QP
Atrium
Left, Ø2Q7
Right, Ø2Q6
Auditory Ossicle
Left, Ø9QA
Right, Ø9Q9
Axilla
Left, ØXQ5
Right, ØXQ4
Back
Lower, ØWQL

Repair — *continued*
- Gland — *continued*
  - Lacrimal
    - Left, Ø8QW
    - Right, Ø8QV
  - Minor Salivary, ØCQJ
  - Parotid
    - Left, ØCQ9
    - Right, ØCQ8
  - Pituitary, ØGQØ
  - Sublingual
    - Left, ØCQF
    - Right, ØCQD
  - Submaxillary
    - Left, ØCQH
    - Right, ØCQG
  - Vestibular, ØUQL
- Glenoid Cavity
  - Left, ØPQ8
  - Right, ØPQ7
- Glomus Jugulare, ØGQC
- Hand
  - Left, ØXQK
  - Right, ØXQJ
- Head, ØWQØ
- Heart, Ø2QA
  - Left, Ø2QC
  - Right, Ø2QB
- Humeral Head
  - Left, ØPQD
  - Right, ØPQC
- Humeral Shaft
  - Left, ØPQG
  - Right, ØPQF
- Hymen, ØUQK
- Hypothalamus, ØØQA
- Ileocecal Valve, ØDQC
- Ileum, ØDQB
- Inguinal Region
  - Bilateral, ØYQA
  - Left, ØYQ6
  - Right, ØYQ5
- Intestine
  - Large, ØDQE
    - Left, ØDQG
    - Right, ØDQF
  - Small, ØDQ8
- Iris
  - Left, Ø8QD3ZZ
  - Right, Ø8QC3ZZ
- Jaw
  - Lower, ØWQ5
  - Upper, ØWQ4
- Jejunum, ØDQA
- Joint
  - Acromioclavicular
    - Left, ØRQH
    - Right, ØRQG
  - Ankle
    - Left, ØSQG
    - Right, ØSQF
  - Carpal
    - Left, ØRQR
    - Right, ØRQQ
  - Carpometacarpal
    - Left, ØRQT
    - Right, ØRQS
  - Cervical Vertebral, ØRQ1
  - Cervicothoracic Vertebral, ØRQ4
  - Coccygeal, ØSQ6
  - Elbow
    - Left, ØRQM
    - Right, ØRQL
  - Finger Phalangeal
    - Left, ØRQX
    - Right, ØRQW
  - Hip
    - Left, ØSQB
    - Right, ØSQ9
  - Knee
    - Left, ØSQD
    - Right, ØSQC
  - Lumbar Vertebral, ØSQØ
  - Lumbosacral, ØSQ3
  - Metacarpophalangeal
    - Left, ØRQV
    - Right, ØRQU
  - Metatarsal-Phalangeal
    - Left, ØSQN

Repair — *continued*
- Joint — *continued*
  - Metatarsal-Phalangeal — *continued*
    - Right, ØSQM
  - Occipital-cervical, ØRQØ
  - Sacrococcygeal, ØSQ5
  - Sacroiliac
    - Left, ØSQ8
    - Right, ØSQ7
  - Shoulder
    - Left, ØRQK
    - Right, ØRQJ
  - Sternoclavicular
    - Left, ØRQF
    - Right, ØRQE
  - Tarsal
    - Left, ØSQJ
    - Right, ØSQH
  - Tarsometatarsal
    - Left, ØSQL
    - Right, ØSQK
  - Temporomandibular
    - Left, ØRQD
    - Right, ØRQC
  - Thoracic Vertebral, ØRQ6
  - Thoracolumbar Vertebral, ØRQA
  - Toe Phalangeal
    - Left, ØSQQ
    - Right, ØSQP
  - Wrist
    - Left, ØRQP
    - Right, ØRQN
- Kidney
  - Left, ØTQ1
  - Right, ØTQØ
- Kidney Pelvis
  - Left, ØTQ4
  - Right, ØTQ3
- Knee Region
  - Left, ØYQG
  - Right, ØYQF
- Larynx, ØCQS
- Leg
  - Lower
    - Left, ØYQJ
    - Right, ØYQH
  - Upper
    - Left, ØYQD
    - Right, ØYQC
- Lens
  - Left, Ø8QK3ZZ
  - Right, Ø8QJ3ZZ
- Lip
  - Lower, ØCQ1
  - Upper, ØCQØ
- Liver, ØFQØ
  - Left Lobe, ØFQ2
  - Right Lobe, ØFQ1
- Lung
  - Bilateral, ØBQM
  - Left, ØBQL
  - Lower Lobe
    - Left, ØBQJ
    - Right, ØBQF
  - Middle Lobe, Right, ØBQD
  - Right, ØBQK
  - Upper Lobe
    - Left, ØBQG
    - Right, ØBQC
- Lung Lingula, ØBQH
- Lymphatic
  - Aortic, Ø7QD
  - Axillary
    - Left, Ø7Q6
    - Right, Ø7Q5
  - Head, Ø7QØ
  - Inguinal
    - Left, Ø7QJ
    - Right, Ø7QH
  - Internal Mammary
    - Left, Ø7Q9
    - Right, Ø7Q8
  - Lower Extremity
    - Left, Ø7QG
    - Right, Ø7QF
  - Mesenteric, Ø7QB
  - Neck
    - Left, Ø7Q2
    - Right, Ø7Q1

Repair — *continued*
- Lymphatic — *continued*
  - Pelvis, Ø7QC
  - Thoracic Duct, Ø7QK
  - Thorax, Ø7Q7
  - Upper Extremity
    - Left, Ø7Q4
    - Right, Ø7Q3
- Mandible
  - Left, ØNQV
  - Right, ØNQT
- Maxilla, ØNQR
- Mediastinum, ØWQC
- Medulla Oblongata, ØØQD
- Mesentery, ØDQV
- Metacarpal
  - Left, ØPQQ
  - Right, ØPQP
- Metatarsal
  - Left, ØQQP
  - Right, ØQQN
- Muscle
  - Abdomen
    - Left, ØKQL
    - Right, ØKQK
  - Extraocular
    - Left, Ø8QM
    - Right, Ø8QL
  - Facial, ØKQ1
  - Foot
    - Left, ØKQW
    - Right, ØKQV
  - Hand
    - Left, ØKQD
    - Right, ØKQC
  - Head, ØKQØ
  - Hip
    - Left, ØKQP
    - Right, ØKQN
  - Lower Arm and Wrist
    - Left, ØKQB
    - Right, ØKQ9
  - Lower Leg
    - Left, ØKQT
    - Right, ØKQS
  - Neck
    - Left, ØKQ3
    - Right, ØKQ2
  - Papillary, Ø2QD
  - Perineum, ØKQM
  - Shoulder
    - Left, ØKQ6
    - Right, ØKQ5
  - Thorax
    - Left, ØKQJ
    - Right, ØKQH
  - Tongue, Palate, Pharynx, ØKQ4
  - Trunk
    - Left, ØKQG
    - Right, ØKQF
  - Upper Arm
    - Left, ØKQ8
    - Right, ØKQ7
  - Upper Leg
    - Left, ØKQR
    - Right, ØKQQ
- Nasal Mucosa and Soft Tissue, Ø9QK
- Nasopharynx, Ø9QN
- Neck, ØWQ6
- Nerve
  - Abdominal Sympathetic, Ø1QM
  - Abducens, ØØQL
  - Accessory, ØØQR
  - Acoustic, ØØQN
  - Brachial Plexus, Ø1Q3
  - Cervical, Ø1Q1
  - Cervical Plexus, Ø1QØ
  - Facial, ØØQM
  - Femoral, Ø1QD
  - Glossopharyngeal, ØØQP
  - Head and Neck Sympathetic, Ø1QK
  - Hypoglossal, ØØQS
  - Lumbar, Ø1QB
  - Lumbar Plexus, Ø1Q9
  - Lumbar Sympathetic, Ø1QN
  - Lumbosacral Plexus, Ø1QA
  - Median, Ø1Q5
  - Oculomotor, ØØQH
  - Olfactory, ØØQF

Repair — continued
 Nerve — continued
 Optic, 00QG
 Peroneal, 01QH
 Phrenic, 01Q2
 Pudendal, 01QC
 Radial, 01Q6
 Sacral, 01QR
 Sacral Plexus, 01QQ
 Sacral Sympathetic, 01QP
 Sciatic, 01QF
 Thoracic, 01Q8
 Thoracic Sympathetic, 01QL
 Tibial, 01QG
 Trigeminal, 00QK
 Trochlear, 00QJ
 Ulnar, 01Q4
 Vagus, 00QQ
 Nipple
 Left, 0HQX
 Right, 0HQW
 Omentum, 0DQU
 Oral Cavity and Throat, 0WQ3
 Orbit
 Left, 0NQQ
 Right, 0NQP
 Ovary
 Bilateral, 0UQ2
 Left, 0UQ1
 Right, 0UQ0
 Palate
 Hard, 0CQ2
 Soft, 0CQ3
 Pancreas, 0FQG
 Para-aortic Body, 0GQ9
 Paraganglion Extremity, 0GQF
 Parathyroid Gland, 0GQR
 Inferior
 Left, 0GQP
 Right, 0GQN
 Multiple, 0GQQ
 Superior
 Left, 0GQM
 Right, 0GQL
 Patella
 Left, 0QQF
 Right, 0QQD
 Penis, 0VQS
 Pericardium, 02QN
 Perineum
 Female, 0WQN
 Male, 0WQM
 Peritoneum, 0DQW
 Phalanx
 Finger
 Left, 0PQV
 Right, 0PQT
 Thumb
 Left, 0PQS
 Right, 0PQR
 Toe
 Left, 0QQR
 Right, 0QQQ
 Pharynx, 0CQM
 Pineal Body, 0GQ1
 Pleura
 Left, 0BQP
 Right, 0BQN
 Pons, 00QB
 Prepuce, 0VQT
 Products of Conception, 10Q0
 Prostate, 0VQ0
 Radius
 Left, 0PQJ
 Right, 0PQH
 Rectum, 0DQP
 Retina
 Left, 08QF3ZZ
 Right, 08QE3ZZ
 Retinal Vessel
 Left, 08QH3ZZ
 Right, 08QG3ZZ
 Ribs
 1 to 2, 0PQ1
 3 or More, 0PQ2
 Sacrum, 0QQ1
 Scapula
 Left, 0PQ6
 Right, 0PQ5

Repair — continued
 Sclera
 Left, 08Q7XZZ
 Right, 08Q6XZZ
 Scrotum, 0VQ5
 Septum
 Atrial, 02Q5
 Nasal, 09QM
 Ventricular, 02QM
 Shoulder Region
 Left, 0XQ3
 Right, 0XQ2
 Sinus
 Accessory, 09QP
 Ethmoid
 Left, 09QV
 Right, 09QU
 Frontal
 Left, 09QT
 Right, 09QS
 Mastoid
 Left, 09QC
 Right, 09QB
 Maxillary
 Left, 09QR
 Right, 09QQ
 Sphenoid
 Left, 09QX
 Right, 09QW
 Skin
 Abdomen, 0HQ7XZZ
 Back, 0HQ6XZZ
 Buttock, 0HQ8XZZ
 Chest, 0HQ5XZZ
 Ear
 Left, 0HQ3XZZ
 Right, 0HQ2XZZ
 Face, 0HQ1XZZ
 Foot
 Left, 0HQNXZZ
 Right, 0HQMXZZ
 Hand
 Left, 0HQGXZZ
 Right, 0HQFXZZ
 Inguinal, 0HQAXZZ
 Lower Arm
 Left, 0HQEXZZ
 Right, 0HQDXZZ
 Lower Leg
 Left, 0HQLXZZ
 Right, 0HQKXZZ
 Neck, 0HQ4XZZ
 Perineum, 0HQ9XZZ
 Scalp, 0HQ0XZZ
 Upper Arm
 Left, 0HQCXZZ
 Right, 0HQBXZZ
 Upper Leg
 Left, 0HQJXZZ
 Right, 0HQHXZZ
 Skull, 0NQ0
 Spinal Cord
 Cervical, 00QW
 Lumbar, 00QY
 Thoracic, 00QX
 Spinal Meninges, 00QT
 Spleen, 07QP
 Sternum, 0PQ0
 Stomach, 0DQ6
 Pylorus, 0DQ7
 Subcutaneous Tissue and Fascia
 Abdomen, 0JQ8
 Back, 0JQ7
 Buttock, 0JQ9
 Chest, 0JQ6
 Face, 0JQ1
 Foot
 Left, 0JQR
 Right, 0JQQ
 Hand
 Left, 0JQK
 Right, 0JQJ
 Lower Arm
 Left, 0JQH
 Right, 0JQG
 Lower Leg
 Left, 0JQP
 Right, 0JQN

Repair — continued
 Subcutaneous Tissue and Fascia — continued
 Neck
 Left, 0JQ5
 Right, 0JQ4
 Pelvic Region, 0JQC
 Perineum, 0JQB
 Scalp, 0JQ0
 Upper Arm
 Left, 0JQF
 Right, 0JQD
 Upper Leg
 Left, 0JQM
 Right, 0JQL
 Tarsal
 Left, 0QQM
 Right, 0QQL
 Tendon
 Abdomen
 Left, 0LQG
 Right, 0LQF
 Ankle
 Left, 0LQT
 Right, 0LQS
 Foot
 Left, 0LQW
 Right, 0LQV
 Hand
 Left, 0LQ8
 Right, 0LQ7
 Head and Neck, 0LQ0
 Hip
 Left, 0LQK
 Right, 0LQJ
 Knee
 Left, 0LQR
 Right, 0LQQ
 Lower Arm and Wrist
 Left, 0LQ6
 Right, 0LQ5
 Lower Leg
 Left, 0LQP
 Right, 0LQN
 Perineum, 0LQH
 Shoulder
 Left, 0LQ2
 Right, 0LQ1
 Thorax
 Left, 0LQD
 Right, 0LQC
 Trunk
 Left, 0LQB
 Right, 0LQ9
 Upper Arm
 Left, 0LQ4
 Right, 0LQ3
 Upper Leg
 Left, 0LQM
 Right, 0LQL
 Testis
 Bilateral, 0VQC
 Left, 0VQB
 Right, 0VQ9
 Thalamus, 00Q9
 Thumb
 Left, 0XQM
 Right, 0XQL
 Thymus, 07QM
 Thyroid Gland, 0GQK
 Left Lobe, 0GQG
 Right Lobe, 0GQH
 Thyroid Gland Isthmus, 0GQJ
 Tibia
 Left, 0QQH
 Right, 0QQG
 Toe
 1st
 Left, 0YQQ
 Right, 0YQP
 2nd
 Left, 0YQS
 Right, 0YQR
 3rd
 Left, 0YQU
 Right, 0YQT
 4th
 Left, 0YQW
 Right, 0YQV

Resection — continued
Tendon — continued
Knee
Left, 0LTR
Right, 0LTQ
Lower Arm and Wrist
Left, 0LT6
Right, 0LT5
Lower Leg
Left, 0LTP
Right, 0LTN
Perineum, 0LTH
Shoulder
Left, 0LT2
Right, 0LT1
Thorax
Left, 0LTD
Right, 0LTC
Trunk
Left, 0LTB
Right, 0LT9
Upper Arm
Left, 0LT4
Right, 0LT3
Upper Leg
Left, 0LTM
Right, 0LTL
Testis
Bilateral, 0VTC
Left, 0VTB
Right, 0VT9
Thymus, 07TM
Thyroid Gland, 0GTK
Left Lobe, 0GTG
Right Lobe, 0GTH
Thyroid Gland Isthmus, 0GTJ
Tibia
Left, 0QTH0ZZ
Right, 0QTG0ZZ
Toe Nail, 0HTRXZZ
Tongue, 0CT7
Tonsils, 0CTP
Tooth
Lower, 0CTX0Z
Upper, 0CTW0Z
Trachea, 0BT1
Tunica Vaginalis
Left, 0VT7
Right, 0VT6
Turbinate, Nasal, 09TL
Tympanic Membrane
Left, 09T8
Right, 09T7
Ulna
Left, 0PTL0ZZ
Right, 0PTK0ZZ
Ureter
Left, 0TT7
Right, 0TT6
Urethra, 0TTD
Uterine Supporting Structure, 0UT4
Uterus, 0UT9
Uvula, 0CTN
Vagina, 0UTG
Valve, Pulmonary, 02TH
Vas Deferens
Bilateral, 0VTQ
Left, 0VTP
Right, 0VTN
Vesicle
Bilateral, 0VT3
Left, 0VT2
Right, 0VT1
Vitreous
Left, 08T53ZZ
Right, 08T43ZZ
Vocal Cord
Left, 0CTV
Right, 0CTT
Vulva, 0UTM
Resection, Left ventricular outflow tract obstruction (LVOT) see Dilation, Ventricle, Left, 027L
Resection, Subaortic membrane (Left ventricular outflow tract obstruction) see Dilation, Ventricle, Left, 027L
Restoration, Cardiac, Single, Rhythm, 5A2204Z

RestoreAdvanced neurostimulator (SureScan) (MRI Safe) use Stimulator Generator, Multiple Array Rechargeable in, 0JH
RestoreSensor neurostimulator (SureScan) (MRI Safe) use Stimulator Generator, Multiple Array Rechargeable in, 0JH
RestoreUltra neurostimulator (SureScan) (MRI Safe) use Stimulator Generator, Multiple Array Rechargeable in, 0JH
Restriction
Ampulla of Vater, 0FVC
Anus, 0DVQ
Aorta
Abdominal, 04V0
Intraluminal Device, Branched or Fenestrated, 04V0
Thoracic
Ascending/Arch, Intraluminal Device, Branched or Fenestrated, 02VX
Descending, Intraluminal Device, Branched or Fenestrated, 02VW
Artery
Anterior Tibial
Left, 04VQ
Right, 04VP
Axillary
Left, 03V6
Right, 03V5
Brachial
Left, 03V8
Right, 03V7
Celiac, 04V1
Colic
Left, 04V7
Middle, 04V8
Right, 04V6
Common Carotid
Left, 03VJ
Right, 03VH
Common Iliac
Left, 04VD
Right, 04VC
External Carotid
Left, 03VN
Right, 03VM
External Iliac
Left, 04VJ
Right, 04VH
Face, 03VR
Femoral
Left, 04VL
Right, 04VK
Foot
Left, 04VW
Right, 04VV
Gastric, 04V2
Hand
Left, 03VF
Right, 03VD
Hepatic, 04V3
Inferior Mesenteric, 04VB
Innominate, 03V2
Internal Carotid
Left, 03VL
Right, 03VK
Internal Iliac
Left, 04VF
Right, 04VE
Internal Mammary
Left, 03V1
Right, 03V0
Intracranial, 03VG
Lower, 04VY
Peroneal
Left, 04VU
Right, 04VT
Popliteal
Left, 04VN
Right, 04VM
Posterior Tibial
Left, 04VS
Right, 04VR
Pulmonary
Left, 02VR
Right, 02VQ
Pulmonary Trunk, 02VP
Radial
Left, 03VC
Right, 03VB

Restriction — continued
Artery — continued
Renal
Left, 04VA
Right, 04V9
Splenic, 04V4
Subclavian
Left, 03V4
Right, 03V3
Superior Mesenteric, 04V5
Temporal
Left, 03VT
Right, 03VS
Thyroid
Left, 03VV
Right, 03VU
Ulnar
Left, 03VA
Right, 03V9
Upper, 03VY
Vertebral
Left, 03VQ
Right, 03VP
Bladder, 0TVB
Bladder Neck, 0TVC
Bronchus
Lingula, 0BV9
Lower Lobe
Left, 0BVB
Right, 0BV6
Main
Left, 0BV7
Right, 0BV3
Middle Lobe, Right, 0BV5
Upper Lobe
Left, 0BV8
Right, 0BV4
Carina, 0BV2
Cecum, 0DVH
Cervix, 0UVC
Cisterna Chyli, 07VL
Colon
Ascending, 0DVK
Descending, 0DVM
Sigmoid, 0DVN
Transverse, 0DVL
Duct
Common Bile, 0FV9
Cystic, 0FV8
Hepatic
Common, 0FV7
Left, 0FV6
Right, 0FV5
Lacrimal
Left, 08VY
Right, 08VX
Pancreatic, 0FVD
Accessory, 0FVF
Parotid
Left, 0CVC
Right, 0CVB
Duodenum, 0DV9
Esophagogastric Junction, 0DV4
Esophagus, 0DV5
Lower, 0DV3
Middle, 0DV2
Upper, 0DV1
Heart, 02VA
Ileocecal Valve, 0DVC
Ileum, 0DVB
Intestine
Large, 0DVE
Left, 0DVG
Right, 0DVF
Small, 0DV8
Jejunum, 0DVA
Kidney Pelvis
Left, 0TV4
Right, 0TV3
Lymphatic
Aortic, 07VD
Axillary
Left, 07V6
Right, 07V5
Head, 07V0
Inguinal
Left, 07VJ
Right, 07VH

Restriction — *continued*
Lymphatic — *continued*
Internal Mammary
Left, 07V9
Right, 07V8
Lower Extremity
Left, 07VG
Right, 07VF
Mesenteric, 07VB
Neck
Left, 07V2
Right, 07V1
Pelvis, 07VC
Thoracic Duct, 07VK
Thorax, 07V7
Upper Extremity
Left, 07V4
Right, 07V3
Rectum, 0DVP
Stomach, 0DV6
Pylorus, 0DV7
Trachea, 0BV1
Ureter
Left, 0TV7
Right, 0TV6
Urethra, 0TVD
Valve, Mitral, 02VG
Vein
Axillary
Left, 05V8
Right, 05V7
Azygos, 05V0
Basilic
Left, 05VC
Right, 05VB
Brachial
Left, 05VA
Right, 05V9
Cephalic
Left, 05VF
Right, 05VD
Colic, 06V7
Common Iliac
Left, 06VD
Right, 06VC
Esophageal, 06V3
External Iliac
Left, 06VG
Right, 06VF
External Jugular
Left, 05VQ
Right, 05VP
Face
Left, 05VV
Right, 05VT
Femoral
Left, 06VN
Right, 06VM
Foot
Left, 06VV
Right, 06VT
Gastric, 06V2
Hand
Left, 05VH
Right, 05VG
Hemiazygos, 05V1
Hepatic, 06V4
Hypogastric
Left, 06VJ
Right, 06VH
Inferior Mesenteric, 06V6
Innominate
Left, 05V4
Right, 05V3
Internal Jugular
Left, 05VN
Right, 05VM
Intracranial, 05VL
Lower, 06VY
Portal, 06V8
Pulmonary
Left, 02VT
Right, 02VS
Renal
Left, 06VB
Right, 06V9
Saphenous
Left, 06VQ
Right, 06VP

Restriction — *continued*
Vein — *continued*
Splenic, 06V1
Subclavian
Left, 05V6
Right, 05V5
Superior Mesenteric, 06V5
Upper, 05VY
Vertebral
Left, 05VS
Right, 05VR
Vena Cava
Inferior, 06V0
Superior, 02VV
Resurfacing Device
Removal of device from
Left, 0SPB0BZ
Right, 0SP90BZ
Revision of device in
Left, 0SWB0BZ
Right, 0SW90BZ
Supplement
Left, 0SUB0BZ
Acetabular Surface, 0SUE0BZ
Femoral Surface, 0SUS0BZ
Right, 0SU90BZ
Acetabular Surface, 0SUA0BZ
Femoral Surface, 0SUR0BZ
Resuscitation
Cardiopulmonary *see* Assistance, Cardiac, 5A02
Cardioversion, 5A2204Z
Defibrillation, 5A2204Z
Endotracheal intubation *see* Insertion of device in,
Trachea, 0BH1
External chest compression, 5A12012
Pulmonary, 5A19054
Resuscitative endovascular balloon occlusion of the
aorta (REBOA)
02LW3DJ
04L03DJ
Resuture, Heart valve prosthesis *see* Revision of device
in, Heart and Great Vessels, 02W
Retained placenta, manual removal *see* Extraction,
Products of Conception, Retained, 10D1
Retraining
Cardiac *see* Motor Treatment, Rehabilitation, F07
Vocational *see* Activities of Daily Living Treatment,
Rehabilitation, F08
Retrogasserian rhizotomy *see* Division, Nerve, Trigemi-
nal, 008K
Retroperitoneal cavity *use* Retroperitoneum
Retroperitoneal lymph node *use* Lymphatic, Aortic
Retroperitoneal space *use* Retroperitoneum
Retropharyngeal lymph node
use Lymphatic, Left Neck
use Lymphatic, Right Neck
Retropubic space *use* Pelvic Cavity
Reveal (DX) (XT) *use* Monitoring Device
Reverse total shoulder replacement *see* Replacement,
Upper Joints, 0RR
Reverse® Shoulder Prosthesis *use* Synthetic Substitute,
Reverse Ball and Socket in, 0RR
Revision
Correcting a portion of existing device *see* Revision
of device in
Removal of device without replacement *see* Removal
of device from
Replacement of existing device
see Removal of device from
see Root operation to place new device, e.g.,
Insertion, Replacement, Supplement
Revision of device in
Abdominal Wall, 0WWF
Acetabulum
Left, 0QW5
Right, 0QW4
Anal Sphincter, 0DWR
Anus, 0DWQ
Artery
Lower, 04WY
Upper, 03WY
Auditory Ossicle
Left, 09WA
Right, 09W9
Back
Lower, 0WWL
Upper, 0WWK
Bladder, 0TWB

Revision of device in — *continued*
Bone
Facial, 0NWW
Lower, 0QWY
Nasal, 0NWB
Pelvic
Left, 0QW3
Right, 0QW2
Upper, 0PWY
Bone Marrow, 07WT
Brain, 00W0
Breast
Left, 0HWU
Right, 0HWT
Bursa and Ligament
Lower, 0MWY
Upper, 0MWX
Carpal
Left, 0PWN
Right, 0PWM
Cavity, Cranial, 0WW1
Cerebral Ventricle, 00W6
Chest Wall, 0WW8
Cisterna Chyli, 07WL
Clavicle
Left, 0PWB
Right, 0PW9
Coccyx, 0QWS
Diaphragm, 0BWT
Disc
Cervical Vertebral, 0RW3
Cervicothoracic Vertebral, 0RW5
Lumbar Vertebral, 0SW2
Lumbosacral, 0SW4
Thoracic Vertebral, 0RW9
Thoracolumbar Vertebral, 0RWB
Duct
Hepatobiliary, 0FWB
Pancreatic, 0FWD
Ear
Inner
Left, 09WE
Right, 09WD
Left, 09WJ
Right, 09WH
Epididymis and Spermatic Cord, 0VWM
Esophagus, 0DW5
Extremity
Lower
Left, 0YWB
Right, 0YW9
Upper
Left, 0XW7
Right, 0XW6
Eye
Left, 08W1
Right, 08W0
Face, 0WW2
Fallopian Tube, 0UW8
Femoral Shaft
Left, 0QW9
Right, 0QW8
Femur
Lower
Left, 0QWC
Right, 0QWB
Upper
Left, 0QW7
Right, 0QW6
Fibula
Left, 0QWK
Right, 0QWJ
Finger Nail, 0HWQX
Gallbladder, 0FW4
Gastrointestinal Tract, 0WWP
Genitourinary Tract, 0WWR
Gland
Adrenal, 0GW5
Endocrine, 0GWS
Pituitary, 0GW0
Salivary, 0CWA
Glenoid Cavity
Left, 0PW8
Right, 0PW7
Great Vessel, 02WY
Hair, 0HWSX
Head, 0WW0
Heart, 02WA

▽ **Subterms under main terms may continue to next column or page**

Right ovarian vein
ICD-10-PCS 2019
Index

Right ovarian vein *use* Inferior Vena Cava
Right second lumbar vein *use* Inferior Vena Cava
Right subclavian trunk *use* Lymphatic, Right Neck
Right subcostal vein *use* Azygos Vein
Right superior pulmonary vein *use* Pulmonary Vein, Right
Right suprarenal vein *use* Inferior Vena Cava
Right testicular vein *use* Inferior Vena Cava
Rima glottidis *use* Larynx
Risorius muscle *use* Facial Muscle
RNS System lead *use* Neurostimulator Lead in Central Nervous System and Cranial Nerves
RNS system neurostimulator generator *use* Neurostimulator Generator in Head and Facial Bones
Robotic Assisted Procedure
Extremity
Lower, 8EØY
Upper, 8EØX
Head and Neck Region, 8EØ9
Trunk Region, 8EØW
Robotic Waterjet Ablation, Destruction, Prostate, XV5Ø8A4
Rotation of fetal head
Forceps, 1ØSØ7ZZ
Manual, 1ØSØXZZ
Round ligament of uterus *use* Uterine Supporting Structure
Round window
use Inner Ear, Left
use Inner Ear, Right
Roux-en-Y operation
see Bypass, Gastrointestinal System, ØD1
see Bypass, Hepatobiliary System and Pancreas, ØF1
Rupture
Adhesions *see* Release
Fluid collection *see* Drainage

S

Sacral ganglion *use* Sacral Sympathetic Nerve
Sacral lymph node *use* Lymphatic, Pelvis
Sacral nerve modulation (SNM) lead *use* Stimulator Lead in Urinary System
Sacral neuromodulation lead *use* Stimulator Lead in Urinary System
Sacral splanchnic nerve *use* Sacral Sympathetic Nerve
Sacrectomy *see* Excision, Lower Bones, ØQB
Sacrococcygeal ligament *use* Lower Spine Bursa and Ligament
Sacrococcygeal symphysis *use* Sacrococcygeal Joint
Sacroiliac ligament *use* Lower Spine Bursa and Ligament
Sacrospinous ligament *use* Lower Spine Bursa and Ligament
Sacrotuberous ligament *use* Lower Spine Bursa and Ligament
Salpingectomy
see Excision, Female Reproductive System, ØUB
see Resection, Female Reproductive System, ØUT
Salpingolysis *see* Release, Female Reproductive System, ØUN
Salpingopexy
see Repair, Female Reproductive System, ØUQ
see Reposition, Female Reproductive System, ØUS
Salpingopharyngeus muscle *use* Tongue, Palate, Pharynx Muscle
Salpingoplasty
see Repair, Female Reproductive System, ØUQ
see Supplement, Female Reproductive System, ØUU
Salpingorrhaphy *see* Repair, Female Reproductive System, ØUQ
Salpingoscopy, ØUJ88ZZ
Salpingostomy *see* Drainage, Female Reproductive System, ØU9
Salpingotomy *see* Drainage, Female Reproductive System, ØU9
Salpinx
use Fallopian Tube, Left
use Fallopian Tube, Right
Saphenous nerve *use* Femoral Nerve
SAPIEN transcatheter aortic valve *use* Zooplastic Tissue in Heart and Great Vessels
Sartorius muscle
use Upper Leg Muscle, Left
use Upper Leg Muscle, Right
Scalene muscle
use Neck Muscle, Left
Scalene muscle — *continued*
use Neck Muscle, Right
Scan
Computerized Tomography (CT) *see* Computerized Tomography (CT Scan)
Radioisotope *see* Planar Nuclear Medicine Imaging
Scaphoid bone
use Carpal, Left
use Carpal, Right
Scapholunate ligament
use Hand Bursa and Ligament, Left
use Hand Bursa and Ligament, Right
Scaphotrapezium ligament
use Hand Bursa and Ligament, Left
use Hand Bursa and Ligament, Right
Scapulectomy
see Excision, Upper Bones, ØPB
see Resection, Upper Bones, ØPT
Scapulopexy
see Repair, Upper Bones, ØPQ
see Reposition, Upper Bones, ØPS
Scarpa's (vestibular) ganglion *use* Acoustic Nerve
Sclerectomy *see* Excision, Eye, Ø8B
Sclerotherapy, mechanical *see* Destruction
Sclerotherapy, via injection of sclerosing agent *see* Introduction, Destructive Agent
Sclerotomy *see* Drainage, Eye, Ø89
Scrotectomy
see Excision, Male Reproductive System, ØVB
see Resection, Male Reproductive System, ØVT
Scrotoplasty
see Repair, Male Reproductive System, ØVQ
see Supplement, Male Reproductive System, ØVU
Scrotorrhaphy *see* Repair, Male Reproductive System, ØVQ
Scrototomy *see* Drainage, Male Reproductive System, ØV9
Sebaceous gland *use* Skin
Second cranial nerve *use* Optic Nerve
Section, cesarean *see* Extraction, Pregnancy, 1ØD
Secura (DR) (VR) *use* Defibrillator Generator in, ØJH
Sella turcica *use* Sphenoid Bone
Semicircular canal
use Inner Ear, Left
use Inner Ear, Right
Semimembranosus muscle
use Upper Leg Muscle, Left
use Upper Leg Muscle, Right
Semitendinosus muscle
use Upper Leg Muscle, Left
use Upper Leg Muscle, Right
Seprafilm *use* Adhesion Barrier
Septal cartilage *use* Nasal Septum
Septectomy
see Excision, Ear, Nose, Sinus, Ø9B
see Excision, Heart and Great Vessels, Ø2B
see Resection, Ear, Nose, Sinus, Ø9T
see Resection, Heart and Great Vessels, Ø2T
Septoplasty
see Repair, Ear, Nose, Sinus, Ø9Q
see Repair, Heart and Great Vessels, Ø2Q
see Replacement, Ear, Nose, Sinus, Ø9R
see Replacement, Heart and Great Vessels, Ø2R
see Reposition, Ear, Nose, Sinus, Ø9S
see Supplement, Ear, Nose, Sinus, Ø9U
see Supplement, Heart and Great Vessels, Ø2U
Septostomy, balloon atrial, Ø2163Z7
Septotomy *see* Drainage, Ear, Nose, Sinus, Ø99
Sequestrectomy, bone *see* Extirpation
Serratus anterior muscle
use Thorax Muscle, Left
use Thorax Muscle, Right
Serratus posterior muscle
use Trunk Muscle, Left
use Trunk Muscle, Right
Seventh cranial nerve *use* Facial Nerve
Sheffield hybrid external fixator
use External Fixation Device, Hybrid in, ØPH
use External Fixation Device, Hybrid in, ØPS
use External Fixation Device, Hybrid in, ØQH
use External Fixation Device, Hybrid in, ØQS
Sheffield ring external fixator
use External Fixation Device, Ring in, ØPH
use External Fixation Device, Ring in, ØPS
use External Fixation Device, Ring in, ØQH
use External Fixation Device, Ring in, ØQS
Shirodkar cervical cerclage, ØUVC7ZZ
Shock Wave Therapy, Musculoskeletal, 6A93
Short gastric artery *use* Splenic Artery
Shortening
see Excision
see Repair
see Reposition
Shunt creation *see* Bypass
Sialoadenectomy
Complete *see* Resection, Mouth and Throat, ØCT
Partial *see* Excision, Mouth and Throat, ØCB
Sialodochoplasty
see Repair, Mouth and Throat, ØCQ
see Replacement, Mouth and Throat, ØCR
see Supplement, Mouth and Throat, ØCU
Sialoectomy
see Excision, Mouth and Throat, ØCB
see Resection, Mouth and Throat, ØCT
Sialography *see* Plain Radiography, Ear, Nose, Mouth and Throat, B9Ø
Sialolithotomy *see* Extirpation, Mouth and Throat, ØCC
Sigmoid artery *use* Inferior Mesenteric Artery
Sigmoid flexure *use* Sigmoid Colon
Sigmoid vein *use* Inferior Mesenteric Vein
Sigmoidectomy
see Excision, Gastrointestinal System, ØDB
see Resection, Gastrointestinal System, ØDT
Sigmoidorrhaphy *see* Repair, Gastrointestinal System, ØDQ
Sigmoidoscopy, ØDJD8ZZ
Sigmoidotomy *see* Drainage, Gastrointestinal System, ØD9
Single lead pacemaker (atrium) (ventricle) *use* Pacemaker, Single Chamber in, ØJH
Single lead rate responsive pacemaker (atrium) (ventricle) *use* Pacemaker, Single Chamber Rate Responsive in, ØJH
Sinoatrial node *use* Conduction Mechanism
Sinogram
Abdominal Wall *see* Fluoroscopy, Abdomen and Pelvis, BW11
Chest Wall *see* Plain Radiography, Chest, BWØ3
Retroperitoneum *see* Fluoroscopy, Abdomen and Pelvis, BW11
Sinus venosus *use* Atrium, Right
Sinusectomy
see Excision, Ear, Nose, Sinus, Ø9B
see Resection, Ear, Nose, Sinus, Ø9T
Sinusoscopy, Ø9JY4ZZ
Sinusotomy *see* Drainage, Ear, Nose, Sinus, Ø99
Sirolimus-eluting coronary stent *use* Intraluminal Device, Drug-eluting in Heart and Great Vessels
Sixth cranial nerve *use* Abducens Nerve
Size reduction, breast *see* Excision, Skin and Breast, ØHB
SJM Biocor® Stented Valve System *use* Zooplastic Tissue in Heart and Great Vessels
Skene's (paraurethral) gland *use* Vestibular Gland
Skin Substitute, Porcine Liver Derived, Replacement, XHRPXL2
Sling
Fascial, orbicularis muscle (mouth) *see* Supplement, Muscle, Facial, ØKU1
Levator muscle, for urethral suspension *see* Reposition, Bladder Neck, ØTSC
Pubococcygeal, for urethral suspension *see* Reposition, Bladder Neck, ØTSC
Rectum *see* Reposition, Rectum, ØDSP
Small bowel series *see* Fluoroscopy, Bowel, Small, BD13
Small saphenous vein
use Saphenous Vein, Left
use Saphenous Vein, Right
Snaring, polyp, colon *see* Excision, Gastrointestinal System, ØDB
Solar (celiac) plexus *use* Abdominal Sympathetic Nerve
Soleus muscle
use Lower Leg Muscle, Left
use Lower Leg Muscle, Right
Spacer
Insertion of device in
Disc
Lumbar Vertebral, ØSH2
Lumbosacral, ØSH4
Joint
Acromioclavicular
Left, ØRHH
Right, ØRHG
Ankle
Left, ØSHG

Right ovarian vein — Spacer

- **Splenic plexus** *use* Abdominal Sympathetic Nerve
- **Splenius capitis muscle** *use* Head Muscle
- **Splenius cervicis muscle**
  - *use* Neck Muscle, Left
  - *use* Neck Muscle, Right
- **Splenolysis** *see* Release, Lymphatic and Hemic Systems, Ø7N
- **Splenopexy**
  - *see* Repair, Lymphatic and Hemic Systems, Ø7Q
  - *see* Reposition, Lymphatic and Hemic Systems, Ø7S
- **Splenoplasty** *see* Repair, Lymphatic and Hemic Systems, Ø7Q
- **Splenorrhaphy** *see* Repair, Lymphatic and Hemic Systems, Ø7Q
- **Splenotomy** *see* Drainage, Lymphatic and Hemic Systems, Ø79
- **Splinting, musculoskeletal** *see* Immobilization, Anatomical Regions, 2W3
- **SPY system intravascular fluorescence angiography** *see* Monitoring, Physiological Systems, 4A1
- **Stapedectomy**
  - *see* Excision, Ear, Nose, Sinus, Ø9B
  - *see* Resection, Ear, Nose, Sinus, Ø9T
- **Stapediolysis** *see* Release, Ear, Nose, Sinus, Ø9N
- **Stapedioplasty**
  - *see* Repair, Ear, Nose, Sinus, Ø9Q
  - *see* Replacement, Ear, Nose, Sinus, Ø9R
  - *see* Supplement, Ear, Nose, Sinus, Ø9U
- **Stapedotomy** *see* Drainage, Ear, Nose, Sinus, Ø99
- **Stapes**
  - *use* Auditory Ossicle, Left
  - *use* Auditory Ossicle, Right
- **Static Spacer (Antibiotic)** *use* Spacer in Lower Joints
- **STELARA®** *use* Other New Technology Therapeutic Substance
- **Stellate ganglion** *use* Head and Neck Sympathetic Nerve
- **Stem cell transplant** *see* Transfusion, Circulatory, 3Ø2
- **Stensen's duct**
  - *use* Parotid Duct, Left
  - *use* Parotid Duct, Right
- **Stent, intraluminal (cardiovascular) (gastrointestinal) (hepatobiliary) (urinary)** *use* Intraluminal Device
- **Stent retriever thrombectomy** *see* Extirpation, Upper Arteries, Ø3C
- **Stented tissue valve** *use* Zooplastic Tissue in Heart and Great Vessels
- **Stereotactic Radiosurgery**
  - Abdomen, DW23
  - Adrenal Gland, DG22
  - Bile Ducts, DF22
  - Bladder, DT22
  - Bone Marrow, D72Ø
  - Brain, DØ2Ø
  - Brain Stem, DØ21
  - Breast
    - Left, DM2Ø
    - Right, DM21
  - Bronchus, DB21
  - Cervix, DU21
  - Chest, DW22
  - Chest Wall, DB27
  - Colon, DD25
  - Diaphragm, DB28
  - Duodenum, DD22
  - Ear, D92Ø
  - Esophagus, DD2Ø
  - Eye, D82Ø
  - Gallbladder, DF21
  - Gamma Beam
    - Abdomen, DW23JZZ
    - Adrenal Gland, DG22JZZ
    - Bile Ducts, DF22JZZ
    - Bladder, DT22JZZ
    - Bone Marrow, D72ØJZZ
    - Brain, DØ2ØJZZ
    - Brain Stem, DØ21JZZ
    - Breast
      - Left, DM2ØJZZ
      - Right, DM21JZZ
    - Bronchus, DB21JZZ
    - Cervix, DU21JZZ
    - Chest, DW22JZZ
    - Chest Wall, DB27JZZ
    - Colon, DD25JZZ
    - Diaphragm, DB28JZZ
    - Duodenum, DD22JZZ
    - Ear, D92ØJZZ
    - Esophagus, DD2ØJZZ

Stereotactic Radiosurgery — *continued*
  - Gamma Beam — *continued*
    - Eye, D82ØJZZ
    - Gallbladder, DF21JZZ
    - Gland
      - Adrenal, DG22JZZ
      - Parathyroid, DG24JZZ
      - Pituitary, DG2ØJZZ
      - Thyroid, DG25JZZ
    - Glands, Salivary, D926JZZ
    - Head and Neck, DW21JZZ
    - Ileum, DD24JZZ
    - Jejunum, DD23JZZ
    - Kidney, DT2ØJZZ
    - Larynx, D92BJZZ
    - Liver, DF2ØJZZ
    - Lung, DB22JZZ
    - Lymphatics
      - Abdomen, D726JZZ
      - Axillary, D724JZZ
      - Inguinal, D728JZZ
      - Neck, D723JZZ
      - Pelvis, D727JZZ
      - Thorax, D725JZZ
    - Mediastinum, DB26JZZ
    - Mouth, D924JZZ
    - Nasopharynx, D92DJZZ
    - Neck and Head, DW21JZZ
    - Nerve, Peripheral, DØ27JZZ
    - Nose, D921JZZ
    - Ovary, DU2ØJZZ
    - Palate
      - Hard, D928JZZ
      - Soft, D929JZZ
    - Pancreas, DF23JZZ
    - Parathyroid Gland, DG24JZZ
    - Pelvic Region, DW26JZZ
    - Pharynx, D92CJZZ
    - Pineal Body, DG21JZZ
    - Pituitary Gland, DG2ØJZZ
    - Pleura, DB25JZZ
    - Prostate, DV2ØJZZ
    - Rectum, DD27JZZ
    - Sinuses, D927JZZ
    - Spinal Cord, DØ26JZZ
    - Spleen, D722JZZ
    - Stomach, DD21JZZ
    - Testis, DV21JZZ
    - Thymus, D721JZZ
    - Thyroid Gland, DG25JZZ
    - Tongue, D925JZZ
    - Trachea, DB2ØJZZ
    - Ureter, DT21JZZ
    - Urethra, DT23JZZ
    - Uterus, DU22JZZ
  - Gland
    - Adrenal, DG22
    - Parathyroid, DG24
    - Pituitary, DG2Ø
    - Thyroid, DG25
  - Glands, Salivary, D926
  - Head and Neck, DW21
  - Ileum, DD24
  - Jejunum, DD23
  - Kidney, DT2Ø
  - Larynx, D92B
  - Liver, DF2Ø
  - Lung, DB22
  - Lymphatics
    - Abdomen, D726
    - Axillary, D724
    - Inguinal, D728
    - Neck, D723
    - Pelvis, D727
    - Thorax, D725
  - Mediastinum, DB26
  - Mouth, D924
  - Nasopharynx, D92D
  - Neck and Head, DW21
  - Nerve, Peripheral, DØ27
  - Nose, D921
  - Other Photon
    - Abdomen, DW23DZZ
    - Adrenal Gland, DG22DZZ
    - Bile Ducts, DF22DZZ
    - Bladder, DT22DZZ
    - Bone Marrow, D72ØDZZ
    - Brain, DØ2ØDZZ
    - Brain Stem, DØ21DZZ

Stereotactic Radiosurgery — *continued*
  - Other Photon — *continued*
    - Breast
      - Left, DM2ØDZZ
      - Right, DM21DZZ
    - Bronchus, DB21DZZ
    - Cervix, DU21DZZ
    - Chest, DW22DZZ
    - Chest Wall, DB27DZZ
    - Colon, DD25DZZ
    - Diaphragm, DB28DZZ
    - Duodenum, DD22DZZ
    - Ear, D92ØDZZ
    - Esophagus, DD2ØDZZ
    - Eye, D82ØDZZ
    - Gallbladder, DF21DZZ
    - Gland
      - Adrenal, DG22DZZ
      - Parathyroid, DG24DZZ
      - Pituitary, DG2ØDZZ
      - Thyroid, DG25DZZ
    - Glands, Salivary, D926DZZ
    - Head and Neck, DW21DZZ
    - Ileum, DD24DZZ
    - Jejunum, DD23DZZ
    - Kidney, DT2ØDZZ
    - Larynx, D92BDZZ
    - Liver, DF2ØDZZ
    - Lung, DB22DZZ
    - Lymphatics
      - Abdomen, D726DZZ
      - Axillary, D724DZZ
      - Inguinal, D728DZZ
      - Neck, D723DZZ
      - Pelvis, D727DZZ
      - Thorax, D725DZZ
    - Mediastinum, DB26DZZ
    - Mouth, D924DZZ
    - Nasopharynx, D92DDZZ
    - Neck and Head, DW21DZZ
    - Nerve, Peripheral, DØ27DZZ
    - Nose, D921DZZ
    - Ovary, DU2ØDZZ
    - Palate
      - Hard, D928DZZ
      - Soft, D929DZZ
    - Pancreas, DF23DZZ
    - Parathyroid Gland, DG24DZZ
    - Pelvic Region, DW26DZZ
    - Pharynx, D92CDZZ
    - Pineal Body, DG21DZZ
    - Pituitary Gland, DG2ØDZZ
    - Pleura, DB25DZZ
    - Prostate, DV2ØDZZ
    - Rectum, DD27DZZ
    - Sinuses, D927DZZ
    - Spinal Cord, DØ26DZZ
    - Spleen, D722DZZ
    - Stomach, DD21DZZ
    - Testis, DV21DZZ
    - Thymus, D721DZZ
    - Thyroid Gland, DG25DZZ
    - Tongue, D925DZZ
    - Trachea, DB2ØDZZ
    - Ureter, DT21DZZ
    - Urethra, DT23DZZ
    - Uterus, DU22DZZ
  - Ovary, DU2Ø
  - Palate
    - Hard, D928
    - Soft, D929
  - Pancreas, DF23
  - Parathyroid Gland, DG24
  - Particulate
    - Abdomen, DW23HZZ
    - Adrenal Gland, DG22HZZ
    - Bile Ducts, DF22HZZ
    - Bladder, DT22HZZ
    - Bone Marrow, D72ØHZZ
    - Brain, DØ2ØHZZ
    - Brain Stem, DØ21HZZ
    - Breast
      - Left, DM2ØHZZ
      - Right, DM21HZZ
    - Bronchus, DB21HZZ
    - Cervix, DU21HZZ
    - Chest, DW22HZZ
    - Chest Wall, DB27HZZ
    - Colon, DD25HZZ

Splenic plexus — Stereotactic Radiosurgery

112

▽ Subterms under main terms may continue to next column or page

Substance Abuse Treatment — *continued*
Counseling — *continued*
 Individual — *continued*
 Infectious Disease — *continued*
 Pre-Test, HZ3CZZZ
 Interpersonal, HZ34ZZZ
 Motivational Enhancement, HZ37ZZZ
 Psychoeducation, HZ36ZZZ
 Spiritual, HZ3BZZZ
 Vocational, HZ35ZZZ
Detoxification Services, for substance abuse, HZ2ZZZZ
Medication Management
 Antabuse, HZ83ZZZ
 Bupropion, HZ87ZZZ
 Clonidine, HZ86ZZZ
 Levo-alpha-acetyl-methadol (LAAM), HZ82ZZZ
 Methadone Maintenance, HZ81ZZZ
 Naloxone, HZ85ZZZ
 Naltrexone, HZ84ZZZ
 Nicotine Replacement, HZ80ZZZ
 Other Replacement Medication, HZ89ZZZ
 Psychiatric Medication, HZ88ZZZ
Pharmacotherapy
 Antabuse, HZ93ZZZ
 Bupropion, HZ97ZZZ
 Clonidine, HZ96ZZZ
 Levo-alpha-acetyl-methadol (LAAM), HZ92ZZZ
 Methadone Maintenance, HZ91ZZZ
 Naloxone, HZ95ZZZ
 Naltrexone, HZ94ZZZ
 Nicotine Replacement, HZ90ZZZ
 Psychiatric Medication, HZ98ZZZ
 Replacement Medication, Other, HZ99ZZZ
Psychotherapy
 12-Step, HZ53ZZZ
 Behavioral, HZ51ZZZ
 Cognitive, HZ50ZZZ
 Cognitive-Behavioral, HZ52ZZZ
 Confrontational, HZ58ZZZ
 Interactive, HZ55ZZZ
 Interpersonal, HZ54ZZZ
 Motivational Enhancement, HZ57ZZZ
 Psychoanalysis, HZ5BZZZ
 Psychodynamic, HZ5CZZZ
 Psychoeducation, HZ56ZZZ
 Psychophysiological, HZ5DZZZ
 Supportive, HZ59ZZZ

Substantia nigra *use* Basal Ganglia

Subtalar (talocalcaneal) joint
 use Tarsal Joint, Left
 use Tarsal Joint, Right

Subtalar ligament
 use Foot Bursa and Ligament, Left
 use Foot Bursa and Ligament, Right

Subthalamic nucleus *use* Basal Ganglia

Suction curettage (D&C), nonobstetric *see* Extraction, Endometrium, ØUDB

Suction curettage, obstetric post-delivery *see* Extraction, Products of Conception, Retained, 10D1

Superficial circumflex iliac vein
 use Saphenous Vein, Left
 use Saphenous Vein, Right

Superficial epigastric artery
 use Femoral Artery, Left
 use Femoral Artery, Right

Superficial epigastric vein
 use Saphenous Vein, Left
 use Saphenous Vein, Right

Superficial Inferior Epigastric Artery Flap
 Replacement
 Bilateral, ØHRVØ78
 Left, ØHRUØ78
 Right, ØHRTØ78
 Transfer
 Left, ØKXG
 Right, ØKXF

Superficial palmar arch
 use Hand Artery, Left
 use Hand Artery, Right

Superficial palmar venous arch
 use Hand Vein, Left
 use Hand Vein, Right

Superficial temporal artery
 use Temporal Artery, Left
 use Temporal Artery, Right

Superficial transverse perineal muscle *use* Perineum Muscle

Superior cardiac nerve *use* Thoracic Sympathetic Nerve

Superior cerebellar vein *use* Intracranial Vein
Superior cerebral vein *use* Intracranial Vein
Superior clunic (cluneal) nerve *use* Lumbar Nerve

Superior epigastric artery
 use Internal Mammary Artery, Left
 use Internal Mammary Artery, Right

Superior genicular artery
 use Popliteal Artery, Left
 use Popliteal Artery, Right

Superior gluteal artery
 use Internal Iliac Artery, Left
 use Internal Iliac Artery, Right

Superior gluteal nerve *use* Lumbar Plexus
Superior hypogastric plexus *use* Abdominal Sympathetic Nerve
Superior labial artery *use* Face Artery

Superior laryngeal artery
 use Thyroid Artery, Left
 use Thyroid Artery, Right

Superior laryngeal nerve *use* Vagus Nerve
Superior longitudinal muscle *use* Tongue, Palate, Pharynx Muscle
Superior mesenteric ganglion *use* Abdominal Sympathetic Nerve
Superior mesenteric lymph node *use* Lymphatic, Mesenteric
Superior mesenteric plexus *use* Abdominal Sympathetic Nerve

Superior oblique muscle
 use Extraocular Muscle, Left
 use Extraocular Muscle, Right

Superior olivary nucleus *use* Pons
Superior rectal artery *use* Inferior Mesenteric Artery
Superior rectal vein *use* Inferior Mesenteric Vein

Superior rectus muscle
 use Extraocular Muscle, Left
 use Extraocular Muscle, Right

Superior tarsal plate
 use Upper Eyelid, Left
 use Upper Eyelid, Right

Superior thoracic artery
 use Axillary Artery, Left
 use Axillary Artery, Right

Superior thyroid artery
 use External Carotid Artery, Left
 use External Carotid Artery, Right
 use Thyroid Artery, Left
 use Thyroid Artery, Right

Superior turbinate *use* Nasal Turbinate

Superior ulnar collateral artery
 use Brachial Artery, Left
 use Brachial Artery, Right

Supersaturated Oxygen therapy, 5AØ512C, 5AØ522C

Supplement
 Abdominal Wall, ØWUF
 Acetabulum
 Left, ØQU5
 Right, ØQU4
 Ampulla of Vater, ØFUC
 Anal Sphincter, ØDUR
 Ankle Region
 Left, ØYUL
 Right, ØYUK
 Anus, ØDUQ
 Aorta
 Abdominal, 04UØ
 Thoracic
 Ascending/Arch, 02UX
 Descending, 02UW
 Arm
 Lower
 Left, ØXUF
 Right, ØXUD
 Upper
 Left, ØXU9
 Right, ØXU8
 Artery
 Anterior Tibial
 Left, 04UQ
 Right, 04UP
 Axillary
 Left, 03U6
 Right, 03U5
 Brachial
 Left, 03U8
 Right, 03U7
 Celiac, 04U1

Supplement — *continued*
 Artery — *continued*
 Colic
 Left, 04U7
 Middle, 04U8
 Right, 04U6
 Common Carotid
 Left, 03UJ
 Right, 03UH
 Common Iliac
 Left, 04UD
 Right, 04UC
 External Carotid
 Left, 03UN
 Right, 03UM
 External Iliac
 Left, 04UJ
 Right, 04UH
 Face, 03UR
 Femoral
 Left, 04UL
 Right, 04UK
 Foot
 Left, 04UW
 Right, 04UV
 Gastric, 04U2
 Hand
 Left, 03UF
 Right, 03UD
 Hepatic, 04U3
 Inferior Mesenteric, 04UB
 Innominate, 03U2
 Internal Carotid
 Left, 03UL
 Right, 03UK
 Internal Iliac
 Left, 04UF
 Right, 04UE
 Internal Mammary
 Left, 03U1
 Right, 03UØ
 Intracranial, 03UG
 Lower, 04UY
 Peroneal
 Left, 04UU
 Right, 04UT
 Popliteal
 Left, 04UN
 Right, 04UM
 Posterior Tibial
 Left, 04US
 Right, 04UR
 Pulmonary
 Left, 02UR
 Right, 02UQ
 Pulmonary Trunk, 02UP
 Radial
 Left, 03UC
 Right, 03UB
 Renal
 Left, 04UA
 Right, 04U9
 Splenic, 04U4
 Subclavian
 Left, 03U4
 Right, 03U3
 Superior Mesenteric, 04U5
 Temporal
 Left, 03UT
 Right, 03US
 Thyroid
 Left, 03UV
 Right, 03UU
 Ulnar
 Left, 03UA
 Right, 03U9
 Upper, 03UY
 Vertebral
 Left, 03UQ
 Right, 03UP
 Atrium
 Left, 02U7
 Right, 02U6
 Auditory Ossicle
 Left, 09UA
 Right, 09U9
 Axilla
 Left, ØXU5
 Right, ØXU4

▽ **Subterms under main terms may continue to next column or page**

Supplement — *continued*
Joint — *continued*
Ankle
 Left, ØSUG
 Right, ØSUF
Carpal
 Left, ØRUR
 Right, ØRUQ
Carpometacarpal
 Left, ØRUT
 Right, ØRUS
Cervical Vertebral, ØRU1
Cervicothoracic Vertebral, ØRU4
Coccygeal, ØSU6
Elbow
 Left, ØRUM
 Right, ØRUL
Finger Phalangeal
 Left, ØRUX
 Right, ØRUW
Hip
 Left, ØSUB
 Acetabular Surface, ØSUE
 Femoral Surface, ØSUS
 Right, ØSU9
 Acetabular Surface, ØSUA
 Femoral Surface, ØSUR
Knee
 Left, ØSUD
 Femoral Surface, ØSUUØ9Z
 Tibial Surface, ØSUWØ9Z
 Right, ØSUC
 Femoral Surface, ØSUTØ9Z
 Tibial Surface, ØSUVØ9Z
Lumbar Vertebral, ØSUØ
Lumbosacral, ØSU3
Metacarpophalangeal
 Left, ØRUV
 Right, ØRUU
Metatarsal-Phalangeal
 Left, ØSUN
 Right, ØSUM
Occipital-cervical, ØRUØ
Sacrococcygeal, ØSU5
Sacroiliac
 Left, ØSU8
 Right, ØSU7
Shoulder
 Left, ØRUK
 Right, ØRUJ
Sternoclavicular
 Left, ØRUF
 Right, ØRUE
Tarsal
 Left, ØSUJ
 Right, ØSUH
Tarsometatarsal
 Left, ØSUL
 Right, ØSUK
Temporomandibular
 Left, ØRUD
 Right, ØRUC
Thoracic Vertebral, ØRU6
Thoracolumbar Vertebral, ØRUA
Toe Phalangeal
 Left, ØSUQ
 Right, ØSUP
Wrist
 Left, ØRUP
 Right, ØRUN
Kidney Pelvis
 Left, ØTU4
 Right, ØTU3
Knee Region
 Left, ØYUG
 Right, ØYUF
Larynx, ØCUS
Leg
 Lower
 Left, ØYUJ
 Right, ØYUH
 Upper
 Left, ØYUD
 Right, ØYUC
Lip
 Lower, ØCU1
 Upper, ØCUØ
Lymphatic
 Aortic, Ø7UD

Supplement — *continued*
Lymphatic — *continued*
Axillary
 Left, Ø7U6
 Right, Ø7U5
Head, Ø7UØ
Inguinal
 Left, Ø7UJ
 Right, Ø7UH
Internal Mammary
 Left, Ø7U9
 Right, Ø7U8
Lower Extremity
 Left, Ø7UG
 Right, Ø7UF
Mesenteric, Ø7UB
Neck
 Left, Ø7U2
 Right, Ø7U1
Pelvis, Ø7UC
Thoracic Duct, Ø7UK
Thorax, Ø7U7
Upper Extremity
 Left, Ø7U4
 Right, Ø7U3
Mandible
 Left, ØNUV
 Right, ØNUT
Maxilla, ØNUR
Mediastinum, ØWUC
Mesentery, ØDUV
Metacarpal
 Left, ØPUQ
 Right, ØPUP
Metatarsal
 Left, ØQUP
 Right, ØQUN
Muscle
 Abdomen
 Left, ØKUL
 Right, ØKUK
 Extraocular
 Left, Ø8UM
 Right, Ø8UL
 Facial, ØKU1
 Foot
 Left, ØKUW
 Right, ØKUV
 Hand
 Left, ØKUD
 Right, ØKUC
 Head, ØKUØ
 Hip
 Left, ØKUP
 Right, ØKUN
 Lower Arm and Wrist
 Left, ØKUB
 Right, ØKU9
 Lower Leg
 Left, ØKUT
 Right, ØKUS
 Neck
 Left, ØKU3
 Right, ØKU2
 Papillary, Ø2UD
 Perineum, ØKUM
 Shoulder
 Left, ØKU6
 Right, ØKU5
 Thorax
 Left, ØKUJ
 Right, ØKUH
 Tongue, Palate, Pharynx, ØKU4
 Trunk
 Left, ØKUG
 Right, ØKUF
 Upper Arm
 Left, ØKU8
 Right, ØKU7
 Upper Leg
 Left, ØKUR
 Right, ØKUQ
Nasal Mucosa and Soft Tissue, Ø9UK
Nasopharynx, Ø9UN
Neck, ØWU6
Nerve
 Abducens, ØØUL
 Accessory, ØØUR
 Acoustic, ØØUN

Supplement — *continued*
Nerve — *continued*
 Cervical, Ø1U1
 Facial, ØØUM
 Femoral, Ø1UD
 Glossopharyngeal, ØØUP
 Hypoglossal, ØØUS
 Lumbar, Ø1UB
 Median, Ø1U5
 Oculomotor, ØØUH
 Olfactory, ØØUF
 Optic, ØØUG
 Peroneal, Ø1UH
 Phrenic, Ø1U2
 Pudendal, Ø1UC
 Radial, Ø1U6
 Sacral, Ø1UR
 Sciatic, Ø1UF
 Thoracic, Ø1U8
 Tibial, Ø1UG
 Trigeminal, ØØUK
 Trochlear, ØØUJ
 Ulnar, Ø1U4
 Vagus, ØØUQ
Nipple
 Left, ØHUX
 Right, ØHUW
Omentum, ØDUU
Orbit
 Left, ØNUQ
 Right, ØNUP
Palate
 Hard, ØCU2
 Soft, ØCU3
Patella
 Left, ØQUF
 Right, ØQUD
Penis, ØVUS
Pericardium, Ø2UN
Perineum
 Female, ØWUN
 Male, ØWUM
Peritoneum, ØDUW
Phalanx
 Finger
 Left, ØPUV
 Right, ØPUT
 Thumb
 Left, ØPUS
 Right, ØPUR
 Toe
 Left, ØQUR
 Right, ØQUQ
Pharynx, ØCUM
Prepuce, ØVUT
Radius
 Left, ØPUJ
 Right, ØPUH
Rectum, ØDUP
Retina
 Left, Ø8UF
 Right, Ø8UE
Retinal Vessel
 Left, Ø8UH
 Right, Ø8UG
Ribs
 1 to 2, ØPU1
 3 or More, ØPU2
Sacrum, ØQU1
Scapula
 Left, ØPU6
 Right, ØPU5
Scrotum, ØVU5
Septum
 Atrial, Ø2U5
 Nasal, Ø9UM
 Ventricular, Ø2UM
Shoulder Region
 Left, ØXU3
 Right, ØXU2
Skull, ØNUØ
Spinal Meninges, ØØUT
Sternum, ØPUØ
Stomach, ØDU6
 Pylorus, ØDU7
Subcutaneous Tissue and Fascia
 Abdomen, ØJU8
 Back, ØJU7
 Buttock, ØJU9

Suspension — *continued*
Uterus *see* Reposition, Uterus, ØUS9
Vagina *see* Reposition, Vagina, ØUSG
Suture
Laceration repair *see* Repair
Ligation *see* Occlusion
Suture Removal
Extremity
Lower, 8EØYXY8
Upper, 8EØXXY8
Head and Neck Region, 8EØ9XY8
Trunk Region, 8EØWXY8
Sutureless valve, Perceval *use* Zooplastic Tissue, Rapid Deployment Technique in New Technology
Sweat gland *use* Skin
Sympathectomy *see* Excision, Peripheral Nervous System, Ø1B
SynCardia Total Artificial Heart *use* Synthetic Substitute
Synchra CRT-P *use* Cardiac Resynchronization Pacemaker Pulse Generator in, ØJH
SynchroMed pump *use* Infusion Device, Pump in Subcutaneous Tissue and Fascia
Synechiotomy, iris *see* Release, Eye, Ø8N
Synovectomy
Lower joint *see* Excision, Lower Joints, ØSB
Upper joint *see* Excision, Upper Joints, ØRB
Synthetic Human Angiotensin II, XWØ
Systemic Nuclear Medicine Therapy
Abdomen, CW7Ø
Anatomical Regions, Multiple, CW7YYZZ
Chest, CW73
Thyroid, CW7G
Whole Body, CW7N

T

Takedown
Arteriovenous shunt *see* Removal of device from, Upper Arteries, Ø3P
Arteriovenous shunt, with creation of new shunt *see* Bypass, Upper Arteries, Ø31
Stoma
see Excision
see Reposition
Talent® Converter *use* Intraluminal Device
Talent® Occluder *use* Intraluminal Device
Talent® Stent Graft (abdominal) (thoracic) *use* Intraluminal Device
Talocalcaneal (subtalar) joint
use Tarsal Joint, Left
use Tarsal Joint, Right
Talocalcaneal ligament
use Foot Bursa and Ligament, Left
use Foot Bursa and Ligament, Right
Talocalcaneonavicular joint
use Tarsal Joint, Left
use Tarsal Joint, Right
Talocalcaneonavicular ligament
use Foot Bursa and Ligament, Left
use Foot Bursa and Ligament, Right
Talocrural joint
use Ankle Joint, Left
use Joint, Ankle, Right
Talofibular ligament
use Ankle Bursa and Ligament, Left
use Ankle Bursa and Ligament, Right
Talus bone
use Tarsal, Left
use Tarsal, Right
TandemHeart® System *use* Short-term External Heart Assist System in Heart and Great Vessels
Tarsectomy
see Excision, Lower Bones, ØQB
see Resection, Lower Bones, ØQT
Tarsometatarsal ligament
use Foot Bursa and Ligament, Left
use Foot Bursa and Ligament, Right
Tarsorrhaphy *see* Repair, Eye, Ø8Q
Tattooing
Cornea, 3EØCXMZ
Skin *see* Introduction of substance in or on, Skin, 3EØØ
TAXUS® Liberté® Paclitaxel-eluting Coronary Stent System *use* Intraluminal Device, Drug-eluting in Heart and Great Vessels
TBNA (transbronchial needle aspiration)
Fluid or gas *see* Drainage, Respiratory System, ØB9
TBNA — *continued*
Tissue biopsy *see* Extraction, Respiratory System, ØBD
Telemetry, 4A12X4Z
Ambulatory, 4A12X45
Temperature gradient study, 4AØZXKZ
Temporal lobe *use* Cerebral Hemisphere
Temporalis muscle *use* Head Muscle
Temporoparietalis muscle *use* Head Muscle
Tendolysis *see* Release, Tendons, ØLN
Tendonectomy
see Excision, Tendons, ØLB
see Resection, Tendons, ØLT
Tendonoplasty, tenoplasty
see Repair, Tendons, ØLQ
see Replacement, Tendons, ØLR
see Supplement, Tendons, ØLU
Tendorrhaphy *see* Repair, Tendons, ØLQ
Tendototomy
see Division, Tendons, ØL8
see Drainage, Tendons, ØL9
Tenectomy, tenonectomy
see Excision, Tendons, ØLB
see Resection, Tendons, ØLT
Tenolysis *see* Release, Tendons, ØLN
Tenontorrhaphy *see* Repair, Tendons, ØLQ
Tenontotomy
see Division, Tendons, ØL8
see Drainage, Tendons, ØL9
Tenorrhaphy *see* Repair, Tendons, ØLQ
Tenosynovectomy
see Excision, Tendons, ØLB
see Resection, Tendons, ØLT
Tenotomy
see Division, Tendons, ØL8
see Drainage, Tendons, ØL9
Tensor fasciae latae muscle
use Hip Muscle, Left
use Hip Muscle, Right
Tensor veli palatini muscle *use* Tongue, Palate, Pharynx Muscle
Tenth cranial nerve *use* Vagus Nerve
Tentorium cerebelli *use* Dura Mater
Teres major muscle
use Shoulder Muscle, Left
use Shoulder Muscle, Right
Teres minor muscle
use Shoulder Muscle, Left
use Shoulder Muscle, Right
Termination of pregnancy
Aspiration curettage, 1ØAØ7ZZ
Dilation and curettage, 1ØAØ7ZZ
Hysterotomy, 1ØAØØZZ
Intra-amniotic injection, 1ØAØ3ZZ
Laminaria, 1ØAØ7ZW
Vacuum, 1ØAØ7Z6
Testectomy
see Excision, Male Reproductive System, ØVB
see Resection, Male Reproductive System, ØVT
Testicular artery *use* Abdominal Aorta
Testing
Glaucoma, 4AØ7XBZ
Hearing *see* Hearing Assessment, Diagnostic Audiology, F13
Mental health *see* Psychological Tests
Muscle function, electromyography (EMG) *see* Measurement, Musculoskeletal, 4AØF
Muscle function, manual *see* Motor Function Assessment, Rehabilitation, FØ1
Neurophysiologic monitoring, intra-operative *see* Monitoring, Physiological Systems, 4A1
Range of motion *see* Motor Function Assessment, Rehabilitation, FØ1
Vestibular function *see* Vestibular Assessment, Diagnostic Audiology, F15
Thalamectomy *see* Excision, Thalamus, ØØB9
Thalamotomy *see* Drainage, Thalamus, ØØ99
Thenar muscle
use Hand Muscle, Left
use Hand Muscle, Right
Therapeutic Massage
Musculoskeletal System, 8EØKX1Z
Reproductive System
Prostate, 8EØVX1C
Rectum, 8EØVX1D
Therapeutic occlusion coil(s) *use* Intraluminal Device
Thermography, 4AØZXKZ
Thermotherapy, prostate *see* Destruction, Prostate, ØV5Ø
Third cranial nerve *use* Oculomotor Nerve
Third occipital nerve *use* Cervical Nerve
Third ventricle *use* Cerebral Ventricle
Thoracectomy *see* Excision, Anatomical Regions, General, ØWB
Thoracentesis *see* Drainage, Anatomical Regions, General, ØW9
Thoracic aortic plexus *use* Thoracic Sympathetic Nerve
Thoracic esophagus *use* Esophagus, Middle
Thoracic facet joint *use* Thoracic Vertebral Joint
Thoracic ganglion *use* Thoracic Sympathetic Nerve
Thoracoacromial artery
use Axillary Artery, Left
use Axillary Artery, Right
Thoracocentesis *see* Drainage, Anatomical Regions, General, ØW9
Thoracolumbar facet joint *use* Thoracolumbar Vertebral Joint
Thoracoplasty
see Repair, Anatomical Regions, General, ØWQ
see Supplement, Anatomical Regions, General, ØWU
Thoracostomy, for lung collapse *see* Drainage, Respiratory System, ØB9
Thoracostomy tube *use* Drainage Device
Thoracotomy *see* Drainage, Anatomical Regions, General, ØW9
Thoratec IVAD (Implantable Ventricular Assist Device) *use* Implantable Heart Assist System in Heart and Great Vessels
Thoratec Paracorporeal Ventricular Assist Device *use* Short-term External Heart Assist System in Heart and Great Vessels
Thrombectomy *see* Extirpation
Thymectomy
see Excision, Lymphatic and Hemic Systems, Ø7B
see Resection, Lymphatic and Hemic Systems, Ø7T
Thymopexy
see Repair, Lymphatic and Hemic Systems, Ø7Q
see Reposition, Lymphatic and Hemic Systems, Ø7S
Thymus gland *use* Thymus
Thyroarytenoid muscle
use Neck Muscle, Left
use Neck Muscle, Right
Thyrocervical trunk
use Thyroid Artery, Left
use Thyroid Artery, Right
Thyroid cartilage *use* Larynx
Thyroidectomy
see Excision, Endocrine System, ØGB
see Resection, Endocrine System, ØGT
Thyroidorrhaphy *see* Repair, Endocrine System, ØGQ
Thyroidoscopy, ØGJK4ZZ
Thyroidotomy *see* Drainage, Endocrine System, ØG9
Tibial insert *use* Liner in Lower Joints
Tibialis anterior muscle
use Lower Leg Muscle, Left
use Lower Leg Muscle, Right
Tibialis posterior muscle
use Lower Leg Muscle, Left
use Lower Leg Muscle, Right
Tibiofemoral joint
use Knee Joint, Left
use Knee Joint, Right
use Knee Joint, Tibial Surface, Left
use Knee Joint, Tibial Surface, Right
Tisagenlecleucel *use* Engineered Autologous Chimeric Antigen Receptor T-cell Immunotherapy
Tissue bank graft *use* Nonautologous Tissue Substitute
Tissue Expander
Insertion of device in
Breast
Bilateral, ØHHV
Left, ØHHU
Right, ØHHT
Nipple
Left, ØHHX
Right, ØHHW
Subcutaneous Tissue and Fascia
Abdomen, ØJH8
Back, ØJH7
Buttock, ØJH9
Chest, ØJH6
Face, ØJH1
Foot
Left, ØJHR

Transfer — *continued*
Bursa and Ligament — *continued*
Upper Extremity — *continued*
Right, 0MX9
Wrist
Left, 0MX6
Right, 0MX5
Finger
Left, 0XXP0ZM
Right, 0XXN0ZL
Gingiva
Lower, 0CX6
Upper, 0CX5
Intestine
Large, 0DXE
Small, 0DX8
Lip
Lower, 0CX1
Upper, 0CX0
Muscle
Abdomen
Left, 0KXL
Right, 0KXK
Extraocular
Left, 08XM
Right, 08XL
Facial, 0KX1
Foot
Left, 0KXW
Right, 0KXV
Hand
Left, 0KXD
Right, 0KXC
Head, 0KX0
Hip
Left, 0KXP
Right, 0KXN
Lower Arm and Wrist
Left, 0KXB
Right, 0KX9
Lower Leg
Left, 0KXT
Right, 0KXS
Neck
Left, 0KX3
Right, 0KX2
Perineum, 0KXM
Shoulder
Left, 0KX6
Right, 0KX5
Thorax
Left, 0KXJ
Right, 0KXH
Tongue, Palate, Pharynx, 0KX4
Trunk
Left, 0KXG
Right, 0KXF
Upper Arm
Left, 0KX8
Right, 0KX7
Upper Leg
Left, 0KXR
Right, 0KXQ
Nerve
Abducens, 00XL
Accessory, 00XR
Acoustic, 00XN
Cervical, 01X1
Facial, 00XM
Femoral, 01XD
Glossopharyngeal, 00XP
Hypoglossal, 00XS
Lumbar, 01XB
Median, 01X5
Oculomotor, 00XH
Olfactory, 00XF
Optic, 00XG
Peroneal, 01XH
Phrenic, 01X2
Pudendal, 01XC
Radial, 01X6
Sciatic, 01XF
Thoracic, 01X8
Tibial, 01XG
Trigeminal, 00XK
Trochlear, 00XJ
Ulnar, 01X4
Vagus, 00XQ
Palate, Soft, 0CX3

Transfer — *continued*
Prepuce, 0VXT
Skin
Abdomen, 0HX7XZZ
Back, 0HX6XZZ
Buttock, 0HX8XZZ
Chest, 0HX5XZZ
Ear
Left, 0HX3XZZ
Right, 0HX2XZZ
Face, 0HX1XZZ
Foot
Left, 0HXNXZZ
Right, 0HXMXZZ
Hand
Left, 0HXGXZZ
Right, 0HXFXZZ
Inguinal, 0HXAXZZ
Lower Arm
Left, 0HXEXZZ
Right, 0HXDXZZ
Lower Leg
Left, 0HXLXZZ
Right, 0HXKXZZ
Neck, 0HX4XZZ
Perineum, 0HX9XZZ
Scalp, 0HX0XZZ
Upper Arm
Left, 0HXCXZZ
Right, 0HXBXZZ
Upper Leg
Left, 0HXJXZZ
Right, 0HXHXZZ
Stomach, 0DX6
Subcutaneous Tissue and Fascia
Abdomen, 0JX8
Back, 0JX7
Buttock, 0JX9
Chest, 0JX6
Face, 0JX1
Foot
Left, 0JXR
Right, 0JXQ
Hand
Left, 0JXK
Right, 0JXJ
Lower Arm
Left, 0JXH
Right, 0JXG
Lower Leg
Left, 0JXP
Right, 0JXN
Neck
Left, 0JX5
Right, 0JX4
Pelvic Region, 0JXC
Perineum, 0JXB
Scalp, 0JX0
Upper Arm
Left, 0JXF
Right, 0JXD
Upper Leg
Left, 0JXM
Right, 0JXL
Tendon
Abdomen
Left, 0LXG
Right, 0LXF
Ankle
Left, 0LXT
Right, 0LXS
Foot
Left, 0LXW
Right, 0LXV
Hand
Left, 0LX8
Right, 0LX7
Head and Neck, 0LX0
Hip
Left, 0LXK
Right, 0LXJ
Knee
Left, 0LXR
Right, 0LXQ
Lower Arm and Wrist
Left, 0LX6
Right, 0LX5
Lower Leg
Left, 0LXP

Transfer — *continued*
Tendon — *continued*
Lower Leg — *continued*
Right, 0LXN
Perineum, 0LXH
Shoulder
Left, 0LX2
Right, 0LX1
Thorax
Left, 0LXD
Right, 0LXC
Trunk
Left, 0LXB
Right, 0LX9
Upper Arm
Left, 0LX4
Right, 0LX3
Upper Leg
Left, 0LXM
Right, 0LXL
Tongue, 0CX7
Transfusion
Artery
Central
Antihemophilic Factors, 3026
Blood
Platelets, 3026
Red Cells, 3026
Frozen, 3026
White Cells, 3026
Whole, 3026
Bone Marrow, 3026
Factor IX, 3026
Fibrinogen, 3026
Globulin, 3026
Plasma
Fresh, 3026
Frozen, 3026
Plasma Cryoprecipitate, 3026
Serum Albumin, 3026
Stem Cells
Cord Blood, 3026
Hematopoietic, 3026
Peripheral
Antihemophilic Factors, 3025
Blood
Platelets, 3025
Red Cells, 3025
Frozen, 3025
White Cells, 3025
Whole, 3025
Bone Marrow, 3025
Factor IX, 3025
Fibrinogen, 3025
Globulin, 3025
Plasma
Fresh, 3025
Frozen, 3025
Plasma Cryoprecipitate, 3025
Serum Albumin, 3025
Stem Cells
Cord Blood, 3025
Hematopoietic, 3025
Products of Conception
Antihemophilic Factors, 3027
Blood
Platelets, 3027
Red Cells, 3027
Frozen, 3027
White Cells, 3027
Whole, 3027
Factor IX, 3027
Fibrinogen, 3027
Globulin, 3027
Plasma
Fresh, 3027
Frozen, 3027
Plasma Cryoprecipitate, 3027
Serum Albumin, 3027
Vein
4-Factor Prothrombin Complex Concentrate, 30280B1
Central
Antihemophilic Factors, 3024
Blood
Platelets, 3024
Red Cells, 3024
Frozen, 3024
White Cells, 3024

Transfusion — *continued*
Vein — *continued*
Central — *continued*
Blood — *continued*
Whole, 3Ø24
Bone Marrow, 3Ø24
Factor IX, 3Ø24
Fibrinogen, 3Ø24
Globulin, 3Ø24
Plasma
Fresh, 3Ø24
Frozen, 3Ø24
Plasma Cryoprecipitate, 3Ø24
Serum Albumin, 3Ø24
Stem Cells
Cord Blood, 3Ø24
Embryonic, 3Ø24
Hematopoietic, 3Ø24
Peripheral
Antihemophilic Factors, 3Ø23
Blood
Platelets, 3Ø23
Red Cells, 3Ø23
Frozen, 3Ø23
White Cells, 3Ø23
Whole, 3Ø23
Bone Marrow, 3Ø23
Factor IX, 3Ø23
Fibrinogen, 3Ø23
Globulin, 3Ø23
Plasma
Fresh, 3Ø23
Frozen, 3Ø23
Plasma Cryoprecipitate, 3Ø23
Serum Albumin, 3Ø23
Stem Cells
Cord Blood, 3Ø23
Embryonic, 3Ø23
Hematopoietic, 3Ø23
Transplant *see* Transplantation
Transplantation
Bone marrow *see* Transfusion, Circulatory, 3Ø2
Esophagus, ØDY5ØZ
Face, ØWY2ØZ
Hand
Left, ØXYKØZ
Right, ØXYJØZ
Heart, Ø2YAØZ
Hematopoietic cell *see* Transfusion, Circulatory, 3Ø2
Intestine
Large, ØDYEØZ
Small, ØDY8ØZ
Kidney
Left, ØTY1ØZ
Right, ØTYØØZ
Liver, ØFYØØZ
Lung
Bilateral, ØBYMØZ
Left, ØBYLØZ
Lower Lobe
Left, ØBYJØZ
Right, ØBYFØZ
Middle Lobe, Right, ØBYDØZ
Right, ØBYKØZ
Upper Lobe
Left, ØBYGØZ
Right, ØBYCØZ
Lung Lingula, ØBYHØZ
Ovary
Left, ØUY1ØZ
Right, ØUYØØZ
Pancreas, ØFYGØZ
Products of Conception, 1ØYØ
Spleen, Ø7YPØZ
Stem cell *see* Transfusion, Circulatory, 3Ø2
Stomach, ØDY6ØZ
Thymus, Ø7YMØZ
Uterus, ØUY9ØZ
Transposition
see Bypass
see Reposition
see Transfer
Transversalis fascia *use* Subcutaneous Tissue and Fascia, Trunk
Transverse acetabular ligament
use Hip Bursa and Ligament, Left
use Hip Bursa and Ligament, Right
Transverse (cutaneous) cervical nerve *use* Cervical Plexus
Transverse facial artery
use Temporal Artery, Left
use Temporal Artery, Right
Transverse foramen *use* Cervical Vertebra
Transverse humeral ligament
use Shoulder Bursa and Ligament, Left
use Shoulder Bursa and Ligament, Right
Transverse ligament of atlas *use* Head and Neck Bursa and Ligament
Transverse process
use Cervical Vertebra
use Lumbar Vertebra
use Thoracic Vertebra
Transverse Rectus Abdominis Myocutaneous Flap
Replacement
Bilateral, ØHRVØ76
Left, ØHRUØ76
Right, ØHRTØ76
Transfer
Left, ØKXL
Right, ØKXK
Transverse scapular ligament
use Shoulder Bursa and Ligament, Left
use Shoulder Bursa and Ligament, Right
Transverse thoracis muscle
use Thorax Muscle, Left
use Thorax Muscle, Right
Transversospinalis muscle
use Trunk Muscle, Left
use Trunk Muscle, Right
Transversus abdominis muscle
use Abdomen Muscle, Left
use Abdomen Muscle, Right
Trapezium bone
use Carpal, Left
use Carpal, Right
Trapezius muscle
use Trunk Muscle, Left
use Trunk Muscle, Right
Trapezoid bone
use Carpal, Left
use Carpal, Right
Triceps brachii muscle
use Upper Arm Muscle, Left
use Upper Arm Muscle, Right
Tricuspid annulus *use* Tricuspid Valve
Trifacial nerve *use* Trigeminal Nerve
Trifecta™ Valve (aortic) *use* Zooplastic Tissue in Heart and Great Vessels
Trigone of bladder *use* Bladder
Trimming, excisional *see* Excision
Triquetral bone
use Carpal, Left
use Carpal, Right
Trochanteric bursa
use Hip Bursa and Ligament, Left
use Hip Bursa and Ligament, Right
TUMT (transurethral microwave thermotherapy of prostate), ØV5Ø7ZZ
TUNA (transurethral needle ablation of prostate), ØV5Ø7ZZ
Tunneled central venous catheter *use* Vascular Access Device, Tunneled in Subcutaneous Tissue and Fascia
Tunneled spinal (intrathecal) catheter *use* Infusion Device
Turbinectomy
see Excision, Ear, Nose, Sinus, Ø9B
see Resection, Ear, Nose, Sinus, Ø9T
Turbinoplasty
see Repair, Ear, Nose, Sinus, Ø9Q
see Replacement, Ear, Nose, Sinus, Ø9R
see Supplement, Ear, Nose, Sinus, Ø9U
Turbinotomy
see Division, Ear, Nose, Sinus, Ø98
see Drainage, Ear, Nose, Sinus, Ø99
TURP (transurethral resection of prostate), ØVBØ7ZZ
see Excision, Prostate, ØVBØ
see Resection, Prostate, ØVTØ
Twelfth cranial nerve *use* Hypoglossal Nerve
Two lead pacemaker *use* Pacemaker, Dual Chamber in, ØJH
Tympanic cavity
use Middle Ear, Left
use Middle Ear, Right
Tympanic nerve *use* Glossopharyngeal Nerve
Tympanic part of temporal bone
use Temporal Bone, Left
use Temporal Bone, Right
Tympanogram *see* Hearing Assessment, Diagnostic Audiology, F13
Tympanoplasty
see Repair, Ear, Nose, Sinus, Ø9Q
see Replacement, Ear, Nose, Sinus, Ø9R
see Supplement, Ear, Nose, Sinus, Ø9U
Tympanosympathectomy *see* Excision, Nerve, Head and Neck Sympathetic, Ø1BK
Tympanotomy *see* Drainage, Ear, Nose, Sinus, Ø99

U

Ulnar collateral carpal ligament
use Wrist Bursa and Ligament, Left
use Wrist Bursa and Ligament, Right
Ulnar collateral ligament
use Elbow Bursa and Ligament, Left
use Elbow Bursa and Ligament, Right
Ulnar notch
use Radius, Left
use Radius, Right
Ulnar vein
use Brachial Vein, Left
use Brachial Vein, Right
Ultrafiltration
Hemodialysis *see* Performance, Urinary, 5A1D
Therapeutic plasmapheresis *see* Pheresis, Circulatory, 6A55
Ultraflex™ Precision Colonic Stent System *use* Intraluminal Device
ULTRAPRO Hernia System (UHS) *use* Synthetic Substitute
ULTRAPRO Partially Absorbable Lightweight Mesh
use Synthetic Substitute
ULTRAPRO Plug *use* Synthetic Substitute
Ultrasonic osteogenic stimulator
use Bone Growth Stimulator in Head and Facial Bones
use Bone Growth Stimulator in Lower Bones
use Bone Growth Stimulator in Upper Bones
Ultrasonography
Abdomen, BW4ØZZZ
Abdomen and Pelvis, BW41ZZZ
Abdominal Wall, BH49ZZZ
Aorta
Abdominal, Intravascular, B44ØZZ3
Thoracic, Intravascular, B34ØZZ3
Appendix, BD48ZZZ
Artery
Brachiocephalic-Subclavian, Right, Intravascular, B341ZZ3
Celiac and Mesenteric, Intravascular, B44KZZ3
Common Carotid
Bilateral, Intravascular, B345ZZ3
Left, Intravascular, B344ZZ3
Right, Intravascular, B343ZZ3
Coronary
Multiple, B241YZZ
Intravascular, B241ZZ3
Transesophageal, B241ZZ4
Single, B24ØYZZ
Intravascular, B24ØZZ3
Transesophageal, B24ØZZ4
Femoral, Intravascular, B44LZZ3
Inferior Mesenteric, Intravascular, B445ZZ3
Internal Carotid
Bilateral, Intravascular, B348ZZ3
Left, Intravascular, B347ZZ3
Right, Intravascular, B346ZZ3
Intra-Abdominal, Other, Intravascular, B44BZZ3
Intracranial, Intravascular, B34RZZ3
Lower Extremity
Bilateral, Intravascular, B44HZZ3
Left, Intravascular, B44GZZ3
Right, Intravascular, B44FZZ3
Mesenteric and Celiac, Intravascular, B44KZZ3
Ophthalmic, Intravascular, B34VZZ3
Penile, Intravascular, B44NZZ3
Pulmonary
Left, Intravascular, B34TZZ3
Right, Intravascular, B34SZZ3
Renal
Bilateral, Intravascular, B448ZZ3
Left, Intravascular, B447ZZ3

Subterms under main terms may continue to next column or page

- **Ultrasonography** — *continued*
  - Artery — *continued*
    - Renal — *continued*
      - Right, Intravascular, B446ZZ3
    - Subclavian, Left, Intravascular, B342ZZ3
    - Superior Mesenteric, Intravascular, B444ZZ3
    - Upper Extremity
      - Bilateral, Intravascular, B34KZZ3
      - Left, Intravascular, B34JZZ3
      - Right, Intravascular, B34HZZ3
  - Bile Duct, BF40ZZZ
  - Bile Duct and Gallbladder, BF43ZZZ
  - Bladder, BT40ZZZ
    - and Kidney, BT4JZZZ
  - Brain, BØ4ØZZZ
  - Breast
    - Bilateral, BH42ZZZ
    - Left, BH41ZZZ
    - Right, BH4ØZZZ
  - Chest Wall, BH4BZZZ
  - Coccyx, BR4FZZZ
  - Connective Tissue
    - Lower Extremity, BL41ZZZ
    - Upper Extremity, BL4ØZZZ
  - Duodenum, BD49ZZZ
  - Elbow
    - Left, Densitometry, BP4HZZ1
    - Right, Densitometry, BP4GZZ1
  - Esophagus, BD41ZZZ
  - Extremity
    - Lower, BH48ZZZ
    - Upper, BH47ZZZ
  - Eye
    - Bilateral, B847ZZZ
    - Left, B846ZZZ
    - Right, B845ZZZ
  - Fallopian Tube
    - Bilateral, BU42
    - Left, BU41
    - Right, BU4Ø
  - Fetal Umbilical Cord, BY47ZZZ
  - Fetus
    - First Trimester, Multiple Gestation, BY4BZZZ
    - Second Trimester, Multiple Gestation, BY4DZZZ
    - Single
      - First Trimester, BY49ZZZ
      - Second Trimester, BY4CZZZ
      - Third Trimester, BY4FZZZ
    - Third Trimester, Multiple Gestation, BY4GZZZ
  - Gallbladder, BF42ZZZ
  - Gallbladder and Bile Duct, BF43ZZZ
  - Gastrointestinal Tract, BD47ZZZ
  - Gland
    - Adrenal
      - Bilateral, BG42ZZZ
      - Left, BG41ZZZ
      - Right, BG4ØZZZ
    - Parathyroid, BG43ZZZ
    - Thyroid, BG44ZZZ
  - Hand
    - Left, Densitometry, BP4PZZ1
    - Right, Densitometry, BP4NZZ1
  - Head and Neck, BH4CZZZ
  - Heart
    - Left, B245YZZ
      - Intravascular, B245ZZ3
      - Transesophageal, B245ZZ4
    - Pediatric, B24DYZZ
      - Intravascular, B24DZZ3
      - Transesophageal, B24DZZ4
    - Right, B244YZZ
      - Intravascular, B244ZZ3
      - Transesophageal, B244ZZ4
    - Right and Left, B246YZZ
      - Intravascular, B246ZZ3
      - Transesophageal, B246ZZ4
  - Heart with Aorta, B24BYZZ
    - Intravascular, B24BZZ3
    - Transesophageal, B24BZZ4
  - Hepatobiliary System, All, BF4CZZZ
  - Hip
    - Bilateral, BQ42ZZZ
    - Left, BQ41ZZZ
    - Right, BQ4ØZZZ
  - Kidney
    - and Bladder, BT4JZZZ
    - Bilateral, BT43ZZZ
    - Left, BT42ZZZ
    - Right, BT41ZZZ
    - Transplant, BT49ZZZ
  - Knee
    - Bilateral, BQ49ZZZ
    - Left, BQ48ZZZ
    - Right, BQ47ZZZ
  - Liver, BF45ZZZ
  - Liver and Spleen, BF46ZZZ
  - Mediastinum, BB4CZZZ
  - Neck, BW4FZZZ
  - Ovary
    - Bilateral, BU45
    - Left, BU44
    - Right, BU43
  - Ovary and Uterus, BU4C
  - Pancreas, BF47ZZZ
  - Pelvic Region, BW4GZZZ
  - Pelvis and Abdomen, BW41ZZZ
  - Penis, BV4BZZZ
  - Pericardium, B24CYZZ
    - Intravascular, B24CZZ3
    - Transesophageal, B24CZZ4
  - Placenta, BY48ZZZ
  - Pleura, BB4BZZZ
  - Prostate and Seminal Vesicle, BV49ZZZ
  - Rectum, BD4CZZZ
  - Sacrum, BR4FZZZ
  - Scrotum, BV44ZZZ
  - Seminal Vesicle and Prostate, BV49ZZZ
  - Shoulder
    - Left, Densitometry, BP49ZZ1
    - Right, Densitometry, BP48ZZ1
  - Spinal Cord, BØ4BZZZ
  - Spine
    - Cervical, BR4ØZZZ
    - Lumbar, BR49ZZZ
    - Thoracic, BR47ZZZ
  - Spleen and Liver, BF46ZZZ
  - Stomach, BD42ZZZ
  - Tendon
    - Lower Extremity, BL43ZZZ
    - Upper Extremity, BL42ZZZ
  - Ureter
    - Bilateral, BT48ZZZ
    - Left, BT47ZZZ
    - Right, BT46ZZZ
  - Urethra, BT45ZZZ
  - Uterus, BU46
  - Uterus and Ovary, BU4C
  - Vein
    - Jugular
      - Left, Intravascular, B544ZZ3
      - Right, Intravascular, B543ZZ3
    - Lower Extremity
      - Bilateral, Intravascular, B54DZZ3
      - Left, Intravascular, B54CZZ3
      - Right, Intravascular, B54BZZ3
    - Portal, Intravascular, B54TZZ3
    - Renal
      - Bilateral, Intravascular, B54LZZ3
      - Left, Intravascular, B54KZZ3
      - Right, Intravascular, B54JZZ3
    - Splanchnic, Intravascular, B54TZZ3
    - Subclavian
      - Left, Intravascular, B547ZZ3
      - Right, Intravascular, B546ZZ3
    - Upper Extremity
      - Bilateral, Intravascular, B54PZZ3
      - Left, Intravascular, B54NZZ3
      - Right, Intravascular, B54MZZ3
  - Vena Cava
    - Inferior, Intravascular, B549ZZ3
    - Superior, Intravascular, B548ZZ3
  - Wrist
    - Left, Densitometry, BP4MZZ1
    - Right, Densitometry, BP4LZZ1
- **Ultrasound bone healing system**
  - *use* Bone Growth Stimulator in Head and Facial Bones
  - *use* Bone Growth Stimulator in Lower Bones
  - *use* Bone Growth Stimulator in Upper Bones
- **Ultrasound Therapy**
  - Heart, 6A75
  - No Qualifier, 6A75
  - Vessels
    - Head and Neck, 6A75
    - Other, 6A75
    - Peripheral, 6A75
- **Ultraviolet Light Therapy, Skin**, 6A8Ø
- **Umbilical artery**
  - *use* Internal Iliac Artery, Left
  - *use* Internal Iliac Artery, Right
  - *use* Lower Artery
- **Uniplanar external fixator**
  - *use* External Fixation Device, Monoplanar in, ØPH
  - *use* External Fixation Device, Monoplanar in, ØPS
  - *use* External Fixation Device, Monoplanar in, ØQH
  - *use* External Fixation Device, Monoplanar in, ØQS
- **Upper GI series** *see* Fluoroscopy, Gastrointestinal, Upper, BD15
- **Ureteral orifice**
  - *use* Ureter
  - *use* Ureter, Left
  - *use* Ureter, Right
  - *use* Ureters, Bilateral
- **Ureterectomy**
  - *see* Excision, Urinary System, ØTB
  - *see* Resection, Urinary System, ØTT
- **Ureterocolostomy** *see* Bypass, Urinary System, ØT1
- **Ureterocystostomy** *see* Bypass, Urinary System, ØT1
- **Ureteroenterostomy** *see* Bypass, Urinary System, ØT1
- **Ureteroileostomy** *see* Bypass, Urinary System, ØT1
- **Ureterolithotomy** *see* Extirpation, Urinary System, ØTC
- **Ureterolysis** *see* Release, Urinary System, ØTN
- **Ureteroneocystostomy**
  - *see* Bypass, Urinary System, ØT1
  - *see* Reposition, Urinary System, ØTS
- **Ureteropelvic junction (UPJ)**
  - *use* Kidney Pelvis, Left
  - *use* Kidney Pelvis, Right
- **Ureteropexy**
  - *see* Repair, Urinary System, ØTQ
  - *see* Reposition, Urinary System, ØTS
- **Ureteroplasty**
  - *see* Repair, Urinary System, ØTQ
  - *see* Replacement, Urinary System, ØTR
  - *see* Supplement, Urinary System, ØTU
- **Ureteroplication** *see* Restriction, Urinary System, ØTV
- **Ureteropyelography** *see* Fluoroscopy, Urinary System, BT1
- **Ureterorrhaphy** *see* Repair, Urinary System, ØTQ
- **Ureteroscopy**, ØTJ98ZZ
- **Ureterostomy**
  - *see* Bypass, Urinary System, ØT1
  - *see* Drainage, Urinary System, ØT9
- **Ureterotomy** *see* Drainage, Urinary System, ØT9
- **Ureteroureterostomy** *see* Bypass, Urinary System, ØT1
- **Ureterovesical orifice**
  - *use* Ureter
  - *use* Ureter, Left
  - *use* Ureter, Right
  - *use* Ureters, Bilateral
- **Urethral catheterization, indwelling**, ØT9B7ØZ
- **Urethrectomy**
  - *see* Excision, Urethra, ØTBD
  - *see* Resection, Urethra, ØTTD
- **Urethrolithotomy** *see* Extirpation, Urethra, ØTCD
- **Urethrolysis** *see* Release, Urethra, ØTND
- **Urethropexy**
  - *see* Repair, Urethra, ØTQD
  - *see* Reposition, Urethra, ØTSD
- **Urethroplasty**
  - *see* Repair, Urethra, ØTQD
  - *see* Replacement, Urethra, ØTRD
  - *see* Supplement, Urethra, ØTUD
- **Urethrorrhaphy** *see* Repair, Urethra, ØTQD
- **Urethroscopy**, ØTJD8ZZ
- **Urethrotomy** *see* Drainage, Urethra, ØT9D
- **Uridine Triacetate**, XWØDX82
- **Urinary incontinence stimulator lead** *use* Stimulator Lead in Urinary System
- **Urography** *see* Fluoroscopy, Urinary System, BT1
- **Ustekinumab** *use* Other New Technology Therapeutic Substance
- **Uterine Artery**
  - *use* Internal Iliac Artery, Left
  - *use* Internal Iliac Artery, Right
- **Uterine artery embolization (UAE)** *see* Occlusion, Lower Arteries, Ø4L
- **Uterine cornu** *use* Uterus
- **Uterine tube**
  - *use* Fallopian Tube, Left
  - *use* Fallopian Tube, Right
- **Uterine vein**
  - *use* Hypogastric Vein, Left

122
Subterms under main terms may continue to next column or page

▽ Subterms under main terms may continue to next column or page

123

Xiphoid process *use* Sternum
XLIF® System *use* Interbody Fusion Device in Lower Joints
X-ray *see* Plain Radiography
X-STOP® Spacer
use Spinal Stabilization Device, Interspinous Process in, ØRH
use Spinal Stabilization Device, Interspinous Process in, ØSH

Y

Yoga Therapy, 8EØZXY4

Z

Zenith AAA Endovascular Graft
use Intraluminal Device
use Intraluminal Device, Branched or Fenestrated, One or Two Arteries in, Ø4V
use Intraluminal Device, Branched or Fenestrated, Three or More Arteries in, Ø4V
Zenith Flex® AAA Endovascular Graft *use* Intraluminal Device
Zenith TX2® TAA Endovascular Graft *use* Intraluminal Device
Zenith® Renu™ AAA Ancillary Graft *use* Intraluminal Device
Zilver® PTX® (paclitaxel) Drug-Eluting Peripheral Stent
use Intraluminal Device, Drug-eluting in Lower Arteries
use Intraluminal Device, Drug-eluting in Upper Arteries
Zimmer® NexGen® LPS Mobile Bearing Knee *use* Synthetic Substitute
Zimmer® NexGen® LPS-Flex Mobile Knee *use* Synthetic Substitute
ZINPLAVA™ use Bezlotoxumab Monoclonal Antibody
Zonule of Zinn
use Lens, Left
use Lens, Right
Zooplastic Tissue, Rapid Deployment Technique, Replacement, X2RF
Zotarolimus-eluting Coronary Stent *use* Intraluminal Device, Drug-eluting in Heart and Great Vessels
Z-plasty, skin for scar contracture *see* Release, Skin and Breast, ØHN
Zygomatic process of frontal bone *use* Frontal Bone
Zygomatic process of temporal bone
use Temporal Bone, Left
use Temporal Bone, Right
Zygomaticus muscle *use* Facial Muscle
Zyvox *use* Oxazolidinones

ICD-10-PCS Tables

Central Nervous System and Cranial Nerves ØØ1–ØØX

Character Meanings

This Character Meaning table is provided as a guide to assist the user in the identification of character members that may be found in this section of code tables. It **SHOULD NOT** be used to build a PCS code.

Operation–Character 3	Body Part–Character 4	Approach–Character 5	Device–Character 6	Qualifier–Character 7
1 Bypass	Ø Brain	Ø Open	Ø Drainage Device	Ø Nasopharynx
2 Change	1 Cerebral Meninges	3 Percutaneous	2 Monitoring Device	1 Mastoid Sinus
5 Destruction	2 Dura Mater	4 Percutaneous Endoscopic	3 Infusion Device	2 Atrium
7 Dilation	3 Epidural Space, Intracranial	X External	4 Radioactive Element, Cesium-131 Collagen Implant	3 Blood Vessel
8 Division	4 Subdural Space, Intracranial		7 Autologous Tissue Substitute	4 Pleural Cavity
9 Drainage	5 Subarachnoid Space, Intracranial		J Synthetic Substitute	5 Intestine
B Excision	6 Cerebral Ventricle		K Nonautologous Tissue Substitute	6 Peritoneal Cavity
C Extirpation	7 Cerebral Hemisphere		M Neurostimulator Lead	7 Urinary Tract
D Extraction	8 Basal Ganglia		Y Other Device	8 Bone Marrow
F Fragmentation	9 Thalamus		Z No Device	9 Fallopian Tube
H Insertion	A Hypothalamus			B Cerebral Cisterns
J Inspection	B Pons			F Olfactory Nerve
K Map	C Cerebellum			G Optic Nerve
N Release	D Medulla Oblongata			H Oculomotor Nerve
P Removal	E Cranial Nerve			J Trochlear Nerve
Q Repair	F Olfactory Nerve			K Trigeminal Nerve
R Replacement	G Optic Nerve			L Abducens Nerve
S Reposition	H Oculomotor Nerve			M Facial Nerve
T Resection	J Trochlear Nerve			N Acoustic Nerve
U Supplement	K Trigeminal Nerve			P Glossopharyngeal Nerve
W Revision	L Abducens Nerve			Q Vagus Nerve
X Transfer	M Facial Nerve			R Accessory Nerve
	N Acoustic Nerve			S Hypoglossal Nerve
	P Glossopharyngeal Nerve			X Diagnostic
	Q Vagus Nerve			Z No Qualifier
	R Accessory Nerve			
	S Hypoglossal Nerve			
	T Spinal Meninges			
	U Spinal Canal			
	V Spinal Cord			
	W Cervical Spinal Cord			
	X Thoracic Spinal Cord			
	Y Lumbar Spinal Cord			

AHA Coding Clinic for table ØØ1

2017, 4Q, 39-41	Dilation and bypass of cerebral ventricle
2015, 2Q, 9	Revision of ventriculoperitoneal (VP) shunt
2013, 2Q, 36	Insertion of ventriculoperitoneal shunt with laparoscopic assistance

AHA Coding Clinic for table ØØ7

2017, 4Q, 39-41	Dilation and bypass of cerebral ventricle

AHA Coding Clinic for table ØØ9

2017, 1Q, 50	Failed lumbar puncture
2015, 3Q, 10	Open evacuation of subdural hematoma
2015, 3Q, 11	Percutaneous drainage of subdural hematoma
2015, 3Q, 12	Subdural evacuation portal system (SEPS) placement
2015, 3Q, 12	Placement of ventriculostomy catheter via burr hole
2015, 2Q, 30	Drainage of syrinx
2015, 1Q, 31	Intrathecal chemotherapy
2014, 1Q, 8	Diagnostic lumbar tap
2014, 1Q, 8	Lumbar drainage port aspiration

AHA Coding Clinic for table ØØB

2017, 3Q, 17	Resection of schwannoma and placement of DuraGen and Lorenz cranial plating system
2016, 2Q, 12	Resection of malignant neoplasm of infratemporal fossa
2016, 2Q, 18	Amygdalohippocampectomy
2014, 4Q, 34	Resection of brain malignancy with implantation of chemotherapeutic wafer
2014, 3Q, 24	Repair of lipomyelomeningocele and tethered cord

AHA Coding Clinic for table ØØC

2017, 4Q, 48	New and revised body part values - Extirpation spinal canal
2016, 2Q, 29	Decompressive craniectomy with cryopreservation and storage of bone flap
2015, 3Q, 10	Open evacuation of subdural hematoma
2015, 3Q, 11	Percutaneous drainage of subdural hematoma
2015, 3Q, 13	Evacuation of intracerebral hematoma

AHA Coding Clinic for table ØØD

2015, 3Q, 13	Nonexcisional debridement of cranial wound with removal and replacement of hardware

AHA Coding Clinic for table ØØH

2017, 4Q, 30-31	Radiotherapeutic brain implant
2017, 3Q, 13	Implantation of bilateral neurostimulator electrodes
2014, 3Q, 19	End of life replacement of Baclofen pump

AHA Coding Clinic for table ØØJ

2017, 1Q, 50	Failed lumbar puncture

AHA Coding Clinic for table ØØN

2017, 3Q, 10	Repair of Chiari malformation
2017, 2Q, 23	Decompression of spinal cord and placement of instrumentation
2016, 2Q, 29	Decompressive craniectomy with cryopreservation and storage of bone flap
2015, 2Q, 20	Cervical laminoplasty
2015, 2Q, 21	Multiple decompressive cervical laminectomies
2015, 2Q, 34	Decompressive laminectomy
2014, 3Q, 24	Repair of lipomyelomeningocele and tethered cord

AHA Coding Clinic for table ØØP

2014, 3Q, 19	End of life replacement of Baclofen pump

AHA Coding Clinic for table ØØQ

2014, 3Q, 7	Hemi-cranioplasty for repair of cranial defect
2013, 3Q, 25	Fracture of frontal bone with repair and coagulation for hemostasis

AHA Coding Clinic for table ØØS

2014, 4Q, 35	Reimplantation of buccal nerve

AHA Coding Clinic for table ØØU

2018, 1Q, 9	Craniectomy with DuraGaurd placement
2017, 4Q, 62	Added and revised device values - Nerve substitutes
2017, 3Q, 10	Repair of Chiari malformation
2017, 3Q, 17	Resection of schwannoma and placement of DuraGen and Lorenz cranial plating system
2015, 4Q, 39	Dural patch graft
2014, 3Q, 24	Repair of lipomyelomeningocele and tethered cord

Brain

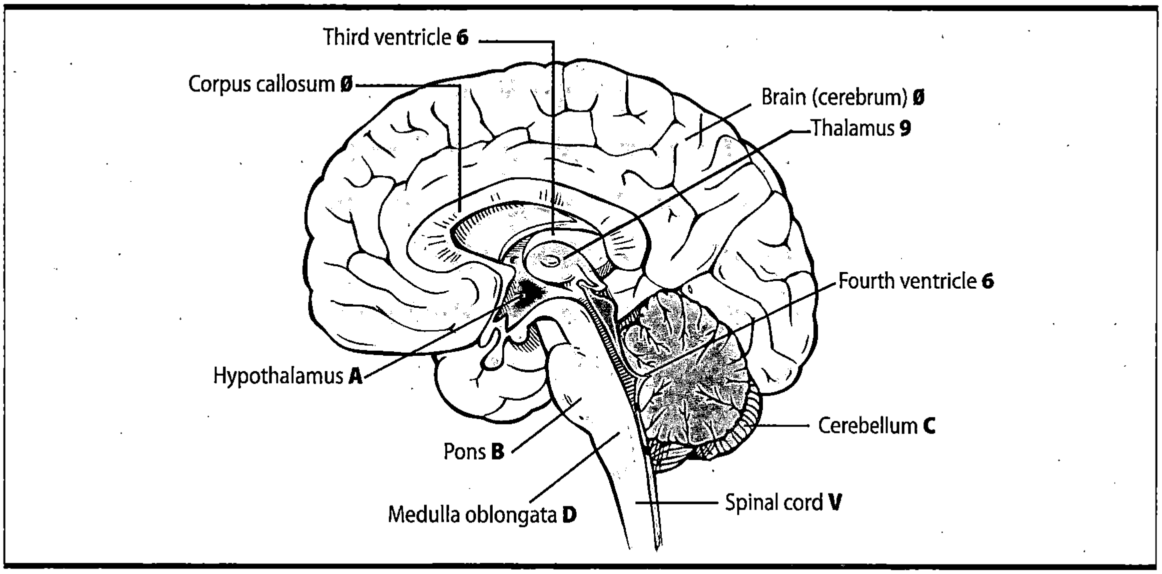

Cranial Nerves

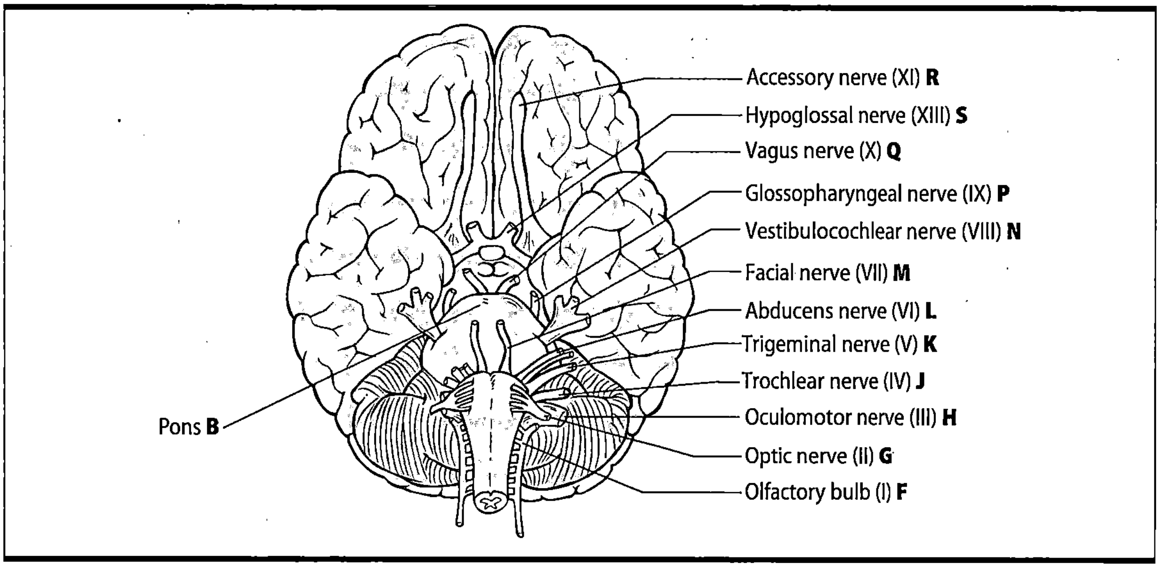

0 Medical and Surgical
0 Central Nervous System and Cranial Nerves
1 Bypass Definition: Altering the route of passage of the contents of a tubular body part

Explanation: Rerouting contents of a body part to a downstream area of the normal route, to a similar route and body part, or to an abnormal route and dissimilar body part. Includes one or more anastomoses, with or without the use of a device.

Body Part Character 4	Approach Character 5	Device Character 6	Qualifier Character 7
6 Cerebral Ventricle Aqueduct of Sylvius Cerebral aqueduct (Sylvius) Choroid plexus Ependyma Foramen of Monro (intraventricular) Fourth ventricle Interventricular foramen (Monro) Left lateral ventricle Right lateral ventricle Third ventricle	0 Open 3 Percutaneous 4 Percutaneous Endoscopic	7 Autologous Tissue Substitute J Synthetic Substitute K Nonautologous Tissue Substitute	0 Nasopharynx 1 Mastoid Sinus 2 Atrium 3 Blood Vessel 4 Pleural Cavity 5 Intestine 6 Peritoneal Cavity 7 Urinary Tract 8 Bone Marrow B Cerebral Cisterns
6 Cerebral Ventricle Aqueduct of Sylvius Cerebral aqueduct (Sylvius) Choroid plexus Ependyma Foramen of Monro (intraventricular) Fourth ventricle Interventricular foramen (Monro) Left lateral ventricle Right lateral ventricle Third ventricle	0 Open 3 Percutaneous 4 Percutaneous Endoscopic	Z No Device	B Cerebral Cisterns
U Spinal Canal Epidural space, spinal Extradural space, spinal Subarachnoid space, spinal Subdural space, spinal Vertebral canal	0 Open 3 Percutaneous 4 Percutaneous Endoscopic	7 Autologous Tissue Substitute J Synthetic Substitute K Nonautologous Tissue Substitute	2 Atrium 4 Pleural Cavity 6 Peritoneal Cavity 7 Urinary Tract 9 Fallopian Tube

0 Medical and Surgical
0 Central Nervous System and Cranial Nerves
2 Change Definition: Taking out or off a device from a body part and putting back an identical or similar device in or on the same body part without cutting or puncturing the skin or a mucous membrane

Explanation: All CHANGE procedures are coded using the approach EXTERNAL

Body Part Character 4	Approach Character 5	Device Character 6	Qualifier Character 7
0 Brain Cerebrum Corpus callosum Encephalon E Cranial Nerve U Spinal Canal Epidural space, spinal Extradural space, spinal Subarachnoid space, spinal Subdural space, spinal Vertebral canal	X External	0 Drainage Device Y Other Device	Z No Qualifier

Non-OR All body part, approach, device, and qualifier values

0 Medical and Surgical
0 Central Nervous System and Cranial Nerves
5 Destruction Definition: Physical eradication of all or a portion of a body part by the direct use of energy, force, or a destructive agent
Explanation: None of the body part is physically taken out

Body Part Character 4	Approach Character 5	Device Character 6	Qualifier Character 7
0 Brain Cerebrum, Corpus callosum, Encephalon **1 Cerebral Meninges** Arachnoid mater, intracranial; Leptomeninges, intracranial; Pia mater, intracranial **2 Dura Mater** Diaphragma sellae; Dura mater, intracranial; Falx cerebri; Tentorium cerebelli **6 Cerebral Ventricle** Aqueduct of Sylvius; Cerebral aqueduct (Sylvius); Choroid plexus; Ependyma; Foramen of Monro (intraventricular); Fourth ventricle; Interventricular foramen (Monro); Left lateral ventricle; Right lateral ventricle; Third ventricle **7 Cerebral Hemisphere** Frontal lobe; Occipital lobe; Parietal lobe; Temporal lobe **8 Basal Ganglia** Basal nuclei; Claustrum; Corpus striatum; Globus pallidus; Substantia nigra; Subthalamic nucleus **9 Thalamus** Epithalamus; Geniculate nucleus; Metathalamus; Pulvinar **A Hypothalamus** Mammillary body **B Pons** Apneustic center; Basis pontis; Locus ceruleus; Pneumotaxic center; Pontine tegmentum; Superior olivary nucleus **C Cerebellum** Culmen **D Medulla Oblongata** Myelencephalon **F Olfactory Nerve** First cranial nerve; Olfactory bulb **G Optic Nerve** Optic chiasma; Second cranial nerve **H Oculomotor Nerve** Third cranial nerve **J Trochlear Nerve** Fourth cranial nerve **K Trigeminal Nerve** Fifth cranial nerve; Gasserian ganglion; Mandibular nerve; Maxillary nerve; Ophthalmic nerve; Trifacial nerve **L Abducens Nerve** Sixth cranial nerve **M Facial Nerve** Chorda tympani; Geniculate ganglion; Greater superficial petrosal nerve; Nerve to the stapedius; Parotid plexus; Posterior auricular nerve; Seventh cranial nerve; Submandibular ganglion **N Acoustic Nerve** Cochlear nerve; Eighth cranial nerve; Scarpa's (vestibular) ganglion; Spiral ganglion; Vestibular (Scarpa's) ganglion; Vestibular nerve; Vestibulocochlear nerve **P Glossopharyngeal Nerve** Carotid sinus nerve; Ninth cranial nerve; Tympanic nerve **Q Vagus Nerve** Anterior vagal trunk; Pharyngeal plexus; Pneumogastric nerve; Posterior vagal trunk; Pulmonary plexus; Recurrent laryngeal nerve; Superior laryngeal nerve; Tenth cranial nerve **R Accessory Nerve** Eleventh cranial nerve **S Hypoglossal Nerve** Twelfth cranial nerve **T Spinal Meninges** Arachnoid mater, spinal; Denticulate (dentate) ligament; Dura mater, spinal; Filum terminale; Leptomeninges, spinal; Pia mater, spinal **W Cervical Spinal Cord** **X Thoracic Spinal Cord** **Y Lumbar Spinal Cord** Cauda equina; Conus medullaris	0 Open 3 Percutaneous 4 Percutaneous Endoscopic	Z No Device	Z No Qualifier

Non-OR 005[F,G,H,J,K,L,M,N,P,Q,R,S][0,3,4]ZZ

0 Medical and Surgical
0 Central Nervous System and Cranial Nerves
7 Dilation Definition: Expanding an orifice or the lumen of a tubular body part

Explanation: The orifice can be a natural orifice or an artificially created orifice. Accomplished by stretching a tubular body part using intraluminal pressure or by cutting part of the orifice or wall of the tubular body part.

Body Part Character 4	Approach Character 5	Device Character 6	Qualifier Character 7
6 Cerebral Ventricle Aqueduct of Sylvius Cerebral aqueduct (Sylvius) Choroid plexus Ependyma Foramen of Monro (intraventricular) Fourth ventricle Interventricular foramen (Monro) Left lateral ventricle Right lateral ventricle Third ventricle	**0 Open** **3 Percutaneous** **4 Percutaneous Endoscopic**	**Z No Device**	**Z No Qualifier**

0 Medical and Surgical
0 Central Nervous System and Cranial Nerves
8 Division Definition: Cutting into a body part, without draining fluids and/or gases from the body part, in order to separate or transect a body part

Explanation: All or a portion of the body part is separated into two or more portions

Body Part Character 4	Approach Character 5	Device Character 6	Qualifier Character 7
0 Brain Cerebrum Corpus callosum Encephalon **7 Cerebral Hemisphere** Frontal lobe Occipital lobe Parietal lobe Temporal lobe **8 Basal Ganglia** Basal nuclei Claustrum Corpus striatum Globus pallidus Substantia nigra Subthalamic nucleus **F Olfactory Nerve** First cranial nerve Olfactory bulb **G Optic Nerve** Optic chiasma Second cranial nerve **H Oculomotor Nerve** Third cranial nerve **J Trochlear Nerve** Fourth cranial nerve **K Trigeminal Nerve** Fifth cranial nerve Gasserian ganglion Mandibular nerve Maxillary nerve Ophthalmic nerve Trifacial nerve **L Abducens Nerve** Sixth cranial nerve **M Facial Nerve** Chorda tympani Geniculate ganglion Greater superficial petrosal nerve Nerve to the stapedius Parotid plexus Posterior auricular nerve Seventh cranial nerve Submandibular ganglion **N Acoustic Nerve** Cochlear nerve Eighth cranial nerve Scarpa's (vestibular) ganglion Spiral ganglion Vestibular (Scarpa's) ganglion Vestibular nerve Vestibulocochlear nerve **P Glossopharyngeal Nerve** Carotid sinus nerve Ninth cranial nerve Tympanic nerve **Q Vagus Nerve** Anterior vagal trunk Pharyngeal plexus Pneumogastric nerve Posterior vagal trunk Pulmonary plexus Recurrent laryngeal nerve Superior laryngeal nerve Tenth cranial nerve **R Accessory Nerve** Eleventh cranial nerve **S Hypoglossal Nerve** Twelfth cranial nerve **W Cervical Spinal Cord** **X Thoracic Spinal Cord** **Y Lumbar Spinal Cord** Cauda equina Conus medullaris	**0 Open** **3 Percutaneous** **4 Percutaneous Endoscopic**	**Z No Device**	**Z No Qualifier**

Ø Medical and Surgical
Ø Central Nervous System and Cranial Nerves
9 Drainage Definition: Taking or letting out fluids and/or gases from a body part
Explanation: The qualifier DIAGNOSTIC is used to identify drainage procedures that are biopsies

Body Part Character 4	Approach Character 5	Device Character 6	Qualifier Character 7
Ø Brain Cerebrum Corpus callosum Encephalon **1 Cerebral Meninges** Arachnoid mater, intracranial Leptomeninges, intracranial Pia mater, intracranial **2 Dura Mater** Diaphragma sellae Dura mater, intracranial Falx cerebri Tentorium cerebelli **3 Epidural Space, Intracranial** Extradural space, intracranial **4 Subdural Space, Intracranial** **5 Subarachnoid Space, Intracranial** **6 Cerebral Ventricle** Aqueduct of Sylvius Cerebral aqueduct (Sylvius) Choroid plexus Ependyma Foramen of Monro (intraventricular) Fourth ventricle Interventricular foramen (Monro) Left lateral ventricle Right lateral ventricle Third ventricle **7 Cerebral Hemisphere** Frontal lobe Occipital lobe Parietal lobe Temporal lobe **8 Basal Ganglia** Basal nuclei Claustrum Corpus striatum Globus pallidus Substantia nigra Subthalamic nucleus **9 Thalamus** Epithalamus Geniculate nucleus Metathalamus Pulvinar **A Hypothalamus** Mammillary body **B Pons** Apneustic center Basis pontis Locus ceruleus Pneumotaxic center Pontine tegmentum Superior olivary nucleus **C Cerebellum** Culmen **D Medulla Oblongata** Myelencephalon **F Olfactory Nerve** First cranial nerve Olfactory bulb **G Optic Nerve** Optic chiasma Second cranial nerve **H Oculomotor Nerve** Third cranial nerve **J Trochlear Nerve** Fourth cranial nerve **K Trigeminal Nerve** Fifth cranial nerve Gasserian ganglion Mandibular nerve Maxillary nerve Ophthalmic nerve Trifacial nerve **L Abducens Nerve** Sixth cranial nerve **M Facial Nerve** Chorda tympani Geniculate ganglion Greater superficial petrosal nerve Nerve to the stapedius Parotid plexus Posterior auricular nerve Seventh cranial nerve Submandibular ganglion **N Acoustic Nerve** Cochlear nerve Eighth cranial nerve Scarpa's (vestibular) ganglion Spiral ganglion Vestibular (Scarpa's) ganglion Vestibular nerve Vestibulocochlear nerve **P Glossopharyngeal Nerve** Carotid sinus nerve Ninth cranial nerve Tympanic nerve **Q Vagus Nerve** Anterior vagal trunk Pharyngeal plexus Pneumogastric nerve Posterior vagal trunk Pulmonary plexus Recurrent laryngeal nerve Superior laryngeal nerve Tenth cranial nerve **R Accessory Nerve** Eleventh cranial nerve **S Hypoglossal Nerve** Twelfth cranial nerve **T Spinal Meninges** Arachnoid mater, spinal Denticulate (dentate) ligament Dura mater, spinal Filum terminale Leptomeninges, spinal Pia mater, spinal **U Spinal Canal** Epidural space, spinal Extradural space, spinal Subarachnoid space, spinal Subdural space, spinal Vertebral canal **W Cervical Spinal Cord** **X Thoracic Spinal Cord** **Y Lumbar Spinal Cord** Cauda equina Conus medullaris	**Ø Open** **3 Percutaneous** **4 Percutaneous Endoscopic**	**Ø Drainage Device**	**Z No Qualifier**

ØØ9 Continued on next page

Non-OR ØØ9[T,W,X,Y]3ØZ
Non-OR ØØ9U[3,4]ØZ

0 Medical and Surgical
0 Central Nervous System and Cranial Nerves
9 Drainage Definition: Taking or letting out fluids and/or gases from a body part
Explanation: The qualifier DIAGNOSTIC is used to identify drainage procedures that are biopsies

009 Continued

Body Part Character 4	Approach Character 5	Device Character 6	Qualifier Character 7
0 **Brain** Cerebrum Corpus callosum Encephalon 1 **Cerebral Meninges** Arachnoid mater, intracranial Leptomeninges, intracranial Pia mater, intracranial 2 **Dura Mater** Diaphragma sellae Dura mater, intracranial Falx cerebri Tentorium cerebelli 3 **Epidural Space, Intracranial** Extradural space, intracranial 4 **Subdural Space, Intracranial** 5 **Subarachnoid Space, Intracranial** 6 **Cerebral Ventricle** Aqueduct of Sylvius Cerebral aqueduct (Sylvius) Choroid plexus Ependyma Foramen of Monro (intraventricular) Fourth ventricle Interventricular foramen (Monro) Left lateral ventricle Right lateral ventricle Third ventricle 7 **Cerebral Hemisphere** Frontal lobe Occipital lobe Parietal lobe Temporal lobe 8 **Basal Ganglia** Basal nuclei Claustrum Corpus striatum Globus pallidus Substantia nigra Subthalamic nucleus 9 **Thalamus** Epithalamus Geniculate nucleus Metathalamus Pulvinar A **Hypothalamus** Mammillary body B **Pons** Apneustic center Basis pontis Locus ceruleus Pneumotaxic center Pontine tegmentum Superior olivary nucleus C **Cerebellum** Culmen D **Medulla Oblongata** Myelencephalon F **Olfactory Nerve** First cranial nerve Olfactory bulb G **Optic Nerve** Optic chiasma Second cranial nerve H **Oculomotor Nerve** Third cranial nerve J **Trochlear Nerve** Fourth cranial nerve K **Trigeminal Nerve** Fifth cranial nerve Gasserian ganglion Mandibular nerve Maxillary nerve Ophthalmic nerve Trifacial nerve L **Abducens Nerve** Sixth cranial nerve M **Facial Nerve** Chorda tympani Geniculate ganglion Greater superficial petrosal nerve Nerve to the stapedius Parotid plexus Posterior auricular nerve Seventh cranial nerve Submandibular ganglion N **Acoustic Nerve** Cochlear nerve Eighth cranial nerve Scarpa's (vestibular) ganglion Spiral ganglion Vestibular (Scarpa's) ganglion Vestibular nerve Vestibulocochlear nerve P **Glossopharyngeal Nerve** Carotid sinus nerve Ninth cranial nerve Tympanic nerve Q **Vagus Nerve** Anterior vagal trunk Pharyngeal plexus Pneumogastric nerve Posterior vagal trunk Pulmonary plexus Recurrent laryngeal nerve Superior laryngeal nerve Tenth cranial nerve R **Accessory Nerve** Eleventh cranial nerve S **Hypoglossal Nerve** Twelfth cranial nerve T **Spinal Meninges** Arachnoid mater, spinal Denticulate (dentate) ligament Dura mater, spinal Filum terminale Leptomeninges, spinal Pia mater, spinal U **Spinal Canal** Epidural space, spinal Extradural space, spinal Subarachnoid space, spinal Subdural space, spinal Vertebral canal W **Cervical Spinal Cord** X **Thoracic Spinal Cord** Y **Lumbar Spinal Cord** Cauda equina Conus medullaris	0 Open 3 Percutaneous 4 Percutaneous Endoscopic	Z No Device	X Diagnostic Z No Qualifier

Non-OR 009[0,1,2,3,4,5,6,7,8,9,A,B,C,D,F,G,H,J,K,L,M,N,P,Q,R,S][3,4]ZX
Non-OR 009[T,W,X,Y]3Z[X,Z]
Non-OR 009U[3,4]Z[X,Z]

Ø Medical and Surgical
Ø Central Nervous System and Cranial Nerves
B Excision Definition: Cutting out or off, without replacement, a portion of a body part
Explanation: The qualifier DIAGNOSTIC is used to identify excision procedures that are biopsies

Body Part Character 4		Approach Character 5	Device Character 6	Qualifier Character 7
Ø Brain Cerebrum Corpus callosum Encephalon **1 Cerebral Meninges** Arachnoid mater, intracranial Leptomeninges, intracranial Pia mater, intracranial **2 Dura Mater** Diaphragma sellae Dura mater, intracranial Falx cerebri Tentorium cerebelli **6 Cerebral Ventricle** Aqueduct of Sylvius Cerebral aqueduct (Sylvius) Choroid plexus Ependyma Foramen of Monro (intraventricular) Fourth ventricle Interventricular foramen (Monro) Left lateral ventricle Right lateral ventricle Third ventricle **7 Cerebral Hemisphere** Frontal lobe Occipital lobe Parietal lobe Temporal lobe **8 Basal Ganglia** Basal nuclei Claustrum Corpus striatum Globus pallidus Substantia nigra Subthalamic nucleus **9 Thalamus** Epithalamus Geniculate nucleus Metathalamus Pulvinar **A Hypothalamus** Mammillary body **B Pons** Apneustic center Basis pontis Locus ceruleus Pneumotaxic center Pontine tegmentum Superior olivary nucleus **C Cerebellum** Culmen **D Medulla Oblongata** Myelencephalon **F Olfactory Nerve** First cranial nerve Olfactory bulb **G Optic Nerve** Optic chiasma Second cranial nerve	**H Oculomotor Nerve** Third cranial nerve **J Trochlear Nerve** Fourth cranial nerve **K Trigeminal Nerve** Fifth cranial nerve Gasserian ganglion Mandibular nerve Maxillary nerve Ophthalmic nerve Trifacial nerve **L Abducens Nerve** Sixth cranial nerve **M Facial Nerve** Chorda tympani Geniculate ganglion Greater superficial petrosal nerve Nerve to the stapedius Parotid plexus Posterior auricular nerve Seventh cranial nerve Submandibular ganglion **N Acoustic Nerve** Cochlear nerve Eighth cranial nerve Scarpa's (vestibular) ganglion Spiral ganglion Vestibular (Scarpa's) ganglion Vestibular nerve Vestibulocochlear nerve **P Glossopharyngeal Nerve** Carotid sinus nerve Ninth cranial nerve Tympanic nerve **Q Vagus Nerve** Anterior vagal trunk Pharyngeal plexus Pneumogastric nerve Posterior vagal trunk Pulmonary plexus Recurrent laryngeal nerve Superior laryngeal nerve Tenth cranial nerve **R Accessory Nerve** Eleventh cranial nerve **S Hypoglossal Nerve** Twelfth cranial nerve **T Spinal Meninges** Arachnoid mater, spinal Denticulate (dentate) ligament Dura mater, spinal Filum terminale Leptomeninges, spinal Pia mater, spinal **W Cervical Spinal Cord** **X Thoracic Spinal Cord** **Y Lumbar Spinal Cord** Cauda equina Conus medullaris	**Ø** Open **3** Percutaneous **4** Percutaneous Endoscopic	**Z** No Device	**X** Diagnostic **Z** No Qualifier

Non-OR ØØB[Ø,1,2,6,7,8,9,A,B,C,D,F,G,H,J,K,L,M,N,P,Q,R,S][3,4]ZX

Ø Medical and Surgical
Ø Central Nervous System and Cranial Nerves
C Extirpation Definition: Taking or cutting out solid matter from a body part

Explanation: The solid matter may be an abnormal byproduct of a biological function or a foreign body; it may be imbedded in a body part or in the lumen of a tubular body part. The solid matter may or may not have been previously broken into pieces.

Body Part Character 4	Approach Character 5	Device Character 6	Qualifier Character 7
Ø Brain Cerebrum Corpus callosum Encephalon **1 Cerebral Meninges** Arachnoid mater, intracranial Leptomeninges, intracranial Pia mater, intracranial **2 Dura Mater** Diaphragma sellae Dura mater, intracranial Falx cerebri Tentorium cerebelli **3 Epidural Space, Intracranial** Extradural space, intracranial **4 Subdural Space, Intracranial** **5 Subarachnoid Space, Intracranial** **6 Cerebral Ventricle** Aqueduct of Sylvius Cerebral aqueduct (Sylvius) Choroid plexus Ependyma Foramen of Monro (intraventricular) Fourth ventricle Interventricular foramen (Monro) Left lateral ventricle Right lateral ventricle Third ventricle **7 Cerebral Hemisphere** Frontal lobe Occipital lobe Parietal lobe Temporal lobe **8 Basal Ganglia** Basal nuclei Claustrum Corpus striatum Globus pallidus Substantia nigra Subthalamic nucleus **9 Thalamus** Epithalamus Geniculate nucleus Metathalamus Pulvinar **A Hypothalamus** Mammillary body **B Pons** Apneustic center Basis pontis Locus ceruleus Pneumotaxic center Pontine tegmentum Superior olivary nucleus **C Cerebellum** Culmen **D Medulla Oblongata** Myelencephalon **F Olfactory Nerve** First cranial nerve Olfactory bulb **G Optic Nerve** Optic chiasma Second cranial nerve **H Oculomotor Nerve** Third cranial nerve **J Trochlear Nerve** Fourth cranial nerve **K Trigeminal Nerve** Fifth cranial nerve Gasserian ganglion Mandibular nerve Maxillary nerve Ophthalmic nerve Trifacial nerve **L Abducens Nerve** Sixth cranial nerve **M Facial Nerve** Chorda tympani Geniculate ganglion Greater superficial petrosal nerve Nerve to the stapedius Parotid plexus Posterior auricular nerve Seventh cranial nerve Submandibular ganglion **N Acoustic Nerve** Cochlear nerve Eighth cranial nerve Scarpa's (vestibular) ganglion Spiral ganglion Vestibular (Scarpa's) ganglion Vestibular nerve Vestibulocochlear nerve **P Glossopharyngeal Nerve** Carotid sinus nerve Ninth cranial nerve Tympanic nerve **Q Vagus Nerve** Anterior vagal trunk Pharyngeal plexus Pneumogastric nerve Posterior vagal trunk Pulmonary plexus Recurrent laryngeal nerve Superior laryngeal nerve Tenth cranial nerve **R Accessory Nerve** Eleventh cranial nerve **S Hypoglossal Nerve** Twelfth cranial nerve **T Spinal Meninges** Arachnoid mater, spinal Denticulate (dentate) ligament Dura mater, spinal Filum terminale Leptomeninges, spinal Pia mater, spinal **U Spinal Canal** **W Cervical Spinal Cord** **X Thoracic Spinal Cord** **Y Lumbar Spinal Cord** Cauda equina Conus medullaris	**Ø Open** **3 Percutaneous** **4 Percutaneous Endoscopic**	**Z No Device**	**Z No Qualifier**

Ø Medical and Surgical
Ø Central Nervous System and Cranial Nerves
D Extraction Definition: Pulling or stripping out or off all or a portion of a body part by the use of force
Explanation: The qualifier DIAGNOSTIC is used to identify extraction procedures that are biopsies

Body Part Character 4		Approach Character 5	Device Character 6	Qualifier Character 7
1 Cerebral Meninges Arachnoid mater, intracranial Leptomeninges, intracranial Pia mater, intracranial **2 Dura Mater** Diaphragma sellae Dura mater, intracranial Falx cerebri Tentorium cerebelli **F Olfactory Nerve** First cranial nerve Olfactory bulb **G Optic Nerve** Optic chiasma Second cranial nerve **H Oculomotor Nerve** Third cranial nerve **J Trochlear Nerve** Fourth cranial nerve **K Trigeminal Nerve** Fifth cranial nerve Gasserian ganglion Mandibular nerve Maxillary nerve Ophthalmic nerve Trifacial nerve **L Abducens Nerve** Sixth cranial nerve **M Facial Nerve** Chorda tympani Geniculate ganglion Greater superficial petrosal nerve Nerve to the stapedius Parotid plexus Posterior auricular nerve Seventh cranial nerve Submandibular ganglion	**N Acoustic Nerve** Cochlear nerve Eighth cranial nerve Scarpa's (vestibular) ganglion Spiral ganglion Vestibular (Scarpa's) ganglion Vestibular nerve Vestibulocochlear nerve **P Glossopharyngeal Nerve** Carotid sinus nerve Ninth cranial nerve Tympanic nerve **Q Vagus Nerve** Anterior vagal trunk Pharyngeal plexus Pneumogastric nerve Posterior vagal trunk Pulmonary plexus Recurrent laryngeal nerve Superior laryngeal nerve Tenth cranial nerve **R Accessory Nerve** Eleventh cranial nerve **S Hypoglossal Nerve** Twelfth cranial nerve **T Spinal Meninges** Arachnoid mater, spinal Denticulate (dentate) ligament Dura mater, spinal Filum terminale Leptomeninges, spinal Pia mater, spinal	**Ø** Open **3** Percutaneous **4** Percutaneous Endoscopic	**Z** No Device	**Z** No Qualifier

Ø Medical and Surgical
Ø Central Nervous System and Cranial Nerves
F Fragmentation Definition: Breaking solid matter in a body part into pieces
Explanation: Physical force (e.g., manual, ultrasonic) applied directly or indirectly is used to break the solid matter into pieces. The solid matter may be an abnormal byproduct of a biological function or a foreign body. The pieces of solid matter are not taken out.

Body Part Character 4	Approach Character 5	Device Character 6	Qualifier Character 7
3 Epidural Space, Intracranial NC Extradural space, intracranial **4 Subdural Space, Intracranial** NC **5 Subarachnoid Space, Intracranial** NC **6 Cerebral Ventricle** NC Aqueduct of Sylvius Cerebral aqueduct (Sylvius) Choroid plexus Ependyma Foramen of Monro (intraventricular) Fourth ventricle Interventricular foramen (Monro) Left lateral ventricle Right lateral ventricle Third ventricle **U Spinal Canal** Epidural space, spinal Extradural space, spinal Subarachnoid space, spinal Subdural space, spinal Vertebral canal	**Ø** Open **3** Percutaneous **4** Percutaneous Endoscopic **X** External	**Z** No Device	**Z** No Qualifier

Non-OR ØØF[3,4,5,6]XZZ
NC ØØF[3,4,5,6]XZZ

Ø Medical and Surgical
Ø Central Nervous System and Cranial Nerves
H Insertion Definition: Putting in a nonbiological appliance that monitors, assists, performs, or prevents a physiological function but does not physically take the place of a body part
Explanation: None

Body Part Character 4		Approach Character 5	Device Character 6	Qualifier Character 7
Ø Brain ⊞ Cerebrum Corpus callosum Encephalon		**Ø Open**	**2 Monitoring Device** **3 Infusion Device** **4 Radioactive Element, Cesium-131 Collagen Implant** **M Neurostimulator Lead** **Y Other Device**	**Z No Qualifier**
Ø Brain ⊞ Cerebrum Corpus callosum Encephalon		**3 Percutaneous** **4 Percutaneous Endoscopic**	**2 Monitoring Device** **3 Infusion Device** **M Neurostimulator Lead** **Y Other Device**	**Z No Qualifier**
6 Cerebral Ventricle ⊞ Aqueduct of Sylvius Cerebral aqueduct (Sylvius) Choroid plexus Ependyma Foramen of Monro (intraventricular) Fourth ventricle Interventricular foramen (Monro) Left lateral ventricle Right lateral ventricle Third ventricle	**E Cranial Nerve** ⊞ **U Spinal Canal** ⊞ Epidural space, spinal Extradural space, spinal Subarachnoid space, spinal Subdural space, spinal Vertebral canal **V Spinal Cord** ⊞	**Ø Open** **3 Percutaneous** **4 Percutaneous Endoscopic**	**2 Monitoring Device** **3 Infusion Device** **M Neurostimulator Lead** **Y Other Device**	**Z No Qualifier**

DRG Non-OR ØØHØØ4Z
Non-OR ØØH[E,U,V]32Z
Non-OR ØØH[E,U][3,4]YZ
Non-OR ØØH[U,V][Ø,3,4]3Z

See Appendix L for Procedure Combinations
⊞ ØØHØØMZ
⊞ ØØHØ[3,4]MZ
⊞ ØØH[6,E,U,V][Ø,3,4]MZ

Ø Medical and Surgical
Ø Central Nervous System and Cranial Nerves
J Inspection Definition: Visually and/or manually exploring a body part
Explanation: Visual exploration may be performed with or without optical instrumentation. Manual exploration may be performed directly or through intervening body layers.

Body Part Character 4		Approach Character 5	Device Character 6	Qualifier Character 7
Ø Brain Cerebrum Corpus callosum Encephalon **E Cranial Nerve**	**U Spinal Canal** Epidural space, spinal Extradural space, spinal Subarachnoid space, spinal Subdural space, spinal Vertebral canal **V Spinal Cord**	**Ø Open** **3 Percutaneous** **4 Percutaneous Endoscopic**	**Z No Device**	**Z No Qualifier**

Non-OR ØØJ[Ø,E,U,V]3ZZ

Ø Medical and Surgical
Ø Central Nervous System and Cranial Nerves
K Map Definition: Locating the route of passage of electrical impulses and/or locating functional areas in a body part
Explanation: Applicable only to the cardiac conduction mechanism and the central nervous system

Body Part Character 4		Approach Character 5	Device Character 6	Qualifier Character 7
Ø Brain Cerebrum Corpus callosum Encephalon **7 Cerebral Hemisphere** Frontal lobe Occipital lobe Parietal lobe Temporal lobe **8 Basal Ganglia** Basal nuclei Claustrum Corpus striatum Globus pallidus Substantia nigra Subthalamic nucleus	**9 Thalamus** Epithalamus Geniculate nucleus Metathalamus Pulvinar **A Hypothalamus** Mammillary body **B Pons** Apneustic center Basis pontis Locus ceruleus Pneumotaxic center Pontine tegmentum Superior olivary nucleus **C Cerebellum** Culmen **D Medulla Oblongata** Myelencephalon	**Ø Open** **3 Percutaneous** **4 Percutaneous Endoscopic**	**Z No Device**	**Z No Qualifier**

Ø Medical and Surgical
Ø Central Nervous System and Cranial Nerves
N Release Definition: Freeing a body part from an abnormal physical constraint by cutting or by the use of force
Explanation: Some of the restraining tissue may be taken out but none of the body part is taken out

Body Part Character 4	Approach Character 5	Device Character 6	Qualifier Character 7
Ø Brain Cerebrum Corpus callosum Encephalon **1 Cerebral Meninges** Arachnoid mater, intracranial Leptomeninges, intracranial Pia mater, intracranial **2 Dura Mater** Diaphragma sellae Dura mater, intracranial Falx cerebri Tentorium cerebelli **6 Cerebral Ventricle** Aqueduct of Sylvius Cerebral aqueduct (Sylvius) Choroid plexus Ependyma Foramen of Monro (intraventricular) Fourth ventricle Interventricular foramen (Monro) Left lateral ventricle Right lateral ventricle Third ventricle **7 Cerebral Hemisphere** Frontal lobe Occipital lobe Parietal lobe Temporal lobe **8 Basal Ganglia** Basal nuclei Claustrum Corpus striatum Globus pallidus Substantia nigra Subthalamic nucleus **9 Thalamus** Epithalamus Geniculate nucleus Metathalamus Pulvinar **A Hypothalamus** Mammillary body **B Pons** Apneustic center Basis pontis Locus ceruleus Pneumotaxic center Pontine tegmentum Superior olivary nucleus **C Cerebellum** Culmen **D Medulla Oblongata** Myelencephalon **F Olfactory Nerve** First cranial nerve Olfactory bulb **G Optic Nerve** Optic chiasma Second cranial nerve **H Oculomotor Nerve** Third cranial nerve **J Trochlear Nerve** Fourth cranial nerve **K Trigeminal Nerve** Fifth cranial nerve Gasserian ganglion Mandibular nerve Maxillary nerve Ophthalmic nerve Trifacial nerve **L Abducens Nerve** Sixth cranial nerve **M Facial Nerve** Chorda tympani Geniculate ganglion Greater superficial petrosal nerve Nerve to the stapedius Parotid plexus Posterior auricular nerve Seventh cranial nerve Submandibular ganglion **N Acoustic Nerve** Cochlear nerve Eighth cranial nerve Scarpa's (vestibular) ganglion Spiral ganglion Vestibular (Scarpa's) ganglion Vestibular nerve Vestibulocochlear nerve **P Glossopharyngeal Nerve** Carotid sinus nerve Ninth cranial nerve Tympanic nerve **Q Vagus Nerve** Anterior vagal trunk Pharyngeal plexus Pneumogastric nerve Posterior vagal trunk Pulmonary plexus Recurrent laryngeal nerve Superior laryngeal nerve Tenth cranial nerve **R Accessory Nerve** Eleventh cranial nerve **S Hypoglossal Nerve** Twelfth cranial nerve **T Spinal Meninges** Arachnoid mater, spinal Denticulate (dentate) ligament Dura mater, spinal Filum terminale Leptomeninges, spinal Pia mater, spinal **W Cervical Spinal Cord** **X Thoracic Spinal Cord** **Y Lumbar Spinal Cord** Cauda equina Conus medullaris	Ø Open 3 Percutaneous 4 Percutaneous Endoscopic	Z No Device	Z No Qualifier

Ø Medical and Surgical
Ø Central Nervous System and Cranial Nerves
P Removal Definition: Taking out or off a device from a body part

Explanation: If a device is taken out and a similar device put in without cutting or puncturing the skin or mucous membrane, the procedure is coded to the root operation CHANGE. Otherwise, the procedure for taking out a device is coded to the root operation REMOVAL.

Body Part Character 4	Approach Character 5	Device Character 6	Qualifier Character 7
Ø Brain Cerebrum Corpus callosum Encephalon **V** Spinal Cord	**Ø** Open **3** Percutaneous **4** Percutaneous Endoscopic	**Ø** Drainage Device **2** Monitoring Device **3** Infusion Device **7** Autologous Tissue Substitute **J** Synthetic Substitute **K** Nonautologous Tissue Substitute **M** Neurostimulator Lead **Y** Other Device	**Z** No Qualifier
Ø Brain Cerebrum Corpus callosum Encephalon **V** Spinal Cord	**X** External	**Ø** Drainage Device **2** Monitoring Device **3** Infusion Device **M** Neurostimulator Lead	**Z** No Qualifier
6 Cerebral Ventricle Aqueduct of Sylvius Cerebral aqueduct (Sylvius) Choroid plexus Ependyma Foramen of Monro (intraventricular) Fourth ventricle Interventricular foramen (Monro) Left lateral ventricle Right lateral ventricle Third ventricle **U** Spinal Canal Epidural space, spinal Extradural space, spinal Subarachnoid space, spinal Subdural space, spinal Vertebral canal	**Ø** Open **3** Percutaneous **4** Percutaneous Endoscopic	**Ø** Drainage Device **2** Monitoring Device **3** Infusion Device **J** Synthetic Substitute **M** Neurostimulator Lead **Y** Other Device	**Z** No Qualifier
6 Cerebral Ventricle Aqueduct of Sylvius Cerebral aqueduct (Sylvius) Choroid plexus Ependyma Foramen of Monro (intraventricular) Fourth ventricle Interventricular foramen (Monro) Left lateral ventricle Right lateral ventricle Third ventricle **U** Spinal Canal Epidural space, spinal Extradural space, spinal Subarachnoid space, spinal Subdural space, spinal Vertebral canal	**X** External	**Ø** Drainage Device **2** Monitoring Device **3** Infusion Device **M** Neurostimulator Lead	**Z** No Qualifier
E Cranial Nerve	**Ø** Open **3** Percutaneous **4** Percutaneous Endoscopic	**Ø** Drainage Device **2** Monitoring Device **3** Infusion Device **7** Autologous Tissue Substitute **M** Neurostimulator Lead **Y** Other Device	**Z** No Qualifier
E Cranial Nerve	**X** External	**Ø** Drainage Device **2** Monitoring Device **3** Infusion Device **M** Neurostimulator Lead	**Z** No Qualifier

Non-OR ØØP[Ø,V]3[Ø,2,3]Z
Non-OR ØØP[Ø,V][3,4]YZ
Non-OR ØØP[Ø,V]X[Ø,2,3,M]Z
Non-OR ØØP[6,U]3[Ø,2,3]Z
Non-OR ØØP[6,U][3,4]YZ
Non-OR ØØP[6,U]X[Ø,2,3,M]Z
Non-OR ØØPE3[Ø,2,3]Z
Non-OR ØØPE[3,4]YZ
Non-OR ØØPEX[Ø,2,3,M]Z

Ø Medical and Surgical
Ø Central Nervous System and Cranial Nerves
Q Repair Definition: Restoring, to the extent possible, a body part to its normal anatomic structure and function
Explanation: Used only when the method to accomplish the repair is not one of the other root operations

Body Part Character 4		Approach Character 5	Device Character 6	Qualifier Character 7
Ø Brain Cerebrum Corpus callosum Encephalon **1 Cerebral Meninges** Arachnoid mater, intracranial Leptomeninges, intracranial Pia mater, intracranial **2 Dura Mater** Diaphragma sellae Dura mater, intracranial Falx cerebri Tentorium cerebelli **6 Cerebral Ventricle** Aqueduct of Sylvius Cerebral aqueduct (Sylvius) Choroid plexus Ependyma Foramen of Monro (intraventricular) Fourth ventricle Interventricular foramen (Monro) Left lateral ventricle Right lateral ventricle Third ventricle **7 Cerebral Hemisphere** Frontal lobe Occipital lobe Parietal lobe Temporal lobe **8 Basal Ganglia** Basal nuclei Claustrum Corpus striatum Globus pallidus Substantia nigra Subthalamic nucleus **9 Thalamus** Epithalamus Geniculate nucleus Metathalamus Pulvinar **A Hypothalamus** Mammillary body **B Pons** Apneustic center Basis pontis Locus ceruleus Pneumotaxic center Pontine tegmentum Superior olivary nucleus **C Cerebellum** Culmen **D Medulla Oblongata** Myelencephalon **F Olfactory Nerve** First cranial nerve Olfactory bulb **G Optic Nerve** Optic chiasma Second cranial nerve	**H Oculomotor Nerve** Third cranial nerve **J Trochlear Nerve** Fourth cranial nerve **K Trigeminal Nerve** Fifth cranial nerve Gasserian ganglion Mandibular nerve Maxillary nerve Ophthalmic nerve Trifacial nerve **L Abducens Nerve** Sixth cranial nerve **M Facial Nerve** Chorda tympani Geniculate ganglion Greater superficial petrosal nerve Nerve to the stapedius Parotid plexus Posterior auricular nerve Seventh cranial nerve Submandibular ganglion **N Acoustic Nerve** Cochlear nerve Eighth cranial nerve Scarpa's (vestibular) ganglion Spiral ganglion Vestibular (Scarpa's) ganglion Vestibular nerve Vestibulocochlear nerve **P Glossopharyngeal Nerve** Carotid sinus nerve Ninth cranial nerve Tympanic nerve **Q Vagus Nerve** Anterior vagal trunk Pharyngeal plexus Pneumogastric nerve Posterior vagal trunk Pulmonary plexus Recurrent laryngeal nerve Superior laryngeal nerve Tenth cranial nerve **R Accessory Nerve** Eleventh cranial nerve **S Hypoglossal Nerve** Twelfth cranial nerve **T Spinal Meninges** Arachnoid mater, spinal Denticulate (dentate) ligament Dura mater, spinal Filum terminale Leptomeninges, spinal Pia mater, spinal **W Cervical Spinal Cord** **X Thoracic Spinal Cord** **Y Lumbar Spinal Cord** Cauda equina Conus medullaris	**Ø Open** **3 Percutaneous** **4 Percutaneous Endoscopic**	**Z No Device**	**Z No Qualifier**

Ø Medical and Surgical
Ø Central Nervous System and Cranial Nerves
R Replacement Definition: Putting in or on biological or synthetic material that physically takes the place and/or function of all or a portion of a body part

Explanation: The body part may have been taken out or replaced, or may be taken out, physically eradicated, or rendered nonfunctional during the REPLACEMENT procedure. A REMOVAL procedure is coded for taking out the device used in a previous replacement procedure.

Body Part Character 4		Approach Character 5	Device Character 6	Qualifier Character 7
1 Cerebral Meninges Arachnoid mater, intracranial; Leptomeninges, intracranial; Pia mater, intracranial **2 Dura Mater** Diaphragma sellae; Dura mater, intracranial; Falx cerebri; Tentorium cerebelli **6 Cerebral Ventricle** Aqueduct of Sylvius; Cerebral aqueduct (Sylvius); Choroid plexus; Ependyma; Foramen of Monro (intraventricular); Fourth ventricle; Interventricular foramen (Monro); Left lateral ventricle; Right lateral ventricle; Third ventricle **F Olfactory Nerve** First cranial nerve; Olfactory bulb **G Optic Nerve** Optic chiasma; Second cranial nerve **H Oculomotor Nerve** Third cranial nerve **J Trochlear Nerve** Fourth cranial nerve **K Trigeminal Nerve** Fifth cranial nerve; Gasserian ganglion; Mandibular nerve; Maxillary nerve; Ophthalmic nerve; Trifacial nerve **L Abducens Nerve** Sixth cranial nerve	**M Facial Nerve** Chorda tympani; Geniculate ganglion; Greater superficial petrosal nerve; Nerve to the stapedius; Parotid plexus; Posterior auricular nerve; Seventh cranial nerve; Submandibular ganglion **N Acoustic Nerve** Cochlear nerve; Eighth cranial nerve; Scarpa's (vestibular) ganglion; Spiral ganglion; Vestibular (Scarpa's) ganglion; Vestibular nerve; Vestibulocochlear nerve **P Glossopharyngeal Nerve** Carotid sinus nerve; Ninth cranial nerve; Tympanic nerve **Q Vagus Nerve** Anterior vagal trunk; Pharyngeal plexus; Pneumogastric nerve; Posterior vagal trunk; Pulmonary plexus; Recurrent laryngeal nerve; Superior laryngeal nerve; Tenth cranial nerve **R Accessory Nerve** Eleventh cranial nerve **S Hypoglossal Nerve** Twelfth cranial nerve **T Spinal Meninges** Arachnoid mater, spinal; Denticulate (dentate) ligament; Dura mater, spinal; Filum terminale; Leptomeninges, spinal; Pia mater, spinal	**Ø Open** **4 Percutaneous Endoscopic**	**7 Autologous Tissue Substitute** **J Synthetic Substitute** **K Nonautologous Tissue Substitute**	**Z No Qualifier**

0 Medical and Surgical
0 Central Nervous System and Cranial Nerves
S Reposition Definition: Moving to its normal location, or other suitable location, all or a portion of a body part

Explanation: The body part is moved to a new location from an abnormal location, or from a normal location where it is not functioning correctly. The body part may or may not be cut out or off to be moved to the new location.

Body Part Character 4		Approach Character 5	Device Character 6	Qualifier Character 7
F Olfactory Nerve First cranial nerve Olfactory bulb **G Optic Nerve** Optic chiasma Second cranial nerve **H Oculomotor Nerve** Third cranial nerve **J Trochlear Nerve** Fourth cranial nerve **K Trigeminal Nerve** Fifth cranial nerve Gasserian ganglion Mandibular nerve Maxillary nerve Ophthalmic nerve Trifacial nerve **L Abducens Nerve** Sixth cranial nerve **M Facial Nerve** Chorda tympani Geniculate ganglion Greater superficial petrosal nerve Nerve to the stapedius Parotid plexus Posterior auricular nerve Seventh cranial nerve Submandibular ganglion	**N Acoustic Nerve** Cochlear nerve Eighth cranial nerve Scarpa's (vestibular) ganglion Spiral ganglion Vestibular (Scarpa's) ganglion Vestibular nerve Vestibulocochlear nerve **P Glossopharyngeal Nerve** Carotid sinus nerve Ninth cranial nerve Tympanic nerve **Q Vagus Nerve** Anterior vagal trunk Pharyngeal plexus Pneumogastric nerve Posterior vagal trunk Pulmonary plexus Recurrent laryngeal nerve Superior laryngeal nerve Tenth cranial nerve **R Accessory Nerve** Eleventh cranial nerve **S Hypoglossal Nerve** Twelfth cranial nerve **W Cervical Spinal Cord** **X Thoracic Spinal Cord** **Y Lumbar Spinal Cord** Cauda equina Conus medullaris	**0 Open** **3 Percutaneous** **4 Percutaneous Endoscopic**	**Z No Device**	**Z No Qualifier**

0 Medical and Surgical
0 Central Nervous System and Cranial Nerves
T Resection Definition: Cutting out or off, without replacement, all of a body part

Explanation: None

Body Part Character 4	Approach Character 5	Device Character 6	Qualifier Character 7
7 Cerebral Hemisphere Frontal lobe Occipital lobe Parietal lobe Temporal lobe	**0 Open** **3 Percutaneous** **4 Percutaneous Endoscopic**	**Z No Device**	**Z No Qualifier**

Central Nervous System and Cranial Nerves

Ø Medical and Surgical
Ø Central Nervous System and Cranial Nerves
U Supplement Definition: Putting in or on biological or synthetic material that physically reinforces and/or augments the function of a portion of a body part

Explanation: The biological material is non-living, or is living and from the same individual. The body part may have been previously replaced, and the SUPPLEMENT procedure is performed to physically reinforce and/or augment the function of the replaced body part.

Body Part Character 4	Approach Character 5	Device Character 6	Qualifier Character 7
1 Cerebral Meninges Arachnoid mater, intracranial Leptomeninges, intracranial Pia mater, intracranial **2 Dura Mater** Diaphragma sellae Dura mater, intracranial Falx cerebri Tentorium cerebelli **6 Cerebral Ventricle** Aqueduct of Sylvius Cerebral aqueduct (Sylvius) Choroid plexus Ependyma Foramen of Monro (intraventricular) Fourth ventricle Interventricular foramen (Monro) Left lateral ventricle Right lateral ventricle Third ventricle **F Olfactory Nerve** First cranial nerve Olfactory bulb **G Optic Nerve** Optic chiasma Second cranial nerve **H Oculomotor Nerve** Third cranial nerve **J Trochlear Nerve** Fourth cranial nerve **K Trigeminal Nerve** Fifth cranial nerve Gasserian ganglion Mandibular nerve Maxillary nerve Ophthalmic nerve Trifacial nerve **L Abducens Nerve** Sixth cranial nerve **M Facial Nerve** Chorda tympani Geniculate ganglion Greater superficial petrosal nerve Nerve to the stapedius Parotid plexus Posterior auricular nerve Seventh cranial nerve Submandibular ganglion **N Acoustic Nerve** Cochlear nerve Eighth cranial nerve Scarpa's (vestibular) ganglion Spiral ganglion Vestibular (Scarpa's) ganglion Vestibular nerve Vestibulocochlear nerve **P Glossopharyngeal Nerve** Carotid sinus nerve Ninth cranial nerve Tympanic nerve **Q Vagus Nerve** Anterior vagal trunk Pharyngeal plexus Pneumogastric nerve Posterior vagal trunk Pulmonary plexus Recurrent laryngeal nerve Superior laryngeal nerve Tenth cranial nerve **R Accessory Nerve** Eleventh cranial nerve **S Hypoglossal Nerve** Twelfth cranial nerve **T Spinal Meninges** Arachnoid mater, spinal Denticulate (dentate) ligament Dura mater, spinal Filum terminale Leptomeninges, spinal Pia mater, spinal	**Ø Open** **3 Percutaneous** **4 Percutaneous Endoscopic**	**7 Autologous Tissue Substitute** **J Synthetic Substitute** **K Nonautologous Tissue Substitute**	**Z No Qualifier**

Ø Medical and Surgical
Ø Central Nervous System and Cranial Nerves
W Revision Definition: Correcting, to the extent possible, a portion of a malfunctioning device or the position of a displaced device

Explanation: Revision can include correcting a malfunctioning or displaced device by taking out or putting in components of the device such as a screw or pin

Body Part Character 4	Approach Character 5	Device Character 6	Qualifier Character 7
Ø Brain Cerebrum Corpus callosum Encephalon V Spinal Cord	Ø Open 3 Percutaneous 4 Percutaneous Endoscopic	Ø Drainage Device 2 Monitoring Device 3 Infusion Device 7 Autologous Tissue Substitute J Synthetic Substitute K Nonautologous Tissue Substitute M Neurostimulator Lead Y Other Device	Z No Qualifier
Ø Brain Cerebrum Corpus callosum Encephalon V Spinal Cord	X External	Ø Drainage Device 2 Monitoring Device 3 Infusion Device 7 Autologous Tissue Substitute J Synthetic Substitute K Nonautologous Tissue Substitute M Neurostimulator Lead	Z No Qualifier
6 Cerebral Ventricle Aqueduct of Sylvius Cerebral aqueduct (Sylvius) Choroid plexus Ependyma Foramen of Monro (intraventricular) Fourth ventricle Interventricular foramen (Monro) Left lateral ventricle Right lateral ventricle Third ventricle U Spinal Canal Epidural space, spinal Extradural space, spinal Subarachnoid space, spinal Subdural space, spinal Vertebral canal	Ø Open 3 Percutaneous 4 Percutaneous Endoscopic	Ø Drainage Device 2 Monitoring Device 3 Infusion Device J Synthetic Substitute M Neurostimulator Lead Y Other Device	Z No Qualifier
6 Cerebral Ventricle Aqueduct of Sylvius Cerebral aqueduct (Sylvius) Choroid plexus Ependyma Foramen of Monro (intraventricular) Fourth ventricle Interventricular foramen (Monro) Left lateral ventricle Right lateral ventricle Third ventricle U Spinal Canal Epidural space, spinal Extradural space, spinal Subarachnoid space, spinal Subdural space, spinal Vertebral canal	X External	Ø Drainage Device 2 Monitoring Device 3 Infusion Device J Synthetic Substitute M Neurostimulator Lead	Z No Qualifier
E Cranial Nerve	Ø Open 3 Percutaneous 4 Percutaneous Endoscopic	Ø Drainage Device 2 Monitoring Device 3 Infusion Device 7 Autologous Tissue Substitute M Neurostimulator Lead Y Other Device	Z No Qualifier
E Cranial Nerve	X External	Ø Drainage Device 2 Monitoring Device 3 Infusion Device 7 Autologous Tissue Substitute M Neurostimulator Lead	Z No Qualifier

Non-OR ØØW[Ø,V][3,4]YZ
Non-OR ØØW[Ø,V]X[Ø,2,3,7,J,K,M]Z
Non-OR ØØW[6,U][3,4]YZ
Non-OR ØØW[6,U]X[Ø,2,3,J,M]Z
Non-OR ØØWE[3,4]YZ
Non-OR ØØWEX[Ø,2,3,7,M]Z

Ø Medical and Surgical
Ø Central Nervous System and Cranial Nerves
X Transfer Definition: Moving, without taking out, all or a portion of a body part to another location to take over the function of all or a portion of a body part
Explanation: The body part transferred remains connected to its vascular and nervous supply

Body Part Character 4	Approach Character 5	Device Character 6	Qualifier Character 7
F Olfactory Nerve First cranial nerve Olfactory bulb **G Optic Nerve** Optic chiasma Second cranial nerve **H Oculomotor Nerve** Third cranial nerve **J Trochlear Nerve** Fourth cranial nerve **K Trigeminal Nerve** Fifth cranial nerve Gasserian ganglion Mandibular nerve Maxillary nerve Ophthalmic nerve Trifacial nerve **L Abducens Nerve** Sixth cranial nerve **M Facial Nerve** Chorda tympani Geniculate ganglion Greater superficial petrosal nerve Nerve to the stapedius Parotid plexus Posterior auricular nerve Seventh cranial nerve Submandibular ganglion **N Acoustic Nerve** Cochlear nerve Eighth cranial nerve Scarpa's (vestibular) ganglion Spiral ganglion Vestibular (Scarpa's) ganglion Vestibular nerve Vestibulocochlear nerve **P Glossopharyngeal Nerve** Carotid sinus nerve Ninth cranial nerve Tympanic nerve **Q Vagus Nerve** Anterior vagal trunk Pharyngeal plexus Pneumogastric nerve Posterior vagal trunk Pulmonary plexus Recurrent laryngeal nerve Superior laryngeal nerve Tenth cranial nerve **R Accessory Nerve** Eleventh cranial nerve **S Hypoglossal Nerve** Twelfth cranial nerve	Ø Open 4 Percutaneous Endoscopic	Z No Device	F Olfactory Nerve G Optic Nerve H Oculomotor Nerve J Trochlear Nerve K Trigeminal Nerve L Abducens Nerve M Facial Nerve N Acoustic Nerve P Glossopharyngeal Nerve Q Vagus Nerve R Accessory Nerve S Hypoglossal Nerve

Peripheral Nervous System Ø12–Ø1X

Character Meanings

This Character Meaning table is provided as a guide to assist the user in the identification of character members that may be found in this section of code tables. It **SHOULD NOT** be used to build a PCS code.

Operation–Character 3	Body Part–Character 4	Approach–Character 5	Device–Character 6	Qualifier–Character 7
2 Change	Ø Cervical Plexus	Ø Open	Ø Drainage Device	1 Cervical Nerve
5 Destruction	1 Cervical Nerve	3 Percutaneous	2 Monitoring Device	2 Phrenic Nerve
8 Division	2 Phrenic Nerve	4 Percutaneous Endoscopic	7 Autologous Tissue Substitute	4 Ulnar Nerve
9 Drainage	3 Brachial Plexus	X External	M Neurostimulator Lead	5 Median Nerve
B Excision	4 Ulnar Nerve		Y Other Device	6 Radial Nerve
C Extirpation	5 Median Nerve		Z No Device	8 Thoracic Nerve
D Extraction	6 Radial Nerve			B Lumbar Nerve
H Insertion	8 Thoracic Nerve			C Perineal Nerve
J Inspection	9 Lumbar Plexus			D Femoral Nerve
N Release	A Lumbosacral Plexus			F Sciatic Nerve
P Removal	B Lumbar Nerve			G Tibial Nerve
Q Repair	C Pudendal Nerve			H Peroneal Nerve
R Replacement	D Femoral Nerve			X Diagnostic
S Reposition	F Sciatic Nerve			Z No Qualifier
U Supplement	G Tibial Nerve			
W Revision	H Peroneal Nerve			
X Transfer	K Head and Neck Sympathetic Nerve			
	L Thoracic Sympathetic Nerve			
	M Abdominal Sympathetic Nerve			
	N Lumbar Sympathetic Nerve			
	P Sacral Sympathetic Nerve			
	Q Sacral Plexus			
	R Sacral Nerve			
	Y Peripheral Nerve			

AHA Coding Clinic for table Ø1B

2018, 2Q, 22 Excision of synovial cyst
2017, 2Q, 19 Thoracic outlet decompression with sympathectomy

AHA Coding Clinic for table Ø1N

2018, 2Q, 22 Excision of synovial cyst
2017, 2Q, 19 Thoracic outlet decompression with sympathectomy
2016, 2Q, 16 Decompressive laminectomy/foraminotomy and lumbar discectomy
2016, 2Q, 17 Removal of longitudinal ligament to decompress cervical nerve root
2016, 2Q, 23 Thoracic outlet syndrome and release of brachial plexus
2015, 2Q, 34 Decompressive laminectomy
2014, 3Q, 33 Radial fracture treatment with open reduction internal fixation, and release of carpal ligament

AHA Coding Clinic for table Ø1U

2017, 4Q, 62 Added and revised device values - Nerve substitutes

Median and Ulnar Nerves

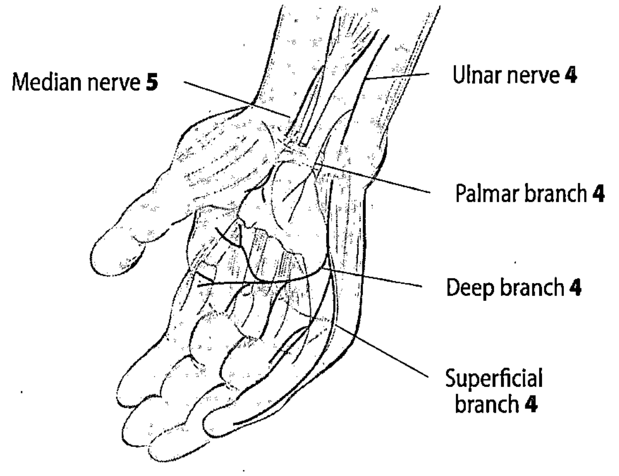

Peripheral Nervous System

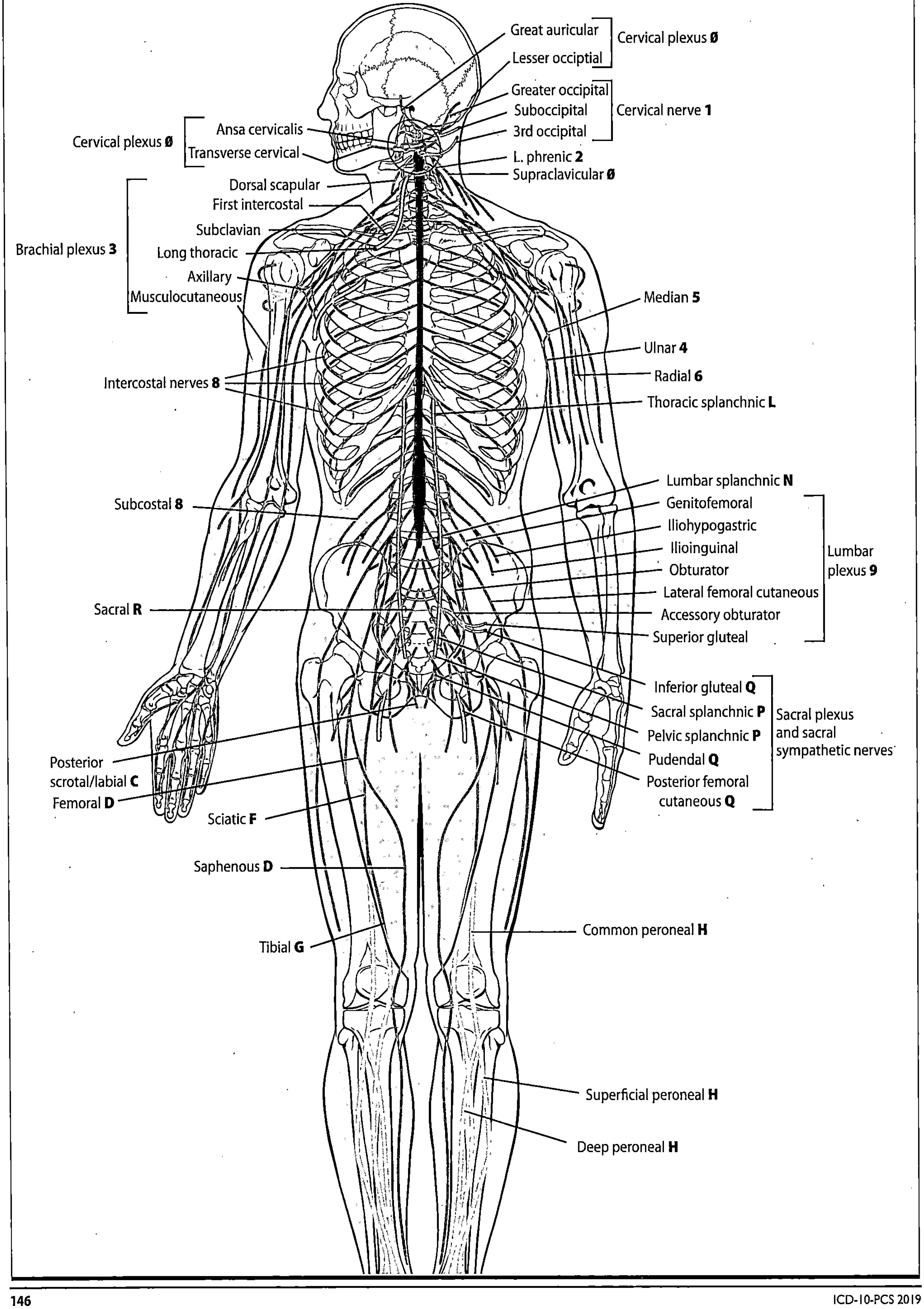
Great auricular
Lesser occiptial
Cervical plexus Ø
Greater occipital
Suboccipital
3rd occipital
Cervical nerve 1
Cervical plexus Ø
Ansa cervicalis
Transverse cervical
L. phrenic 2
Supraclavicular Ø
Dorsal scapular
First intercostal
Subclavian
Brachial plexus 3
Long thoracic
Axillary
Musculocutaneous
Median 5
Ulnar 4
Radial 6
Intercostal nerves 8
Thoracic splanchnic L
Lumbar splanchnic N
Genitofemoral
Iliohypogastric
Ilioinguinal
Obturator
Lateral femoral cutaneous
Accessory obturator
Superior gluteal
Lumbar plexus 9
Subcostal 8
Sacral R
Inferior gluteal Q
Sacral splanchnic P
Pelvic splanchnic P
Pudendal Q
Posterior femoral cutaneous Q
Sacral plexus and sacral sympathetic nerves
Posterior scrotal/labial C
Femoral D
Sciatic F
Saphenous D
Common peroneal H
Tibial G
Superficial peroneal H
Deep peroneal H

Ø Medical and Surgical
1 Peripheral Nervous System
2 Change Definition: Taking out or off a device from a body part and putting back an identical or similar device in or on the same body part without cutting or puncturing the skin or a mucous membrane

Explanation: All CHANGE procedures are coded using the approach EXTERNAL

Body Part Character 4	Approach Character 5	Device Character 6	Qualifier Character 7
Y Peripheral Nerve	X External	Ø Drainage Device Y Other Device	Z No Qualifier

Non-OR All body part, approach, device, and qualifier values

Ø Medical and Surgical
1 Peripheral Nervous System
5 Destruction

Definition: Physical eradication of all or a portion of a body part by the direct use of energy, force, or a destructive agent

Explanation: None of the body part is physically taken out

Body Part Character 4	Approach Character 5	Device Character 6	Qualifier Character 7
Ø Cervical Plexus Ansa cervicalis Cutaneous (transverse) cervical nerve Great auricular nerve Lesser occipital nerve Supraclavicular nerve Transverse (cutaneous) cervical nerve **1 Cervical Nerve** Greater occipital nerve Spinal nerve, cervical Suboccipital nerve Third occipital nerve **2 Phrenic Nerve** Accessory phrenic nerve **3 Brachial Plexus** Axillary nerve Dorsal scapular nerve First intercostal nerve Long thoracic nerve Musculocutaneous nerve Subclavius nerve Suprascapular nerve **4 Ulnar Nerve** Cubital nerve **5 Median Nerve** Anterior interosseous nerve Palmar cutaneous nerve **6 Radial Nerve** Dorsal digital nerve Musculospiral nerve Palmar cutaneous nerve Posterior interosseous nerve **8 Thoracic Nerve** Intercostal nerve Intercostobrachial nerve Spinal nerve, thoracic Subcostal nerve **9 Lumbar Plexus** Accessory obturator nerve Genitofemoral nerve Iliohypogastric nerve Ilioinguinal nerve Lateral femoral cutaneous nerve Obturator nerve Superior gluteal nerve **A Lumbosacral Plexus** **B Lumbar Nerve** Lumbosacral trunk Spinal nerve, lumbar Superior clunic (cluneal) nerve **C Pudendal Nerve** Posterior labial nerve Posterior scrotal nerve **D Femoral Nerve** Anterior crural nerve Saphenous nerve **F Sciatic Nerve** Ischiatic nerve **G Tibial Nerve** Lateral plantar nerve Medial plantar nerve Medial popliteal nerve Medial sural cutaneous nerve **H Peroneal Nerve** Common fibular nerve Common peroneal nerve External popliteal nerve Lateral sural cutaneous nerve **K Head and Neck Sympathetic Nerve** Cavernous plexus Cervical ganglion Ciliary ganglion Internal carotid plexus Otic ganglion Pterygopalatine (sphenopalatine) ganglion Sphenopalatine (pterygopalatine) ganglion Stellate ganglion Submandibular ganglion Submaxillary ganglion **L Thoracic Sympathetic Nerve** Cardiac plexus Esophageal plexus Greater splanchnic nerve Inferior cardiac nerve Least splanchnic nerve Lesser splanchnic nerve Middle cardiac nerve Pulmonary plexus Superior cardiac nerve Thoracic aortic plexus Thoracic ganglion **M Abdominal Sympathetic Nerve** Abdominal aortic plexus Auerbach's (myenteric) plexus Celiac (solar) plexus Celiac ganglion Gastric plexus Hepatic plexus Inferior hypogastric plexus Inferior mesenteric ganglion Inferior mesenteric plexus Meissner's (submucous) plexus Myenteric (Auerbach's) plexus Pancreatic plexus Pelvic splanchnic nerve Renal plexus Solar (celiac) plexus Splenic plexus Submucous (Meissner's) plexus Superior hypogastric plexus Superior mesenteric ganglion Superior mesenteric plexus Suprarenal plexus **N Lumbar Sympathetic Nerve** Lumbar ganglion Lumbar splanchnic nerve **P Sacral Sympathetic Nerve** Ganglion impar (ganglion of Walther) Pelvic splanchnic nerve Sacral ganglion Sacral splanchnic nerve **Q Sacral Plexus** Inferior gluteal nerve Posterior femoral cutaneous nerve Pudendal nerve **R Sacral Nerve** Spinal nerve, sacral	Ø Open 3 Percutaneous 4 Percutaneous Endoscopic	Z No Device	Z No Qualifier

Non-OR Ø15[Ø,2,3,4,5,6,9,A,C,D,F,G,H,Q][Ø,3,4]ZZ Non-OR Ø15[1,8,B,R]3ZZ

0 Medical and Surgical
1 Peripheral Nervous System
8 Division Definition: Cutting into a body part, without draining fluids and/or gases from the body part, in order to separate or transect a body part
Explanation: All or a portion of the body part is separated into two or more portions

Body Part Character 4	Approach Character 5	Device Character 6	Qualifier Character 7
0 Cervical Plexus Ansa cervicalis Cutaneous (transverse) cervical nerve Great auricular nerve Lesser occipital nerve Supraclavicular nerve Transverse (cutaneous) cervical nerve **1 Cervical Nerve** Greater occipital nerve Spinal nerve, cervical Suboccipital nerve Third occipital nerve **2 Phrenic Nerve** Accessory phrenic nerve **3 Brachial Plexus** Axillary nerve Dorsal scapular nerve First intercostal nerve Long thoracic nerve Musculocutaneous nerve Subclavius nerve Suprascapular nerve **4 Ulnar Nerve** Cubital nerve **5 Median Nerve** Anterior interosseous nerve Palmar cutaneous nerve **6 Radial Nerve** Dorsal digital nerve Musculospiral nerve Palmar cutaneous nerve Posterior interosseous nerve **8 Thoracic Nerve** Intercostal nerve Intercostobrachial nerve Spinal nerve, thoracic Subcostal nerve **9 Lumbar Plexus** Accessory obturator nerve Genitofemoral nerve Iliohypogastric nerve Ilioinguinal nerve Lateral femoral cutaneous nerve Obturator nerve Superior gluteal nerve **A Lumbosacral Plexus** **B Lumbar Nerve** Lumbosacral trunk Spinal nerve, lumbar Superior clunic (cluneal) nerve **C Pudendal Nerve** Posterior labial nerve Posterior scrotal nerve **D Femoral Nerve** Anterior crural nerve Saphenous nerve **F Sciatic Nerve** Ischiatic nerve **G Tibial Nerve** Lateral plantar nerve Medial plantar nerve Medial popliteal nerve Medial sural cutaneous nerve **H Peroneal Nerve** Common fibular nerve Common peroneal nerve External popliteal nerve Lateral sural cutaneous nerve **K Head and Neck Sympathetic Nerve** Cavernous plexus Cervical ganglion Ciliary ganglion Internal carotid plexus Otic ganglion Pterygopalatine (sphenopalatine) ganglion Sphenopalatine (pterygopalatine) ganglion Stellate ganglion Submandibular ganglion Submaxillary ganglion **L Thoracic Sympathetic Nerve** Cardiac plexus Esophageal plexus Greater splanchnic nerve Inferior cardiac nerve Least splanchnic nerve Lesser splanchnic nerve Middle cardiac nerve Pulmonary plexus Superior cardiac nerve Thoracic aortic plexus Thoracic ganglion **M Abdominal Sympathetic Nerve** Abdominal aortic plexus Auerbach's (myenteric) plexus Celiac (solar) plexus Celiac ganglion Gastric plexus Hepatic plexus Inferior hypogastric plexus Inferior mesenteric ganglion Inferior mesenteric plexus Meissner's (submucous) plexus Myenteric (Auerbach's) plexus Pancreatic plexus Pelvic splanchnic nerve Renal plexus Solar (celiac) plexus Splenic plexus Submucous (Meissner's) plexus Superior hypogastric plexus Superior mesenteric ganglion Superior mesenteric plexus Suprarenal plexus **N Lumbar Sympathetic Nerve** Lumbar ganglion Lumbar splanchnic nerve **P Sacral Sympathetic Nerve** Ganglion impar (ganglion of Walther) Pelvic splanchnic nerve Sacral ganglion Sacral splanchnic nerve **Q Sacral Plexus** Inferior gluteal nerve Posterior femoral cutaneous nerve Pudendal nerve **R Sacral Nerve** Spinal nerve, sacral	**0 Open** **3 Percutaneous** **4 Percutaneous Endoscopic**	**Z No Device**	**Z No Qualifier**

Ø Medical and Surgical
1 Peripheral Nervous System
9 Drainage Definition: Taking or letting out fluids and/or gases from a body part
Explanation: The qualifier DIAGNOSTIC is used to identify drainage procedures that are biopsies

Body Part Character 4	Approach Character 5	Device Character 6	Qualifier Character 7
Ø Cervical Plexus Ansa cervicalis; Cutaneous (transverse) cervical nerve; Great auricular nerve; Lesser occipital nerve; Supraclavicular nerve; Transverse (cutaneous) cervical nerve **1 Cervical Nerve** Greater occipital nerve; Spinal nerve, cervical; Suboccipital nerve; Third occipital nerve **2 Phrenic Nerve** Accessory phrenic nerve **3 Brachial Plexus** Axillary nerve; Dorsal scapular nerve; First intercostal nerve; Long thoracic nerve; Musculocutaneous nerve; Subclavius nerve; Suprascapular nerve **4 Ulnar Nerve** Cubital nerve **5 Median Nerve** Anterior interosseous nerve; Palmar cutaneous nerve **6 Radial Nerve** Dorsal digital nerve; Musculospiral nerve; Palmar cutaneous nerve; Posterior interosseous nerve **8 Thoracic Nerve** Intercostal nerve; Intercostobrachial nerve; Spinal nerve, thoracic; Subcostal nerve **9 Lumbar Plexus** Accessory obturator nerve; Genitofemoral nerve; Iliohypogastric nerve; Ilioinguinal nerve; Lateral femoral cutaneous nerve; Obturator nerve; Superior gluteal nerve **A Lumbosacral Plexus** **B Lumbar Nerve** Lumbosacral trunk; Spinal nerve, lumbar; Superior clunic (cluneal) nerve **C Pudendal Nerve** Posterior labial nerve; Posterior scrotal nerve **D Femoral Nerve** Anterior crural nerve; Saphenous nerve **F Sciatic Nerve** Ischiatic nerve **G Tibial Nerve** Lateral plantar nerve; Medial plantar nerve; Medial popliteal nerve; Medial sural cutaneous nerve **H Peroneal Nerve** Common fibular nerve; Common peroneal nerve; External popliteal nerve; Lateral sural cutaneous nerve **K Head and Neck Sympathetic Nerve** Cavernous plexus; Cervical ganglion; Ciliary ganglion; Internal carotid plexus; Otic ganglion; Pterygopalatine (sphenopalatine) ganglion; Sphenopalatine (pterygopalatine) ganglion; Stellate ganglion; Submandibular ganglion; Submaxillary ganglion **L Thoracic Sympathetic Nerve** Cardiac plexus; Esophageal plexus; Greater splanchnic nerve; Inferior cardiac nerve; Least splanchnic nerve; Lesser splanchnic nerve; Middle cardiac nerve; Pulmonary plexus; Superior cardiac nerve; Thoracic aortic plexus; Thoracic ganglion **M Abdominal Sympathetic Nerve** Abdominal aortic plexus; Auerbach's (myenteric) plexus; Celiac (solar) plexus; Celiac ganglion; Gastric plexus; Hepatic plexus; Inferior hypogastric plexus; Inferior mesenteric ganglion; Inferior mesenteric plexus; Meissner's (submucous) plexus; Myenteric (Auerbach's) plexus; Pancreatic plexus; Pelvic splanchnic nerve; Renal plexus; Solar (celiac) plexus; Splenic plexus; Submucous (Meissner's) plexus; Superior hypogastric plexus; Superior mesenteric ganglion; Superior mesenteric plexus; Suprarenal plexus **N Lumbar Sympathetic Nerve** Lumbar ganglion; Lumbar splanchnic nerve **P Sacral Sympathetic Nerve** Ganglion impar (ganglion of Walther); Pelvic splanchnic nerve; Sacral ganglion; Sacral splanchnic nerve **Q Sacral Plexus** Inferior gluteal nerve; Posterior femoral cutaneous nerve; Pudendal nerve **R Sacral Nerve** Spinal nerve, sacral	Ø Open 3 Percutaneous 4 Percutaneous Endoscopic	Ø Drainage Device	Z No Qualifier

Ø19 Continued on next page

Non-OR Ø19[Ø,1,2,3,4,5,6,8,9,A,B,C,D,F,G,H,K,L,M,N,P,Q,R]3ØZ

Peripheral Nervous System

Ø19 Continued

Ø Medical and Surgical
1 Peripheral Nervous System
9 Drainage Definition: Taking or letting out fluids and/or gases from a body part
Explanation: The qualifier DIAGNOSTIC is used to identify drainage procedures that are biopsies

Body Part Character 4	Approach Character 5	Device Character 6	Qualifier Character 7
Ø Cervical Plexus Ansa cervicalis Cutaneous (transverse) cervical nerve Great auricular nerve Lesser occipital nerve Supraclavicular nerve Transverse (cutaneous) cervical nerve **1 Cervical Nerve** Greater occipital nerve Spinal nerve, cervical Suboccipital nerve Third occipital nerve **2 Phrenic Nerve** Accessory phrenic nerve **3 Brachial Plexus** Axillary nerve Dorsal scapular nerve First intercostal nerve Long thoracic nerve Musculocutaneous nerve Subclavius nerve Suprascapular nerve **4 Ulnar Nerve** Cubital nerve **5 Median Nerve** Anterior interosseous nerve Palmar cutaneous nerve **6 Radial Nerve** Dorsal digital nerve Musculospiral nerve Palmar cutaneous nerve Posterior interosseous nerve **8 Thoracic Nerve** Intercostal nerve Intercostobrachial nerve Spinal nerve, thoracic Subcostal nerve **9 Lumbar Plexus** Accessory obturator nerve Genitofemoral nerve Iliohypogastric nerve Ilioinguinal nerve Lateral femoral cutaneous nerve Obturator nerve Superior gluteal nerve **A Lumbosacral Plexus** **B Lumbar Nerve** Lumbosacral trunk Spinal nerve, lumbar Superior clunic (cluneal) nerve **C Pudendal Nerve** Posterior labial nerve Posterior scrotal nerve **D Femoral Nerve** Anterior crural nerve Saphenous nerve **F Sciatic Nerve** Ischiatic nerve **G Tibial Nerve** Lateral plantar nerve Medial plantar nerve Medial popliteal nerve Medial sural cutaneous nerve **H Peroneal Nerve** Common fibular nerve Common peroneal nerve External popliteal nerve Lateral sural cutaneous nerve **K Head and Neck Sympathetic Nerve** Cavernous plexus Cervical ganglion Ciliary ganglion Internal carotid plexus Otic ganglion Pterygopalatine (sphenopalatine) ganglion Sphenopalatine (pterygopalatine) ganglion Stellate ganglion Submandibular ganglion Submaxillary ganglion **L Thoracic Sympathetic Nerve** Cardiac plexus Esophageal plexus Greater splanchnic nerve Inferior cardiac nerve Least splanchnic nerve Lesser splanchnic nerve Middle cardiac nerve Pulmonary plexus Superior cardiac nerve Thoracic aortic plexus Thoracic ganglion **M Abdominal Sympathetic Nerve** Abdominal aortic plexus Auerbach's (myenteric) plexus Celiac (solar) plexus Celiac ganglion Gastric plexus Hepatic plexus Inferior hypogastric plexus Inferior mesenteric ganglion Inferior mesenteric plexus Meissner's (submucous) plexus Myenteric (Auerbach's) plexus Pancreatic plexus Pelvic splanchnic nerve Renal plexus Solar (celiac) plexus Splenic plexus Submucous (Meissner's) plexus Superior hypogastric plexus Superior mesenteric ganglion Superior mesenteric plexus Suprarenal plexus **N Lumbar Sympathetic Nerve** Lumbar ganglion Lumbar splanchnic nerve **P Sacral Sympathetic Nerve** Ganglion impar (ganglion of Walther) Pelvic splanchnic nerve Sacral ganglion Sacral splanchnic nerve **Q Sacral Plexus** Inferior gluteal nerve Posterior femoral cutaneous nerve Pudendal nerve **R Sacral Nerve** Spinal nerve, sacral	**Ø Open** **3 Percutaneous** **4 Percutaneous Endoscopic**	**Z No Device**	**X Diagnostic** **Z No Qualifier**

Non-OR Ø19[Ø,1,2,3,4,5,6,8,9,A,B,C,D,F,G,H,Q,R][3,4]ZX
Non-OR Ø19[Ø,1,2,3,4,5,6,8,9,A,B,C,D,F,G,H,K,L,M,N,P,Q,R]3ZZ

Ø19–Ø19

Ø Medical and Surgical
1 Peripheral Nervous System
B Excision Definition: Cutting out or off, without replacement, a portion of a body part
Explanation: The qualifier DIAGNOSTIC is used to identify excision procedures that are biopsies

Body Part Character 4	Approach Character 5	Device Character 6	Qualifier Character 7
Ø Cervical Plexus Ansa cervicalis Cutaneous (transverse) cervical nerve Great auricular nerve Lesser occipital nerve Supraclavicular nerve Transverse (cutaneous) cervical nerve **1 Cervical Nerve** Greater occipital nerve Spinal nerve, cervical Suboccipital nerve Third occipital nerve **2 Phrenic Nerve** Accessory phrenic nerve **3 Brachial Plexus** Axillary nerve Dorsal scapular nerve First intercostal nerve Long thoracic nerve Musculocutaneous nerve Subclavius nerve Suprascapular nerve **4 Ulnar Nerve** Cubital nerve **5 Median Nerve** Anterior interosseous nerve Palmar cutaneous nerve **6 Radial Nerve** Dorsal digital nerve Musculospiral nerve Palmar cutaneous nerve Posterior interosseous nerve **8 Thoracic Nerve** Intercostal nerve Intercostobrachial nerve Spinal nerve, thoracic Subcostal nerve **9 Lumbar Plexus** Accessory obturator nerve Genitofemoral nerve Iliohypogastric nerve Ilioinguinal nerve Lateral femoral cutaneous nerve Obturator nerve Superior gluteal nerve **A Lumbosacral Plexus** **B Lumbar Nerve** Lumbosacral trunk Spinal nerve, lumbar Superior clunic (cluneal) nerve **C Pudendal Nerve** Posterior labial nerve Posterior scrotal nerve **D Femoral Nerve** Anterior crural nerve Saphenous nerve **F Sciatic Nerve** Ischiatic nerve **G Tibial Nerve** Lateral plantar nerve Medial plantar nerve Medial popliteal nerve Medial sural cutaneous nerve **H Peroneal Nerve** Common fibular nerve Common peroneal nerve External popliteal nerve Lateral sural cutaneous nerve **K Head and Neck Sympathetic Nerve** Cavernous plexus Cervical ganglion Ciliary ganglion Internal carotid plexus Otic ganglion Pterygopalatine (sphenopalatine) ganglion Sphenopalatine (pterygopalatine) ganglion Stellate ganglion Submandibular ganglion Submaxillary ganglion **L Thoracic Sympathetic Nerve** Cardiac plexus Esophageal plexus Greater splanchnic nerve Inferior cardiac nerve Least splanchnic nerve Lesser splanchnic nerve Middle cardiac nerve Pulmonary plexus Superior cardiac nerve Thoracic aortic plexus Thoracic ganglion **M Abdominal Sympathetic Nerve** Abdominal aortic plexus Auerbach's (myenteric) plexus Celiac (solar) plexus Celiac ganglion Gastric plexus Hepatic plexus Inferior hypogastric plexus Inferior mesenteric ganglion Inferior mesenteric plexus Meissner's (submucous) plexus Myenteric (Auerbach's) plexus Pancreatic plexus Pelvic splanchnic nerve Renal plexus Solar (celiac) plexus Splenic plexus Submucous (Meissner's) plexus Superior hypogastric plexus Superior mesenteric ganglion Superior mesenteric plexus Suprarenal plexus **N Lumbar Sympathetic Nerve** Lumbar ganglion Lumbar splanchnic nerve **P Sacral Sympathetic Nerve** Ganglion impar (ganglion of Walther) Pelvic splanchnic nerve Sacral ganglion Sacral splanchnic nerve **Q Sacral Plexus** Inferior gluteal nerve Posterior femoral cutaneous nerve Pudendal nerve **R Sacral Nerve** Spinal nerve, sacral	**Ø Open** **3 Percutaneous** **4 Percutaneous Endoscopic**	**Z No Device**	**X Diagnostic** **Z No Qualifier**

Non-OR Ø1B[Ø,1,2,3,4,5,6,8,9,A,B,C,D,F,G,H,Q,R][3,4]ZX

Ø Medical and Surgical
1 Peripheral Nervous System
C Extirpation Definition: Taking or cutting out solid matter from a body part

Explanation: The solid matter may be an abnormal byproduct of a biological function or a foreign body; it may be imbedded in a body part or in the lumen of a tubular body part. The solid matter may or may not have been previously broken into pieces.

Body Part Character 4	Approach Character 5	Device Character 6	Qualifier Character 7
Ø Cervical Plexus Ansa cervicalis Cutaneous (transverse) cervical nerve Great auricular nerve Lesser occipital nerve Supraclavicular nerve Transverse (cutaneous) cervical nerve **1 Cervical Nerve** Greater occipital nerve Spinal nerve, cervical Suboccipital nerve Third occipital nerve **2 Phrenic Nerve** Accessory phrenic nerve **3 Brachial Plexus** Axillary nerve Dorsal scapular nerve First intercostal nerve Long thoracic nerve Musculocutaneous nerve Subclavius nerve Suprascapular nerve **4 Ulnar Nerve** Cubital nerve **5 Median Nerve** Anterior interosseous nerve Palmar cutaneous nerve **6 Radial Nerve** Dorsal digital nerve Musculospiral nerve Palmar cutaneous nerve Posterior interosseous nerve **8 Thoracic Nerve** Intercostal nerve Intercostobrachial nerve Spinal nerve, thoracic Subcostal nerve **9 Lumbar Plexus** Accessory obturator nerve Genitofemoral nerve Iliohypogastric nerve Ilioinguinal nerve Lateral femoral cutaneous nerve Obturator nerve Superior gluteal nerve **A Lumbosacral Plexus** **B Lumbar Nerve** Lumbosacral trunk Spinal nerve, lumbar Superior clunic (cluneal) nerve **C Pudendal Nerve** Posterior labial nerve Posterior scrotal nerve **D Femoral Nerve** Anterior crural nerve Saphenous nerve **F Sciatic Nerve** Ischiatic nerve **G Tibial Nerve** Lateral plantar nerve Medial plantar nerve Medial popliteal nerve Medial sural cutaneous nerve **H Peroneal Nerve** Common fibular nerve Common peroneal nerve External popliteal nerve Lateral sural cutaneous nerve **K Head and Neck Sympathetic Nerve** Cavernous plexus Cervical ganglion Ciliary ganglion Internal carotid plexus Otic ganglion Pterygopalatine (sphenopalatine) ganglion Sphenopalatine (pterygopalatine) ganglion Stellate ganglion Submandibular ganglion Submaxillary ganglion **L Thoracic Sympathetic Nerve** Cardiac plexus Esophageal plexus Greater splanchnic nerve Inferior cardiac nerve Least splanchnic nerve Lesser splanchnic nerve Middle cardiac nerve Pulmonary plexus Superior cardiac nerve Thoracic aortic plexus Thoracic ganglion **M Abdominal Sympathetic Nerve** Abdominal aortic plexus Auerbach's (myenteric) plexus Celiac (solar) plexus Celiac ganglion Gastric plexus Hepatic plexus Inferior hypogastric plexus Inferior mesenteric ganglion Inferior mesenteric plexus Meissner's (submucous) plexus Myenteric (Auerbach's) plexus Pancreatic plexus Pelvic splanchnic nerve Renal plexus Solar (celiac) plexus Splenic plexus Submucous (Meissner's) plexus Superior hypogastric plexus Superior mesenteric ganglion Superior mesenteric plexus Suprarenal plexus **N Lumbar Sympathetic Nerve** Lumbar ganglion Lumbar splanchnic nerve **P Sacral Sympathetic Nerve** Ganglion impar (ganglion of Walther) Pelvic splanchnic nerve Sacral ganglion Sacral splanchnic nerve **Q Sacral Plexus** Inferior gluteal nerve Posterior femoral cutaneous nerve Pudendal nerve **R Sacral Nerve** Spinal nerve, sacral	**Ø Open** **3 Percutaneous** **4 Percutaneous Endoscopic**	**Z No Device**	**Z No Qualifier**

Ø Medical and Surgical
1 Peripheral Nervous System
D Extraction Definition: Pulling or stripping out or off all or a portion of a body part by the use of force
Explanation: The qualifier DIAGNOSTIC is used to identify extraction procedures that are biopsies

Body Part Character 4	Approach Character 5	Device Character 6	Qualifier Character 7
Ø Cervical Plexus Ansa cervicalis; Cutaneous (transverse) cervical nerve; Great auricular nerve; Lesser occipital nerve; Supraclavicular nerve; Transverse (cutaneous) cervical nerve **1 Cervical Nerve** Greater occipital nerve; Spinal nerve, cervical; Suboccipital nerve; Third occipital nerve **2 Phrenic Nerve** Accessory phrenic nerve **3 Brachial Plexus** Axillary nerve; Dorsal scapular nerve; First intercostal nerve; Long thoracic nerve; Musculocutaneous nerve; Subclavius nerve; Suprascapular nerve **4 Ulnar Nerve** Cubital nerve **5 Median Nerve** Anterior interosseous nerve; Palmar cutaneous nerve **6 Radial Nerve** Dorsal digital nerve; Musculospiral nerve; Palmar cutaneous nerve; Posterior interosseous nerve **8 Thoracic Nerve** Intercostal nerve; Intercostobrachial nerve; Spinal nerve, thoracic; Subcostal nerve **9 Lumbar Plexus** Accessory obturator nerve; Genitofemoral nerve; Iliohypogastric nerve; Ilioinguinal nerve; Lateral femoral cutaneous nerve; Obturator nerve; Superior gluteal nerve **A Lumbosacral Plexus** **B Lumbar Nerve** Lumbosacral trunk; Spinal nerve, lumbar; Superior clunic (cluneal) nerve **C Pudendal Nerve]** Posterior labial nerve; Posterior scrotal nerve **D Femoral Nerve** Anterior crural nerve; Saphenous nerve **F Sciatic Nerve** Ischiatic nerve **G Tibial Nerve** Lateral plantar nerve; Medial plantar nerve; Medial popliteal nerve; Medial sural cutaneous nerve **H Peroneal Nerve** Common fibular nerve; Common peroneal nerve; External popliteal nerve; Lateral sural cutaneous nerve **K Head and Neck Sympathetic Nerve** Cavernous plexus; Cervical ganglion; Ciliary ganglion; Internal carotid plexus; Otic ganglion; Pterygopalatine (sphenopalatine) ganglion; Sphenopalatine (pterygopalatine) ganglion; Stellate ganglion; Submandibular ganglion; Submaxillary ganglion **L Thoracic Sympathetic Nerve** Cardiac plexus; Esophageal plexus; Greater splanchnic nerve; Inferior cardiac nerve; Least splanchnic nerve; Lesser splanchnic nerve; Middle cardiac nerve; Pulmonary plexus; Superior cardiac nerve; Thoracic aortic plexus; Thoracic ganglion **M Abdominal Sympathetic Nerve** Abdominal aortic plexus; Auerbach's (myenteric) plexus; Celiac (solar) plexus; Celiac ganglion; Gastric plexus; Hepatic plexus; Inferior hypogastric plexus; Inferior mesenteric ganglion; Inferior mesenteric plexus; Meissner's (submucous) plexus; Myenteric (Auerbach's) plexus; Pancreatic plexus; Pelvic splanchnic nerve; Renal plexus; Solar (celiac) plexus; Splenic plexus; Submucous (Meissner's) plexus; Superior hypogastric plexus; Superior mesenteric ganglion; Superior mesenteric plexus; Suprarenal plexus **N Lumbar Sympathetic Nerve** Lumbar ganglion; Lumbar splanchnic nerve **P Sacral Sympathetic Nerve** Ganglion impar (ganglion of Walther); Pelvic splanchnic nerve; Sacral ganglion; Sacral splanchnic nerve **Q Sacral Plexus** Inferior gluteal nerve; Posterior femoral cutaneous nerve; Pudendal nerve **R Sacral Nerve** Spinal nerve, sacral	Ø Open 3 Percutaneous 4 Percutaneous Endoscopic	Z No Device	Z No Qualifier

Ø Medical and Surgical
1 Peripheral Nervous System
H Insertion Definition: Putting in a nonbiological appliance that monitors, assists, performs, or prevents a physiological function but does not physically take the place of a body part

Explanation: None

Body Part Character 4	Approach Character 5	Device Character 6	Qualifier Character 7
Y Peripheral Nerve ⊞	Ø Open 3 Percutaneous 4 Percutaneous Endoscopic	2 Monitoring Device M Neurostimulator Lead Y Other Device	Z No Qualifier

Non-OR Ø1HY[3,4]YZ

See Appendix L for Procedure Combinations
⊞ Ø1HY[Ø,3,4]MZ

Ø Medical and Surgical
1 Peripheral Nervous System
J Inspection Definition: Visually and/or manually exploring a body part

Explanation: Visual exploration may be performed with or without optical instrumentation. Manual exploration may be performed directly or through intervening body layers.

Body Part Character 4	Approach Character 5	Device Character 6	Qualifier Character 7
Y Peripheral Nerve	Ø Open 3 Percutaneous 4 Percutaneous Endoscopic	Z No Device	Z No Qualifier

Non-OR Ø1JY3ZZ

Ø Medical and Surgical
1 Peripheral Nervous System
N Release Definition: Freeing a body part from an abnormal physical constraint by cutting or by the use of force
Explanation: Some of the restraining tissue may be taken out but none of the body part is taken out

Body Part Character 4	Approach Character 5	Device Character 6	Qualifier Character 7
Ø Cervical Plexus Ansa cervicalis Cutaneous (transverse) cervical nerve Great auricular nerve Lesser occipital nerve Supraclavicular nerve Transverse (cutaneous) cervical nerve **1 Cervical Nerve** Greater occipital nerve Spinal nerve, cervical Suboccipital nerve Third occipital nerve **2 Phrenic Nerve** Accessory phrenic nerve **3 Brachial Plexus** Axillary nerve Dorsal scapular nerve First intercostal nerve Long thoracic nerve Musculocutaneous nerve Subclavius nerve Suprascapular nerve **4 Ulnar Nerve** Cubital nerve **5 Median Nerve** Anterior interosseous nerve Palmar cutaneous nerve **6 Radial Nerve** Dorsal digital nerve Musculospiral nerve Palmar cutaneous nerve Posterior interosseous nerve **8 Thoracic Nerve** Intercostal nerve Intercostobrachial nerve Spinal nerve, thoracic Subcostal nerve **9 Lumbar Plexus** Accessory obturator nerve Genitofemoral nerve Iliohypogastric nerve Ilioinguinal nerve Lateral femoral cutaneous nerve Obturator nerve Superior gluteal nerve **A Lumbosacral Plexus** **B Lumbar Nerve** Lumbosacral trunk Spinal nerve, lumbar Superior clunic (cluneal) nerve **C Pudendal Nerve** Posterior labial nerve Posterior scrotal nerve **D Femoral Nerve** Anterior crural nerve Saphenous nerve **F Sciatic Nerve** Ischiatic nerve **G Tibial Nerve** Lateral plantar nerve Medial plantar nerve Medial popliteal nerve Medial sural cutaneous nerve **H Peroneal Nerve** Common fibular nerve Common peroneal nerve External popliteal nerve Lateral sural cutaneous nerve **K Head and Neck Sympathetic Nerve** Cavernous plexus Cervical ganglion Ciliary ganglion Internal carotid plexus Otic ganglion Pterygopalatine (sphenopalatine) ganglion Sphenopalatine (pterygopalatine) ganglion Stellate ganglion Submandibular ganglion Submaxillary ganglion **L Thoracic Sympathetic Nerve** Cardiac plexus Esophageal plexus Greater splanchnic nerve Inferior cardiac nerve Least splanchnic nerve Lesser splanchnic nerve Middle cardiac nerve Pulmonary plexus Superior cardiac nerve Thoracic aortic plexus Thoracic ganglion **M Abdominal Sympathetic Nerve** Abdominal aortic plexus Auerbach's (myenteric) plexus Celiac (solar) plexus Celiac ganglion Gastric plexus Hepatic plexus Inferior hypogastric plexus Inferior mesenteric ganglion Inferior mesenteric plexus Meissner's (submucous) plexus Myenteric (Auerbach's) plexus Pancreatic plexus Pelvic splanchnic nerve Renal plexus Solar (celiac) plexus Splenic plexus Submucous (Meissner's) plexus Superior hypogastric plexus Superior mesenteric ganglion Superior mesenteric plexus Suprarenal plexus **N Lumbar Sympathetic Nerve** Lumbar ganglion Lumbar splanchnic nerve **P Sacral Sympathetic Nerve** Ganglion impar (ganglion of Walther) Pelvic splanchnic nerve Sacral ganglion Sacral splanchnic nerve **Q Sacral Plexus** Inferior gluteal nerve Posterior femoral cutaneous nerve Pudendal nerve **R Sacral Nerve** Spinal nerve, sacral	**Ø** Open **3** Percutaneous **4** Percutaneous Endoscopic	**Z** No Device	**Z** No Qualifier

Ø Medical and Surgical
1 Peripheral Nervous System
P Removal Definition: Taking out or off a device from a body part

Explanation: If a device is taken out and a similar device put in without cutting or puncturing the skin or mucous membrane, the procedure is coded to the root operation CHANGE. Otherwise, the procedure for taking out a device is coded to the root operation REMOVAL.

Body Part Character 4	Approach Character 5	Device Character 6	Qualifier Character 7
Y Peripheral Nerve	Ø Open 3 Percutaneous 4 Percutaneous Endoscopic	Ø Drainage Device 2 Monitoring Device 7 Autologous Tissue Substitute M Neurostimulator Lead Y Other Device	Z No Qualifier
Y Peripheral Nerve	X External	Ø Drainage Device 2 Monitoring Device M Neurostimulator Lead	Z No Qualifier

Non-OR Ø1PY3[Ø,2]Z
Non-OR Ø1PY[3,4]YZ
Non-OR Ø1PYX[Ø,2,M]Z

Ø Medical and Surgical
1 Peripheral Nervous System
Q Repair Definition: Restoring, to the extent possible, a body part to its normal anatomic structure and function
Explanation: Used only when the method to accomplish the repair is not one of the other root operations

Body Part Character 4	Approach Character 5	Device Character 6	Qualifier Character 7
Ø Cervical Plexus Ansa cervicalis; Cutaneous (transverse) cervical nerve; Great auricular nerve; Lesser occipital nerve; Supraclavicular nerve; Transverse (cutaneous) cervical nerve **1 Cervical Nerve** Greater occipital nerve; Spinal nerve, cervical; Suboccipital nerve; Third occipital nerve **2 Phrenic Nerve** Accessory phrenic nerve **3 Brachial Plexus** Axillary nerve; Dorsal scapular nerve; First intercostal nerve; Long thoracic nerve; Musculocutaneous nerve; Subclavius nerve; Suprascapular nerve **4 Ulnar Nerve** Cubital nerve **5 Median Nerve** Anterior interosseous nerve; Palmar cutaneous nerve **6 Radial Nerve** Dorsal digital nerve; Musculospiral nerve; Palmar cutaneous nerve; Posterior interosseous nerve **8 Thoracic Nerve** Intercostal nerve; Intercostobrachial nerve; Spinal nerve, thoracic; Subcostal nerve **9 Lumbar Plexus** Accessory obturator nerve; Genitofemoral nerve; Iliohypogastric nerve; Ilioinguinal nerve; Lateral femoral cutaneous nerve; Obturator nerve; Superior gluteal nerve **A Lumbosacral Plexus** **B Lumbar Nerve** Lumbosacral trunk; Spinal nerve, lumbar; Superior clunic (cluneal) nerve **C Pudendal Nerve** Posterior labial nerve; Posterior scrotal nerve **D Femoral Nerve** Anterior crural nerve; Saphenous nerve **F Sciatic Nerve** Ischiatic nerve **G Tibial Nerve** Lateral plantar nerve; Medial plantar nerve; Medial popliteal nerve; Medial sural cutaneous nerve **H Peroneal Nerve** Common fibular nerve; Common peroneal nerve; External popliteal nerve; Lateral sural cutaneous nerve **K Head and Neck Sympathetic Nerve** Cavernous plexus; Cervical ganglion; Ciliary ganglion; Internal carotid plexus; Otic ganglion; Pterygopalatine (sphenopalatine) ganglion; Sphenopalatine (pterygopalatine) ganglion; Stellate ganglion; Submandibular ganglion; Submaxillary ganglion **L Thoracic Sympathetic Nerve** Cardiac plexus; Esophageal plexus; Greater splanchnic nerve; Inferior cardiac nerve; Least splanchnic nerve; Lesser splanchnic nerve; Middle cardiac nerve; Pulmonary plexus; Superior cardiac nerve; Thoracic aortic plexus; Thoracic ganglion **M Abdominal Sympathetic Nerve** Abdominal aortic plexus; Auerbach's (myenteric) plexus; Celiac (solar) plexus; Celiac ganglion; Gastric plexus; Hepatic plexus; Inferior hypogastric plexus; Inferior mesenteric ganglion; Inferior mesenteric plexus; Meissner's (submucous) plexus; Myenteric (Auerbach's) plexus; Pancreatic plexus; Pelvic splanchnic nerve; Renal plexus; Solar (celiac) plexus; Splenic plexus; Submucous (Meissner's) plexus; Superior hypogastric plexus; Superior mesenteric ganglion; Superior mesenteric plexus; Suprarenal plexus **N Lumbar Sympathetic Nerve** Lumbar ganglion; Lumbar splanchnic nerve **P Sacral Sympathetic Nerve** Ganglion impar (ganglion of Walther); Pelvic splanchnic nerve; Sacral ganglion; Sacral splanchnic nerve **Q Sacral Plexus** Inferior gluteal nerve; Posterior femoral cutaneous nerve; Pudendal nerve **R Sacral Nerve** Spinal nerve, sacral	**Ø** Open **3** Percutaneous **4** Percutaneous Endoscopic	**Z** No Device	**Z** No Qualifier

Peripheral Nervous System
Ø1Q–Ø1Q

0 Medical and Surgical
1 Peripheral Nervous System
R Replacement Definition: Putting in or on biological or synthetic material that physically takes the place and/or function of all or a portion of a body part

Explanation: The body part may have been taken out or replaced, or may be taken out, physically eradicated, or rendered nonfunctional during the REPLACEMENT procedure. A REMOVAL procedure is coded for taking out the device used in a previous replacement procedure.

Body Part Character 4	Approach Character 5	Device Character 6	Qualifier Character 7
1 Cervical Nerve Greater occipital nerve Spinal nerve, cervical Suboccipital nerve Third occipital nerve **2 Phrenic Nerve** Accessory phrenic nerve **4 Ulnar Nerve** Cubital nerve **5 Median Nerve** Anterior interosseous nerve Palmar cutaneous nerve **6 Radial Nerve** Dorsal digital nerve Musculospiral nerve Palmar cutaneous nerve Posterior interosseous nerve **8 Thoracic Nerve** Intercostal nerve Intercostobrachial nerve Spinal nerve, thoracic Subcostal nerve **B Lumbar Nerve** Lumbosacral trunk Spinal nerve, lumbar Superior clunic (cluneal) nerve **C Pudendal Nerve** Posterior labial nerve Posterior scrotal nerve **D Femoral Nerve** Anterior crural nerve Saphenous nerve **F Sciatic Nerve** Ischiatic nerve **G Tibial Nerve** Lateral plantar nerve Medial plantar nerve Medial popliteal nerve Medial sural cutaneous nerve **H Peroneal Nerve** Common fibular nerve Common peroneal nerve External popliteal nerve Lateral sural cutaneous nerve **R Sacral Nerve** Spinal nerve, sacral	**0 Open** **4 Percutaneous Endoscopic**	**7 Autologous Tissue Substitute** **J Synthetic Substitute** **K Nonautologous Tissue Substitute**	**Z No Qualifier**

Ø Medical and Surgical
1 Peripheral Nervous System
S Reposition Definition: Moving to its normal location, or other suitable location, all or a portion of a body part

Explanation: The body part is moved to a new location from an abnormal location, or from a normal location where it is not functioning correctly. The body part may or may not be cut out or off to be moved to the new location.

Body Part Character 4	Approach Character 5	Device Character 6	Qualifier Character 7
Ø Cervical Plexus Ansa cervicalis Cutaneous (transverse) cervical nerve Great auricular nerve Lesser occipital nerve Supraclavicular nerve Transverse (cutaneous) cervical nerve **1 Cervical Nerve** Greater occipital nerve Spinal nerve, cervical Suboccipital nerve Third occipital nerve **2 Phrenic Nerve** Accessory phrenic nerve **3 Brachial Plexus** Axillary nerve Dorsal scapular nerve First intercostal nerve Long thoracic nerve Musculocutaneous nerve Subclavius nerve Suprascapular nerve **4 Ulnar Nerve** Cubital nerve **5 Median Nerve** Anterior interosseous nerve Palmar cutaneous nerve **6 Radial Nerve** Dorsal digital nerve Musculospiral nerve Palmar cutaneous nerve Posterior interosseous nerve **8 Thoracic Nerve** Intercostal nerve Intercostobrachial nerve Spinal nerve, thoracic Subcostal nerve **9 Lumbar Plexus** Accessory obturator nerve Genitofemoral nerve Iliohypogastric nerve Ilioinguinal nerve Lateral femoral cutaneous nerve Obturator nerve Superior gluteal nerve **A Lumbosacral Plexus** **B Lumbar Nerve** Lumbosacral trunk Spinal nerve, lumbar Superior clunic (cluneal) nerve **C Pudendal Nerve** Posterior labial nerve Posterior scrotal nerve **D Femoral Nerve** Anterior crural nerve Saphenous nerve **F Sciatic Nerve** Ischiatic nerve **G Tibial Nerve** Lateral plantar nerve Medial plantar nerve Medial popliteal nerve Medial sural cutaneous nerve **H Peroneal Nerve** Common fibular nerve Common peroneal nerve External popliteal nerve Lateral sural cutaneous nerve **Q Sacral Plexus** Inferior gluteal nerve Posterior femoral cutaneous nerve Pudendal nerve **R Sacral Nerve** Spinal nerve, sacral	**Ø** Open **3** Percutaneous **4** Percutaneous Endoscopic	**Z** No Device	**Z** No Qualifier

0 Medical and Surgical
1 Peripheral Nervous System
U Supplement Definition: Putting in or on biological or synthetic material that physically reinforces and/or augments the function of a portion of a body part

Explanation: The biological material is non-living, or is living and from the same individual. The body part may have been previously replaced, and the SUPPLEMENT procedure is performed to physically reinforce and/or augment the function of the replaced body part.

Body Part Character 4	Approach Character 5	Device Character 6	Qualifier Character 7
1 Cervical Nerve Greater occipital nerve Spinal nerve, cervical Suboccipital nerve Third occipital nerve **2 Phrenic Nerve** Accessory phrenic nerve **4 Ulnar Nerve** Cubital nerve **5 Median Nerve** Anterior interosseous nerve Palmar cutaneous nerve **6 Radial Nerve** Dorsal digital nerve Musculospiral nerve Palmar cutaneous nerve Posterior interosseous nerve **8 Thoracic Nerve** Intercostal nerve Intercostobrachial nerve Spinal nerve, thoracic Subcostal nerve **B Lumbar Nerve** Lumbosacral trunk Spinal nerve, lumbar Superior clunic (cluneal) nerve **C Pudendal Nerve** Posterior labial nerve Posterior scrotal nerve **D Femoral Nerve** Anterior crural nerve Saphenous nerve **F Sciatic Nerve** Ischiatic nerve **G Tibial Nerve** Lateral plantar nerve Medial plantar nerve Medial popliteal nerve Medial sural cutaneous nerve **H Peroneal Nerve** Common fibular nerve Common peroneal nerve External popliteal nerve Lateral sural cutaneous nerve **R Sacral Nerve** Spinal nerve, sacral	0 Open 3 Percutaneous 4 Percutaneous Endoscopic	7 Autologous Tissue Substitute J Synthetic Substitute K Nonautologous Tissue Substitute	Z No Qualifier

0 Medical and Surgical
1 Peripheral Nervous System
W Revision Definition: Correcting, to the extent possible, a portion of a malfunctioning device or the position of a displaced device

Explanation: Revision can include correcting a malfunctioning or displaced device by taking out or putting in components of the device such as a screw or pin

Body Part Character 4	Approach Character 5	Device Character 6	Qualifier Character 7
Y Peripheral Nerve	0 Open 3 Percutaneous 4 Percutaneous Endoscopic	0 Drainage Device 2 Monitoring Device 7 Autologous Tissue Substitute M Neurostimulator Lead Y Other Device	Z No Qualifier
Y Peripheral Nerve	X External	0 Drainage Device 2 Monitoring Device 7 Autologous Tissue Substitute M Neurostimulator Lead	Z No Qualifier

Non-OR 01WY[3,4]YZ
Non-OR 01WYX[0,2,7,M]Z

Ø Medical and Surgical
1 Peripheral Nervous System
X Transfer Definition: Moving, without taking out, all or a portion of a body part to another location to take over the function of all or a portion of a body part
Explanation: The body part transferred remains connected to its vascular and nervous supply

Body Part Character 4	Approach Character 5	Device Character 6	Qualifier Character 7
1 Cervical Nerve Greater occipital nerve Spinal nerve, cervical Suboccipital nerve Third occipital nerve **2 Phrenic Nerve** Accessory phrenic nerve	**Ø Open** **4 Percutaneous Endoscopic**	**Z No Device**	**1 Cervical Nerve** **2 Phrenic Nerve**
4 Ulnar Nerve Cubital nerve **5 Median Nerve** Anterior interosseous nerve Palmar cutaneous nerve **6 Radial Nerve** Dorsal digital nerve Musculospiral nerve Palmar cutaneous nerve Posterior interosseous nerve	**Ø Open** **4 Percutaneous Endoscopic**	**Z No Device**	**4 Ulnar Nerve** **5 Median Nerve** **6 Radial Nerve**
8 Thoracic Nerve Intercostal nerve Intercostobrachial nerve Spinal nerve, thoracic Subcostal nerve	**Ø Open** **4 Percutaneous Endoscopic**	**Z No Device**	**8 Thoracic Nerve**
B Lumbar Nerve Lumbosacral trunk Spinal nerve, lumbar Superior clunic (cluneal) nerve **C Pudendal Nerve** Posterior labial nerve Posterior scrotal nerve	**Ø Open** **4 Percutaneous Endoscopic**	**Z No Device**	**B Lumbar Nerve** **C Perineal Nerve**
D Femoral Nerve Anterior crural nerve Saphenous nerve **F Sciatic Nerve** Ischiatic nerve **G Tibial Nerve** Lateral plantar nerve Medial plantar nerve Medial popliteal nerve Medial sural cutaneous nerve **H Peroneal Nerve** Common fibular nerve Common peroneal nerve External popliteal nerve Lateral sural cutaneous nerve	**Ø Open** **4 Percutaneous Endoscopic**	**Z No Device**	**D Femoral Nerve** **F Sciatic Nerve** **G Tibial Nerve** **H Peroneal Nerve**

Heart and Great Vessels Ø21–Ø2Y

Character Meanings

This Character Meaning table is provided as a guide to assist the user in the identification of character members that may be found in this section of code tables. It **SHOULD NOT** be used to build a PCS code.

Operation–Character 3	Body Part–Character 4	Approach–Character 5	Device–Character 6	Qualifier–Character 7
1 Bypass	Ø Coronary Artery, One Artery	Ø Open	Ø Monitoring Device, Pressure Sensor	Ø Allogeneic
4 Creation	1 Coronary Artery, Two Arteries	3 Percutaneous	2 Monitoring Device	1 Syngeneic
5 Destruction	2 Coronary Artery, Three Arteries	4 Percutaneous Endoscopic	3 Infusion Device	2 Zooplastic OR Common Atrioventricular Valve
7 Dilation	3 Coronary Artery, Four or More Arteries	X External	4 Intraluminal Device, Drug-eluting	3 Coronary Artery
8 Division	4 Coronary Vein		5 Intraluminal Device, Drug-eluting, Two	4 Coronary Vein
B Excision	5 Atrial Septum		6 Intraluminal Device, Drug-eluting, Three	5 Coronary Circulation
C Extirpation	6 Atrium, Right		7 Intraluminal Device, Drug-eluting, Four or More OR Autologous Tissue Substitute	6 Bifurcation
F Fragmentation	7 Atrium, Left		8 Zooplastic Tissue	7 Atrium, Left
H Insertion	8 Conduction Mechanism		9 Autologous Venous Tissue	8 Internal Mammary, Right
J Inspection	9 Chordae Tendineae		A Autologous Arterial Tissue	9 Internal Mammary, Left
K Map	A Heart		C Extraluminal Device	A Innominate Artery
L Occlusion	B Heart, Right		D Intraluminal Device	B Subclavian
N Release	C Heart, Left		E Intraluminal Device, Two OR Intraluminal Device, Branched or Fenestrated, One or Two Arteries	C Thoracic Artery
P Removal	D Papillary Muscle		F Intraluminal Device, Three OR Intraluminal Device, Branched or Fenestrated, Three or More Arteries	D Carotid
Q Repair	F Aortic Valve		G Intraluminal Device, Four or More	E Atrioventricular Valve, Left
R Replacement	G Mitral Valve		J Synthetic Substitute OR Cardiac Lead, Pacemaker	F Abdominal Artery
S Reposition	H Pulmonary Valve		K Nonautologous Tissue Substitute OR Cardiac Lead, Defibrillator	G Atrioventricular Valve, Right OR Axillary Artery
T Resection	J Tricuspid Valve		M Cardiac Lead	H Transapical OR Brachial Artery
U Supplement	K Ventricle, Right		N Intracardiac Pacemaker	J Truncal Valve OR Temporary OR Intraoperative
V Restriction	L Ventricle, Left		Q Implantable Heart Assist System	K Left Atrial Appendage
W Revision	M Ventricular Septum		R Short-term External Heart Assist System	P Pulmonary Trunk
Y Transplantation	N Pericardium		T Intraluminal Device, Radioactive	Q Pulmonary Artery, Right
	P Pulmonary Trunk		Y Other Device	R Pulmonary Artery, Left
	Q Pulmonary Artery, Right		Z No Device	S Pulmonary Vein, Right OR Biventricular
	R Pulmonary Artery, Left			T Pulmonary Vein, Left OR Ductus Arteriosus

Continued on next page

Continued from previous page

Operation–Character 3	Body Part–Character 4	Approach–Character 5	Device–Character 6	Qualifier–Character 7
	S Pulmonary Vein, Right			U Pulmonary Vein, Confluence
	T Pulmonary Vein, Left			V Lower Extremity Artery
	V Superior Vena Cava			W Aorta
	W Thoracic Aorta, Descending			X Diagnostic
	X Thoracic Aorta, Ascending/ Arch			Z No Qualifier
	Y Great Vessel			

AHA Coding Clinic for table Ø21

2017, 4Q, 56 Added approach values - Percutaneous heart valve procedures
2017, 1Q, 19 Norwood Sano procedure
2016, 4Q, 80-81 Thoracic aorta, ascending/arch and descending
2016, 4Q, 82-83 Coronary artery, number of arteries
2016, 4Q, 102-109 Correction of congenital heart defects
2016, 4Q, 144 Repair of atrial septal defect and anomalous pulmonary venous return
2016, 4Q, 145 Modified Warden procedure for repair of septal defect and right partial anomalous pulmonary venous return
2016, 1Q, 27 Aortocoronary bypass graft utilizing Y-graft
2015, 4Q, 22, 24 Congenital heart corrective procedures
2015, 3Q, 16 Revision of previous truncus arteriosus surgery with ventricle to pulmonary artery conduit
2014, 3Q, 3 Blalock-Taussig shunt procedure
2014, 3Q, 8 Coronary artery bypass graft utilizing internal mammary as pedicle graft
2014, 3Q, 20 MAZE procedure performed with coronary artery bypass graft
2014, 3Q, 29 Fontan completion procedure stage II
2014, 3Q, 30 Creation of conduit from right ventricle to pulmonary artery
2014, 1Q, 10 Repair of thoracic aortic aneurysm & coronary artery bypass graft
2013, 2Q, 37 Coronary artery release performed during coronary artery bypass graft

AHA Coding Clinic for table Ø24

2016, 4Q, 101 Root operation Creation
2016, 4Q, 102-109 Correction of congenital heart defects

AHA Coding Clinic for table Ø25

2016, 4Q, 80-81 Thoracic aorta, ascending/arch and descending
2016, 3Q, 43-44 Peri-pulmonary catheter ablation
2016, 3Q, 44-45 Maze procedure
2016, 2Q, 17 Photodynamic therapy for treatment of malignant mesothelioma
2014, 4Q, 47 Catheter ablation of peripulmonary veins
2014, 3Q, 19 Ablation of ventricular tachycardia with Impella® support
2014, 3Q, 20 MAZE procedure performed with coronary artery bypass graft
2013, 2Q, 38 Catheter ablation to treat atrial fibrillation

AHA Coding Clinic for table Ø27

2018, 2Q, 24 Coronary artery bifurcation
2017, 4Q, 32-33 Corrective surgery of left ventricular outflow tract obstruction
2016, 4Q, 80-81 Thoracic aorta, ascending/arch and descending
2016, 4Q, 82-83 Coronary artery, number of arteries
2016, 4Q, 84-85 Coronary Artery, number of stents
2016, 4Q, 86-88 Coronary and peripheral artery bifurcation
2016, 1Q, 16 Pulmonary valvotomy and dilation of annulus
2015, 4Q, 13 New Section X codes—New Technology procedures
2015, 3Q, 9 Failed attempt to treat coronary artery occlusion
2015, 3Q, 10 Coronary angioplasty with unsuccessful stent insertion
2015, 3Q, 16 Revision of previous truncus arteriosus surgery with ventricle to pulmonary artery conduit
2015, 2Q, 3-5 Coronary artery intervention site
2014, 2Q, 4 Coronary angioplasty of bypassed vessel

AHA Coding Clinic for table Ø2B

2017, 1Q, 38 Mitral valve repair and chordae tendineae transfer
2016, 4Q, 80-81 Thoracic aorta, ascending/arch and descending
2015, 2Q, 23 Annuloplasty ring

AHA Coding Clinic for table Ø2C

2018, 2Q, 24 Coronary artery bifurcation
2017, 2Q, 23 Thrombectomy via Fogarty catheter
2016, 4Q, 80-81 Thoracic aorta, ascending/arch and descending
2016, 4Q, 82-83 Coronary artery, number of arteries
2016, 4Q, 86-87 Coronary and peripheral artery bifurcation
2016, 2Q, 24 Repair/decalcification of mitral valve
2016, 2Q, 25 Aortic valve surgery with excision of calcium deposits

AHA Coding Clinic for table Ø2H

2018, 2Q, 3-5 Intra-aortic balloon pump
2018, 2Q, 19 Pacing lead attached to automatic implantable cardioverter defibrillator
2017, 4Q, 42-45 Insertion of external heart assist devices
2017, 4Q, 63-64 Added and revised device values - Vascular access reservoir
2017, 4Q, 104 Placement of Watchman ™ left atrial appendage device
2017, 3Q, 11 Placement of peripherally inserted central catheter using 3CG ECG technology
2017, 2Q, 24 Tunneled catheter versus totally implantable catheter
2017, 2Q, 26 Exchange of tunneled catheter
2017, 1Q, 10-11 External heart assist device
2016, 4Q, 80-81 Thoracic aorta, ascending/arch and descending
2016, 4Q, 95 Intracardiac pacemaker
2016, 4Q, 137-138 Heart assist device systems
2016, 2Q, 15 Removal and replacement of tunneled internal jugular catheter
2015, 4Q, 14 New Section X codes—New Technology procedures
2015, 4Q, 26-31 Vascular access devices
2015, 3Q, 35 Swan Ganz catheterization
2015, 2Q, 31 Leadless pacemaker insertion
2015, 2Q, 33 Totally implantable central venous access device (Port-a-Cath)
2013, 3Q, 18 Placement of peripherally inserted central catheter (PICC)

AHA Coding Clinic for table Ø2J

2015, 3Q, 9 Failed attempt to treat coronary artery occlusion

AHA Coding Clinic for table Ø2L

2017, 4Q, 31 Resuscitative endovascular balloon occlusion of the aorta
2017, 4Q, 33-34 Occlusion/ligation of pulmonary trunk & right pulmonary artery
2016, 4Q, 102-109 Correction of congenital heart defects
2016, 2Q, 26 Embolization of pulmonary arteriovenous fistula
2015, 4Q, 23 Congenital heart corrective procedures
2014, 3Q, 20 MAZE procedure performed with coronary artery bypass graft

AHA Coding Clinic for table Ø2N

2017, 4Q, 35 Release of myocardial bridge
2016, 4Q, 80-81 Thoracic aorta, ascending/arch and descending
2014, 3Q, 16 Repair of Tetralogy of Fallot

AHA Coding Clinic for table Ø2P

2018, 2Q, 3-5 Intra-aortic balloon pump
2017, 4Q, 42-45 Insertion of external heart assist devices
2017, 4Q, 104 Placement of Watchman ™ left atrial appendage device
2017, 3Q, 18 Intra-aortic balloon pump removal
2017, 2Q, 24 Tunneled catheter versus totally implantable catheter
2017, 2Q, 26 Exchange of tunneled catheter
2017, 1Q, 11 External heart assist device
2017, 1Q, 13 SynCardia total artificial heart
2016, 4Q, 95-96 Intracardiac pacemaker
2016, 4Q, 137-139 Heart assist device systems
2016, 3Q, 19 Nonoperative removal of peripherally inserted central catheter
2016, 2Q, 15 Removal and replacement of tunneled internal jugular catheter
2015, 4Q, 31 Vascular access devices
2015, 3Q, 33 Approach values for repositioning and removal of cardiac lead

AHA Coding Clinic for table Ø2Q

2018, 1Q, 12 Percutaneous balloon valvuloplasty & cardiac catheterization with ventriculogram
2017, 1Q, 18 Sutureless repair of pulmonary vein stenosis
2016, 4Q, 80-81 Thoracic aorta, ascending/arch and descending
2016, 4Q, 82-83 Coronary artery, number of arteries
2016, 4Q, 101 Root operation Creation
2016, 4Q, 102-109 Correction of congenital heart defects
2015, 4Q, 23 Congenital heart corrective procedures
2015, 3Q, 16 Vascular ring surgery and double aortic arch
2015, 2Q, 23 Annuloplasty ring
2013, 3Q, 26 Transcatheter replacement of heart valve (TAVR) with measurements

AHA Coding Clinic for table Ø2R

2018, 1Q, 12 Percutaneous balloon valvuloplasty & cardiac catheterization with ventriculogram
2017, 4Q, 55-56 Added approach values - Percutaneous heart valve procedures
2017, 1Q, 13 SynCardia total artificial heart
2016, 4Q, 80-81 Thoracic aorta, ascending/arch and descending
2016, 3Q, 32 Transcatheter tricuspid valve replacement
2014, 1Q, 10 Repair of thoracic aortic aneurysm & coronary artery bypass graft

AHA Coding Clinic for table Ø2S

2016, 4Q, 80-81 Thoracic aorta, ascending/arch and descending
2016, 4Q, 82-83 Coronary artery, number of arteries
2016, 4Q, 102-109 Correction of congenital heart defects
2015, 4Q, 23 Congenital heart corrective procedures

AHA Coding Clinic for table Ø2U

2018, 1Q, 12 Percutaneous balloon valvuloplasty & cardiac catheterization with ventriculogram
2017, 4Q, 36 Alfieri stitch procedure
2017, 3Q, 7 Senning procedure (arterial switch)
2017, 1Q, 19 Norwood Sano procedure
2016, 4Q, 80-81 Thoracic aorta, ascending/arch and descending
2016, 4Q, 101 Root operation Creation
2016, 4Q, 102-109 Correction of congenital heart defects
2016, 2Q, 23 Repair of tetralogy of Fallot with autologous pericardial patch graft
2016, 2Q, 26 Aortic valve replacement with aortic root enlargement
2015, 4Q, 22-24 Congenital heart corrective procedures
2015, 3Q, 16 Revision of previous truncus arteriosus surgery with ventricle to pulmonary artery conduit
2015, 2Q, 23 Annuloplasty ring
2014, 3Q, 16 Repair of Tetralogy of Fallot

AHA Coding Clinic for table Ø2V

2017, 4Q, 35-36 Alfieri stitch procedure
2016, 4Q, 80-81 Thoracic aorta, ascending/arch and descending
2016, 4Q, 89-92 Branched and fenestrated endograft repair of aneurysms

AHA Coding Clinic for table Ø2W

2018, 1Q, 17 Repositioning of Impella short-term external heart assist device
2017, 4Q, 42-45 Insertion of external heart assist devices
2017, 4Q, 55-56 Added approach values - Percutaneous heart valve procedures
2016, 4Q, 85 Coronary Artery, number of stents
2016, 4Q, 95-96 Intracardiac pacemaker
2015, 3Q, 32 Approach values for repositioning and removal of cardiac lead
2014, 3Q, 31 Closure of paravalvular leak using Amplatzer® vascular plug

AHA Coding Clinic for table Ø2Y

2013, 3Q, 18 Heart transplant surgery

Coronary Arteries

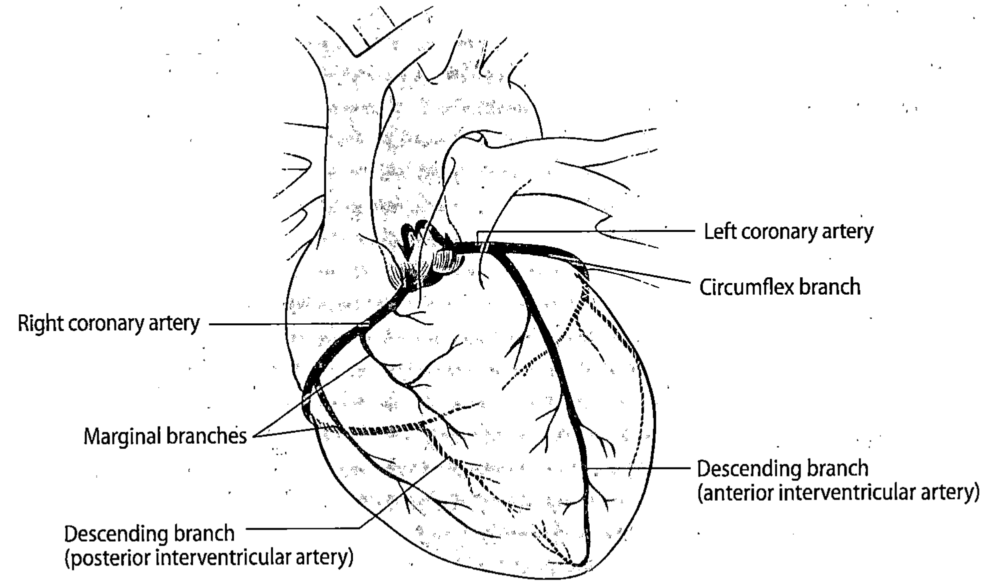
Left coronary artery
Circumflex branch
Right coronary artery
Marginal branches
Descending branch
(anterior interventricular artery)
Descending branch
(posterior interventricular artery)

Heart Anatomy

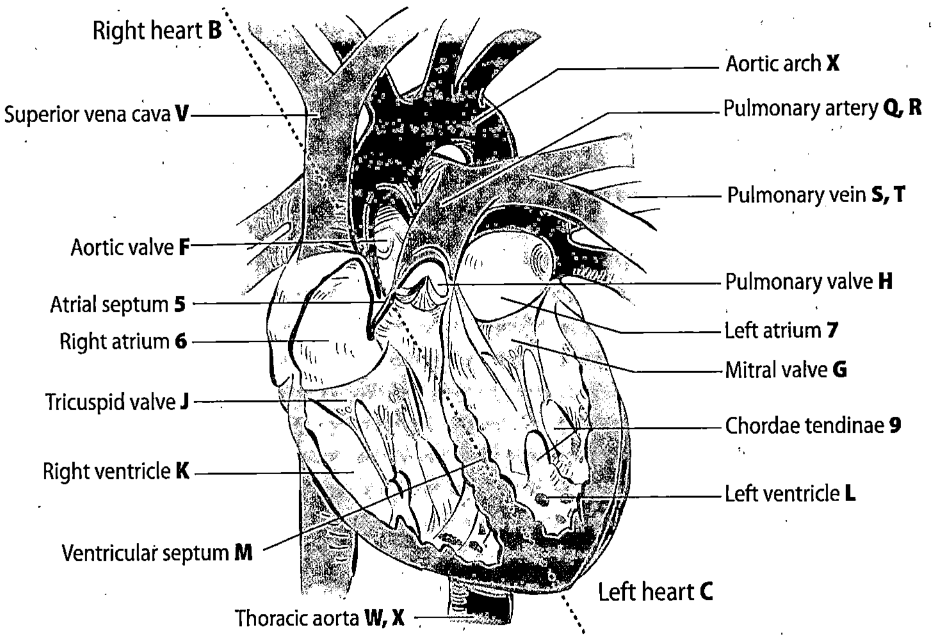
Right heart **B**
Superior vena cava **V**
Aortic arch **X**
Pulmonary artery **Q, R**
Pulmonary vein **S, T**
Aortic valve **F**
Pulmonary valve **H**
Atrial septum **5**
Left atrium **7**
Right atrium **6**
Mitral valve **G**
Tricuspid valve **J**
Chordae tendinae **9**
Right ventricle **K**
Left ventricle **L**
Ventricular septum **M**
Left heart **C**
Thoracic aorta **W, X**

0 Medical and Surgical
2 Heart and Great Vessels
1 Bypass Definition: Altering the route of passage of the contents of a tubular body part

Explanation: Rerouting contents of a body part to a downstream area of the normal route, to a similar route and body part, or to an abnormal route and dissimilar body part. Includes one or more anastomoses, with or without the use of a device.

Body Part Character 4	Approach Character 5	Device Character 6	Qualifier Character 7
0 Coronary Artery, One Artery 1 Coronary Artery, Two Arteries 2 Coronary Artery, Three Arteries 3 Coronary Artery, Four or More Arteries	0 Open	8 Zooplastic Tissue 9 Autologous Venous Tissue A Autologous Arterial Tissue J Synthetic Substitute K Nonautologous Tissue Substitute	3 Coronary Artery 8 Internal Mammary, Right 9 Internal Mammary, Left C Thoracic Artery F Abdominal Artery W Aorta
0 Coronary Artery, One Artery 1 Coronary Artery, Two Arteries 2 Coronary Artery, Three Arteries 3 Coronary Artery, Four or More Arteries	0 Open	Z No Device	3 Coronary Artery 8 Internal Mammary, Right 9 Internal Mammary, Left C Thoracic Artery F Abdominal Artery
0 Coronary Artery, One Artery 1 Coronary Artery, Two Arteries 2 Coronary Artery, Three Arteries 3 Coronary Artery, Four or More Arteries	3 Percutaneous	4 Intraluminal Device, Drug-eluting D Intraluminal Device	4 Coronary Vein
0 Coronary Artery, One Artery 1 Coronary Artery, Two Arteries 2 Coronary Artery, Three Arteries 3 Coronary Artery, Four or More Arteries	4 Percutaneous Endoscopic	4 Intraluminal Device, Drug-eluting D Intraluminal Device	4 Coronary Vein
0 Coronary Artery, One Artery 1 Coronary Artery, Two Arteries 2 Coronary Artery, Three Arteries 3 Coronary Artery, Four or More Arteries	4 Percutaneous Endoscopic	8 Zooplastic Tissue 9 Autologous Venous Tissue A Autologous Arterial Tissue J Synthetic Substitute K Nonautologous Tissue Substitute	3 Coronary Artery 8 Internal Mammary, Right 9 Internal Mammary, Left C Thoracic Artery F Abdominal Artery W Aorta
0 Coronary Artery, One Artery 1 Coronary Artery, Two Arteries 2 Coronary Artery, Three Arteries 3 Coronary Artery, Four or More Arteries	4 Percutaneous Endoscopic	Z No Device	3 Coronary Artery 8 Internal Mammary, Right 9 Internal Mammary, Left C Thoracic Artery F Abdominal Artery
6 Atrium, Right Atrium dextrum cordis Right auricular appendix Sinus venosus	0 Open 4 Percutaneous Endoscopic	8 Zooplastic Tissue 9 Autologous Venous Tissue A Autologous Arterial Tissue J Synthetic Substitute K Nonautologous Tissue Substitute	P Pulmonary Trunk Q Pulmonary Artery, Right R Pulmonary Artery, Left
6 Atrium, Right Atrium dextrum cordis Right auricular appendix Sinus venosus	0 Open 4 Percutaneous Endoscopic	Z No Device	7 Atrium, Left P Pulmonary Trunk Q Pulmonary Artery, Right R Pulmonary Artery, Left
6 Atrium, Right Atrium dextrum cordis Right auricular appendix Sinus venosus	3 Percutaneous	Z No Device	7 Atrium, Left
7 Atrium, Left Atrium pulmonale Left auricular appendix V Superior Vena Cava Precava	0 Open 4 Percutaneous Endoscopic	8 Zooplastic Tissue 9 Autologous Venous Tissue A Autologous Arterial Tissue J Synthetic Substitute K Nonautologous Tissue Substitute Z No Device	P Pulmonary Trunk Q Pulmonary Artery, Right R Pulmonary Artery, Left S Pulmonary Vein, Right T Pulmonary Vein, Left U Pulmonary Vein, Confluence
K Ventricle, Right Conus arteriosus L Ventricle, Left	0 Open 4 Percutaneous Endoscopic	8 Zooplastic Tissue 9 Autologous Venous Tissue A Autologous Arterial Tissue J Synthetic Substitute K Nonautologous Tissue Substitute	P Pulmonary Trunk Q Pulmonary Artery, Right R Pulmonary Artery, Left

021 Continued on next page

HAC 021[0,1,2,3]0[8,9,A,J,K][3,8,9,C,F,W] when reported with SDx J98.51 or J98.59
HAC 021[0,1,2,3]0Z[3,8,9,C,F] when reported with SDx J98.51 or J98.59
HAC 021[0,1,2,3]4[8,9,A,J,K][3,8,9,C,F,W] when reported with SDx J98.51 or J98.59
HAC 021[0,1,2,3]4Z[3,8,9,C,F] when reported with SDx J98.51 or J98.59=

Ø21 Continued

Ø Medical and Surgical
2 Heart and Great Vessels
1 Bypass Definition: Altering the route of passage of the contents of a tubular body part

Explanation: Rerouting contents of a body part to a downstream area of the normal route, to a similar route and body part, or to an abnormal route and dissimilar body part. Includes one or more anastomoses, with or without the use of a device.

Body Part Character 4	Approach Character 5	Device Character 6	Qualifier Character 7
K Ventricle, Right Conus arteriosus L Ventricle, Left	Ø Open 4 Percutaneous Endoscopic	Z No Device	5 Coronary Circulation 8 Internal Mammary, Right 9 Internal Mammary, Left C Thoracic Artery F Abdominal Artery P Pulmonary Trunk Q Pulmonary Artery, Right R Pulmonary Artery, Left W Aorta
P Pulmonary Trunk Q Pulmonary Artery, Right R Pulmonary Artery, Left Arterial canal (duct) Botallo's duct Pulmoaortic canal	Ø Open 4 Percutaneous Endoscopic	8 Zooplastic Tissue 9 Autologous Venous Tissue A Autologous Arterial Tissue J Synthetic Substitute K Nonautologous Tissue Substitute Z No Device	A Innominate Artery B Subclavian D Carotid
W Thoracic Aorta, Descending	Ø Open	8 Zooplastic Tissue 9 Autologous Venous Tissue A Autologous Arterial Tissue J Synthetic Substitute K Nonautologous Tissue Substitute	B Subclavian D Carotid F Abdominal Artery G Axillary Artery H Brachial Artery P Pulmonary Trunk Q Pulmonary Artery, Right R Pulmonary Artery, Left V Lower Extremity Artery
W Thoracic Aorta, Descending	Ø Open	Z No Device	B Subclavian D Carotid P Pulmonary Trunk Q Pulmonary Artery, Right R Pulmonary Artery, Left
W Thoracic Aorta, Descending	4 Percutaneous Endoscopic	8 Zooplastic Tissue 9 Autologous Venous Tissue A Autologous Arterial Tissue J Synthetic Substitute K Nonautologous Tissue Substitute Z No Device	B Subclavian D Carotid P Pulmonary Trunk Q Pulmonary Artery, Right R Pulmonary Artery, Left
X Thoracic Aorta, Ascending/Arch Aortic arch Ascending aorta	Ø Open 4 Percutaneous Endoscopic	8 Zooplastic Tissue 9 Autologous Venous Tissue A Autologous Arterial Tissue J Synthetic Substitute K Nonautologous Tissue Substitute Z No Device	B Subclavian D Carotid P Pulmonary Trunk Q Pulmonary Artery, Right R Pulmonary Artery, Left

Ø Medical and Surgical
2 Heart and Great Vessels
4 Creation Definition: Putting in or on biological or synthetic material to form a new body part that to the extent possible replicates the anatomic structure or function of an absent body part

Explanation: Used for gender reassignment surgery and corrective procedures in individuals with congenital anomalies

Body Part Character 4	Approach Character 5	Device Character 6	Qualifier Character 7
F Aortic Valve Aortic annulus	Ø Open	7 Autologous Tissue 8 Zooplastic Tissue J Synthetic Substitute K Nonautologous Tissue Substitute	J Truncal Valve
G Mitral Valve Bicuspid valve Left atrioventricular valve Mitral annulus J Tricuspid Valve Right atrioventricular valve Tricuspid annulus	Ø Open	7 Autologous Tissue 8 Zooplastic Tissue J Synthetic Substitute K Nonautologous Tissue Substitute	2 Common Atrioventricular Valve

Ø Medical and Surgical
2 Heart and Great Vessels
5 Destruction Definition: Physical eradication of all or a portion of a body part by the direct use of energy, force, or a destructive agent
Explanation: None of the body part is physically taken out

Body Part Character 4	Approach Character 5	Device Character 6	Qualifier Character 7
4 Coronary Vein **5 Atrial Septum** Interatrial septum **6 Atrium, Right** Atrium dextrum cordis Right auricular appendix Sinus venosus **8 Conduction Mechanism** Atrioventricular node Bundle of His Bundle of Kent Sinoatrial node **9 Chordae Tendineae** **D Papillary Muscle** **F Aortic Valve** Aortic annulus **G Mitral Valve** Bicuspid valve Left atrioventricular valve Mitral annulus **H Pulmonary Valve** Pulmonary annulus Pulmonic valve **J Tricuspid Valve** Right atrioventricular valve Tricuspid annulus **K Ventricle, Right** Conus arteriosus **L Ventricle, Left** **M Ventricular Septum** Interventricular septum **N Pericardium** **P Pulmonary Trunk** **Q Pulmonary Artery, Right** **R Pulmonary Artery, Left** Arterial canal (duct) Botallo's duct Pulmoaortic canal **S Pulmonary Vein, Right** Right inferior pulmonary vein Right superior pulmonary vein **T Pulmonary Vein, Left** Left inferior pulmonary vein Left superior pulmonary vein **V Superior Vena Cava** Precava **W Thoracic Aorta, Descending** **X Thoracic Aorta, Ascending/Arch** Aortic arch Ascending aorta	**Ø Open** **3 Percutaneous** **4 Percutaneous Endoscopic**	**Z No Device**	**Z No Qualifier**
7 Atrium, Left Atrium pulmonale Left auricular appendix	**Ø Open** **3 Percutaneous** **4 Percutaneous Endoscopic**	**Z No Device**	**K Left Atrial Appendage** **Z No Qualifier**

DRG Non-OR Ø257[Ø,3,4]ZK

Ø Medical and Surgical
2 Heart and Great Vessels
7 Dilation Definition: Expanding an orifice or the lumen of a tubular body part

Explanation: The orifice can be a natural orifice or an artificially created orifice. Accomplished by stretching a tubular body part using intraluminal pressure or by cutting part of the orifice or wall of the tubular body part.

Body Part Character 4	Approach Character 5	Device Character 6	Qualifier Character 7
Ø Coronary Artery, One Artery **1** Coronary Artery, Two Arteries **2** Coronary Artery, Three Arteries **3** Coronary Artery, Four or More Arteries	**Ø** Open **3** Percutaneous **4** Percutaneous Endoscopic	**4** Intraluminal Device, Drug-eluting **5** Intraluminal Device, Drug-eluting, Two **6** Intraluminal Device, Drug-eluting, Three **7** Intraluminal Device, Drug-eluting, Four or More **D** Intraluminal Device **E** Intraluminal Device, Two **F** Intraluminal Device, Three **G** Intraluminal Device, Four or More **T** Intraluminal Device, Radioactive **Z** No Device	**6** Bifurcation **Z** No Qualifier
F Aortic Valve Aortic annulus **G** Mitral Valve Bicuspid valve Left atrioventricular valve Mitral annulus **H** Pulmonary Valve Pulmonary annulus Pulmonic valve **J** Tricuspid Valve Right atrioventricular valve Tricuspid annulus **K** Ventricle, Right Conus arteriosus **L** Ventricle, Left **P** Pulmonary Trunk **Q** Pulmonary Artery, Right **S** Pulmonary Vein, Right Right inferior pulmonary vein Right superior pulmonary vein **T** Pulmonary Vein, Left Left inferior pulmonary vein Left superior pulmonary vein **V** Superior Vena Cava Precava **W** Thoracic Aorta, Descending **X** Thoracic Aorta, Ascending/Arch Aortic arch Ascending aorta	**Ø** Open **3** Percutaneous **4** Percutaneous Endoscopic	**4** Intraluminal Device, Drug-eluting **D** Intraluminal Device **Z** No Device	**Z** No Qualifier
R Pulmonary Artery, Left Arterial canal (duct) Botallo's duct Pulmoaortic canal	**Ø** Open **3** Percutaneous **4** Percutaneous Endoscopic	**4** Intraluminal Device, Drug-eluting **D** Intraluminal Device **Z** No Device	**T** Ductus Arteriosus **Z** No Qualifier

Ø Medical and Surgical
2 Heart and Great Vessels
8 Division Definition: Cutting into a body part, without draining fluids and/or gases from the body part, in order to separate or transect a body part

Explanation: All or a portion of the body part is separated into two or more portions

Body Part Character 4	Approach Character 5	Device Character 6	Qualifier Character 7
8 Conduction Mechanism Atrioventricular node Bundle of His Bundle of Kent Sinoatrial node **9** Chordae Tendineae **D** Papillary Muscle	**Ø** Open **3** Percutaneous **4** Percutaneous Endoscopic	**Z** No Device	**Z** No Qualifier

0 Medical and Surgical
2 Heart and Great Vessels
B Excision Definition: Cutting out or off, without replacement, a portion of a body part
Explanation: The qualifier DIAGNOSTIC is used to identify excision procedures that are biopsies

Body Part Character 4	Approach Character 5	Device Character 6	Qualifier Character 7
4 Coronary Vein 5 Atrial Septum Interatrial septum 6 Atrium, Right Atrium dextrum cordis Right auricular appendix Sinus venosus 8 Conduction Mechanism Atrioventricular node Bundle of His Bundle of Kent Sinoatrial node 9 Chordae Tendineae D Papillary Muscle F Aortic Valve Aortic annulus G Mitral Valve Bicuspid valve Left atrioventricular valve Mitral annulus H Pulmonary Valve Pulmonary annulus Pulmonic valve J Tricuspid Valve Right atrioventricular valve Tricuspid annulus K Ventricle, Right NC Conus arteriosus L Ventricle, Left NC M Ventricular Septum Interventricular septum N Pericardium P Pulmonary Trunk Q Pulmonary Artery, Right R Pulmonary Artery, Left Arterial canal (duct) Botallo's duct Pulmoaortic canal S Pulmonary Vein, Right Right inferior pulmonary vein Right superior pulmonary vein T Pulmonary Vein, Left Left inferior pulmonary vein Left superior pulmonary vein V Superior Vena Cava Precava W Thoracic Aorta, Descending X Thoracic Aorta, Ascending/Arch Aortic arch Ascending aorta	0 Open 3 Percutaneous 4 Percutaneous Endoscopic	Z No Device	X Diagnostic Z No Qualifier
7 Atrium, Left Atrium pulmonale Left auricular appendix	0 Open 3 Percutaneous 4 Percutaneous Endoscopic	Z No Device	K Left Atrial Appendage X Diagnostic Z No Qualifier

DRG Non-OR 02B7[0,3,4]ZK
Non-OR 02B[4,5,6,8,9,D,F,G,H,J,K,L,M][0,3,4]ZX
NC 02B[K,L][0,3,4]ZZ

Ø Medical and Surgical
2 Heart and Great Vessels
C Extirpation Definition: Taking or cutting out solid matter from a body part

Explanation: The solid matter may be an abnormal byproduct of a biological function or a foreign body; it may be imbedded in a body part or in the lumen of a tubular body part. The solid matter may or may not have been previously broken into pieces.

Body Part Character 4	Approach Character 5	Device Character 6	Qualifier Character 7
Ø Coronary Artery, One Artery **1** Coronary Artery, Two Arteries **2** Coronary Artery, Three Arteries **3** Coronary Artery, Four or More Arteries	**Ø** Open **3** Percutaneous **4** Percutaneous Endoscopic	**Z** No Device	**6** Bifurcation **Z** No Qualifier
4 Coronary Vein **5** Atrial Septum Interatrial septum **6** Atrium, Right Atrium dextrum cordis Right auricular appendix Sinus venosus **7** Atrium, Left Atrium pulmonale Left auricular appendix **8** Conduction Mechanism Atrioventricular node Bundle of His Bundle of Kent Sinoatrial node **9** Chordae Tendineae **D** Papillary Muscle **F** Aortic Valve Aortic annulus **G** Mitral Valve Bicuspid valve Left atrioventricular valve Mitral annulus **H** Pulmonary Valve Pulmonary annulus Pulmonic valve **J** Tricuspid Valve Right atrioventricular valve Tricuspid annulus **K** Ventricle, Right Conus arteriosus **L** Ventricle, Left **M** Ventricular Septum Interventricular septum **N** Pericardium **P** Pulmonary Trunk **Q** Pulmonary Artery, Right **R** Pulmonary Artery, Left Arterial canal (duct) Botallo's duct Pulmoaortic canal **S** Pulmonary Vein, Right Right inferior pulmonary vein Right superior pulmonary vein **T** Pulmonary Vein, Left Left inferior pulmonary vein Left superior pulmonary vein **V** Superior Vena Cava Precava **W** Thoracic Aorta, Descending **X** Thoracic Aorta, Ascending/Arch Aortic arch Ascending aorta	**Ø** Open **3** Percutaneous **4** Percutaneous Endoscopic	**Z** No Device	**Z** No Qualifier

Ø Medical and Surgical
2 Heart and Great Vessels
F Fragmentation Definition: Breaking solid matter in a body part into pieces

Explanation: Physical force (e.g., manual, ultrasonic) applied directly or indirectly is used to break the solid matter into pieces. The solid matter may be an abnormal byproduct of a biological function or a foreign body. The pieces of solid matter are not taken out.

Body Part Character 4	Approach Character 5	Device Character 6	Qualifier Character 7
N Pericardium NC	**Ø** Open **3** Percutaneous **4** Percutaneous Endoscopic **X** External	**Z** No Device	**Z** No Qualifier

Non-OR Ø2FNXZZ
NC Ø2FNXZZ

Ø Medical and Surgical
2 Heart and Great Vessels
H Insertion Definition: Putting in a nonbiological appliance that monitors, assists, performs, or prevents a physiological function but does not physically take the place of a body part

Explanation: None

Body Part Character 4	Approach Character 5	Device Character 6	Qualifier Character 7
4 Coronary Vein ⊞ 6 Atrium, Right ⊞ Atrium dextrum cordis Right auricular appendix Sinus venosus 7 Atrium, Left ⊞ Atrium pulmonale Left auricular appendix K Ventricle, Right ⊞ Conus arteriosus L Ventricle, Left ⊞	Ø Open 3 Percutaneous 4 Percutaneous Endoscopic	Ø Monitoring Device, Pressure Sensor 2 Monitoring Device 3 Infusion Device D Intraluminal Device J Cardiac Lead, Pacemaker K Cardiac Lead, Defibrillator M Cardiac Lead N Intracardiac Pacemaker Y Other Device	Z No Qualifier
A Heart LC NC	Ø Open 3 Percutaneous 4 Percutaneous Endoscopic	Q Implantable Heart Assist System Y Other Device	Z No Qualifier
A Heart ⊞	Ø Open 3 Percutaneous 4 Percutaneous Endoscopic	R Short-term External Heart Assist System	J Intraoperative S Biventricular Z No Qualifier
N Pericardium ⊞	Ø Open 3 Percutaneous 4 Percutaneous Endoscopic	Ø Monitoring Device, Pressure Sensor 2 Monitoring Device J Cardiac Lead, Pacemaker K Cardiac Lead, Defibrillator M Cardiac Lead Y Other Device	Z No Qualifier
P Pulmonary Trunk Q Pulmonary Artery, Right R Pulmonary Artery, Left Arterial canal (duct) Botallo's duct Pulmoaortic canal S Pulmonary Vein, Right Right inferior pulmonary vein Right superior pulmonary vein T Pulmonary Vein, Left Left inferior pulmonary vein Left superior pulmonary vein V Superior Vena Cava Precava W Thoracic Aorta, Descending	Ø Open 3 Percutaneous 4 Percutaneous Endoscopic	Ø Monitoring Device, Pressure Sensor 2 Monitoring Device 3 Infusion Device D Intraluminal Device Y Other Device	Z No Qualifier
X Thoracic Aorta, Ascending/Arch Aortic arch Ascending aorta	Ø Open 3 Percutaneous 4 Percutaneous Endoscopic	Ø Monitoring Device, Pressure Sensor 2 Monitoring Device 3 Infusion Device D Intraluminal Device	Z No Qualifier

DRG Non-OR Ø2H[4,6,7][Ø,4][J,M]Z
DRG Non-OR Ø2H[6,7]3JZ
DRG Non-OR Ø2H[K,L][Ø,3,4][J,M]Z
DRG Non-OR Ø2HK32Z
Non-OR Ø2H[4,6,7,L]3[2,3]Z
Non-OR Ø2H[6,7]3MZ
Non-OR Ø2HK3[Ø,3]Z
Non-OR Ø2HN32Z
Non-OR Ø2HP[Ø,3,4][Ø,2,3]Z
Non-OR Ø2H[Q,R][Ø,3,4][2,3]Z
Non-OR Ø2H[S,T,V,W][Ø,3,4]3Z
Non-OR Ø2H[S,T,V,W]32Z
Non-OR Ø2HW[Ø,3]ØZ
Non-OR Ø2HX[Ø,3,4][Ø,3]Z

HAC Ø2H43[J,K,M]Z when reported with SDx K68.11 or T81.4XXA or T82.6XXA or T82.7XXA
HAC Ø2H[6,K]33Z when reported with SDx J95.811
HAC Ø2H[6,7]3[J,M]Z when reported with SDx K68.11 or T81.4XXA or T82.6XXA or T82.7XXA
HAC Ø2H[K,L]3JZ when reported with SDx K68.11 or T81.4XXA or T82.6XXA or T82.7XXA
HAC Ø2HN[Ø,3,4][J,M]Z when reported with SDx K68.11 or T81.4XXA or T82.6XXA or T82.7XXA
HAC Ø2H[S,T,V][3,4]3Z when reported with SDx J95.811
LC Ø2HAØQZ
NC Ø2HA[3,4]QZ

See Appendix L for Procedure Combinations
⊞ Ø2H[4,6,7,K,L][Ø,3,4]KZ
⊞ Ø2H43[J,M]Z
⊞ Ø2HA[Ø,4]R[S,Z]
⊞ Ø2HA3RS
⊞ Ø2HN[Ø,3,4][J,K,M]Z

Ø Medical and Surgical
2 Heart and Great Vessels
J Inspection Definition: Visually and/or manually exploring a body part
Explanation: Visual exploration may be performed with or without optical instrumentation. Manual exploration may be performed directly or through intervening body layers.

Body Part Character 4	Approach Character 5	Device Character 6	Qualifier Character 7
A Heart Y Great Vessel	Ø Open 3 Percutaneous 4 Percutaneous Endoscopic	Z No Device	Z No Qualifier

Non-OR Ø2J[A,Y]3ZZ

Ø Medical and Surgical
2 Heart and Great Vessels
K Map Definition: Locating the route of passage of electrical impulses and/or locating functional areas in a body part
Explanation: Applicable only to the cardiac conduction mechanism and the central nervous system

Body Part Character 4	Approach Character 5	Device Character 6	Qualifier Character 7
8 Conduction Mechanism Atrioventricular node Bundle of His Bundle of Kent Sinoatrial node	Ø Open 3 Percutaneous 4 Percutaneous Endoscopic	Z No Device	Z No Qualifier

DRG Non-OR Ø2K8[Ø,3,4]ZZ

Ø Medical and Surgical
2 Heart and Great Vessels
L Occlusion Definition: Completely closing an orifice or the lumen of a tubular body part
Explanation: The orifice can be a natural orifice or an artificially created orifice

Body Part Character 4	Approach Character 5	Device Character 6	Qualifier Character 7
7 Atrium, Left Atrium pulmonale Left auricular appendix	Ø Open 3 Percutaneous 4 Percutaneous Endoscopic	C Extraluminal Device D Intraluminal Device Z No Device	K Left Atrial Appendage
H Pulmonary Valve Pulmonary annulus Pulmonic valve P Pulmonary Trunk Q Pulmonary Artery, Right S Pulmonary Vein, Right Right inferior pulmonary vein Right superior pulmonary vein T Pulmonary Vein, Left Left inferior pulmonary vein Left superior pulmonary vein V Superior Vena Cava Precava	Ø Open 3 Percutaneous 4 Percutaneous Endoscopic	C Extraluminal Device D Intraluminal Device Z No Device	Z No Qualifier
R Pulmonary Artery, Left Arterial canal (duct) Botallo's duct Pulmoaortic canal	Ø Open 3 Percutaneous 4 Percutaneous Endoscopic	C Extraluminal Device D Intraluminal Device Z No Device	T Ductus Arteriosus Z No Qualifier
W Thoracic Aorta, Descending	3 Percutaneous	D Intraluminal Device	J Temporary

DRG Non-OR Ø2L7[Ø,3,4][C,D,Z]K

0 Medical and Surgical
2 Heart and Great Vessels
N Release Definition: Freeing a body part from an abnormal physical constraint by cutting or by the use of force
Explanation: Some of the restraining tissue may be taken out but none of the body part is taken out

Body Part Character 4	Approach Character 5	Device Character 6	Qualifier Character 7
0 Coronary Artery, One Artery **1 Coronary Artery, Two Arteries** **2 Coronary Artery, Three Arteries** **3 Coronary Artery, Four or More Arteries** **4 Coronary Vein** **5 Atrial Septum** Interatrial septum **6 Atrium, Right** Atrium dextrum cordis Right auricular appendix Sinus venosus **7 Atrium, Left** Atrium pulmonale Left auricular appendix **8 Conduction Mechanism** Atrioventricular node Bundle of His Bundle of Kent Sinoatrial node **9 Chordae Tendineae** **D Papillary Muscle** **F Aortic Valve** Aortic annulus **G Mitral Valve** Bicuspid valve Left atrioventricular valve Mitral annulus **H Pulmonary Valve** Pulmonary annulus Pulmonic valve **J Tricuspid Valve** Right atrioventricular valve Tricuspid annulus **K Ventricle, Right** Conus arteriosus **L Ventricle, Left** **M Ventricular Septum** Interventricular septum **N Pericardium** **P Pulmonary Trunk** **Q Pulmonary Artery, Right** **R Pulmonary Artery, Left** Arterial canal (duct) Botallo's duct Pulmoaortic canal **S Pulmonary Vein, Right** Right inferior pulmonary vein Right superior pulmonary vein **T Pulmonary Vein, Left** Left inferior pulmonary vein Left superior pulmonary vein **V Superior Vena Cava** Precava **W Thoracic Aorta, Descending** **X Thoracic Aorta, Ascending/Arch** Aortic arch Ascending aorta	0 Open 3 Percutaneous 4 Percutaneous Endoscopic	Z No Device	Z No Qualifier

Ø Medical and Surgical
2 Heart and Great Vessels
P Removal Definition: Taking out or off a device from a body part

Explanation: If a device is taken out and a similar device put in without cutting or puncturing the skin or mucous membrane, the procedure is coded to the root operation CHANGE. Otherwise, the procedure for taking out a device is coded to the root operation REMOVAL.

Body Part Character 4	Approach Character 5	Device Character 6	Qualifier Character 7
A Heart	Ø Open 3 Percutaneous 4 Percutaneous Endoscopic	2 Monitoring Device 3 Infusion Device 7 Autologous Tissue Substitute 8 Zooplastic Tissue C Extraluminal Device D Intraluminal Device J Synthetic Substitute K Nonautologous Tissue Substitute M Cardiac Lead N Intracardiac Pacemaker Q Implantable Heart Assist System Y Other Device	Z No Qualifier
A Heart ⊞	Ø Open 3 Percutaneous 4 Percutaneous Endoscopic	R Short-term External Heart Assist System	S Biventricular Z No Qualifier
A Heart	X External	2 Monitoring Device 3 Infusion Device D Intraluminal Device M Cardiac Lead	Z No Qualifier
Y Great Vessel	Ø Open 3 Percutaneous 4 Percutaneous Endoscopic	2 Monitoring Device 3 Infusion Device 7 Autologous Tissue Substitute 8 Zooplastic Tissue C Extraluminal Device D Intraluminal Device J Synthetic Substitute K Nonautologous Tissue Substitute Y Other Device	Z No Qualifier
Y Great Vessel	X External	2 Monitoring Device 3 Infusion Device D Intraluminal Device	Z No Qualifier

Non-OR Ø2PA3[2,3,D]Z
Non-OR Ø2PA[3,4]YZ
Non-OR Ø2PAX[2,3,D,M]Z
Non-OR Ø2PY3[2,3,D]Z
Non-OR Ø2PY[3,4]YZ
Non-OR Ø2PYX[2,3,D]Z
HAC Ø2PA[Ø,3,4]MZ when reported with SDx K68.11 or T81.4XXA or T82.6XXA or T82.7XXA
HAC Ø2PAXMZ when reported with SDx K68.11 or T81.4XXA or T82.6XXA or T82.7XXA

See Appendix L for Procedure Combinations
⊞ Ø2PA[Ø,3,4]RZ

Ø Medical and Surgical
2 Heart and Great Vessels
Q Repair Definition: Restoring, to the extent possible, a body part to its normal anatomic structure and function
Explanation: Used only when the method to accomplish the repair is not one of the other root operations

Body Part Character 4	Approach Character 5	Device Character 6	Qualifier Character 7
Ø Coronary Artery, One Artery **1 Coronary Artery, Two Arteries** **2 Coronary Artery, Three Arteries** **3 Coronary Artery, Four or More Arteries** **4 Coronary Vein** **5 Atrial Septum** Interatrial septum **6 Atrium, Right** Atrium dextrum cordis Right auricular appendix Sinus venosus **7 Atrium, Left** Atrium pulmonale Left auricular appendix **8 Conduction Mechanism** Atrioventricular node Bundle of His Bundle of Kent Sinoatrial node **9 Chordae Tendineae** **A Heart** **B Heart, Right** Right coronary sulcus **C Heart, Left** Left coronary sulcus Obtuse margin **D Papillary Muscle** **H Pulmonary Valve** Pulmonary annulus Pulmonic valve **K Ventricle, Right** Conus arteriosus **L Ventricle, Left** **M Ventricular Septum** Interventricular septum **N Pericardium** **P Pulmonary Trunk** **Q Pulmonary Artery, Right** **R Pulmonary Artery, Left** Arterial canal (duct) Botallo's duct Pulmoaortic canal **S Pulmonary Vein, Right** Right inferior pulmonary vein Right superior pulmonary vein **T Pulmonary Vein, Left** Left inferior pulmonary vein Left superior pulmonary vein **V Superior Vena Cava** Precava **W Thoracic Aorta, Descending** **X Thoracic Aorta, Ascending/Arch** Aortic arch Ascending aorta	Ø Open 3 Percutaneous 4 Percutaneous Endoscopic	Z No Device	Z No Qualifier
F Aortic Valve Aortic annulus	Ø Open 3 Percutaneous 4 Percutaneous Endoscopic	Z No Device	J Truncal Valve Z No Qualifier
G Mitral Valve Bicuspid valve Left atrioventricular valve Mitral annulus	Ø Open 3 Percutaneous 4 Percutaneous Endoscopic	Z No Device	E Atrioventricular Valve, Left Z No Qualifier
J Tricuspid Valve Right atrioventricular valve Tricuspid annulus	Ø Open 3 Percutaneous 4 Percutaneous Endoscopic	Z No Device	G Atrioventricular Valve, Right Z No Qualifier

Ø Medical and Surgical
2 Heart and Great Vessels
R Replacement Definition: Putting in or on biological or synthetic material that physically takes the place and/or function of all or a portion of a body part

Explanation: The body part may have been taken out or replaced, or may be taken out, physically eradicated, or rendered nonfunctional during the REPLACEMENT procedure. A REMOVAL procedure is coded for taking out the device used in a previous replacement procedure.

Body Part Character 4	Approach Character 5	Device Character 6	Qualifier Character 7
5 Atrial Septum Interatrial septum **6 Atrium, Right** Atrium dextrum cordis Right auricular appendix Sinus venosus **7 Atrium, Left** Atrium pulmonale Left auricular appendix **9 Chordae Tendineae** **D Papillary Muscle** **K Ventricle, Right** ⊞ LC NC Conus arteriosus **L Ventricle, Left** ⊞ LC NC **M Ventricular Septum** Interventricular septum **N Pericardium** **P Pulmonary Trunk** **Q Pulmonary Artery, Right** **R Pulmonary Artery, Left** Arterial canal (duct) Botallo's duct Pulmoaortic canal **S Pulmonary Vein, Right** Right inferior pulmonary vein Right superior pulmonary vein **T Pulmonary Vein, Left** Left inferior pulmonary vein Left superior pulmonary vein **V Superior Vena Cava** Precava **W Thoracic Aorta, Descending** **X Thoracic Aorta, Ascending/Arch** Aortic arch Ascending aorta	**Ø Open** **4 Percutaneous Endoscopic**	**7 Autologous Tissue Substitute** **8 Zooplastic Tissue** **J Synthetic Substitute** **K Nonautologous Tissue Substitute**	**Z No Qualifier**
F Aortic Valve Aortic annulus **G Mitral Valve** Bicuspid valve Left atrioventricular valve Mitral annulus **H Pulmonary Valve** Pulmonary annulus Pulmonic valve **J Tricuspid Valve** Right atrioventricular valve Tricuspid annulus	**Ø Open** **4 Percutaneous Endoscopic**	**7 Autologous Tissue Substitute** **8 Zooplastic Tissue** **J Synthetic Substitute** **K Nonautologous Tissue Substitute**	**Z No Qualifier**
F Aortic Valve Aortic annulus **G Mitral Valve** Bicuspid valve Left atrioventricular valve Mitral annulus **H Pulmonary Valve** Pulmonary annulus Pulmonic valve **J Tricuspid Valve** Right atrioventricular valve Tricuspid annulus	**3 Percutaneous**	**7 Autologous Tissue Substitute** **8 Zooplastic Tissue** **J Synthetic Substitute** **K Nonautologous Tissue Substitute**	**H Transapical** **Z No Qualifier**

LC Ø2RKØJZ with Ø2RLØJZ with diagnosis code ZØØ.6
NC Ø2RKØJZ with Ø2RLØJZ without diagnosis code ZØØ.6

See Appendix L for Procedure Combinations
⊞ Ø2R[K,L]ØJZ

Ø Medical and Surgical
2 Heart and Great Vessels
S Reposition Definition: Moving to its normal location, or other suitable location, all or a portion of a body part

Explanation: The body part is moved to a new location from an abnormal location, or from a normal location where it is not functioning correctly. The body part may or may not be cut out or off to be moved to the new location.

Body Part Character 4	Approach Character 5	Device Character 6	Qualifier Character 7
Ø Coronary Artery, One Artery **1 Coronary Artery, Two Arteries** **P Pulmonary Trunk** **Q Pulmonary Artery, Right** **R Pulmonary Artery, Left** Arterial canal (duct) Botallo's duct Pulmoaortic canal **S Pulmonary Vein, Right** Right inferior pulmonary vein Right superior pulmonary vein **T Pulmonary Vein, Left** Left inferior pulmonary vein Left superior pulmonary vein **V Superior Vena Cava** Precava **W Thoracic Aorta, Descending** **X Thoracic Aorta, Ascending/Arch** Aortic arch Ascending aorta	Ø Open	Z No Device	Z No Qualifier

Ø Medical and Surgical
2 Heart and Great Vessels
T Resection Definition: Cutting out or off, without replacement, all of a body part

Explanation: None

Body Part Character 4	Approach Character 5	Device Character 6	Qualifier Character 7
5 Atrial Septum Interatrial septum **8 Conduction Mechanism** Atrioventricular node Bundle of His Bundle of Kent Sinoatrial node **9 Chordae Tendineae** **D Papillary Muscle** **H Pulmonary Valve** Pulmonary annulus Pulmonic valve **M Ventricular Septum** Interventricular septum **N Pericardium**	Ø Open 3 Percutaneous 4 Percutaneous Endoscopic	Z No Device	Z No Qualifier

Ø Medical and Surgical
2 Heart and Great Vessels
U Supplement Definition: Putting in or on biological or synthetic material that physically reinforces and/or augments the function of a portion of a body part
Explanation: The biological material is non-living, or is living and from the same individual. The body part may have been previously replaced, and the SUPPLEMENT procedure is performed to physically reinforce and/or augment the function of the replaced body part.

Body Part Character 4	Approach Character 5	Device Character 6	Qualifier Character 7
5 Atrial Septum Interatrial septum **6 Atrium, Right** Atrium dextrum cordis Right auricular appendix Sinus venosus **7 Atrium, Left** Atrium pulmonale Left auricular appendix **9 Chordae Tendineae** **A Heart** **D Papillary Muscle** **H Pulmonary Valve** Pulmonary annulus Pulmonic valve **K Ventricle, Right** Conus arteriosus **L Ventricle, Left** **M Ventricular Septum** Interventricular septum **N Pericardium** **P Pulmonary Trunk** **Q Pulmonary Artery, Right** **R Pulmonary Artery, Left** Arterial canal (duct) Botallo's duct Pulmoaortic canal **S Pulmonary Vein, Right** Right inferior pulmonary vein Right superior pulmonary vein **T Pulmonary Vein, Left** Left inferior pulmonary vein Left superior pulmonary vein **V Superior Vena Cava** Precava **W Thoracic Aorta, Descending** **X Thoracic Aorta, Ascending/Arch** Aortic arch Ascending aorta	**Ø Open** **3 Percutaneous** **4 Percutaneous Endoscopic**	**7 Autologous Tissue Substitute** **8 Zooplastic Tissue** **J Synthetic Substitute** **K Nonautologous Tissue Substitute**	**Z No Qualifier**
F Aortic Valve Aortic annulus	**Ø Open** **3 Percutaneous** **4 Percutaneous Endoscopic**	**7 Autologous Tissue Substitute** **8 Zooplastic Tissue** **J Synthetic Substitute** **K Nonautologous Tissue Substitute**	**J Truncal Valve** **Z No Qualifier**
G Mitral Valve Bicuspid valve Left atrioventricular valve Mitral annulus	**Ø Open** **3 Percutaneous** **4 Percutaneous Endoscopic**	**7 Autologous Tissue Substitute** **8 Zooplastic Tissue** **J Synthetic Substitute** **K Nonautologous Tissue Substitute**	**E Atrioventricular Valve, Left** **Z No Qualifier**
J Tricuspid Valve Right atrioventricular valve Tricuspid annulus	**Ø Open** **3 Percutaneous** **4 Percutaneous Endoscopic**	**7 Autologous Tissue Substitute** **8 Zooplastic Tissue** **J Synthetic Substitute** **K Nonautologous Tissue Substitute**	**G Atrioventricular Valve, Right** **Z No Qualifier**

DRG Non-OR Ø2U7[3,4]JZ

Ø Medical and Surgical
2 Heart and Great Vessels
V Restriction Definition: Partially closing an orifice or the lumen of a tubular body part
Explanation: The orifice can be a natural orifice or an artificially created orifice

Body Part Character 4	Approach Character 5	Device Character 6	Qualifier Character 7
A Heart	Ø Open 3 Percutaneous 4 Percutaneous Endoscopic	C Extraluminal Device Z No Device	Z No Qualifier
G Mitral Valve Bicuspid valve Left atrioventricular valve Mitral annulus	Ø Open 3 Percutaneous 4 Percutaneous Endoscopic	Z No Device	Z No Qualifier
P Pulmonary Trunk Q Pulmonary Artery, Right S Pulmonary Vein, Right Right inferior pulmonary vein Right superior pulmonary vein T Pulmonary Vein, Left Left inferior pulmonary vein Left superior pulmonary vein V Superior Vena Cava Precava	Ø Open 3 Percutaneous 4 Percutaneous Endoscopic	C Extraluminal Device D Intraluminal Device Z No Device	Z No Qualifier
R Pulmonary Artery, Left Arterial canal (duct) Botallo's duct Pulmoaortic canal	Ø Open 3 Percutaneous 4 Percutaneous Endoscopic	C Extraluminal Device D Intraluminal Device Z No Device	T Ductus Arteriosus Z No Qualifier
W Thoracic Aorta, Descending X Thoracic Aorta, Ascending/Arch Aortic arch Ascending aorta	Ø Open 3 Percutaneous 4 Percutaneous Endoscopic	C Extraluminal Device D Intraluminal Device E Intraluminal Device, Branched or Fenestrated, One or Two Arteries F Intraluminal Device, Branched or Fenestrated, Three or More Arteries Z No Device	Z No Qualifier

Ø Medical and Surgical
2 Heart and Great Vessels
W Revision Definition: Correcting, to the extent possible, a portion of a malfunctioning device or the position of a displaced device
Explanation: Revision can include correcting a malfunctioning or displaced device by taking out or putting in components of the device such as a screw or pin

Body Part Character 4	Approach Character 5	Device Character 6	Qualifier Character 7
5 Atrial Septum Interatrial septum M Ventricular Septum Interventricular septum	Ø Open 4 Percutaneous Endoscopic	J Synthetic Substitute	Z No Qualifier
A Heart ⊞ LC NC	Ø Open 3 Percutaneous 4 Percutaneous Endoscopic	2 Monitoring Device 3 Infusion Device 7 Autologous Tissue Substitute 8 Zooplastic Tissue C Extraluminal Device D Intraluminal Device J Synthetic Substitute K Nonautologous Tissue Substitute M Cardiac Lead N Intracardiac Pacemaker Q Implantable Heart Assist System Y Other Device	Z No Qualifier
A Heart ⊞	Ø Open 3 Percutaneous 4 Percutaneous Endoscopic	R Short-term External Heart Assist System	S Biventricular Z No Qualifier
A Heart	X External	2 Monitoring Device 3 Infusion Device 7 Autologous Tissue Substitute 8 Zooplastic Tissue C Extraluminal Device D Intraluminal Device J Synthetic Substitute K Nonautologous Tissue Substitute M Cardiac Lead N Intracardiac Pacemaker Q Implantable Heart Assist System	Z No Qualifier
A Heart	X External	R Short-term External Heart Assist System	S Biventricular Z No Qualifier
F Aortic Valve Aortic annulus G Mitral Valve Bicuspid valve Left atrioventricular valve Mitral annulus H Pulmonary Valve Pulmonary annulus Pulmonic valve J Tricuspid Valve Right atrioventricular valve Tricuspid annulus	Ø Open 3 Percutaneous 4 Percutaneous Endoscopic	7 Autologous Tissue Substitute 8 Zooplastic Tissue J Synthetic Substitute K Nonautologous Tissue Substitute	Z No Qualifier
Y Great Vessel	Ø Open 3 Percutaneous 4 Percutaneous Endoscopic	2 Monitoring Device 3 Infusion Device 7 Autologous Tissue Substitute 8 Zooplastic Tissue C Extraluminal Device D Intraluminal Device J Synthetic Substitute K Nonautologous Tissue Substitute Y Other Device	Z No Qualifier
Y Great Vessel	X External	2 Monitoring Device 3 Infusion Device 7 Autologous Tissue Substitute 8 Zooplastic Tissue C Extraluminal Device D Intraluminal Device J Synthetic Substitute K Nonautologous Tissue Substitute	Z No Qualifier

Non-OR Ø2WA3[2,3,D]Z
Non-OR Ø2WA[3,4]YZ
Non-OR Ø2WAX[2,3,7,8,C,D,J,K,M,N,Q]Z
Non-OR Ø2WAXRZ
Non-OR Ø2WY3[2,3,D]Z
Non-OR Ø2WY[3,4]YZ
Non-OR Ø2WYX[2,3,7,8,C,D,J,K]Z

HAC Ø2WA[Ø,3,4]MZ when reported with SDx K68.11 or T81.4XXA or T82.6XXA or T82.7XXA
LC Ø2WAØ[J,Q]Z
NC Ø2WA[3,4]QZ

See Appendix L for Procedure Combinations
⊞ Ø2WA[Ø,3,4]QZ
⊞ Ø2WA[Ø,3,4]RZ

Ø Medical and Surgical
2 Heart and Great Vessels
Y Transplantation Definition: Putting in or on all or a portion of a living body part taken from another individual or animal to physically take the place and/or function of all or a portion of a similar body part

Explanation: The native body part may or may not be taken out, and the transplanted body part may take over all or a portion of its function

Body Part Character 4	Approach Character 5	Device Character 6	Qualifier Character 7
A Heart LC	Ø Open	Z No Device	Ø Allogeneic 1 Syngeneic 2 Zooplastic

LC Ø2YAØZ[Ø,1,2]

Upper Arteries Ø31–Ø3W

Character Meanings

This Character Meaning table is provided as a guide to assist the user in the identification of character members that may be found in this section of code tables. It **SHOULD NOT** be used to build a PCS code.

Operation–Character 3	Body Part–Character 4	Approach–Character 5	Device–Character 6	Qualifier–Character 7
1 Bypass	Ø Internal Mammary Artery, Right	Ø Open	Ø Drainage Device	Ø Upper Arm Artery, Right
5 Destruction	1 Internal Mammary Artery, Left	3 Percutaneous	2 Monitoring Device	1 Upper Arm Artery, Left OR Drug-Coated Balloon
7 Dilation	2 Innominate Artery	4 Percutaneous Endoscopic	3 Infusion Device	2 Upper Arm Artery, Bilateral
9 Drainage	3 Subclavian Artery, Right	X External	4 Intraluminal Device, Drug-eluting	3 Lower Arm Artery, Right
B Excision	4 Subclavian Artery, Left		5 Intraluminal Device, Drug-eluting, Two	4 Lower Arm Artery, Left
C Extirpation	5 Axillary Artery, Right		6 Intraluminal Device, Drug-eluting, Three	5 Lower Arm Artery, Bilateral
H Insertion	6 Axillary Artery, Left		7 Intraluminal Device, Drug-eluting, Four or More OR Autologous Tissue Substitute	6 Upper Leg Artery, Right OR Bifurcation
J Inspection	7 Brachial Artery, Right		9 Autologous Venous Tissue	7 Upper Leg Artery, Left OR Stent Retriever
L Occlusion	8 Brachial Artery, Left		A Autologous Arterial Tissue	8 Upper Leg Artery, Bilateral
N Release	9 Ulnar Artery, Right		B Intraluminal Device, Bioactive	9 Lower Leg Artery, Right
P Removal	A Ulnar Artery, Left		C Extraluminal Device	B Lower Leg Artery, Left
Q Repair	B Radial Artery, Right		D Intraluminal Device	C Lower Leg Artery, Bilateral
R Replacement	C Radial Artery, Left		E Intraluminal Device, Two	D Upper Arm Vein
S Reposition	D Hand Artery, Right		F Intraluminal Device, Three	F Lower Arm Vein
U Supplement	F Hand Artery, Left		G Intraluminal Device, Four or More	G Intracranial Artery
V Restriction	G Intracranial Artery		J Synthetic Substitute	J Extracranial Artery, Right
W Revision	H Common Carotid Artery, Right		K Nonautologous Tissue Substitute	K Extracranial Artery, Left
	J Common Carotid Artery, Left		M Stimulator Lead	M Pulmonary Artery, Right
	K Internal Carotid Artery, Right		Y Other Device	N Pulmonary Artery, Left
	L Internal Carotid Artery, Left		Z No Device	T Abdominal Artery
	M External Carotid Artery, Right			V Superior Vena Cava
	N External Carotid Artery, Left			X Diagnostic
	P Vertebral Artery, Right			Y Upper Artery
	Q Vertebral Artery, Left			Z No Qualifier
	R Face Artery			
	S Temporal Artery, Right			
	T Temporal Artery, Left			
	U Thyroid Artery, Right			
	V Thyroid Artery, Left			
	Y Upper Artery			

AHA Coding Clinic for table Ø31

2017, 4Q, 64-65	New qualifier values - Left to right carotid bypass
2017, 2Q, 22	Carotid artery to subclavian artery transposition
2017, 1Q, 31	Left to right common carotid artery bypass
2016, 3Q, 37	Insertion of arteriovenous graft using HeRO device
2016, 3Q, 39	Revision of arteriovenous graft
2013, 4Q, 125	Stage II cephalic vein transposition (superficialization) of arteriovenous fistula
2013, 1Q, 27	Creation of radial artery fistula

AHA Coding Clinic for table Ø37

2018, 2Q, 24	Coronary artery bifurcation
2016, 4Q, 86	Peripheral artery, number of stents
2016, 4Q, 86-87	Coronary and peripheral artery bifurcation
2015, 1Q, 32	Deployment of stent for herniated/migrated coil in basilar artery

AHA Coding Clinic for table Ø3B

2016, 2Q, 12	Resection of malignant neoplasm of infratemporal fossa

AHA Coding Clinic for table Ø3C

2018, 2Q, 24	Coronary artery bifurcation
2017, 4Q, 64-65	New qualifier values - Left to right carotid bypass
2017, 2Q, 23	Thrombectomy via Fogarty catheter
2016, 4Q, 86-87	Coronary and peripheral artery bifurcation
2016, 2Q, 11	Carotid endarterectomy with patch angioplasty
2015, 1Q, 29	Discontinued carotid endarterectomy

AHA Coding Clinic for table Ø3H

2016, 2Q, 32	Arterial catheter placement

AHA Coding Clinic for table Ø3J

2015, 1Q, 29	Discontinued carotid endarterectomy

AHA Coding Clinic for table Ø3L

2016, 2Q, 30	Clipping (occlusion) of cerebral artery, decompressive craniectomy and storage of bone flap in abdominal wall
2014, 4Q, 20	Control of epistaxis
2014, 4Q, 37	Endovascular embolization of arteriovenous malformation using Onyx-18 liquid

AHA Coding Clinic for table Ø3Q

2017, 1Q, 31	Left to right common carotid artery bypass

AHA Coding Clinic for table Ø3S

2017, 2Q, 22	Carotid artery to subclavian artery transposition
2015, 3Q, 27	Moyamoya disease and hemispheric pial synagiosis with craniotomy

AHA Coding Clinic for table Ø3U

2016, 2Q, 11	Carotid endarterectomy with patch angioplasty

AHA Coding Clinic for table Ø3V

2016, 1Q, 19	Embolization of superior hypophyseal aneurysm using stent-assisted coil

AHA Coding Clinic for table Ø3W

2016, 3Q, 39	Revision of arteriovenous graft
2015, 1Q, 32	Deployment of stent for herniated/migrated coil in basilar artery

Upper Arteries

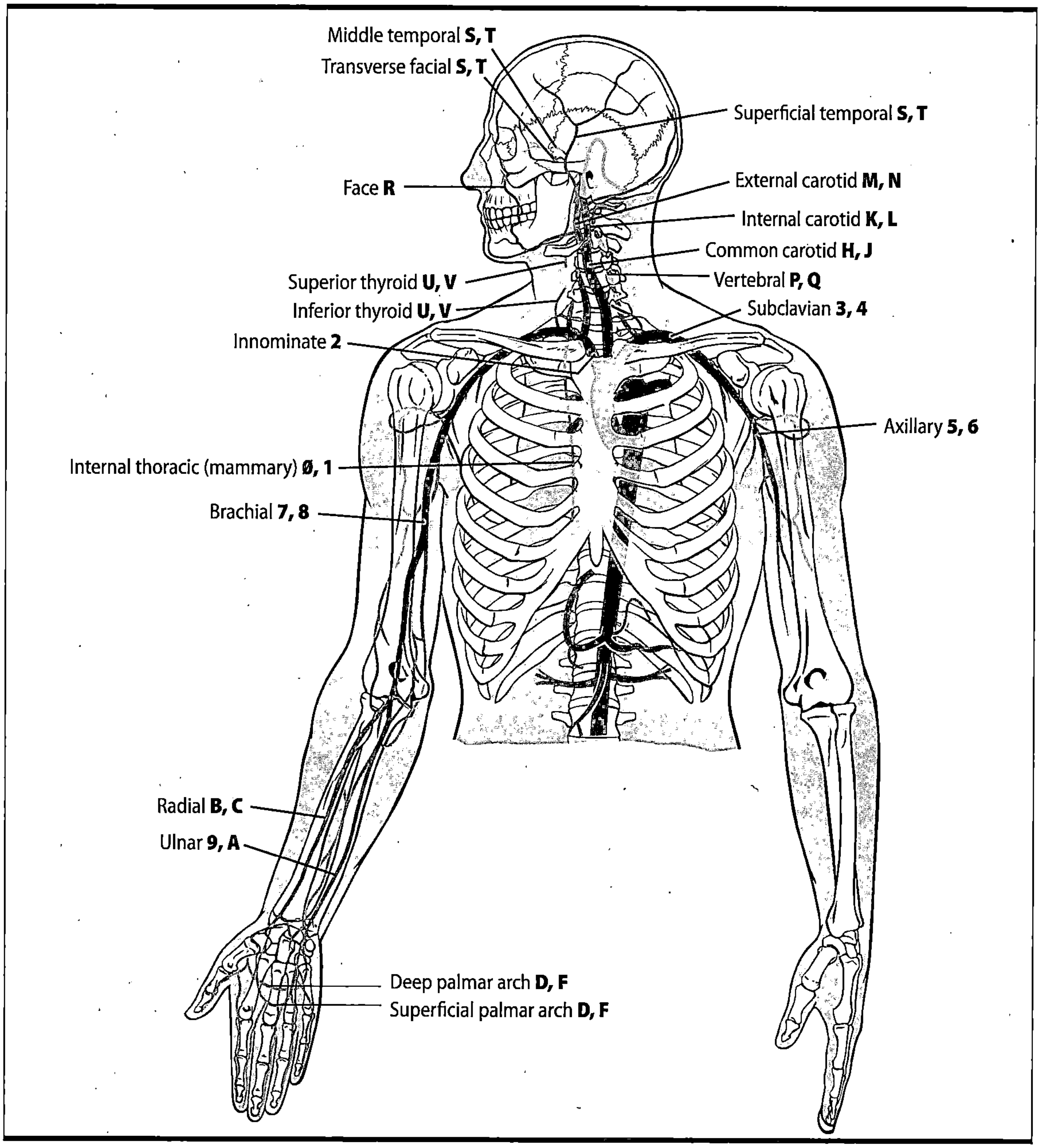
Middle temporal **S, T**
Transverse facial **S, T**
Superficial temporal **S, T**
Face **R**
External carotid **M, N**
Internal carotid **K, L**
Common carotid **H, J**
Superior thyroid **U, V**
Vertebral **P, Q**
Inferior thyroid **U, V**
Subclavian **3, 4**
Innominate **2**
Axillary **5, 6**
Internal thoracic (mammary) **Ø, 1**
Brachial **7, 8**
Radial **B, C**
Ulnar **9, A**
Deep palmar arch **D, F**
Superficial palmar arch **D, F**

Head and Neck Arteries

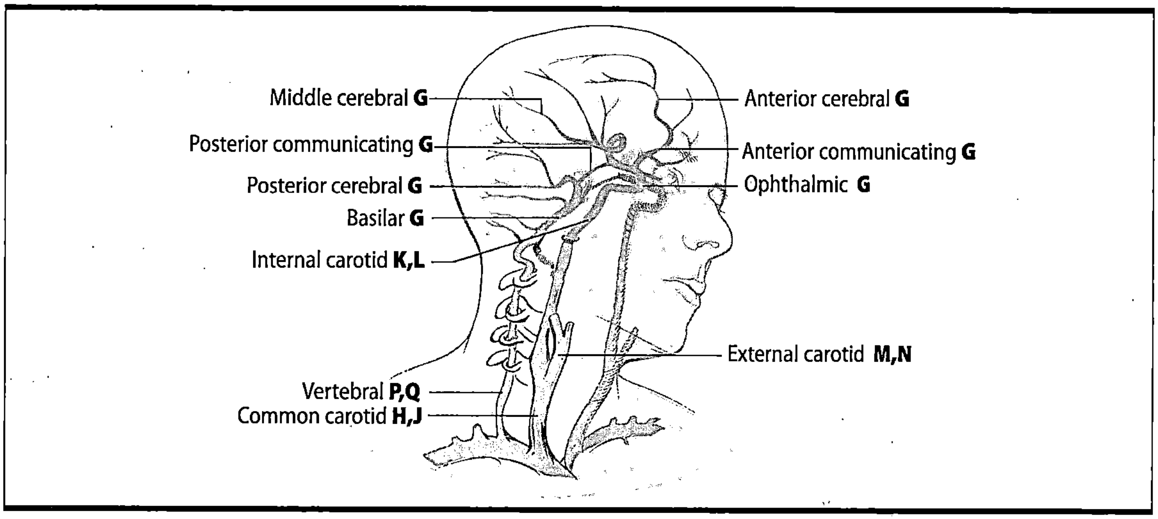
Middle cerebral **G**
Anterior cerebral **G**
Posterior communicating **G**
Anterior communicating **G**
Posterior cerebral **G**
Ophthalmic **G**
Basilar **G**
Internal carotid **K,L**
External carotid **M,N**
Vertebral **P,Q**
Common carotid **H,J**

Ø Medical and Surgical
3 Upper Arteries
1 Bypass Definition: Altering the route of passage of the contents of a tubular body part

Explanation: Rerouting contents of a body part to a downstream area of the normal route, to a similar route and body part, or to an abnormal route and dissimilar body part. Includes one or more anastomoses, with or without the use of a device.

Body Part Character 4	Approach Character 5	Device Character 6	Qualifier Character 7
2 Innominate Artery Brachiocephalic artery Brachiocephalic trunk	**Ø Open**	**9 Autologous Venous Tissue** **A Autologous Arterial Tissue** **J Synthetic Substitute** **K Nonautologous Tissue Substitute** **Z No Device**	**Ø Upper Arm Artery, Right** **1 Upper Arm Artery, Left** **2 Upper Arm Artery, Bilateral** **3 Lower Arm Artery, Right** **4 Lower Arm Artery, Left** **5 Lower Arm Artery, Bilateral** **6 Upper Leg Artery, Right** **7 Upper Leg Artery, Left** **8 Upper Leg Artery, Bilateral** **9 Lower Leg Artery, Right** **B Lower Leg Artery, Left** **C Lower Leg Artery, Bilateral** **D Upper Arm Vein** **F Lower Arm Vein** **J Extracranial Artery, Right** **K Extracranial Artery, Left**
3 Subclavian Artery, Right Costocervical trunk Dorsal scapular artery Internal thoracic artery **4 Subclavian Artery, Left** *See 3 Subclavian Artery, Right*	**Ø Open**	**9 Autologous Venous Tissue** **A Autologous Arterial Tissue** **J Synthetic Substitute** **K Nonautologous Tissue Substitute** **Z No Device**	**Ø Upper Arm Artery, Right** **1 Upper Arm Artery, Left** **2 Upper Arm Artery, Bilateral** **3 Lower Arm Artery, Right** **4 Lower Arm Artery, Left** **5 Lower Arm Artery, Bilateral** **6 Upper Leg Artery, Right** **7 Upper Leg Artery, Left** **8 Upper Leg Artery, Bilateral** **9 Lower Leg Artery, Right** **B Lower Leg Artery, Left** **C Lower Leg Artery, Bilateral** **D Upper Arm Vein** **F Lower Arm Vein** **J Extracranial Artery, Right** **K Extracranial Artery, Left** **M Pulmonary Artery, Right** **N Pulmonary Artery, Left**
5 Axillary Artery, Right Anterior circumflex humeral artery Lateral thoracic artery Posterior circumflex humeral artery Subscapular artery Superior thoracic artery Thoracoacromial artery **6 Axillary Artery, Left** *See 5 Axillary Artery, Right*	**Ø Open**	**9 Autologous Venous Tissue** **A Autologous Arterial Tissue** **J Synthetic Substitute** **K Nonautologous Tissue Substitute** **Z No Device**	**Ø Upper Arm Artery, Right** **1 Upper Arm Artery, Left** **2 Upper Arm Artery, Bilateral** **3 Lower Arm Artery, Right** **4 Lower Arm Artery, Left** **5 Lower Arm Artery, Bilateral** **6 Upper Leg Artery, Right** **7 Upper Leg Artery, Left** **8 Upper Leg Artery, Bilateral** **9 Lower Leg Artery, Right** **B Lower Leg Artery, Left** **C Lower Leg Artery, Bilateral** **D Upper Arm Vein** **F Lower Arm Vein** **J Extracranial Artery, Right** **K Extracranial Artery, Left** **T Abdominal Artery** **V Superior Vena Cava**
7 Brachial Artery, Right Inferior ulnar collateral artery Profunda brachii Superior ulnar collateral artery	**Ø Open**	**9 Autologous Venous Tissue** **A Autologous Arterial Tissue** **J Synthetic Substitute** **K Nonautologous Tissue Substitute** **Z No Device**	**Ø Upper Arm Artery, Right** **3 Lower Arm Artery, Right** **D Upper Arm Vein** **F Lower Arm Vein** **V Superior Vena Cava**
8 Brachial Artery, Left Inferior ulnar collateral artery Profunda brachii Superior ulnar collateral artery	**Ø Open**	**9 Autologous Venous Tissue** **A Autologous Arterial Tissue** **J Synthetic Substitute** **K Nonautologous Tissue Substitute** **Z No Device**	**1 Upper Arm Artery, Left** **4 Lower Arm Artery, Left** **D Upper Arm Vein** **F Lower Arm Vein** **V Superior Vena Cava**

Ø31 Continued on next page

Ø Medical and Surgical
3 Upper Arteries
1 Bypass Definition: Altering the route of passage of the contents of a tubular body part

Explanation: Rerouting contents of a body part to a downstream area of the normal route, to a similar route and body part, or to an abnormal route and dissimilar body part. Includes one or more anastomoses, with or without the use of a device.

Ø31 Continued

Body Part Character 4	Approach Character 5	Device Character 6	Qualifier Character 7
9 Ulnar Artery, Right Anterior ulnar recurrent artery Common interosseous artery Posterior ulnar recurrent artery **B Radial Artery, Right** Radial recurrent artery	**Ø Open**	**9 Autologous Venous Tissue** **A Autologous Arterial Tissue** **J Synthetic Substitute** **K Nonautologous Tissue Substitute** **Z No Device**	**3 Lower Arm Artery, Right** **F Lower Arm Vein**
A Ulnar Artery, Left Anterior ulnar recurrent artery Common interosseous artery Posterior ulnar recurrent artery **C Radial Artery, Left** Radial recurrent artery	**Ø Open**	**9 Autologous Venous Tissue** **A Autologous Arterial Tissue** **J Synthetic Substitute** **K Nonautologous Tissue Substitute** **Z No Device**	**4 Lower Arm Artery, Left** **F Lower Arm Vein**
G Intracranial Artery Anterior cerebral artery Anterior choroidal artery Anterior communicating artery Basilar artery Circle of Willis Internal carotid artery, intracranial portion Middle cerebral artery Ophthalmic artery Posterior cerebral artery Posterior communicating artery Posterior inferior cerebellar artery (PICA) **S Temporal Artery, Right** Middle temporal artery Superficial temporal artery Transverse facial artery **T Temporal Artery, Left** *See S Temporal Artery, Right*	**Ø Open**	**9 Autologous Venous Tissue** **A Autologous Arterial Tissue** **J Synthetic Substitute** **K Nonautologous Tissue Substitute** **Z No Device**	**G Intracranial Artery**
H Common Carotid Artery, Right **J Common Carotid Artery, Left**	**Ø Open**	**9 Autologous Venous Tissue** **A Autologous Arterial Tissue** **J Synthetic Substitute** **K Nonautologous Tissue Substitute** **Z No Device**	**G Intracranial Artery** **J Extracranial Artery, Right** **K Extracranial Artery, Left** **Y Upper Artery**
K Internal Carotid Artery, Right Caroticotympanic artery Carotid sinus **L Internal Carotid Artery, Left** Caroticotympanic artery Carotid sinus **M External Carotid Artery, Right** Ascending pharyngeal artery Internal maxillary artery Lingual artery Maxillary artery Occipital artery Posterior auricular artery Superior thyroid artery **N External Carotid Artery, Left** Ascending pharyngeal artery Internal maxillary artery Lingual artery Maxillary artery Occipital artery Posterior auricular artery Superior thyroid artery	**Ø Open**	**9 Autologous Venous Tissue** **A Autologous Arterial Tissue** **J Synthetic Substitute** **K Nonautologous Tissue Substitute** **Z No Device**	**J Extracranial Artery, Right** **K Extracranial Artery, Left**

Upper Arteries

Ø31–Ø31

Ø Medical and Surgical
3 Upper Arteries
5 Destruction Definition: Physical eradication of all or a portion of a body part by the direct use of energy, force, or a destructive agent
Explanation: None of the body part is physically taken out

Body Part Character 4	Approach Character 5	Device Character 6	Qualifier Character 7
Ø Internal Mammary Artery, Right Anterior intercostal artery Internal thoracic artery Musculophrenic artery Pericardiophrenic artery Superior epigastric artery **1 Internal Mammary Artery, Left** *See Ø Internal Mammary Artery, Right* **2 Innominate Artery** Brachiocephalic artery Brachiocephalic trunk **3 Subclavian Artery, Right** Costocervical trunk Dorsal scapular artery Internal thoracic artery **4 Subclavian Artery, Left** *See 3 Subclavian Artery, Right* **5 Axillary Artery, Right** Anterior circumflex humeral artery Lateral thoracic artery Posterior circumflex humeral artery Subscapular artery Superior thoracic artery Thoracoacromial artery **6 Axillary Artery, Left** *See 5 Axillary Artery, Right* **7 Brachial Artery, Right** Inferior ulnar collateral artery Profunda brachii Superior ulnar collateral artery **8 Brachial Artery, Left** *See 7 Brachial Artery, Right* **9 Ulnar Artery, Right** Anterior ulnar recurrent artery Common interosseous artery Posterior ulnar recurrent artery **A Ulnar Artery, Left** *See 9 Ulnar Artery, Right* **B Radial Artery, Right** Radial recurrent artery **C Radial Artery, Left** *See B Radial Artery, Right* **D Hand Artery, Right** Deep palmar arch Princeps pollicis artery Radialis indicis Superficial palmar arch **F Hand Artery, Left** *See D Hand Artery, Right* **G Intracranial Artery** Anterior cerebral artery Anterior choroidal artery Anterior communicating artery Basilar artery Circle of Willis Internal carotid artery, intracranial portion Middle cerebral artery Ophthalmic artery Posterior cerebral artery Posterior communicating artery Posterior inferior cerebellar artery (PICA) **H Common Carotid Artery, Right** **J Common Carotid Artery, Left** **K Internal Carotid Artery, Right** Caroticotympanic artery Carotid sinus **L Internal Carotid Artery, Left** *See K Internal Carotid Artery, Right* **M External Carotid Artery, Right** Ascending pharyngeal artery Internal maxillary artery Lingual artery Maxillary artery Occipital artery Posterior auricular artery Superior thyroid artery **N External Carotid Artery, Left** *See M External Carotid Artery, Right* **P Vertebral Artery, Right** Anterior spinal artery Posterior spinal artery **Q Vertebral Artery, Left** *See P Vertebral Artery, Right* **R Face Artery** Angular artery Ascending palatine artery External maxillary artery Facial artery Inferior labial artery Submental artery Superior labial artery **S Temporal Artery, Right** Middle temporal artery Superficial temporal artery Transverse facial artery **T Temporal Artery, Left** *See S Temporal Artery, Right* **U Thyroid Artery, Right** Cricothyroid artery Hyoid artery Sternocleidomastoid artery Superior laryngeal artery Superior thyroid artery Thyrocervical trunk **V Thyroid Artery, Left** *See U Thyroid Artery, Right* **Y Upper Artery** Aortic intercostal artery Bronchial artery Esophageal artery Subcostal artery	**Ø Open** **3 Percutaneous** **4 Percutaneous Endoscopic**	**Z No Device**	**Z No Qualifier**

Ø Medical and Surgical
3 Upper Arteries
7 Dilation Definition: Expanding an orifice or the lumen of a tubular body part

Explanation: The orifice can be a natural orifice or an artificially created orifice. Accomplished by stretching a tubular body part using intraluminal pressure or by cutting part of the orifice or wall of the tubular body part.

Body Part Character 4		Approach Character 5	Device Character 6	Qualifier Character 7
Ø Internal Mammary Artery, Right Anterior intercostal artery Internal thoracic artery Musculophrenic artery Pericardiophrenic artery Superior epigastric artery **1 Internal Mammary Artery, Left** *See Ø Internal Mammary Artery, Right* **2 Innominate Artery** Brachiocephalic artery Brachiocephalic trunk **3 Subclavian Artery, Right** Costocervical trunk Dorsal scapular artery Internal thoracic artery **4 Subclavian Artery, Left** *See 3 Subclavian Artery, Right* **5 Axillary Artery, Right** Anterior circumflex humeral artery Lateral thoracic artery Posterior circumflex humeral artery Subscapular artery Superior thoracic artery Thoracoacromial artery	**6 Axillary Artery, Left** *See 5 Axillary Artery, Right* **7 Brachial Artery, Right** Inferior ulnar collateral artery Profunda brachii Superior ulnar collateral artery **8 Brachial Artery, Left** *See 7 Brachial Artery, Right* **9 Ulnar Artery, Right** Anterior ulnar recurrent artery Common interosseous artery Posterior ulnar recurrent artery **A Ulnar Artery, Left** *See 9 Ulnar Artery, Right* **B Radial Artery, Right** Radial recurrent artery **C Radial Artery, Left** *See B Radial Artery, Right*	**Ø** Open **3** Percutaneous **4** Percutaneous Endoscopic	**4** Intraluminal Device, Drug-eluting **5** Intraluminal Device, Drug-eluting, Two **6** Intraluminal Device, Drug-eluting, Three **7** Intraluminal Device, Drug-eluting, Four or More **E** Intraluminal Device, Two **F** Intraluminal Device, Three **G** Intraluminal Device, Four or More	**6** Bifurcation **Z** No Qualifier
Ø Internal Mammary Artery, Right Anterior intercostal artery Internal thoracic artery Musculophrenic artery Pericardiophrenic artery Superior epigastric artery **1 Internal Mammary Artery, Left** *See Ø Internal Mammary Artery, Right* **2 Innominate Artery** Brachiocephalic artery Brachiocephalic trunk **3 Subclavian Artery, Right** Costocervical trunk Dorsal scapular artery Internal thoracic artery **4 Subclavian Artery, Left** *See 3 Subclavian Artery, Right* **5 Axillary Artery, Right** Anterior circumflex humeral artery Lateral thoracic artery Posterior circumflex humeral artery Subscapular artery Superior thoracic artery Thoracoacromial artery	**6 Axillary Artery, Left** *See 5 Axillary Artery, Right* **7 Brachial Artery, Right** Inferior ulnar collateral artery Profunda brachii Superior ulnar collateral artery **8 Brachial Artery, Left** *See 7 Brachial Artery, Right* **9 Ulnar Artery, Right** Anterior ulnar recurrent artery Common interosseous artery Posterior ulnar recurrent artery **A Ulnar Artery, Left** *See 9 Ulnar Artery, Right* **B Radial Artery, Right** Radial recurrent artery **C Radial Artery, Left** *See B Radial Artery, Right*	**Ø** Open **3** Percutaneous **4** Percutaneous Endoscopic	**D** Intraluminal Device **Z** No Device	**1** Drug-Coated Balloon **6** Bifurcation **Z** No Qualifier

Ø37 Continued on next page

Ø37 Continued

Ø Medical and Surgical
3 Upper Arteries
7 Dilation Definition: Expanding an orifice or the lumen of a tubular body part

Explanation: The orifice can be a natural orifice or an artificially created orifice. Accomplished by stretching a tubular body part using intraluminal pressure or by cutting part of the orifice or wall of the tubular body part.

Body Part Character 4		Approach Character 5	Device Character 6	Qualifier Character 7
D Hand Artery, Right Deep palmar arch Princeps pollicis artery Radialis indicis Superficial palmar arch **F Hand Artery, Left** *See D Hand Artery, Right* **G Intracranial Artery** NC Anterior cerebral artery Anterior choroidal artery Anterior communicating artery Basilar artery Circle of Willis Internal carotid artery, intracranial portion Middle cerebral artery Ophthalmic artery Posterior cerebral artery Posterior communicating artery Posterior inferior cerebellar artery (PICA) **H Common Carotid Artery, Right** **J Common Carotid Artery, Left** **K Internal Carotid Artery, Right** Caroticotympanic artery Carotid sinus **L Internal Carotid Artery, Left** *See K Internal Carotid Artery, Right* **M External Carotid Artery, Right** Ascending pharyngeal artery Internal maxillary artery Lingual artery Maxillary artery Occipital artery Posterior auricular artery Superior thyroid artery	**N External Carotid Artery, Left** *See M External Carotid Artery, Right* **P Vertebral Artery, Right** Anterior spinal artery Posterior spinal artery **Q Vertebral Artery, Left** *See P Vertebral Artery, Right* **R Face Artery** Angular artery Ascending palatine artery External maxillary artery Facial artery Inferior labial artery Submental artery Superior labial artery **S Temporal Artery, Right** Middle temporal artery Superficial temporal artery Transverse facial artery **T Temporal Artery, Left** *See S Temporal Artery, Right* **U Thyroid Artery, Right** Cricothyroid artery Hyoid artery Sternocleidomastoid artery Superior laryngeal artery Superior thyroid artery Thyrocervical trunk **V Thyroid Artery, Left** *See U Thyroid Artery, Right* **Y Upper Artery** Aortic intercostal artery Bronchial artery Esophageal artery Subcostal artery	**Ø** Open **3** Percutaneous **4** Percutaneous Endoscopic	**4** Intraluminal Device, Drug-eluting **5** Intraluminal Device, Drug-eluting, Two **6** Intraluminal Device, Drug-eluting, Three **7** Intraluminal Device, Drug-eluting, Four or More **D** Intraluminal Device **E** Intraluminal Device, Two **F** Intraluminal Device, Three **G** Intraluminal Device, Four or More **Z** No Device	**6** Bifurcation **Z** No Qualifier

NC Ø37G[3,4]Z[6,Z]

Ø Medical and Surgical
3 Upper Arteries
9 Drainage Definition: Taking or letting out fluids and/or gases from a body part
Explanation: The qualifier DIAGNOSTIC is used to identify drainage procedures that are biopsies

Body Part Character 4	Approach Character 5	Device Character 6	Qualifier Character 7
Ø Internal Mammary Artery, Right Anterior intercostal artery Internal thoracic artery Musculophrenic artery Pericardiophrenic artery Superior epigastric artery **1 Internal Mammary Artery, Left** *See Ø Internal Mammary Artery, Right above* **2 Innominate Artery** Brachiocephalic artery Brachiocephalic trunk **3 Subclavian Artery, Right** Costocervical trunk Dorsal scapular artery Internal thoracic artery **4 Subclavian Artery, Left** *See 3 Subclavian Artery, Right* **5 Axillary Artery, Right** Anterior circumflex humeral artery Lateral thoracic artery Posterior circumflex humeral artery Subscapular artery Superior thoracic artery Thoracoacromial artery **6 Axillary Artery, Left** *See 5 Axillary Artery, Right* **7 Brachial Artery, Right** Inferior ulnar collateral artery Profunda brachii Superior ulnar collateral artery **8 Brachial Artery, Left** *See 7 Brachial Artery, Right* **9 Ulnar Artery, Right** Anterior ulnar recurrent artery Common interosseous artery Posterior ulnar recurrent artery **A Ulnar Artery, Left** *See 9 Ulnar Artery, Right* **B Radial Artery, Right** Radial recurrent artery **C Radial Artery, Left** *See B Radial Artery, Right* **D Hand Artery, Right** Deep palmar arch Princeps pollicis artery Radialis indicis Superficial palmar arch **F Hand Artery, Left** *See D Hand Artery, Right* **G Intracranial Artery** Anterior cerebral artery Anterior choroidal artery Anterior communicating artery Basilar artery Circle of Willis Internal carotid artery, intracranial portion Middle cerebral artery Ophthalmic artery Posterior cerebral artery Posterior communicating artery Posterior inferior cerebellar artery (PICA) **H Common Carotid Artery, Right** **J Common Carotid Artery, Left** **K Internal Carotid Artery, Right** Caroticotympanic artery Carotid sinus **L Internal Carotid Artery, Left** *See K Internal Carotid Artery, Right* **M External Carotid Artery, Right** Ascending pharyngeal artery Internal maxillary artery Lingual artery Maxillary artery Occipital artery Posterior auricular artery Superior thyroid artery **N External Carotid Artery, Left** *See M External Carotid Artery, Right* **P Vertebral Artery, Right** Anterior spinal artery Posterior spinal artery **Q Vertebral Artery, Left** *See P Vertebral Artery, Right* **R Face Artery** Angular artery Ascending palatine artery External maxillary artery Facial artery Inferior labial artery Submental artery Superior labial artery **S Temporal Artery, Right** Middle temporal artery Superficial temporal artery Transverse facial artery **T Temporal Artery, Left** *See S Temporal Artery, Right* **U Thyroid Artery, Right** Cricothyroid artery Hyoid artery Sternocleidomastoid artery Superior laryngeal artery Superior thyroid artery Thyrocervical trunk **V Thyroid Artery, Left** *See U Thyroid Artery, Right* **Y Upper Artery** Aortic intercostal artery Bronchial artery Esophageal artery Subcostal artery	Ø Open 3 Percutaneous 4 Percutaneous Endoscopic	Ø Drainage Device	Z No Qualifier

Ø39 Continued on next page

Non-OR Ø39[Ø,1,2,3,4,5,6,7,8,9,A,B,C,D,F,G,H,J,K,L,M,N,P,Q,R,S,T,U,V,Y][Ø,3,4]ØZ

Ø39 Continued

Ø Medical and Surgical
3 Upper Arteries
9 Drainage Definition: Taking or letting out fluids and/or gases from a body part
Explanation: The qualifier DIAGNOSTIC is used to identify drainage procedures that are biopsies

Body Part Character 4	Approach Character 5	Device Character 6	Qualifier Character 7
Ø Internal Mammary Artery, Right Anterior intercostal artery Internal thoracic artery Musculophrenic artery Pericardiophrenic artery Superior epigastric artery **1 Internal Mammary Artery, Left** *See Ø Internal Mammary Artery, Right* **2 Innominate Artery** Brachiocephalic artery Brachiocephalic trunk **3 Subclavian Artery, Right** Costocervical trunk Dorsal scapular artery Internal thoracic artery **4 Subclavian Artery, Left** *See 3 Subclavian Artery, Right* **5 Axillary Artery, Right** Anterior circumflex humeral artery Lateral thoracic artery Posterior circumflex humeral artery Subscapular artery Superior thoracic artery Thoracoacromial artery **6 Axillary Artery, Left** *See 5 Axillary Artery, Right* **7 Brachial Artery, Right** Inferior ulnar collateral artery Profunda brachii Superior ulnar collateral artery **8 Brachial Artery, Left** *See 7 Brachial Artery, Right* **9 Ulnar Artery, Right** Anterior ulnar recurrent artery Common interosseous artery Posterior ulnar recurrent artery **A Ulnar Artery, Left** *See 9 Ulnar Artery, Right* **B Radial Artery, Right** Radial recurrent artery **C Radial Artery, Left** *See B Radial Artery, Right* **D Hand Artery, Right** Deep palmar arch Princeps pollicis artery Radialis indicis Superficial palmar arch **F Hand Artery, Left** *See D Hand Artery, Right* **G Intracranial Artery** Anterior cerebral artery Anterior choroidal artery Anterior communicating artery Basilar artery Circle of Willis Internal carotid artery, intracranial portion Middle cerebral artery Ophthalmic artery Posterior cerebral artery Posterior communicating artery Posterior inferior cerebellar artery (PICA) **H Common Carotid Artery, Right** **J Common Carotid Artery, Left** **K Internal Carotid Artery, Right** Caroticotympanic artery Carotid sinus **L Internal Carotid Artery, Left** *See K Internal Carotid Artery, Right* **M External Carotid Artery, Right** Ascending pharyngeal artery Internal maxillary artery Lingual artery Maxillary artery Occipital artery Posterior auricular artery Superior thyroid artery **N External Carotid Artery, Left** *See M External Carotid Artery, Right* **P Vertebral Artery, Right** Anterior spinal artery Posterior spinal artery **Q Vertebral Artery, Left** *See P Vertebral Artery, Right* **R Face Artery** Angular artery Ascending palatine artery External maxillary artery Facial artery Inferior labial artery Submental artery Superior labial artery **S Temporal Artery, Right** Middle temporal artery Superficial temporal artery Transverse facial artery **T Temporal Artery, Left** *See S Temporal Artery, Right* **U Thyroid Artery, Right** Cricothyroid artery Hyoid artery Sternocleidomastoid artery Superior laryngeal artery Superior thyroid artery Thyrocervical trunk **V Thyroid Artery, Left** *See U Thyroid Artery, Right* **Y Upper Artery** Aortic intercostal artery Bronchial artery Esophageal artery Subcostal artery	Ø Open 3 Percutaneous 4 Percutaneous Endoscopic	Z No Device	X Diagnostic Z No Qualifier

Non-OR Ø39[Ø,1,2,3,4,5,6,7,8,9,A,B,C,D,F,G,H,J,K,L,M,N,P,Q,R,S,T,U,V,Y]3ZX
Non-OR Ø39[Ø,1,2,3,4,5,6,7,8,9,A,B,C,D,F,G,H,J,K,L,M,N,P,Q,R,S,T,U,V,Y][Ø,3,4]ZZ

Ø Medical and Surgical
3 Upper Arteries
B Excision Definition: Cutting out or off, without replacement, a portion of a body part
Explanation: The qualifier DIAGNOSTIC is used to identify excision procedures that are biopsies

Body Part Character 4	Approach Character 5	Device Character 6	Qualifier Character 7
Ø Internal Mammary Artery, Right Anterior intercostal artery Internal thoracic artery Musculophrenic artery Pericardiophrenic artery Superior epigastric artery **1 Internal Mammary Artery, Left** *See Ø Internal Mammary Artery, Right* **2 Innominate Artery** Brachiocephalic artery Brachiocephalic trunk **3 Subclavian Artery, Right** Costocervical trunk Dorsal scapular artery Internal thoracic artery **4 Subclavian Artery, Left** *See 3 Subclavian Artery, Right* **5 Axillary Artery, Right** Anterior circumflex humeral artery Lateral thoracic artery Posterior circumflex humeral artery Subscapular artery Superior thoracic artery Thoracoacromial artery **6 Axillary Artery, Left** *See 5 Axillary Artery, Right* **7 Brachial Artery, Right** Inferior ulnar collateral artery Profunda brachii Superior ulnar collateral artery **8 Brachial Artery, Left** *See 7 Brachial Artery, Right* **9 Ulnar Artery, Right** Anterior ulnar recurrent artery Common interosseous artery Posterior ulnar recurrent artery **A Ulnar Artery, Left** *See 9 Ulnar Artery, Right* **B Radial Artery, Right** Radial recurrent artery **C Radial Artery, Left** *See B Radial Artery, Right* **D Hand Artery, Right** Deep palmar arch Princeps pollicis artery Radialis indicis Superficial palmar arch **F Hand Artery, Left** *See D Hand Artery, Right* **G Intracranial Artery** Anterior cerebral artery Anterior choroidal artery Anterior communicating artery Basilar artery Circle of Willis Internal carotid artery, intracranial portion Middle cerebral artery Ophthalmic artery Posterior cerebral artery Posterior communicating artery Posterior inferior cerebellar artery (PICA) **H Common Carotid Artery, Right** **J Common Carotid Artery, Left** **K Internal Carotid Artery, Right** Caroticotympanic artery Carotid sinus **L Internal Carotid Artery, Left** *See K Internal Carotid Artery, Right* **M External Carotid Artery, Right** Ascending pharyngeal artery Internal maxillary artery Lingual artery Maxillary artery Occipital artery Posterior auricular artery Superior thyroid artery **N External Carotid Artery, Left** *See M External Carotid Artery, Right* **P Vertebral Artery, Right** Anterior spinal artery Posterior spinal artery **Q Vertebral Artery, Left** *See P Vertebral Artery, Right* **R Face Artery** Angular artery Ascending palatine artery External maxillary artery Facial artery Inferior labial artery Submental artery Superior labial artery **S Temporal Artery, Right** Middle temporal artery Superficial temporal artery Transverse facial artery **T Temporal Artery, Left** *See S Temporal Artery, Right* **U Thyroid Artery, Right** Cricothyroid artery Hyoid artery Sternocleidomastoid artery Superior laryngeal artery Superior thyroid artery Thyrocervical trunk **V Thyroid Artery, Left** *See U Thyroid Artery, Right* **Y Upper Artery** Aortic intercostal artery Bronchial artery Esophageal artery Subcostal artery	Ø Open 3 Percutaneous 4 Percutaneous Endoscopic	Z No Device	X Diagnostic Z No Qualifier

Ø Medical and Surgical
3 Upper Arteries
C Extirpation Definition: Taking or cutting out solid matter from a body part

Explanation: The solid matter may be an abnormal byproduct of a biological function or a foreign body; it may be imbedded in a body part or in the lumen of a tubular body part. The solid matter may or may not have been previously broken into pieces.

Body Part Character 4	Approach Character 5	Device Character 6	Qualifier Character 7
Ø Internal Mammary Artery, Right Anterior intercostal artery Internal thoracic artery Musculophrenic artery Pericardiophrenic artery Superior epigastric artery **1** Internal Mammary Artery, Left *See Ø Internal Mammary Artery, Right* **2** Innominate Artery Brachiocephalic artery Brachiocephalic trunk **3** Subclavian Artery, Right Costocervical trunk Dorsal scapular artery Internal thoracic artery **4** Subclavian Artery, Left *See 3 Subclavian Artery, Right* **5** Axillary Artery, Right Anterior circumflex humeral artery Lateral thoracic artery Posterior circumflex humeral artery Subscapular artery Superior thoracic artery Thoracoacromial artery **6** Axillary Artery, Left *See 5 Axillary Artery, Right* **7** Brachial Artery, Right Inferior ulnar collateral artery Profunda brachii Superior ulnar collateral artery **8** Brachial Artery, Left *See 7 Brachial Artery, Right* **9** Ulnar Artery, Right Anterior ulnar recurrent artery Common interosseous artery Posterior ulnar recurrent artery **A** Ulnar Artery, Left *See 9 Ulnar Artery, Right* **B** Radial Artery, Right Radial recurrent artery **C** Radial Artery, Left *See B Radial Artery, Right* **D** Hand Artery, Right Deep palmar arch Princeps pollicis artery Radialis indicis Superficial palmar arch **F** Hand Artery, Left *See D Hand Artery, Right* **R** Face Artery Angular artery Ascending palatine artery External maxillary artery Facial artery Inferior labial artery Submental artery Superior labial artery **S** Temporal Artery, Right Middle temporal artery Superficial temporal artery Transverse facial artery **T** Temporal Artery, Left *See S Temporal Artery, Right* **U** Thyroid Artery, Right Cricothyroid artery Hyoid artery Sternocleidomastoid artery Superior laryngeal artery Superior thyroid artery Thyrocervical trunk **V** Thyroid Artery, Left *See U Thyroid Artery, Right* **Y** Upper Artery Aortic intercostal artery Bronchial artery Esophageal artery Subcostal artery	**Ø** Open **3** Percutaneous **4** Percutaneous Endoscopic	**Z** No Device	**6** Bifurcation **Z** No Qualifier
G Intracranial Artery Anterior cerebral artery Anterior choroidal artery Anterior communicating artery Basilar artery Circle of Willis Internal carotid artery, intracranial portion Middle cerebral artery Ophthalmic artery Posterior cerebral artery Posterior communicating artery Posterior inferior cerebellar artery (PICA) **H** Common Carotid Artery, Right **J** Common Carotid Artery, Left **K** Internal Carotid Artery, Right Caroticotympanic artery Carotid sinus **L** Internal Carotid Artery, Left *See K Internal Carotid Artery, Right* **M** External Carotid Artery, Right Ascending pharyngeal artery Internal maxillary artery Lingual artery Maxillary artery Occipital artery Posterior auricular artery Superior thyroid artery **N** External Carotid Artery, Left *See M External Carotid Artery, Right* **P** Vertebral Artery, Right Anterior spinal artery Posterior spinal artery **Q** Vertebral Artery, Left *See P Vertebral Artery, Right*	**Ø** Open **4** Percutaneous Endoscopic	**Z** No Device	**6** Bifurcation **Z** No Qualifier

Ø3C Continued on next page

Ø Medical and Surgical
3 Upper Arteries
C Extirpation Definition: Taking or cutting out solid matter from a body part

Ø3C Continued

Explanation: The solid matter may be an abnormal byproduct of a biological function or a foreign body; it may be imbedded in a body part or in the lumen of a tubular body part. The solid matter may or may not have been previously broken into pieces.

Body Part Character 4	Approach Character 5	Device Character 6	Qualifier Character 7
G Intracranial Artery Anterior cerebral artery Anterior choroidal artery Anterior communicating artery Basilar artery Circle of Willis Internal carotid artery, intracranial portion Middle cerebral artery Ophthalmic artery Posterior cerebral artery Posterior communicating artery Posterior inferior cerebellar artery (PICA) **H Common Carotid Artery, Right** **J Common Carotid Artery, Left** **K Internal Carotid Artery, Right** Caroticotympanic artery Carotid sinus **L Internal Carotid Artery, Left** *See K Internal Carotid Artery, Right* **M External Carotid Artery, Right** Ascending pharyngeal artery Internal maxillary artery Lingual artery Maxillary artery Occipital artery Posterior auricular artery Superior thyroid artery **N External Carotid Artery, Left** *See M External Carotid Artery, Right* **P Vertebral Artery, Right** Anterior spinal artery Posterior spinal artery **Q Vertebral Artery, Left** *See P Vertebral Artery, Right*	**3** Percutaneous	**Z** No Device	**6** Bifurcation **7** Stent Retriever **Z** No Qualifier

Ø Medical and Surgical
3 Upper Arteries
H Insertion Definition: Putting in a nonbiological appliance that monitors, assists, performs, or prevents a physiological function but does not physically take the place of a body part
Explanation: None

Body Part Character 4	Approach Character 5	Device Character 6	Qualifier Character 7
Ø Internal Mammary Artery, Right Anterior intercostal artery Internal thoracic artery Musculophrenic artery Pericardiophrenic artery Superior epigastric artery **1 Internal Mammary Artery, Left** *See Ø Internal Mammary Artery, Right* **2 Innominate Artery** Brachiocephalic artery Brachiocephalic trunk **3 Subclavian Artery, Right** Costocervical trunk Dorsal scapular artery Internal thoracic artery **4 Subclavian Artery, Left** *See 3 Subclavian Artery, Right* **5 Axillary Artery, Right** Anterior circumflex humeral artery Lateral thoracic artery Posterior circumflex humeral artery Subscapular artery Superior thoracic artery Thoracoacromial artery **6 Axillary Artery, Left** *See 5 Axillary Artery, Right* **7 Brachial Artery, Right** Inferior ulnar collateral artery Profunda brachii Superior ulnar collateral artery **8 Brachial Artery, Left** *See 7 Brachial Artery, Right* **9 Ulnar Artery, Right** Anterior ulnar recurrent artery Common interosseous artery Posterior ulnar recurrent artery **A Ulnar Artery, Left** *See 9 Ulnar Artery, Right* **B Radial Artery, Right** Radial recurrent artery **C Radial Artery, Left** *See B Radial Artery, Right* **D Hand Artery, Right** Deep palmar arch Princeps pollicis artery Radialis indicis Superficial palmar arch **F Hand Artery, Left** *See D Hand Artery, Right* **G Intracranial Artery** Anterior cerebral artery Anterior choroidal artery Anterior communicating artery Basilar artery Circle of Willis Internal carotid artery, intracranial portion Middle cerebral artery Ophthalmic artery Posterior cerebral artery Posterior communicating artery Posterior inferior cerebellar artery (PICA) **H Common Carotid Artery, Right** **J Common Carotid Artery, Left** **M External Carotid Artery, Right** Ascending pharyngeal artery Internal maxillary artery Lingual artery Maxillary artery Occipital artery Posterior auricular artery Superior thyroid artery **N External Carotid Artery, Left** *See M External Carotid Artery, Right* **P Vertebral Artery, Right** Anterior spinal artery Posterior spinal artery **Q Vertebral Artery, Left** *See P Vertebral Artery, Right* **R Face Artery** Angular artery Ascending palatine artery External maxillary artery Facial artery Inferior labial artery Submental artery Superior labial artery **S Temporal Artery, Right** Middle temporal artery Superficial temporal artery Transverse facial artery **T Temporal Artery, Left** *See S Temporal Artery, Right* **U Thyroid Artery, Right** Cricothyroid artery Hyoid artery Sternocleidomastoid artery Superior laryngeal artery Superior thyroid artery Thyrocervical trunk **V Thyroid Artery, Left** *See U Thyroid Artery, Right*	**Ø Open** **3 Percutaneous** **4 Percutaneous Endoscopic**	**3 Infusion Device** **D Intraluminal Device**	**Z No Qualifier**
K Internal Carotid Artery, Right Caroticotympanic artery Carotid sinus **L Internal Carotid Artery, Left** *See K Internal Carotid Artery, Right*	**Ø Open** **3 Percutaneous** **4 Percutaneous Endoscope**	**3 Infusion Device** **D Intraluminal Device** **M Stimulator Lead**	**Z No Qualifier**
Y Upper Artery Aortic intercostal artery Bronchial artery Esophageal artery Subcostal artery	**Ø Open** **3 Percutaneous** **4 Percutaneous Endoscopic**	**2 Monitoring Device** **3 Infusion Device** **D Intraluminal Device** **Y Other Device**	**Z No Qualifier**

Non-OR Ø3H[Ø,1,2,3,4,5,6,7,8,9,A,B,C,D,F,G,H,J,M,N,P,Q,R,S,T,U,V][Ø,3,4]3Z
Non-OR Ø3H[K,L][Ø,3,4]3Z
Non-OR Ø3HY[Ø,3,4]3Z
Non-OR Ø3HY32Z
Non-OR Ø3HY[3,4]YZ

Ø Medical and Surgical
3 Upper Arteries
J Inspection Definition: Visually and/or manually exploring a body part

Explanation: Visual exploration may be performed with or without optical instrumentation. Manual exploration may be performed directly or through intervening body layers.

Body Part Character 4	Approach Character 5	Device Character 6	Qualifier Character 7
Y Upper Artery Aortic intercostal artery Bronchial artery Esophageal artery Subcostal artery	Ø Open 3 Percutaneous 4 Percutaneous Endoscopic X External	Z No Device	Z No Qualifier

Non-OR Ø3JY[3,4,X]ZZ

Ø Medical and Surgical
3 Upper Arteries
L Occlusion Definition: Completely closing an orifice or the lumen of a tubular body part
Explanation: The orifice can be a natural orifice or an artificially created orifice

Body Part Character 4		Approach Character 5	Device Character 6	Qualifier Character 7
Ø Internal Mammary Artery, Right Anterior intercostal artery Internal thoracic artery Musculophrenic artery Pericardiophrenic artery Superior epigastric artery **1 Internal Mammary Artery, Left** *See Ø Internal Mammary Artery, Left* **2 Innominate Artery** Brachiocephalic artery Brachiocephalic trunk **3 Subclavian Artery, Right** Costocervical trunk Dorsal scapular artery Internal thoracic artery **4 Subclavian Artery, Left** *See 3 Subclavian Artery, Right* **5 Axillary Artery, Right** Anterior circumflex humeral artery Lateral thoracic artery Posterior circumflex humeral artery Subscapular artery Superior thoracic artery Thoracoacromial artery **6 Axillary Artery, Left** *See 5 Axillary Artery, Right* **7 Brachial Artery, Right** Inferior ulnar collateral artery Profunda brachii Superior ulnar collateral artery **8 Brachial Artery, Left** *See 7 Brachial Artery, Right* **9 Ulnar Artery, Right** Anterior ulnar recurrent artery Common interosseous artery Posterior ulnar recurrent artery	**A Ulnar Artery, Left** *See 9 Ulnar Artery, Right* **B Radial Artery, Right** Radial recurrent artery **C Radial Artery, Left** *See B Radial Artery, Right* **D Hand Artery, Right** Deep palmar arch Princeps pollicis artery Radialis indicis Superficial palmar arch **F Hand Artery, Left** *See D Hand Artery, Right* **R Face Artery** Angular artery Ascending palatine artery External maxillary artery Facial artery Inferior labial artery Submental artery Superior labial artery **S Temporal Artery, Right** Middle temporal artery Superficial temporal artery Transverse facial artery **T Temporal Artery, Left** *See S Temporal Artery, Right* **U Thyroid Artery, Right** Cricothyroid artery Hyoid artery Sternocleidomastoid artery Superior laryngeal artery Superior thyroid artery Thyrocervical trunk **V Thyroid Artery, Left** *See U Thyroid Artery, Right* **Y Upper Artery** Aortic intercostal artery Bronchial artery Esophageal artery Subcostal artery	**Ø Open** **3 Percutaneous** **4 Percutaneous Endoscopic**	**C Extraluminal Device** **D Intraluminal Device** **Z No Device**	**Z No Qualifier**
G Intracranial Artery Anterior cerebral artery Anterior choroidal artery Anterior communicating artery Basilar artery Circle of Willis Internal carotid artery, intracranial portion Middle cerebral artery Ophthalmic artery Posterior cerebral artery Posterior communicating artery Posterior inferior cerebellar artery (PICA) **H Common Carotid Artery, Right** **J Common Carotid Artery, Left** **K Internal Carotid Artery, Right** Caroticotympanic artery Carotid sinus	**L Internal Carotid Artery, Left** *See K Internal Carotid Artery, Right* **M External Carotid Artery, Right** Ascending pharyngeal artery Internal maxillary artery Lingual artery Maxillary artery Occipital artery Posterior auricular artery Superior thyroid artery **N External Carotid Artery, Left** *See M External Carotid Artery, Right* **P Vertebral Artery, Right** Anterior spinal artery Posterior spinal artery **Q Vertebral Artery, Left** *See P Vertebral Artery, Right*	**Ø Open** **3 Percutaneous** **4 Percutaneous Endoscopic**	**B Intraluminal Device, Bioactive** **C Extraluminal Device** **D Intraluminal Device** **Z No Device**	**Z No Qualifier**

Ø Medical and Surgical
3 Upper Arteries
N Release Definition: Freeing a body part from an abnormal physical constraint by cutting or by the use of force
Explanation: Some of the restraining tissue may be taken out but none of the body part is taken out

Body Part Character 4	Approach Character 5	Device Character 6	Qualifier Character 7
Ø Internal Mammary Artery, Right Anterior intercostal artery Internal thoracic artery Musculophrenic artery Pericardiophrenic artery Superior epigastric artery **1 Internal Mammary Artery, Left** *See Ø Internal Mammary Artery, Right* **2 Innominate Artery** Brachiocephalic artery Brachiocephalic trunk **3 Subclavian Artery, Right** Costocervical trunk Dorsal scapular artery Internal thoracic artery **4 Subclavian Artery, Left** *See 3 Subclavian Artery, Right* **5 Axillary Artery, Right** Anterior circumflex humeral artery Lateral thoracic artery Posterior circumflex humeral artery Subscapular artery Superior thoracic artery Thoracoacromial artery **6 Axillary Artery, Left** *See 5 Axillary Artery, Right* **7 Brachial Artery, Right** Inferior ulnar collateral artery Profunda brachii Superior ulnar collateral artery **8 Brachial Artery, Left** *See 7 Brachial Artery, Right* **9 Ulnar Artery, Right** Anterior ulnar recurrent artery Common interosseous artery Posterior ulnar recurrent artery **A Ulnar Artery, Left** *See 9 Ulnar Artery, Right* **B Radial Artery, Right** Radial recurrent artery **C Radial Artery, Left** *See B Radial Artery, Right* **D Hand Artery, Right** Deep palmar arch Princeps pollicis artery Radialis indicis Superficial palmar arch **F Hand Artery, Left** *See D Hand Artery, Right* **G Intracranial Artery** Anterior cerebral artery Anterior choroidal artery Anterior communicating artery Basilar artery Circle of Willis Internal carotid artery, intracranial portion Middle cerebral artery Ophthalmic artery Posterior cerebral artery Posterior communicating artery Posterior inferior cerebellar artery (PICA) **H Common Carotid Artery, Right** **J Common Carotid Artery, Left** **K Internal Carotid Artery, Right** Caroticotympanic artery Carotid sinus **L Internal Carotid Artery, Left** *See K Internal Carotid Artery, Right* **M External Carotid Artery, Right** Ascending pharyngeal artery Internal maxillary artery Lingual artery Maxillary artery Occipital artery Posterior auricular artery Superior thyroid artery **N External Carotid Artery, Left** *See M External Carotid Artery, Right* **P Vertebral Artery, Right** Anterior spinal artery Posterior spinal artery **Q Vertebral Artery, Left** *See P Vertebral Artery, Right* **R Face Artery** Angular artery Ascending palatine artery External maxillary artery Facial artery Inferior labial artery Submental artery Superior labial artery **S Temporal Artery, Right** Middle temporal artery Superficial temporal artery Transverse facial artery **T Temporal Artery, Left** *See S Temporal Artery, Right* **U Thyroid Artery, Right** Cricothyroid artery Hyoid artery Sternocleidomastoid artery Superior laryngeal artery Superior thyroid artery Thyrocervical trunk **V Thyroid Artery, Left** *See U Thyroid Artery, Right* **Y Upper Artery** Aortic intercostal artery Bronchial artery Esophageal artery Subcostal artery	Ø Open 3 Percutaneous 4 Percutaneous Endoscopic	Z No Device	Z No Qualifier

Ø Medical and Surgical
3 Upper Arteries
P Removal Definition: Taking out or off a device from a body part

Explanation: If a device is taken out and a similar device put in without cutting or puncturing the skin or mucous membrane, the procedure is coded to the root operation CHANGE. Otherwise, the procedure for taking out a device is coded to the root operation REMOVAL.

Body Part Character 4	Approach Character 5	Device Character 6	Qualifier Character 7
Y Upper Artery Aortic intercostal artery Bronchial artery Esophageal artery Subcostal artery	**Ø** Open **3** Percutaneous **4** Percutaneous Endoscopic	**Ø** Drainage Device **2** Monitoring Device **3** Infusion Device **7** Autologous Tissue Substitute **C** Extraluminal Device **D** Intraluminal Device **J** Synthetic Substitute **K** Nonautologous Tissue Substitute **M** Stimulator Lead **Y** Other Device	**Z** No Qualifier
Y Upper Artery Aortic intercostal artery Bronchial artery Esophageal artery Subcostal artery	**X** External	**Ø** Drainage Device **2** Monitoring Device **3** Infusion Device **D** Intraluminal Device **M** Stimulator Lead	**Z** No Qualifier

Non-OR Ø3PY3[Ø,2,3,D]Z
Non-OR Ø3PY[3,4]YZ
Non-OR Ø3PYX[Ø,2,3,D,M]Z

Ø Medical and Surgical
3 Upper Arteries
Q Repair Definition: Restoring, to the extent possible, a body part to its normal anatomic structure and function
Explanation: Used only when the method to accomplish the repair is not one of the other root operations

Body Part Character 4	Approach Character 5	Device Character 6	Qualifier Character 7
Ø Internal Mammary Artery, Right Anterior intercostal artery Internal thoracic artery Musculophrenic artery Pericardiophrenic artery Superior epigastric artery **1 Internal Mammary Artery, Left** *See Ø Internal Mammary Artery, Right* **2 Innominate Artery** Brachiocephalic artery Brachiocephalic trunk **3 Subclavian Artery, Right** Costocervical trunk Dorsal scapular artery Internal thoracic artery **4 Subclavian Artery, Left** *See 3 Subclavian Artery, Right* **5 Axillary Artery, Right** Anterior circumflex humeral artery Lateral thoracic artery Posterior circumflex humeral artery Subscapular artery Superior thoracic artery Thoracoacromial artery **6 Axillary Artery, Left** *See 5 Axillary Artery, Right* **7 Brachial Artery, Right** Inferior ulnar collateral artery Profunda brachii Superior ulnar collateral artery **8 Brachial Artery, Left** *See 7 Brachial Artery, Right* **9 Ulnar Artery, Right** Anterior ulnar recurrent artery Common interosseous artery Posterior ulnar recurrent artery **A Ulnar Artery, Left** *See 9 Ulnar Artery, Right* **B Radial Artery, Right** Radial recurrent artery **C Radial Artery, Left** *See B Radial Artery, Right* **D Hand Artery, Right** Deep palmar arch Princeps pollicis artery Radialis indicis Superficial palmar arch **F Hand Artery, Left** *See D Hand Artery, Right* **G Intracranial Artery** Anterior cerebral artery Anterior choroidal artery Anterior communicating artery Basilar artery Circle of Willis Internal carotid artery, intracranial portion Middle cerebral artery Ophthalmic artery Posterior cerebral artery Posterior communicating artery Posterior inferior cerebellar artery (PICA) **H Common Carotid Artery, Right** **J Common Carotid Artery, Left** **K Internal Carotid Artery, Right** Caroticotympanic artery Carotid sinus **L Internal Carotid Artery, Left** *See K Internal Carotid Artery, Right* **M External Carotid Artery, Right** Ascending pharyngeal artery Internal maxillary artery Lingual artery Maxillary artery Occipital artery Posterior auricular artery Superior thyroid artery **N External Carotid Artery, Left** *See M External Carotid Artery, Right* **P Vertebral Artery, Right** Anterior spinal artery Posterior spinal artery **Q Vertebral Artery, Left** *See P Vertebral Artery, Right* **R Face Artery** Angular artery Ascending palatine artery External maxillary artery Facial artery Inferior labial artery Submental artery Superior labial artery **S Temporal Artery, Right** Middle temporal artery Superficial temporal artery Transverse facial artery **T Temporal Artery, Left** *See S Temporal Artery, Right* **U Thyroid Artery, Right** Cricothyroid artery Hyoid artery Sternocleidomastoid artery Superior laryngeal artery Superior thyroid artery Thyrocervical trunk **V Thyroid Artery, Left** *See U Thyroid Artery, Right* **Y Upper Artery** Aortic intercostal artery Bronchial artery Esophageal artery Subcostal artery	**Ø** Open **3** Percutaneous **4** Percutaneous Endoscopic	**Z** No Device	**Z** No Qualifier

Ø Medical and Surgical
3 Upper Arteries
R Replacement Definition: Putting in or on biological or synthetic material that physically takes the place and/or function of all or a portion of a body part

Explanation: The body part may have been taken out or replaced, or may be taken out, physically eradicated, or rendered nonfunctional during the REPLACEMENT procedure. A REMOVAL procedure is coded for taking out the device used in a previous replacement procedure.

Body Part Character 4		Approach Character 5	Device Character 6	Qualifier Character 7
Ø Internal Mammary Artery, Right Anterior intercostal artery Internal thoracic artery Musculophrenic artery Pericardiophrenic artery Superior epigastric artery **1 Internal Mammary Artery, Left** *See Ø Internal Mammary Artery, Right* **2 Innominate Artery** Brachiocephalic artery Brachiocephalic trunk **3 Subclavian Artery, Right** Costocervical trunk Dorsal scapular artery Internal thoracic artery **4 Subclavian Artery, Left** *See 3 Subclavian Artery, Right* **5 Axillary Artery, Right** Anterior circumflex humeral artery Lateral thoracic artery Posterior circumflex humeral artery Subscapular artery Superior thoracic artery Thoracoacromial artery **6 Axillary Artery, Left** *See 5 Axillary Artery, Right* **7 Brachial Artery, Right** Inferior ulnar collateral artery Profunda brachii Superior ulnar collateral artery **8 Brachial Artery, Left** *See 7 Brachial Artery, Right* **9 Ulnar Artery, Right** Anterior ulnar recurrent artery Common interosseous artery Posterior ulnar recurrent artery **A Ulnar Artery, Left** *See 9 Ulnar Artery, Right* **B Radial Artery, Right** Radial recurrent artery **C Radial Artery, Left** *See B Radial Artery, Right* **D Hand Artery, Right** Deep palmar arch Princeps pollicis artery Radialis indicis Superficial palmar arch **F Hand Artery, Left** *See D Hand Artery, Right* **G Intracranial Artery** Anterior cerebral artery Anterior choroidal artery Anterior communicating artery Basilar artery Circle of Willis Internal carotid artery, intracranial portion Middle cerebral artery Ophthalmic artery Posterior cerebral artery Posterior communicating artery Posterior inferior cerebellar artery (PICA)	**H Common Carotid Artery, Right** **J Common Carotid Artery, Left** **K Internal Carotid Artery, Right** Caroticotympanic artery Carotid sinus **L Internal Carotid Artery, Left** *See K Internal Carotid Artery, Right* **M External Carotid Artery, Right** Ascending pharyngeal artery Internal maxillary artery Lingual artery Maxillary artery Occipital artery Posterior auricular artery Superior thyroid artery **N External Carotid Artery, Left** *See M External Carotid Artery, Right* **P Vertebral Artery, Right** Anterior spinal artery Posterior spinal artery **Q Vertebral Artery, Left** *See P Vertebral Artery, Right* **R Face Artery** Angular artery Ascending palatine artery External maxillary artery Facial artery Inferior labial artery Submental artery Superior labial artery **S Temporal Artery, Right** Middle temporal artery Superficial temporal artery Transverse facial artery **T Temporal Artery, Left** *See S Temporal Artery, Right* **U Thyroid Artery, Right** Cricothyroid artery Hyoid artery Sternocleidomastoid artery Superior laryngeal artery Superior thyroid artery Thyrocervical trunk **V Thyroid Artery, Left** *See U Thyroid Artery, Right* **Y Upper Artery** Aortic intercostal artery Bronchial artery Esophageal artery Subcostal artery	Ø Open 4 Percutaneous Endoscopic	7 Autologous Tissue Substitute J Synthetic Substitute K Nonautologous Tissue Substitute	Z No Qualifier

Ø Medical and Surgical
3 Upper Arteries
S Reposition Definition: Moving to its normal location, or other suitable location, all or a portion of a body part

Explanation: The body part is moved to a new location from an abnormal location, or from a normal location where it is not functioning correctly. The body part may or may not be cut out or off to be moved to the new location.

Body Part Character 4	Approach Character 5	Device Character 6	Qualifier Character 7
Ø Internal Mammary Artery, Right Anterior intercostal artery Internal thoracic artery Musculophrenic artery Pericardiophrenic artery Superior epigastric artery **1 Internal Mammary Artery, Left** *See Ø Internal Mammary Artery, Right* **2 Innominate Artery** Brachiocephalic artery Brachiocephalic trunk **3 Subclavian Artery, Right** Costocervical trunk Dorsal scapular artery Internal thoracic artery **4 Subclavian Artery, Left** *See 3 Subclavian Artery, Right* **5 Axillary Artery, Right** Anterior circumflex humeral artery Lateral thoracic artery Posterior circumflex humeral artery Subscapular artery Superior thoracic artery Thoracoacromial artery **6 Axillary Artery, Left** *See 5 Axillary Artery, Right* **7 Brachial Artery, Right** Inferior ulnar collateral artery Profunda brachii Superior ulnar collateral artery **8 Brachial Artery, Left** *See 7 Brachial Artery, Right* **9 Ulnar Artery, Right** Anterior ulnar recurrent artery Common interosseous artery Posterior ulnar recurrent artery **A Ulnar Artery, Left** *See 9 Ulnar Artery, Right* **B Radial Artery, Right** Radial recurrent artery **C Radial Artery, Left** *See B Radial Artery, Right* **D Hand Artery, Right** Deep palmar arch Princeps pollicis artery Radialis indicis Superficial palmar arch **F Hand Artery, Left** *See D Hand Artery, Right* **G Intracranial Artery** Anterior cerebral artery Anterior choroidal artery Anterior communicating artery Basilar artery Circle of Willis Internal carotid artery, intracranial portion Middle cerebral artery Ophthalmic artery Posterior cerebral artery Posterior communicating artery Posterior inferior cerebellar artery (PICA) **H Common Carotid Artery, Right** **J Common Carotid Artery, Left** **K Internal Carotid Artery, Right** Caroticotympanic artery Carotid sinus **L Internal Carotid Artery, Left** *See K Internal Carotid Artery, Right* **M External Carotid Artery, Right** Ascending pharyngeal artery Internal maxillary artery Lingual artery Maxillary artery Occipital artery Posterior auricular artery Superior thyroid artery **N External Carotid Artery, Left** *See M External Carotid Artery, Right* **P Vertebral Artery, Right** Anterior spinal artery Posterior spinal artery **Q Vertebral Artery, Left** *See P Vertebral Artery, Right* **R Face Artery** Angular artery Ascending palatine artery External maxillary artery Facial artery Inferior labial artery Submental artery Superior labial artery **S Temporal Artery, Right** Middle temporal artery Superficial temporal artery Transverse facial artery **T Temporal Artery, Left** *See S Temporal Artery, Right* **U Thyroid Artery, Right** Cricothyroid artery Hyoid artery Sternocleidomastoid artery Superior laryngeal artery Superior thyroid artery Thyrocervical trunk **V Thyroid Artery, Left** *See U Thyroid Artery, Right* **Y Upper Artery** Aortic intercostal artery Bronchial artery Esophageal artery Subcostal artery	**Ø Open** **3 Percutaneous** **4 Percutaneous Endoscopic**	**Z No Device**	**Z No Qualifier**

Upper Arteries

Ø3S–Ø3S

LC Limited Coverage NC Noncovered ⊞ Combination Member HAC associated procedure Combination Only DRG Non-OR Non-OR New/Revised in GREEN

Ø Medical and Surgical
3 Upper Arteries
U Supplement Definition: Putting in or on biological or synthetic material that physically reinforces and/or augments the function of a portion of a body part

Explanation: The biological material is non-living, or is living and from the same individual. The body part may have been previously replaced, and the SUPPLEMENT procedure is performed to physically reinforce and/or augment the function of the replaced body part.

Body Part Character 4	Approach Character 5	Device Character 6	Qualifier Character 7
Ø Internal Mammary Artery, Right Anterior intercostal artery Internal thoracic artery Musculophrenic artery Pericardiophrenic artery Superior epigastric artery **1 Internal Mammary Artery, Left** *See Ø Internal Mammary Artery, Right* **2 Innominate Artery** Brachiocephalic artery Brachiocephalic trunk **3 Subclavian Artery, Right** Costocervical trunk Dorsal scapular artery Internal thoracic artery **4 Subclavian Artery, Left** *See 3 Subclavian Artery, Right* **5 Axillary Artery, Right** Anterior circumflex humeral artery Lateral thoracic artery Posterior circumflex humeral artery Subscapular artery Superior thoracic artery Thoracoacromial artery **6 Axillary Artery, Left** *See 5 Axillary Artery, Right* **7 Brachial Artery, Right** Inferior ulnar collateral artery Profunda brachii Superior ulnar collateral artery **8 Brachial Artery, Left** *See 7 Brachial Artery, Right* **9 Ulnar Artery, Right** Anterior ulnar recurrent artery Common interosseous artery Posterior ulnar recurrent artery **A Ulnar Artery, Left** *See 9 Ulnar Artery, Right* **B Radial Artery, Right** Radial recurrent artery **C Radial Artery, Left** *See B Radial Artery, Right* **D Hand Artery, Right** Deep palmar arch Princeps pollicis artery Radialis indicis Superficial palmar arch **F Hand Artery, Left** *See D Hand Artery, Right* **G Intracranial Artery** Anterior cerebral artery Anterior choroidal artery Anterior communicating artery Basilar artery Circle of Willis Internal carotid artery, intracranial portion Middle cerebral artery Ophthalmic artery Posterior cerebral artery Posterior communicating artery Posterior inferior cerebellar artery (PICA) **H Common Carotid Artery, Right** **J Common Carotid Artery, Left** **K Internal Carotid Artery, Right** Caroticotympanic artery Carotid sinus **L Internal Carotid Artery, Left** *See K Internal Carotid Artery, Right* **M External Carotid Artery, Right** Ascending pharyngeal artery Internal maxillary artery Lingual artery Maxillary artery Occipital artery Posterior auricular artery Superior thyroid artery **N External Carotid Artery, Left** *See M External Carotid Artery, Right* **P Vertebral Artery, Right** Anterior spinal artery Posterior spinal artery **Q Vertebral Artery, Left** *See P Vertebral Artery, Right* **R Face Artery** Angular artery Ascending palatine artery External maxillary artery Facial artery Inferior labial artery Submental artery Superior labial artery **S Temporal Artery, Right** Middle temporal artery Superficial temporal artery Transverse facial artery **T Temporal Artery, Left** *See S Temporal Artery, Right* **U Thyroid Artery, Right** Cricothyroid artery Hyoid artery Sternocleidomastoid artery Superior laryngeal artery Superior thyroid artery Thyrocervical trunk **V Thyroid Artery, Left** *See U Thyroid Artery, Right* **Y Upper Artery** Aortic intercostal artery Bronchial artery Esophageal artery Subcostal artery	Ø Open 3 Percutaneous 4 Percutaneous Endoscopic	7 Autologous Tissue Substitute J Synthetic Substitute K Nonautologous Tissue Substitute	Z No Qualifier

Ø Medical and Surgical
3 Upper Arteries
V Restriction Definition: Partially closing an orifice or the lumen of a tubular body part
Explanation: The orifice can be a natural orifice or an artificially created orifice

Body Part Character 4	Approach Character 5	Device Character 6	Qualifier Character 7
Ø Internal Mammary Artery, Right Anterior intercostal artery Internal thoracic artery Musculophrenic artery Pericardiophrenic artery Superior epigastric artery **1 Internal Mammary Artery, Left** *See Ø Internal Mammary Artery, Right* **2 Innominate Artery** Brachiocephalic artery Brachiocephalic trunk **3 Subclavian Artery, Right** Costocervical trunk Dorsal scapular artery Internal thoracic artery **4 Subclavian Artery, Left** *See 3 Subclavian Artery, Right* **5 Axillary Artery, Right** Anterior circumflex humeral artery Lateral thoracic artery Posterior circumflex humeral artery Subscapular artery Superior thoracic artery Thoracoacromial artery **6 Axillary Artery, Left** *See 5 Axillary Artery, Right* **7 Brachial Artery, Right** Inferior ulnar collateral artery Profunda brachii Superior ulnar collateral artery **8 Brachial Artery, Left** *See 7 Brachial Artery, Right* **9 Ulnar Artery, Right** Anterior ulnar recurrent artery Common interosseous artery Posterior ulnar recurrent artery **A Ulnar Artery, Left** *See 9 Ulnar Artery, Right* **B Radial Artery, Right** Radial recurrent artery **C Radial Artery, Left** *See B Radial Artery, Right* **D Hand Artery, Right** Deep palmar arch Princeps pollicis artery Radialis indicis Superficial palmar arch **F Hand Artery, Left** *See D Hand Artery, Right* **R Face Artery** Angular artery Ascending palatine artery External maxillary artery Facial artery Inferior labial artery Submental artery Superior labial artery **S Temporal Artery, Right** Middle temporal artery Superficial temporal artery Transverse facial artery **T Temporal Artery, Left** *See S Temporal Artery, Right* **U Thyroid Artery, Right** Cricothyroid artery Hyoid artery Sternocleidomastoid artery Superior laryngeal artery Superior thyroid artery Thyrocervical trunk **V Thyroid Artery, Left** *See U Thyroid Artery, Right* **Y Upper Artery** Aortic intercostal artery Bronchial artery Esophageal artery Subcostal artery	**Ø Open** **3 Percutaneous** **4 Percutaneous Endoscopic**	**C Extraluminal Device** **D Intraluminal Device** **Z No Device**	**Z No Qualifier**
G Intracranial Artery Anterior cerebral artery Anterior choroidal artery Anterior communicating artery Basilar artery Circle of Willis Internal carotid artery, intracranial portion Middle cerebral artery Ophthalmic artery Posterior cerebral artery Posterior communicating artery Posterior inferior cerebellar artery (PICA) **H Common Carotid Artery, Right** **J Common Carotid Artery, Left** **K Internal Carotid Artery, Right** Caroticotympanic artery Carotid sinus **L Internal Carotid Artery, Left** *See K Internal Carotid Artery, Right* **M External Carotid Artery, Right** Ascending pharyngeal artery Internal maxillary artery Lingual artery Maxillary artery Occipital artery Posterior auricular artery Superior thyroid artery **N External Carotid Artery, Left** *See M External Carotid Artery, Right* **P Vertebral Artery, Right** Anterior spinal artery Posterior spinal artery **Q Vertebral Artery, Left** *See P Vertebral Artery, Right*	**Ø Open** **3 Percutaneous** **4 Percutaneous Endoscopic**	**B Intraluminal Device, Bioactive** **C Extraluminal Device** **D Intraluminal Device** **Z No Device**	**Z No Qualifier**

Ø Medical and Surgical
3 Upper Arteries
W Revision Definition: Correcting, to the extent possible, a portion of a malfunctioning device or the position of a displaced device

Explanation: Revision can include correcting a malfunctioning or displaced device by taking out or putting in components of the device such as a screw or pin

Body Part Character 4	Approach Character 5	Device Character 6	Qualifier Character 7
Y Upper Artery Aortic intercostal artery Bronchial artery Esophageal artery Subcostal artery	**Ø** Open **3** Percutaneous **4** Percutaneous Endoscopic	**Ø** Drainage Device **2** Monitoring Device **3** Infusion Device **7** Autologous Tissue Substitute **C** Extraluminal Device **D** Intraluminal Device **J** Synthetic Substitute **K** Nonautologous Tissue Substitute **M** Stimulator Lead **Y** Other Device	**Z** No Qualifier
Y Upper Artery Aortic intercostal artery Bronchial artery Esophageal artery Subcostal artery	**X** External	**Ø** Drainage Device **2** Monitoring Device **3** Infusion Device **7** Autologous Tissue Substitute **C** Extraluminal Device **D** Intraluminal Device **J** Synthetic Substitute **K** Nonautologous Tissue Substitute **M** Stimulator Lead	**Z** No Qualifier

Non-OR Ø3WY3[Ø,2,3,D]Z
Non-OR Ø3WY[3,4]YZ
Non-OR Ø3WYX[Ø,2,3,7,C,D,J,K,M]Z

Lower Arteries Ø41–Ø4W

Character Meanings

This Character Meaning table is provided as a guide to assist the user in the identification of character members that may be found in this section of code tables. It **SHOULD NOT** be used to build a PCS code.

Operation–Character 3	Body Part–Character 4	Approach–Character 5	Device–Character 6	Qualifier–Character 7
1 Bypass	Ø Abdominal Aorta	Ø Open	Ø Drainage Device	Ø Abdominal Aorta
5 Destruction	1 Celiac Artery	3 Percutaneous	1 Radioactive Element	1 Celiac Artery OR Drug-Coated Balloon
7 Dilation	2 Gastric Artery	4 Percutaneous Endoscopic	2 Monitoring Device	2 Mesenteric Artery
9 Drainage	3 Hepatic Artery	X External	3 Infusion Device	3 Renal Artery, Right
B Excision	4 Splenic Artery		4 Intraluminal Device, Drug-eluting	4 Renal Artery, Left
C Extirpation	5 Superior Mesenteric Artery		5 Intraluminal Device, Drug-eluting, Two	5 Renal Artery, Bilateral
H Insertion	6 Colic Artery, Right		6 Intraluminal Device, Drug-eluting, Three	6 Common Iliac Artery, Right OR Bifurcation
J Inspection	7 Colic Artery, Left		7 Intraluminal Device, Drug-eluting, Four or More OR Autologous Tissue Substitute	7 Common Iliac Artery, Left
L Occlusion	8 Colic Artery, Middle		9 Autologous Venous Tissue	8 Common Iliac Arteries, Bilateral
N Release	9 Renal Artery, Right		A Autologous Arterial Tissue	9 Internal Iliac Artery, Right
P Removal	A Renal Artery, Left		C Extraluminal Device	B Internal Iliac Artery, Left
Q Repair	B Inferior Mesenteric Artery		D Intraluminal Device	C Internal Iliac Arteries, Bilateral
R Replacement	C Common Iliac Artery, Right		E Intraluminal Device, Two OR Intraluminal Device, Branched or Fenestrated, One or Two Arteries	D External Iliac Artery, Right
S Reposition	D Common Iliac Artery, Left		F Intraluminal Device, Three OR Intraluminal Device, Branched or Fenestrated, Three or More Arteries	F External Iliac Artery, Left
U Supplement	E Internal Iliac Artery, Right		G Intraluminal Device, Four or More	G External Iliac Arteries, Bilateral
V Restriction	F Internal Iliac Artery, Left		J Synthetic Substitute	H Femoral Artery, Right
W Revision	H External Iliac Artery, Right		K Nonautologous Tissue Substitute	J Femoral Artery, Left OR Temporary
	J External Iliac Artery, Left		Y Other Device	K Femoral Arteries, Bilateral
	K Femoral Artery, Right		Z No Device	L Popliteal Artery
	L Femoral Artery, Left			M Peroneal Artery
	M Popliteal Artery, Right			N Posterior Tibial Artery
	N Popliteal Artery, Left			P Foot Artery
	P Anterior Tibial Artery, Right			Q Lower Extremity Artery
	Q Anterior Tibial Artery, Left			R Lower Artery
	R Posterior Tibial Artery, Right			S Lower Extremity Vein
	S Posterior Tibial Artery, Left			T Uterine Artery, Right
	T Peroneal Artery, Right			U Uterine Artery, Left
	U Peroneal Artery, Left			X Diagnostic
	V Foot Artery, Right			Z No Qualifier
	W Foot Artery, Left			
	Y Lower Artery			

AHA Coding Clinic for table Ø41

2017, 4Q, 46-47	New and revised body part values - Bypass hepatic artery to renal artery
2017, 3Q, 5	Femoral artery to posterior tibial artery bypass using autologous and synthetic grafts
2017, 3Q, 16	Abdominal aortic debranching with bypass of external iliac artery to bilateral renal arteries and superior mesenteric artery
2017, 1Q, 32	Peroneal artery to dorsalis pedis artery bypass using saphenous vein graft
2016, 2Q, 18	Femoral-tibial artery bypass and saphenous vein graft
2015, 3Q, 28	Bilateral renal artery bypass

AHA Coding Clinic for table Ø47

2018, 2Q, 24	Coronary artery bifurcation
2016, 4Q, 86	Peripheral artery, number of stents
2016, 4Q, 86-88	Coronary and peripheral artery bifurcation
2016, 3Q, 39	Infrarenal abdominal aortic aneurysm repair with iliac graft extension
2015, 4Q, 4-7, 15	Drug-coated balloon angioplasty in peripheral vessels
2015, 3Q, 9	Aborted endovascular stenting of superficial femoral artery

AHA Coding Clinic for table Ø4C

2018, 2Q, 24	Coronary artery bifurcation
2017, 2Q, 23	Thrombectomy via Fogarty catheter
2016, 4Q, 86-88	Coronary and peripheral artery bifurcation
2016, 1Q, 31	Iliofemoral endarterectomy with patch repair
2015, 1Q, 29	Discontinued carotid endarterectomy
2015, 1Q, 36	Percutaneous mechanical thrombectomy of femoropopliteal bypass graft

AHA Coding Clinic for table Ø4H

2017, 1Q, 30	Insertion of umbilical artery catheter

AHA Coding Clinic for table Ø4L

2018, 2Q, 18	Transverse rectus abdominis myocutaneous (TRAM) delay
2017, 4Q, 31	Resuscitative endovascular balloon occlusion of the aorta
2015, 2Q, 27	Uterine artery embolization using Gelfoam
2014, 3Q, 26	Coil embolization of gastroduodenal artery with chemoembolization of hepatic artery
2014, 1Q, 24	Endovascular embolization for gastrointestinal bleeding

AHA Coding Clinic for table Ø4N

2015, 2Q, 28	Release and replacement of celiac artery

AHA Coding Clinic for table Ø4Q

2014, 1Q, 21	Repair of femoral artery pseudoaneurysm

AHA Coding Clinic for table Ø4R

2015, 2Q, 28	Release and replacement of celiac artery

AHA Coding Clinic for table Ø4U

2016, 2Q, 18	Femoral-tibial artery bypass and saphenous vein graft
2016, 1Q, 31	Iliofemoral endarterectomy with patch repair
2014, 4Q, 37	Bovine patch arterioplasty
2014, 1Q, 22	Repair of pseudoaneurysm of femoral-popliteal bypass graft

AHA Coding Clinic for table Ø4V

2018, 2Q, 24	Coronary artery bifurcation
2016, 4Q, 86-87	Coronary and peripheral artery bifurcation
2016, 4Q, 89-93	Branched and fenestrated endograft repair of aneurysms
2016, 3Q, 39	Infrarenal abdominal aortic aneurysm repair with iliac graft extension
2014, 1Q, 9	Endovascular repair of abdominal aortic aneurysm

AHA Coding Clinic for table Ø4W

2015, 1Q, 36	Revision of femoropopliteal bypass graft
2014, 1Q, 9	Endovascular repair of endoleak
2014, 1Q, 22	Repair of pseudoaneurysm of femoral-popliteal bypass graft

Lower Arteries

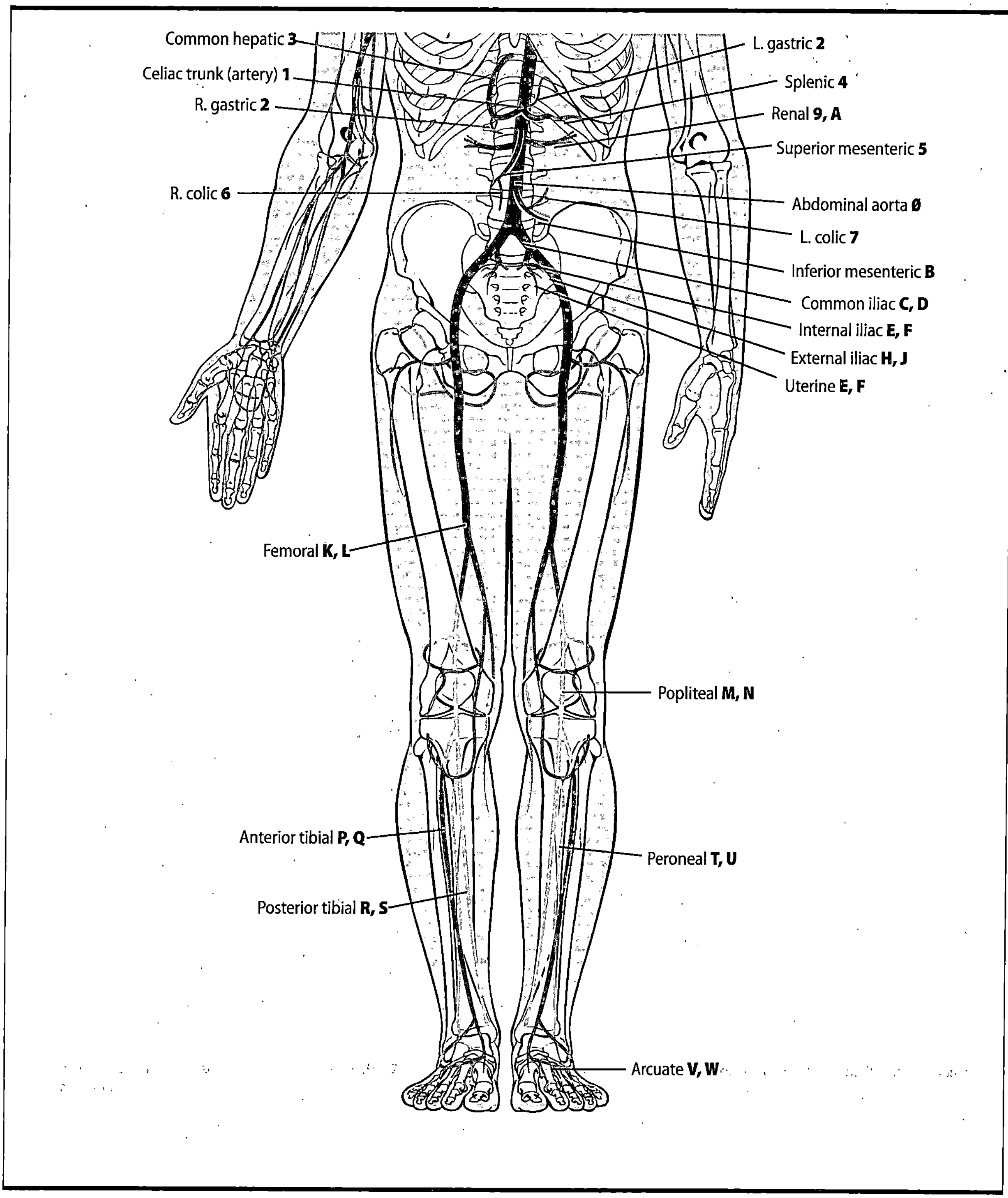
Common hepatic **3**
Celiac trunk (artery) **1**
R. gastric **2**
R. colic **6**
L. gastric **2**
Splenic **4**
Renal **9, A**
Superior mesenteric **5**
Abdominal aorta **Ø**
L. colic **7**
Inferior mesenteric **B**
Common iliac **C, D**
Internal iliac **E, F**
External iliac **H, J**
Uterine **E, F**
Femoral **K, L**
Popliteal **M, N**
Anterior tibial **P, Q**
Peroneal **T, U**
Posterior tibial **R, S**
Arcuate **V, W**

0 Medical and Surgical
4 Lower Arteries
1 Bypass Definition: Altering the route of passage of the contents of a tubular body part

Explanation: Rerouting contents of a body part to a downstream area of the normal route, to a similar route and body part, or to an abnormal route and dissimilar body part. Includes one or more anastomoses, with or without the use of a device.

Body Part Character 4	Approach Character 5	Device Character 6	Qualifier Character 7
0 Abdominal Aorta Inferior phrenic artery Lumbar artery Median sacral artery Middle suprarenal artery Ovarian artery Testicular artery **C Common Iliac Artery, Right** **D Common Iliac Artery, Left**	**0 Open** **4 Percutaneous Endoscopic**	**9 Autologous Venous Tissue** **A Autologous Arterial Tissue** **J Synthetic Substitute** **K Nonautologous Tissue Substitute** **Z No Device**	**0 Abdominal Aorta** **1 Celiac Artery** **2 Mesenteric Artery** **3 Renal Artery, Right** **4 Renal Artery, Left** **5 Renal Artery, Bilateral** **6 Common Iliac Artery, Right** **7 Common Iliac Artery, Left** **8 Common Iliac Arteries, Bilateral** **9 Internal Iliac Artery, Right** **B Internal Iliac Artery, Left** **C Internal Iliac Arteries, Bilateral** **D External Iliac Artery, Right** **F External Iliac Artery, Left** **G External Iliac Arteries, Bilateral** **H Femoral Artery, Right** **J Femoral Artery, Left** **K Femoral Arteries, Bilateral** **Q Lower Extremity Artery** **R Lower Artery**
3 Hepatic Artery Common hepatic artery Gastroduodenal artery Hepatic artery proper **4 Splenic Artery** Left gastroepiploic artery Pancreatic artery Short gastric artery	**0 Open** **4 Percutaneous Endoscopic**	**9 Autologous Venous Tissue** **A Autologous Arterial Tissue** **J Synthetic Substitute** **K Nonautologous Tissue Substitute** **Z No Device**	**3 Renal Artery, Right** **4 Renal Artery, Left** **5 Renal Artery, Bilateral**
E Internal Iliac Artery, Right Deferential artery Hypogastric artery Iliolumbar artery Inferior gluteal artery Inferior vesical artery Internal pudendal artery Lateral sacral artery Middle rectal artery Obturator artery Superior gluteal artery Umbilical artery Uterine artery Vaginal artery **F Internal Iliac Artery, Left** *See E Internal Iliac Artery, Right* **H External Iliac Artery, Right** Deep circumflex iliac artery Inferior epigastric artery **J External Iliac Artery, Left** *See H External Iliac Artery, Right*	**0 Open** **4 Percutaneous Endoscopic**	**9 Autologous Venous Tissue** **A Autologous Arterial Tissue** **J Synthetic Substitute** **K Nonautologous Tissue Substitute** **Z No Device**	**9 Internal Iliac Artery, Right** **B Internal Iliac Artery, Left** **C Internal Iliac Arteries, Bilateral** **D External Iliac Artery, Right** **F External Iliac Artery, Left** **G External Iliac Arteries, Bilateral** **H Femoral Artery, Right** **J Femoral Artery, Left** **K Femoral Arteries, Bilateral** **P Foot Artery** **Q Lower Extremity Artery**
K Femoral Artery, Right Circumflex iliac artery Deep femoral artery Descending genicular artery External pudendal artery Superficial epigastric artery **L Femoral Artery, Left** *See K Femoral Artery, Right*	**0 Open** **4 Percutaneous Endoscopic**	**9 Autologous Venous Tissue** **A Autologous Arterial Tissue** **J Synthetic Substitute** **K Nonautologous Tissue Substitute** **Z No Device**	**H Femoral Artery, Right** **J Femoral Artery, Left** **K Femoral Arteries, Bilateral** **L Popliteal Artery** **M Peroneal Artery** **N Posterior Tibial Artery** **P Foot Artery** **Q Lower Extremity Artery** **S Lower Extremity Vein**
K Femoral Artery, Right Circumflex iliac artery Deep femoral artery Descending genicular artery External pudendal artery Superficial epigastric artery **L Femoral Artery, Left** *See K Femoral Artery, Right*	**3 Percutaneous**	**J Synthetic Substitute**	**Q Lower Extremity Artery** **S Lower Extremity Vein**
M Popliteal Artery, Right Inferior genicular artery Middle genicular artery Superior genicular artery Sural artery **N Popliteal Artery, Left** *See M Popliteal Artery, Right*	**0 Open** **4 Percutaneous Endoscopic**	**9 Autologous Venous Tissue** **A Autologous Arterial Tissue** **J Synthetic Substitute** **K Nonautologous Tissue Substitute** **Z No Device**	**L Popliteal Artery** **M Peroneal Artery** **P Foot Artery** **Q Lower Extremity Artery** **S Lower Extremity Vein**

041 Continued on next page

Ø Medical and Surgical
4 Lower Arteries
1 Bypass Definition: Altering the route of passage of the contents of a tubular body part

Explanation: Rerouting contents of a body part to a downstream area of the normal route, to a similar route and body part, or to an abnormal route and dissimilar body part. Includes one or more anastomoses, with or without the use of a device.

Ø41 Continued

Body Part Character 4		Approach Character 5	Device Character 6	Qualifier Character 7
M Popliteal Artery, Right Inferior genicular artery Middle genicular artery Superior genicular artery Sural artery	**N Popliteal Artery, Left** *See M Popliteal Artery, Right*	3 Percutaneous	J Synthetic Substitute	Q Lower Extremity Artery S Lower Extremity Vein
P Anterior Tibial Artery, Right Anterior lateral malleolar artery Anterior medial malleolar artery Anterior tibial recurrent artery Dorsalis pedis artery Posterior tibial recurrent artery	**Q Anterior Tibial Artery, Left** *See P Anterior Tibial Artery, Right* **R Posterior Tibial Artery, Right** **S Posterior Tibial Artery, Left**	Ø Open 3 Percutaneous 4 Percutaneous Endoscopic	J Synthetic Substitute	Q Lower Extremity Artery S Lower Extremity Vein
T Peroneal Artery, Right Fibular artery **U Peroneal Artery, Left** *See T Peroneal Artery, Right*	**V Foot Artery, Right** Arcuate artery Dorsal metatarsal artery Lateral plantar artery Lateral tarsal artery Medial plantar artery **W Foot Artery, Left** *See V Foot Artery, Right*	Ø Open 4 Percutaneous Endoscopic	9 Autologous Venous Tissue A Autologous Arterial Tissue J Synthetic Substitute K Nonautologous Tissue Substitute Z No Device	P Foot Artery Q Lower Extremity Artery S Lower Extremity Vein
T Peroneal Artery, Right Fibular artery **U Peroneal Artery, Left** *See T Peroneal Artery, Right*	**V Foot Artery, Right** Arcuate artery Dorsal metatarsal artery Lateral plantar artery Lateral tarsal artery Medial plantar artery **W Foot Artery, Left** *See V Foot Artery, Right*	3 Percutaneous	J Synthetic Substitute	Q Lower Extremity Artery S Lower Extremity Vein

Ø Medical and Surgical
4 Lower Arteries
5 Destruction Definition: Physical eradication of all or a portion of a body part by the direct use of energy, force, or a destructive agent
Explanation: None of the body part is physically taken out

Body Part Character 4		Approach Character 5	Device Character 6	Qualifier Character 7
Ø Abdominal Aorta Inferior phrenic artery Lumbar artery Median sacral artery Middle suprarenal artery Ovarian artery Testicular artery **1 Celiac Artery** Celiac trunk **2 Gastric Artery** Left gastric artery Right gastric artery **3 Hepatic Artery** Common hepatic artery Gastroduodenal artery Hepatic artery proper **4 Splenic Artery** Left gastroepiploic artery Pancreatic artery Short gastric artery **5 Superior Mesenteric Artery** Ileal artery Ileocolic artery Inferior pancreaticoduodenal artery Jejunal artery **6 Colic Artery, Right** **7 Colic Artery, Left** **8 Colic Artery, Middle** **9 Renal Artery, Right** Inferior suprarenal artery Renal segmental artery **A Renal Artery, Left** *See 9 Renal Artery, Right* **B Inferior Mesenteric Artery** Sigmoid artery Superior rectal artery **C Common Iliac Artery, Right** **D Common Iliac Artery, Left** **E Internal Iliac Artery, Right** Deferential artery Hypogastric artery Iliolumbar artery Inferior gluteal artery Inferior vesical artery Internal pudendal artery Lateral sacral artery Middle rectal artery Obturator artery Superior gluteal artery Umbilical artery Uterine artery Vaginal artery	**F Internal Iliac Artery, Left** *See E Internal Iliac Artery, Right* **H External Iliac Artery, Right** Deep circumflex iliac artery Inferior epigastric artery **J External Iliac Artery, Left** *See H External Iliac Artery, Right* **K Femoral Artery, Right** Circumflex iliac artery Deep femoral artery Descending genicular artery External pudendal artery Superficial epigastric artery **L Femoral Artery, Left** *See K Femoral Artery, Right* **M Popliteal Artery, Right** Inferior genicular artery Middle genicular artery Superior genicular artery Sural artery **N Popliteal Artery, Left** *See M Popliteal Artery, Right* **P Anterior Tibial Artery, Right** Anterior lateral malleolar artery Anterior medial malleolar artery Anterior tibial recurrent artery Dorsalis pedis artery Posterior tibial recurrent artery **Q Anterior Tibial Artery, Left** *See P Anterior Tibial Artery, Right* **R Posterior Tibial Artery, Right** **S Posterior Tibial Artery, Left** **T Peroneal Artery, Right** Fibular artery **U Peroneal Artery, Left** *See T Peroneal Artery, Right* **V Foot Artery, Right** Arcuate artery Dorsal metatarsal artery Lateral plantar artery Lateral tarsal artery Medial plantar artery **W Foot Artery, Left** *See V Foot Artery, Right* **Y Lower Artery** Umbilical artery	Ø Open 3 Percutaneous 4 Percutaneous Endoscopic	Z No Device	Z No Qualifier

Ø Medical and Surgical
4 Lower Arteries
7 Dilation Definition: Expanding an orifice or the lumen of a tubular body part

Explanation: The orifice can be a natural orifice or an artificially created orifice. Accomplished by stretching a tubular body part using intraluminal pressure or by cutting part of the orifice or wall of the tubular body part.

Body Part Character 4	Approach Character 5	Device Character 6	Qualifier Character 7
Ø Abdominal Aorta Inferior phrenic artery Lumbar artery Median sacral artery Middle suprarenal artery Ovarian artery Testicular artery **1 Celiac Artery** Celiac trunk **2 Gastric Artery** Left gastric artery Right gastric artery **3 Hepatic Artery** Common hepatic artery Gastroduodenal artery Hepatic artery proper **4 Splenic Artery** Left gastroepiploic artery Pancreatic artery Short gastric artery **5 Superior Mesenteric Artery** Ileal artery Ileocolic artery Inferior pancreaticoduodenal artery Jejunal artery **6 Colic Artery, Right** **7 Colic Artery, Left** **8 Colic Artery, Middle** **9 Renal Artery, Right** Inferior suprarenal artery Renal segmental artery **A Renal Artery, Left** *See 9 Renal Artery, Right* **B Inferior Mesenteric Artery** Sigmoid artery Superior rectal artery **C Common Iliac Artery, Right** **D Common Iliac Artery, Left** **E Internal Iliac Artery, Right** Deferential artery Hypogastric artery Iliolumbar artery Inferior gluteal artery Inferior vesical artery Internal pudendal artery Lateral sacral artery Middle rectal artery Obturator artery Superior gluteal artery Umbilical artery Uterine artery Vaginal artery **F Internal Iliac Artery, Left** *See E Internal Iliac Artery, Right* **H External Iliac Artery, Right** Deep circumflex iliac artery Inferior epigastric artery **J External Iliac Artery, Left** *See H External Iliac Artery, Right* **K Femoral Artery, Right** Circumflex iliac artery Deep femoral artery Descending genicular artery External pudendal artery Superficial epigastric artery **L Femoral Artery, Left** *See K Femoral Artery, Right* **M Popliteal Artery, Right** Inferior genicular artery Middle genicular artery Superior genicular artery Sural artery **N Popliteal Artery, Left** *See M Popliteal Artery, Right* **P Anterior Tibial Artery, Right** Anterior lateral malleolar artery Anterior medial malleolar artery Anterior tibial recurrent artery Dorsalis pedis artery Posterior tibial recurrent artery **Q Anterior Tibial Artery, Left** *See P Anterior Tibial Artery, Right* **R Posterior Tibial Artery, Right** **S Posterior Tibial Artery, Left** **T Peroneal Artery, Right** Fibular artery **U Peroneal Artery, Left** *See T Peroneal Artery, Right* **V Foot Artery, Right** Arcuate artery Dorsal metatarsal artery Lateral plantar artery Lateral tarsal artery Medial plantar artery **W Foot Artery, Left** *See V Foot Artery, Right* **Y Lower Artery** Umbilical artery	Ø Open 3 Percutaneous 4 Percutaneous Endoscopic	4 Intraluminal Device, Drug-eluting D Intraluminal Device Z No Device	1 Drug-Coated Balloon 6 Bifurcation Z No Qualifier

Ø47 Continued on next page

Ø47 Continued

Ø Medical and Surgical
4 Lower Arteries
7 Dilation Definition: Expanding an orifice or the lumen of a tubular body part

Explanation: The orifice can be a natural orifice or an artificially created orifice. Accomplished by stretching a tubular body part using intraluminal pressure or by cutting part of the orifice or wall of the tubular body part.

Body Part Character 4		Approach Character 5	Device Character 6	Qualifier Character 7
Ø Abdominal Aorta Inferior phrenic artery Lumbar artery Median sacral artery Middle suprarenal artery Ovarian artery Testicular artery **1 Celiac Artery** Celiac trunk **2 Gastric Artery** Left gastric artery Right gastric artery **3 Hepatic Artery** Common hepatic artery Gastroduodenal artery Hepatic artery proper **4 Splenic Artery** Left gastroepiploic artery Pancreatic artery Short gastric artery **5 Superior Mesenteric Artery** Ileal artery Ileocolic artery Inferior pancreaticoduodenal artery Jejunal artery **6 Colic Artery, Right** **7 Colic Artery, Left** **8 Colic Artery, Middle** **9 Renal Artery, Right** Inferior suprarenal artery Renal segmental artery **A Renal Artery, Left** *See 9 Renal Artery, Right* **B Inferior Mesenteric Artery** Sigmoid artery Superior rectal artery **C Common Iliac Artery, Right** **D Common Iliac Artery, Left** **E Internal Iliac Artery, Right** Deferential artery Hypogastric artery Iliolumbar artery Inferior gluteal artery Inferior vesical artery Internal pudendal artery Lateral sacral artery Middle rectal artery Obturator artery Superior gluteal artery Umbilical artery Uterine artery Vaginal artery	**F Internal Iliac Artery, Left** *See E Internal Iliac Artery, Right* **H External Iliac Artery, Right** Deep circumflex iliac artery Inferior epigastric artery **J External Iliac Artery, Left** *See H External Iliac Artery, Right* **K Femoral Artery, Right** Circumflex iliac artery Deep femoral artery Descending genicular artery External pudendal artery Superficial epigastric artery **L Femoral Artery, Left** *See K Femoral Artery, Right* **M Popliteal Artery, Right** Inferior genicular artery Middle genicular artery Superior genicular artery Sural artery **N Popliteal Artery, Left** *See M Popliteal Artery, Right* **P Anterior Tibial Artery, Right** Anterior lateral malleolar artery Anterior medial malleolar artery Anterior tibial recurrent artery Dorsalis pedis artery Posterior tibial recurrent artery **Q Anterior Tibial Artery, Left** *See P Anterior Tibial Artery, Right* **R Posterior Tibial Artery, Right** **S Posterior Tibial Artery, Left** **T Peroneal Artery, Right** Fibular artery **U Peroneal Artery, Left** *See T Peroneal Artery, Right* **V Foot Artery, Right** Arcuate artery Dorsal metatarsal artery Lateral plantar artery Lateral tarsal artery Medial plantar artery **W Foot Artery, Left** *See V Foot Artery, Right* **Y Lower Artery** Umbilical artery	**Ø** Open **3** Percutaneous **4** Percutaneous Endoscopic	**5** Intraluminal Device, Drug-eluting, Two **6** Intraluminal Device, Drug-eluting, Three **7** Intraluminal Device, Drug-eluting, Four or More **E** Intraluminal Device, Two **F** Intraluminal Device, Three **G** Intraluminal Device, Four or More	**6** Bifurcation **Z** No Qualifier

Ø Medical and Surgical
4 Lower Arteries
9 Drainage Definition: Taking or letting out fluids and/or gases from a body part
Explanation: The qualifier DIAGNOSTIC is used to identify drainage procedures that are biopsies

Body Part Character 4		Approach Character 5	Device Character 6	Qualifier Character 7
Ø Abdominal Aorta Inferior phrenic artery Lumbar artery Median sacral artery Middle suprarenal artery Ovarian artery Testicular artery **1 Celiac Artery** Celiac trunk **2 Gastric Artery** Left gastric artery Right gastric artery **3 Hepatic Artery** Common hepatic artery Gastroduodenal artery Hepatic artery proper **4 Splenic Artery** Left gastroepiploic artery Pancreatic artery Short gastric artery **5 Superior Mesenteric Artery** Ileal artery Ileocolic artery Inferior pancreaticoduodenal artery Jejunal artery **6 Colic Artery, Right** **7 Colic Artery, Left** **8 Colic Artery, Middle** **9 Renal Artery, Right** Inferior suprarenal artery Renal segmental artery **A Renal Artery, Left** *See 9 Renal Artery, Right* **B Inferior Mesenteric Artery** Sigmoid artery Superior rectal artery **C Common Iliac Artery, Right** **D Common Iliac Artery, Left** **E Internal Iliac Artery, Right** Deferential artery Hypogastric artery Iliolumbar artery Inferior gluteal artery Inferior vesical artery Internal pudendal artery Lateral sacral artery Middle rectal artery Obturator artery Superior gluteal artery Umbilical artery Uterine artery Vaginal artery	**F Internal Iliac Artery, Left** *See E Internal Iliac Artery, Right* **H External Iliac Artery, Right** Deep circumflex iliac artery Inferior epigastric artery **J External Iliac Artery, Left** *See H External Iliac Artery, Right* **K Femoral Artery, Right** Circumflex iliac artery Deep femoral artery Descending genicular artery External pudendal artery Superficial epigastric artery **L Femoral Artery, Left** *See K Femoral Artery, Right* **M Popliteal Artery, Right** Inferior genicular artery Middle genicular artery Superior genicular artery Sural artery **N Popliteal Artery, Left** *See M Popliteal Artery, Right* **P Anterior Tibial Artery, Right** Anterior lateral malleolar artery Anterior medial malleolar artery Anterior tibial recurrent artery Dorsalis pedis artery Posterior tibial recurrent artery **Q Anterior Tibial Artery, Left** *See P Anterior Tibial Artery, Right* **R Posterior Tibial Artery, Right** **S Posterior Tibial Artery, Left** **T Peroneal Artery, Right** Fibular artery **U Peroneal Artery, Left** *See T Peroneal Artery, Right* **V Foot Artery, Right** Arcuate artery Dorsal metatarsal artery Lateral plantar artery Lateral tarsal artery Medial plantar artery **W Foot Artery, Left** *See V Foot Artery, Right* **Y Lower Artery** Umbilical artery	**Ø** Open **3** Percutaneous **4** Percutaneous Endoscopic	**Ø** Drainage Device	**Z** No Qualifier

Ø49 Continued on next page

Non-OR Ø49[Ø,1,2,3,4,5,6,7,8,9,A,B,C,D,E,F,H,J,K,L,M,N,P,Q,R,S,T,U,V,W,Y][Ø,3,4]ØZ

Ø49–Ø49

Ø49 Continued

Ø Medical and Surgical
4 Lower Arteries
9 Drainage Definition: Taking or letting out fluids and/or gases from a body part
Explanation: The qualifier DIAGNOSTIC is used to identify drainage procedures that are biopsies

Body Part Character 4		Approach Character 5	Device Character 6	Qualifier Character 7
Ø Abdominal Aorta Inferior phrenic artery Lumbar artery Median sacral artery Middle suprarenal artery Ovarian artery Testicular artery **1 Celiac Artery** Celiac trunk **2 Gastric Artery** Left gastric artery Right gastric artery **3 Hepatic Artery** Common hepatic artery Gastroduodenal artery Hepatic artery proper **4 Splenic Artery** Left gastroepiploic artery Pancreatic artery Short gastric artery **5 Superior Mesenteric Artery** Ileal artery Ileocolic artery Inferior pancreaticoduodenal artery Jejunal artery **6 Colic Artery, Right** **7 Colic Artery, Left** **8 Colic Artery, Middle** **9 Renal Artery, Right** Inferior suprarenal artery Renal segmental artery **A Renal Artery, Left** *See 9 Renal Artery, Right* **B Inferior Mesenteric Artery** Sigmoid artery Superior rectal artery **C Common Iliac Artery, Right** **D Common Iliac Artery, Left** **E Internal Iliac Artery, Right** Deferential artery Hypogastric artery Iliolumbar artery Inferior gluteal artery Inferior vesical artery Internal pudendal artery Lateral sacral artery Middle rectal artery Obturator artery Superior gluteal artery Umbilical artery Uterine artery Vaginal artery	**F Internal Iliac Artery, Left** *See E Internal Iliac Artery, Right* **H External Iliac Artery, Right** Deep circumflex iliac artery Inferior epigastric artery **J External Iliac Artery, Left** *See H External Iliac Artery, Right* **K Femoral Artery, Right** Circumflex iliac artery Deep femoral artery Descending genicular artery External pudendal artery Superficial epigastric artery **L Femoral Artery, Left** *See K Femoral Artery, Right* **M Popliteal Artery, Right** Inferior genicular artery Middle genicular artery Superior genicular artery Sural artery **N Popliteal Artery, Left** *See M Popliteal Artery, Right* **P Anterior Tibial Artery, Right** Anterior lateral malleolar artery Anterior medial malleolar artery Anterior tibial recurrent artery Dorsalis pedis artery Posterior tibial recurrent artery **Q Anterior Tibial Artery, Left** *See P Anterior Tibial Artery, Right* **R Posterior Tibial Artery, Right** **S Posterior Tibial Artery, Left** **T Peroneal Artery, Right** Fibular artery **U Peroneal Artery, Left** *See T Peroneal Artery, Right* **V Foot Artery, Right** Arcuate artery Dorsal metatarsal artery Lateral plantar artery Lateral tarsal artery Medial plantar artery **W Foot Artery, Left** *See V Foot Artery, Right* **Y Lower Artery** Umbilical artery	**Ø Open** **3 Percutaneous** **4 Percutaneous Endoscopic**	**Z No Device**	**X Diagnostic** **Z No Qualifier**

Non-OR Ø49[Ø,1,2,3,4,5,6,7,8,9,A,B,C,D,E,F,H,J,K,L,M,N,P,Q,R,S,T,U,V,W,Y]3ZX
Non-OR Ø49[Ø,1,2,3,4,5,6,7,8,9,A,B,C,D,E,F,H,J,K,L,M,N,P,Q,R,S,T,U,V,W,Y][Ø,3,4]ZZ

Ø Medical and Surgical
4 Lower Arteries
B Excision Definition: Cutting out or off, without replacement, a portion of a body part
Explanation: The qualifier DIAGNOSTIC is used to identify excision procedures that are biopsies

Body Part Character 4	Approach Character 5	Device Character 6	Qualifier Character 7
Ø Abdominal Aorta Inferior phrenic artery Lumbar artery Median sacral artery Middle suprarenal artery Ovarian artery Testicular artery **1 Celiac Artery** Celiac trunk **2 Gastric Artery** Left gastric artery Right gastric artery **3 Hepatic Artery** Common hepatic artery Gastroduodenal artery Hepatic artery proper **4 Splenic Artery** Left gastroepiploic artery Pancreatic artery Short gastric artery **5 Superior Mesenteric Artery** Ileal artery Ileocolic artery Inferior pancreaticoduodenal artery Jejunal artery **6 Colic Artery, Right** **7 Colic Artery, Left** **8 Colic Artery, Middle** **9 Renal Artery, Right** Inferior suprarenal artery Renal segmental artery **A Renal Artery, Left** *See 9 Renal Artery, Right* **B Inferior Mesenteric Artery** Sigmoid artery Superior rectal artery **C Common Iliac Artery, Right** **D Common Iliac Artery, Left** **E Internal Iliac Artery, Right** Deferential artery Hypogastric artery Iliolumbar artery Inferior gluteal artery Inferior vesical artery Internal pudendal artery Lateral sacral artery Middle rectal artery Obturator artery Superior gluteal artery Umbilical artery Uterine artery Vaginal artery **F Internal Iliac Artery, Left** *See E Internal Iliac Artery, Right* **H External Iliac Artery, Right** Deep circumflex iliac artery Inferior epigastric artery **J External Iliac Artery, Left** *See H External Iliac Artery, Right* **K Femoral Artery, Right** Circumflex iliac artery Deep femoral artery Descending genicular artery External pudendal artery Superficial epigastric artery **L Femoral Artery, Left** *See K Femoral Artery, Right* **M Popliteal Artery, Right** Inferior genicular artery Middle genicular artery Superior genicular artery Sural artery **N Popliteal Artery, Left** *See M Popliteal Artery, Right* **P Anterior Tibial Artery, Right** Anterior lateral malleolar artery Anterior medial malleolar artery Anterior tibial recurrent artery Dorsalis pedis artery Posterior tibial recurrent artery **Q Anterior Tibial Artery, Left** *See P Anterior Tibial Artery, Right* **R Posterior Tibial Artery, Right** **S Posterior Tibial Artery, Left** **T Peroneal Artery, Right** Fibular artery **U Peroneal Artery, Left** *See T Peroneal Artery, Right* **V Foot Artery, Right** Arcuate artery Dorsal metatarsal artery Lateral plantar artery Lateral tarsal artery Medial plantar artery **W Foot Artery, Left** *See V Foot Artery, Right* **Y Lower Artery** Umbilical artery	Ø Open 3 Percutaneous 4 Percutaneous Endoscopic	Z No Device	X Diagnostic Z No Qualifier

Ø Medical and Surgical
4 Lower Arteries
C Extirpation Definition: Taking or cutting out solid matter from a body part

Explanation: The solid matter may be an abnormal byproduct of a biological function or a foreign body; it may be imbedded in a body part or in the lumen of a tubular body part. The solid matter may or may not have been previously broken into pieces.

Body Part Character 4		Approach Character 5	Device Character 6	Qualifier Character 7
Ø Abdominal Aorta Inferior phrenic artery Lumbar artery Median sacral artery Middle suprarenal artery Ovarian artery Testicular artery **1 Celiac Artery** Celiac trunk **2 Gastric Artery** Left gastric artery Right gastric artery **3 Hepatic Artery** Common hepatic artery Gastroduodenal artery Hepatic artery proper **4 Splenic Artery** Left gastroepiploic artery Pancreatic artery Short gastric artery **5 Superior Mesenteric Artery** Ileal artery Ileocolic artery Inferior pancreaticoduodenal artery Jejunal artery **6 Colic Artery, Right** **7 Colic Artery, Left** **8 Colic Artery, Middle** **9 Renal Artery, Right** Inferior suprarenal artery Renal segmental artery **A Renal Artery, Left** *See 9 Renal Artery, Right* **B Inferior Mesenteric Artery** Sigmoid artery Superior rectal artery **C Common Iliac Artery, Right** **D Common Iliac Artery, Left** **E Internal Iliac Artery, Right** Deferential artery Hypogastric artery Iliolumbar artery Inferior gluteal artery Inferior vesical artery Internal pudendal artery Lateral sacral artery Middle rectal artery Obturator artery Superior gluteal artery Umbilical artery Uterine artery Vaginal artery	**F Internal Iliac Artery, Left** *See E Internal Iliac Artery, Right* **H External Iliac Artery, Right** Deep circumflex iliac artery Inferior epigastric artery **J External Iliac Artery, Left** *See H External Iliac Artery, Right* **K Femoral Artery, Right** Circumflex iliac artery Deep femoral artery Descending genicular artery External pudendal artery Superficial epigastric artery **L Femoral Artery, Left** *See K Femoral Artery, Right* **M Popliteal Artery, Right** Inferior genicular artery Middle genicular artery Superior genicular artery Sural artery **N Popliteal Artery, Left** *See M Popliteal Artery, Right* **P Anterior Tibial Artery, Right** Anterior lateral malleolar artery Anterior medial malleolar artery Anterior tibial recurrent artery Dorsalis pedis artery Posterior tibial recurrent artery **Q Anterior Tibial Artery, Left** *See P Anterior Tibial Artery, Right* **R Posterior Tibial Artery, Right** **S Posterior Tibial Artery, Left** **T Peroneal Artery, Right** Fibular artery **U Peroneal Artery, Left** *See T Peroneal Artery, Right* **V Foot Artery, Right** Arcuate artery Dorsal metatarsal artery Lateral plantar artery Lateral tarsal artery Medial plantar artery **W Foot Artery, Left** *See V Foot Artery, Right* **Y Lower Artery** Umbilical artery	**Ø Open** **3 Percutaneous** **4 Percutaneous Endoscopic**	**Z No Device**	**6 Bifurcation** **Z No Qualifier**

Ø Medical and Surgical
4 Lower Arteries
H Insertion Definition: Putting in a nonbiological appliance that monitors, assists, performs, or prevents a physiological function but does not physically take the place of a body part

Explanation: None

Body Part Character 4	Approach Character 5	Device Character 6	Qualifier Character 7
Ø Abdominal Aorta Inferior phrenic artery Lumbar artery Median sacral artery Middle suprarenal artery Ovarian artery Testicular artery	**Ø** Open **3** Percutaneous **4** Percutaneous Endoscopic	**2** Monitoring Device **3** Infusion Device **D** Intraluminal Device	**Z** No Qualifier
1 Celiac Artery Celiac trunk **2 Gastric Artery** Left gastric artery Right gastric artery **3 Hepatic Artery** Common hepatic artery Gastroduodenal artery Hepatic artery proper **4 Splenic Artery** Left gastroepiploic artery Pancreatic artery Short gastric artery **5 Superior Mesenteric Artery** Ileal artery Ileocolic artery Inferior pancreaticoduodenal artery Jejunal artery **6 Colic Artery, Right** **7 Colic Artery, Left** **8 Colic Artery, Middle** **9 Renal Artery, Right** Inferior suprarenal artery Renal segmental artery **A Renal Artery, Left** *See 9 Renal Artery, Right* **B Inferior Mesenteric Artery** Sigmoid artery Superior rectal artery **C Common Iliac Artery, Right** **D Common Iliac Artery, Left** **E Internal Iliac Artery, Right** Deferential artery Hypogastric artery Iliolumbar artery Inferior gluteal artery Inferior vesical artery Internal pudendal artery Lateral sacral artery Middle rectal artery Obturator artery Superior gluteal artery Umbilical artery Uterine artery Vaginal artery **F Internal Iliac Artery, Left** *See E Internal Iliac Artery, Right* **H External Iliac Artery, Right** Deep circumflex iliac artery Inferior epigastric artery **J External Iliac Artery, Left** *See H External Iliac Artery, Right* **K Femoral Artery, Right** Circumflex iliac artery Deep femoral artery Descending genicular artery External pudendal artery Superficial epigastric artery **L Femoral Artery, Left** *See K Femoral Artery, Right* **M Popliteal Artery, Right** Inferior genicular artery Middle genicular artery Superior genicular artery Sural artery **N Popliteal Artery, Left** *See M Popliteal Artery, Right* **P Anterior Tibial Artery, Right** Anterior lateral malleolar artery Anterior medial malleolar artery Anterior tibial recurrent artery Dorsalis pedis artery Posterior tibial recurrent artery **Q Anterior Tibial Artery, Left** *See P Anterior Tibial Artery, Right* **R Posterior Tibial Artery, Right** **S Posterior Tibial Artery, Left** **T Peroneal Artery, Right** Fibular artery **U Peroneal Artery, Left** *See T Peroneal Artery, Right* **V Foot Artery, Right** Arcuate artery Dorsal metatarsal artery Lateral plantar artery Lateral tarsal artery Medial plantar artery **W Foot Artery, Left** *See V Foot Artery, Right*	**Ø** Open **3** Percutaneous **4** Percutaneous Endoscopic	**3** Infusion Device **D** Intraluminal Device	**Z** No Qualifier
Y Lower Artery Umbilical artery	**Ø** Open **3** Percutaneous **4** Percutaneous Endoscopic	**2** Monitoring Device **3** Infusion Device **D** Intraluminal Device **Y** Other Device	**Z** No Qualifier

Non-OR Ø4HØ[Ø,3,4][2,3]Z
Non-OR Ø4H[1,2,3,4,5,6,7,8,9,A,B,C,D,E,F,H,J,K,L,M,N,P,Q,R,S,T,U,V,W][Ø,3,4]3Z
Non-OR Ø4HY32Z
Non-OR Ø4HY[Ø,3,4]3Z
Non-OR Ø4HY[3,4]YZ

Ø Medical and Surgical
4 Lower Arteries
J Inspection Definition: Visually and/or manually exploring a body part

Explanation: Visual exploration may be performed with or without optical instrumentation. Manual exploration may be performed directly or through intervening body layers.

Body Part Character 4	Approach Character 5	Device Character 6	Qualifier Character 7
Y Lower Artery Umbilical artery	Ø Open 3 Percutaneous 4 Percutaneous Endoscopic X External	Z No Device	Z No Qualifier

Non-OR Ø4JY[3,4,X]ZZ

Ø Medical and Surgical
4 Lower Arteries
L Occlusion Definition: Completely closing an orifice or the lumen of a tubular body part

Explanation: The orifice can be a natural orifice or an artificially created orifice

Body Part Character 4	Approach Character 5	Device Character 6	Qualifier Character 7
Ø Abdominal Aorta Inferior phrenic artery Lumbar artery Median sacral artery Middle suprarenal artery Ovarian artery Testicular artery	Ø Open 4 Percutaneous Endoscopic	C Extraluminal Device D Intraluminal Device Z No Device	Z No Qualifier
Ø Abdominal Aorta Inferior phrenic artery Lumbar artery Median sacral artery Middle suprarenal artery Ovarian artery Testicular artery	3 Percutaneous	C Extraluminal Device Z No Device	Z No Qualifier
Ø Abdominal Aorta Inferior phrenic artery Lumbar artery Median sacral artery Middle suprarenal artery Ovarian artery Testicular artery	3 Percutaneous	D Intraluminal Device	J Temporary Z No Qualifier

Ø4L Continued on next page

Ø Medical and Surgical
4 Lower Arteries
L Occlusion Definition: Completely closing an orifice or the lumen of a tubular body part
Explanation: The orifice can be a natural orifice or an artificially created orifice

Ø4L Continued

Body Part Character 4	Approach Character 5	Device Character 6	Qualifier Character 7
1 Celiac Artery Celiac trunk **2 Gastric Artery** Left gastric artery Right gastric artery **3 Hepatic Artery** Common hepatic artery Gastroduodenal artery Hepatic artery proper **4 Splenic Artery** Left gastroepiploic artery Pancreatic artery Short gastric artery **5 Superior Mesenteric Artery** Ileal artery Ileocolic artery Inferior pancreaticoduodenal artery Jejunal artery **6 Colic Artery, Right** **7 Colic Artery, Left** **8 Colic Artery, Middle** **9 Renal Artery, Right** Inferior suprarenal artery Renal segmental artery **A Renal Artery, Left** *See 9 Renal Artery, Right* **B Inferior Mesenteric Artery** Sigmoid artery Superior rectal artery **C Common Iliac Artery, Right** **D Common Iliac Artery, Left** **H External Iliac Artery, Right** Deep circumflex iliac artery Inferior epigastric artery **J External Iliac Artery, Left** *See H External Iliac Artery, Right* **K Femoral Artery, Right** Circumflex iliac artery Deep femoral artery Descending genicular artery External pudendal artery Superficial epigastric artery **L Femoral Artery, Left** *See K Femoral Artery, Right* **M Popliteal Artery, Right** Inferior genicular artery Middle genicular artery Superior genicular artery Sural artery **N Popliteal Artery, Left** *See M Popliteal Artery, Right* **P Anterior Tibial Artery, Right** Anterior lateral malleolar artery Anterior medial malleolar artery Anterior tibial recurrent artery Dorsalis pedis artery Posterior tibial recurrent artery **Q Anterior Tibial Artery, Left** *See P Anterior Tibial Artery, Right* **R Posterior Tibial Artery, Right** **S Posterior Tibial Artery, Left** **T Peroneal Artery, Right** Fibular artery **U Peroneal Artery, Left** *See T Peroneal Artery, Right* **V Foot Artery, Right** Arcuate artery Dorsal metatarsal artery Lateral plantar artery Lateral tarsal artery Medial plantar artery **W Foot Artery, Left** *See V Foot Artery, Right* **Y Lower Artery** Umbilical artery	**Ø Open** **3 Percutaneous** **4 Percutaneous Endoscopic**	**C Extraluminal Device** **D Intraluminal Device** **Z No Device**	**Z No Qualifier**
E Internal Iliac Artery, Right Deferential artery Hypogastric artery Iliolumbar artery Inferior gluteal artery Inferior vesical artery Internal pudendal artery Lateral sacral artery Middle rectal artery Obturator artery Superior gluteal artery Umbilical artery Uterine artery Vaginal artery	**Ø Open** **3 Percutaneous** **4 Percutaneous Endoscopic**	**C Extraluminal Device** **D Intraluminal Device** **Z No Device**	**T Uterine Artery, Right** ♀ **Z No Qualifier**
F Internal Iliac Artery, Left Deferential artery Hypogastric artery Iliolumbar artery Inferior gluteal artery Inferior vesical artery Internal pudendal artery Lateral sacral artery Middle rectal artery Obturator artery Superior gluteal artery Umbilical artery Uterine Artery Vaginal artery	**Ø Open** **3 Percutaneous** **4 Percutaneous Endoscopic**	**C Extraluminal Device** **D Intraluminal Device** **Z No Device**	**U Uterine Artery, Left** ♀ **Z No Qualifier**

Non-OR Ø4L23DZ
♀ Ø4LE[Ø,3,4][C,D,Z]T
♀ Ø4LF[Ø,3,4][C,D,Z]U

Ø Medical and Surgical
4 Lower Arteries
N Release Definition: Freeing a body part from an abnormal physical constraint by cutting or by the use of force
Explanation: Some of the restraining tissue may be taken out but none of the body part is taken out

Body Part Character 4	Approach Character 5	Device Character 6	Qualifier Character 7
Ø Abdominal Aorta Inferior phrenic artery Lumbar artery Median sacral artery Middle suprarenal artery Ovarian artery Testicular artery **1 Celiac Artery** Celiac trunk **2 Gastric Artery** Left gastric artery Right gastric artery **3 Hepatic Artery** Common hepatic artery Gastroduodenal artery Hepatic artery proper **4 Splenic Artery** Left gastroepiploic artery Pancreatic artery Short gastric artery **5 Superior Mesenteric Artery** Ileal artery Ileocolic artery Inferior pancreaticoduodenal artery Jejunal artery **6 Colic Artery, Right** **7 Colic Artery, Left** **8 Colic Artery, Middle** **9 Renal Artery, Right** Inferior suprarenal artery Renal segmental artery **A Renal Artery, Left** *See 9 Renal Artery, Right* **B Inferior Mesenteric Artery** Sigmoid artery Superior rectal artery **C Common Iliac Artery, Right** **D Common Iliac Artery, Left** **E Internal Iliac Artery, Right** Deferential artery Hypogastric artery Iliolumbar artery Inferior gluteal artery Inferior vesical artery Internal pudendal artery Lateral sacral artery Middle rectal artery Obturator artery Superior gluteal artery Umbilical artery Uterine artery Vaginal artery **F Internal Iliac Artery, Left** *See E Internal Iliac Artery, Right* **H External Iliac Artery, Right** Deep circumflex iliac artery Inferior epigastric artery **J External Iliac Artery, Left** *See H External Iliac Artery, Right* **K Femoral Artery, Right** Circumflex iliac artery Deep femoral artery Descending genicular artery External pudendal artery Superficial epigastric artery **L Femoral Artery, Left** *See K Femoral Artery, Right* **M Popliteal Artery, Right** Inferior genicular artery Middle genicular artery Superior genicular artery Sural artery **N Popliteal Artery, Left** *See M Popliteal Artery, Right* **P Anterior Tibial Artery, Right** Anterior lateral malleolar artery Anterior medial malleolar artery Anterior tibial recurrent artery Dorsalis pedis artery Posterior tibial recurrent artery **Q Anterior Tibial Artery, Left** *See P Anterior Tibial Artery, Right* **R Posterior Tibial Artery, Right** **S Posterior Tibial Artery, Left** **T Peroneal Artery, Right** Fibular artery **U Peroneal Artery, Left** *See T Peroneal Artery, Right* **V Foot Artery, Right** Arcuate artery Dorsal metatarsal artery Lateral plantar artery Lateral tarsal artery Medial plantar artery **W Foot Artery, Left** *See V Foot Artery, Right* **Y Lower Artery** Umbilical artery	**Ø** Open **3** Percutaneous **4** Percutaneous Endoscopic	**Z** No Device	**Z** No Qualifier

Ø Medical and Surgical
4 Lower Arteries
P Removal Definition: Taking out or off a device from a body part

Explanation: If a device is taken out and a similar device put in without cutting or puncturing the skin or mucous membrane, the procedure is coded to the root operation CHANGE. Otherwise, the procedure for taking out a device is coded to the root operation REMOVAL.

Body Part Character 4	Approach Character 5	Device Character 6	Qualifier Character 7
Y Lower Artery Umbilical artery	**Ø** Open **3** Percutaneous **4** Percutaneous Endoscopic	**Ø** Drainage Device **2** Monitoring Device **3** Infusion Device **7** Autologous Tissue Substitute **C** Extraluminal Device **D** Intraluminal Device **J** Synthetic Substitute **K** Nonautologous Tissue Substitute **Y** Other Device	**Z** No Qualifier
Y Lower Artery Umbilical artery	**X** External	**Ø** Drainage Device **1** Radioactive Element **2** Monitoring Device **3** Infusion Device **D** Intraluminal Device	**Z** No Qualifier

Non-OR Ø4PY3[Ø,2,3,D]Z
Non-OR Ø4PY[3,4]YZ
Non-OR Ø4PYX[Ø,1,2,3,D]Z

Ø Medical and Surgical
4 Lower Arteries
Q Repair Definition: Restoring, to the extent possible, a body part to its normal anatomic structure and function
Explanation: Used only when the method to accomplish the repair is not one of the other root operations

Body Part Character 4	Approach Character 5	Device Character 6	Qualifier Character 7
Ø Abdominal Aorta Inferior phrenic artery Lumbar artery Median sacral artery Middle suprarenal artery Ovarian artery Testicular artery **1 Celiac Artery** Celiac trunk **2 Gastric Artery** Left gastric artery Right gastric artery **3 Hepatic Artery** Common hepatic artery Gastroduodenal artery Hepatic artery proper **4 Splenic Artery** Left gastroepiploic artery Pancreatic artery Short gastric artery **5 Superior Mesenteric Artery** Ileal artery Ileocolic artery Inferior pancreaticoduodenal artery Jejunal artery **6 Colic Artery, Right** **7 Colic Artery, Left** **8 Colic Artery, Middle** **9 Renal Artery, Right** Inferior suprarenal artery Renal segmental artery **A Renal Artery, Left** *See 9 Renal Artery, Right* **B Inferior Mesenteric Artery** Sigmoid artery Superior rectal artery **C Common Iliac Artery, Right** **D Common Iliac Artery, Left** **E Internal Iliac Artery, Right** Deferential artery Hypogastric artery Iliolumbar artery Inferior gluteal artery Inferior vesical artery Internal pudendal artery Lateral sacral artery Middle rectal artery Obturator artery Superior gluteal artery Umbilical artery Uterine artery Vaginal artery **F Internal Iliac Artery, Left** *See E Internal Iliac Artery, Right* **H External Iliac Artery, Right** Deep circumflex iliac artery Inferior epigastric artery **J External Iliac Artery, Left** *See H External Iliac Artery, Right* **K Femoral Artery, Right** Circumflex iliac artery Deep femoral artery Descending genicular artery External pudendal artery Superficial epigastric artery **L Femoral Artery, Left** *See K Femoral Artery, Right* **M Popliteal Artery, Right** Inferior genicular artery Middle genicular artery Superior genicular artery Sural artery **N Popliteal Artery, Left** *See M Popliteal Artery, Right* **P Anterior Tibial Artery, Right** Anterior lateral malleolar artery Anterior medial malleolar artery Anterior tibial recurrent artery Dorsalis pedis artery Posterior tibial recurrent artery **Q Anterior Tibial Artery, Left** *See P Anterior Tibial Artery, Right* **R Posterior Tibial Artery, Right** **S Posterior Tibial Artery, Left** **T Peroneal Artery, Right** Fibular artery **U Peroneal Artery, Left** *See T Peroneal Artery, Right* **V Foot Artery, Right** Arcuate artery Dorsal metatarsal artery Lateral plantar artery Lateral tarsal artery Medial plantar artery **W Foot Artery, Left** *See V Foot Artery, Right* **Y Lower Artery** Umbilical artery	**Ø Open** **3 Percutaneous** **4 Percutaneous Endoscopic**	**Z No Device**	**Z No Qualifier**

Ø Medical and Surgical
4 Lower Arteries
R Replacement Definition: Putting in or on biological or synthetic material that physically takes the place and/or function of all or a portion of a body part

Explanation: The body part may have been taken out or replaced, or may be taken out, physically eradicated, or rendered nonfunctional during the REPLACEMENT procedure. A REMOVAL procedure is coded for taking out the device used in a previous replacement procedure.

Body Part Character 4		Approach Character 5	Device Character 6	Qualifier Character 7
Ø Abdominal Aorta Inferior phrenic artery Lumbar artery Median sacral artery Middle suprarenal artery Ovarian artery Testicular artery **1 Celiac Artery** Celiac trunk **2 Gastric Artery** Left gastric artery Right gastric artery **3 Hepatic Artery** Common hepatic artery Gastroduodenal artery Hepatic artery proper **4 Splenic Artery** Left gastroepiploic artery Pancreatic artery Short gastric artery **5 Superior Mesenteric Artery** Ileal artery Ileocolic artery Inferior pancreaticoduodenal artery Jejunal artery **6 Colic Artery, Right** **7 Colic Artery, Left** **8 Colic Artery, Middle** **9 Renal Artery, Right** Inferior suprarenal artery Renal segmental artery **A Renal Artery, Left** *See 9 Renal Artery, Right* **B Inferior Mesenteric Artery** Sigmoid artery Superior rectal artery **C Common Iliac Artery, Right** **D Common Iliac Artery, Left** **E Internal Iliac Artery, Right** Deferential artery Hypogastric artery Iliolumbar artery Inferior gluteal artery Inferior vesical artery Internal pudendal artery Lateral sacral artery Middle rectal artery Obturator artery Superior gluteal artery Umbilical artery Uterine artery Vaginal artery	**F Internal Iliac Artery, Left** *See E Internal Iliac Artery, Right* **H External Iliac Artery, Right** Deep circumflex iliac artery Inferior epigastric artery **J External Iliac Artery, Left** *See H External Iliac Artery, Right* **K Femoral Artery, Right** Circumflex iliac artery Deep femoral artery Descending genicular artery External pudendal artery Superficial epigastric artery **L Femoral Artery, Left** *See K Femoral Artery, Right* **M Popliteal Artery, Right** Inferior genicular artery Middle genicular artery Superior genicular artery Sural artery **N Popliteal Artery, Left** *See M Popliteal Artery, Right* **P Anterior Tibial Artery, Right** Anterior lateral malleolar artery Anterior medial malleolar artery Anterior tibial recurrent artery Dorsalis pedis artery Posterior tibial recurrent artery **Q Anterior Tibial Artery, Left** *See P Anterior Tibial Artery, Right* **R Posterior Tibial Artery, Right** **S Posterior Tibial Artery, Left** **T Peroneal Artery, Right** Fibular artery **U Peroneal Artery, Left** *See T Peroneal Artery, Right* **V Foot Artery, Right** Arcuate artery Dorsal metatarsal artery Lateral plantar artery Lateral tarsal artery Medial plantar artery **W Foot Artery, Left** *See V Foot Artery, Right* **Y Lower Artery** Umbilical artery	**Ø Open** **4 Percutaneous Endoscopic**	**7 Autologous Tissue Substitute** **J Synthetic Substitute** **K Nonautologous Tissue Substitute**	**Z No Qualifier**

Ø Medical and Surgical
4 Lower Arteries
S Reposition Definition: Moving to its normal location, or other suitable location, all or a portion of a body part

Explanation: The body part is moved to a new location from an abnormal location, or from a normal location where it is not functioning correctly. The body part may or may not be cut out or off to be moved to the new location.

Body Part Character 4	Approach Character 5	Device Character 6	Qualifier Character 7
Ø Abdominal Aorta Inferior phrenic artery Lumbar artery Median sacral artery Middle suprarenal artery Ovarian artery Testicular artery **1 Celiac Artery** Celiac trunk **2 Gastric Artery** Left gastric artery Right gastric artery **3 Hepatic Artery** Common hepatic artery Gastroduodenal artery Hepatic artery proper **4 Splenic Artery** Left gastroepiploic artery Pancreatic artery Short gastric artery **5 Superior Mesenteric Artery** Ileal artery Ileocolic artery Inferior pancreaticoduodenal artery Jejunal artery **6 Colic Artery, Right** **7 Colic Artery, Left** **8 Colic Artery, Middle** **9 Renal Artery, Right** Inferior suprarenal artery Renal segmental artery **A Renal Artery, Left** *See 9 Renal Artery, Right* **B Inferior Mesenteric Artery** Sigmoid artery Superior rectal artery **C Common Iliac Artery, Right** **D Common Iliac Artery, Left** **E Internal Iliac Artery, Right** Deferential artery Hypogastric artery Iliolumbar artery Inferior gluteal artery Inferior vesical artery Internal pudendal artery Lateral sacral artery Middle rectal artery Obturator artery Superior gluteal artery Umbilical artery Uterine artery Vaginal artery **F Internal Iliac Artery, Left** *See E Internal Iliac Artery, Right* **H External Iliac Artery, Right** Deep circumflex iliac artery Inferior epigastric artery **J External Iliac Artery, Left** *See H External Iliac Artery, Right* **K Femoral Artery, Right** Circumflex iliac artery Deep femoral artery Descending genicular artery External pudendal artery Superficial epigastric artery **L Femoral Artery, Left** *See K Femoral Artery, Right* **M Popliteal Artery, Right** Inferior genicular artery Middle genicular artery Superior genicular artery Sural artery **N Popliteal Artery, Left** *See M Popliteal Artery, Right* **P Anterior Tibial Artery, Right** Anterior lateral malleolar artery Anterior medial malleolar artery Anterior tibial recurrent artery Dorsalis pedis artery Posterior tibial recurrent artery **Q Anterior Tibial Artery, Left** *See P Anterior Tibial Artery, Right* **R Posterior Tibial Artery, Right** **S Posterior Tibial Artery, Left** **T Peroneal Artery, Right** Fibular artery **U Peroneal Artery, Left** *See T Peroneal Artery, Right* **V Foot Artery, Right** Arcuate artery Dorsal metatarsal artery Lateral plantar artery Lateral tarsal artery Medial plantar artery **W Foot Artery, Left** *See V Foot Artery, Right* **Y Lower Artery** Umbilical artery	**Ø** Open **3** Percutaneous **4** Percutaneous Endoscopic	**Z** No Device	**Z** No Qualifier

0 Medical and Surgical
4 Lower Arteries
U Supplement Definition: Putting in or on biological or synthetic material that physically reinforces and/or augments the function of a portion of a body part

Explanation: The biological material is non-living, or is living and from the same individual. The body part may have been previously replaced, and the SUPPLEMENT procedure is performed to physically reinforce and/or augment the function of the replaced body part.

Body Part Character 4		Approach Character 5	Device Character 6	Qualifier Character 7
0 Abdominal Aorta Inferior phrenic artery Lumbar artery Median sacral artery Middle suprarenal artery Ovarian artery Testicular artery **1 Celiac Artery** Celiac trunk **2 Gastric Artery** Left gastric artery Right gastric artery **3 Hepatic Artery** Common hepatic artery Gastroduodenal artery Hepatic artery proper **4 Splenic Artery** Left gastroepiploic artery Pancreatic artery Short gastric artery **5 Superior Mesenteric Artery** Ileal artery Ileocolic artery Inferior pancreaticoduodenal artery Jejunal artery **6 Colic Artery, Right** **7 Colic Artery, Left** **8 Colic Artery, Middle** **9 Renal Artery, Right** Inferior suprarenal artery Renal segmental artery **A Renal Artery, Left** *See 9 Renal Artery, Right* **B Inferior Mesenteric Artery** Sigmoid artery Superior rectal artery **C Common Iliac Artery, Right** **D Common Iliac Artery, Left** **E Internal Iliac Artery, Right** Deferential artery Hypogastric artery Iliolumbar artery Inferior gluteal artery Inferior vesical artery Internal pudendal artery Lateral sacral artery Middle rectal artery Obturator artery Superior gluteal artery Umbilical artery Uterine artery Vaginal artery	**F Internal Iliac Artery, Left** *See E Internal Iliac Artery, Right* **H External Iliac Artery, Right** Deep circumflex iliac artery Inferior epigastric artery **J External Iliac Artery, Left** *See H External Iliac Artery, Right* **K Femoral Artery, Right** Circumflex iliac artery Deep femoral artery Descending genicular artery External pudendal artery Superficial epigastric artery **L Femoral Artery, Left** *See K Femoral Artery, Right* **M Popliteal Artery, Right** Inferior genicular artery Middle genicular artery Superior genicular artery Sural artery **N Popliteal Artery, Left** *See M Popliteal Artery, Right* **P Anterior Tibial Artery, Right** Anterior lateral malleolar artery Anterior medial malleolar artery Anterior tibial recurrent artery Dorsalis pedis artery Posterior tibial recurrent artery **Q Anterior Tibial Artery, Left** *See P Anterior Tibial Artery, Right* **R Posterior Tibial Artery, Right** **S Posterior Tibial Artery, Left** **T Peroneal Artery, Right** Fibular artery **U Peroneal Artery, Left** *See T Peroneal Artery, Right* **V Foot Artery, Right** Arcuate artery Dorsal metatarsal artery Lateral plantar artery Lateral tarsal artery Medial plantar artery **W Foot Artery, Left** *See V Foot Artery, Right* **Y Lower Artery** Umbilical artery	**0** Open **3** Percutaneous **4** Percutaneous Endoscopic	**7** Autologous Tissue Substitute **J** Synthetic Substitute **K** Nonautologous Tissue Substitute	**Z** No Qualifier

0 Medical and Surgical
4 Lower Arteries
V Restriction Definition: Partially closing an orifice or the lumen of a tubular body part
Explanation: The orifice can be a natural orifice or an artificially created orifice

Body Part Character 4	Approach Character 5	Device Character 6	Qualifier Character 7
0 Abdominal Aorta Inferior phrenic artery Lumbar artery Median sacral artery Middle suprarenal artery Ovarian artery Testicular artery	**0 Open** **3 Percutaneous** **4 Percutaneous Endoscopic**	**C Extraluminal Device** **E Intraluminal Device, Branched or Fenestrated, One or Two Arteries** **F Intraluminal Device, Branched or Fenestrated, Three or More Arteries** **Z No Device**	**6 Bifurcation** **Z No Qualifier**
0 Abdominal Aorta Inferior phrenic artery Lumbar artery Median sacral artery Middle suprarenal artery Ovarian artery Testicular artery	**0 Open** **3 Percutaneous** **4 Percutaneous Endoscopic**	**D Intraluminal Device**	**6 Bifurcation** **J Temporary** **Z No Qualifier**
1 Celiac Artery Celiac trunk **2 Gastric Artery** Left gastric artery Right gastric artery **3 Hepatic Artery** Common hepatic artery Gastroduodenal artery Hepatic artery proper **4 Splenic Artery** Left gastroepiploic artery Pancreatic artery Short gastric artery **5 Superior Mesenteric Artery** Ileal artery Ileocolic artery Inferior pancreaticoduodenal artery Jejunal artery **6 Colic Artery, Right** **7 Colic Artery, Left** **8 Colic Artery, Middle** **9 Renal Artery, Right** Inferior suprarenal artery Renal segmental artery **A Renal Artery, Left** *See 9 Renal Artery, Right* **B Inferior Mesenteric Artery** Sigmoid artery Superior rectal artery **E Internal Iliac Artery, Right** Deferential artery Hypogastric artery Iliolumbar artery Inferior gluteal artery Inferior vesical artery Internal pudendal artery Lateral sacral artery Middle rectal artery Obturator artery Superior gluteal artery Umbilical artery Uterine artery Vaginal artery **F Internal Iliac Artery, Left** *See E Internal Iliac Artery, Right* **H External Iliac Artery, Right** Deep circumflex iliac artery Inferior epigastric artery **J External Iliac Artery, Left** *See H External Iliac Artery, Right* **K Femoral Artery, Right** Circumflex iliac artery Deep femoral artery Descending genicular artery External pudendal artery Superficial epigastric artery **L Femoral Artery, Left** *See K Femoral Artery, Right* **M Popliteal Artery, Right** Inferior genicular artery Middle genicular artery Superior genicular artery Sural artery **N Popliteal Artery, Left** *See M Popliteal Artery, Right* **P Anterior Tibial Artery, Right** Anterior lateral malleolar artery Anterior medial malleolar artery Anterior tibial recurrent artery Dorsalis pedis artery Posterior tibial recurrent artery **Q Anterior Tibial Artery, Left** *See P Anterior Tibial Artery, Right* **R Posterior Tibial Artery, Right** **S Posterior Tibial Artery, Left** **T Peroneal Artery, Right** Fibular artery **U Peroneal Artery, Left** *See T Peroneal Artery, Right* **V Foot Artery, Right** Arcuate artery Dorsal metatarsal artery Lateral plantar artery Lateral tarsal artery Medial plantar artery **W Foot Artery, Left** *See V Foot Artery, Right* **Y Lower Artery** Umbilical artery	**0 Open** **3 Percutaneous** **4 Percutaneous Endoscopic**	**C Extraluminal Device** **D Intraluminal Device** **Z No Device**	**Z No Qualifier**
C Common Iliac Artery, Right **D Common Iliac Artery, Left**	**0 Open** **3 Percutaneous** **4 Percutaneous Endoscopic**	**C Extraluminal Device** **D Intraluminal Device** **E Intraluminal Device, Branched or Fenestrated, One or Two Arteries** **Z No Device**	**Z No Qualifier**

Ø Medical and Surgical
4 Lower Arteries
W Revision Definition: Correcting, to the extent possible, a portion of a malfunctioning device or the position of a displaced device

Explanation: Revision can include correcting a malfunctioning or displaced device by taking out or putting in components of the device such as a screw or pin

Body Part Character 4	Approach Character 5	Device Character 6	Qualifier Character 7
Y Lower Artery Umbilical artery	**Ø** Open **3** Percutaneous **4** Percutaneous Endoscopic	**Ø** Drainage Device **2** Monitoring Device **3** Infusion Device **7** Autologous Tissue Substitute **C** Extraluminal Device **D** Intraluminal Device **J** Synthetic Substitute **K** Nonautologous Tissue Substitute **Y** Other Device	**Z** No Qualifier
Y Lower Artery Umbilical artery	**X** External	**Ø** Drainage Device **2** Monitoring Device **3** Infusion Device **7** Autologous Tissue Substitute **C** Extraluminal Device **D** Intraluminal Device **J** Synthetic Substitute **K** Nonautologous Tissue Substitute	**Z** No Qualifier

Non-OR Ø4WY3[Ø,2,3,D]Z
Non-OR Ø4WY[3,4]YZ
Non-OR Ø4WYX[Ø,2,3,7,C,D,J,K]Z

Upper Veins Ø51–Ø5W

Character Meanings

This Character Meaning table is provided as a guide to assist the user in the identification of character members that may be found in this section of code tables. It **SHOULD NOT** be used to build a PCS code.

Operation–Character 3		Body Part–Character 4		Approach–Character 5		Device–Character 6		Qualifier–Character 7	
1	Bypass	Ø	Azygos Vein	Ø	Open	Ø	Drainage Device	1	Drug-Coated Balloon
5	Destruction	1	Hemiazygos Vein	3	Percutaneous	2	Monitoring Device	X	Diagnostic
7	Dilation	3	Innominate Vein, Right	4	Percutaneous Endoscopic	3	Infusion Device	Y	Upper Vein
9	Drainage	4	Innominate Vein, Left	X	External	7	Autologous Tissue Substitute	Z	No Qualifier
B	Excision	5	Subclavian Vein, Right			9	Autologous Venous Tissue		
C	Extirpation	6	Subclavian Vein, Left			A	Autologous Arterial Tissue		
D	Extraction	7	Axillary Vein, Right			C	Extraluminal Device		
H	Insertion	8	Axillary Vein, Left			D	Intraluminal Device		
J	Inspection	9	Brachial Vein, Right			J	Synthetic Substitute		
L	Occlusion	A	Brachial Vein, Left			K	Nonautologous Tissue Substitute		
N	Release	B	Basilic Vein, Right			M	Neurostimulator Lead		
P	Removal	C	Basilic Vein, Left			Y	Other Device		
Q	Repair	D	Cephalic Vein, Right			Z	No Device		
R	Replacement	F	Cephalic Vein, Left						
S	Reposition	G	Hand Vein, Right						
U	Supplement	H	Hand Vein, Left						
V	Restriction	L	Intracranial Vein						
W	Revision	M	Internal Jugular Vein, Right						
		N	Internal Jugular Vein, Left						
		P	External Jugular Vein, Right						
		Q	External Jugular Vein, Left						
		R	Vertebral Vein, Right						
		S	Vertebral Vein, Left						
		T	Face Vein, Right						
		V	Face Vein, Left						
		Y	Upper Vein						

AHA Coding Clinic for table Ø51
2017, 3Q, 15 Bypass of innominate vein to atrial appendage

AHA Coding Clinic for table Ø5B
2016, 2Q, 12 Resection of malignant neoplasm of infratemporal fossa

AHA Coding Clinic for table Ø5H
2016, 4Q, 97-98 Phrenic neurostimulator

AHA Coding Clinic for table Ø5P
2016, 4Q, 97-98 Phrenic neurostimulator

AHA Coding Clinic for table Ø5Q
2017, 3Q, 15 Bypass of innominate vein to atrial appendage

AHA Coding Clinic for table Ø5S
2013, 4Q, 125 Stage II cephalic vein transposition (superficialization) of arteriovenous fistula

AHA Coding Clinic for table Ø5W
2016, 4Q, 97-98 Phrenic neurostimulator

Head and Neck Veins

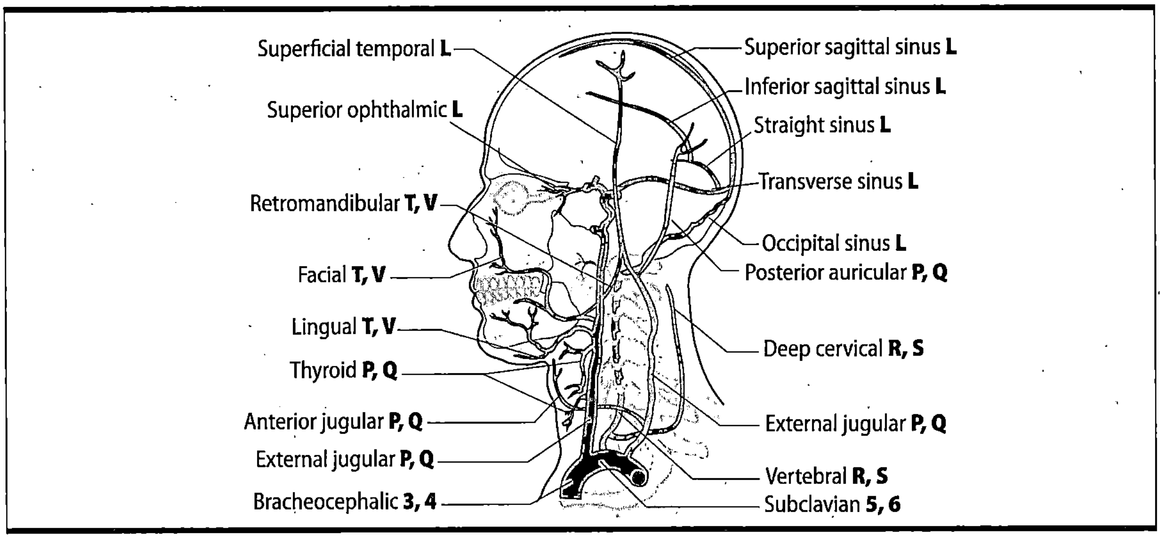
Superficial temporal **L**
Superior ophthalmic **L**
Retromandibular **T, V**
Facial **T, V**
Lingual **T, V**
Thyroid **P, Q**
Anterior jugular **P, Q**
External jugular **P, Q**
Bracheocephalic **3, 4**
Superior sagittal sinus **L**
Inferior sagittal sinus **L**
Straight sinus **L**
Transverse sinus **L**
Occipital sinus **L**
Posterior auricular **P, Q**
Deep cervical **R, S**
External jugular **P, Q**
Vertebral **R, S**
Subclavian **5, 6**

Upper Veins

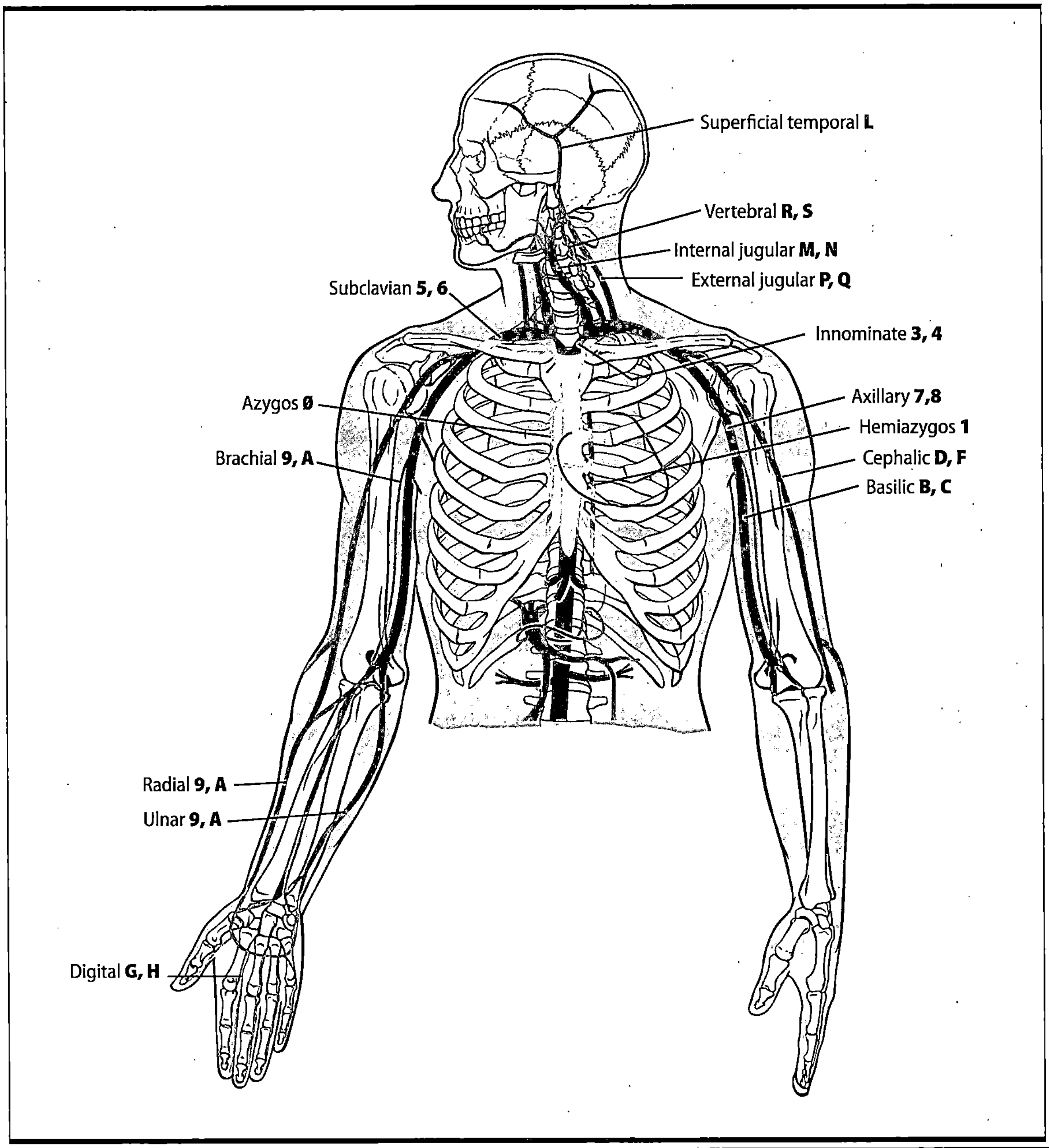
Superficial temporal **L**
Vertebral **R, S**
Internal jugular **M, N**
External jugular **P, Q**
Subclavian **5, 6**
Innominate **3, 4**
Azygos **Ø**
Axillary **7,8**
Hemiazygos **1**
Brachial **9, A**
Cephalic **D, F**
Basilic **B, C**
Radial **9, A**
Ulnar **9, A**
Digital **G, H**

Ø Medical and Surgical
5 Upper Veins
1 Bypass

Definition: Altering the route of passage of the contents of a tubular body part

Explanation: Rerouting contents of a body part to a downstream area of the normal route, to a similar route and body part, or to an abnormal route and dissimilar body part. Includes one or more anastomoses, with or without the use of a device.

Body Part Character 4	Approach Character 5	Device Character 6	Qualifier Character 7
Ø Azygos Vein Right ascending lumbar vein Right subcostal vein **1 Hemiazygos Vein** Left ascending lumbar vein Left subcostal vein **3 Innominate Vein, Right** Brachiocephalic vein Inferior thyroid vein **4 Innominate Vein, Left** *See 3 Innominate Vein, Right* **5 Subclavian Vein, Right** **6 Subclavian Vein, Left** **7 Axillary Vein, Right** **8 Axillary Vein, Left** **9 Brachial Vein, Right** Radial vein Ulnar vein **A Brachial Vein, Left** *See 9 Brachial Vein, Right* **B Basilic Vein, Right** Median antebrachial vein Median cubital vein **C Basilic Vein, Left** *See B Basilic Vein, Right* **D Cephalic Vein, Right** Accessory cephalic vein **F Cephalic Vein, Left** *See D Cephalic Vein, Right* **G Hand Vein, Right** Dorsal metacarpal vein Palmar (volar) digital vein Palmar (volar) metacarpal vein Superficial palmar venous arch Volar (palmar) digital vein Volar (palmar) metacarpal vein **H Hand Vein, Left** *See G Hand Vein, Right* **L Intracranial Vein** Anterior cerebral vein Basal (internal) cerebral vein Dural venous sinus Great cerebral vein Inferior cerebellar vein Inferior cerebral vein Internal (basal) cerebral vein Middle cerebral vein Ophthalmic vein Superior cerebellar vein Superior cerebral vein **M Internal Jugular Vein, Right** **N Internal Jugular Vein, Left** **P External Jugular Vein, Right** Posterior auricular vein **Q External Jugular Vein, Left** *See P External Jugular Vein, Right* **R Vertebral Vein, Right** Deep cervical vein Suboccipital venous plexus **S Vertebral Vein, Left** *See R Vertebral Vein, Right* **T Face Vein, Right** Angular vein Anterior facial vein Common facial vein Deep facial vein Frontal vein Posterior facial (retromandibular) vein Supraorbital vein **V Face Vein, Left** *See T Face Vein, Right*	**Ø Open** **4 Percutaneous Endoscopic**	**7 Autologous Tissue Substitute** **9 Autologous Venous Tissue** **A Autologous Arterial Tissue** **J Synthetic Substitute** **K Nonautologous Tissue Substitute** **Z No Device**	**Y Upper Vein**

Ø Medical and Surgical
5 Upper Veins
5 Destruction Definition: Physical eradication of all or a portion of a body part by the direct use of energy, force, or a destructive agent
Explanation: None of the body part is physically taken out

Body Part Character 4		Approach Character 5	Device Character 6	Qualifier Character 7
Ø Azygos Vein Right ascending lumbar vein Right subcostal vein **1 Hemiazygos Vein** Left ascending lumbar vein Left subcostal vein **3 Innominate Vein, Right** Brachiocephalic vein Inferior thyroid vein **4 Innominate Vein, Left** *See 3 Innominate Vein, Right* **5 Subclavian Vein, Right** **6 Subclavian Vein, Left** **7 Axillary Vein, Right** **8 Axillary Vein, Left** **9 Brachial Vein, Right** Radial vein Ulnar vein **A Brachial Vein, Left** *See 9 Brachial Vein, Right* **B Basilic Vein, Right** Median antebrachial vein Median cubital vein **C Basilic Vein, Left** *See B Basilic Vein, Right* **D Cephalic Vein, Right** Accessory cephalic vein **F Cephalic Vein, Left** *See D Cephalic Vein, Right* **G Hand Vein, Right** Dorsal metacarpal vein Palmar (volar) digital vein Palmar (volar) metacarpal vein Superficial palmar venous arch Volar (palmar) digital vein Volar (palmar) metacarpal vein	**H Hand Vein, Left** *See G Hand Vein, Right* **L Intracranial Vein** Anterior cerebral vein Basal (internal) cerebral vein Dural venous sinus Great cerebral vein Inferior cerebellar vein Inferior cerebral vein Internal (basal) cerebral vein Middle cerebral vein Ophthalmic vein Superior cerebellar vein Superior cerebral vein **M Internal Jugular Vein, Right** **N Internal Jugular Vein, Left** **P External Jugular Vein, Right** Posterior auricular vein **Q External Jugular Vein, Left** *See P External Jugular Vein, Right* **R Vertebral Vein, Right** Deep cervical vein Suboccipital venous plexus **S Vertebral Vein, Left** *See R Vertebral Vein, Right* **T Face Vein, Right** Angular vein Anterior facial vein Common facial vein Deep facial vein Frontal vein Posterior facial (retromandibular) vein Supraorbital vein **V Face Vein, Left** *See T Face Vein, Right* **Y Upper Vein**	**Ø Open** **3 Percutaneous** **4 Percutaneous Endoscopic**	**Z No Device**	**Z No Qualifier**

Ø Medical and Surgical
5 Upper Veins
7 Dilation Definition: Expanding an orifice or the lumen of a tubular body part

Explanation: The orifice can be a natural orifice or an artificially created orifice. Accomplished by stretching a tubular body part using intraluminal pressure or by cutting part of the orifice or wall of the tubular body part.

Body Part Character 4		Approach Character 5	Device Character 6	Qualifier Character 7
Ø Azygos Vein Right ascending lumbar vein Right subcostal vein **1 Hemiazygos Vein** Left ascending lumbar vein Left subcostal vein **G Hand Vein, Right** Dorsal metacarpal vein Palmar (volar) digital vein Palmar (volar) metacarpal vein Superficial palmar venous arch Volar (palmar) digital vein Volar (palmar) metacarpal vein **H Hand Vein, Left** *See G Hand Vein, Right* **L Intracranial Vein** NC Anterior cerebral vein Basal (internal) cerebral vein Dural venous sinus Great cerebral vein Inferior cerebellar vein Inferior cerebral vein Internal (basal) cerebral vein Middle cerebral vein Ophthalmic vein Superior cerebellar vein Superior cerebral vein	**M Internal Jugular Vein, Right** **N Internal Jugular Vein, Left** **P External Jugular Vein, Right** Posterior auricular vein **Q External Jugular Vein, Left** *See P External Jugular Vein, Right* **R Vertebral Vein, Right** Deep cervical vein Suboccipital venous plexus **S Vertebral Vein, Left** *See R Vertebral Vein, Right* **T Face Vein, Right** Angular vein Anterior facial vein Common facial vein Deep facial vein Frontal vein Posterior facial (retromandibular) vein Supraorbital vein **V Face Vein, Left** *See T Face Vein, Right* **Y Upper Vein**	Ø Open 3 Percutaneous 4 Percutaneous Endoscopic	D Intraluminal Device Z No Device	Z No Qualifier
3 Innominate Vein, Right Brachiocephalic vein Inferior thyroid vein **4 Innominate Vein, Left** *See 3 Innominate Vein, Right* **5 Subclavian Vein, Right** **6 Subclavian Vein, Left** **7 Axillary Vein, Right** **8 Axillary Vein, Left** **9 Brachial Vein, Right** Radial vein Ulnar vein	**A Brachial Vein, Left** *See 9 Brachial Vein, Right* **B Basilic Vein, Right** Median antebrachial vein Median cubital vein **C Basilic Vein, Left** *See B Basilic Vein, Right* **D Cephalic Vein, Right** Accessory cephalic vein **F Cephalic Vein, Left** *See D Cephalic Vein, Right*	Ø Open 3 Percutaneous 4 Percutaneous Endoscopic	D Intraluminal Device Z No Device	1 Drug-Coated Balloon Z No Qualifier

NC Ø57L[3,4]ZZ

0 Medical and Surgical
5 Upper Veins
9 Drainage Definition: Taking or letting out fluids and/or gases from a body part
Explanation: The qualifier DIAGNOSTIC is used to identify drainage procedures that are biopsies

Body Part Character 4	Approach Character 5	Device Character 6	Qualifier Character 7
0 Azygos Vein Right ascending lumbar vein Right subcostal vein **1 Hemiazygos Vein** Left ascending lumbar vein Left subcostal vein **3 Innominate Vein, Right** Brachiocephalic vein Inferior thyroid vein **4 Innominate Vein, Left** *See 3 Innominate Vein, Right* **5 Subclavian Vein, Right** **6 Subclavian Vein, Left** **7 Axillary Vein, Right** **8 Axillary Vein, Left** **9 Brachial Vein, Right** Radial vein Ulnar vein **A Brachial Vein, Left** *See 9 Brachial Vein, Right* **B Basilic Vein, Right** Median antebrachial vein Median cubital vein **C Basilic Vein, Left** *See B Basilic Vein, Right* **D Cephalic Vein, Right** Accessory cephalic vein **F Cephalic Vein, Left** *See D Cephalic Vein, Right* **G Hand Vein, Right** Dorsal metacarpal vein Palmar (volar) digital vein Palmar (volar) metacarpal vein Superficial palmar venous arch Volar (palmar) digital vein Volar (palmar) metacarpal vein **H Hand Vein, Left** *See G Hand Vein, Right* **L Intracranial Vein** Anterior cerebral vein Basal (internal) cerebral vein Dural venous sinus Great cerebral vein Inferior cerebellar vein Inferior cerebral vein Internal (basal) cerebral vein Middle cerebral vein Ophthalmic vein Superior cerebellar vein Superior cerebral vein **M Internal Jugular Vein, Right** **N Internal Jugular Vein, Left** **P External Jugular Vein, Right** Posterior auricular vein **Q External Jugular Vein, Left** *See P External Jugular Vein, Right* **R Vertebral Vein, Right** Deep cervical vein Suboccipital venous plexus **S Vertebral Vein, Left** *See R Vertebral Vein, Right* **T Face Vein, Right** Angular vein Anterior facial vein Common facial vein Deep facial vein Frontal vein Posterior facial (retromandibular) vein Supraorbital vein **V Face Vein, Left** *See T Face Vein, Right* **Y Upper Vein**	**0 Open** **3 Percutaneous** **4 Percutaneous Endoscopic**	**0 Drainage Device**	**Z No Qualifier**
0 Azygos Vein Right ascending lumbar vein Right subcostal vein **1 Hemiazygos Vein** Left ascending lumbar vein Left subcostal vein **3 Innominate Vein, Right** Brachiocephalic vein Inferior thyroid vein **4 Innominate Vein, Left** *See 3 Innominate Vein, Right* **5 Subclavian Vein, Right** **6 Subclavian Vein, Left** **7 Axillary Vein, Right** **8 Axillary Vein, Left** **9 Brachial Vein, Right** Radial vein Ulnar vein **A Brachial Vein, Left** *See 9 Brachial Vein, Right* **B Basilic Vein, Right** Median antebrachial vein Median cubital vein **C Basilic Vein, Left** *See B Basilic Vein, Right* **D Cephalic Vein, Right** Accessory cephalic vein **F Cephalic Vein, Left** *See D Cephalic Vein, Right* **G Hand Vein, Right** Dorsal metacarpal vein Palmar (volar) digital vein Palmar (volar) metacarpal vein Superficial palmar venous arch Volar (palmar) digital vein Volar (palmar) metacarpal vein **H Hand Vein, Left** *See G Hand Vein, Right* **L Intracranial Vein** Anterior cerebral vein Basal (internal) cerebral vein Dural venous sinus Great cerebral vein Inferior cerebellar vein Inferior cerebral vein Internal (basal) cerebral vein Middle cerebral vein Ophthalmic vein Superior cerebellar vein Superior cerebral vein **M Internal Jugular Vein, Right** **N Internal Jugular Vein, Left** **P External Jugular Vein, Right** Posterior auricular vein **Q External Jugular Vein, Left** *See P External Jugular Vein, Right* **R Vertebral Vein, Right** Deep cervical vein Suboccipital venous plexus **S Vertebral Vein, Left** *See R Vertebral Vein, Right* **T Face Vein, Right** Angular vein Anterior facial vein Common facial vein Deep facial vein Frontal vein Posterior facial (retromandibular) vein Supraorbital vein **V Face Vein, Left** *See T Face Vein, Right* **Y Upper Vein**	**0 Open** **3 Percutaneous** **4 Percutaneous Endoscopic**	**Z No Device**	**X Diagnostic** **Z No Qualifier**

Non-OR 059[0,1,3,4,5,6,7,8,9,A,B,C,D,F,G,H,L,M,N,P,Q,R,S,T,V,Y][0,3,4]0Z
Non-OR 059[0,1,3,4,5,6,7,8,9,A,B,C,D,F,G,H,L,M,N,P,Q,R,S,T,V,Y]3ZX
Non-OR 059[0,1,3,4,5,6,7,8,9,A,B,C,D,F,G,H,L,M,N,P,Q,R,S,T,V,Y][0,3,4]ZZ

Ø Medical and Surgical
5 Upper Veins
B Excision Definition: Cutting out or off, without replacement, a portion of a body part
Explanation: The qualifier DIAGNOSTIC is used to identify excision procedures that are biopsies

Body Part Character 4		Approach Character 5	Device Character 6	Qualifier Character 7
Ø Azygos Vein Right ascending lumbar vein Right subcostal vein **1 Hemiazygos Vein** Left ascending lumbar vein Left subcostal vein **3 Innominate Vein, Right** Brachiocephalic vein Inferior thyroid vein **4 Innominate Vein, Left** *See 3 Innominate Vein, Right* **5 Subclavian Vein, Right** **6 Subclavian Vein, Left** **7 Axillary Vein, Right** **8 Axillary Vein, Left** **9 Brachial Vein, Right** Radial vein Ulnar vein **A Brachial Vein, Left** *See 9 Brachial Vein, Right* **B Basilic Vein, Right** Median antebrachial vein Median cubital vein **C Basilic Vein, Left** *See B Basilic Vein, Right* **D Cephalic Vein, Right** Accessory cephalic vein **F Cephalic Vein, Left** *See D Cephalic Vein, Right* **G Hand Vein, Right** Dorsal metacarpal vein Palmar (volar) digital vein Palmar (volar) metacarpal vein Superficial palmar venous arch Volar (palmar) digital vein Volar (palmar) metacarpal vein	**H Hand Vein, Left** *See G Hand Vein, Right* **L Intracranial Vein** Anterior cerebral vein Basal (internal) cerebral vein Dural venous sinus Great cerebral vein Inferior cerebellar vein Inferior cerebral vein Internal (basal) cerebral vein Middle cerebral vein Ophthalmic vein Superior cerebellar vein Superior cerebral vein **M Internal Jugular Vein, Right** **N Internal Jugular Vein, Left** **P External Jugular Vein, Right** Posterior auricular vein **Q External Jugular Vein, Left** *See P External Jugular Vein, Right* **R Vertebral Vein, Right** Deep cervical vein Suboccipital venous plexus **S Vertebral Vein, Left** *See R Vertebral Vein, Right* **T Face Vein, Right** Angular vein Anterior facial vein Common facial vein Deep facial vein Frontal vein Posterior facial (retromandibular) vein Supraorbital vein **V Face Vein, Left** *See T Face Vein, Right* **Y Upper Vein**	**Ø** Open **3** Percutaneous **4** Percutaneous Endoscopic	**Z** No Device	**X** Diagnostic **Z** No Qualifier

Ø Medical and Surgical
5 Upper Veins
C Extirpation Definition: Taking or cutting out solid matter from a body part

Explanation: The solid matter may be an abnormal byproduct of a biological function or a foreign body; it may be imbedded in a body part or in the lumen of a tubular body part. The solid matter may or may not have been previously broken into pieces.

Body Part Character 4		Approach Character 5	Device Character 6	Qualifier Character 7
Ø Azygos Vein Right ascending lumbar vein Right subcostal vein **1 Hemiazygos Vein** Left ascending lumbar vein Left subcostal vein **3 Innominate Vein, Right** Brachiocephalic vein Inferior thyroid vein **4 Innominate Vein, Left** *See 3 Innominate Vein, Right* **5 Subclavian Vein, Right** **6 Subclavian Vein, Left** **7 Axillary Vein, Right** **8 Axillary Vein, Left** **9 Brachial Vein, Right** Radial vein Ulnar vein **A Brachial Vein, Left** *See 9 Brachial Vein, Right* **B Basilic Vein, Right** Median antebrachial vein Median cubital vein **C Basilic Vein, Left** *See B Basilic Vein, Right* **D Cephalic Vein, Right** Accessory cephalic vein **F Cephalic Vein, Left** *See D Cephalic Vein, Right* **G Hand Vein, Right** Dorsal metacarpal vein Palmar (volar) digital vein Palmar (volar) metacarpal vein Superficial palmar venous arch Volar (palmar) digital vein Volar (palmar) metacarpal vein	**H Hand Vein, Left** *See G Hand Vein, Right* **L Intracranial Vein** Anterior cerebral vein Basal (internal) cerebral vein Dural venous sinus Great cerebral vein Inferior cerebellar vein Inferior cerebral vein Internal (basal) cerebral vein Middle cerebral vein Ophthalmic vein Superior cerebellar vein Superior cerebral vein **M Internal Jugular Vein, Right** **N Internal Jugular Vein, Left** **P External Jugular Vein, Right** Posterior auricular vein **Q External Jugular Vein, Left** *See P External Jugular Vein, Right* **R Vertebral Vein, Right** Deep cervical vein Suboccipital venous plexus **S Vertebral Vein, Left** *See R Vertebral Vein, Right* **T Face Vein, Right** Angular vein Anterior facial vein Common facial vein Deep facial vein Frontal vein Posterior facial (retromandibular) vein Supraorbital vein **V Face Vein, Left** *See T Face Vein, Right* **Y Upper Vein**	**Ø** Open **3** Percutaneous **4** Percutaneous Endoscopic	**Z** No Device	**Z** No Qualifier

Ø Medical and Surgical
5 Upper Veins
D Extraction Definition: Pulling or stripping out or off all or a portion of a body part by the use of force

Explanation: The qualifier DIAGNOSTIC is used to identify extraction procedures that are biopsies

Body Part Character 4		Approach Character 5	Device Character 6	Qualifier Character 7
9 Brachial Vein, Right Radial vein Ulnar vein **A Brachial Vein, Left** *See 9 Brachial Vein, Right* **B Basilic Vein, Right** Median antebrachial vein Median cubital vein **C Basilic Vein, Left** *See B Basilic Vein, Right* **D Cephalic Vein, Right** Accessory cephalic vein	**F Cephalic Vein, Left** *See D Cephalic Vein, Right* **G Hand Vein, Right** Dorsal metacarpal vein Palmar (volar) digital vein Palmar (volar) metacarpal vein Superficial palmar venous arch Volar (palmar) digital vein Volar (palmar) metacarpal vein **H Hand Vein, Left** *See G Hand Vein, Right* **Y Upper Vein**	**Ø** Open **3** Percutaneous	**Z** No Device	**Z** No Qualifier

Ø Medical and Surgical
5 Upper Veins
H Insertion Definition: Putting in a nonbiological appliance that monitors, assists, performs, or prevents a physiological function but does not physically take the place of a body part

Explanation: None

Body Part Character 4	Approach Character 5	Device Character 6	Qualifier Character 7
Ø Azygos Vein ⊞ Right ascending lumbar vein Right subcostal vein	**Ø** Open **3** Percutaneous **4** Percutaneous Endoscopic	**2** Monitoring Device **3** Infusion Device **D** Intraluminal Device **M** Neurostimulator Lead	**Z** No Qualifier
1 Hemiazygos Vein Left ascending lumbar vein Left subcostal vein **5 Subclavian Vein, Right** **6 Subclavian Vein, Left** **7 Axillary Vein, Right** **8 Axillary Vein, Left** **9 Brachial Vein, Right** Radial vein Ulnar vein **A Brachial Vein, Left** *See 9 Brachial Vein, Right* **B Basilic Vein, Right** Median antebrachial vein Median cubital vein **C Basilic Vein, Left** *See B Basilic Vein, Right* **D Cephalic Vein, Right** Accessory cephalic vein **F Cephalic Vein, Left** *See D Cephalic Vein, Right* **G Hand Vein, Right** Dorsal metacarpal vein Palmar (volar) digital vein Palmar (volar) metacarpal vein Superficial palmar venous arch Volar (palmar) digital vein Volar (palmar) metacarpal vein **H Hand Vein, Left** *See G Hand Vein, Right* **L Intracranial Vein** Anterior cerebral vein Basal (internal) cerebral vein Dural venous sinus Great cerebral vein Inferior cerebellar vein Inferior cerebral vein Internal (basal) cerebral vein Middle cerebral vein Ophthalmic vein Superior cerebellar vein Superior cerebral vein **M Internal Jugular Vein, Right** **N Internal Jugular Vein, Left** **P External Jugular Vein, Right** Posterior auricular vein **Q External Jugular Vein, Left** *See P External Jugular Vein, Right* **R Vertebral Vein, Right** Deep cervical vein Suboccipital venous plexus **S Vertebral Vein, Left** *See R Vertebral Vein, Right* **T Face Vein, Right** Angular vein Anterior facial vein Common facial vein Deep facial vein Frontal vein Posterior facial (retromandibular) vein Supraorbital vein **V Face Vein, Left** *See T Face Vein, Right*	**Ø** Open **3** Percutaneous **4** Percutaneous Endoscopic	**3** Infusion Device **D** Intraluminal Device	**Z** No Qualifier
3 Innominate Vein, Right ⊞ Brachiocephalic vein Inferior thyroid vein **4 Innominate Vein, Left** ⊞ *See 3 Innominate Vein, Right*	**Ø** Open **3** Percutaneous **4** Percutaneous Endoscopic	**3** Infusion Device **D** Intraluminal Device **M** Neurostimulator Lead	**Z** No Qualifier
Y Upper Vein	**Ø** Open **3** Percutaneous **4** Percutaneous Endoscopic	**2** Monitoring Device **3** Infusion Device **D** Intraluminal Device **Y** Other Device	**Z** No Qualifier

Non-OR Ø5HØ[Ø,3,4]3Z
Non-OR Ø5H[1,5,6,7,8,9,A,B,C,D,F,G,H,L,M,N,P,Q,R,S,T,V][Ø,3,4]3Z
Non-OR Ø5H[3,4][Ø,3,4]3Z
Non-OR Ø5HY[Ø,3,4]3Z
Non-OR Ø5HY32Z
Non-OR Ø5HY[3,4]YZ
HAC Ø5HØ[3,4]3Z when reported with SDx J95.811
HAC Ø5H[1,5,6][3,4]3Z when reported with SDx J95.811
HAC Ø5H[M,N,P,Q]33Z when reported with SDx J95.811
HAC Ø5H[3,4][3,4]3Z when reported with SDx J95.811

See Appendix L for Procedure Combinations
⊞ Ø5HØ[Ø,3,4]MZ
⊞ Ø5H[3,4][Ø,3,4]MZ

Ø Medical and Surgical
5 Upper Veins
J Inspection Definition: Visually and/or manually exploring a body part

Explanation: Visual exploration may be performed with or without optical instrumentation. Manual exploration may be performed directly or through intervening body layers.

Body Part Character 4	Approach Character 5	Device Character 6	Qualifier Character 7
Y Upper Vein	**Ø** Open **3** Percutaneous **4** Percutaneous Endoscopic **X** External	**Z** No Device	**Z** No Qualifier

Non-OR Ø5JY[3,X]ZZ

Ø Medical and Surgical
5 Upper Veins
L Occlusion Definition: Completely closing an orifice or the lumen of a tubular body part
Explanation: The orifice can be a natural orifice or an artificially created orifice

Body Part Character 4		Approach Character 5	Device Character 6	Qualifier Character 7
Ø Azygos Vein Right ascending lumbar vein Right subcostal vein **1 Hemiazygos Vein** Left ascending lumbar vein Left subcostal vein **3 Innominate Vein, Right** Brachiocephalic vein Inferior thyroid vein **4 Innominate Vein, Left** *See 3 Innominate Vein, Right* **5 Subclavian Vein, Right** **6 Subclavian Vein, Left** **7 Axillary Vein, Right** **8 Axillary Vein, Left** **9 Brachial Vein, Right** Radial vein Ulnar vein **A Brachial Vein, Left** *See 9 Brachial Vein, Right* **B Basilic Vein, Right** Median antebrachial vein Median cubital vein **C Basilic Vein, Left** *See B Basilic Vein, Right* **D Cephalic Vein, Right** Accessory cephalic vein **F Cephalic Vein, Left** *See D Cephalic Vein, Right* **G Hand Vein, Right** Dorsal metacarpal vein Palmar (volar) digital vein Palmar (volar) metacarpal vein Superficial palmar venous arch Volar (palmar) digital vein Volar (palmar) metacarpal vein	**H Hand Vein, Left** *See G Hand Vein, Right* **L Intracranial Vein** Anterior cerebral vein Basal (internal) cerebral vein Dural venous sinus Great cerebral vein Inferior cerebellar vein Inferior cerebral vein Internal (basal) cerebral vein Middle cerebral vein Ophthalmic vein Superior cerebellar vein Superior cerebral vein **M Internal Jugular Vein, Right** **N Internal Jugular Vein, Left** **P External Jugular Vein, Right** Posterior auricular vein **Q External Jugular Vein, Left** *See P External Jugular Vein, Right* **R Vertebral Vein, Right** Deep cervical vein Suboccipital venous plexus **S Vertebral Vein, Left** *See R Vertebral Vein, Right* **T Face Vein, Right** Angular vein Anterior facial vein Common facial vein Deep facial vein Frontal vein Posterior facial (retromandibular) vein Supraorbital vein **V Face Vein, Left** *See T Face Vein, Right* **Y Upper Vein**	**Ø Open** **3 Percutaneous** **4 Percutaneous Endoscopic**	**C Extraluminal Device** **D Intraluminal Device** **Z No Device**	**Z No Qualifier**

Ø Medical and Surgical
5 Upper Veins
N Release Definition: Freeing a body part from an abnormal physical constraint by cutting or by the use of force
Explanation: Some of the restraining tissue may be taken out but none of the body part is taken out

Body Part Character 4	Approach Character 5	Device Character 6	Qualifier Character 7
Ø Azygos Vein Right ascending lumbar vein Right subcostal vein **1 Hemiazygos Vein** Left ascending lumbar vein Left subcostal vein **3 Innominate Vein, Right** Brachiocephalic vein Inferior thyroid vein **4 Innominate Vein, Left** *See 3 Innominate Vein, Right* **5 Subclavian Vein, Right** **6 Subclavian Vein, Left** **7 Axillary Vein, Right** **8 Axillary Vein, Left** **9 Brachial Vein, Right** Radial vein Ulnar vein **A Brachial Vein, Left** *See 9 Brachial Vein, Right* **B Basilic Vein, Right** Median antebrachial vein Median cubital vein **C Basilic Vein, Left** *See B Basilic Vein, Right* **D Cephalic Vein, Right** Accessory cephalic vein **F Cephalic Vein, Left** *See D Cephalic Vein, Right* **G Hand Vein, Right** Dorsal metacarpal vein Palmar (volar) digital vein Palmar (volar) metacarpal vein Superficial palmar venous arch Volar (palmar) digital vein Volar (palmar) metacarpal vein **H Hand Vein, Left** *See G Hand Vein, Right* **L Intracranial Vein** Anterior cerebral vein Basal (internal) cerebral vein Dural venous sinus Great cerebral vein Inferior cerebellar vein Inferior cerebral vein Internal (basal) cerebral vein Middle cerebral vein Ophthalmic vein Superior cerebellar vein Superior cerebral vein **M Internal Jugular Vein, Right** **N Internal Jugular Vein, Left** **P External Jugular Vein, Right** Posterior auricular vein **Q External Jugular Vein, Left** *See P External Jugular Vein, Right* **R Vertebral Vein, Right** Deep cervical vein Suboccipital venous plexus **S Vertebral Vein, Left** *See R Vertebral Vein, Right* **T Face Vein, Right** Angular vein Anterior facial vein Common facial vein Deep facial vein Frontal vein Posterior facial (retromandibular) vein Supraorbital vein **V Face Vein, Left** *See T Face Vein, Right* **Y Upper Vein**	**Ø Open** **3 Percutaneous** **4 Percutaneous Endoscopic**	**Z No Device**	**Z No Qualifier**

Ø Medical and Surgical
5 Upper Veins
P Removal Definition: Taking out or off a device from a body part

Explanation: If a device is taken out and a similar device put in without cutting or puncturing the skin or mucous membrane, the procedure is coded to the root operation CHANGE. Otherwise, the procedure for taking out a device is coded to the root operation REMOVAL.

Body Part Character 4	Approach Character 5	Device Character 6	Qualifier Character 7
Ø Azygos Vein Right ascending lumbar vein Right subcostal vein	**Ø** Open **3** Percutaneous **4** Percutaneous Endoscopic **X** External	**2** Monitoring Device **M** Neurostimulator Lead	**Z** No Qualifier
3 Innominate Vein, Right Brachiocephalic vein Inferior thyroid vein **4** Innominate Vein, Left *See 3 Innominate Vein, Right*	**Ø** Open **3** Percutaneous **4** Percutaneous Endoscopic **X** External	**M** Neurostimulator Lead	**Z** No Qualifier
Y Upper Vein	**Ø** Open **3** Percutaneous **4** Percutaneous Endoscopic	**Ø** Drainage Device **2** Monitoring Device **3** Infusion Device **7** Autologous Tissue Substitute **C** Extraluminal Device **D** Intraluminal Device **J** Synthetic Substitute **K** Nonautologous Tissue Substitute **Y** Other Device	**Z** No Qualifier
Y Upper Vein	**X** External	**Ø** Drainage Device **2** Monitoring Device **3** Infusion Device **D** Intraluminal Device	**Z** No Qualifier

Non-OR Ø5PØ[Ø,3,4,X]2Z
Non-OR Ø5PY3[Ø,2,3]Z
Non-OR Ø5PY[3,4]YZ
Non-OR Ø5PYX[Ø,2,3,D]Z

Ø Medical and Surgical
5 Upper Veins
Q Repair Definition: Restoring, to the extent possible, a body part to its normal anatomic structure and function
Explanation: Used only when the method to accomplish the repair is not one of the other root operations

Body Part Character 4		Approach Character 5	Device Character 6	Qualifier Character 7
Ø Azygos Vein Right ascending lumbar vein Right subcostal vein **1 Hemiazygos Vein** Left ascending lumbar vein Left subcostal vein **3 Innominate Vein, Right** Brachiocephalic vein Inferior thyroid vein **4 Innominate Vein, Left** *See 3 Innominate Vein, Right* **5 Subclavian Vein, Right** **6 Subclavian Vein, Left** **7 Axillary Vein, Right** **8 Axillary Vein, Left** **9 Brachial Vein, Right** Radial vein Ulnar vein **A Brachial Vein, Left** *See 9 Brachial Vein, Right* **B Basilic Vein, Right** Median antebrachial vein Median cubital vein **C Basilic Vein, Left** *See B Basilic Vein, Right* **D Cephalic Vein, Right** Accessory cephalic vein **F Cephalic Vein, Left** *See D Cephalic Vein, Right* **G Hand Vein, Right** Dorsal metacarpal vein Palmar (volar) digital vein Palmar (volar) metacarpal vein Superficial palmar venous arch Volar (palmar) digital vein Volar (palmar) metacarpal vein	**H Hand Vein, Left** *See G Hand Vein, Right* **L Intracranial Vein** Anterior cerebral vein Basal (internal) cerebral vein Dural venous sinus Great cerebral vein Inferior cerebellar vein Inferior cerebral vein Internal (basal) cerebral vein Middle cerebral vein Ophthalmic vein Superior cerebellar vein Superior cerebral vein **M Internal Jugular Vein, Right** **N Internal Jugular Vein, Left** **P External Jugular Vein, Right** Posterior auricular vein **Q External Jugular Vein, Left** *See P External Jugular Vein, Right* **R Vertebral Vein, Right** Deep cervical vein Suboccipital venous plexus **S Vertebral Vein, Left** *See R Vertebral Vein, Right* **T Face Vein, Right** Angular vein Anterior facial vein Common facial vein Deep facial vein Frontal vein Posterior facial (retromandibular) vein Supraorbital vein **V Face Vein, Left** *See T Face Vein, Right* **Y Upper Vein**	**Ø Open** **3 Percutaneous** **4 Percutaneous Endoscopic**	**Z No Device**	**Z No Qualifier**

Ø Medical and Surgical
5 Upper Veins
R Replacement Definition: Putting in or on biological or synthetic material that physically takes the place and/or function of all or a portion of a body part

Explanation: The body part may have been taken out or replaced, or may be taken out, physically eradicated, or rendered nonfunctional during the REPLACEMENT procedure. A REMOVAL procedure is coded for taking out the device used in a previous replacement procedure.

Body Part Character 4		Approach Character 5	Device Character 6	Qualifier Character 7
Ø Azygos Vein Right ascending lumbar vein Right subcostal vein **1 Hemiazygos Vein** Left ascending lumbar vein Left subcostal vein **3 Innominate Vein, Right** Brachiocephalic vein Inferior thyroid vein **4 Innominate Vein, Left** *See 3 Innominate Vein, Right* **5 Subclavian Vein, Right** **6 Subclavian Vein, Left** **7 Axillary Vein, Right** **8 Axillary Vein, Left** **9 Brachial Vein, Right** Radial vein Ulnar vein **A Brachial Vein, Left** *See 9 Brachial Vein, Right* **B Basilic Vein, Right** Median antebrachial vein Median cubital vein **C Basilic Vein, Left** *See B Basilic Vein, Right* **D Cephalic Vein, Right** Accessory cephalic vein **F Cephalic Vein, Left** *See D Cephalic Vein, Right* **G Hand Vein, Right** Dorsal metacarpal vein Palmar (volar) digital vein Palmar (volar) metacarpal vein Superficial palmar venous arch Volar (palmar) digital vein Volar (palmar) metacarpal vein	**H Hand Vein, Left** *See G Hand Vein, Right* **L Intracranial Vein** Anterior cerebral vein Basal (internal) cerebral vein Dural venous sinus Great cerebral vein Inferior cerebellar vein Inferior cerebral vein Internal (basal) cerebral vein Middle cerebral vein Ophthalmic vein Superior cerebellar vein Superior cerebral vein **M Internal Jugular Vein, Right** **N Internal Jugular Vein, Left** **P External Jugular Vein, Right** Posterior auricular vein **Q External Jugular Vein, Left** *See P External Jugular Vein, Right* **R Vertebral Vein, Right** Deep cervical vein Suboccipital venous plexus **S Vertebral Vein, Left** *See R Vertebral Vein, Right* **T Face Vein, Right** Angular vein Anterior facial vein Common facial vein Deep facial vein Frontal vein Posterior facial (retromandibular) vein Supraorbital vein **V Face Vein, Left** *See T Face Vein, Right* **Y Upper Vein**	**Ø Open** **4 Percutaneous Endoscopic**	**7 Autologous Tissue Substitute** **J Synthetic Substitute** **K Nonautologous Tissue Substitute**	**Z No Qualifier**

Ø Medical and Surgical
5 Upper Veins
S Reposition Definition: Moving to its normal location, or other suitable location, all or a portion of a body part

Explanation: The body part is moved to a new location from an abnormal location, or from a normal location where it is not functioning correctly. The body part may or may not be cut out or off to be moved to the new location.

Body Part Character 4		Approach Character 5	Device Character 6	Qualifier Character 7
Ø Azygos Vein Right ascending lumbar vein Right subcostal vein **1 Hemiazygos Vein** Left ascending lumbar vein Left subcostal vein **3 Innominate Vein, Right** Brachiocephalic vein Inferior thyroid vein **4 Innominate Vein, Left** *See 3 Innominate Vein, Right* **5 Subclavian Vein, Right** **6 Subclavian Vein, Left** **7 Axillary Vein, Right** **8 Axillary Vein, Left** **9 Brachial Vein, Right** Radial vein Ulnar vein **A Brachial Vein, Left** *See 9 Brachial Vein, Right* **B Basilic Vein, Right** Median antebrachial vein Median cubital vein **C Basilic Vein, Left** *See B Basilic Vein, Right* **D Cephalic Vein, Right** Accessory cephalic vein **F Cephalic Vein, Left** *See D Cephalic Vein, Right* **G Hand Vein, Right** Dorsal metacarpal vein Palmar (volar) digital vein Palmar (volar) metacarpal vein Superficial palmar venous arch Volar (palmar) digital vein Volar (palmar) metacarpal vein	**H Hand Vein, Left** *See G Hand Vein, Right* **L Intracranial Vein** Anterior cerebral vein Basal (internal) cerebral vein Dural venous sinus Great cerebral vein Inferior cerebellar vein Inferior cerebral vein Internal (basal) cerebral vein Middle cerebral vein Ophthalmic vein Superior cerebellar vein Superior cerebral vein **M Internal Jugular Vein, Right** **N Internal Jugular Vein, Left** **P External Jugular Vein, Right** Posterior auricular vein **Q External Jugular Vein, Left** *See P External Jugular Vein, Right* **R Vertebral Vein, Right** Deep cervical vein Suboccipital venous plexus **S Vertebral Vein, Left** *See R Vertebral Vein, Right* **T Face Vein, Right** Angular vein Anterior facial vein Common facial vein Deep facial vein Frontal vein Posterior facial (retromandibular) vein Supraorbital vein **V Face Vein, Left** *See T Face Vein, Right* **Y Upper Vein**	**Ø Open** **3 Percutaneous** **4 Percutaneous Endoscopic**	**Z No Device**	**Z No Qualifier**

Ø Medical and Surgical
5 Upper Veins
U Supplement Definition: Putting in or on biological or synthetic material that physically reinforces and/or augments the function of a portion of a body part

Explanation: The biological material is non-living, or is living and from the same individual. The body part may have been previously replaced, and the SUPPLEMENT procedure is performed to physically reinforce and/or augment the function of the replaced body part.

Body Part Character 4	Approach Character 5	Device Character 6	Qualifier Character 7
Ø Azygos Vein Right ascending lumbar vein Right subcostal vein **1 Hemiazygos Vein** Left ascending lumbar vein Left subcostal vein **3 Innominate Vein, Right** Brachiocephalic vein Inferior thyroid vein **4 Innominate Vein, Left** *See 3 Innominate Vein, Right* **5 Subclavian Vein, Right** **6 Subclavian Vein, Left** **7 Axillary Vein, Right** **8 Axillary Vein, Left** **9 Brachial Vein, Right** Radial vein Ulnar vein **A Brachial Vein, Left** *See 9 Brachial Vein, Right* **B Basilic Vein, Right** Median antebrachial vein Median cubital vein **C Basilic Vein, Left** *See B Basilic Vein, Right* **D Cephalic Vein, Right** Accessory cephalic vein **F Cephalic Vein, Left** *See D Cephalic Vein, Right* **G Hand Vein, Right** Dorsal metacarpal vein Palmar (volar) digital vein Palmar (volar) metacarpal vein Superficial palmar venous arch Volar (palmar) digital vein Volar (palmar) metacarpal vein **H Hand Vein, Left** *See G Hand Vein, Right* **L Intracranial Vein** Anterior cerebral vein Basal (internal) cerebral vein Dural venous sinus Great cerebral vein Inferior cerebellar vein Inferior cerebral vein Internal (basal) cerebral vein Middle cerebral vein Ophthalmic vein Superior cerebellar vein Superior cerebral vein **M Internal Jugular Vein, Right** **N Internal Jugular Vein, Left** **P External Jugular Vein, Right** Posterior auricular vein **Q External Jugular Vein, Left** *See P External Jugular Vein, Right* **R Vertebral Vein, Right** Deep cervical vein Suboccipital venous plexus **S Vertebral Vein, Left** *See R Vertebral Vein, Right* **T Face Vein, Right** Angular vein Anterior facial vein Common facial vein Deep facial vein Frontal vein Posterior facial (retromandibular) vein Supraorbital vein **V Face Vein, Left** *See T Face Vein, Right* **Y Upper Vein**	**Ø** Open **3** Percutaneous **4** Percutaneous Endoscopic	**7** Autologous Tissue Substitute **J** Synthetic Substitute **K** Nonautologous Tissue Substitute	**Z** No Qualifier

Ø Medical and Surgical
5 Upper Veins
V Restriction Definition: Partially closing an orifice or the lumen of a tubular body part
Explanation: The orifice can be a natural orifice or an artificially created orifice

Body Part Character 4	Approach Character 5	Device Character 6	Qualifier Character 7
Ø Azygos Vein Right ascending lumbar vein Right subcostal vein **1 Hemiazygos Vein** Left ascending lumbar vein Left subcostal vein **3 Innominate Vein, Right** Brachiocephalic vein Inferior thyroid vein **4 Innominate Vein, Left** *See 3 Innominate Vein, Right* **5 Subclavian Vein, Right** **6 Subclavian Vein, Left** **7 Axillary Vein, Right** **8 Axillary Vein, Left** **9 Brachial Vein, Right** Radial vein Ulnar vein **A Brachial Vein, Left** *See 9 Brachial Vein, Right* **B Basilic Vein, Right** Median antebrachial vein Median cubital vein **C Basilic Vein, Left** *See B Basilic Vein, Right* **D Cephalic Vein, Right** Accessory cephalic vein **F Cephalic Vein, Left** *See D Cephalic Vein, Right* **G Hand Vein, Right** Dorsal metacarpal vein Palmar (volar) digital vein Palmar (volar) metacarpal vein Superficial palmar venous arch Volar (palmar) digital vein Volar (palmar) metacarpal vein **H Hand Vein, Left** *See G Hand Vein, Right* **L Intracranial Vein** Anterior cerebral vein Basal (internal) cerebral vein Dural venous sinus Great cerebral vein Inferior cerebellar vein Inferior cerebral vein Internal (basal) cerebral vein Middle cerebral vein Ophthalmic vein Superior cerebellar vein Superior cerebral vein **M Internal Jugular Vein, Right** **N Internal Jugular Vein, Left** **P External Jugular Vein, Right** Posterior auricular vein **Q External Jugular Vein, Left** *See P External Jugular Vein, Right* **R Vertebral Vein, Right** Deep cervical vein Suboccipital venous plexus **S Vertebral Vein, Left** *See R Vertebral Vein, Right* **T Face Vein, Right** Angular vein Anterior facial vein Common facial vein Deep facial vein Frontal vein Posterior facial (retromandibular) vein Supraorbital vein **V Face Vein, Left** *See T Face Vein, Right* **Y Upper Vein**	**Ø** Open **3** Percutaneous **4** Percutaneous Endoscopic	**C** Extraluminal Device **D** Intraluminal Device **Z** No Device	**Z** No Qualifier

Ø Medical and Surgical
5 Upper Veins
W Revision Definition: Correcting, to the extent possible, a portion of a malfunctioning device or the position of a displaced device

Explanation: Revision can include correcting a malfunctioning or displaced device by taking out or putting in components of the device such as a screw or pin

Body Part Character 4	Approach Character 5	Device Character 6	Qualifier Character 7
Ø Azygos Vein Right ascending lumbar vein Right subcostal vein	**Ø Open** **3 Percutaneous** **4 Percutaneous Endoscopic** **X External**	**2 Monitoring Device** **M Neurostimulator Lead**	**Z No Qualifier**
3 Innominate Vein, Right Brachiocephalic vein Inferior thyroid vein **4 Innominate Vein, Left** *See 3 Innominate Vein, Right*	**Ø Open** **3 Percutaneous** **4 Percutaneous Endoscopic** **X External**	**M Neurostimulator Lead**	**Z No Qualifier**
Y Upper Vein	**Ø Open** **3 Percutaneous** **4 Percutaneous Endoscopic**	**Ø Drainage Device** **2 Monitoring Device** **3 Infusion Device** **7 Autologous Tissue Substitute** **C Extraluminal Device** **D Intraluminal Device** **J Synthetic Substitute** **K Nonautologous Tissue Substitute** **Y Other Device**	**Z No Qualifier**
Y Upper Vein	**X External**	**Ø Drainage Device** **2 Monitoring Device** **3 Infusion Device** **7 Autologous Tissue Substitute** **C Extraluminal Device** **D Intraluminal Device** **J Synthetic Substitute** **K Nonautologous Tissue Substitute**	**Z No Qualifier**

Non-OR Ø5WØXMZ
Non-OR Ø5W[3,4]XMZ
Non-OR Ø5WY3[Ø,2,3,D]Z
Non-OR Ø5WY[3,4]YZ
Non-OR Ø5WYX[Ø,2,3,7,C,D,J,K]Z

Lower Veins Ø61–Ø6W

Character Meanings

This Character Meaning table is provided as a guide to assist the user in the identification of character members that may be found in this section of code tables. It **SHOULD NOT** be used to build a PCS code.

Operation–Character 3	Body Part–Character 4	Approach–Character 5	Device–Character 6	Qualifier–Character 7
1 Bypass	Ø Inferior Vena Cava	Ø Open	Ø Drainage Device	4 Hepatic Vein
5 Destruction	1 Splenic Vein	3 Percutaneous	2 Monitoring Device	5 Superior Mesenteric Vein
7 Dilation	2 Gastric Vein	4 Percutaneous Endoscopic	3 Infusion Device	6 Inferior Mesenteric Vein
9 Drainage	3 Esophageal Vein	7 Via Natural or Artificial Opening	7 Autologous Tissue Substitute	9 Renal Vein, Right
B Excision	4 Hepatic Vein	8 Via Natural or Artificial Opening Endoscopic	9 Autologous Venous Tissue	B Renal Vein, Left
C Extirpation	5 Superior Mesenteric Vein	X External	A Autologous Arterial Tissue	C Hemorrhoidal Plexus
D Extraction	6 Inferior Mesenteric Vein		C Extraluminal Device	P Pulmonary Trunk
H Insertion	7 Colic Vein		D Intraluminal Device	Q Pulmonary Artery, Right
J Inspection	8 Portal Vein		J Synthetic Substitute	R Pulmonary Artery, Left
L Occlusion	9 Renal Vein, Right		K Nonautologous Tissue Substitute	T Via Umbilical Vein
N Release	B Renal Vein, Left		Y Other Device	X Diagnostic
P Removal	C Common Iliac Vein, Right		Z No Device	Y Lower Vein
Q Repair	D Common Iliac Vein, Left			Z No Qualifier
R Replacement	F External Iliac Vein, Right			
S Reposition	G External Iliac Vein, Left			
U Supplement	H Hypogastric Vein, Right			
V Restriction	J Hypogastric Vein, Left			
W Revision	M Femoral Vein, Right			
	N Femoral Vein, Left			
	P Saphenous Vein, Right			
	Q Saphenous Vein, Left			
	T Foot Vein, Right			
	V Foot Vein, Left			
	Y Lower Vein			

AHA Coding Clinic for table Ø61
2017, 4Q, 36-38 Fontan completion procedure
2017, 4Q, 66-67 New qualifier values - Portal to hepatic shunt

AHA Coding Clinic for table Ø6B
2017, 3Q, 5 Femoral artery to posterior tibial artery bypass using autologous and synthetic grafts
2017, 1Q, 31 Left to right common carotid artery bypass
2017, 1Q, 32 Peroneal artery to dorsalis pedis artery bypass using saphenous vein graft
2016, 3Q, 31 Femoral to peroneal artery bypass with in-situ saphenous vein graft and lysis of valves
2016, 2Q, 18 Femoral-tibial artery bypass and saphenous vein graft
2016, 1Q, 27 Aortocoronary bypass graft utilizing Y-graft
2014, 3Q, 8 Excision of saphenous vein for coronary artery bypass graft
2014, 3Q, 20 MAZE procedure performed with coronary artery bypass graft
2014, 1Q, 10 Repair of thoracic aortic aneurysm & coronary artery bypass graft

AHA Coding Clinic for table Ø6H
2017, 3Q, 11 Placement of peripherally inserted central catheter using 3CG ECG technology
2017, 1Q, 31 Umbilical vein catheterization
2017, 1Q, 31 Central catheter placement in femoral vein
2013, 3Q, 18 Heart transplant surgery

AHA Coding Clinic for table Ø6L
2018, 2Q, 18 Transverse rectus abdominis myocutaneous (TRAM) delay
2017, 4Q, 57-58 Added approach values - Transorifice esophageal vein banding
2013, 4Q, 112 Endoscopic banding of esophageal varices

AHA Coding Clinic for table Ø6V
2018, 1Q, 10 Revision of transjugular intrahepatic portosystemic shunt

AHA Coding Clinic for table Ø6W
2018, 1Q, 10 Revision of transjugular intrahepatic portosystemic shunt
2014, 3Q, 25 Revision of transjugular intrahepatic portosystemic shunt (TIPS)

Lower Veins

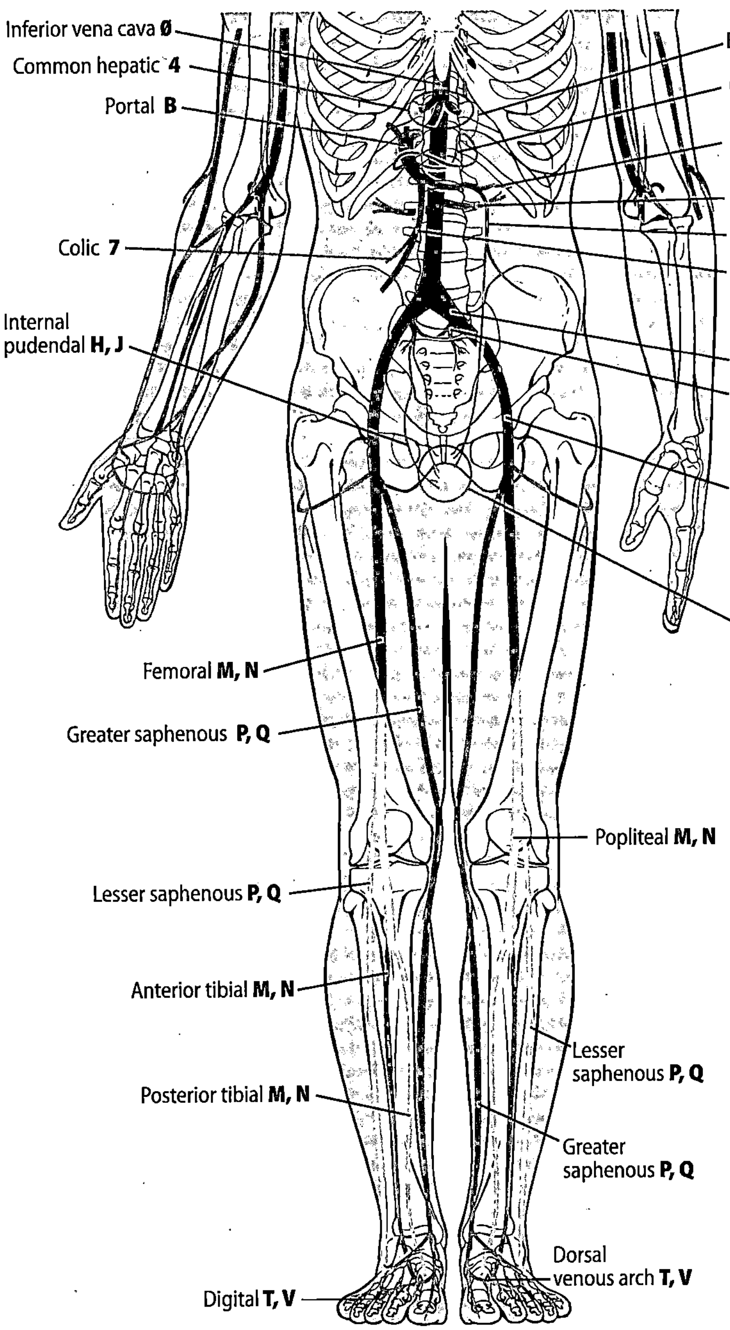
Inferior vena cava Ø
Common hepatic 4
Portal B
Colic 7
Internal pudendal H, J
Esophageal 3
Gastric 2
Splenic 1
Renal 9, B
Inferior mesenteric 6
Superior mesenteric 5
Common iliac C, D
Internal iliac (Hypogastric) H, J
External iliac F, G
Rectal venous plexus H, J
Femoral M, N
Greater saphenous P, Q
Popliteal M, N
Lesser saphenous P, Q
Anterior tibial M, N
Posterior tibial M, N
Lesser saphenous P, Q
Greater saphenous P, Q
Dorsal venous arch T, V
Digital T, V

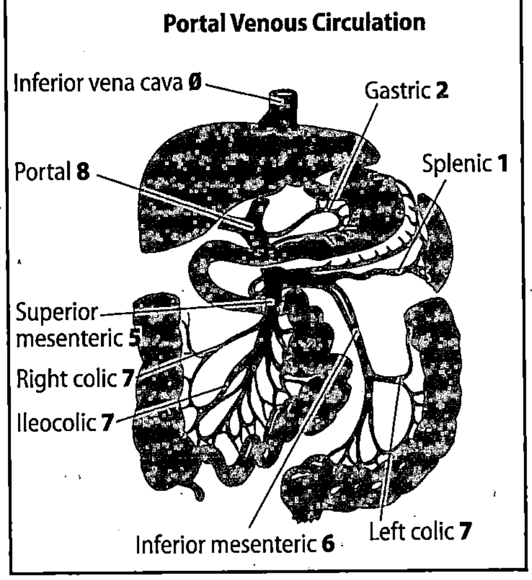
Portal Venous Circulation
Inferior vena cava Ø
Gastric 2
Portal 8
Splenic 1
Superior mesenteric 5
Right colic 7
Ileocolic 7
Inferior mesenteric 6
Left colic 7

Ø Medical and Surgical
6 Lower Veins
1 Bypass Definition: Altering the route of passage of the contents of a tubular body part

Explanation: Rerouting contents of a body part to a downstream area of the normal route, to a similar route and body part, or to an abnormal route and dissimilar body part. Includes one or more anastomoses, with or without the use of a device.

Body Part Character 4	Approach Character 5	Device Character 6	Qualifier Character 7
Ø Inferior Vena Cava Postcava Right inferior phrenic vein Right ovarian vein Right second lumbar vein Right suprarenal vein Right testicular vein	**Ø Open** **4 Percutaneous Endoscopic**	**7 Autologous Tissue Substitute** **9 Autologous Venous Tissue** **A Autologous Arterial Tissue** **J Synthetic Substitute** **K Nonautologous Tissue Substitute** **Z No Device**	**5 Superior Mesenteric Vein** **6 Inferior Mesenteric Vein** **P Pulmonary Trunk** **Q Pulmonary Artery, Right** **R Pulmonary Artery, Left** **Y Lower Vein**
1 Splenic Vein Left gastroepiploic vein Pancreatic vein	**Ø Open** **4 Percutaneous Endoscopic**	**7 Autologous Tissue Substitute** **9 Autologous Venous Tissue** **A Autologous Arterial Tissue** **J Synthetic Substitute** **K Nonautologous Tissue Substitute** **Z No Device**	**9 Renal Vein, Right** **B Renal Vein, Left** **Y Lower Vein**
2 Gastric Vein **3 Esophageal Vein** **4 Hepatic Vein** **5 Superior Mesenteric Vein** Right gastroepiploic vein **6 Inferior Mesenteric Vein** Sigmoid vein Superior rectal vein **7 Colic Vein** Ileocolic vein Left colic vein Middle colic vein Right colic vein **9 Renal Vein, Right** **B Renal Vein, Left** Left inferior phrenic vein Left ovarian vein Left second lumbar vein Left suprarenal vein Left testicular vein **C Common Iliac Vein, Right** **D Common Iliac Vein, Left** **F External Iliac Vein, Right** **G External Iliac Vein, Left** **H Hypogastric Vein, Right** Gluteal vein Internal iliac vein Internal pudendal vein Lateral sacral vein Middle hemorrhoidal vein Obturator vein Uterine vein Vaginal vein Vesical vein **J Hypogastric Vein, Left** *See H Hypogastric Vein, Right* **M Femoral Vein, Right** Deep femoral (profunda femoris) vein Popliteal vein Profunda femoris (deep femoral) vein **N Femoral Vein, Left** *See M Femoral Vein, Right* **P Saphenous Vein, Right** External pudendal vein Great(er) saphenous vein Lesser saphenous vein Small saphenous vein Superficial circumflex iliac vein Superficial epigastric vein **Q Saphenous Vein, Left** *See P Saphenous Vein, Right* **T Foot Vein, Right** Common digital vein Dorsal metatarsal vein Dorsal venous arch Plantar digital vein Plantar metatarsal vein Plantar venous arch **V Foot Vein, Left** *See T Foot Vein, Right*	**Ø Open** **4 Percutaneous Endoscopic**	**7 Autologous Tissue Substitute** **9 Autologous Venous Tissue** **A Autologous Arterial Tissue** **J Synthetic Substitute** **K Nonautologous Tissue Substitute** **Z No Device**	**Y Lower Vein**
8 Portal Vein Hepatic portal vein	**Ø Open**	**7 Autologous Tissue Substitute** **9 Autologous Venous Tissue** **A Autologous Arterial Tissue** **J Synthetic Substitute** **K Nonautologous Tissue Substitute** **Z No Device**	**9 Renal Vein, Right** **B Renal Vein, Left** **Y Lower Vein**
8 Portal Vein Hepatic portal vein	**3 Percutaneous**	**J Synthetic Substitute**	**4 Hepatic Vein** **Y Lower Vein**
8 Portal Vein Hepatic portal vein	**4 Percutaneous Endoscopic**	**7 Autologous Tissue Substitute** **9 Autologous Venous Tissue** **A Autologous Arterial Tissue** **K Nonautologous Tissue Substitute** **Z No Device**	**9 Renal Vein, Right** **B Renal Vein, Left** **Y Lower Vein**
8 Portal Vein Hepatic portal vein	**4 Percutaneous Endoscopic**	**J Synthetic Substitute**	**4 Hepatic Vein** **9 Renal Vein, Right** **B Renal Vein, Left** **Y Lower Vein**

Ø Medical and Surgical
6 Lower Veins
5 Destruction Definition: Physical eradication of all or a portion of a body part by the direct use of energy, force, or a destructive agent
Explanation: None of the body part is physically taken out

Body Part Character 4	Approach Character 5	Device Character 6	Qualifier Character 7
Ø Inferior Vena Cava Postcava Right inferior phrenic vein Right ovarian vein Right second lumbar vein Right suprarenal vein Right testicular vein **1 Splenic Vein** Left gastroepiploic vein Pancreatic vein **2 Gastric Vein** **3 Esophageal Vein** **4 Hepatic Vein** **5 Superior Mesenteric Vein** Right gastroepiploic vein **6 Inferior Mesenteric Vein** Sigmoid vein Superior rectal vein **7 Colic Vein** Ileocolic vein Left colic vein Middle colic vein Right colic vein **8 Portal Vein** Hepatic portal vein **9 Renal Vein, Right** **B Renal Vein, Left** Left inferior phrenic vein Left ovarian vein Left second lumbar vein Left suprarenal vein Left testicular vein **C Common Iliac Vein, Right** **D Common Iliac Vein, Left** **F External Iliac Vein, Right** **G External Iliac Vein, Left** **H Hypogastric Vein, Right** Gluteal vein Internal iliac vein Internal pudendal vein Lateral sacral vein Middle hemorrhoidal vein Obturator vein Uterine vein Vaginal vein Vesical vein **J Hypogastric Vein, Left** *See H Hypogastric Vein, Right* **M Femoral Vein, Right** Deep femoral (profunda femoris) vein Popliteal vein Profunda femoris (deep femoral) vein **N Femoral Vein, Left** *See M Femoral Vein, Right* **P Saphenous Vein, Right** External pudendal vein Great(er) saphenous vein Lesser saphenous vein Small saphenous vein Superficial circumflex iliac vein Superficial epigastric vein **Q Saphenous Vein, Left** *See P Saphenous Vein, Right* **T Foot Vein, Right** Common digital vein Dorsal metatarsal vein Dorsal venous arch Plantar digital vein Plantar metatarsal vein Plantar venous arch **V Foot Vein, Left** *See T Foot Vein, Right*	**Ø Open** **3 Percutaneous** **4 Percutaneous Endoscopic**	**Z No Device**	**Z No Qualifier**
Y Lower Vein	**Ø Open** **3 Percutaneous** **4 Percutaneous Endoscopic**	**Z No Device**	**C Hemorrhoidal Plexus** **Z No Qualifier**

Ø Medical and Surgical
6 Lower Veins
7 Dilation Definition: Expanding an orifice or the lumen of a tubular body part

Explanation: The orifice can be a natural orifice or an artificially created orifice. Accomplished by stretching a tubular body part using intraluminal pressure or by cutting part of the orifice or wall of the tubular body part.

Body Part Character 4	Approach Character 5	Device Character 6	Qualifier Character 7
Ø Inferior Vena Cava Postcava Right inferior phrenic vein Right ovarian vein Right second lumbar vein Right suprarenal vein Right testicular vein **1 Splenic Vein** Left gastroepiploic vein Pancreatic vein **2 Gastric Vein** **3 Esophageal Vein** **4 Hepatic Vein** **5 Superior Mesenteric Vein** Right gastroepiploic vein **6 Inferior Mesenteric Vein** Sigmoid vein Superior rectal vein **7 Colic Vein** Ileocolic vein Left colic vein Middle colic vein Right colic vein **8 Portal Vein** Hepatic portal vein **9 Renal Vein, Right** **B Renal Vein, Left** Left inferior phrenic vein Left ovarian vein Left second lumbar vein Left suprarenal vein Left testicular vein **C Common Iliac Vein, Right** **D Common Iliac Vein, Left** **F External Iliac Vein, Right** **G External Iliac Vein, Left** **H Hypogastric Vein, Right** Gluteal vein Internal iliac vein Internal pudendal vein Lateral sacral vein Middle hemorrhoidal vein Obturator vein Uterine vein Vaginal vein Vesical vein **J Hypogastric Vein, Left** *See H Hypogastric Vein, Right* **M Femoral Vein, Right** Deep femoral (profunda femoris) vein Popliteal vein Profunda femoris (deep femoral) vein **N Femoral Vein, Left** *See M Femoral Vein, Right* **P Saphenous Vein, Right** External pudendal vein Great(er) saphenous vein Lesser saphenous vein Small saphenous vein Superficial circumflex iliac vein Superficial epigastric vein **Q Saphenous Vein, Left** *See P Saphenous Vein, Right* **T Foot Vein, Right** Common digital vein Dorsal metatarsal vein Dorsal venous arch Plantar digital vein Plantar metatarsal vein Plantar venous arch **V Foot Vein, Left** *See T Foot Vein, Right* **Y Lower Vein**	Ø Open 3 Percutaneous 4 Percutaneous Endoscopic	D Intraluminal Device Z No Device	Z No Qualifier

Ø Medical and Surgical
6 Lower Veins
9 Drainage Definition: Taking or letting out fluids and/or gases from a body part
Explanation: The qualifier DIAGNOSTIC is used to identify drainage procedures that are biopsies

Body Part Character 4	Approach Character 5	Device Character 6	Qualifier Character 7
Ø Inferior Vena Cava Postcava Right inferior phrenic vein Right ovarian vein Right second lumbar vein Right suprarenal vein Right testicular vein **1 Splenic Vein** Left gastroepiploic vein Pancreatic vein **2 Gastric Vein** **3 Esophageal Vein** **4 Hepatic Vein** **5 Superior Mesenteric Vein** Right gastroepiploic vein **6 Inferior Mesenteric Vein** Sigmoid vein Superior rectal vein **7 Colic Vein** Ileocolic vein Left colic vein Middle colic vein Right colic vein **8 Portal Vein** Hepatic portal vein **9 Renal Vein, Right** **B Renal Vein, Left** Left inferior phrenic vein Left ovarian vein Left second lumbar vein Left suprarenal vein Left testicular vein **C Common Iliac Vein, Right** **D Common Iliac Vein, Left** **F External Iliac Vein, Right** **G External Iliac Vein, Left** **H Hypogastric Vein, Right** Gluteal vein Internal iliac vein Internal pudendal vein Lateral sacral vein Middle hemorrhoidal vein Obturator vein Uterine vein Vaginal vein Vesical vein **J Hypogastric Vein, Left** *See H Hypogastric Vein, Right* **M Femoral Vein, Right** Deep femoral (profunda femoris) vein Popliteal vein Profunda femoris (deep femoral) vein **N Femoral Vein, Left** *See M Femoral Vein, Right* **P Saphenous Vein, Right** External pudendal vein Great(er) saphenous vein Lesser saphenous vein Small saphenous vein Superficial circumflex iliac vein Superficial epigastric vein **Q Saphenous Vein, Left** *See P Saphenous Vein, Right* **T Foot Vein, Right** Common digital vein Dorsal metatarsal vein Dorsal venous arch Plantar digital vein Plantar metatarsal vein Plantar venous arch **V Foot Vein, Left** *See T Foot Vein, Right* **Y Lower Vein**	**Ø Open** **3 Percutaneous** **4 Percutaneous Endoscopic**	**Ø Drainage Device**	**Z No Qualifier**

Ø69 Continued on next page

Non-OR Ø69[Ø,1,2,4,5,6,7,8,9,B,C,D,F,G,H,J,M,N,P,Q,T,V,Y][Ø,3,4]ØZ
Non-OR Ø6933ØZ

Ø Medical and Surgical
6 Lower Veins
9 Drainage Definition: Taking or letting out fluids and/or gases from a body part
Explanation: The qualifier DIAGNOSTIC is used to identify drainage procedures that are biopsies

Ø69 Continued

Body Part Character 4	Approach Character 5	Device Character 6	Qualifier Character 7
Ø Inferior Vena Cava Postcava Right inferior phrenic vein Right ovarian vein Right second lumbar vein Right suprarenal vein Right testicular vein **1 Splenic Vein** Left gastroepiploic vein Pancreatic vein **2 Gastric Vein** **3 Esophageal Vein** **4 Hepatic Vein** **5 Superior Mesenteric Vein** Right gastroepiploic vein **6 Inferior Mesenteric Vein** Sigmoid vein Superior rectal vein **7 Colic Vein** Ileocolic vein Left colic vein Middle colic vein Right colic vein **8 Portal Vein** Hepatic portal vein **9 Renal Vein, Right** **B Renal Vein, Left** Left inferior phrenic vein Left ovarian vein Left second lumbar vein Left suprarenal vein Left testicular vein **C Common Iliac Vein, Right** **D Common Iliac Vein, Left** **F External Iliac Vein, Right** **G External Iliac Vein, Left** **H Hypogastric Vein, Right** Gluteal vein Internal iliac vein Internal pudendal vein Lateral sacral vein Middle hemorrhoidal vein Obturator vein Uterine vein Vaginal vein Vesical vein **J Hypogastric Vein, Left** *See H Hypogastric Vein, Right* **M Femoral Vein, Right** Deep femoral (profunda femoris) vein Popliteal vein Profunda femoris (deep femoral) vein **N Femoral Vein, Left** *See M Femoral Vein, Right* **P Saphenous Vein, Right** External pudendal vein Great(er) saphenous vein Lesser saphenous vein Small saphenous vein Superficial circumflex iliac vein Superficial epigastric vein **Q Saphenous Vein, Left** *See P Saphenous Vein, Right* **T Foot Vein, Right** Common digital vein Dorsal metatarsal vein Dorsal venous arch Plantar digital vein Plantar metatarsal vein Plantar venous arch **V Foot Vein, Left** *See T Foot Vein, Right* **Y Lower Vein**	**Ø Open** **3 Percutaneous** **4 Percutaneous Endoscopic**	**Z No Device**	**X Diagnostic** **Z No Qualifier**

Non-OR Ø69[Ø,1,2,3,4,5,6,7,8,9,B,C,D,F,G,H,J,M,N,P,Q,T,V,Y]3ZX
Non-OR Ø69[Ø,1,2,4,5,6,7,8,9,B,C,D,F,G,H,J,M,N,P,Q,T,V,Y][Ø,3,4]ZZ
Non-OR Ø6933ZZ

Ø Medical and Surgical
6 Lower Veins
B Excision Definition: Cutting out or off, without replacement, a portion of a body part

Explanation: The qualifier DIAGNOSTIC is used to identify excision procedures that are biopsies

Body Part Character 4	Approach Character 5	Device Character 6	Qualifier Character 7
Ø Inferior Vena Cava Postcava Right inferior phrenic vein Right ovarian vein Right second lumbar vein Right suprarenal vein Right testicular vein **1 Splenic Vein** Left gastroepiploic vein Pancreatic vein **2 Gastric Vein** **3 Esophageal Vein** **4 Hepatic Vein** **5 Superior Mesenteric Vein** Right gastroepiploic vein **6 Inferior Mesenteric Vein** Sigmoid vein Superior rectal vein **7 Colic Vein** Ileocolic vein Left colic vein Middle colic vein Right colic vein **8 Portal Vein** Hepatic portal vein **9 Renal Vein, Right** **B Renal Vein, Left** Left inferior phrenic vein Left ovarian vein Left second lumbar vein Left suprarenal vein Left testicular vein **C Common Iliac Vein, Right** **D Common Iliac Vein, Left** **F External Iliac Vein, Right** **G External Iliac Vein, Left** **H Hypogastric Vein, Right** Gluteal vein Internal iliac vein Internal pudendal vein Lateral sacral vein Middle hemorrhoidal vein Obturator vein Uterine vein Vaginal vein Vesical vein **J Hypogastric Vein, Left** *See H Hypogastric Vein, Right* **M Femoral Vein, Right** Deep femoral (profunda femoris) vein Popliteal vein Profunda femoris (deep femoral) vein **N Femoral Vein, Left** *See M Femoral Vein, Right* **P Saphenous Vein, Right** External pudendal vein Great(er) saphenous vein Lesser saphenous vein Small saphenous vein Superficial circumflex iliac vein Superficial epigastric vein **Q Saphenous Vein, Left** *See P Saphenous Vein, Right* **T Foot Vein, Right** Common digital vein Dorsal metatarsal vein Dorsal venous arch Plantar digital vein Plantar metatarsal vein Plantar venous arch **V Foot Vein, Left** *See T Foot Vein, Right*	**Ø** Open **3** Percutaneous **4** Percutaneous Endoscopic	**Z** No Device	**X** Diagnostic **Z** No Qualifier
Y Lower Vein	**Ø** Open **3** Percutaneous **4** Percutaneous Endoscopic	**Z** No Device	**C** Hemorrhoidal Plexus **X** Diagnostic **Z** No Qualifier

Ø Medical and Surgical
6 Lower Veins
C Extirpation Definition: Taking or cutting out solid matter from a body part

Explanation: The solid matter may be an abnormal byproduct of a biological function or a foreign body; it may be imbedded in a body part or in the lumen of a tubular body part. The solid matter may or may not have been previously broken into pieces.

Body Part Character 4	Approach Character 5	Device Character 6	Qualifier Character 7
Ø Inferior Vena Cava Postcava Right inferior phrenic vein Right ovarian vein Right second lumbar vein Right suprarenal vein Right testicular vein **1 Splenic Vein** Left gastroepiploic vein Pancreatic vein **2 Gastric Vein** **3 Esophageal Vein** **4 Hepatic Vein** **5 Superior Mesenteric Vein** Right gastroepiploic vein **6 Inferior Mesenteric Vein** Sigmoid vein Superior rectal vein **7 Colic Vein** Ileocolic vein Left colic vein Middle colic vein Right colic vein **8 Portal Vein** Hepatic portal vein **9 Renal Vein, Right** **B Renal Vein, Left** Left inferior phrenic vein Left ovarian vein Left second lumbar vein Left suprarenal vein Left testicular vein **C Common Iliac Vein, Right** **D Common Iliac Vein, Left** **F External Iliac Vein, Right** **G External Iliac Vein, Left** **H Hypogastric Vein, Right** Gluteal vein Internal iliac vein Internal pudendal vein Lateral sacral vein Middle hemorrhoidal vein Obturator vein Uterine vein Vaginal vein Vesical vein **J Hypogastric Vein, Left** *See H Hypogastric Vein, Right* **M Femoral Vein, Right** Deep femoral (profunda femoris) vein Popliteal vein Profunda femoris (deep femoral) vein **N Femoral Vein, Left** *See M Femoral Vein, Right* **P Saphenous Vein, Right** External pudendal vein Great(er) saphenous vein Lesser saphenous vein Small saphenous vein Superficial circumflex iliac vein Superficial epigastric vein **Q Saphenous Vein, Left** *See P Saphenous Vein, Right* **T Foot Vein, Right** Common digital vein Dorsal metatarsal vein Dorsal venous arch Plantar digital vein Plantar metatarsal vein Plantar venous arch **V Foot Vein, Left** *See T Foot Vein, Right* **Y Lower Vein**	**Ø Open** **3 Percutaneous** **4 Percutaneous Endoscopic**	**Z No Device**	**Z No Qualifier**

Ø Medical and Surgical
6 Lower Veins
D Extraction Definition: Pulling or stripping out or off all or a portion of a body part by the use of force

Explanation: The qualifier DIAGNOSTIC is used to identify extraction procedures that are biopsies

Body Part Character 4	Approach Character 5	Device Character 6	Qualifier Character 7
M Femoral Vein, Right Deep femoral (profunda femoris) vein Popliteal vein Profunda femoris (deep femoral) vein **N Femoral Vein, Left** *See M Femoral Vein, Right* **P Saphenous Vein, Right** External pudendal vein Great(er) saphenous vein Lesser saphenous vein Small saphenous vein Superficial circumflex iliac vein Superficial epigastric vein **Q Saphenous Vein, Left** *See P Saphenous Vein, Right* **T Foot Vein, Right** Common digital vein Dorsal metatarsal vein Dorsal venous arch Plantar digital vein Plantar metatarsal vein Plantar venous arch **V Foot Vein, Left** *See T Foot Vein, Right* **Y Lower Vein**	**Ø Open** **3 Percutaneous** **4 Percutaneous Endoscopic**	**Z No Device**	**Z No Qualifier**

Ø Medical and Surgical
6 Lower Veins
H Insertion Definition: Putting in a nonbiological appliance that monitors, assists, performs, or prevents a physiological function but does not physically take the place of a body part

Explanation: None

Body Part Character 4	Approach Character 5	Device Character 6	Qualifier Character 7
Ø Inferior Vena Cava Postcava Right inferior phrenic vein Right ovarian vein Right second lumbar vein Right suprarenal vein Right testicular vein	Ø Open 3 Percutaneous	3 Infusion Device	T Via Umbilical Vein Z No Qualifier
Ø Inferior Vena Cava Postcava Right inferior phrenic vein Right ovarian vein Right second lumbar vein Right suprarenal vein Right testicular vein	Ø Open 3 Percutaneous	D Intraluminal Device	Z No Qualifier
Ø Inferior Vena Cava Postcava Right inferior phrenic vein Right ovarian vein Right second lumbar vein Right suprarenal vein Right testicular vein	4 Percutaneous Endoscopic	3 Infusion Device D Intraluminal Device	Z No Qualifier
1 Splenic Vein Left gastroepiploic vein Pancreatic vein **2 Gastric Vein** **3 Esophageal Vein** **4 Hepatic Vein** **5 Superior Mesenteric Vein** Right gastroepiploic vein **6 Inferior Mesenteric Vein** Sigmoid vein Superior rectal vein **7 Colic Vein** Ileocolic vein Left colic vein Middle colic vein Right colic vein **8 Portal Vein** Hepatic portal vein **9 Renal Vein, Right** **B Renal Vein, Left** Left inferior phrenic vein Left ovarian vein Left second lumbar vein Left suprarenal vein Left testicular vein **C Common Iliac Vein, Right** **D Common Iliac Vein, Left** **F External Iliac Vein, Right** **G External Iliac Vein, Left** **H Hypogastric Vein, Right** Gluteal vein Internal iliac vein Internal pudendal vein Lateral sacral vein Middle hemorrhoidal vein Obturator vein Uterine vein Vaginal vein Vesical vein **J Hypogastric Vein, Left** *See H Hypogastric Vein, Right* **M Femoral Vein, Right** Deep femoral (profunda femoris) vein Popliteal vein Profunda femoris (deep femoral) vein **N Femoral Vein, Left** *See M Femoral Vein, Right* **P Saphenous Vein, Right** External pudendal vein Great(er) saphenous vein Lesser saphenous vein Small saphenous vein Superficial circumflex iliac vein Superficial epigastric vein **Q Saphenous Vein, Left** *See P Saphenous Vein, Right* **T Foot Vein, Right** Common digital vein Dorsal metatarsal vein Dorsal venous arch Plantar digital vein Plantar metatarsal vein Plantar venous arch **V Foot Vein, Left** *See T Foot Vein, Right*	Ø Open 3 Percutaneous 4 Percutaneous Endoscopic	3 Infusion Device D Intraluminal Device	Z No Qualifier
Y Lower Vein	Ø Open 3 Percutaneous 4 Percutaneous Endoscopic	2 Monitoring Device 3 Infusion Device D Intraluminal Device Y Other Device	Z No Qualifier

Non-OR	Ø6HØ[Ø,3]3[T,Z]
Non-OR	Ø6HØ3DZ
Non-OR	Ø6HØ43Z
Non-OR	Ø6H[1,2,3,4,5,6,7,8,9,B,C,D,F,G,H,J,M,N,P,Q,T,V][Ø,3,4]3Z
Non-OR	Ø6HY[Ø,3,4]3Z
Non-OR	Ø6HY32Z
Non-OR	Ø6HY[3,4]YZ

Ø Medical and Surgical
6 Lower Veins
J Inspection Definition: Visually and/or manually exploring a body part

Explanation: Visual exploration may be performed with or without optical instrumentation. Manual exploration may be performed directly or through intervening body layers.

Body Part Character 4	Approach Character 5	Device Character 6	Qualifier Character 7
Y Lower Vein	Ø Open 3 Percutaneous 4 Percutaneous Endoscopic X External	Z No Device	Z No Qualifier

Non-OR Ø6JY[3,X]ZZ

Ø Medical and Surgical
6 Lower Veins
L Occlusion Definition: Completely closing an orifice or the lumen of a tubular body part

Explanation: The orifice can be a natural orifice or an artificially created orifice

Body Part Character 4	Approach Character 5	Device Character 6	Qualifier Character 7
Ø Inferior Vena Cava Postcava Right inferior phrenic vein Right ovarian vein Right second lumbar vein Right suprarenal vein Right testicular vein 1 Splenic Vein Left gastroepiploic vein Pancreatic vein 2 Gastric Vein 4 Hepatic Vein 5 Superior Mesenteric Vein Right gastroepiploic vein 6 Inferior Mesenteric Vein Sigmoid vein Superior rectal vein 7 Colic Vein Ileocolic vein Left colic vein Middle colic vein Right colic vein 8 Portal Vein Hepatic portal vein 9 Renal Vein, Right B Renal Vein, Left Left inferior phrenic vein Left ovarian vein Left second lumbar vein Left suprarenal vein Left testicular vein C Common Iliac Vein, Right D Common Iliac Vein, Left F External Iliac Vein, Right G External Iliac Vein, Left H Hypogastric Vein, Right Gluteal vein Internal iliac vein Internal pudendal vein Lateral sacral vein Middle hemorrhoidal vein Obturator vein Uterine vein Vaginal vein Vesical vein J Hypogastric Vein, Left *See H Hypogastric Vein, Right* M Femoral Vein, Right Deep femoral (profunda femoris) vein Popliteal vein Profunda femoris (deep femoral) vein N Femoral Vein, Left *See M Femoral Vein, Right* P Saphenous Vein, Right External pudendal vein Great(er) saphenous vein Lesser saphenous vein Small saphenous vein Superficial circumflex iliac vein Superficial epigastric vein Q Saphenous Vein, Left *See P Saphenous Vein, Right* T Foot Vein, Right Common digital vein Dorsal metatarsal vein Dorsal venous arch Plantar digital vein Plantar metatarsal vein Plantar venous arch V Foot Vein, Left *See T Foot Vein, Right*	Ø Open 3 Percutaneous 4 Percutaneous Endoscopic	C Extraluminal Device D Intraluminal Device Z No Device	Z No Qualifier
3 Esophageal Vein	Ø Open 3 Percutaneous 4 Percutaneous Endoscopic 7 Via Natural or Artificial Opening 8 Via Natural or Artificial Opening Endoscopic	C Extraluminal Device D Intraluminal Device Z No Device	Z No Qualifier
Y Lower Vein	Ø Open 3 Percutaneous 4 Percutaneous Endoscopic	C Extraluminal Device D Intraluminal Device Z No Device	C Hemorrhoidal Plexus Z No Qualifier

Non-OR Ø6L3[3,4,7,8][C,D,Z]Z

Ø Medical and Surgical
6 Lower Veins
N Release Definition: Freeing a body part from an abnormal physical constraint by cutting or by the use of force
Explanation: Some of the restraining tissue may be taken out but none of the body part is taken out

Body Part Character 4		Approach Character 5	Device Character 6	Qualifier Character 7
Ø Inferior Vena Cava Postcava Right inferior phrenic vein Right ovarian vein Right second lumbar vein Right suprarenal vein Right testicular vein **1 Splenic Vein** Left gastroepiploic vein Pancreatic vein **2 Gastric Vein** **3 Esophageal Vein** **4 Hepatic Vein** **5 Superior Mesenteric Vein** Right gastroepiploic vein **6 Inferior Mesenteric Vein** Sigmoid vein Superior rectal vein **7 Colic Vein** Ileocolic vein Left colic vein Middle colic vein Right colic vein **8 Portal Vein** Hepatic portal vein **9 Renal Vein, Right** **B Renal Vein, Left** Left inferior phrenic vein Left ovarian vein Left second lumbar vein Left suprarenal vein Left testicular vein **C Common Iliac Vein, Right** **D Common Iliac Vein, Left** **F External Iliac Vein, Right** **G External Iliac Vein, Left**	**H Hypogastric Vein, Right** Gluteal vein Internal iliac vein Internal pudendal vein Lateral sacral vein Middle hemorrhoidal vein Obturator vein Uterine vein Vaginal vein Vesical vein **J Hypogastric Vein, Left** *See H Hypogastric Vein, Right* **M Femoral Vein, Right** Deep femoral (profunda femoris) vein Popliteal vein Profunda femoris (deep femoral) vein **N Femoral Vein, Left** *See M Femoral Vein, Right* **P Saphenous Vein, Right** External pudendal vein Great(er) saphenous vein Lesser saphenous vein Small saphenous vein Superficial circumflex iliac vein Superficial epigastric vein **Q Saphenous Vein, Left** *See P Saphenous Vein, Right* **T Foot Vein, Right** Common digital vein Dorsal metatarsal vein Dorsal venous arch Plantar digital vein Plantar metatarsal vein Plantar venous arch **V Foot Vein, Left** *See T Foot Vein, Right* **Y Lower Vein**	**Ø Open** **3 Percutaneous** **4 Percutaneous Endoscopic**	**Z No Device**	**Z No Qualifier**

Ø Medical and Surgical
6 Lower Veins
P Removal Definition: Taking out or off a device from a body part
Explanation: If a device is taken out and a similar device put in without cutting or puncturing the skin or mucous membrane, the procedure is coded to the root operation CHANGE. Otherwise, the procedure for taking out a device is coded to the root operation REMOVAL.

Body Part Character 4	Approach Character 5	Device Character 6	Qualifier Character 7
Y Lower Vein	**Ø Open** **3 Percutaneous** **4 Percutaneous Endoscopic**	**Ø Drainage Device** **2 Monitoring Device** **3 Infusion Device** **7 Autologous Tissue Substitute** **C Extraluminal Device** **D Intraluminal Device** **J Synthetic Substitute** **K Nonautologous Tissue Substitute** **Y Other Device**	**Z No Qualifier**
Y Lower Vein	**X External**	**Ø Drainage Device** **2 Monitoring Device** **3 Infusion Device** **D Intraluminal Device**	**Z No Qualifier**

Non-OR Ø6PY3[Ø,2,3]Z
Non-OR Ø6PY[3,4]YZ
Non-OR Ø6PYX[Ø,2,3,D]Z

Ø Medical and Surgical
6 Lower Veins
Q Repair Definition: Restoring, to the extent possible, a body part to its normal anatomic structure and function
Explanation: Used only when the method to accomplish the repair is not one of the other root operations

Body Part Character 4	Approach Character 5	Device Character 6	Qualifier Character 7
Ø Inferior Vena Cava Postcava Right inferior phrenic vein Right ovarian vein Right second lumbar vein Right suprarenal vein Right testicular vein **1 Splenic Vein** Left gastroepiploic vein Pancreatic vein **2 Gastric Vein** **3 Esophageal Vein** **4 Hepatic Vein** **5 Superior Mesenteric Vein** Right gastroepiploic vein **6 Inferior Mesenteric Vein** Sigmoid vein Superior rectal vein **7 Colic Vein** Ileocolic vein Left colic vein Middle colic vein Right colic vein **8 Portal Vein** Hepatic portal vein **9 Renal Vein, Right** **B Renal Vein, Left** Left inferior phrenic vein Left ovarian vein Left second lumbar vein Left suprarenal vein Left testicular vein **C Common Iliac Vein, Right** **D Common Iliac Vein, Left** **F External Iliac Vein, Right** **G External Iliac Vein, Left** **H Hypogastric Vein, Right** Gluteal vein Internal iliac vein Internal pudendal vein Lateral sacral vein Middle hemorrhoidal vein Obturator vein Uterine vein Vaginal vein Vesical vein **J Hypogastric Vein, Left** *See H Hypogastric Vein, Right* **M Femoral Vein, Right** Deep femoral (profunda femoris) vein Popliteal vein Profunda femoris (deep femoral) vein **N Femoral Vein, Left** *See M Femoral Vein, Right* **P Saphenous Vein, Right** External pudendal vein Great(er) saphenous vein Lesser saphenous vein Small saphenous vein Superficial circumflex iliac vein Superficial epigastric vein **Q Saphenous Vein, Left** *See P Saphenous Vein, Right* **T Foot Vein, Right** Common digital vein Dorsal metatarsal vein Dorsal venous arch Plantar digital vein Plantar metatarsal vein Plantar venous arch **V Foot Vein, Left** *See T Foot Vein, Right* **Y Lower Vein**	Ø Open 3 Percutaneous 4 Percutaneous Endoscopic	Z No Device	Z No Qualifier

Ø Medical and Surgical
6 Lower Veins
R Replacement Definition: Putting in or on biological or synthetic material that physically takes the place and/or function of all or a portion of a body part

Explanation: The body part may have been taken out or replaced, or may be taken out, physically eradicated, or rendered nonfunctional during the REPLACEMENT procedure. A REMOVAL procedure is coded for taking out the device used in a previous replacement procedure.

Body Part Character 4	Approach Character 5	Device Character 6	Qualifier Character 7
Ø Inferior Vena Cava Postcava Right inferior phrenic vein Right ovarian vein Right second lumbar vein Right suprarenal vein Right testicular vein **1 Splenic Vein** Left gastroepiploic vein Pancreatic vein **2 Gastric Vein** **3 Esophageal Vein** **4 Hepatic Vein** **5 Superior Mesenteric Vein** Right gastroepiploic vein **6 Inferior Mesenteric Vein** Sigmoid vein Superior rectal vein **7 Colic Vein** Ileocolic vein Left colic vein Middle colic vein Right colic vein **8 Portal Vein** Hepatic portal vein **9 Renal Vein, Right** **B Renal Vein, Left** Left inferior phrenic vein Left ovarian vein Left second lumbar vein Left suprarenal vein Left testicular vein **C Common Iliac Vein, Right** **D Common Iliac Vein, Left** **F External Iliac Vein, Right** **G External Iliac Vein, Left** **H Hypogastric Vein, Right** Gluteal vein Internal iliac vein Internal pudendal vein Lateral sacral vein Middle hemorrhoidal vein Obturator vein Uterine vein Vaginal vein Vesical vein **J Hypogastric Vein, Left** *See H Hypogastric Vein, Right* **M Femoral Vein, Right** Deep femoral (profunda femoris) vein Popliteal vein Profunda femoris (deep femoral) vein **N Femoral Vein, Left** *See M Femoral Vein, Right* **P Saphenous Vein, Right** External pudendal vein Great(er) saphenous vein Lesser saphenous vein Small saphenous vein Superficial circumflex iliac vein Superficial epigastric vein **Q Saphenous Vein, Left** *See P Saphenous Vein, Right* **T Foot Vein, Right** Common digital vein Dorsal metatarsal vein Dorsal venous arch Plantar digital vein Plantar metatarsal vein Plantar venous arch **V Foot Vein, Left** *See T Foot Vein, Right* **Y Lower Vein**	**Ø Open** **4 Percutaneous Endoscopic**	**7 Autologous Tissue Substitute** **J Synthetic Substitute** **K Nonautologous Tissue Substitute**	**Z No Qualifier**

Ø Medical and Surgical
6 Lower Veins
S Reposition Definition: Moving to its normal location, or other suitable location, all or a portion of a body part

Explanation: The body part is moved to a new location from an abnormal location, or from a normal location where it is not functioning correctly. The body part may or may not be cut out or off to be moved to the new location.

Body Part Character 4	Approach Character 5	Device Character 6	Qualifier Character 7
Ø Inferior Vena Cava Postcava Right inferior phrenic vein Right ovarian vein Right second lumbar vein Right suprarenal vein Right testicular vein **1 Splenic Vein** Left gastroepiploic vein Pancreatic vein **2 Gastric Vein** **3 Esophageal Vein** **4 Hepatic Vein** **5 Superior Mesenteric Vein** Right gastroepiploic vein **6 Inferior Mesenteric Vein** Sigmoid vein Superior rectal vein **7 Colic Vein** Ileocolic vein Left colic vein Middle colic vein Right colic vein **8 Portal Vein** Hepatic portal vein **9 Renal Vein, Right** **B Renal Vein, Left** Left inferior phrenic vein Left ovarian vein Left second lumbar vein Left suprarenal vein Left testicular vein **C Common Iliac Vein, Right** **D Common Iliac Vein, Left** **F External Iliac Vein, Right** **G External Iliac Vein, Left** **H Hypogastric Vein, Right** Gluteal vein Internal iliac vein Internal pudendal vein Lateral sacral vein Middle hemorrhoidal vein Obturator vein Uterine vein Vaginal vein Vesical vein **J Hypogastric Vein, Left** *See H Hypogastric Vein, Right* **M Femoral Vein, Right** Deep femoral (profunda femoris) vein Popliteal vein Profunda femoris (deep femoral) vein **N Femoral Vein, Left** *See M Femoral Vein, Right* **P Saphenous Vein, Right** External pudendal vein Great(er) saphenous vein Lesser saphenous vein Small saphenous vein Superficial circumflex iliac vein Superficial epigastric vein **Q Saphenous Vein, Left** *See P Saphenous Vein, Right* **T Foot Vein, Right** Common digital vein Dorsal metatarsal vein Dorsal venous arch Plantar digital vein Plantar metatarsal vein Plantar venous arch **V Foot Vein, Left** *See T Foot Vein, Right* **Y Lower Vein**	**Ø Open** **3 Percutaneous** **4 Percutaneous Endoscopic**	**Z No Device**	**Z No Qualifier**

Ø Medical and Surgical
6 Lower Veins
U Supplement Definition: Putting in or on biological or synthetic material that physically reinforces and/or augments the function of a portion of a body part
Explanation: The biological material is non-living, or is living and from the same individual. The body part may have been previously replaced, and the SUPPLEMENT procedure is performed to physically reinforce and/or augment the function of the replaced body part.

Body Part Character 4	Approach Character 5	Device Character 6	Qualifier Character 7
Ø Inferior Vena Cava Postcava Right inferior phrenic vein Right ovarian vein Right second lumbar vein Right suprarenal vein Right testicular vein **1 Splenic Vein** Left gastroepiploic vein Pancreatic vein **2 Gastric Vein** **3 Esophageal Vein** **4 Hepatic Vein** **5 Superior Mesenteric Vein** Right gastroepiploic vein **6 Inferior Mesenteric Vein** Sigmoid vein Superior rectal vein **7 Colic Vein** Ileocolic vein Left colic vein Middle colic vein Right colic vein **8 Portal Vein** Hepatic portal vein **9 Renal Vein, Right** **B Renal Vein, Left** Left inferior phrenic vein Left ovarian vein Left second lumbar vein Left suprarenal vein Left testicular vein **C Common Iliac Vein, Right** **D Common Iliac Vein, Left** **F External Iliac Vein, Right** **G External Iliac Vein, Left** **H Hypogastric Vein, Right** Gluteal vein Internal iliac vein Internal pudendal vein Lateral sacral vein Middle hemorrhoidal vein Obturator vein Uterine vein Vaginal vein Vesical vein **J Hypogastric Vein, Left** *See H Hypogastric Vein, Right* **M Femoral Vein, Right** Deep femoral (profunda femoris) vein Popliteal vein Profunda femoris (deep femoral) vein **N Femoral Vein, Left** *See M Femoral Vein, Right* **P Saphenous Vein, Right** External pudendal vein Great(er) saphenous vein Lesser saphenous vein Small saphenous vein Superficial circumflex iliac vein Superficial epigastric vein **Q Saphenous Vein, Left** *See P Saphenous Vein, Right* **T Foot Vein, Right** Common digital vein Dorsal metatarsal vein Dorsal venous arch Plantar digital vein Plantar metatarsal vein Plantar venous arch **V Foot Vein, Left** *See T Foot Vein, Right* **Y Lower Vein**	**Ø Open** **3 Percutaneous** **4 Percutaneous Endoscopic**	**7 Autologous Tissue Substitute** **J Synthetic Substitute** **K Nonautologous Tissue Substitute**	**Z No Qualifier**

Ø Medical and Surgical
6 Lower Veins
V Restriction Definition: Partially closing an orifice or the lumen of a tubular body part
Explanation: The orifice can be a natural orifice or an artificially created orifice

Body Part Character 4	Approach Character 5	Device Character 6	Qualifier Character 7
Ø Inferior Vena Cava Postcava Right inferior phrenic vein Right ovarian vein Right second lumbar vein Right suprarenal vein Right testicular vein **1 Splenic Vein** Left gastroepiploic vein Pancreatic vein **2 Gastric Vein** **3 Esophageal Vein** **4 Hepatic Vein** **5 Superior Mesenteric Vein** Right gastroepiploic vein **6 Inferior Mesenteric Vein** Sigmoid vein Superior rectal vein **7 Colic Vein** Ileocolic vein Left colic vein Middle colic vein Right colic vein **8 Portal Vein** Hepatic portal vein **9 Renal Vein, Right** **B Renal Vein, Left** Left inferior phrenic vein Left ovarian vein Left second lumbar vein Left suprarenal vein Left testicular vein **C Common Iliac Vein, Right** **D Common Iliac Vein, Left** **F External Iliac Vein, Right** **G External Iliac Vein, Left** **H Hypogastric Vein, Right** Gluteal vein Internal iliac vein Internal pudendal vein Lateral sacral vein Middle hemorrhoidal vein Obturator vein Uterine vein Vaginal vein Vesical vein **J Hypogastric Vein, Left** *See H Hypogastric Vein, Right* **M Femoral Vein, Right** Deep femoral (profunda femoris) vein Popliteal vein Profunda femoris (deep femoral) vein **N Femoral Vein, Left** *See M Femoral Vein, Right* **P Saphenous Vein, Right** External pudendal vein Great(er) saphenous vein Lesser saphenous vein Small saphenous vein Superficial circumflex iliac vein Superficial epigastric vein **Q Saphenous Vein, Left** *See P Saphenous Vein, Right* **T Foot Vein, Right** Common digital vein Dorsal metatarsal vein Dorsal venous arch Plantar digital vein Plantar metatarsal vein Plantar venous arch **V Foot Vein, Left** *See T Foot Vein, Right* **Y Lower Vein**	**Ø Open** **3 Percutaneous** **4 Percutaneous Endoscopic**	**C Extraluminal Device** **D Intraluminal Device** **Z No Device**	**Z No Qualifier**

Ø Medical and Surgical
6 Lower Veins
W Revision

Definition: Correcting, to the extent possible, a portion of a malfunctioning device or the position of a displaced device

Explanation: Revision can include correcting a malfunctioning or displaced device by taking out or putting in components of the device such as a screw or pin

Body Part Character 4	Approach Character 5	Device Character 6	Qualifier Character 7
Y Lower Vein	Ø Open 3 Percutaneous 4 Percutaneous Endoscopic	Ø Drainage Device 2 Monitoring Device 3 Infusion Device 7 Autologous Tissue Substitute C Extraluminal Device D Intraluminal Device J Synthetic Substitute K Nonautologous Tissue Substitute Y Other Device	Z No Qualifier
Y Lower Vein	X External	Ø Drainage Device 2 Monitoring Device 3 Infusion Device 7 Autologous Tissue Substitute C Extraluminal Device D Intraluminal Device J Synthetic Substitute K Nonautologous Tissue Substitute	Z No Qualifier

Non-OR Ø6WY3[Ø,2,3,D]Z
Non-OR Ø6WY[3,4]YZ
Non-OR Ø6WYX[Ø,2,3,7,C,D,J,K]Z

Lymphatic and Hemic Systems Ø72–Ø7Y

Character Meanings*

This Character Meaning table is provided as a guide to assist the user in the identification of character members that may be found in this section of code tables. It **SHOULD NOT** be used to build a PCS code.

Operation–Character 3	Body Part–Character 4	Approach–Character 5	Device–Character 6	Qualifier–Character 7
2 Change	Ø Lymphatic, Head	Ø Open	Ø Drainage Device	Ø Allogeneic
5 Destruction	1 Lymphatic, Right Neck	3 Percutaneous	3 Infusion Device	1 Syngeneic
9 Drainage	2 Lymphatic, Left Neck	4 Percutaneous Endoscopic	7 Autologous Tissue Substitute	2 Zooplastic
B Excision	3 Lymphatic, Right Upper Extremity	8 Via Natural or Artificial Opening Endoscopic	C Extraluminal Device	X Diagnostic
C Extirpation	4 Lymphatic, Left Upper Extremity	X External	D Intraluminal Device	Z No Qualifier
D Extraction	5 Lymphatic, Right Axillary		J Synthetic Substitute	
H Insertion	6 Lymphatic, Left Axillary		K Nonautologous Tissue Substitute	
J Inspection	7 Lymphatic, Thorax		Y Other Device	
L Occlusion	8 Lymphatic, Internal Mammary, Right		Z No Device	
N Release	9 Lymphatic, Internal Mammary, Left			
P Removal	B Lymphatic, Mesenteric			
Q Repair	C Lymphatic, Pelvis			
S Reposition	D Lymphatic, Aortic			
T Resection	F Lymphatic, Right Lower Extremity			
U Supplement	G Lymphatic, Left Lower Extremity			
V Restriction	H Lymphatic, Right Inguinal			
W Revision	J Lymphatic, Left Inguinal			
Y Transplantation	K Thoracic Duct			
	L Cisterna Chyli			
	M Thymus			
	N Lymphatic			
	P Spleen			
	Q Bone Marrow, Sternum			
	R Bone Marrow, Iliac			
	S Bone Marrow, Vertebral			
	T Bone Marrow			

* Includes lymph vessels and lymph nodes.

AHA Coding Clinic for table Ø79
2017, 1Q, 34 Lymphovenous bypass following mastectomy
2014, 1Q, 26 Transbronchial needle aspiration lymph node biopsy
2013, 4Q, 111 Transbronchial needle aspiration lymph node biopsy

AHA Coding Clinic for table Ø7B
2018, 1Q, 22 Resection of lymph node chains
2016, 1Q, 30 Axillary lymph node resection with modified radical mastectomy
2014, 3Q, 10 Selective excision of paratracheal lymph nodes
2014, 1Q, 20 Fiducial marker placement
2014, 1Q, 26 Transbronchial endoscopic lymph node aspiration biopsy

AHA Coding Clinic for table Ø7D
2013, 4Q, 111 Root operation for bone marrow biopsy

AHA Coding Clinic for table Ø7Q
2017, 1Q, 34 Lymphovenous bypass following mastectomy

AHA Coding Clinic for table Ø7T
2018, 1Q, 22 Resection of lymph node chains
2016, 2Q, 12 Resection of malignant neoplasm of infratemporal fossa
2016, 1Q, 30 Axillary lymph node resection with modified radical mastectomy
2015, 4Q, 13 New Section X codes—New Technology procedures
2014, 3Q, 9 Radical resection of level I lymph nodes
2014, 3Q, 16 Repair of Tetralogy of Fallot

Lymphatic System

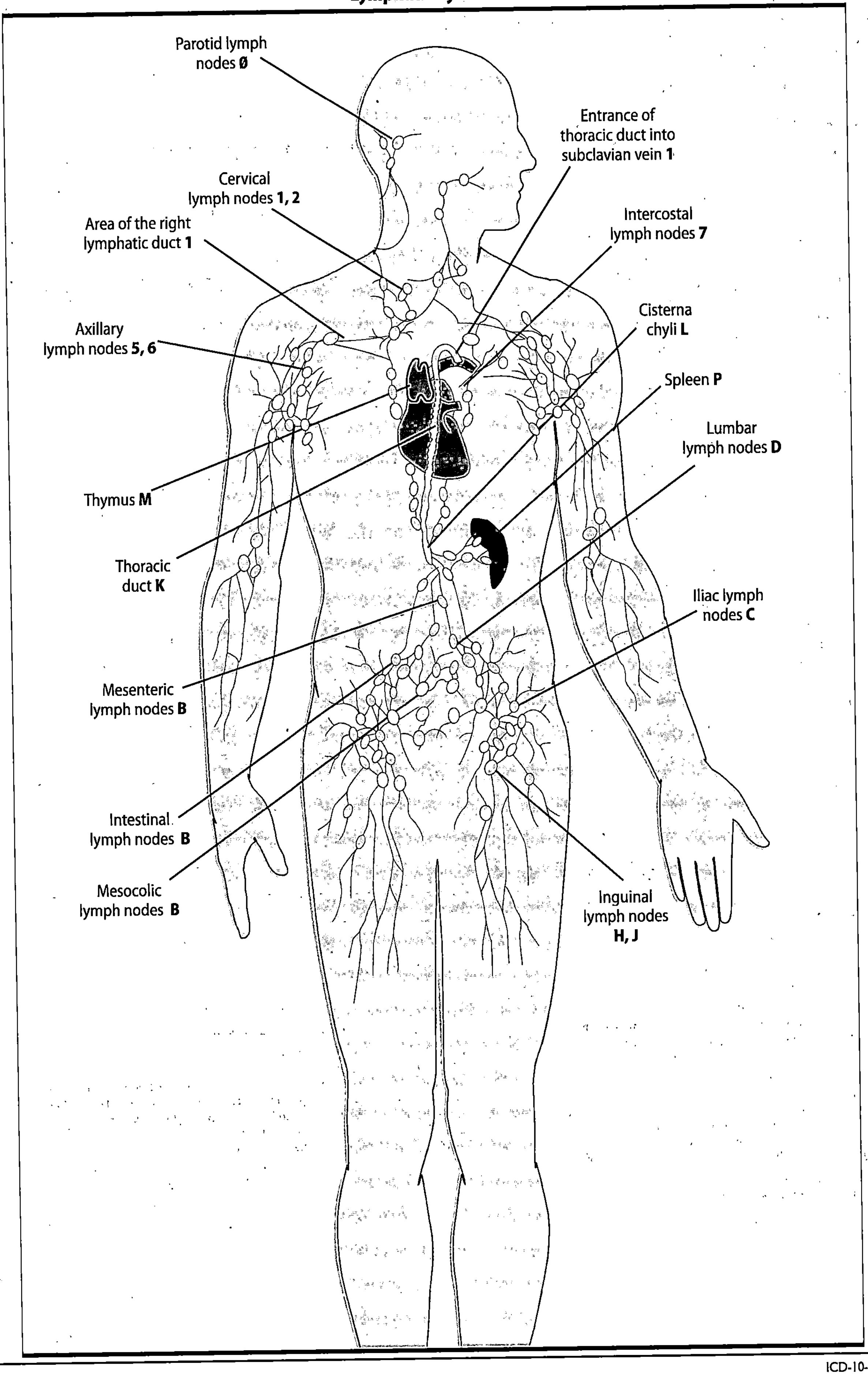
Parotid lymph nodes Ø
Entrance of thoracic duct into subclavian vein 1
Cervical lymph nodes 1, 2
Area of the right lymphatic duct 1
Intercostal lymph nodes 7
Cisterna chyli L
Axillary lymph nodes 5, 6
Spleen P
Lumbar lymph nodes D
Thymus M
Thoracic duct K
Iliac lymph nodes C
Mesenteric lymph nodes B
Intestinal lymph nodes B
Mesocolic lymph nodes B
Inguinal lymph nodes H, J

Ø Medical and Surgical
7 Lymphatic and Hemic Systems
2 Change Definition: Taking out or off a device from a body part and putting back an identical or similar device in or on the same body part without cutting or puncturing the skin or a mucous membrane

Explanation: All CHANGE procedures are coded using the approach EXTERNAL

Body Part Character 4		Approach Character 5	Device Character 6	Qualifier Character 7
K Thoracic Duct Left jugular trunk Left subclavian trunk **L** Cisterna Chyli Intestinal lymphatic trunk Lumbar lymphatic trunk	**M** Thymus Thymus gland **N** Lymphatic **P** Spleen Accessory spleen **T** Bone Marrow	**X** External	**Ø** Drainage Device **Y** Other Device	**Z** No Qualifier

Non-OR All body part, approach, device, and qualifier values

Ø Medical and Surgical
7 Lymphatic and Hemic Systems
5 Destruction Definition: Physical eradication of all or a portion of a body part by the direct use of energy, force, or a destructive agent

Explanation: None of the body part is physically taken out

Body Part Character 4		Approach Character 5	Device Character 6	Qualifier Character 7
Ø **Lymphatic, Head** Buccinator lymph node Infraauricular lymph node Infraparotid lymph node Parotid lymph node Preauricular lymph node Submandibular lymph node Submaxillary lymph node Submental lymph node Subparotid lymph node Suprahyoid lymph node **1** **Lymphatic, Right Neck** Cervical lymph node Jugular lymph node Mastoid (postauricular) lymph node Occipital lymph node Postauricular (mastoid) lymph node Retropharyngeal lymph node Right jugular trunk Right lymphatic duct Right subclavian trunk Supraclavicular (Virchow's) lymph node Virchow's (supraclavicular) lymph node **2** **Lymphatic, Left Neck** Cervical lymph node Jugular lymph node Mastoid (postauricular) lymph node Occipital lymph node Postauricular (mastoid) lymph node Retropharyngeal lymph node Supraclavicular (Virchow's) lymph node Virchow's (supraclavicular) lymph node **3** **Lymphatic, Right Upper Extremity** Cubital lymph node Deltopectoral (infraclavicular) lymph node Epitrochlear lymph node Infraclavicular (deltopectoral) lymph node Supratrochlear lymph node **4** **Lymphatic, Left Upper Extremity** *See 3 Lymphatic, Right Upper Extremity* **5** **Lymphatic, Right Axillary** Anterior (pectoral) lymph node Apical (subclavicular) lymph node Brachial (lateral) lymph node Central axillary lymph node Lateral (brachial) lymph node Pectoral (anterior) lymph node Posterior (subscapular) lymph node Subclavicular (apical) lymph node Subscapular (posterior) lymph node	**6** **Lymphatic, Left Axillary** *See 5 Lymphatic, Right Axillary* **7** **Lymphatic, Thorax** Intercostal lymph node Mediastinal lymph node Parasternal lymph node Paratracheal lymph node Tracheobronchial lymph node **8** **Lymphatic, Internal Mammary, Right** **9** **Lymphatic, Internal Mammary, Left** **B** **Lymphatic, Mesenteric** Inferior mesenteric lymph node Pararectal lymph node Superior mesenteric lymph node **C** **Lymphatic, Pelvis** Common iliac (subaortic) lymph node Gluteal lymph node Iliac lymph node Inferior epigastric lymph node Obturator lymph node Sacral lymph node Subaortic (common iliac) lymph node Suprainguinal lymph node **D** **Lymphatic, Aortic** Celiac lymph node Gastric lymph node Hepatic lymph node Lumbar lymph node Pancreaticosplenic lymph node Paraaortic lymph node Retroperitoneal lymph node **F** **Lymphatic, Right Lower Extremity** Femoral lymph node Popliteal lymph node **G** **Lymphatic, Left Lower Extremity** *See F Lymphatic, Right Lower Extremity* **H** **Lymphatic, Right Inguinal** **J** **Lymphatic, Left Inguinal** **K** **Thoracic Duct** Left jugular trunk Left subclavian trunk **L** **Cisterna Chyli** Intestinal lymphatic trunk Lumbar lymphatic trunk **M** **Thymus** Thymus gland **P** **Spleen** Accessory spleen	**Ø** Open **3** Percutaneous **4** Percutaneous Endoscopic	**Z** No Device	**Z** No Qualifier

Ø Medical and Surgical
7 Lymphatic and Hemic Systems
9 Drainage Definition: Taking or letting out fluids and/or gases from a body part
Explanation: The qualifier DIAGNOSTIC is used to identify drainage procedures that are biopsies

Body Part Character 4	Approach Character 5	Device Character 6	Qualifier Character 7
Ø Lymphatic, Head Buccinator lymph node Infraauricular lymph node Infraparotid lymph node Parotid lymph node Preauricular lymph node Submandibular lymph node Submaxillary lymph node Submental lymph node Subparotid lymph node Suprahyoid lymph node **1 Lymphatic, Right Neck** Cervical lymph node Jugular lymph node Mastoid (postauricular) lymph node Occipital lymph node Postauricular (mastoid) lymph node Retropharyngeal lymph node Right jugular trunk Right lymphatic duct Right subclavian trunk Supraclavicular (Virchow's) lymph node Virchow's (supraclavicular) lymph node **2 Lymphatic, Left Neck** Cervical lymph node Jugular lymph node Mastoid (postauricular) lymph node Occipital lymph node Postauricular (mastoid) lymph node Retropharyngeal lymph node Supraclavicular (Virchow's) lymph node Virchow's (supraclavicular) lymph node **3 Lymphatic, Right Upper Extremity** Cubital lymph node Deltopectoral (infraclavicular) lymph node Epitrochlear lymph node Infraclavicular (deltopectoral) lymph node Supratrochlear lymph node **4 Lymphatic, Left Upper Extremity** *See 3 Lymphatic, Right Upper Extremity* **5 Lymphatic, Right Axillary** Anterior (pectoral) lymph node Apical (subclavicular) lymph node Brachial (lateral) lymph node Central axillary lymph node Lateral (brachial) lymph node Pectoral (anterior) lymph node Posterior (subscapular) lymph node Subclavicular (apical) lymph node Subscapular (posterior) lymph node **6 Lymphatic, Left Axillary** *See 5 Lymphatic, Right Axillary* **7 Lymphatic, Thorax** Intercostal lymph node Mediastinal lymph node Parasternal lymph node Paratracheal lymph node Tracheobronchial lymph node **8 Lymphatic, Internal Mammary, Right** **9 Lymphatic, Internal Mammary, Left** **B Lymphatic, Mesenteric** Inferior mesenteric lymph node Pararectal lymph node Superior mesenteric lymph node **C Lymphatic, Pelvis** Common iliac (subaortic) lymph node Gluteal lymph node Iliac lymph node Inferior epigastric lymph node Obturator lymph node Sacral lymph node Subaortic (common iliac) lymph node Suprainguinal lymph node **D Lymphatic, Aortic** Celiac lymph node Gastric lymph node Hepatic lymph node Lumbar lymph node Pancreaticosplenic lymph node Paraaortic lymph node Retroperitoneal lymph node **F Lymphatic, Right Lower Extremity** Femoral lymph node Popliteal lymph node **G Lymphatic, Left Lower Extremity** *See F Lymphatic, Right Lower Extremity* **H Lymphatic, Right Inguinal** **J Lymphatic, Left Inguinal** **K Thoracic Duct** Left jugular trunk Left subclavian trunk **L Cisterna Chyli** Intestinal lymphatic trunk Lumbar lymphatic trunk	**Ø Open** **3 Percutaneous** **4 Percutaneous Endoscopic** **8 Via Natural or Artificial Opening Endoscopic**	**Ø Drainage Device**	**Z No Qualifier**

Ø79 Continued on next page

Non-OR Ø79[Ø,1,2,3,4,5,6,7,8,9,B,C,D,F,G,H,J,K,L][3,8]ØZ

Ø Medical and Surgical
7 Lymphatic and Hemic Systems
9 Drainage Definition: Taking or letting out fluids and/or gases from a body part
Explanation: The qualifier DIAGNOSTIC is used to identify drainage procedures that are biopsies

Ø79 Continued

Body Part Character 4	Approach Character 5	Device Character 6	Qualifier Character 7
Ø Lymphatic, Head Buccinator lymph node Infraauricular lymph node Infraparotid lymph node Parotid lymph node Preauricular lymph node Submandibular lymph node Submaxillary lymph node Submental lymph node Subparotid lymph node Suprahyoid lymph node **1 Lymphatic, Right Neck** Cervical lymph node Jugular lymph node Mastoid (postauricular) lymph node Occipital lymph node Postauricular (mastoid) lymph node Retropharyngeal lymph node Right jugular trunk Right lymphatic duct Right subclavian trunk Supraclavicular (Virchow's) lymph node Virchow's (supraclavicular) lymph node **2 Lymphatic, Left Neck** Cervical lymph node Jugular lymph node Mastoid (postauricular) lymph node Occipital lymph node Postauricular (mastoid) lymph node Retropharyngeal lymph node Supraclavicular (Virchow's) lymph node Virchow's (supraclavicular) lymph node **3 Lymphatic, Right Upper Extremity** Cubital lymph node Deltopectoral (infraclavicular) lymph node Epitrochlear lymph node Infraclavicular (deltopectoral) lymph node Supratrochlear lymph node **4 Lymphatic, Left Upper Extremity** *See 3 Lymphatic, Right Upper Extremity* **5 Lymphatic, Right Axillary** Anterior (pectoral) lymph node Apical (subclavicular) lymph node Brachial (lateral) lymph node Central axillary lymph node Lateral (brachial) lymph node Pectoral (anterior) lymph node Posterior (subscapular) lymph node Subclavicular (apical) lymph node Subscapular (posterior) lymph node **6 Lymphatic, Left Axillary** *See 5 Lymphatic, Right Axillary* **7 Lymphatic, Thorax** Intercostal lymph node Mediastinal lymph node Parasternal lymph node Paratracheal lymph node Tracheobronchial lymph node **8 Lymphatic, Internal Mammary, Right** **9 Lymphatic, Internal Mammary, Left** **B Lymphatic, Mesenteric** Inferior mesenteric lymph node Pararectal lymph node Superior mesenteric lymph node **C Lymphatic, Pelvis** Common iliac (subaortic) lymph node Gluteal lymph node Iliac lymph node Inferior epigastric lymph node Obturator lymph node Sacral lymph node Subaortic (common iliac) lymph node Suprainguinal lymph node **D Lymphatic, Aortic** Celiac lymph node Gastric lymph node Hepatic lymph node Lumbar lymph node Pancreaticosplenic lymph node Paraaortic lymph node Retroperitoneal lymph node **F Lymphatic, Right Lower Extremity** Femoral lymph node Popliteal lymph node **G Lymphatic, Left Lower Extremity** *See F Lymphatic, Right Lower Extremity* **H Lymphatic, Right Inguinal** **J Lymphatic, Left Inguinal** **K Thoracic Duct** Left jugular trunk Left subclavian trunk **L Cisterna Chyli** Intestinal lymphatic trunk Lumbar lymphatic trunk	**Ø** Open **3** Percutaneous **4** Percutaneous Endoscopic **8** Via Natural or Artificial Opening Endoscopic	**Z** No Device	**X** Diagnostic **Z** No Qualifier
M Thymus Thymus gland **P Spleen** Accessory spleen **T Bone Marrow**	**Ø** Open **3** Percutaneous **4** Percutaneous Endoscopic	**Ø** Drainage Device	**Z** No Qualifier
M Thymus Thymus gland **P Spleen** Accessory spleen **T Bone Marrow**	**Ø** Open **3** Percutaneous **4** Percutaneous Endoscopic	**Z** No Device	**X** Diagnostic **Z** No Qualifier

Non-OR Ø79[Ø,1,2,3,4,5,6,7,8,9,B,C,D,F,G,H,J,K,L]8ZX
Non-OR Ø79[Ø,1,2,3,4,5,6,7,8,9,B,C,D,F,G,H,J,K,L][3,8]ZZ
Non-OR Ø79M3ØZ
Non-OR Ø79P[3,4]ØZ
Non-OR Ø79T[Ø,3,4]ØZ
Non-OR Ø79M3ZZ
Non-OR Ø79P[3,4]Z[X,Z]
Non-OR Ø79T[Ø,3,4]Z[X,Z]

Ø Medical and Surgical
7 Lymphatic and Hemic Systems
B Excision Definition: Cutting out or off, without replacement, a portion of a body part
Explanation: The qualifier DIAGNOSTIC is used to identify excision procedures that are biopsies

Body Part Character 4	Approach Character 5	Device Character 6	Qualifier Character 7
Ø Lymphatic, Head Buccinator lymph node Infraauricular lymph node Infraparotid lymph node Parotid lymph node Preauricular lymph node Submandibular lymph node Submaxillary lymph node Submental lymph node Subparotid lymph node Suprahyoid lymph node **1 Lymphatic, Right Neck** Cervical lymph node Jugular lymph node Mastoid (postauricular) lymph node Occipital lymph node Postauricular (mastoid) lymph node Retropharyngeal lymph node Right jugular trunk Right lymphatic duct Right subclavian trunk Supraclavicular (Virchow's) lymph node Virchow's (supraclavicular) lymph node **2 Lymphatic, Left Neck** Cervical lymph node Jugular lymph node Mastoid (postauricular) lymph node Occipital lymph node Postauricular (mastoid) lymph node Retropharyngeal lymph node Supraclavicular (Virchow's) lymph node Virchow's (supraclavicular) lymph node **3 Lymphatic, Right Upper Extremity** Cubital lymph node Deltopectoral (infraclavicular) lymph node Epitrochlear lymph node Infraclavicular (deltopectoral) lymph node Supratrochlear lymph node **4 Lymphatic, Left Upper Extremity** *See 3 Lymphatic, Right Upper Extremity* **5 Lymphatic, Right Axillary** Anterior (pectoral) lymph node Apical (subclavicular) lymph node Brachial (lateral) lymph node Central axillary lymph node Lateral (brachial) lymph node Pectoral (anterior) lymph node Posterior (subscapular) lymph node Subclavicular (apical) lymph node Subscapular (posterior) lymph node **6 Lymphatic, Left Axillary** *See 5 Lymphatic, Right Axillary* **7 Lymphatic, Thorax** Intercostal lymph node Mediastinal lymph node Parasternal lymph node Paratracheal lymph node Tracheobronchial lymph node **8 Lymphatic, Internal Mammary, Right** **9 Lymphatic, Internal Mammary, Left** **B Lymphatic, Mesenteric** Inferior mesenteric lymph node Pararectal lymph node Superior mesenteric lymph node **C Lymphatic, Pelvis** Common iliac (subaortic) lymph node Gluteal lymph node Iliac lymph node Inferior epigastric lymph node Obturator lymph node Sacral lymph node Subaortic (common iliac) lymph node Suprainguinal lymph node **D Lymphatic, Aortic** Celiac lymph node Gastric lymph node Hepatic lymph node Lumbar lymph node Pancreaticosplenic lymph node Paraaortic lymph node Retroperitoneal lymph node **F Lymphatic, Right Lower Extremity** Femoral lymph node Popliteal lymph node **G Lymphatic, Left Lower Extremity** *See F Lymphatic, Right Lower Extremity* **H Lymphatic, Right Inguinal** ⊞ **J Lymphatic, Left Inguinal** ⊞ **K Thoracic Duct** Left jugular trunk Left subclavian trunk **L Cisterna Chyli** Intestinal lymphatic trunk Lumbar lymphatic trunk **M Thymus** Thymus gland **P Spleen** Accessory spleen	**Ø Open** **3 Percutaneous** **4 Percutaneous Endoscopic**	**Z No Device**	**X Diagnostic** **Z No Qualifier**

Non-OR Ø7BP[3,4]ZX

See Appendix L for Procedure Combinations
⊞ Ø7B[H,J][Ø,4]ZZ

Ø Medical and Surgical
7 Lymphatic and Hemic Systems
C Extirpation Definition: Taking or cutting out solid matter from a body part

Explanation: The solid matter may be an abnormal byproduct of a biological function or a foreign body; it may be imbedded in a body part or in the lumen of a tubular body part. The solid matter may or may not have been previously broken into pieces.

Body Part Character 4	Approach Character 5	Device Character 6	Qualifier Character 7
Ø Lymphatic, Head Buccinator lymph node Infraauricular lymph node Infraparotid lymph node Parotid lymph node Preauricular lymph node Submandibular lymph node Submaxillary lymph node Submental lymph node Subparotid lymph node Suprahyoid lymph node **1 Lymphatic, Right Neck** Cervical lymph node Jugular lymph node Mastoid (postauricular) lymph node Occipital lymph node Postauricular (mastoid) lymph node Retropharyngeal lymph node Right jugular trunk Right lymphatic duct Right subclavian trunk Supraclavicular (Virchow's) lymph node Virchow's (supraclavicular) lymph node **2 Lymphatic, Left Neck** Cervical lymph node Jugular lymph node Mastoid (postauricular) lymph node Occipital lymph node Postauricular (mastoid) lymph node Retropharyngeal lymph node Supraclavicular (Virchow's) lymph node Virchow's (supraclavicular) lymph node **3 Lymphatic, Right Upper Extremity** Cubital lymph node Deltopectoral (infraclavicular) lymph node Epitrochlear lymph node Infraclavicular (deltopectoral) lymph node Supratrochlear lymph node **4 Lymphatic, Left Upper Extremity** *See 3 Lymphatic, Right Upper Extremity* **5 Lymphatic, Right Axillary** Anterior (pectoral) lymph node Apical (subclavicular) lymph node Brachial (lateral) lymph node Central axillary lymph node Lateral (brachial) lymph node Pectoral (anterior) lymph node Posterior (subscapular) lymph node Subclavicular (apical) lymph node Subscapular (posterior) lymph node **6 Lymphatic, Left Axillary** *See 5 Lymphatic, Right Axillary* **7 Lymphatic, Thorax** Intercostal lymph node Mediastinal lymph node Parasternal lymph node Paratracheal lymph node Tracheobronchial lymph node **8 Lymphatic, Internal Mammary, Right** **9 Lymphatic, Internal Mammary, Left** **B Lymphatic, Mesenteric** Inferior mesenteric lymph node Pararectal lymph node Superior mesenteric lymph node **C Lymphatic, Pelvis** Common iliac (subaortic) lymph node Gluteal lymph node Iliac lymph node Inferior epigastric lymph node Obturator lymph node Sacral lymph node Subaortic (common iliac) lymph node Suprainguinal lymph node **D Lymphatic, Aortic** Celiac lymph node Gastric lymph node Hepatic lymph node Lumbar lymph node Pancreaticosplenic lymph node Paraaortic lymph node Retroperitoneal lymph node **F Lymphatic, Right Lower Extremity** Femoral lymph node Popliteal lymph node **G Lymphatic, Left Lower Extremity** *See F Lymphatic, Right Lower Extremity* **H Lymphatic, Right Inguinal** **J Lymphatic, Left Inguinal** **K Thoracic Duct** Left jugular trunk Left subclavian trunk **L Cisterna Chyli** Intestinal lymphatic trunk Lumbar lymphatic trunk **M Thymus** Thymus gland **P Spleen** Accessory spleen	Ø Open 3 Percutaneous 4 Percutaneous Endoscopic	Z No Device	Z No Qualifier

Non-OR Ø7CP[3,4]ZZ

Ø Medical and Surgical
7 Lymphatic and Hemic Systems
D Extraction Definition: Pulling or stripping out or off all or a portion of a body part by the use of force
Explanation: The qualifier DIAGNOSTIC is used to identify extraction procedures that are biopsies

Body Part Character 4	Approach Character 5	Device Character 6	Qualifier Character 7
Ø Lymphatic, Head Buccinator lymph node Infraauricular lymph node Infraparotid lymph node Parotid lymph node Preauricular lymph node Submandibular lymph node Submaxillary lymph node Submental lymph node Subparotid lymph node Suprahyoid lymph node **1 Lymphatic, Right Neck** Cervical lymph node Jugular lymph node Mastoid (postauricular) lymph node Occipital lymph node Postauricular (mastoid) lymph node Retropharyngeal lymph node Right jugular trunk Right lymphatic duct Right subclavian trunk Supraclavicular (Virchow's) lymph node Virchow's (supraclavicular) lymph node **2 Lymphatic, Left Neck** Cervical lymph node Jugular lymph node Mastoid (postauricular) lymph node Occipital lymph node Postauricular (mastoid) lymph node Retropharyngeal lymph node Supraclavicular (Virchow's) lymph node Virchow's (supraclavicular) lymph node **3 Lymphatic, Right Upper Extremity** Cubital lymph node Deltopectoral (infraclavicular) lymph node Epitrochlear lymph node Infraclavicular (deltopectoral) lymph node Supratrochlear lymph node **4 Lymphatic, Left Upper Extremity** *See 3 Lymphatic, Right Upper Extremity* **5 Lymphatic, Right Axillary** Anterior (pectoral) lymph node Apical (subclavicular) lymph node Brachial (lateral) lymph node Central axillary lymph node Lateral (brachial) lymph node Pectoral (anterior) lymph node Posterior (subscapular) lymph node Subclavicular (apical) lymph node Subscapular (posterior) lymph node **6 Lymphatic, Left Axillary** *See 5 Lymphatic, Right Axillary* **7 Lymphatic, Thorax** Intercostal lymph node Mediastinal lymph node Parasternal lymph node Paratracheal lymph node Tracheobronchial lymph node **8 Lymphatic, Internal Mammary, Right** **9 Lymphatic, Internal Mammary, Left** **B Lymphatic, Mesenteric** Inferior mesenteric lymph node Pararectal lymph node Superior mesenteric lymph node **C Lymphatic, Pelvis** Common iliac (subaortic) lymph node Gluteal lymph node Iliac lymph node Inferior epigastric lymph node Obturator lymph node Sacral lymph node Subaortic (common iliac) lymph node Suprainguinal lymph node **D Lymphatic, Aortic** Celiac lymph node Gastric lymph node Hepatic lymph node Lumbar lymph node Pancreaticosplenic lymph node Paraaortic lymph node Retroperitoneal lymph node **F Lymphatic, Right Lower Extremity** Femoral lymph node Popliteal lymph node **G Lymphatic, Left Lower Extremity** *See F Lymphatic, Right Lower Extremity* **H Lymphatic, Right Inguinal** **J Lymphatic, Left Inguinal** **K Thoracic Duct** Left jugular trunk Left subclavian trunk **L Cisterna Chyli** Intestinal lymphatic trunk Lumbar lymphatic trunk	**3 Percutaneous** **4 Percutaneous Endoscopic** **8 Via Natural or Artificial Opening Endoscopic**	**Z No Device**	**X Diagnostic**
M Thymus Thymus gland **P Spleen** Accessory spleen	**3 Percutaneous** **4 Percutaneous Endoscopic**	**Z No Device**	**X Diagnostic**
Q Bone Marrow, Sternum **R Bone Marrow, Iliac** **S Bone Marrow, Vertebral**	**Ø Open** **3 Percutaneous**	**Z No Device**	**X Diagnostic** **Z No Qualifier**

Non-OR All body part, approach, device, and qualifier values

Ø Medical and Surgical
7 Lymphatic and Hemic Systems
H Insertion Definition: Putting in a nonbiological appliance that monitors, assists, performs, or prevents a physiological function but does not physically take the place of a body part

Explanation: None

Body Part Character 4	Approach Character 5	Device Character 6	Qualifier Character 7
K Thoracic Duct Left jugular trunk Left subclavian trunk **L** Cisterna Chyli Intestinal lymphatic trunk Lumbar lymphatic trunk **M** Thymus Thymus gland **N** Lymphatic **P** Spleen Accessory spleen	**Ø** Open **3** Percutaneous **4** Percutaneous Endoscopic	**3** Infusion Device **Y** Other Device	**Z** No Qualifier

Non-OR Ø7H[K,L,M,N,P][Ø,3,4]3Z
Non-OR Ø7H[K,L,M]3YZ
Non-OR Ø7H[N,P][3,4]YZ

Ø Medical and Surgical
7 Lymphatic and Hemic Systems
J Inspection Definition: Visually and/or manually exploring a body part

Explanation: Visual exploration may be performed with or without optical instrumentation. Manual exploration may be performed directly or through intervening body layers.

Body Part Character 4	Approach Character 5	Device Character 6	Qualifier Character 7
K Thoracic Duct Left jugular trunk Left subclavian trunk **L** Cisterna Chyli Intestinal lymphatic trunk Lumbar lymphatic trunk **M** Thymus Thymus gland **T** Bone Marrow	**Ø** Open **3** Percutaneous **4** Percutaneous Endoscopic	**Z** No Device	**Z** No Qualifier
N Lymphatic	**Ø** Open **3** Percutaneous **4** Percutaneous Endoscopic **8** Via Natural or Artificial Opening Endoscopic **X** External	**Z** No Device	**Z** No Qualifier
P Spleen Accessory spleen	**Ø** Open **3** Percutaneous **4** Percutaneous Endoscopic **X** External	**Z** No Device	**Z** No Qualifier

Non-OR Ø7J[K,L,M]3ZZ
Non-OR Ø7JT[Ø,3,4]ZZ
Non-OR Ø7JN[3,8,X]ZZ
Non-OR Ø7JP[3,4,X]ZZ

Ø Medical and Surgical
7 Lymphatic and Hemic Systems
L Occlusion Definition: Completely closing an orifice or the lumen of a tubular body part
Explanation: The orifice can be a natural orifice or an artificially created orifice

Body Part Character 4	Approach Character 5	Device Character 6	Qualifier Character 7
Ø Lymphatic, Head Buccinator lymph node Infraauricular lymph node Infraparotid lymph node Parotid lymph node Preauricular lymph node Submandibular lymph node Submaxillary lymph node Submental lymph node Subparotid lymph node Suprahyoid lymph node **1 Lymphatic, Right Neck** Cervical lymph node Jugular lymph node Mastoid (postauricular) lymph node Occipital lymph node Postauricular (mastoid) lymph node Retropharyngeal lymph node Right jugular trunk Right lymphatic duct Right subclavian trunk Supraclavicular (Virchow's) lymph node Virchow's (supraclavicular) lymph node **2 Lymphatic, Left Neck** Cervical lymph node Jugular lymph node Mastoid (postauricular) lymph node Occipital lymph node Postauricular (mastoid) lymph node Retropharyngeal lymph node Supraclavicular (Virchow's) lymph node Virchow's (supraclavicular) lymph node **3 Lymphatic, Right Upper Extremity** Cubital lymph node Deltopectoral (infraclavicular) lymph node Epitrochlear lymph node Infraclavicular (deltopectoral) lymph node Supratrochlear lymph node **4 Lymphatic, Left Upper Extremity** *See 3 Lymphatic, Right Upper Extremity* **5 Lymphatic, Right Axillary** Anterior (pectoral) lymph node Apical (subclavicular) lymph node Brachial (lateral) lymph node Central axillary lymph node Lateral (brachial) lymph node Pectoral (anterior) lymph node Posterior (subscapular) lymph node Subclavicular (apical) lymph node Subscapular (posterior) lymph node **6 Lymphatic, Left Axillary** *See 5 Lymphatic, Right Axillary* **7 Lymphatic, Thorax** Intercostal lymph node Mediastinal lymph node Parasternal lymph node Paratracheal lymph node Tracheobronchial lymph node **8 Lymphatic, Internal Mammary, Right** **9 Lymphatic, Internal Mammary, Left** **B Lymphatic, Mesenteric** Inferior mesenteric lymph node Pararectal lymph node Superior mesenteric lymph node **C Lymphatic, Pelvis** Common iliac (subaortic) lymph node Gluteal lymph node Iliac lymph node Inferior epigastric lymph node Obturator lymph node Sacral lymph node Subaortic (common iliac) lymph node Suprainguinal lymph node **D Lymphatic, Aortic** Celiac lymph node Gastric lymph node Hepatic lymph node Lumbar lymph node Pancreaticosplenic lymph node Paraaortic lymph node Retroperitoneal lymph node **F Lymphatic, Right Lower Extremity** Femoral lymph node Popliteal lymph node **G Lymphatic, Left Lower Extremity** *See F Lymphatic, Right Lower Extremity* **H Lymphatic, Right Inguinal** **J Lymphatic, Left Inguinal** **K Thoracic Duct** Left jugular trunk Left subclavian trunk **L Cisterna Chyli** Intestinal lymphatic trunk Lumbar lymphatic trunk	**Ø** Open **3** Percutaneous **4** Percutaneous Endoscopic	**C** Extraluminal Device **D** Intraluminal Device **Z** No Device	**Z** No Qualifier

Ø Medical and Surgical
7 Lymphatic and Hemic Systems
N Release Definition: Freeing a body part from an abnormal physical constraint by cutting or by the use of force
Explanation: Some of the restraining tissue may be taken out but none of the body part is taken out

Body Part Character 4	Approach Character 5	Device Character 6	Qualifier Character 7
Ø Lymphatic, Head Buccinator lymph node Infraauricular lymph node Infraparotid lymph node Parotid lymph node Preauricular lymph node Submandibular lymph node Submaxillary lymph node Submental lymph node Subparotid lymph node Suprahyoid lymph node **1 Lymphatic, Right Neck** Cervical lymph node Jugular lymph node Mastoid (postauricular) lymph node Occipital lymph node Postauricular (mastoid) lymph node Retropharyngeal lymph node Right jugular trunk Right lymphatic duct Right subclavian trunk Supraclavicular (Virchow's) lymph node Virchow's (supraclavicular) lymph node **2 Lymphatic, Left Neck** Cervical lymph node Jugular lymph node Mastoid (postauricular) lymph node Occipital lymph node Postauricular (mastoid) lymph node Retropharyngeal lymph node Supraclavicular (Virchow's) lymph node Virchow's (supraclavicular) lymph node **3 Lymphatic, Right Upper Extremity** Cubital lymph node Deltopectoral (infraclavicular) lymph node Epitrochlear lymph node Infraclavicular (deltopectoral) lymph node Supratrochlear lymph node **4 Lymphatic, Left Upper Extremity** *See 3 Lymphatic, Right Upper Extremity* **5 Lymphatic, Right Axillary** Anterior (pectoral) lymph node Apical (subclavicular) lymph node Brachial (lateral) lymph node Central axillary lymph node Lateral (brachial) lymph node Pectoral (anterior) lymph node Posterior (subscapular) lymph node Subclavicular (apical) lymph node Subscapular (posterior) lymph node **6 Lymphatic, Left Axillary** *See 5 Lymphatic, Right Axillary* **7 Lymphatic, Thorax** Intercostal lymph node Mediastinal lymph node Parasternal lymph node Paratracheal lymph node Tracheobronchial lymph node **8 Lymphatic, Internal Mammary, Right** **9 Lymphatic, Internal Mammary, Left** **B Lymphatic, Mesenteric** Inferior mesenteric lymph node Pararectal lymph node Superior mesenteric lymph node **C Lymphatic, Pelvis** Common iliac (subaortic) lymph node Gluteal lymph node Iliac lymph node Inferior epigastric lymph node Obturator lymph node Sacral lymph node Subaortic (common iliac) lymph node Suprainguinal lymph node **D Lymphatic, Aortic** Celiac lymph node Gastric lymph node Hepatic lymph node Lumbar lymph node Pancreaticosplenic lymph node Paraaortic lymph node Retroperitoneal lymph node **F Lymphatic, Right Lower Extremity** Femoral lymph node Popliteal lymph node **G Lymphatic, Left Lower Extremity** *See F Lymphatic, Right Lower Extremity* **H Lymphatic, Right Inguinal** **J Lymphatic, Left Inguinal** **K Thoracic Duct** Left jugular trunk Left subclavian trunk **L Cisterna Chyli** Intestinal lymphatic trunk Lumbar lymphatic trunk **M Thymus** Thymus gland **P Spleen** Accessory spleen	**Ø Open** **3 Percutaneous** **4 Percutaneous Endoscopic**	**Z No Device**	**Z No Qualifier**

Ø Medical and Surgical
7 Lymphatic and Hemic Systems
P Removal Definition: Taking out or off a device from a body part

Explanation: If a device is taken out and a similar device put in without cutting or puncturing the skin or mucous membrane, the procedure is coded to the root operation CHANGE. Otherwise, the procedure for taking out a device is coded to the root operation REMOVAL.

Body Part Character 4	Approach Character 5	Device Character 6	Qualifier Character 7
K Thoracic Duct Left jugular trunk Left subclavian trunk **L** Cisterna Chyli Intestinal lymphatic trunk Lumbar lymphatic trunk **N** Lymphatic	**Ø** Open **3** Percutaneous **4** Percutaneous Endoscopic	**Ø** Drainage Device **3** Infusion Device **7** Autologous Tissue Substitute **C** Extraluminal Device **D** Intraluminal Device **J** Synthetic Substitute **K** Nonautologous Tissue Substitute **Y** Other Device	**Z** No Qualifier
K Thoracic Duct Left jugular trunk Left subclavian trunk **L** Cisterna Chyli Intestinal lymphatic trunk Lumbar lymphatic trunk **N** Lymphatic	**X** External	**Ø** Drainage Device **3** Infusion Device **D** Intraluminal Device	**Z** No Qualifier
M Thymus Thymus gland **P** Spleen Accessory spleen	**Ø** Open **3** Percutaneous **4** Percutaneous Endoscopic	**Ø** Drainage Device **3** Infusion Device **Y** Other Device	**Z** No Qualifier
M Thymus Thymus gland **P** Spleen Accessory spleen	**X** External	**Ø** Drainage Device **3** Infusion Device	**Z** No Qualifier
T Bone Marrow	**Ø** Open **3** Percutaneous **4** Percutaneous Endoscopic **X** External	**Ø** Drainage Device	**Z** No Qualifier

Non-OR Ø7P[K,L,N][3,4]YZ
Non-OR Ø7P[K,L,N]X[Ø,3,D]Z
Non-OR Ø7P[M,P][3,4]YZ
Non-OR Ø7P[M,P]X[Ø,3]Z
Non-OR Ø7PT[Ø,3,4,X]ØZ

Ø Medical and Surgical
7 Lymphatic and Hemic Systems
Q Repair Definition: Restoring, to the extent possible, a body part to its normal anatomic structure and function
Explanation: Used only when the method to accomplish the repair is not one of the other root operations

Body Part Character 4	Approach Character 5	Device Character 6	Qualifier Character 7
Ø Lymphatic, Head Buccinator lymph node Infraauricular lymph node Infraparotid lymph node Parotid lymph node Preauricular lymph node Submandibular lymph node Submaxillary lymph node Submental lymph node Subparotid lymph node Suprahyoid lymph node **1 Lymphatic, Right Neck** Cervical lymph node Jugular lymph node Mastoid (postauricular) lymph node Occipital lymph node Postauricular (mastoid) lymph node Retropharyngeal lymph node Right jugular trunk Right lymphatic duct Right subclavian trunk Supraclavicular (Virchow's) lymph node Virchow's (supraclavicular) lymph node **2 Lymphatic, Left Neck** Cervical lymph node Jugular lymph node Mastoid (postauricular) lymph node Occipital lymph node Postauricular (mastoid) lymph node Retropharyngeal lymph node Supraclavicular (Virchow's) lymph node Virchow's (supraclavicular) lymph node **3 Lymphatic, Right Upper Extremity** Cubital lymph node Deltopectoral (infraclavicular) lymph node Epitrochlear lymph node Infraclavicular (deltopectoral) lymph node Supratrochlear lymph node **4 Lymphatic, Left Upper Extremity** *See 3 Lymphatic, Right Upper Extremity* **5 Lymphatic, Right Axillary** Anterior (pectoral) lymph node Apical (subclavicular) lymph node Brachial (lateral) lymph node Central axillary lymph node Lateral (brachial) lymph node Pectoral (anterior) lymph node Posterior (subscapular) lymph node Subclavicular (apical) lymph node Subscapular (posterior) lymph node **6 Lymphatic, Left Axillary** *See 5 Lymphatic, Right Axillary* **7 Lymphatic, Thorax** Intercostal lymph node Mediastinal lymph node Parasternal lymph node Paratracheal lymph node Tracheobronchial lymph node **8 Lymphatic, Internal Mammary, Right** **9 Lymphatic, Internal Mammary, Left** **B Lymphatic, Mesenteric** Inferior mesenteric lymph node Pararectal lymph node Superior mesenteric lymph node **C Lymphatic, Pelvis** Common iliac (subaortic) lymph node Gluteal lymph node Iliac lymph node Inferior epigastric lymph node Obturator lymph node Sacral lymph node Subaortic (common iliac) lymph node Suprainguinal lymph node **D Lymphatic, Aortic** Celiac lymph node Gastric lymph node Hepatic lymph node Lumbar lymph node Pancreaticosplenic lymph node Paraaortic lymph node Retroperitoneal lymph node **F Lymphatic, Right Lower Extremity** Femoral lymph node Popliteal lymph node **G Lymphatic, Left Lower Extremity** *See F Lymphatic, Right Lower Extremity* **H Lymphatic, Right Inguinal** **J Lymphatic, Left Inguinal** **K Thoracic Duct** Left jugular trunk Left subclavian trunk **L Cisterna Chyli** Intestinal lymphatic trunk Lumbar lymphatic trunk	**Ø Open** **3 Percutaneous** **4 Percutaneous Endoscopic** **8 Via Natural or Artificial Opening Endoscopic**	**Z No Device**	**Z No Qualifier**
M Thymus Thymus gland **P Spleen** Accessory spleen	**Ø Open** **3 Percutaneous** **4 Percutaneous Endoscopic**	**Z No Device**	**Z No Qualifier**

Lymphatic and Hemic Systems

Ø7Q–Ø7Q

Ø Medical and Surgical
7 Lymphatic and Hemic Systems
S Reposition Definition: Moving to its normal location, or other suitable location, all or a portion of a body part

Explanation: The body part is moved to a new location from an abnormal location, or from a normal location where it is not functioning correctly. The body part may or may not be cut out or off to be moved to the new location.

Body Part Character 4	Approach Character 5	Device Character 6	Qualifier Character 7
M Thymus Thymus gland **P** Spleen Accessory spleen	**Ø** Open	**Z** No Device	**Z** No Qualifier

Ø Medical and Surgical
7 Lymphatic and Hemic Systems
T Resection Definition: Cutting out or off, without replacement, all of a body part

Explanation: None

Body Part Character 4	Approach Character 5	Device Character 6	Qualifier Character 7
Ø **Lymphatic, Head** Buccinator lymph node Infraauricular lymph node Infraparotid lymph node Parotid lymph node Preauricular lymph node Submandibular lymph node Submaxillary lymph node Submental lymph node Subparotid lymph node Suprahyoid lymph node **1** **Lymphatic, Right Neck** Cervical lymph node Jugular lymph node Mastoid (postauricular) lymph node Occipital lymph node Postauricular (mastoid) lymph node Retropharyngeal lymph node Right jugular trunk Right lymphatic duct Right subclavian trunk Supraclavicular (Virchow's) lymph node Virchow's (supraclavicular) lymph node **2** **Lymphatic, Left Neck** Cervical lymph node Jugular lymph node Mastoid (postauricular) lymph node Occipital lymph node Postauricular (mastoid) lymph node Retropharyngeal lymph node Supraclavicular (Virchow's) lymph node Virchow's (supraclavicular) lymph node **3** **Lymphatic, Right Upper Extremity** Cubital lymph node Deltopectoral (infraclavicular) lymph node Epitrochlear lymph node Infraclavicular (deltopectoral) lymph node Supratrochlear lymph node **4** **Lymphatic, Left Upper Extremity** *See 3 Lymphatic, Right Upper Extremity* **5** **Lymphatic, Right Axillary** ⊞ Anterior (pectoral) lymph node Apical (subclavicular) lymph node Brachial (lateral) lymph node Central axillary lymph node Lateral (brachial) lymph node Pectoral (anterior) lymph node Posterior (subscapular) lymph node Subclavicular (apical) lymph node Subscapular (posterior) lymph node **6** **Lymphatic, Left Axillary** ⊞ *See 5 Lymphatic, Right Axillary* **7** **Lymphatic, Thorax** ⊞ Intercostal lymph node Mediastinal lymph node Parasternal lymph node Paratracheal lymph node Tracheobronchial lymph node **8** **Lymphatic, Internal Mammary, Right** ⊞ **9** **Lymphatic, Internal Mammary, Left** ⊞ **B** **Lymphatic, Mesenteric** Inferior mesenteric lymph node Pararectal lymph node Superior mesenteric lymph node **C** **Lymphatic, Pelvis** Common iliac (subaortic) lymph node Gluteal lymph node Iliac lymph node Inferior epigastric lymph node Obturator lymph node Sacral lymph node Subaortic (common iliac) lymph node Suprainguinal lymph node **D** **Lymphatic, Aortic** Celiac lymph node Gastric lymph node Hepatic lymph node Lumbar lymph node Pancreaticosplenic lymph node Paraaortic lymph node Retroperitoneal lymph node **F** **Lymphatic, Right Lower Extremity** Femoral lymph node Popliteal lymph node **G** **Lymphatic, Left Lower Extremity** *See F Lymphatic, Right Lower Extremity* **H** **Lymphatic, Right Inguinal** **J** **Lymphatic, Left Inguinal** **K** **Thoracic Duct** Left jugular trunk Left subclavian trunk **L** **Cisterna Chyli** Intestinal lymphatic trunk Lumbar lymphatic trunk **M** **Thymus** Thymus gland **P** **Spleen** Accessory spleen	**Ø** Open **4** Percutaneous Endoscopic	**Z** No Device	**Z** No Qualifier

See Appendix L for Procedure Combinations

⊞ Ø7T[5,6,7,8,9]ØZZ

Ø Medical and Surgical
7 Lymphatic and Hemic Systems
U Supplement Definition: Putting in or on biological or synthetic material that physically reinforces and/or augments the function of a portion of a body part
Explanation: The biological material is non-living, or is living and from the same individual. The body part may have been previously replaced, and the SUPPLEMENT procedure is performed to physically reinforce and/or augment the function of the replaced body part.

Body Part Character 4		Approach Character 5	Device Character 6	Qualifier Character 7
Ø Lymphatic, Head Buccinator lymph node Infraauricular lymph node Infraparotid lymph node Parotid lymph node Preauricular lymph node Submandibular lymph node Submaxillary lymph node Submental lymph node Subparotid lymph node Suprahyoid lymph node **1 Lymphatic, Right Neck** Cervical lymph node Jugular lymph node Mastoid (postauricular) lymph node Occipital lymph node Postauricular (mastoid) lymph node Retropharyngeal lymph node Right jugular trunk Right lymphatic duct Right subclavian trunk Supraclavicular (Virchow's) lymph node Virchow's (supraclavicular) lymph node **2 Lymphatic, Left Neck** Cervical lymph node Jugular lymph node Mastoid (postauricular) lymph node Occipital lymph node Postauricular (mastoid) lymph node Retropharyngeal lymph node Supraclavicular (Virchow's) lymph node Virchow's (supraclavicular) lymph node **3 Lymphatic, Right Upper Extremity** Cubital lymph node Deltopectoral (infraclavicular) lymph node Epitrochlear lymph node Infraclavicular (deltopectoral) lymph node Supratrochlear lymph node **4 Lymphatic, Left Upper Extremity** *See 3 Lymphatic, Right Upper Extremity* **5 Lymphatic, Right Axillary** Anterior (pectoral) lymph node Apical (subclavicular) lymph node Brachial (lateral) lymph node Central axillary lymph node Lateral (brachial) lymph node Pectoral (anterior) lymph node Posterior (subscapular) lymph node Subclavicular (apical) lymph node Subscapular (posterior) lymph node	**6 Lymphatic, Left Axillary** *See 5 Lymphatic, Right Axillary* **7 Lymphatic, Thorax** Intercostal lymph node Mediastinal lymph node Parasternal lymph node Paratracheal lymph node Tracheobronchial lymph node **8 Lymphatic, Internal Mammary, Right** **9 Lymphatic, Internal Mammary, Left** **B Lymphatic, Mesenteric** Inferior mesenteric lymph node Pararectal lymph node Superior mesenteric lymph node **C Lymphatic, Pelvis** Common iliac (subaortic) lymph node Gluteal lymph node Iliac lymph node Inferior epigastric lymph node Obturator lymph node Sacral lymph node Subaortic (common iliac) lymph node Suprainguinal lymph node **D Lymphatic, Aortic** Celiac lymph node Gastric lymph node Hepatic lymph node Lumbar lymph node Pancreaticosplenic lymph node Paraaortic lymph node Retroperitoneal lymph node **F Lymphatic, Right Lower Extremity** Femoral lymph node Popliteal lymph node **G Lymphatic, Left Lower Extremity** *See F Lymphatic, Right Lower Extremity* **H Lymphatic, Right Inguinal** **J Lymphatic, Left Inguinal** **K Thoracic Duct** Left jugular trunk Left subclavian trunk **L Cisterna Chyli** Intestinal lymphatic trunk Lumbar lymphatic trunk	**Ø Open** **4 Percutaneous Endoscopic**	**7 Autologous Tissue Substitute** **J Synthetic Substitute** **K Nonautologous Tissue Substitute**	**Z No Qualifier**

Ø Medical and Surgical
7 Lymphatic and Hemic Systems
V Restriction Definition: Partially closing an orifice or the lumen of a tubular body part
Explanation: The orifice can be a natural orifice or an artificially created orifice

Body Part Character 4	Approach Character 5	Device Character 6	Qualifier Character 7
Ø Lymphatic, Head Buccinator lymph node Infraauricular lymph node Infraparotid lymph node Parotid lymph node Preauricular lymph node Submandibular lymph node Submaxillary lymph node Submental lymph node Subparotid lymph node Suprahyoid lymph node **1 Lymphatic, Right Neck** Cervical lymph node Jugular lymph node Mastoid (postauricular) lymph node Occipital lymph node Postauricular (mastoid) lymph node Retropharyngeal lymph node Right jugular trunk Right lymphatic duct Right subclavian trunk Supraclavicular (Virchow's) lymph node Virchow's (supraclavicular) lymph node **2 Lymphatic, Left Neck** Cervical lymph node Jugular lymph node Mastoid (postauricular) lymph node Occipital lymph node Postauricular (mastoid) lymph node Retropharyngeal lymph node Supraclavicular (Virchow's) lymph node Virchow's (supraclavicular) lymph node **3 Lymphatic, Right Upper Extremity** Cubital lymph node Deltopectoral (infraclavicular) lymph node Epitrochlear lymph node Infraclavicular (deltopectoral) lymph node Supratrochlear lymph node **4 Lymphatic, Left Upper Extremity** *See 3 Lymphatic, Right Upper Extremity* **5 Lymphatic, Right Axillary** Anterior (pectoral) lymph node Apical (subclavicular) lymph node Brachial (lateral) lymph node Central axillary lymph node Lateral (brachial) lymph node Pectoral (anterior) lymph node Posterior (subscapular) lymph node Subclavicular (apical) lymph node Subscapular (posterior) lymph node **6 Lymphatic, Left Axillary** *See 5 Lymphatic, Right Axillary* **7 Lymphatic, Thorax** Intercostal lymph node Mediastinal lymph node Parasternal lymph node Paratracheal lymph node Tracheobronchial lymph node **8 Lymphatic, Internal Mammary, Right** **9 Lymphatic, Internal Mammary, Left** **B Lymphatic, Mesenteric** Inferior mesenteric lymph node Pararectal lymph node Superior mesenteric lymph node **C Lymphatic, Pelvis** Common iliac (subaortic) lymph node Gluteal lymph node Iliac lymph node Inferior epigastric lymph node Obturator lymph node Sacral lymph node Subaortic (common iliac) lymph node Suprainguinal lymph node **D Lymphatic, Aortic** Celiac lymph node Gastric lymph node Hepatic lymph node Lumbar lymph node Pancreaticosplenic lymph node Paraaortic lymph node Retroperitoneal lymph node **F Lymphatic, Right Lower Extremity** Femoral lymph node Popliteal lymph node **G Lymphatic, Left Lower Extremity** *See F Lymphatic, Right Lower Extremity* **H Lymphatic, Right Inguinal** **J Lymphatic, Left Inguinal** **K Thoracic Duct** Left jugular trunk Left subclavian trunk **L Cisterna Chyli** Intestinal lymphatic trunk Lumbar lymphatic trunk	**Ø Open** **3 Percutaneous** **4 Percutaneous Endoscopic**	**C Extraluminal Device** **D Intraluminal Device** **Z No Device**	**Z No Qualifier**

Ø Medical and Surgical
7 Lymphatic and Hemic Systems
W Revision Definition: Correcting, to the extent possible, a portion of a malfunctioning device or the position of a displaced device

Explanation: Revision can include correcting a malfunctioning or displaced device by taking out or putting in components of the device such as a screw or pin

Body Part Character 4	Approach Character 5	Device Character 6	Qualifier Character 7
K Thoracic Duct Left jugular trunk Left subclavian trunk L Cisterna Chyli Intestinal lymphatic trunk Lumbar lymphatic trunk N Lymphatic	Ø Open 3 Percutaneous 4 Percutaneous Endoscopic	Ø Drainage Device 3 Infusion Device 7 Autologous Tissue Substitute C Extraluminal Device D Intraluminal Device J Synthetic Substitute K Nonautologous Tissue Substitute Y Other Device	Z No Qualifier
K Thoracic Duct Left jugular trunk Left subclavian trunk L Cisterna Chyli Intestinal lymphatic trunk Lumbar lymphatic trunk N Lymphatic	X External	Ø Drainage Device 3 Infusion Device 7 Autologous Tissue Substitute C Extraluminal Device D Intraluminal Device J Synthetic Substitute K Nonautologous Tissue Substitute	Z No Qualifier
M Thymus Thymus gland P Spleen Accessory spleen	Ø Open 3 Percutaneous 4 Percutaneous Endoscopic	Ø Drainage Device 3 Infusion Device Y Other Device	Z No Qualifier
M Thymus Thymus gland P Spleen Accessory spleen	X External	Ø Drainage Device 3 Infusion Device	Z No Qualifier
T Bone Marrow	Ø Open 3 Percutaneous 4 Percutaneous Endoscopic X External	Ø Drainage Device	Z No Qualifier

Non-OR Ø7W[K,L,N][3,4]YZ
Non-OR Ø7W[K,L,N]X[Ø,3,7,C,D,J,K]Z
Non-OR Ø7W[M,P][3,4]YZ
Non-OR Ø7W[M,P]X[Ø,3]Z
Non-OR Ø7WT[Ø,3,4,X]ØZ

Ø Medical and Surgical
7 Lymphatic and Hemic Systems
Y Transplantation Definition: Putting in or on all or a portion of a living body part taken from another individual or animal to physically take the place and/or function of all or a portion of a similar body part

Explanation: The native body part may or may not be taken out, and the transplanted body part may take over all or a portion of its function

Body Part Character 4	Approach Character 5	Device Character 6	Qualifier Character 7
M Thymus Thymus gland P Spleen Accessory spleen	Ø Open	Z No Device	Ø Allogeneic 1 Syngeneic 2 Zooplastic

Eye Ø8Ø–Ø8X

Character Meanings

This Character Meaning table is provided as a guide to assist the user in the identification of character members that may be found in this section of code tables. It **SHOULD NOT** be used to build a PCS code.

Operation–Character 3		Body Part–Character 4		Approach–Character 5		Device–Character 6		Qualifier–Character 7	
Ø	Alteration	Ø	Eye, Right	Ø	Open	Ø	Drainage Device OR Synthetic Substitute, Intraocular Telescope	3	Nasal Cavity
1	Bypass	1	Eye, Left	3	Percutaneous	1	Radioactive Element	4	Sclera
2	Change	2	Anterior Chamber, Right	7	Via Natural or Artificial Opening	3	Infusion Device	X	Diagnostic
5	Destruction	3	Anterior Chamber, Left	8	Via Natural or Artificial Opening Endoscopic	5	Epiretinal Visual Prosthesis	Z	No Qualifier
7	Dilation	4	Vitreous, Right	X	External	7	Autologous Tissue Substitute		
9	Drainage	5	Vitreous, Left			C	Extraluminal Device		
B	Excision	6	Sclera, Right			D	Intraluminal Device		
C	Extirpation	7	Sclera, Left			J	Synthetic Substitute		
D	Extraction	8	Cornea, Right			K	Nonautologous Tissue Substitute		
F	Fragmentation	9	Cornea, Left			Y	Other Device		
H	Insertion	A	Choroid, Right			Z	No Device		
J	Inspection	B	Choroid, Left						
L	Occlusion	C	Iris, Right						
M	Reattachment	D	Iris, Left						
N	Release	E	Retina, Right						
P	Removal	F	Retina, Left						
Q	Repair	G	Retinal Vessel, Right						
R	Replacement	H	Retinal Vessel, Left						
S	Reposition	J	Lens, Right						
T	Resection	K	Lens, Left						
U	Supplement	L	Extraocular Muscle, Right						
V	Restriction	M	Extraocular Muscle, Left						
W	Revision	N	Upper Eyelid, Right						
X	Transfer	P	Upper Eyelid, Left						
		Q	Lower Eyelid, Right						
		R	Lower Eyelid, Left						
		S	Conjunctiva, Right						
		T	Conjunctiva, Left						
		V	Lacrimal Gland, Right						
		W	Lacrimal Gland, Left						
		X	Lacrimal Duct, Right						
		Y	Lacrimal Duct, Left						

AHA Coding Clinic for table Ø89
2016, 2Q, 21 Laser trabeculoplasty

AHA Coding Clinic for table Ø8B
2014, 4Q, 35 Vitrectomy with air/fluid exchange
2014, 4Q, 36 Pars plans vitrectomy without mention of instillation of oil, air or fluid

AHA Coding Clinic for table Ø8J
2015, 1Q, 35 Attempted removal of foreign body from cornea

AHA Coding Clinic for table Ø8N
2015, 2Q, 24 Penetrating keratoplasty and anterior segment reconstruction

AHA Coding Clinic for table Ø8R
2015, 2Q, 24 Penetrating keratoplasty and anterior segment reconstruction
2015, 2Q, 25 Penetrating keratoplasty and placement of viscoelastic eye with paracentesis

AHA Coding Clinic for table Ø8T
2015, 2Q, 12 Orbital exenteration

AHA Coding Clinic for table Ø8U
2014, 3Q, 31 Corneal amniotic membrane transplantation

Eye

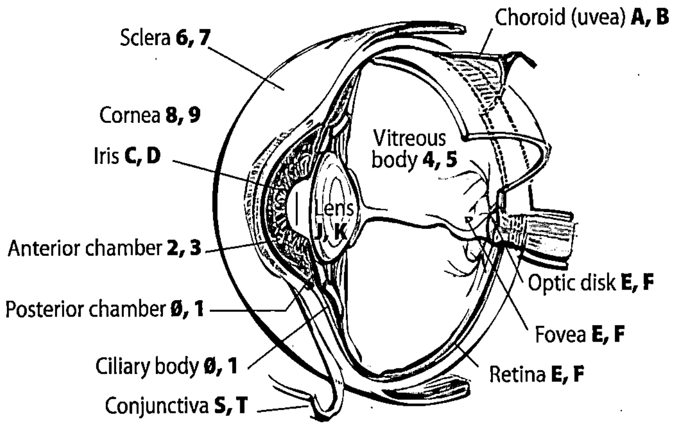

Eye Musculature

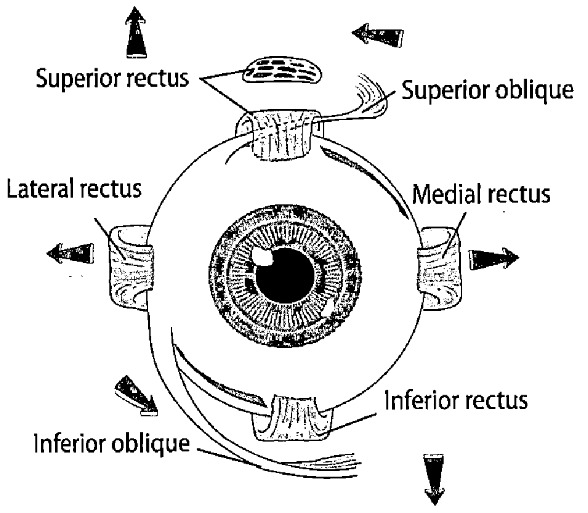

Muscles and actions (right eye) **L, M**

Lacrimal System

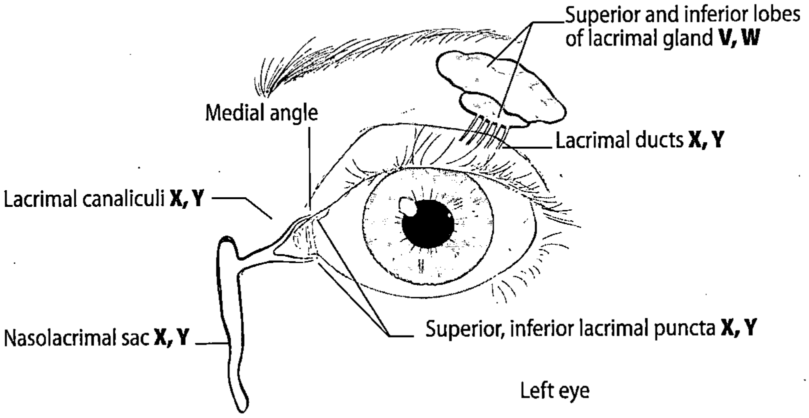

Left eye

Ø Medical and Surgical
8 Eye
Ø Alteration Definition: Modifying the anatomic structure of a body part without affecting the function of the body part
Explanation: Principal purpose is to improve appearance

Body Part Character 4	Approach Character 5	Device Character 6	Qualifier Character 7
N Upper Eyelid, Right Lateral canthus Levator palpebrae superioris muscle Orbicularis oculi muscle Superior tarsal plate **P** Upper Eyelid, Left *See N Upper Eyelid, Right* **Q** Lower Eyelid, Right Inferior tarsal plate Medial canthus **R** Lower Eyelid, Left *See Q Lower Eyelid, Right*	**Ø** Open **3** Percutaneous **X** External	**7** Autologous Tissue Substitute **J** Synthetic Substitute **K** Nonautologous Tissue Substitute **Z** No Device	**Z** No Qualifier

Non-OR All body part, approach, device, and qualifier values

Ø Medical and Surgical
8 Eye
1 Bypass Definition: Altering the route of passage of the contents of a tubular body part
Explanation: Rerouting contents of a body part to a downstream area of the normal route, to a similar route and body part, or to an abnormal route and dissimilar body part. Includes one or more anastomoses, with or without the use of a device.

Body Part Character 4	Approach Character 5	Device Character 6	Qualifier Character 7
2 Anterior Chamber, Right Aqueous humour **3** Anterior Chamber, Left *See 2 Anterior Chamber, Right*	**3** Percutaneous	**J** Synthetic Substitute **K** Nonautologous Tissue Substitute **Z** No Device	**4** Sclera
X Lacrimal Duct, Right Lacrimal canaliculus Lacrimal punctum Lacrimal sac Nasolacrimal duct **Y** Lacrimal Duct, Left *See X Lacrimal Duct, Right*	**Ø** Open **3** Percutaneous	**J** Synthetic Substitute **K** Nonautologous Tissue Substitute **Z** No Device	**3** Nasal Cavity

Ø Medical and Surgical
8 Eye
2 Change Definition: Taking out or off a device from a body part and putting back an identical or similar device in or on the same body part without cutting or puncturing the skin or a mucous membrane
Explanation: All CHANGE procedures are coded using the approach EXTERNAL

Body Part Character 4	Approach Character 5	Device Character 6	Qualifier Character 7
Ø Eye, Right Ciliary body Posterior chamber **1** Eye, Left *See Ø Eye, Right*	**X** External	**Ø** Drainage Device **Y** Other Device	**Z** No Qualifier

Non-OR All body part, approach, device, and qualifier values

Ø Medical and Surgical
8 Eye
5 Destruction Definition: Physical eradication of all or a portion of a body part by the direct use of energy, force, or a destructive agent
Explanation: None of the body part is physically taken out

Body Part Character 4		Approach Character 5	Device Character 6	Qualifier Character 7
Ø Eye, Right Ciliary body Posterior chamber **1 Eye, Left** *See Ø Eye, Right* **6 Sclera, Right** **7 Sclera, Left**	**8 Cornea, Right** **9 Cornea, Left** **S Conjunctiva, Right** Plica semilunaris **T Conjunctiva, Left** *See S Conjunctiva, Right*	**X External**	**Z No Device**	**Z No Qualifier**
2 Anterior Chamber, Right Aqueous humour **3 Anterior Chamber, Left** *See 2 Anterior Chamber, Right* **4 Vitreous, Right** Vitreous body **5 Vitreous, Left** *See 4 Vitreous, Right* **C Iris, Right** **D Iris, Left**	**E Retina, Right** Fovea Macula Optic disc **F Retina, Left** *See E Retina, Right* **G Retinal Vessel, Right** **H Retinal Vessel, Left** **J Lens, Right** Zonule of Zinn **K Lens, Left** *See J Lens, Right*	**3 Percutaneous**	**Z No Device**	**Z No Qualifier**
A Choroid, Right **B Choroid, Left** **L Extraocular Muscle, Right** Inferior oblique muscle Inferior rectus muscle Lateral rectus muscle Medial rectus muscle Superior oblique muscle Superior rectus muscle	**M Extraocular Muscle, Left** *See L Extraocular Muscle, Right* **V Lacrimal Gland, Right** **W Lacrimal Gland, Left**	**Ø Open** **3 Percutaneous**	**Z No Device**	**Z No Qualifier**
N Upper Eyelid, Right Lateral canthus Levator palpebrae superioris muscle Orbicularis oculi muscle Superior tarsal plate **P Upper Eyelid, Left** *See N Upper Eyelid, Right*	**Q Lower Eyelid, Right** Inferior tarsal plate Medial canthus **R Lower Eyelid, Left** *See Q Lower Eyelid, Right*	**Ø Open** **3 Percutaneous** **X External**	**Z No Device**	**Z No Qualifier**
X Lacrimal Duct, Right Lacrimal canaliculus Lacrimal punctum Lacrimal sac Nasolacrimal duct	**Y Lacrimal Duct, Left** *See X Lacrimal Duct, Right*	**Ø Open** **3 Percutaneous** **7 Via Natural or Artificial Opening** **8 Via Natural or Artificial Opening Endoscopic**	**Z No Device**	**Z No Qualifier**

Non-OR Ø85[E,F]3ZZ

Ø Medical and Surgical
8 Eye
7 Dilation Definition: Expanding an orifice or the lumen of a tubular body part
Explanation: The orifice can be a natural orifice or an artificially created orifice. Accomplished by stretching a tubular body part using intraluminal pressure or by cutting part of the orifice or wall of the tubular body part.

Body Part Character 4	Approach Character 5	Device Character 6	Qualifier Character 7
X Lacrimal Duct, Right Lacrimal canaliculus Lacrimal punctum Lacrimal sac Nasolacrimal duct **Y Lacrimal Duct, Left** *See X Lacrimal Duct, Right*	**Ø Open** **3 Percutaneous** **7 Via Natural or Artificial Opening** **8 Via Natural or Artificial Opening Endoscopic**	**D Intraluminal Device** **Z No Device**	**Z No Qualifier**

Ø Medical and Surgical
8 Eye
9 Drainage Definition: Taking or letting out fluids and/or gases from a body part
Explanation: The qualifier DIAGNOSTIC is used to identify drainage procedures that are biopsies

Body Part Character 4		Approach Character 5	Device Character 6	Qualifier Character 7
Ø Eye, Right Ciliary body Posterior chamber **1 Eye, Left** *See Ø Eye, Right* **6 Sclera, Right** **7 Sclera, Left**	**8 Cornea, Right** **9 Cornea, Left** **S Conjunctiva, Right** Plica semilunaris **T Conjunctiva, Left** *See S Conjunctiva, Right*	**X External**	**Ø Drainage Device**	**Z No Qualifier**
Ø Eye, Right Ciliary body Posterior chamber **1 Eye, Left** *See Ø Eye, Right* **6 Sclera, Right** **7 Sclera, Left**	**8 Cornea, Right** **9 Cornea, Left** **S Conjunctiva, Right** Plica semilunaris **T Conjunctiva, Left** *See S Conjunctiva, Right*	**X External**	**Z No Device**	**X Diagnostic** **Z No Qualifier**
2 Anterior Chamber, Right Aqueous humour **3 Anterior Chamber, Left** *See 2 Anterior Chamber, Right* **4 Vitreous, Right** Vitreous body **5 Vitreous, Left** *See 4 Vitreous, Right* **C Iris, Right** **D Iris, Left**	**E Retina, Right** Fovea Macula Optic disc **F Retina, Left** *See E Retina, Right* **G Retinal Vessel, Right** **H Retinal Vessel, Left** **J Lens, Right** Zonule of Zinn **K Lens, Left** *See J Lens, Right*	**3 Percutaneous**	**Ø Drainage Device**	**Z No Qualifier**
2 Anterior Chamber, Right Aqueous humour **3 Anterior Chamber, Left** *See 2 Anterior Chamber, Right* **4 Vitreous, Right** Vitreous body **5 Vitreous, Left** *See 4 Vitreous, Right* **C Iris, Right** **D Iris, Left**	**E Retina, Right** Fovea Macula Optic disc **F Retina, Left** *See E Retina, Right* **G Retinal Vessel, Right** **H Retinal Vessel, Left** **J Lens, Right** Zonule of Zinn **K Lens, Left** *See J Lens, Right*	**3 Percutaneous**	**Z No Device**	**X Diagnostic** **Z No Qualifier**
A Choroid, Right **B Choroid, Left** **L Extraocular Muscle, Right** Inferior oblique muscle Inferior rectus muscle Lateral rectus muscle Medial rectus muscle Superior oblique muscle Superior rectus muscle	**M Extraocular Muscle, Left** *See L Extraocular Muscle, Right* **V Lacrimal Gland, Right** **W Lacrimal Gland, Left**	**Ø Open** **3 Percutaneous**	**Ø Drainage Device**	**Z No Qualifier**
A Choroid, Right **B Choroid, Left** **L Extraocular Muscle, Right** Inferior oblique muscle Inferior rectus muscle Lateral rectus muscle Medial rectus muscle Superior oblique muscle Superior rectus muscle	**M Extraocular Muscle, Left** *See L Extraocular Muscle, Right* **V Lacrimal Gland, Right** **W Lacrimal Gland, Left**	**Ø Open** **3 Percutaneous**	**Z No Device**	**X Diagnostic** **Z No Qualifier**
N Upper Eyelid, Right Lateral canthus Levator palpebrae superioris muscle Orbicularis oculi muscle Superior tarsal plate **P Upper Eyelid, Left** *See N Upper Eyelid, Right*	**Q Lower Eyelid, Right** Inferior tarsal plate Medial canthus **R Lower Eyelid, Left** *See Q Lower Eyelid, Right*	**Ø Open** **3 Percutaneous** **X External**	**Ø Drainage Device**	**Z No Qualifier**

Ø89 Continued on next page

Non-OR Ø89[Ø,1,6,7,8,9,S,T]XZ[X,Z]
Non-OR Ø89[N,P,Q,R][Ø,3,X]ØZ

Ø Medical and Surgical
8 Eye
9 Drainage Definition: Taking or letting out fluids and/or gases from a body part
Explanation: The qualifier DIAGNOSTIC is used to identify drainage procedures that are biopsies

Ø89 Continued

Body Part Character 4		Approach Character 5	Device Character 6	Qualifier Character 7
N Upper Eyelid, Right Lateral canthus Levator palpebrae superioris muscle Orbicularis oculi muscle Superior tarsal plate **P Upper Eyelid, Left** *See N Upper Eyelid, Right*	**Q Lower Eyelid, Right** Inferior tarsal plate Medial canthus **R Lower Eyelid, Left** *See Q Lower Eyelid, Right*	**Ø Open** **3 Percutaneous** **X External**	**Z No Device**	**X Diagnostic** **Z No Qualifier**
X Lacrimal Duct, Right Lacrimal canaliculus Lacrimal punctum Lacrimal sac Nasolacrimal duct	**Y Lacrimal Duct, Left** *See X Lacrimal Duct, Right*	**Ø Open** **3 Percutaneous** **7 Via Natural or Artificial Opening** **8 Via Natural or Artificial Opening Endoscopic**	**Ø Drainage Device**	**Z No Qualifier**
X Lacrimal Duct, Right Lacrimal canaliculus Lacrimal punctum Lacrimal sac Nasolacrimal duct	**Y Lacrimal Duct, Left** *See X Lacrimal Duct, Right*	**Ø Open** **3 Percutaneous** **7 Via Natural or Artificial Opening** **8 Via Natural or Artificial Opening Endoscopic**	**Z No Device**	**X Diagnostic** **Z No Qualifier**

Non-OR Ø89[N,P,Q,R]ØZZ
Non-OR Ø89[N,P,Q,R][3,X]Z[X,Z]

Ø Medical and Surgical
8 Eye
B Excision Definition: Cutting out or off, without replacement, a portion of a body part
Explanation: The qualifier DIAGNOSTIC is used to identify excision procedures that are biopsies

Body Part Character 4		Approach Character 5	Device Character 6	Qualifier Character 7
Ø Eye, Right Ciliary body Posterior chamber **1 Eye, Left** *See Ø Eye, Right* **N Upper Eyelid, Right** Lateral canthus Levator palpebrae superioris muscle Orbicularis oculi muscle Superior tarsal plate	**P Upper Eyelid, Left** *See N Upper Eyelid, Right* **Q Lower Eyelid, Right** Inferior tarsal plate Medial canthus **R Lower Eyelid, Left** *See Q Lower Eyelid, Right*	**Ø Open** **3 Percutaneous** **X External**	**Z No Device**	**X Diagnostic** **Z No Qualifier**
4 Vitreous, Right Vitreous body **5 Vitreous, Left** *See 4 Vitreous, Right* **C Iris, Right** **D Iris, Left** **E Retina, Right** Fovea Macula Optic disc	**F Retina, Left** *See E Retina, Right* **J Lens, Right** Zonule of Zinn **K Lens, Left** *See J Lens, Right*	**3 Percutaneous**	**Z No Device**	**X Diagnostic** **Z No Qualifier**
6 Sclera, Right **7 Sclera, Left** **8 Cornea, Right** **9 Cornea, Left**	**S Conjunctiva, Right** Plica semilunaris **T Conjunctiva, Left** *See S Conjunctiva, Right*	**X External**	**Z No Device**	**X Diagnostic** **Z No Qualifier**
A Choroid, Right **B Choroid, Left** **L Extraocular Muscle, Right** Inferior oblique muscle Inferior rectus muscle Lateral rectus muscle Medial rectus muscle Superior oblique muscle Superior rectus muscle	**M Extraocular Muscle, Left** *See L Extraocular Muscle, Right* **V Lacrimal Gland, Right** **W Lacrimal Gland, Left**	**Ø Open** **3 Percutaneous**	**Z No Device**	**X Diagnostic** **Z No Qualifier**
X Lacrimal Duct, Right Lacrimal canaliculus Lacrimal punctum Lacrimal sac Nasolacrimal duct	**Y Lacrimal Duct, Left** *See X Lacrimal Duct, Right*	**Ø Open** **3 Percutaneous** **7 Via Natural or Artificial Opening** **8 Via Natural or Artificial Opening Endoscopic**	**Z No Device**	**X Diagnostic** **Z No Qualifier**

Ø Medical and Surgical
8 Eye
C Extirpation Definition: Taking or cutting out solid matter from a body part

Explanation: The solid matter may be an abnormal byproduct of a biological function or a foreign body; it may be imbedded in a body part or in the lumen of a tubular body part. The solid matter may or may not have been previously broken into pieces.

Body Part Character 4	Approach Character 5	Device Character 6	Qualifier Character 7
Ø Eye, Right Ciliary body Posterior chamber **1 Eye, Left** *See Ø Eye, Right* **6 Sclera, Right** **7 Sclera, Left** **8 Cornea, Right** **9 Cornea, Left** **S Conjunctiva, Right** Plica semilunaris **T Conjunctiva, Left** *See S Conjunctiva, Right*	**X External**	**Z No Device**	**Z No Qualifier**
2 Anterior Chamber, Right Aqueous humour **3 Anterior Chamber, Left** *See 2 Anterior Chamber, Right* **4 Vitreous, Right** Vitreous body **5 Vitreous, Left** *See 4 Vitreous, Right* **C Iris, Right** **D Iris, Left** **E Retina, Right** Fovea Macula Optic disc **F Retina, Left** *See* E Retina, Right **G Retinal Vessel, Right** **H Retinal Vessel, Left** **J Lens, Right** Zonule of Zinn **K Lens, Left** *See J Lens, Right*	**3 Percutaneous** **X External**	**Z No Device**	**Z No Qualifier**
A Choroid, Right **B Choroid, Left** **L Extraocular Muscle, Right** Inferior oblique muscle Inferior rectus muscle Lateral rectus muscle Medial rectus muscle Superior oblique muscle Superior rectus muscle **M Extraocular Muscle, Left** *See L Extraocular Muscle, Right* **N Upper Eyelid, Right** Lateral canthus Levator palpebrae superioris muscle Orbicularis oculi muscle Superior tarsal plate **P Upper Eyelid, Left** *See N Upper Eyelid, Right* **Q Lower Eyelid, Right** Inferior tarsal plate Medial canthus **R Lower Eyelid, Left** *See Q Lower Eyelid, Right* **V Lacrimal Gland, Right** **W Lacrimal Gland, Left**	**Ø Open** **3 Percutaneous** **X External**	**Z No Device**	**Z No Qualifier**
X Lacrimal Duct, Right Lacrimal canaliculus Lacrimal punctum Lacrimal sac Nasolacrimal duct **Y Lacrimal Duct, Left** *See X Lacrimal Duct, Right*	**Ø Open** **3 Percutaneous** **7 Via Natural or Artificial Opening** **8 Via Natural or Artificial Opening Endoscopic**	**Z No Device**	**Z No Qualifier**

Non-OR Ø8C[Ø,1,6,7,S,T]XZZ
Non-OR Ø8C[2,3]XZZ
Non-OR Ø8C[N,P,Q,R][Ø,3,X]ZZ

Ø Medical and Surgical
8 Eye
D Extraction Definition: Pulling or stripping out or off all or a portion of a body part by the use of force
Explanation: The qualifier DIAGNOSTIC is used to identify extraction procedures that are biopsies

Body Part Character 4	Approach Character 5	Device Character 6	Qualifier Character 7
8 Cornea, Right **9** Cornea, Left	**X** External	**Z** No Device	**X** Diagnostic **Z** No Qualifier
J Lens, Right Zonule of Zinn **K** Lens, Left *See J Lens, Right*	**3** Percutaneous	**Z** No Device	**Z** No Qualifier

Ø Medical and Surgical
8 Eye
F Fragmentation Definition: Breaking solid matter in a body part into pieces
Explanation: Physical force (e.g., manual, ultrasonic) applied directly or indirectly is used to break the solid matter into pieces. The solid matter may be an abnormal byproduct of a biological function or a foreign body. The pieces of solid matter are not taken out.

Body Part Character 4	Approach Character 5	Device Character 6	Qualifier Character 7
4 Vitreous, Right NC Vitreous body **5** Vitreous, Left NC *See 4 Vitreous, Right*	**3** Percutaneous **X** External	**Z** No Device	**Z** No Qualifier

Non-OR Ø8F[4,5]XZZ
NC Ø8F[4,5]XZZ

Ø Medical and Surgical
8 Eye
H Insertion Definition: Putting in a nonbiological appliance that monitors, assists, performs, or prevents a physiological function but does not physically take the place of a body part
Explanation: None

Body Part Character 4	Approach Character 5	Device Character 6	Qualifier Character 7
Ø Eye, Right Ciliary body Posterior chamber **1** Eye, Left *See Ø Eye, Right*	**Ø** Open	**5** Epiretinal Visual Prosthesis **Y** Other Device	**Z** No Qualifier
Ø Eye, Right Ciliary body Posterior chamber **1** Eye, Left *See Ø Eye, Right*	**3** Percutaneous	**1** Radioactive Element **3** Infusion Device **Y** Other Device	**Z** No Qualifier
Ø Eye, Right Ciliary body Posterior chamber **1** Eye, Left *See Ø Eye, Right*	**7** Via Natural or Artificial Opening **8** Via Natural or Artificial Opening Endoscopic	**Y** Other Device	**Z** No Qualifier
Ø Eye, Right Ciliary body Posterior chamber **1** Eye, Left *See Ø Eye, Right*	**X** External	**1** Radioactive Element **3** Infusion Device	**Z** No Qualifier

Non-OR Ø8H[Ø,1]3YZ
Non-OR Ø8H[Ø,1][7,8]YZ

Ø Medical and Surgical
8 Eye
J Inspection Definition: Visually and/or manually exploring a body part

Explanation: Visual exploration may be performed with or without optical instrumentation. Manual exploration may be performed directly or through intervening body layers.

Body Part Character 4	Approach Character 5	Device Character 6	Qualifier Character 7
Ø Eye, Right Ciliary body Posterior chamber **1 Eye, Left** *See Ø Eye, Right* **J Lens, Right** Zonule of Zinn **K Lens, Left** *See J Lens, Right*	**X External**	**Z No Device**	**Z No Qualifier**
L Extraocular Muscle, Right Inferior oblique muscle Inferior rectus muscle Lateral rectus muscle Medial rectus muscle Superior oblique muscle Superior rectus muscle **M Extraocular Muscle, Left** *See L Extraocular Muscle, Right*	**Ø Open** **X External**	**Z No Device**	**Z No Qualifier**

Non-OR Ø8J[Ø,1,J,K]XZZ
Non-OR Ø8J[L,M]XZZ

Ø Medical and Surgical
8 Eye
L Occlusion Definition: Completely closing an orifice or the lumen of a tubular body part

Explanation: The orifice can be a natural orifice or an artificially created orifice

Body Part Character 4	Approach Character 5	Device Character 6	Qualifier Character 7
X Lacrimal Duct, Right Lacrimal canaliculus Lacrimal punctum Lacrimal sac Nasolacrimal duct **Y Lacrimal Duct, Left** *See X Lacrimal Duct, Right*	**Ø Open** **3 Percutaneous**	**C Extraluminal Device** **D Intraluminal Device** **Z No Device**	**Z No Qualifier**
X Lacrimal Duct, Right Lacrimal canaliculus Lacrimal punctum Lacrimal sac Nasolacrimal duct **Y Lacrimal Duct, Left** *See X Lacrimal Duct, Right*	**7 Via Natural or Artificial Opening** **8 Via Natural or Artificial Opening Endoscopic**	**D Intraluminal Device** **Z No Device**	**Z No Qualifier**

Ø Medical and Surgical
8 Eye
M Reattachment Definition: Putting back in or on all or a portion of a separated body part to its normal location or other suitable location

Explanation: Vascular circulation and nervous pathways may or may not be reestablished

Body Part Character 4	Approach Character 5	Device Character 6	Qualifier Character 7
N Upper Eyelid, Right Lateral canthus Levator palpebrae superioris muscle Orbicularis oculi muscle Superior tarsal plate **P Upper Eyelid, Left** *See N Upper Eyelid, Right* **Q Lower Eyelid, Right** Inferior tarsal plate Medial canthus **R Lower Eyelid, Left** *See Q Lower Eyelid, Right*	**X External**	**Z No Device**	**Z No Qualifier**

Ø Medical and Surgical
8 Eye
N Release Definition: Freeing a body part from an abnormal physical constraint by cutting or by the use of force
Explanation: Some of the restraining tissue may be taken out but none of the body part is taken out

Body Part Character 4	Approach Character 5	Device Character 6	Qualifier Character 7
Ø Eye, Right Ciliary body Posterior chamber **1 Eye, Left** *See Ø Eye, Right* **6 Sclera, Right** **7 Sclera, Left** **8 Cornea, Right** **9 Cornea, Left** **S Conjunctiva, Right** Plica semilunaris **T Conjunctiva, Left** *See S Conjunctiva, Right*	**X External**	**Z No Device**	**Z No Qualifier**
2 Anterior Chamber, Right Aqueous humour **3 Anterior Chamber, Left** *See 2 Anterior Chamber, Right* **4 Vitreous, Right** Vitreous body **5 Vitreous, Left** *See 4 Vitreous, Right* **C Iris, Right** **D Iris, Left** **E Retina, Right** Fovea Macula Optic disc **F Retina, Left** *See E Retina, Right* **G Retinal Vessel, Right** **H Retinal Vessel, Left** **J Lens, Right** Zonule of Zinn **K Lens, Left** *See J Lens, Right*	**3 Percutaneous**	**Z No Device**	**Z No Qualifier**
A Choroid, Right **B Choroid, Left** **L Extraocular Muscle, Right** Inferior oblique muscle Inferior rectus muscle Lateral rectus muscle Medial rectus muscle Superior oblique muscle Superior rectus muscle **M Extraocular Muscle, Left** *See L Extraocular Muscle, Right* **V Lacrimal Gland, Right** **W Lacrimal Gland, Left**	**Ø Open** **3 Percutaneous**	**Z No Device**	**Z No Qualifier**
N Upper Eyelid, Right Lateral canthus Levator palpebrae superioris muscle Orbicularis oculi muscle Superior tarsal plate **P Upper Eyelid, Left** *See N Upper Eyelid, Right* **Q Lower Eyelid, Right** Inferior tarsal plate Medial canthus **R Lower Eyelid, Left** *See Q Lower Eyelid, Right*	**Ø Open** **3 Percutaneous** **X External**	**Z No Device**	**Z No Qualifier**
X Lacrimal Duct, Right Lacrimal canaliculus Lacrimal punctum Lacrimal sac Nasolacrimal duct **Y Lacrimal Duct, Left** *See X Lacrimal Duct, Right*	**Ø Open** **3 Percutaneous** **7 Via Natural or Artificial Opening** **8 Via Natural or Artificial Opening Endoscopic**	**Z No Device**	**Z No Qualifier**

Ø Medical and Surgical
8 Eye
P Removal Definition: Taking out or off a device from a body part

Explanation: If a device is taken out and a similar device put in without cutting or puncturing the skin or mucous membrane, the procedure is coded to the root operation CHANGE. Otherwise, the procedure for taking out a device is coded to the root operation REMOVAL.

Body Part Character 4	Approach Character 5	Device Character 6	Qualifier Character 7
Ø Eye, Right Ciliary body Posterior chamber **1** Eye, Left *See Ø Eye, Right*	**Ø** Open **3** Percutaneous **7** Via Natural or Artificial Opening **8** Via Natural or Artificial Opening Endoscopic	**Ø** Drainage Device **1** Radioactive Element **3** Infusion Device **7** Autologous Tissue Substitute **C** Extraluminal Device **D** Intraluminal Device **J** Synthetic Substitute **K** Nonautologous Tissue Substitute **Y** Other Device	**Z** No Qualifier
Ø Eye, Right Ciliary body Posterior chamber **1** Eye, Left *See Ø Eye, Right*	**X** External	**Ø** Drainage Device **1** Radioactive Element **3** Infusion Device **7** Autologous Tissue Substitute **C** Extraluminal Device **D** Intraluminal Device **J** Synthetic Substitute **K** Nonautologous Tissue Substitute	**Z** No Qualifier
J Lens, Right Zonule of Zinn **K** Lens, Left *See J Lens, Right*	**3** Percutaneous	**J** Synthetic Substitute **Y** Other Device	**Z** No Qualifier
L Extraocular Muscle, Right Inferior oblique muscle Inferior rectus muscle Lateral rectus muscle Medial rectus muscle Superior oblique muscle Superior rectus muscle **M** Extraocular Muscle, Left *See L Extraocular Muscle, Right*	**Ø** Open **3** Percutaneous	**Ø** Drainage Device **7** Autologous Tissue Substitute **J** Synthetic Substitute **K** Nonautologous Tissue Substitute **Y** Other Device	**Z** No Qualifier

Non-OR Ø8P[Ø,1]3YZ
Non-OR Ø8P[Ø,1][7,8][Ø,3,D,Y]Z
Non-OR Ø8P[Ø,1]X[Ø,1,3,C,D,J]Z
Non-OR Ø8P[J,K]3YZ
Non-OR Ø8P[L,M]3YZ

Ø Medical and Surgical
8 Eye
Q Repair Definition: Restoring, to the extent possible, a body part to its normal anatomic structure and function
Explanation: Used only when the method to accomplish the repair is not one of the other root operations

Body Part Character 4	Approach Character 5	Device Character 6	Qualifier Character 7
Ø Eye, Right Ciliary body Posterior chamber **1 Eye, Left** *See Ø Eye, Right* **6 Sclera, Right** **7 Sclera, Left** **8 Cornea, Right** NC **9 Cornea, Left** NC **S Conjunctiva, Right** Plica semilunaris **T Conjunctiva, Left** *See S Conjunctiva, Right*	**X External**	**Z No Device**	**Z No Qualifier**
2 Anterior Chamber, Right Aqueous humour **3 Anterior Chamber, Left** *See 2 Anterior Chamber, Right* **4 Vitreous, Right** Vitreous body **5 Vitreous, Left** *See 4 Vitreous, Right* **C Iris, Right** **D Iris, Left** **E Retina, Right** Fovea Macula Optic disc **F Retina, Left** *See E Retina, Right* **G Retinal Vessel, Right** **H Retinal Vessel, Left** **J Lens, Right** Zonule of Zinn **K Lens, Left** *See J Lens, Right*	**3 Percutaneous**	**Z No Device**	**Z No Qualifier**
A Choroid, Right **B Choroid, Left** **L Extraocular Muscle, Right** Inferior oblique muscle Inferior rectus muscle Lateral rectus muscle Medial rectus muscle Superior oblique muscle Superior rectus muscle **M Extraocular Muscle, Left** *See L Extraocular Muscle, Right* **V Lacrimal Gland, Right** **W Lacrimal Gland, Left**	**Ø Open** **3 Percutaneous**	**Z No Device**	**Z No Qualifier**
N Upper Eyelid, Right Lateral canthus Levator palpebrae superioris muscle Orbicularis oculi muscle Superior tarsal plate **P Upper Eyelid, Left** *See N Upper Eyelid, Right* **Q Lower Eyelid, Right** Inferior tarsal plate Medial canthus **R Lower Eyelid, Left** *See Q Lower Eyelid, Right*	**Ø Open** **3 Percutaneous** **X External**	**Z No Device**	**Z No Qualifier**
X Lacrimal Duct, Right Lacrimal canaliculus Lacrimal punctum Lacrimal sac Nasolacrimal duct **Y Lacrimal Duct, Left** *See X Lacrimal Duct, Right*	**Ø Open** **3 Percutaneous** **7 Via Natural or Artificial Opening** **8 Via Natural or Artificial Opening Endoscopic**	**Z No Device**	**Z No Qualifier**

Non-OR Ø8Q[N,P,Q,R][Ø,3,X]ZZ
NC Ø8Q[8,9]XZZ

Ø Medical and Surgical
8 Eye
R Replacement Definition: Putting in or on biological or synthetic material that physically takes the place and/or function of all or a portion of a body part
Explanation: The body part may have been taken out or replaced, or may be taken out, physically eradicated, or rendered nonfunctional during the REPLACEMENT procedure. A REMOVAL procedure is coded for taking out the device used in a previous replacement procedure.

Body Part Character 4	Approach Character 5	Device Character 6	Qualifier Character 7
Ø Eye, Right Ciliary body Posterior chamber **1 Eye, Left** *See Ø Eye, Right* **A Choroid, Right** **B Choroid, Left**	**Ø Open** **3 Percutaneous**	**7 Autologous Tissue Substitute** **J Synthetic Substitute** **K Nonautologous Tissue Substitute**	**Z No Qualifier**
4 Vitreous, Right Vitreous body **5 Vitreous, Left** *See 4 Vitreous, Right* **C Iris, Right** **D Iris, Left** **G Retinal Vessel, Right** **H Retinal Vessel, Left**	**3 Percutaneous**	**7 Autologous Tissue Substitute** **J Synthetic Substitute** **K Nonautologous Tissue Substitute**	**Z No Qualifier**
6 Sclera, Right **7 Sclera, Left** **S Conjunctiva, Right** Plica semilunaris **T Conjunctiva, Left** *See S Conjunctiva, Right*	**X External**	**7 Autologous Tissue Substitute** **J Synthetic Substitute** **K Nonautologous Tissue Substitute**	**Z No Qualifier**
8 Cornea, Right **9 Cornea, Left**	**3 Percutaneous** **X External**	**7 Autologous Tissue Substitute** **J Synthetic Substitute** **K Nonautologous Tissue Substitute**	**Z No Qualifier**
J Lens, Right Zonule of Zinn **K Lens, Left** *See J Lens, Right*	**3 Percutaneous**	**Ø Synthetic Substitute, Intraocular Telescope** **7 Autologous Tissue Substitute** **J Synthetic Substitute** **K Nonautologous Tissue Substitute**	**Z No Qualifier**
N Upper Eyelid, Right Lateral canthus Levator palpebrae superioris muscle Orbicularis oculi muscle Superior tarsal plate **P Upper Eyelid, Left** *See N Upper Eyelid, Right* **Q Lower Eyelid, Right** Inferior tarsal plate Medial canthus **R Lower Eyelid, Left** *See Q Lower Eyelid, Right*	**Ø Open** **3 Percutaneous** **X External**	**7 Autologous Tissue Substitute** **J Synthetic Substitute** **K Nonautologous Tissue Substitute**	**Z No Qualifier**
X Lacrimal Duct, Right Lacrimal canaliculus Lacrimal punctum Lacrimal sac Nasolacrimal duct **Y Lacrimal Duct, Left** *See X Lacrimal Duct, Right*	**Ø Open** **3 Percutaneous** **7 Via Natural or Artificial Opening** **8 Via Natural or Artificial Opening Endoscopic**	**7 Autologous Tissue Substitute** **J Synthetic Substitute** **K Nonautologous Tissue Substitute**	**Z No Qualifier**

Ø Medical and Surgical
8 Eye
S Reposition Definition: Moving to its normal location, or other suitable location, all or a portion of a body part

Explanation: The body part is moved to a new location from an abnormal location, or from a normal location where it is not functioning correctly. The body part may or may not be cut out or off to be moved to the new location.

Body Part Character 4	Approach Character 5	Device Character 6	Qualifier Character 7
C Iris, Right **D** Iris, Left **G** Retinal Vessel, Right **H** Retinal Vessel, Left **J** Lens, Right Zonule of Zinn **K** Lens, Left *See J Lens, Right*	**3** Percutaneous	**Z** No Device	**Z** No Qualifier
L Extraocular Muscle, Right Inferior oblique muscle Inferior rectus muscle Lateral rectus muscle Medial rectus muscle Superior oblique muscle Superior rectus muscle **M** Extraocular Muscle, Left *See L Extraocular Muscle, Right* **V** Lacrimal Gland, Right **W** Lacrimal Gland, Left	**Ø** Open **3** Percutaneous	**Z** No Device	**Z** No Qualifier
N Upper Eyelid, Right Lateral canthus Levator palpebrae superioris muscle Orbicularis oculi muscle Superior tarsal plate **P** Upper Eyelid, Left *See N Upper Eyelid, Right* **Q** Lower Eyelid, Right Inferior tarsal plate Medial canthus **R** Lower Eyelid, Left *See Q Lower Eyelid, Right*	**Ø** Open **3** Percutaneous **X** External	**Z** No Device	**Z** No Qualifier
X Lacrimal Duct, Right Lacrimal canaliculus Lacrimal punctum Lacrimal sac Nasolacrimal duct **Y** Lacrimal Duct, Left *See X Lacrimal Duct, Right*	**Ø** Open **3** Percutaneous **7** Via Natural or Artificial Opening **8** Via Natural or Artificial Opening Endoscopic	**Z** No Device	**Z** No Qualifier

Ø Medical and Surgical
8 Eye
T Resection Definition: Cutting out or off, without replacement, all of a body part
Explanation: None

Body Part Character 4	Approach Character 5	Device Character 6	Qualifier Character 7
Ø Eye, Right Ciliary body Posterior chamber **1 Eye, Left** *See Ø Eye, Right* **8 Cornea, Right** **9 Cornea, Left**	**X External**	**Z No Device**	**Z No Qualifier**
4 Vitreous, Right Vitreous body **5 Vitreous, Left** *See 4 Vitreous, Right* **C Iris, Right** **D Iris, Left** **J Lens, Right** Zonule of Zinn **K Lens, Left** *See J Lens, Right*	**3 Percutaneous**	**Z No Device**	**Z No Qualifier**
L Extraocular Muscle, Right Inferior oblique muscle Inferior rectus muscle Lateral rectus muscle Medial rectus muscle Superior oblique muscle Superior rectus muscle **M Extraocular Muscle, Left** *See L Extraocular Muscle, Right* **V Lacrimal Gland, Right** **W Lacrimal Gland, Left**	**Ø Open** **3 Percutaneous**	**Z No Device**	**Z No Qualifier**
N Upper Eyelid, Right Lateral canthus Levator palpebrae superioris muscle Orbicularis oculi muscle Superior tarsal plate **P Upper Eyelid, Left** *See N Upper Eyelid, Right* **Q Lower Eyelid, Right** Inferior tarsal plate Medial canthus **R Lower Eyelid, Left** *See Q Lower Eyelid, Right*	**Ø Open** **X External**	**Z No Device**	**Z No Qualifier**
X Lacrimal Duct, Right Lacrimal canaliculus Lacrimal punctum Lacrimal sac Nasolacrimal duct **Y Lacrimal Duct, Left** *See X Lacrimal Duct, Right*	**Ø Open** **3 Percutaneous** **7 Via Natural or Artificial Opening** **8 Via Natural or Artificial Opening Endoscopic**	**Z No Device**	**Z No Qualifier**

Ø Medical and Surgical
8 Eye
U Supplement Definition: Putting in or on biological or synthetic material that physically reinforces and/or augments the function of a portion of a body part
Explanation: The biological material is non-living, or is living and from the same individual. The body part may have been previously replaced, and the SUPPLEMENT procedure is performed to physically reinforce and/or augment the function of the replaced body part.

Body Part Character 4	Approach Character 5	Device Character 6	Qualifier Character 7
Ø Eye, Right Ciliary body Posterior chamber **1 Eye, Left** *See Ø Eye, Right* **C Iris, Right** **D Iris, Left** **E Retina, Right** Fovea Macula Optic disc **F Retina, Left** *See E Retina, Right* **G Retinal Vessel, Right** **H Retinal Vessel, Left** **L Extraocular Muscle, Right** Inferior oblique muscle Inferior rectus muscle Lateral rectus muscle Medial rectus muscle Superior oblique muscle Superior rectus muscle **M Extraocular Muscle, Left** *See L Extraocular Muscle, Right*	**Ø Open** **3 Percutaneous**	**7 Autologous Tissue Substitute** **J Synthetic Substitute** **K Nonautologous Tissue Substitute**	**Z No Qualifier**
8 Cornea, Right NC **9 Cornea, Left** NC **N Upper Eyelid, Right** Lateral canthus Levator palpebrae superioris muscle Orbicularis oculi muscle Superior tarsal plate **P Upper Eyelid, Left** *See N Upper Eyelid, Right* **Q Lower Eyelid, Right** Inferior tarsal plate Medial canthus **R Lower Eyelid, Left** *See Q Lower Eyelid, Right*	**Ø Open** **3 Percutaneous** **X External**	**7 Autologous Tissue Substitute** **J Synthetic Substitute** **K Nonautologous Tissue Substitute**	**Z No Qualifier**
X Lacrimal Duct, Right Lacrimal canaliculus Lacrimal punctum Lacrimal sac Nasolacrimal duct **Y Lacrimal Duct, Left** *See X Lacrimal Duct, Right*	**Ø Open** **3 Percutaneous** **7 Via Natural or Artificial Opening** **8 Via Natural or Artificial Opening Endoscopic**	**7 Autologous Tissue Substitute** **J Synthetic Substitute** **K Nonautologous Tissue Substitute**	**Z No Qualifier**

NC Ø8U[8,9][Ø,3,X]KZ

Ø Medical and Surgical
8 Eye
V Restriction Definition: Partially closing an orifice or the lumen of a tubular body part
Explanation: The orifice can be a natural orifice or an artificially created orifice

Body Part Character 4	Approach Character 5	Device Character 6	Qualifier Character 7
X Lacrimal Duct, Right Lacrimal canaliculus Lacrimal punctum Lacrimal sac Nasolacrimal duct **Y Lacrimal Duct, Left** *See X Lacrimal Duct, Right*	**Ø Open** **3 Percutaneous**	**C Extraluminal Device** **D Intraluminal Device** **Z No Device**	**Z No Qualifier**
X Lacrimal Duct, Right Lacrimal canaliculus Lacrimal punctum Lacrimal sac Nasolacrimal duct **Y Lacrimal Duct, Left** *See X Lacrimal Duct, Right*	**7 Via Natural or Artificial Opening** **8 Via Natural or Artificial Opening Endoscopic**	**D Intraluminal Device** **Z No Device**	**Z No Qualifier**

Ø Medical and Surgical
8 Eye
W Revision Definition: Correcting, to the extent possible, a portion of a malfunctioning device or the position of a displaced device

Explanation: Revision can include correcting a malfunctioning or displaced device by taking out or putting in components of the device such as a screw or pin

Body Part Character 4	Approach Character 5	Device Character 6	Qualifier Character 7
Ø Eye, Right Ciliary body Posterior chamber **1** Eye, Left *See Ø Eye, Right*	**Ø** Open **3** Percutaneous **7** Via Natural or Artificial Opening **8** Via Natural or Artificial Opening Endoscopic	**Ø** Drainage Device **3** Infusion Device **7** Autologous Tissue Substitute **C** Extraluminal Device **D** Intraluminal Device **J** Synthetic Substitute **K** Nonautologous Tissue Substitute **Y** Other Device	**Z** No Qualifier
Ø Eye, Right Ciliary body Posterior chamber **1** Eye, Left *See Ø Eye, Right*	**X** External	**Ø** Drainage Device **3** Infusion Device **7** Autologous Tissue Substitute **C** Extraluminal Device **D** Intraluminal Device **J** Synthetic Substitute **K** Nonautologous Tissue Substitute	**Z** No Qualifier
J Lens, Right Zonule of Zinn **K** Lens, Left *See J Lens, Right*	**3** Percutaneous	**J** Synthetic Substitute **Y** Other Device	**Z** No Qualifier
J Lens, Right Zonule of Zinn **K** Lens, Left *See J Lens, Right*	**X** External	**J** Synthetic Substitute	**Z** No Qualifier
L Extraocular Muscle, Right Inferior oblique muscle Inferior rectus muscle Lateral rectus muscle Medial rectus muscle Superior oblique muscle Superior rectus muscle **M** Extraocular Muscle, Left *See L Extraocular Muscle, Right*	**Ø** Open **3** Percutaneous	**Ø** Drainage Device **7** Autologous Tissue Substitute **J** Synthetic Substitute **K** Nonautologous Tissue Substitute **Y** Other Device	**Z** No Qualifier

Non-OR Ø8W[Ø,1][3,7,8]YZ
Non-OR Ø8W[Ø,1]X[Ø,3,7,C,D,J,K]Z
Non-OR Ø8W[J,K]3YZ
Non-OR Ø8W[J,K]XJZ
Non-OR Ø8W[L,M]3YZ

Ø Medical and Surgical
8 Eye
X Transfer Definition: Moving, without taking out, all or a portion of a body part to another location to take over the function of all or a portion of a body part

Explanation: The body part transferred remains connected to its vascular and nervous supply

Body Part Character 4	Approach Character 5	Device Character 6	Qualifier Character 7
L Extraocular Muscle, Right Inferior oblique muscle Inferior rectus muscle Lateral rectus muscle Medial rectus muscle Superior oblique muscle Superior rectus muscle **M** Extraocular Muscle, Left *See L Extraocular Muscle, Right*	**Ø** Open **3** Percutaneous	**Z** No Device	**Z** No Qualifier

Ear, Nose, Sinus Ø9Ø–Ø9W

Character Meanings*

This Character Meaning table is provided as a guide to assist the user in the identification of character members that may be found in this section of code tables. It **SHOULD NOT** be used to build a PCS code.

Operation–Character 3	Body Part–Character 4	Approach–Character 5	Device–Character 6	Qualifier–Character 7
Ø Alteration	Ø External Ear, Right	Ø Open	Ø Drainage Device	Ø Endolymphatic
1 Bypass	1 External Ear, Left	3 Percutaneous	4 Hearing Device, Bone Conduction	X Diagnostic
2 Change	2 External Ear, Bilateral	4 Percutaneous Endoscopic	5 Hearing Device, Single Channel Cochlear Prosthesis	Z No Qualifier
3 Control	3 External Auditory Canal, Right	7 Via Natural or Artificial Opening	6 Hearing Device, Multiple Channel Cochlear Prosthesis	
5 Destruction	4 External Auditory Canal, Left	8 Via Natural or Artificial Opening Endoscopic	7 Autologous Tissue Substitute	
7 Dilation	5 Middle Ear, Right	X External	B Intraluminal Device, Airway	
8 Division	6 Middle Ear, Left		D Intraluminal Device	
9 Drainage	7 Tympanic Membrane, Right		J Synthetic Substitute	
B Excision	8 Tympanic Membrane, Left		K Nonautologous Tissue Substitute	
C Extirpation	9 Auditory Ossicle, Right		S Hearing Device	
D Extraction	A Auditory Ossicle, Left		Y Other Device	
H Insertion	B Mastoid Sinus, Right		Z No Device	
J Inspection	C Mastoid Sinus, Left			
M Reattachment	D Inner Ear, Right			
N Release	E Inner Ear, Left			
P Removal	F Eustachian Tube, Right			
Q Repair	G Eustachian Tube, Left			
R Replacement	H Ear, Right			
S Reposition	J Ear, Left			
T Resection	K Nasal Mucosa and Soft Tissue			
U Supplement	L Nasal Turbinate			
W Revision	M Nasal Septum			
	N Nasopharynx			
	P Accessory Sinus			
	Q Maxillary Sinus, Right			
	R Maxillary Sinus, Left			
	S Frontal Sinus, Right			
	T Frontal Sinus, Left			
	U Ethmoid Sinus, Right			
	V Ethmoid Sinus, Left			
	W Sphenoid Sinus, Right			
	X Sphenoid Sinus, Left			
	Y Sinus			

* Includes sinus ducts.

AHA Coding Clinic for table Ø95
2018, 1Q, 19 Control of epistaxis via silver nitrate cauterization

AHA Coding Clinic for table Ø9Q
2018, 1Q, 19 Control of epistaxis via silver nitrate cauterization
2017, 4Q, 106 Control of bleeding of external naris using suture
2014, 4Q, 20 Control of epistaxis
2014, 3Q, 22 Transsphenoidal removal of pituitary tumor and fat graft placement
2013, 4Q, 114 Balloon sinuplasty

Ear Anatomy

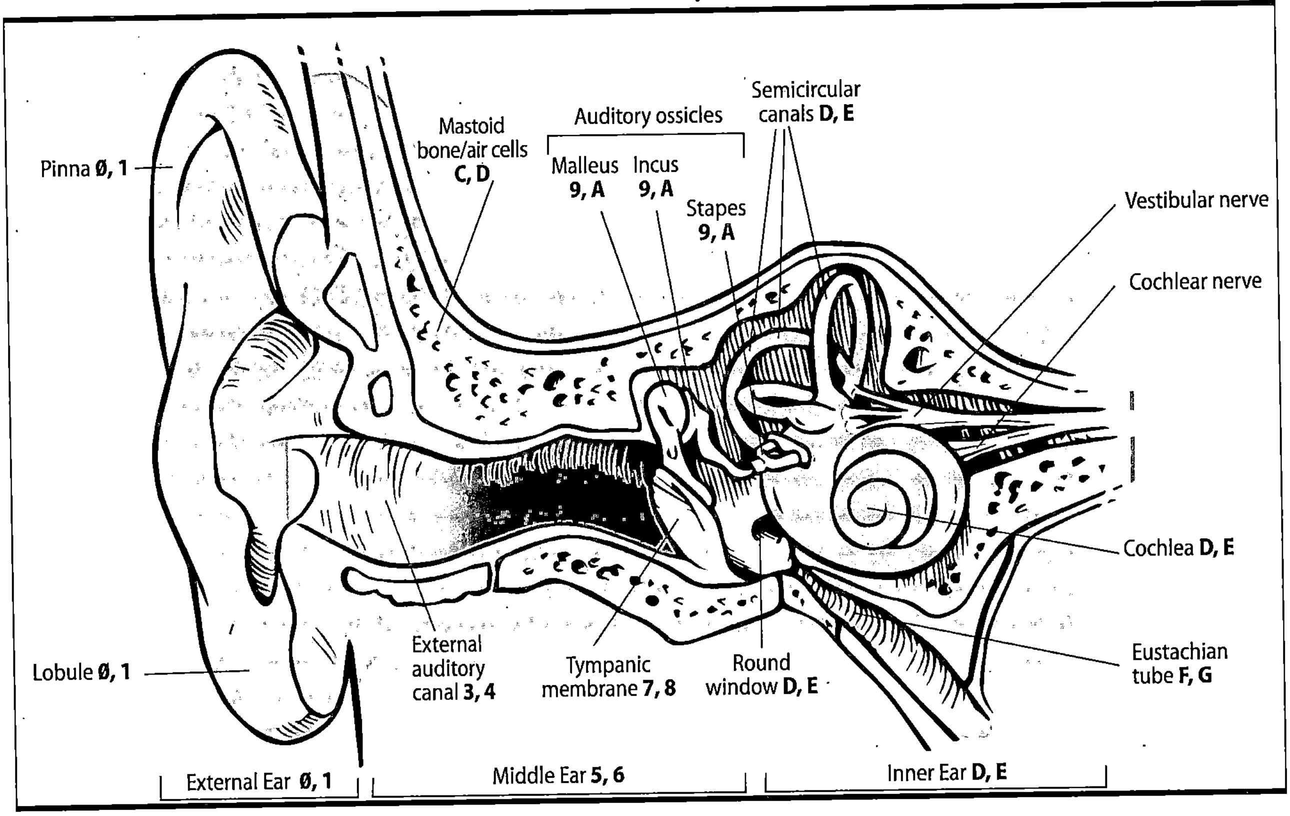
Pinna Ø, 1
Mastoid bone/air cells C, D
Auditory ossicles
Malleus 9, A
Incus 9, A
Stapes 9, A
Semicircular canals D, E
Vestibular nerve
Cochlear nerve
Cochlea D, E
Eustachian tube F, G
Lobule Ø, 1
External auditory canal 3, 4
Tympanic membrane 7, 8
Round window D, E
External Ear Ø, 1
Middle Ear 5, 6
Inner Ear D, E

Nasal Turbinates

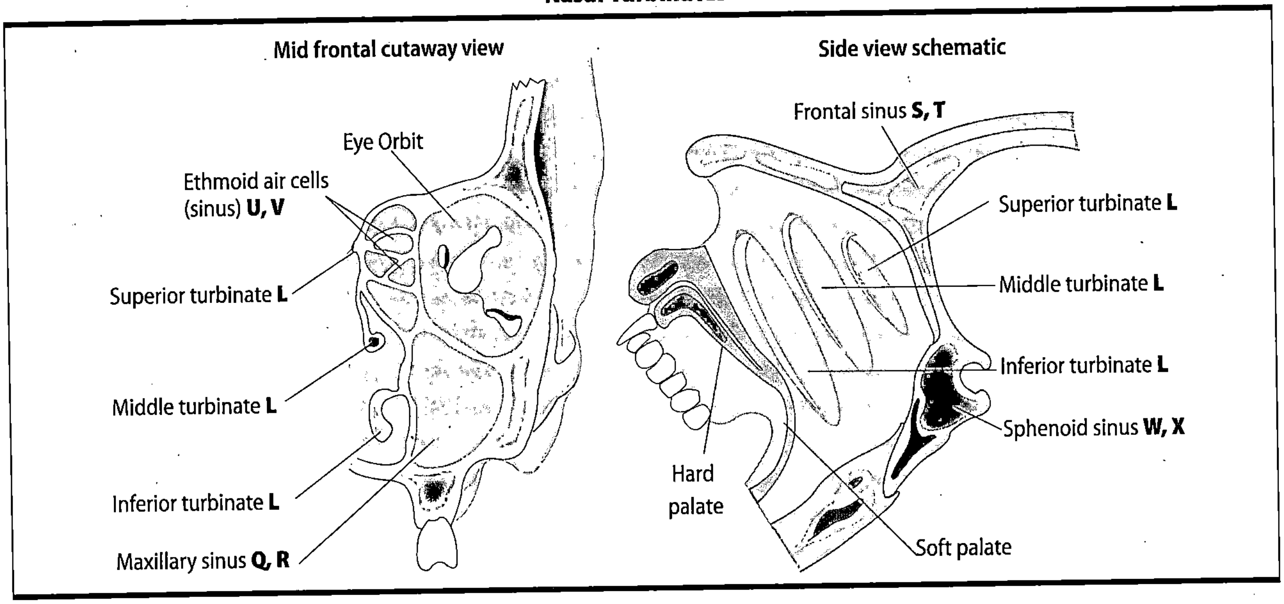
Mid frontal cutaway view
Eye Orbit
Ethmoid air cells (sinus) U, V
Superior turbinate L
Middle turbinate L
Inferior turbinate L
Maxillary sinus Q, R
Side view schematic
Frontal sinus S, T
Superior turbinate L
Middle turbinate L
Inferior turbinate L
Sphenoid sinus W, X
Hard palate
Soft palate

Paranasal Sinuses

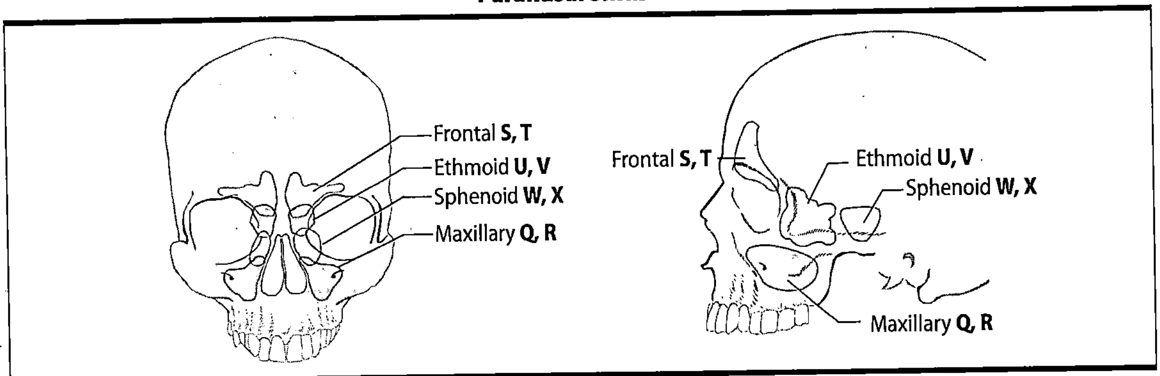
Frontal S, T
Ethmoid U, V
Sphenoid W, X
Maxillary Q, R
Frontal S, T
Ethmoid U, V
Sphenoid W, X
Maxillary Q, R

Ø Medical and Surgical
9 Ear, Nose, Sinus
Ø Alteration Definition: Modifying the anatomic structure of a body part without affecting the function of the body part
Explanation: Principal purpose is to improve appearance

Body Part Character 4		Approach Character 5	Device Character 6	Qualifier Character 7
Ø External Ear, Right Antihelix Antitragus Auricle Earlobe Helix Pinna Tragus **1 External Ear, Left** *See Ø External Ear, Right*	**2 External Ear, Bilateral** *See Ø External Ear, Right* **K Nasal Mucosa and Soft Tissue** Columella External naris Greater alar cartilage Internal naris Lateral nasal cartilage Lesser alar cartilage Nasal cavity Nostril	**Ø Open** **3 Percutaneous** **4 Percutaneous Endoscopic** **X External**	**7 Autologous Tissue Substitute** **J Synthetic Substitute** **K Nonautologous Tissue Substitute** **Z No Device**	**Z No Qualifier**

Ø Medical and Surgical
9 Ear, Nose, Sinus
1 Bypass Definition: Altering the route of passage of the contents of a tubular body part
Explanation: Rerouting contents of a body part to a downstream area of the normal route, to a similar route and body part, or to an abnormal route and dissimilar body part. Includes one or more anastomoses, with or without the use of a device.

Body Part Character 4	Approach Character 5	Device Character 6	Qualifier Character 7
D Inner Ear, Right Bony labyrinth Bony vestibule Cochlea Round window Semicircular canal **E Inner Ear, Left** *See D Inner Ear, Right*	**Ø Open**	**7 Autologous Tissue Substitute** **J Synthetic Substitute** **K Nonautologous Tissue Substitute** **Z No Device**	**Ø Endolymphatic**

Ø Medical and Surgical
9 Ear, Nose, Sinus
2 Change Definition: Taking out or off a device from a body part and putting back an identical or similar device in or on the same body part without cutting or puncturing the skin or a mucous membrane
Explanation: All CHANGE procedures are coded using the approach EXTERNAL

Body Part Character 4	Approach Character 5	Device Character 6	Qualifier Character 7
H Ear, Right **J Ear, Left** **K Nasal Mucosa and Soft Tissue** Columella External naris Greater alar cartilage Internal naris Lateral nasal cartilage Lesser alar cartilage Nasal cavity Nostril **Y Sinus**	**X External**	**Ø Drainage Device** **Y Other Device**	**Z No Qualifier**
Non-OR All body part, approach, device, and qualifier values			

Ø Medical and Surgical
9 Ear, Nose, Sinus
3 Control Definition: Stopping, or attempting to stop, postprocedural or other acute bleeding
Explanation: The site of the bleeding is coded as an anatomical region and not to a specific body part

Body Part Character 4	Approach Character 5	Device Character 6	Qualifier Character 7
K Nasal Mucosa and Soft Tissue Columella External naris Greater alar cartilage Internal naris Lateral nasal cartilage Lesser alar cartilage Nasal cavity Nostril	**7 Via Natural or Artificial Opening** **8 Via Natural or Artificial Opening Endoscopic**	**Z No Device**	**Z No Qualifier**

Ø Medical and Surgical
9 Ear, Nose, Sinus
5 Destruction Definition: Physical eradication of all or a portion of a body part by the direct use of energy, force, or a destructive agent
Explanation: None of the body part is physically taken out

Body Part Character 4		Approach Character 5	Device Character 6	Qualifier Character 7
Ø External Ear, Right Antihelix Antitragus Auricle Earlobe Helix Pinna Tragus	**1 External Ear, Left** *See Ø External Ear, Right*	**Ø Open** **3 Percutaneous** **4 Percutaneous Endoscopic** **X External**	**Z No Device**	**Z No Qualifier**
3 External Auditory Canal, Right External auditory meatus	**4 External Auditory Canal, Left** *See 3 External Auditory Canal, Right*	**Ø Open** **3 Percutaneous** **4 Percutaneous Endoscopic** **7 Via Natural or Artificial Opening** **8 Via Natural or Artificial Opening Endoscopic** **X External**	**Z No Device**	**Z No Qualifier**
5 Middle Ear, Right Oval window Tympanic cavity **6 Middle Ear, Left** *See 5 Middle Ear, Right* **9 Auditory Ossicle, Right** Incus Malleus Stapes **A Auditory Ossicle, Left** *See 9 Auditory Ossicle, Right*	**D Inner Ear, Right** Bony labyrinth Bony vestibule Cochlea Round window Semicircular canal **E Inner Ear, Left** *See D Inner Ear, Right*	**Ø Open** **8 Via Natural or Artificial Opening Endoscopic**	**Z No Device**	**Z No Qualifier**
7 Tympanic Membrane, Right Pars flaccida **8 Tympanic Membrane, Left** *See 7 Tympanic Membrane, Right* **F Eustachian Tube, Right** Auditory tube Pharyngotympanic tube **G Eustachian Tube, Left** *See F Eustachian Tube, Right*	**L Nasal Turbinate** Inferior turbinate Middle turbinate Nasal concha Superior turbinate **N Nasopharynx** Choana Fossa of Rosenmuller Pharyngeal recess Rhinopharynx	**Ø Open** **3 Percutaneous** **4 Percutaneous Endoscopic** **7 Via Natural or Artificial Opening** **8 Via Natural or Artificial Opening Endoscopic**	**Z No Device**	**Z No Qualifier**
B Mastoid Sinus, Right Mastoid air cells **C Mastoid Sinus, Left** *See B Mastoid Sinus, Right* **M Nasal Septum** Quadrangular cartilage Septal cartilage Vomer bone **P Accessory Sinus** **Q Maxillary Sinus, Right** Antrum of Highmore	**R Maxillary Sinus, Left** *See Q Maxillary Sinus, Right* **S Frontal Sinus, Right** **T Frontal Sinus, Left** **U Ethmoid Sinus, Right** Ethmoidal air cell **V Ethmoid Sinus, Left** *See U Ethmoid Sinus, Right* **W Sphenoid Sinus, Right** **X Sphenoid Sinus, Left**	**Ø Open** **3 Percutaneous** **4 Percutaneous Endoscopic** **8 Via Natural or Artificial Opening Endoscopic**	**Z No Device**	**Z No Qualifier**
K Nasal Mucosa and Soft Tissue Columella External naris Greater alar cartilage Internal naris Lateral nasal cartilage Lesser alar cartilage Nasal cavity Nostril		**Ø Open** **3 Percutaneous** **4 Percutaneous Endoscopic** **8 Via Natural or Artificial Opening Endoscopic** **X External**	**Z No Device**	**Z No Qualifier**

Non-OR Ø95[Ø,1][Ø,3,4,X]ZZ
Non-OR Ø95[3,4][Ø,3,4,7,8,X]ZZ
Non-OR Ø95[F,G][Ø,3,4,7,8]ZZ
Non-OR Ø95M[Ø,3,4,8]ZZ
Non-OR Ø95K[Ø,3,4,8,X]ZZ

Ø Medical and Surgical
9 Ear, Nose, Sinus
7 Dilation Definition: Expanding an orifice or the lumen of a tubular body part

Explanation: The orifice can be a natural orifice or an artificially created orifice. Accomplished by stretching a tubular body part using intraluminal pressure or by cutting part of the orifice or wall of the tubular body part.

Body Part Character 4	Approach Character 5	Device Character 6	Qualifier Character 7
F Eustachian Tube, Right Auditory tube Pharyngotympanic tube **G** Eustachian Tube, Left *See F Eustachian Tube, Right*	**Ø** Open **7** Via Natural or Artificial Opening **8** Via Natural or Artificial Opening Endoscopic	**D** Intraluminal Device **Z** No Device	**Z** No Qualifier
F Eustachian Tube, Right Auditory tube Pharyngotympanic tube **G** Eustachian Tube, Left *See F Eustachian Tube, Right*	**3** Percutaneous **4** Percutaneous Endoscopic	**Z** No Device	**Z** No Qualifier

Non-OR All body part, approach, device, and qualifier values

Ø Medical and Surgical
9 Ear, Nose, Sinus
8 Division Definition: Cutting into a body part, without draining fluids and/or gases from the body part, in order to separate or transect a body part

Explanation: All or a portion of the body part is separated into two or more portions

Body Part Character 4	Approach Character 5	Device Character 6	Qualifier Character 7
L Nasal Turbinate Inferior turbinate Middle turbinate Nasal concha Superior turbinate	**Ø** Open **3** Percutaneous **4** Percutaneous Endoscopic **7** Via Natural or Artificial Opening **8** Via Natural or Artificial Opening Endoscopic	**Z** No Device	**Z** No Qualifier

Ø Medical and Surgical
9 Ear, Nose, Sinus
9 Drainage Definition: Taking or letting out fluids and/or gases from a body part
Explanation: The qualifier DIAGNOSTIC is used to identify drainage procedures that are biopsies

Body Part Character 4		Approach Character 5	Device Character 6	Qualifier Character 7
Ø External Ear, Right Antihelix Antitragus Auricle Earlobe Helix Pinna Tragus	**1 External Ear, Left** *See Ø External Ear, Right*	**Ø Open** **3 Percutaneous** **4 Percutaneous Endoscopic** **X External**	**Ø Drainage Device**	**Z No Qualifier**
Ø External Ear, Right Antihelix Antitragus Auricle Earlobe Helix Pinna Tragus	**1 External Ear, Left** *See Ø External Ear, Right*	**Ø Open** **3 Percutaneous** **4 Percutaneous Endoscopic** **X External**	**Z No Device**	**X Diagnostic** **Z No Qualifier**
3 External Auditory Canal, Right External auditory meatus **4 External Auditory Canal, Left** *See 3 External Auditory Canal, Right*	**K Nasal Mucosa and Soft Tissue** Columella External naris Greater alar cartilage Internal naris Lateral nasal cartilage Lesser alar cartilage Nasal cavity Nostril	**Ø Open** **3 Percutaneous** **4 Percutaneous Endoscopic** **7 Via Natural or Artificial Opening** **8 Via Natural or Artificial Opening Endoscopic** **X External**	**Ø Drainage Device**	**Z No Qualifier**
3 External Auditory Canal, Right External auditory meatus **4 External Auditory Canal, Left** *See 3 External Auditory Canal, Right*	**K Nasal Mucosa and Soft Tissue** Columella External naris Greater alar cartilage Internal naris Lateral nasal cartilage Lesser alar cartilage Nasal cavity Nostril	**Ø Open** **3 Percutaneous** **4 Percutaneous Endoscopic** **7 Via Natural or Artificial Opening** **8 Via Natural or Artificial Opening Endoscopic** **X External**	**Z No Device**	**X Diagnostic** **Z No Qualifier**
5 Middle Ear, Right Oval window Tympanic cavity **6 Middle Ear, Left** *See 5 Middle Ear, Right* **9 Auditory Ossicle, Right** Incus Malleus Stapes	**A Auditory Ossicle, Left** *See 9 Auditory Ossicle, Right* **D Inner Ear, Right** Bony labyrinth Bony vestibule Cochlea Round window Semicircular canal **E Inner Ear, Left** *See D Inner Ear, Right*	**Ø Open** **7 Via Natural or Artificial Opening** **8 Via Natural or Artificial Opening Endoscopic**	**Ø Drainage Device**	**Z No Qualifier**
5 Middle Ear, Right Oval window Tympanic cavity **6 Middle Ear, Left** *See 5 Middle Ear, Right* **9 Auditory Ossicle, Right** Incus Malleus Stapes	**A Auditory Ossicle, Left** *See 9 Auditory Ossicle, Right* **D Inner Ear, Right** Bony labyrinth Bony vestibule Cochlea Round window Semicircular canal **E Inner Ear, Left** *See D Inner Ear, Right*	**Ø Open** **7 Via Natural or Artificial Opening** **8 Via Natural or Artificial Opening Endoscopic**	**Z No Device**	**X Diagnostic** **Z No Qualifier**

Ø99 Continued on next page

Non-OR Ø99[Ø,1][Ø,3,4,X]ØZ
Non-OR Ø99[Ø,1][Ø,3,4,X]Z[X,Z]
Non-OR Ø99[3,4,K][Ø,3,4,7,8,X]ØZ
Non-OR Ø99[3,4,K][Ø,3,4,7,8,X]Z[X,Z]
Non-OR Ø9958ØZ
Non-OR Ø99[6,9,A,D,E][7,8]ØZ
Non-OR Ø99[5,6]ØZZ
Non-OR Ø99[5,6,9,A,D,E][7,8]Z[X,Z]

Ø Medical and Surgical
9 Ear, Nose, Sinus
9 Drainage Definition: Taking or letting out fluids and/or gases from a body part
Explanation: The qualifier DIAGNOSTIC is used to identify drainage procedures that are biopsies

Ø99 Continued

Body Part Character 4	Approach Character 5	Device Character 6	Qualifier Character 7
7 Tympanic Membrane, Right Pars flaccida **8** Tympanic Membrane, Left *See 7 Tympanic Membrane, Right* **B** Mastoid Sinus, Right Mastoid air cells **C** Mastoid Sinus, Left *See B Mastoid Sinus, Right* **F** Eustachian Tube, Right Auditory tube Pharyngotympanic tube **G** Eustachian Tube, Left *See F Eustachian Tube, Right* **L** Nasal Turbinate Inferior turbinate Middle turbinate Nasal concha Superior turbinate **M** Nasal Septum Quadrangular cartilage Septal cartilage Vomer bone **N** Nasopharynx Choana Fossa of Rosenmuller Pharyngeal recess Rhinopharynx **P** Accessory Sinus **Q** Maxillary Sinus, Right Antrum of Highmore **R** Maxillary Sinus, Left *See Q Maxillary Sinus, Right* **S** Frontal Sinus, Right **T** Frontal Sinus, Left **U** Ethmoid Sinus, Right Ethmoidal air cell **V** Ethmoid Sinus, Left *See U Ethmoid Sinus, Right* **W** Sphenoid Sinus, Right **X** Sphenoid Sinus, Left	**Ø** Open **3** Percutaneous **4** Percutaneous Endoscopic **7** Via Natural or Artificial Opening **8** Via Natural or Artificial Opening Endoscopic	**Ø** Drainage Device	**Z** No Qualifier
7 Tympanic Membrane, Right Pars flaccida **8** Tympanic Membrane, Left *See 7 Tympanic Membrane, Right* **B** Mastoid Sinus, Right Mastoid air cells **C** Mastoid Sinus, Left *See B Mastoid Sinus, Right* **F** Eustachian Tube, Right Auditory tube Pharyngotympanic tube **G** Eustachian Tube, Left *See F Eustachian Tube, Right* **L** Nasal Turbinate Inferior turbinate Middle turbinate Nasal concha Superior turbinate **M** Nasal Septum Quadrangular cartilage Septal cartilage Vomer bone **N** Nasopharynx Choana Fossa of Rosenmuller Pharyngeal recess Rhinopharynx **P** Accessory Sinus **Q** Maxillary Sinus, Right Antrum of Highmore **R** Maxillary Sinus, Left *See Q Maxillary Sinus, Right* **S** Frontal Sinus, Right **T** Frontal Sinus, Left **U** Ethmoid Sinus, Right Ethmoidal air cell **V** Ethmoid Sinus, Left *See U Ethmoid Sinus, Right* **W** Sphenoid Sinus, Right **X** Sphenoid Sinus, Left	**Ø** Open **3** Percutaneous **4** Percutaneous Endoscopic **7** Via Natural or Artificial Opening **8** Via Natural or Artificial Opening Endoscopic	**Z** No Device	**X** Diagnostic **Z** No Qualifier

Non-OR Ø99[B,C][3,7,8]ØZ
Non-OR Ø99[F,G,L,M][Ø,3,4,7,8]ØZ
Non-OR Ø99N3ØZ
Non-OR Ø99[P,Q,R,S,T,U,V,W,X][3,4,7,8]ØZ
Non-OR Ø99[7,8][Ø,3,4,7,8]ZZ
Non-OR Ø99[7,8][7,8]ZX
Non-OR Ø99[B,C]3ZZ
Non-OR Ø99[B,C][7,8]Z[X,Z]
Non-OR Ø99[F,G][Ø,3,4,7,8]ZZ
Non-OR Ø99[F,G][7,8]ZX
Non-OR Ø99[L,M][Ø,3,4,7,8]Z[X,Z]
Non-OR Ø99N[Ø,3,4,7,8]ZX
Non-OR Ø99N3ZZ
Non-OR Ø99[P,Q,R,S,T,U,V,W,X][3,4,7,8]Z[X,Z]

Ear, Nose, Sinus
Ø99–Ø99

Ø Medical and Surgical
9 Ear, Nose, Sinus
B Excision Definition: Cutting out or off, without replacement, a portion of a body part
Explanation: The qualifier DIAGNOSTIC is used to identify excision procedures that are biopsies

Body Part Character 4		Approach Character 5	Device Character 6	Qualifier Character 7
Ø External Ear, Right Antihelix Antitragus Auricle Earlobe Helix Pinna Tragus	**1 External Ear, Left** *See Ø External Ear, Right*	**Ø Open** **3 Percutaneous** **4 Percutaneous Endoscopic** **X External**	**Z No Device**	**X Diagnostic** **Z No Qualifier**
3 External Auditory Canal, Right External auditory meatus	**4 External Auditory Canal, Left** *See 3 External Auditory Canal, Right*	**Ø Open** **3 Percutaneous** **4 Percutaneous Endoscopic** **7 Via Natural or Artificial Opening** **8 Via Natural or Artificial Opening Endoscopic** **X External**	**Z No Device**	**X Diagnostic** **Z No Qualifier**
5 Middle Ear, Right Oval window Tympanic cavity **6 Middle Ear, Left** *See 5 Middle Ear, Right* **9 Auditory Ossicle, Right** Incus Malleus Stapes	**A Auditory Ossicle, Left** *See 9 Auditory Ossicle, Right* **D Inner Ear, Right** Bony labyrinth Bony vestibule Cochlea Round window Semicircular canal **E Inner Ear, Left** *See D Inner Ear, Right*	**Ø Open** **8 Via Natural or Artificial Opening Endoscopic**	**Z No Device**	**X Diagnostic** **Z No Qualifier**
7 Tympanic Membrane, Right Pars flaccida **8 Tympanic Membrane, Left** *See 7 Tympanic Membrane, Right* **F Eustachian Tube, Right** Auditory tube Pharyngotympanic tube **G Eustachian Tube, Left** *See F Eustachian Tube, Right*	**L Nasal Turbinate** Inferior turbinate Middle turbinate Nasal concha Superior turbinate **N Nasopharynx** Choana Fossa of Rosenmuller Pharyngeal recess Rhinopharynx	**Ø Open** **3 Percutaneous** **4 Percutaneous Endoscopic** **7 Via Natural or Artificial Opening** **8 Via Natural or Artificial Opening Endoscopic**	**Z No Device**	**X Diagnostic** **Z No Qualifier**
B Mastoid Sinus, Right Mastoid air cells **C Mastoid Sinus, Left** *See B Mastoid Sinus, Right* **M Nasal Septum** Quadrangular cartilage Septal cartilage Vomer bone **P Accessory Sinus** **Q Maxillary Sinus, Right** Antrum of Highmore	**R Maxillary Sinus, Left** *See Q Maxillary Sinus, Right* **S Frontal Sinus, Right** **T Frontal Sinus, Left** **U Ethmoid Sinus, Right** Ethmoidal air cell **V Ethmoid Sinus, Left** *See U Ethmoid Sinus, Right* **W Sphenoid Sinus, Right** **X Sphenoid Sinus, Left**	**Ø Open** **3 Percutaneous** **4 Percutaneous Endoscopic** **8 Via Natural or Artificial Opening Endoscopic**	**Z No Device**	**X Diagnostic** **Z No Qualifier**
K Nasal Mucosa and Soft Tissue Columella External naris Greater alar cartilage Internal naris Lateral nasal cartilage Lesser alar cartilage Nasal cavity Nostril		**Ø Open** **3 Percutaneous** **4 Percutaneous Endoscopic** **8 Via Natural or Artificial Opening Endoscopic** **X External**	**Z No Device**	**X Diagnostic** **Z No Qualifier**

Non-OR Ø9B[Ø,1][Ø,3,4,X]Z[X,Z]
Non-OR Ø9B[3,4][Ø,3,4,7,8,X]Z[X,Z]
Non-OR Ø9B[F,G,L,N][Ø,3,4,7,8]Z[X,Z]
Non-OR Ø9BM[Ø,3,4,8]ZX
Non-OR Ø9B[P,Q,R,S,T,U,V,W,X][3,4,8]ZX
Non-OR Ø9BK8Z[X,Z]

Ø Medical and Surgical
9 Ear, Nose, Sinus
C Extirpation Definition: Taking or cutting out solid matter from a body part

Explanation: The solid matter may be an abnormal byproduct of a biological function or a foreign body; it may be imbedded in a body part or in the lumen of a tubular body part. The solid matter may or may not have been previously broken into pieces.

Body Part Character 4		Approach Character 5	Device Character 6	Qualifier Character 7
Ø External Ear, Right Antihelix Antitragus Auricle Earlobe Helix Pinna Tragus	**1 External Ear, Left** *See Ø External Ear, Right*	**Ø** Open **3** Percutaneous **4** Percutaneous Endoscopic **X** External	**Z** No Device	**Z** No Qualifier
3 External Auditory Canal, Right External auditory meatus	**4 External Auditory Canal, Left** *See 3 External Auditory Canal, Right*	**Ø** Open **3** Percutaneous **4** Percutaneous Endoscopic **7** Via Natural or Artificial Opening **8** Via Natural or Artificial Opening Endoscopic **X** External	**Z** No Device	**Z** No Qualifier
5 Middle Ear, Right Oval window Tympanic cavity **6 Middle Ear, Left** *See 5 Middle Ear, Right* **9 Auditory Ossicle, Right** Incus Malleus Stapes	**A Auditory Ossicle, Left** *See 9 Auditory Ossicle, Right* **D Inner Ear, Right** Bony labyrinth Bony vestibule Cochlea Round window Semicircular canal **E Inner Ear, Left** *See D Inner Ear, Right*	**Ø** Open **8** Via Natural or Artificial Opening Endoscopic	**Z** No Device	**Z** No Qualifier
7 Tympanic Membrane, Right Pars flaccida **8 Tympanic Membrane, Left** *See 7 Tympanic Membrane, Right* **F Eustachian Tube, Right** Auditory tube Pharyngotympanic tube **G Eustachian Tube, Left** *See F Eustachian Tube, Right*	**L Nasal Turbinate** Inferior turbinate Middle turbinate Nasal concha Superior turbinate **N Nasopharynx** Choana Fossa of Rosenmuller Pharyngeal recess Rhinopharynx	**Ø** Open **3** Percutaneous **4** Percutaneous Endoscopic **7** Via Natural or Artificial Opening **8** Via Natural or Artificial Opening Endoscopic	**Z** No Device	**Z** No Qualifier
B Mastoid Sinus, Right Mastoid air cells **C Mastoid Sinus, Left** *See B Mastoid Sinus, Right* **M Nasal Septum** Quadrangular cartilage Septal cartilage Vomer bone **P Accessory Sinus** **Q Maxillary Sinus, Right** Antrum of Highmore	**R Maxillary Sinus, Left** *See Q Maxillary Sinus, Right* **S Frontal Sinus, Right** **T Frontal Sinus, Left** **U Ethmoid Sinus, Right** Ethmoidal air cell **V Ethmoid Sinus, Left** *See U Ethmoid Sinus, Right* **W Sphenoid Sinus, Right** **X Sphenoid Sinus, Left**	**Ø** Open **3** Percutaneous **4** Percutaneous Endoscopic **8** Via Natural or Artificial Opening Endoscopic	**Z** No Device	**Z** No Qualifier
K Nasal Mucosa and Soft Tissue Columella External naris Greater alar cartilage Internal naris Lateral nasal cartilage Lesser alar cartilage Nasal cavity Nostril		**Ø** Open **3** Percutaneous **4** Percutaneous Endoscopic **8** Via Natural or Artificial Opening Endoscopic **X** External	**Z** No Device	**Z** No Qualifier

Non-OR Ø9C[Ø,1][Ø,3,4,X]ZZ
Non-OR Ø9C[3,4][Ø,3,4,7,8,X]ZZ
Non-OR Ø9C[7,8,F,G,L][Ø,3,4,7,8]ZZ
Non-OR Ø9CM[Ø,3,4,8]ZZ
Non-OR Ø9CK8ZZ

Ø Medical and Surgical
9 Ear, Nose, Sinus
D Extraction Definition: Pulling or stripping out or off all or a portion of a body part by the use of force
Explanation: The qualifier DIAGNOSTIC is used to identify extraction procedures that are biopsies

Body Part Character 4	Approach Character 5	Device Character 6	Qualifier Character 7
7 Tympanic Membrane, Right Pars flaccida **8 Tympanic Membrane, Left** *See 7 Tympanic Membrane, Right* **L Nasal Turbinate** Inferior turbinate Middle turbinate Nasal concha Superior turbinate	**Ø Open** **3 Percutaneous** **4 Percutaneous Endoscopic** **7 Via Natural or Artificial Opening** **8 Via Natural or Artificial Opening Endoscopic**	**Z No Device**	**Z No Qualifier**
9 Auditory Ossicle, Right Incus Malleus Stapes **A Auditory Ossicle, Left** *See 9 Auditory Ossicle, Right*	**Ø Open**	**Z No Device**	**Z No Qualifier**
B Mastoid Sinus, Right Mastoid air cells **C Mastoid Sinus, Left** *See B Mastoid Sinus, Right* **M Nasal Septum** Quadrangular cartilage Septal cartilage Vomer bone **P Accessory Sinus** **Q Maxillary Sinus, Right** Antrum of Highmore **R Maxillary Sinus, Left** *See Q Maxillary Sinus, Right* **S Frontal Sinus, Right** **T Frontal Sinus, Left** **U Ethmoid Sinus, Right** Ethmoidal air cell **V Ethmoid Sinus, Left** *See U Ethmoid Sinus, Right* **W Sphenoid Sinus, Right** **X Sphenoid Sinus, Left**	**Ø Open** **3 Percutaneous** **4 Percutaneous Endoscopic**	**Z No Device**	**Z No Qualifier**

Ø Medical and Surgical
9 Ear, Nose, Sinus
H Insertion Definition: Putting in a nonbiological appliance that monitors, assists, performs, or prevents a physiological function but does not physically take the place of a body part
Explanation: None

Body Part Character 4	Approach Character 5	Device Character 6	Qualifier Character 7
D Inner Ear, Right Bony labyrinth Bony vestibule Cochlea Round window Semicircular canal **E Inner Ear, Left** *See D Inner Ear, Right*	**Ø Open** **3 Percutaneous** **4 Percutaneous Endoscopic**	**4 Hearing Device, Bone Conduction** **5 Hearing Device, Single Channel Cochlear Prosthesis** **6 Hearing Device, Multiple Channel Cochlear Prosthesis** **S Hearing Device**	**Z No Qualifier**
H Ear, Right **J Ear, Left** **K Nasal Mucosa and Soft Tissue** Columella External naris Greater alar cartilage Internal naris Lateral nasal cartilage Lesser alar cartilage Nasal cavity Nostril **Y Sinus**	**Ø Open** **3 Percutaneous** **4 Percutaneous Endoscopic** **7 Via Natural or Artificial Opening** **8 Via Natural or Artificial Opening Endoscopic**	**Y Other Device**	**Z No Qualifier**
N Nasopharynx Choana Fossa of Rosenmuller Pharyngeal recess Rhinopharynx	**7 Via Natural or Artificial Opening** **8 Via Natural or Artificial Opening Endoscopic**	**B Intraluminal Device, Airway**	**Z No Qualifier**

Non-OR Ø9H[H,J][3,4,7,8]YZ
Non-OR Ø9H[K,Y][Ø,3,4,7,8]YZ
Non-OR Ø9HN[7,8]BZ

Ø Medical and Surgical
9 Ear, Nose, Sinus
J Inspection Definition: Visually and/or manually exploring a body part

Explanation: Visual exploration may be performed with or without optical instrumentation. Manual exploration may be performed directly or through intervening body layers.

Body Part Character 4	Approach Character 5	Device Character 6	Qualifier Character 7
7 Tympanic Membrane, Right Pars flaccida 8 Tympanic Membrane, Left *See 7 Tympanic Membrane, Right* H Ear, Right J Ear, Left	Ø Open 3 Percutaneous 4 Percutaneous Endoscopic 7 Via Natural or Artificial Opening 8 Via Natural or Artificial Opening Endoscopic X External	Z No Device	Z No Qualifier
D Inner Ear, Right Bony labyrinth Bony vestibule Cochlea Round window Semicircular canal E Inner Ear, Left *See D Inner Ear, Right* K Nasal Mucosa and Soft Tissue Columella External naris Greater alar cartilage Internal naris Lateral nasal cartilage Lesser alar cartilage Nasal cavity Nostril Y Sinus	Ø Open 3 Percutaneous 4 Percutaneous Endoscopic 8 Via Natural or Artificial Opening Endoscopic X External	Z No Device	Z No Qualifier

Non-OR Ø9J[7,8][3,7,8,X]ZZ
Non-OR Ø9J[H,J][Ø,3,4,7,8,X]ZZ
Non-OR Ø9J[D,E][3,8,X]ZZ
Non-OR Ø9J[K,Y][Ø,3,4,8,X]ZZ

Ø Medical and Surgical
9 Ear, Nose, Sinus
M Reattachment Definition: Putting back in or on all or a portion of a separated body part to its normal location or other suitable location

Explanation: Vascular circulation and nervous pathways may or may not be reestablished

Body Part Character 4	Approach Character 5	Device Character 6	Qualifier Character 7
Ø External Ear, Right Antihelix Antitragus Auricle Earlobe Helix Pinna Tragus 1 External Ear, Left *See Ø External Ear, Right* K Nasal Mucosa and Soft Tissue Columella External naris Greater alar cartilage Internal naris Lateral nasal cartilage Lesser alar cartilage Nasal cavity Nostril	X External	Z No Device	Z No Qualifier

Ø Medical and Surgical
9 Ear, Nose, Sinus
N Release Definition: Freeing a body part from an abnormal physical constraint by cutting or by the use of force
Explanation: Some of the restraining tissue may be taken out but none of the body part is taken out

Body Part Character 4	Approach Character 5	Device Character 6	Qualifier Character 7
Ø External Ear, Right Antihelix Antitragus Auricle Earlobe Helix Pinna Tragus **1 External Ear, Left** *See Ø External Ear, Right*	**Ø Open** **3 Percutaneous** **4 Percutaneous Endoscopic** **X External**	**Z No Device**	**Z No Qualifier**
3 External Auditory Canal, Right External auditory meatus **4 External Auditory Canal, Left** *See 3 External Auditory Canal, Right*	**Ø Open** **3 Percutaneous** **4 Percutaneous Endoscopic** **7 Via Natural or Artificial Opening** **8 Via Natural or Artificial Opening Endoscopic** **X External**	**Z No Device**	**Z No Qualifier**
5 Middle Ear, Right Oval window Tympanic cavity **6 Middle Ear, Left** *See 5 Middle Ear, Right* **9 Auditory Ossicle, Right** Incus Malleus Stapes **A Auditory Ossicle, Left** *See 9 Auditory Ossicle, Right* **D Inner Ear, Right** Bony labyrinth Bony vestibule Cochlea Round window Semicircular canal **E Inner Ear, Left** *See D Inner Ear, Right*	**Ø Open** **8 Via Natural or Artificial Opening Endoscopic**	**Z No Device**	**Z No Qualifier**
7 Tympanic Membrane, Right Pars flaccida **8 Tympanic Membrane, Left** *See 7 Tympanic Membrane, Right* **F Eustachian Tube, Right** Auditory tube Pharyngotympanic tube **G Eustachian Tube, Left** *See F Eustachian Tube, Right* **L Nasal Turbinate** Inferior turbinate Middle turbinate Nasal concha Superior turbinate **N Nasopharynx** Choana Fossa of Rosenmuller Pharyngeal recess Rhinopharynx	**Ø Open** **3 Percutaneous** **4 Percutaneous Endoscopic** **7 Via Natural or Artificial Opening** **8 Via Natural or Artificial Opening Endoscopic**	**Z No Device**	**Z No Qualifier**
B Mastoid Sinus, Right Mastoid air cells **C Mastoid Sinus, Left** *See B Mastoid Sinus, Right* **M Nasal Septum** Quadrangular cartilage Septal cartilage Vomer bone **P Accessory Sinus** **Q Maxillary Sinus, Right** Antrum of Highmore **R Maxillary Sinus, Left** *See Q Maxillary Sinus, Right* **S Frontal Sinus, Right** **T Frontal Sinus, Left** **U Ethmoid Sinus, Right** Ethmoidal air cell **V Ethmoid Sinus, Left** *See U Ethmoid Sinus, Right* **W Sphenoid Sinus, Right** **X Sphenoid Sinus, Left**	**Ø Open** **3 Percutaneous** **4 Percutaneous Endoscopic** **8 Via Natural or Artificial Opening Endoscopic**	**Z No Device**	**Z No Qualifier**
K Nasal Mucosa and Soft Tissue Columella External naris Greater alar cartilage Internal naris Lateral nasal cartilage Lesser alar cartilage Nasal cavity Nostril	**Ø Open** **3 Percutaneous** **4 Percutaneous Endoscopic** **8 Via Natural or Artificial Opening Endoscopic** **X External**	**Z No Device**	**Z No Qualifier**

Non-OR Ø9N[Ø,1]XZZ
Non-OR Ø9N[3,4]XZZ
Non-OR Ø9N[F,G,L][Ø,3,4,7,8]ZZ
Non-OR Ø9NM[Ø,3,4,8]ZZ
Non-OR Ø9NK[Ø,3,4,8,X]ZZ

Ø Medical and Surgical
9 Ear, Nose, Sinus
P Removal Definition: Taking out or off a device from a body part

Explanation: If a device is taken out and a similar device put in without cutting or puncturing the skin or mucous membrane, the procedure is coded to the root operation CHANGE. Otherwise, the procedure for taking out a device is coded to the root operation REMOVAL.

Body Part Character 4	Approach Character 5	Device Character 6	Qualifier Character 7
7 Tympanic Membrane, Right Pars flaccida **8** Tympanic Membrane, Left *See 7 Tympanic Membrane, Right*	**Ø** Open **7** Via Natural or Artificial Opening **8** Via Natural or Artificial Opening Endoscopic **X** External	**Ø** Drainage Device	**Z** No Qualifier
D Inner Ear, Right Bony labyrinth Bony vestibule Cochlea Round window Semicircular canal **E** Inner Ear, Left *See D Inner Ear, Right*	**Ø** Open **7** Via Natural or Artificial Opening **8** Via Natural or Artificial Opening Endoscopic	**S** Hearing Device	**Z** No Qualifier
H Ear, Right **J** Ear, Left **K** Nasal Mucosa and Soft Tissue Columella External naris Greater alar cartilage Internal naris Lateral nasal cartilage Lesser alar cartilage Nasal cavity Nostril	**Ø** Open **3** Percutaneous **4** Percutaneous Endoscopic **7** Via Natural or Artificial Opening **8** Via Natural or Artificial Opening Endoscopic	**Ø** Drainage Device **7** Autologous Tissue Substitute **D** Intraluminal Device **J** Synthetic Substitute **K** Nonautologous Tissue Substitute **Y** Other Device	**Z** No Qualifier
H Ear, Right **J** Ear, Left **K** Nasal Mucosa and Soft Tissue Columella External naris Greater alar cartilage Internal naris Lateral nasal cartilage Lesser alar cartilage Nasal cavity Nostril	**X** External	**Ø** Drainage Device **7** Autologous Tissue Substitute **D** Intraluminal Device **J** Synthetic Substitute **K** Nonautologous Tissue Substitute	**Z** No Qualifier
Y Sinus	**Ø** Open **3** Percutaneous **4** Percutaneous Endoscopic	**Ø** Drainage Device **Y** Other Device	**Z** No Qualifier
Y Sinus	**7** Via Natural or Artificial Opening **8** Via Natural or Artificial Opening Endoscopic	**Y** Other Device	**Z** No Qualifier
Y Sinus	**X** External	**Ø** Drainage Device	**Z** No Qualifier

Non-OR Ø9P[7,8][Ø,7,8,X]ØZ
Non-OR Ø9P[H,J][3,4][Ø,J,K,Y]Z
Non-OR Ø9P[H,J][7,8][Ø,D,Y]Z
Non-OR Ø9PK[Ø,3,4,7,8][Ø,7,D,J,K,Y]Z
Non-OR Ø9P[H,J]X[Ø,7,D,J,K]Z
Non-OR Ø9PKX[Ø,7,D,J,K]Z
Non-OR Ø9PY[3,4]YZ
Non-OR Ø9PY[7,8]YZ
Non-OR Ø9PYXØZ

Ø Medical and Surgical
9 Ear, Nose, Sinus
Q Repair Definition: Restoring, to the extent possible, a body part to its normal anatomic structure and function
Explanation: Used only when the method to accomplish the repair is not one of the other root operations

Body Part Character 4		Approach Character 5	Device Character 6	Qualifier Character 7
Ø External Ear, Right Antihelix Antitragus Auricle Earlobe Helix Pinna Tragus	**1 External Ear, Left** *See Ø External Ear, Right* **2 External Ear, Bilateral** *See Ø External Ear, Right*	**Ø Open** **3 Percutaneous** **4 Percutaneous Endoscopic** **X External**	**Z No Device**	**Z No Qualifier**
3 External Auditory Canal, Right External auditory meatus **4 External Auditory Canal, Left** *See 3 External Auditory Canal, Right*	**F Eustachian Tube, Right** Auditory tube Pharyngotympanic tube **G Eustachian Tube, Left** *See F Eustachian Tube, Right*	**Ø Open** **3 Percutaneous** **4 Percutaneous Endoscopic** **7 Via Natural or Artificial Opening** **8 Via Natural or Artificial Opening Endoscopic** **X External**	**Z No Device**	**Z No Qualifier**
5 Middle Ear, Right Oval window Tympanic cavity **6 Middle Ear, Left** *See 5 Middle Ear, Right* **9 Auditory Ossicle, Right** Incus Malleus Stapes	**A Auditory Ossicle, Left** *See 9 Auditory Ossicle, Right* **D Inner Ear, Right** Bony labyrinth Bony vestibule Cochlea Round window Semicircular canal **E Inner Ear, Left** *See D Inner Ear, Right*	**Ø Open** **8 Via Natural or Artificial Opening Endoscopic**	**Z No Device**	**Z No Qualifier**
7 Tympanic Membrane, Right Pars flaccida **8 Tympanic Membrane, Left** *See 7 Tympanic Membrane, Right* **L Nasal Turbinate** Inferior turbinate Middle turbinate Nasal concha Superior turbinate	**N Nasopharynx** Choana Fossa of Rosenmuller Pharyngeal recess Rhinopharynx	**Ø Open** **3 Percutaneous** **4 Percutaneous Endoscopic** **7 Via Natural or Artificial Opening** **8 Via Natural or Artificial Opening Endoscopic**	**Z No Device**	**Z No Qualifier**
B Mastoid Sinus, Right Mastoid air cells **C Mastoid Sinus, Left** *See B Mastoid Sinus, Right* **M Nasal Septum** Quadrangular cartilage Septal cartilage Vomer bone **P Accessory Sinus** **Q Maxillary Sinus, Right** Antrum of Highmore	**R Maxillary Sinus, Left** *See Q Maxillary Sinus, Right* **S Frontal Sinus, Right** **T Frontal Sinus, Left** **U Ethmoid Sinus, Right** Ethmoidal air cell **V Ethmoid Sinus, Left** *See U Ethmoid Sinus, Right* **W Sphenoid Sinus, Right** **X Sphenoid Sinus, Left**	**Ø Open** **3 Percutaneous** **4 Percutaneous Endoscopic** **8 Via Natural or Artificial Opening Endoscopic**	**Z No Device**	**Z No Qualifier**
K Nasal Mucosa and Soft Tissue Columella External naris Greater alar cartilage Internal naris Lateral nasal cartilage Lesser alar cartilage Nasal cavity Nostril		**Ø Open** **3 Percutaneous** **4 Percutaneous Endoscopic** **8 Via Natural or Artificial Opening Endoscopic** **X External**	**Z No Device**	**Z No Qualifier**

Non-OR Ø9Q[Ø,1,2]XZZ
Non-OR Ø9Q[3,4]XZZ
Non-OR Ø9Q[F,G][Ø,3,4,7,8,X]ZZ
Non-OR Ø9QKXZZ

Ø Medical and Surgical
9 Ear, Nose, Sinus
R Replacement Definition: Putting in or on biological or synthetic material that physically takes the place and/or function of all or a portion of a body part
Explanation: The body part may have been taken out or replaced, or may be taken out, physically eradicated, or rendered nonfunctional during the REPLACEMENT procedure. A REMOVAL procedure is coded for taking out the device used in a previous replacement procedure.

Body Part Character 4	Approach Character 5	Device Character 6	Qualifier Character 7
Ø External Ear, Right Antihelix Antitragus Auricle Earlobe Helix Pinna Tragus **1 External Ear, Left** *See Ø External Ear, Right* **2 External Ear, Bilateral** *See Ø External Ear, Right* **K Nasal Mucosa and Soft Tissue** Columella External naris Greater alar cartilage Internal naris Lateral nasal cartilage Lesser alar cartilage Nasal cavity Nostril	**Ø Open** **X External**	**7 Autologous Tissue Substitute** **J Synthetic Substitute** **K Nonautologous Tissue Substitute**	**Z No Qualifier**
5 Middle Ear, Right Oval window Tympanic cavity **6 Middle Ear, Left** *See 5 Middle Ear, Right* **9 Auditory Ossicle, Right** Incus Malleus Stapes **A Auditory Ossicle, Left** *See 9 Auditory Ossicle, Right* **D Inner Ear, Right** Bony labyrinth Bony vestibule Cochlea Round window Semicircular canal **E Inner Ear, Left** *See D Inner Ear, Right*	**Ø Open**	**7 Autologous Tissue Substitute** **J Synthetic Substitute** **K Nonautologous Tissue Substitute**	**Z No Qualifier**
7 Tympanic Membrane, Right Pars flaccida **8 Tympanic Membrane, Left** *See 7 Tympanic Membrane, Right* **N Nasopharynx** Choana Fossa of Rosenmuller Pharyngeal recess Rhinopharynx	**Ø Open** **7 Via Natural or Artificial Opening** **8 Via Natural or Artificial Opening Endoscopic**	**7 Autologous Tissue Substitute** **J Synthetic Substitute** **K Nonautologous Tissue Substitute**	**Z No Qualifier**
L Nasal Turbinate Inferior turbinate Middle turbinate Nasal concha Superior turbinate	**Ø Open** **3 Percutaneous** **4 Percutaneous Endoscopic** **7 Via Natural or Artificial Opening** **8 Via Natural or Artificial Opening Endoscopic**	**7 Autologous Tissue Substitute** **J Synthetic Substitute** **K Nonautologous Tissue Substitute**	**Z No Qualifier**
M Nasal Septum Quadrangular cartilage Septal cartilage Vomer bone	**Ø Open** **3 Percutaneous** **4 Percutaneous Endoscopic**	**7 Autologous Tissue Substitute** **J Synthetic Substitute** **K Nonautologous Tissue Substitute**	**Z No Qualifier**

Ø Medical and Surgical
9 Ear, Nose, Sinus
S Reposition Definition: Moving to its normal location, or other suitable location, all or a portion of a body part

Explanation: The body part is moved to a new location from an abnormal location, or from a normal location where it is not functioning correctly. The body part may or may not be cut out or off to be moved to the new location.

Body Part Character 4	Approach Character 5	Device Character 6	Qualifier Character 7
Ø External Ear, Right Antihelix Antitragus Auricle Earlobe Helix Pinna Tragus **1 External Ear, Left** *See Ø External Ear, Right* **2 External Ear, Bilateral** *See Ø External Ear, Right* **K Nasal Mucosa and Soft Tissue** Columella External naris Greater alar cartilage Internal naris Lateral nasal cartilage Lesser alar cartilage Nasal cavity Nostril	**Ø Open** **4 Percutaneous Endoscopic** **X External**	**Z No Device**	**Z No Qualifier**
7 Tympanic Membrane, Right Pars flaccida **8 Tympanic Membrane, Left** *See 7 Tympanic Membrane, Right* **F Eustachian Tube, Right** Auditory tube Pharyngotympanic tube **G Eustachian Tube, Left** *See F Eustachian Tube, Right* **L Nasal Turbinate** Inferior turbinate Middle turbinate Nasal concha Superior turbinate	**Ø Open** **4 Percutaneous Endoscopic** **7 Via Natural or Artificial Opening** **8 Via Natural or Artificial Opening Endoscopic**	**Z No Device**	**Z No Qualifier**
9 Auditory Ossicle, Right Incus Malleus Stapes **A Auditory Ossicle, Left** *See 9 Auditory Ossicle, Right* **M Nasal Septum** Quadrangular cartilage Septal cartilage Vomer bone	**Ø Open** **4 Percutaneous Endoscopic**	**Z No Device**	**Z No Qualifier**

Non-OR Ø9S[F,G][Ø,4,7,8]ZZ

Ø Medical and Surgical
9 Ear, Nose, Sinus
T Resection Definition: Cutting out or off, without replacement, all of a body part
Explanation: None

Body Part Character 4		Approach Character 5	Device Character 6	Qualifier Character 7
Ø External Ear, Right Antihelix Antitragus Auricle Earlobe Helix Pinna Tragus	**1 External Ear, Left** *See Ø External Ear, Right*	**Ø Open** **4 Percutaneous Endoscopic** **X External**	**Z No Device**	**Z No Qualifier**
5 Middle Ear, Right Oval window Tympanic cavity **6 Middle Ear, Left** *See 5 Middle Ear, Right* **9 Auditory Ossicle, Right** Incus Malleus Stapes	**A Auditory Ossicle, Left** *See 9 Auditory Ossicle, Right* **D Inner Ear, Right** Bony labyrinth Bony vestibule Cochlea Round window Semicircular canal **E Inner Ear, Left** *See D Inner Ear, Right*	**Ø Open** **8 Via Natural or Artificial Opening Endoscopic**	**Z No Device**	**Z No Qualifier**
7 Tympanic Membrane, Right Pars flaccida **8 Tympanic Membrane, Left** *See 7 Tympanic Membrane, Right* **F Eustachian Tube, Right** Auditory tube Pharyngotympanic tube **G Eustachian Tube, Left** *See F Eustachian Tube, Right*	**L Nasal Turbinate** Inferior turbinate Middle turbinate Nasal concha Superior turbinate **N Nasopharynx** Choana Fossa of Rosenmuller Pharyngeal recess Rhinopharynx	**Ø Open** **4 Percutaneous Endoscopic** **7 Via Natural or Artificial Opening** **8 Via Natural or Artificial Opening Endoscopic**	**Z No Device**	**Z No Qualifier**
B Mastoid Sinus, Right Mastoid air cells **C Mastoid Sinus, Left** *See B Mastoid Sinus, Right* **M Nasal Septum** Quadrangular cartilage Septal cartilage Vomer bone **P Accessory Sinus** **Q Maxillary Sinus, Right** Antrum of Highmore	**R Maxillary Sinus, Left** *See Q Maxillary Sinus, Right* **S Frontal Sinus, Right** **T Frontal Sinus, Left** **U Ethmoid Sinus, Right** Ethmoidal air cell **V Ethmoid Sinus, Left** *See U Ethmoid Sinus, Right* **W Sphenoid Sinus, Right** **X Sphenoid Sinus, Left**	**Ø Open** **4 Percutaneous Endoscopic** **8 Via Natural or Artificial Opening Endoscopic**	**Z No Device**	**Z No Qualifier**
K Nasal Mucosa and Soft Tissue Columella External naris Greater alar cartilage Internal naris Lateral nasal cartilage Lesser alar cartilage Nasal cavity Nostril		**Ø Open** **4 Percutaneous Endoscopic** **8 Via Natural or Artificial Opening Endoscopic** **X External**	**Z No Device**	**Z No Qualifier**

Non-OR Ø9T[F,G][Ø,4,7,8]ZZ

Ø Medical and Surgical
9 Ear, Nose, Sinus
U Supplement Definition: Putting in or on biological or synthetic material that physically reinforces and/or augments the function of a portion of a body part
Explanation: The biological material is non-living, or is living and from the same individual. The body part may have been previously replaced, and the SUPPLEMENT procedure is performed to physically reinforce and/or augment the function of the replaced body part.

Body Part Character 4	Approach Character 5	Device Character 6	Qualifier Character 7
Ø External Ear, Right Antihelix Antitragus Auricle Earlobe Helix Pinna Tragus **1 External Ear, Left** *See Ø External Ear, Right* **2 External Ear, Bilateral** *See Ø External Ear, Right*	**Ø** Open **X** External	**7** Autologous Tissue Substitute **J** Synthetic Substitute **K** Nonautologous Tissue Substitute	**Z** No Qualifier
5 Middle Ear, Right Oval window Tympanic cavity **6 Middle Ear, Left** *See 5 Middle Ear, Right* **9 Auditory Ossicle, Right** Incus Malleus Stapes **A Auditory Ossicle, Left** *See 9 Auditory Ossicle, Right* **D Inner Ear, Right** Bony labyrinth Bony vestibule Cochlea Round window Semicircular canal **E Inner Ear, Left** *See D Inner Ear, Right*	**Ø** Open **8** Via Natural or Artificial Opening Endoscopic	**7** Autologous Tissue Substitute **J** Synthetic Substitute **K** Nonautologous Tissue Substitute	**Z** No Qualifier
7 Tympanic Membrane, Right Pars flaccida **8 Tympanic Membrane, Left** *See 7 Tympanic Membrane, Right* **N Nasopharynx** Choana Fossa of Rosenmuller Pharyngeal recess Rhinopharynx	**Ø** Open **7** Via Natural or Artificial Opening **8** Via Natural or Artificial Opening Endoscopic	**7** Autologous Tissue Substitute **J** Synthetic Substitute **K** Nonautologous Tissue Substitute	**Z** No Qualifier
K Nasal Mucosa and Soft Tissue Columella External naris Greater alar cartilage Internal naris Lateral nasal cartilage Lesser alar cartilage Nasal cavity Nostril	**Ø** Open **8** Via Natural or Artificial Opening Endoscopic **X** External	**7** Autologous Tissue Substitute **J** Synthetic Substitute **K** Nonautologous Tissue Substitute	**Z** No Qualifier
L Nasal Turbinate Inferior turbinate Middle turbinate Nasal concha Superior turbinate	**Ø** Open **3** Percutaneous **4** Percutaneous Endoscopic **7** Via Natural or Artificial Opening **8** Via Natural or Artificial Opening Endoscopic	**7** Autologous Tissue Substitute **J** Synthetic Substitute **K** Nonautologous Tissue Substitute	**Z** No Qualifier
M Nasal Septum Quadrangular cartilage Septal cartilage Vomer bone	**Ø** Open **3** Percutaneous **4** Percutaneous Endoscopic **8** Via Natural or Artificial Opening Endoscopic	**7** Autologous Tissue Substitute **J** Synthetic Substitute **K** Nonautologous Tissue Substitute	**Z** No Qualifier

Ø Medical and Surgical
9 Ear, Nose, Sinus
W Revision Definition: Correcting, to the extent possible, a portion of a malfunctioning device or the position of a displaced device

Explanation: Revision can include correcting a malfunctioning or displaced device by taking out or putting in components of the device such as a screw or pin

Body Part Character 4	Approach Character 5	Device Character 6	Qualifier Character 7
7 Tympanic Membrane, Right Pars flaccida **8 Tympanic Membrane, Left** *See 7 Tympanic Membrane, Right* **9 Auditory Ossicle, Right** Incus Malleus Stapes **A Auditory Ossicle, Left** *See 9 Auditory Ossicle, Right*	**Ø Open** **7 Via Natural or Artificial Opening** **8 Via Natural or Artificial Opening Endoscopic**	**7 Autologous Tissue Substitute** **J Synthetic Substitute** **K Nonautologous Tissue Substitute**	**Z No Qualifier**
D Inner Ear, Right Bony labyrinth Bony vestibule Cochlea Round window Semicircular canal **E Inner Ear, Left** *See D Inner Ear, Right*	**Ø Open** **7 Via Natural or Artificial Opening** **8 Via Natural or Artificial Opening Endoscopic**	**S Hearing Device**	**Z No Qualifier**
H Ear, Right **J Ear, Left** **K Nasal Mucosa and Soft Tissue** Columella External naris Greater alar cartilage Internal naris Lateral nasal cartilage Lesser alar cartilage Nasal cavity Nostril	**Ø Open** **3 Percutaneous** **4 Percutaneous Endoscopic** **7 Via Natural or Artificial Opening** **8 Via Natural or Artificial Opening Endoscopic**	**Ø Drainage Device** **7 Autologous Tissue Substitute** **D Intraluminal Device** **J Synthetic Substitute** **K Nonautologous Tissue Substitute** **Y Other Device**	**Z No Qualifier**
H Ear, Right **J Ear, Left** **K Nasal Mucosa and Soft Tissue** Columella External naris Greater alar cartilage Internal naris Lateral nasal cartilage Lesser alar cartilage Nasal cavity Nostril	**X External**	**Ø Drainage Device** **7 Autologous Tissue Substitute** **D Intraluminal Device** **J Synthetic Substitute** **K Nonautologous Tissue Substitute**	**Z No Qualifier**
Y Sinus	**Ø Open** **3 Percutaneous** **4 Percutaneous Endoscopic**	**Ø Drainage Device** **Y Other Device**	**Z No Qualifier**
Y Sinus	**7 Via Natural or Artificial Opening** **8 Via Natural or Artificial Opening Endoscopic**	**Y Other Device**	**Z No Qualifier**
Y Sinus	**X External**	**Ø Drainage Device**	**Z No Qualifier**

Non-OR Ø9W[H,J][3,4][J,K,Y]Z
Non-OR Ø9W[H,J][7,8][D,Y]Z
Non-OR Ø9WK[Ø,3,4,7,8][Ø,7,D,J,K,Y]Z
Non-OR Ø9W[H,J,K]X[Ø,7,D,J,K]Z
Non-OR Ø9WY[3,4]YZ
Non-OR Ø9WY[7,8]YZ
Non-OR Ø9WYXØZ

Respiratory System ØB1–ØBY

Character Meanings

This Character Meaning table is provided as a guide to assist the user in the identification of character members that may be found in this section of code tables. It **SHOULD NOT** be used to build a PCS code.

Operation–Character 3		Body Part–Character 4		Approach–Character 5		Device–Character 6		Qualifier–Character 7	
1	Bypass	Ø	Tracheobronchial Tree	Ø	Open	Ø	Drainage Device	Ø	Allogeneic
2	Change	1	Trachea	3	Percutaneous	1	Radioactive Element	1	Syngeneic
5	Destruction	2	Carina	4	Percutaneous Endoscopic	2	Monitoring Device	2	Zooplastic
7	Dilation	3	Main Bronchus, Right	7	Via Natural or Artificial Opening	3	Infusion Device	4	Cutaneous
9	Drainage	4	Upper Lobe Bronchus, Right	8	Via Natural or Artificial Opening Endoscopic	7	Autologous Tissue Substitute	6	Esophagus
B	Excision	5	Middle Lobe Bronchus, Right	X	External	C	Extraluminal Device	X	Diagnostic
C	Extirpation	6	Lower Lobe Bronchus, Right			D	Intraluminal Device	Z	No Qualifier
D	Extraction	7	Main Bronchus, Left			E	Intraluminal Device, Endotracheal Airway		
F	Fragmentation	8	Upper Lobe Bronchus, Left			F	Tracheostomy Device		
H	Insertion	9	Lingula Bronchus			G	Intraluminal Device, Endobronchial Valve		
J	Inspection	B	Lower Lobe Bronchus, Left			J	Synthetic Substitute		
L	Occlusion	C	Upper Lung Lobe, Right			K	Nonautologous Tissue Substitute		
M	Reattachment	D	Middle Lung Lobe, Right			M	Diaphragmatic Pacemaker Lead		
N	Release	F	Lower Lung Lobe, Right			Y	Other Device		
P	Removal	G	Upper Lung Lobe, Left			Z	No Device		
Q	Repair	H	Lung Lingula						
R	Replacement	J	Lower Lung Lobe, Left						
S	Reposition	K	Lung, Right						
T	Resection	L	Lung, Left						
U	Supplement	M	Lungs, Bilateral						
V	Restriction	N	Pleura, Right						
W	Revision	P	Pleura, Left						
Y	Transplantation	Q	Pleura						
		T	Diaphragm						

AHA Coding Clinic for table ØB5
2016, 2Q, 17 Photodynamic therapy for treatment of malignant mesothelioma
2015, 2Q, 31 Thoracoscopic talc pleurodesis

AHA Coding Clinic for table ØB9
2017, 3Q, 15 Bronchoscopy with suctioning for removal of retained secretions
2017, 1Q, 51 Bronchoalveolar lavage
2016, 1Q, 26 Bronchoalveolar lavage, endobronchial biopsy and transbronchial biopsy
2016, 1Q, 27 Fiberoptic bronchoscopy with brushings and bronchoalveolar lavage

AHA Coding Clinic for table ØBB
2016, 1Q, 26 Bronchoalveolar lavage, endobronchial biopsy and transbronchial biopsy
2016, 1Q, 27 Fiberoptic bronchoscopy with brushings and bronchoalveolar lavage
2014, 1Q, 20 Fiducial marker placement

AHA Coding Clinic for table ØBC
2017, 3Q, 14 Bronchoscopy with suctioning and washings for removal of mucus plug

AHA Coding Clinic for table ØBH
2014, 4Q, 3-10 Mechanical ventilation

AHA Coding Clinic for table ØBJ
2015, 2Q, 31 Thoracoscopic talc pleurodesis
2014, 1Q, 20 Fiducial marker placement

AHA Coding Clinic for table ØBN
2015, 3Q, 15 Vascular ring surgery with release of esophagus and trachea

AHA Coding Clinic for table ØBQ
2016, 2Q, 22 Esophageal lengthening Collis gastroplasty with Nissen fundoplication and hiatal hernia
2014, 3Q, 28 Laparoscopic Nissen fundoplication and diaphragmatic hernia repair

AHA Coding Clinic for table ØBU
2015, 1Q, 28 Repair of bronchopleural fistula using omental pedicle graft

Respiratory System

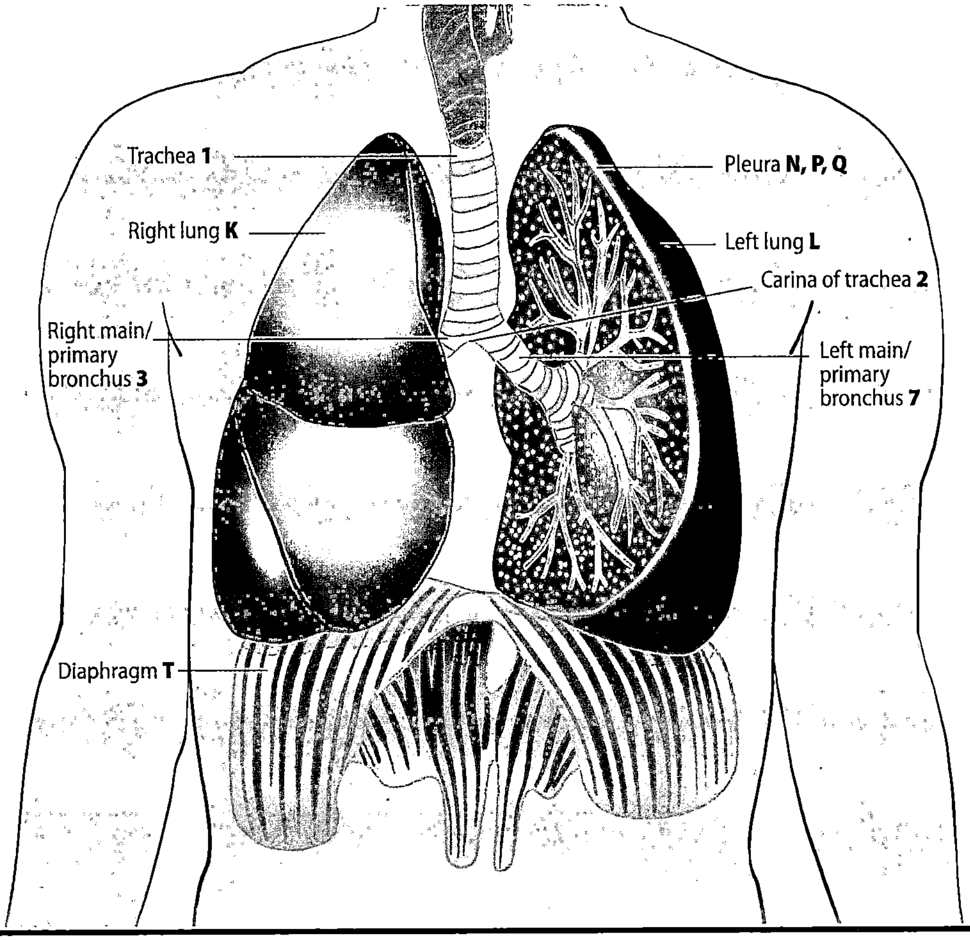

Right Lung Bronchi

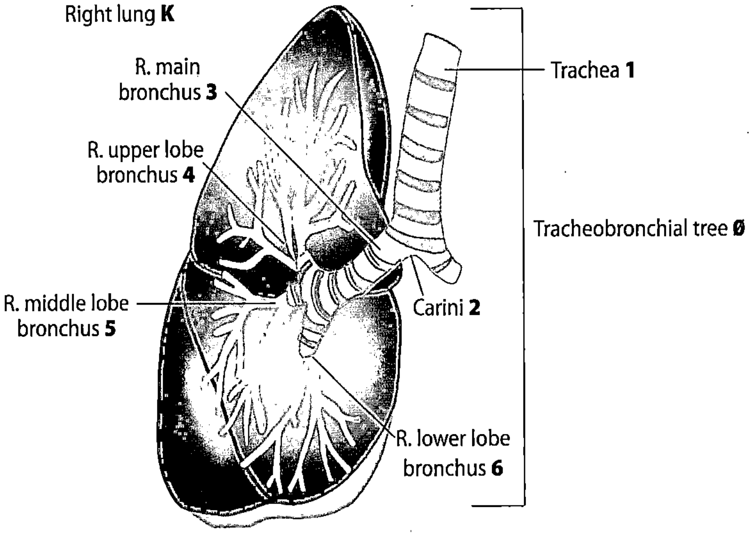

Ø Medical and Surgical
B Respiratory System
1 Bypass Definition: Altering the route of passage of the contents of a tubular body part

Explanation: Rerouting contents of a body part to a downstream area of the normal route, to a similar route and body part, or to an abnormal route and dissimilar body part. Includes one or more anastomoses, with or without the use of a device.

Body Part Character 4	Approach Character 5	Device Character 6	Qualifier Character 7
1 Trachea Cricoid cartilage	Ø Open	D Intraluminal Device	6 Esophagus
1 Trachea Cricoid cartilage	Ø Open	F Tracheostomy Device Z No Device	4 Cutaneous
1 Trachea Cricoid cartilage	3 Percutaneous 4 Percutaneous Endoscopic	F Tracheostomy Device Z No Device	4 Cutaneous

DRG Non-OR ØB113[F,Z]4
Non-OR ØB11ØD6

Ø Medical and Surgical
B Respiratory System
2 Change Definition: Taking out or off a device from a body part and putting back an identical or similar device in or on the same body part without cutting or puncturing the skin or a mucous membrane

Explanation: All CHANGE procedures are coded using the approach EXTERNAL

Body Part Character 4	Approach Character 5	Device Character 6	Qualifier Character 7
Ø Tracheobronchial Tree K Lung, Right L Lung, Left Q Pleura T Diaphragm	X External	Ø Drainage Device Y Other Device	Z No Qualifier
1 Trachea Cricoid cartilage	X External	Ø Drainage Device E Intraluminal Device, Endotracheal Airway F Tracheostomy Device Y Other Device	Z No Qualifier

Non-OR All body part, approach, device, and qualifier values

Ø Medical and Surgical
B Respiratory System
5 Destruction Definition: Physical eradication of all or a portion of a body part by the direct use of energy, force, or a destructive agent

Explanation: None of the body part is physically taken out

Body Part Character 4	Approach Character 5	Device Character 6	Qualifier Character 7
1 Trachea Cricoid cartilage 2 Carina 3 Main Bronchus, Right Bronchus intermedius Intermediate bronchus 4 Upper Lobe Bronchus, Right 5 Middle Lobe Bronchus, Right 6 Lower Lobe Bronchus, Right 7 Main Bronchus, Left 8 Upper Lobe Bronchus, Left 9 Lingula Bronchus B Lower Lobe Bronchus, Left C Upper Lung Lobe, Right D Middle Lung Lobe, Right F Lower Lung Lobe, Right G Upper Lung Lobe, Left H Lung Lingula J Lower Lung Lobe, Left K Lung, Right L Lung, Left M Lungs, Bilateral	Ø Open 3 Percutaneous 4 Percutaneous Endoscopic 7 Via Natural or Artificial Opening 8 Via Natural or Artificial Opening Endoscopic	Z No Device	Z No Qualifier
N Pleura, Right P Pleura, Left T Diaphragm	Ø Open 3 Percutaneous 4 Percutaneous Endoscopic	Z No Device	Z No Qualifier

Non-OR ØB5[3,4,5,6,7,8,9,B][4,8]ZZ
Non-OR ØB5[C,D,F,G,H,J,K,L,M]8ZZ

Ø Medical and Surgical
B Respiratory System
7 Dilation Definition: Expanding an orifice or the lumen of a tubular body part

Explanation: The orifice can be a natural orifice or an artificially created orifice. Accomplished by stretching a tubular body part using intraluminal pressure or by cutting part of the orifice or wall of the tubular body part.

Body Part Character 4	Approach Character 5	Device Character 6	Qualifier Character 7
1 Trachea Cricoid cartilage **2** Carina **3** Main Bronchus, Right Bronchus intermedius Intermediate bronchus **4** Upper Lobe Bronchus, Right **5** Middle Lobe Bronchus, Right **6** Lower Lobe Bronchus, Right **7** Main Bronchus, Left **8** Upper Lobe Bronchus, Left **9** Lingula Bronchus **B** Lower Lobe Bronchus, Left	**Ø** Open **3** Percutaneous **4** Percutaneous Endoscopic **7** Via Natural or Artificial Opening **8** Via Natural or Artificial Opening Endoscopic	**D** Intraluminal Device **Z** No Device	**Z** No Qualifier

Non-OR ØB7[3,4,5,6,7,8,9,B][Ø,3,4,7,8][D,Z]Z

Ø Medical and Surgical
B Respiratory System
9 Drainage Definition: Taking or letting out fluids and/or gases from a body part

Explanation: The qualifier DIAGNOSTIC is used to identify drainage procedures that are biopsies

Body Part Character 4	Approach Character 5	Device Character 6	Qualifier Character 7
1 Trachea Cricoid cartilage **2** Carina **3** Main Bronchus, Right Bronchus intermedius Intermediate bronchus **4** Upper Lobe Bronchus, Right **5** Middle Lobe Bronchus, Right **6** Lower Lobe Bronchus, Right **7** Main Bronchus, Left **8** Upper Lobe Bronchus, Left **9** Lingula Bronchus **B** Lower Lobe Bronchus, Left **C** Upper Lung Lobe, Right **D** Middle Lung Lobe, Right **F** Lower Lung Lobe, Right **G** Upper Lung Lobe, Left **H** Lung Lingula **J** Lower Lung Lobe, Left **K** Lung, Right **L** Lung, Left **M** Lungs, Bilateral	**Ø** Open **3** Percutaneous **4** Percutaneous Endoscopic **7** Via Natural or Artificial Opening **8** Via Natural or Artificial Opening Endoscopic	**Ø** Drainage Device	**Z** No Qualifier
1 Trachea Cricoid cartilage **2** Carina **3** Main Bronchus, Right Bronchus intermedius Intermediate bronchus **4** Upper Lobe Bronchus, Right **5** Middle Lobe Bronchus, Right **6** Lower Lobe Bronchus, Right **7** Main Bronchus, Left **8** Upper Lobe Bronchus, Left **9** Lingula Bronchus **B** Lower Lobe Bronchus, Left **C** Upper Lung Lobe, Right **D** Middle Lung Lobe, Right **F** Lower Lung Lobe, Right **G** Upper Lung Lobe, Left **H** Lung Lingula **J** Lower Lung Lobe, Left **K** Lung, Right **L** Lung, Left **M** Lungs, Bilateral	**Ø** Open **3** Percutaneous **4** Percutaneous Endoscopic **7** Via Natural or Artificial Opening **8** Via Natural or Artificial Opening Endoscopic	**Z** No Device	**X** Diagnostic **Z** No Qualifier
N Pleura, Right **P** Pleura, Left	**Ø** Open **3** Percutaneous **4** Percutaneous Endoscopic **8** Via Natural or Artificial Opening Endoscopic	**Ø** Drainage Device	**Z** No Qualifier
N Pleura, Right **P** Pleura, Left	**Ø** Open **3** Percutaneous **4** Percutaneous Endoscopic **8** Via Natural or Artificial Opening Endoscopic	**Z** No Device	**X** Diagnostic **Z** No Qualifier
T Diaphragm	**Ø** Open **3** Percutaneous **4** Percutaneous Endoscopic	**Ø** Drainage Device	**Z** No Qualifier
T Diaphragm	**Ø** Open **3** Percutaneous **4** Percutaneous Endoscopic	**Z** No Device	**X** Diagnostic **Z** No Qualifier

Non-OR ØB9[1,2,3,4,5,6,7,8,9,B][7,8]ØZ
Non-OR ØB9[1,2,3,4,5,6,7,8,9,B][3,4]ZX
Non-OR ØB9[1,2,3,4,5,6,7,8,9,B][7,8]Z[X,Z]
Non-OR ØB9[C,D,F,G,H,J,K,L,M][3,4,7]ZX
Non-OR ØB9[N,P][Ø,3,8]ØZ
Non-OR ØB9[N,P][Ø,3,8]Z[X,Z]
Non-OR ØB9[N,P]4ZX
Non-OR ØB9T[3,4]ØZ
Non-OR ØB9T[3,4]Z[X,Z]

Ø Medical and Surgical
B Respiratory System
B Excision Definition: Cutting out or off, without replacement, a portion of a body part
Explanation: The qualifier DIAGNOSTIC is used to identify excision procedures that are biopsies

Body Part Character 4	Approach Character 5	Device Character 6	Qualifier Character 7
1 Trachea Cricoid cartilage 2 Carina 3 Main Bronchus, Right Bronchus intermedius Intermediate bronchus 4 Upper Lobe Bronchus, Right 5 Middle Lobe Bronchus, Right 6 Lower Lobe Bronchus, Right 7 Main Bronchus, Left 8 Upper Lobe Bronchus, Left 9 Lingula Bronchus B Lower Lobe Bronchus, Left C Upper Lung Lobe, Right D Middle Lung Lobe, Right F Lower Lung Lobe, Right G Upper Lung Lobe, Left H Lung Lingula J Lower Lung Lobe, Left K Lung, Right L Lung, Left M Lungs, Bilateral	Ø Open 3 Percutaneous 4 Percutaneous Endoscopic 7 Via Natural or Artificial Opening 8 Via Natural or Artificial Opening Endoscopic	Z No Device	X Diagnostic Z No Qualifier
N Pleura, Right P Pleura, Left	Ø Open 3 Percutaneous 4 Percutaneous Endoscopic 8 Via Natural or Artificial Opening Endoscopic	Z No Device	X Diagnostic Z No Qualifier
T Diaphragm	Ø Open 3 Percutaneous 4 Percutaneous Endoscopic	Z No Device	X Diagnostic Z No Qualifier

Non-OR ØBB[1,2,3,4,5,6,7,8,9,B][3,4,7,8]ZX
Non-OR ØBB[3,4,5,6,7,8,9,B,M][4,8]ZZ
Non-OR ØBB[C,D,F,G,H,J,K,L,M]3ZX
Non-OR ØBB[C,D,F,G,H,J,K,L]8ZZ
Non-OR ØBB[N,P][Ø,3]ZX

Ø Medical and Surgical
B Respiratory System
C Extirpation Definition: Taking or cutting out solid matter from a body part
Explanation: The solid matter may be an abnormal byproduct of a biological function or a foreign body; it may be imbedded in a body part or in the lumen of a tubular body part. The solid matter may or may not have been previously broken into pieces.

Body Part Character 4	Approach Character 5	Device Character 6	Qualifier Character 7
1 Trachea Cricoid cartilage 2 Carina 3 Main Bronchus, Right Bronchus intermedius Intermediate bronchus 4 Upper Lobe Bronchus, Right 5 Middle Lobe Bronchus, Right 6 Lower Lobe Bronchus, Right 7 Main Bronchus, Left 8 Upper Lobe Bronchus, Left 9 Lingula Bronchus B Lower Lobe Bronchus, Left C Upper Lung Lobe, Right D Middle Lung Lobe, Right F Lower Lung Lobe, Right G Upper Lung Lobe, Left H Lung Lingula J Lower Lung Lobe, Left K Lung, Right L Lung, Left M Lungs, Bilateral	Ø Open 3 Percutaneous 4 Percutaneous Endoscopic 7 Via Natural or Artificial Opening 8 Via Natural or Artificial Opening Endoscopic	Z No Device	Z No Qualifier
N Pleura, Right P Pleura, Left T Diaphragm	Ø Open 3 Percutaneous 4 Percutaneous Endoscopic	Z No Device	Z No Qualifier

Non-OR ØBC[1,2,3,4,5,6,7,8,9,B][7,8]ZZ
Non-OR ØBC[N,P][Ø,3,4]ZZ

Ø Medical and Surgical
B Respiratory System
D Extraction Definition: Pulling or stripping out or off all or a portion of a body part by the use of force
Explanation: The qualifier DIAGNOSTIC is used to identify extraction procedures that are biopsies

Body Part Character 4	Approach Character 5	Device Character 6	Qualifier Character 7
1 Trachea Cricoid cartilage 2 Carina 3 Main Bronchus, Right Bronchus intermedius Intermediate bronchus 4 Upper Lobe Bronchus, Right 5 Middle Lobe Bronchus, Right 6 Lower Lobe Bronchus, Right 7 Main Bronchus, Left 8 Upper Lobe Bronchus, Left 9 Lingula Bronchus B Lower Lobe Bronchus, Left C Upper Lung Lobe, Right D Middle Lung Lobe, Right F Lower Lung Lobe, Right G Upper Lung Lobe, Left H Lung Lingula J Lower Lung Lobe, Left K Lung, Right L Lung, Left M Lungs, Bilateral	4 Percutaneous Endoscopic 8 Via Natural or Artificial Opening Endoscopic	Z No Device	X Diagnostic
N Pleura, Right P Pleura, Left	Ø Open 3 Percutaneous 4 Percutaneous Endoscopic	Z No Device	X Diagnostic Z No Qualifier

Non-OR ØBD[1,2,3,4,5,6,7,8,9,B,C,D,F,G,H,J,K,L,M][4,8]ZX

Ø Medical and Surgical
B Respiratory System
F Fragmentation Definition: Breaking solid matter in a body part into pieces
Explanation: Physical force (e.g., manual, ultrasonic) applied directly or indirectly is used to break the solid matter into pieces. The solid matter may be an abnormal byproduct of a biological function or a foreign body. The pieces of solid matter are not taken out.

Body Part Character 4	Approach Character 5	Device Character 6	Qualifier Character 7
1 Trachea NC Cricoid cartilage 2 Carina NC 3 Main Bronchus, Right NC Bronchus intermedius Intermediate bronchus 4 Upper Lobe Bronchus, Right NC 5 Middle Lobe Bronchus, Right NC 6 Lower Lobe Bronchus, Right NC 7 Main Bronchus, Left NC 8 Upper Lobe Bronchus, Left NC 9 Lingula Bronchus NC B Lower Lobe Bronchus, Left NC	Ø Open 3 Percutaneous 4 Percutaneous Endoscopic 7 Via Natural or Artificial Opening 8 Via Natural or Artificial Opening Endoscopic X External	Z No Device	Z No Qualifier

Non-OR ØBF[1,2,3,4,5,6,7,8,9,B]XZZ
Non-OR ØBF[3,4,5,6,7,8,9,B][7,8]ZZ
NC ØBF[1,2,3,4,5,6,7,8,9,B]XZZ

Ø Medical and Surgical
B Respiratory System
H Insertion Definition: Putting in a nonbiological appliance that monitors, assists, performs, or prevents a physiological function but does not physically take the place of a body part
Explanation: None

Body Part Character 4	Approach Character 5	Device Character 6	Qualifier Character 7
Ø Tracheobronchial Tree	Ø Open 3 Percutaneous 4 Percutaneous Endoscopic 7 Via Natural or Artificial Opening 8 Via Natural or Artificial Opening Endoscopic	1 Radioactive Element 2 Monitoring Device 3 Infusion Device D Intraluminal Device Y Other Device	Z No Qualifier
1 Trachea Cricoid cartilage	Ø Open	2 Monitoring Device D Intraluminal Device Y Other Device	Z No Qualifier
1 Trachea Cricoid cartilage	3 Percutaneous	D Intraluminal Device E Intraluminal Device, Endotracheal Airway Y Other Device	Z No Qualifier
1 Trachea Cricoid cartilage	4 Percutaneous Endoscopic	D Intraluminal Device Y Other Device	Z No Qualifier
1 Trachea Cricoid cartilage	7 Via Natural or Artificial Opening 8 Via Natural or Artificial Opening Endoscopic	2 Monitoring Device D Intraluminal Device E Intraluminal Device, Endotracheal Airway Y Other Device	Z No Qualifier
3 Main Bronchus, Right Bronchus intermedius Intermediate bronchus 4 Upper Lobe Bronchus, Right 5 Middle Lobe Bronchus, Right 6 Lower Lobe Bronchus, Right 7 Main Bronchus, Left 8 Upper Lobe Bronchus, Left 9 Lingula Bronchus B Lower Lobe Bronchus, Left	Ø Open 3 Percutaneous 4 Percutaneous Endoscopic 7 Via Natural or Artificial Opening 8 Via Natural or Artificial Opening Endoscopic	G Intraluminal Device, Endobronchial Valve	Z No Qualifier
K Lung, Right L Lung, Left	Ø Open 3 Percutaneous 4 Percutaneous Endoscopic 7 Via Natural or Artificial Opening 8 Via Natural or Artificial Opening Endoscopic	1 Radioactive Element 2 Monitoring Device 3 Infusion Device Y Other Device	Z No Qualifier
Q Pleura	Ø Open 3 Percutaneous 4 Percutaneous Endoscopic 7 Via Natural or Artificial Opening 8 Via Natural or Artificial Opening Endoscopic	Y Other Device	Z No Qualifier
T Diaphragm	Ø Open 3 Percutaneous 4 Percutaneous Endoscopic	2 Monitoring Device M Diaphragmatic Pacemaker Lead Y Other Device	Z No Qualifier
T Diaphragm	7 Via Natural or Artificial Opening 8 Via Natural or Artificial Opening Endoscopic	Y Other Device	Z No Qualifier

Non-OR ØBHØ3YZ
Non-OR ØBHØ[7,8][2,3,D,Y]Z
Non-OR ØBH13[E,Y]Z
Non-OR ØBH1[7,8][2,D,E,Y]Z
Non-OR ØBH[3,4,5,6,7,8,9,B]8GZ
Non-OR ØBH[K,L]3YZ
Non-OR ØBH[K,L]7[2,3,Y]Z
Non-OR ØBH[K,L]8[2,3]Z
Non-OR ØBHQ[3,7]YZ
Non-OR ØBHT3YZ
Non-OR ØBHT[7,8]YZ

Ø Medical and Surgical
B Respiratory System
J Inspection Definition: Visually and/or manually exploring a body part

Explanation: Visual exploration may be performed with or without optical instrumentation. Manual exploration may be performed directly or through intervening body layers.

Body Part Character 4	Approach Character 5	Device Character 6	Qualifier Character 7
Ø Tracheobronchial Tree 1 Trachea Cricoid cartilage K Lung, Right L Lung, Left Q Pleura T Diaphragm	Ø Open 3 Percutaneous 4 Percutaneous Endoscopic 7 Via Natural or Artificial Opening 8 Via Natural or Artificial Opening Endoscopic X External	Z No Device	Z No Qualifier

Non-OR ØBJ[Ø,K,L,Q,T][3,7,8,X]ZZ
Non-OR ØBJ1[3,4,7,8,X]ZZ

Ø Medical and Surgical
B Respiratory System
L Occlusion Definition: Completely closing an orifice or the lumen of a tubular body part

Explanation: The orifice can be a natural orifice or an artificially created orifice

Body Part Character 4	Approach Character 5	Device Character 6	Qualifier Character 7
1 Trachea Cricoid cartilage 2 Carina 3 Main Bronchus, Right Bronchus intermedius Intermediate bronchus 4 Upper Lobe Bronchus, Right 5 Middle Lobe Bronchus, Right 6 Lower Lobe Bronchus, Right 7 Main Bronchus, Left 8 Upper Lobe Bronchus, Left 9 Lingula Bronchus B Lower Lobe Bronchus, Left	Ø Open 3 Percutaneous 4 Percutaneous Endoscopic	C Extraluminal Device D Intraluminal Device Z No Device	Z No Qualifier
1 Trachea Cricoid cartilage 2 Carina 3 Main Bronchus, Right Bronchus intermedius Intermediate bronchus 4 Upper Lobe Bronchus, Right 5 Middle Lobe Bronchus, Right 6 Lower Lobe Bronchus, Right 7 Main Bronchus, Left 8 Upper Lobe Bronchus, Left 9 Lingula Bronchus B Lower Lobe Bronchus, Left	7 Via Natural or Artificial Opening 8 Via Natural or Artificial Opening Endoscopic	D Intraluminal Device Z No Device	Z No Qualifier

Ø Medical and Surgical
B Respiratory System
M Reattachment Definition: Putting back in or on all or a portion of a separated body part to its normal location or other suitable location
Explanation: Vascular circulation and nervous pathways may or may not be reestablished

Body Part Character 4	Approach Character 5	Device Character 6	Qualifier Character 7
1 Trachea Cricoid cartilage 2 Carina 3 Main Bronchus, Right Bronchus intermedius Intermediate bronchus 4 Upper Lobe Bronchus, Right 5 Middle Lobe Bronchus, Right 6 Lower Lobe Bronchus, Right 7 Main Bronchus, Left 8 Upper Lobe Bronchus, Left 9 Lingula Bronchus B Lower Lobe Bronchus, Left C Upper Lung Lobe, Right D Middle Lung Lobe, Right F Lower Lung Lobe, Right G Upper Lung Lobe, Left H Lung Lingula J Lower Lung Lobe, Left K Lung, Right L Lung, Left T Diaphragm	Ø Open	Z No Device	Z No Qualifier

Ø Medical and Surgical
B Respiratory System
N Release Definition: Freeing a body part from an abnormal physical constraint by cutting or by the use of force
Explanation: Some of the restraining tissue may be taken out but none of the body part is taken out

Body Part Character 4	Approach Character 5	Device Character 6	Qualifier Character 7
1 Trachea Cricoid cartilage 2 Carina 3 Main Bronchus, Right Bronchus intermedius Intermediate bronchus 4 Upper Lobe Bronchus, Right 5 Middle Lobe Bronchus, Right 6 Lower Lobe Bronchus, Right 7 Main Bronchus, Left 8 Upper Lobe Bronchus, Left 9 Lingula Bronchus B Lower Lobe Bronchus, Left C Upper Lung Lobe, Right D Middle Lung Lobe, Right F Lower Lung Lobe, Right G Upper Lung Lobe, Left H Lung Lingula J Lower Lung Lobe, Left K Lung, Right L Lung, Left M Lungs, Bilateral	Ø Open 3 Percutaneous 4 Percutaneous Endoscopic 7 Via Natural or Artificial Opening 8 Via Natural or Artificial Opening Endoscopic	Z No Device	Z No Qualifier
N Pleura, Right P Pleura, Left T Diaphragm	Ø Open 3 Percutaneous 4 Percutaneous Endoscopic	Z No Device	Z No Qualifier

Respiratory System

Ø Medical and Surgical
B Respiratory System
P Removal Definition: Taking out or off a device from a body part

Explanation: If a device is taken out and a similar device put in without cutting or puncturing the skin or mucous membrane, the procedure is coded to the root operation CHANGE. Otherwise, the procedure for taking out a device is coded to the root operation REMOVAL.

Body Part Character 4	Approach Character 5	Device Character 6	Qualifier Character 7
Ø Tracheobronchial Tree	Ø Open 3 Percutaneous 4 Percutaneous Endoscopic 7 Via Natural or Artificial Opening 8 Via Natural or Artificial Opening Endoscopic	Ø Drainage Device 1 Radioactive Element 2 Monitoring Device 3 Infusion Device 7 Autologous Tissue Substitute C Extraluminal Device D Intraluminal Device J Synthetic Substitute K Nonautologous Tissue Substitute Y Other Device	Z No Qualifier
Ø Tracheobronchial Tree	X External	Ø Drainage Device 1 Radioactive Element 2 Monitoring Device 3 Infusion Device D Intraluminal Device	Z No Qualifier
1 Trachea Cricoid cartilage	Ø Open 3 Percutaneous 4 Percutaneous Endoscopic 7 Via Natural or Artificial Opening 8 Via Natural or Artificial Opening Endoscopic	Ø Drainage Device 2 Monitoring Device 7 Autologous Tissue Substitute C Extraluminal Device D Intraluminal Device F Tracheostomy Device J Synthetic Substitute K Nonautologous Tissue Substitute	Z No Qualifier
1 Trachea Cricoid cartilage	X External	Ø Drainage Device 2 Monitoring Device D Intraluminal Device F Tracheostomy Device	Z No Qualifier
K Lung, Right L Lung, Left	Ø Open 3 Percutaneous 4 Percutaneous Endoscopic 7 Via Natural or Artificial Opening 8 Via Natural or Artificial Opening Endoscopic	Ø Drainage Device 1 Radioactive Element 2 Monitoring Device 3 Infusion Device Y Other Device	Z No Qualifier
K Lung, Right L Lung, Left	X External	Ø Drainage Device 1 Radioactive Element 2 Monitoring Device 3 Infusion Device	Z No Qualifier
Q Pleura	Ø Open 3 Percutaneous 4 Percutaneous Endoscopic 7 Via Natural or Artificial Opening 8 Via Natural or Artificial Opening Endoscopic	Ø Drainage Device 1 Radioactive Element 2 Monitoring Device Y Other Device	Z No Qualifier
Q Pleura	X External	Ø Drainage Device 1 Radioactive Element 2 Monitoring Device	Z No Qualifier
T Diaphragm	Ø Open 3 Percutaneous 4 Percutaneous Endoscopic 7 Via Natural or Artificial Opening 8 Via Natural or Artificial Opening Endoscopic	Ø Drainage Device 2 Monitoring Device 7 Autologous Tissue Substitute J Synthetic Substitute K Nonautologous Tissue Substitute M Diaphragmatic Pacemaker Lead Y Other Device	Z No Qualifier
T Diaphragm	X External	Ø Drainage Device 2 Monitoring Device M Diaphragmatic Pacemaker Lead	Z No Qualifier

Non-OR ØBPØ[3,4]YZ
Non-OR ØBPØ[7,8][Ø,2,3,D,Y]Z
Non-OR ØBPØX[Ø,1,2,3,D]Z
Non-OR ØBP1[Ø,3,4]FZ
Non-OR ØBP1[7,8][Ø,2,D,F]Z
Non-OR ØBP1X[Ø,2,D,F]Z
Non-OR ØBP[K,L]3YZ
Non-OR ØBPK7[Ø,1,2,3,Y]Z
Non-OR ØBPK8[Ø,1,2,3]Z
Non-OR ØBPL7[Ø,2,3,Y]Z
Non-OR ØBPL8[Ø,2,3]Z
Non-OR ØBP[K,L]X[Ø,1,2,3]Z
Non-OR ØBPQ[Ø,3,4,7,8][Ø,1,2,]Z
Non-OR ØBPQ[3,7]YZ
Non-OR ØBPQX[Ø,1,2]Z
Non-OR ØBPT3YZ
Non-OR ØBPT[7,8][Ø,2,Y]Z
Non-OR ØBPTX[Ø,2,M]Z

Ø Medical and Surgical
B Respiratory System
Q Repair Definition: Restoring, to the extent possible, a body part to its normal anatomic structure and function
Explanation: Used only when the method to accomplish the repair is not one of the other root operations

Body Part Character 4	Approach Character 5	Device Character 6	Qualifier Character 7
1 Trachea Cricoid cartilage **2** Carina **3** Main Bronchus, Right Bronchus intermedius Intermediate bronchus **4** Upper Lobe Bronchus, Right **5** Middle Lobe Bronchus, Right **6** Lower Lobe Bronchus, Right **7** Main Bronchus, Left **8** Upper Lobe Bronchus, Left **9** Lingula Bronchus **B** Lower Lobe Bronchus, Left **C** Upper Lung Lobe, Right **D** Middle Lung Lobe, Right **F** Lower Lung Lobe, Right **G** Upper Lung Lobe, Left **H** Lung Lingula **J** Lower Lung Lobe, Left **K** Lung, Right **L** Lung, Left **M** Lungs, Bilateral	**Ø** Open **3** Percutaneous **4** Percutaneous Endoscopic **7** Via Natural or Artificial Opening **8** Via Natural or Artificial Opening Endoscopic	**Z** No Device	**Z** No Qualifier
N Pleura, Right **P** Pleura, Left **T** Diaphragm	**Ø** Open **3** Percutaneous **4** Percutaneous Endoscopic	**Z** No Device	**Z** No Qualifier

Ø Medical and Surgical
B Respiratory System
R Replacement Definition: Putting in or on biological or synthetic material that physically takes the place and/or function of all or a portion of a body part

Explanation: The body part may have been taken out or replaced, or may be taken out, physically eradicated, or rendered nonfunctional during the REPLACEMENT procedure. A REMOVAL procedure is coded for taking out the device used in a previous replacement procedure.

Body Part Character 4	Approach Character 5	Device Character 6	Qualifier Character 7
1 Trachea Cricoid cartilage **2 Carina** **3 Main Bronchus, Right** Bronchus intermedius Intermediate bronchus **4 Upper Lobe Bronchus, Right** **5 Middle Lobe Bronchus, Right** **6 Lower Lobe Bronchus, Right** **7 Main Bronchus, Left** **8 Upper Lobe Bronchus, Left** **9 Lingula Bronchus** **B Lower Lobe Bronchus, Left** **T Diaphragm**	**Ø Open** **4 Percutaneous Endoscopic**	**7 Autologous Tissue Substitute** **J Synthetic Substitute** **K Nonautologous Tissue Substitute**	**Z No Qualifier**

Ø Medical and Surgical
B Respiratory System
S Reposition Definition: Moving to its normal location, or other suitable location, all or a portion of a body part

Explanation: The body part is moved to a new location from an abnormal location, or from a normal location where it is not functioning correctly. The body part may or may not be cut out or off to be moved to the new location.

Body Part Character 4	Approach Character 5	Device Character 6	Qualifier Character 7
1 Trachea Cricoid cartilage **2 Carina** **3 Main Bronchus, Right** Bronchus intermedius Intermediate bronchus **4 Upper Lobe Bronchus, Right** **5 Middle Lobe Bronchus, Right** **6 Lower Lobe Bronchus, Right** **7 Main Bronchus, Left** **8 Upper Lobe Bronchus, Left** **9 Lingula Bronchus** **B Lower Lobe Bronchus, Left** **C Upper Lung Lobe, Right** **D Middle Lung Lobe, Right** **F Lower Lung Lobe, Right** **G Upper Lung Lobe, Left** **H Lung Lingula** **J Lower Lung Lobe, Left** **K Lung, Right** **L Lung, Left** **T Diaphragm**	**Ø Open**	**Z No Device**	**Z No Qualifier**

Ø Medical and Surgical
B Respiratory System
T Resection Definition: Cutting out or off, without replacement, all of a body part
Explanation: None

Body Part Character 4	Approach Character 5	Device Character 6	Qualifier Character 7
1 Trachea Cricoid cartilage **2** Carina **3** Main Bronchus, Right Bronchus intermedius Intermediate bronchus **4** Upper Lobe Bronchus, Right **5** Middle Lobe Bronchus, Right **6** Lower Lobe Bronchus, Right **7** Main Bronchus, Left **8** Upper Lobe Bronchus, Left **9** Lingula Bronchus **B** Lower Lobe Bronchus, Left **C** Upper Lung Lobe, Right **D** Middle Lung Lobe, Right **F** Lower Lung Lobe, Right **G** Upper Lung Lobe, Left **H** Lung Lingula **J** Lower Lung Lobe, Left **K** Lung, Right **L** Lung, Left **M** Lungs, Bilateral **T** Diaphragm	**Ø** Open **4** Percutaneous Endoscopic	**Z** No Device	**Z** No Qualifier

Ø Medical and Surgical
B Respiratory System
U Supplement Definition: Putting in or on biological or synthetic material that physically reinforces and/or augments the function of a portion of a body part
Explanation: The biological material is non-living, or is living and from the same individual. The body part may have been previously replaced, and the SUPPLEMENT procedure is performed to physically reinforce and/or augment the function of the replaced body part.

Body Part Character 4	Approach Character 5	Device Character 6	Qualifier Character 7
1 Trachea Cricoid cartilage **2** Carina **3** Main Bronchus, Right Bronchus intermedius Intermediate bronchus **4** Upper Lobe Bronchus, Right **5** Middle Lobe Bronchus, Right **6** Lower Lobe Bronchus, Right **7** Main Bronchus, Left **8** Upper Lobe Bronchus, Left **9** Lingula Bronchus **B** Lower Lobe Bronchus, Left	**Ø** Open **4** Percutaneous Endoscopic **8** Via Natural or Artificial Opening Endoscopic	**7** Autologous Tissue Substitute **J** Synthetic Substitute **K** Nonautologous Tissue Substitute	**Z** No Qualifier
T Diaphragm	**Ø** Open **4** Percutaneous Endoscopic	**7** Autologous Tissue Substitute **J** Synthetic Substitute **K** Nonautologous Tissue Substitute	**Z** No Qualifier

Ø Medical and Surgical
B Respiratory System
V Restriction Definition: Partially closing an orifice or the lumen of a tubular body part
Explanation: The orifice can be a natural orifice or an artificially created orifice

Body Part Character 4	Approach Character 5	Device Character 6	Qualifier Character 7
1 Trachea Cricoid cartilage **2** Carina **3** Main Bronchus, Right Bronchus intermedius Intermediate bronchus **4** Upper Lobe Bronchus, Right **5** Middle Lobe Bronchus, Right **6** Lower Lobe Bronchus, Right **7** Main Bronchus, Left **8** Upper Lobe Bronchus, Left **9** Lingula Bronchus **B** Lower Lobe Bronchus, Left	**Ø** Open **3** Percutaneous **4** Percutaneous Endoscopic	**C** Extraluminal Device **D** Intraluminal Device **Z** No Device	**Z** No Qualifier
1 Trachea Cricoid cartilage **2** Carina **3** Main Bronchus, Right Bronchus intermedius Intermediate bronchus **4** Upper Lobe Bronchus, Right **5** Middle Lobe Bronchus, Right **6** Lower Lobe Bronchus, Right **7** Main Bronchus, Left **8** Upper Lobe Bronchus, Left **9** Lingula Bronchus **B** Lower Lobe Bronchus, Left	**7** Via Natural or Artificial Opening **8** Via Natural or Artificial Opening Endoscopic	**D** Intraluminal Device **Z** No Device	**Z** No Qualifier

Ø Medical and Surgical
B Respiratory System
W Revision Definition: Correcting, to the extent possible, a portion of a malfunctioning device or the position of a displaced device

Explanation: Revision can include correcting a malfunctioning or displaced device by taking out or putting in components of the device such as a screw or pin

Body Part Character 4	Approach Character 5	Device Character 6	Qualifier Character 7
Ø Tracheobronchial Tree	Ø Open 3 Percutaneous 4 Percutaneous Endoscopic 7 Via Natural or Artificial Opening 8 Via Natural or Artificial Opening Endoscopic	Ø Drainage Device 2 Monitoring Device 3 Infusion Device 7 Autologous Tissue Substitute C Extraluminal Device D Intraluminal Device J Synthetic Substitute K Nonautologous Tissue Substitute Y Other Device	Z No Qualifier
Ø Tracheobronchial Tree	X External	Ø Drainage Device 2 Monitoring Device 3 Infusion Device 7 Autologous Tissue Substitute C Extraluminal Device D Intraluminal Device J Synthetic Substitute K Nonautologous Tissue Substitute	Z No Qualifier
1 Trachea Cricoid cartilage	Ø Open 3 Percutaneous 4 Percutaneous Endoscopic 7 Via Natural or Artificial Opening 8 Via Natural or Artificial Opening Endoscopic X External	Ø Drainage Device 2 Monitoring Device 7 Autologous Tissue Substitute C Extraluminal Device D Intraluminal Device F Tracheostomy Device J Synthetic Substitute K Nonautologous Tissue Substitute	Z No Qualifier
K Lung, Right L Lung, Left	Ø Open 3 Percutaneous 4 Percutaneous Endoscopic 7 Via Natural or Artificial Opening 8 Via Natural or Artificial Opening Endoscopic	Ø Drainage Device 2 Monitoring Device 3 Infusion Device Y Other Device	Z No Qualifier
K Lung, Right L Lung, Left	X External	Ø Drainage Device 2 Monitoring Device 3 Infusion Device	Z No Qualifier
Q Pleura	Ø Open 3 Percutaneous 4 Percutaneous Endoscopic 7 Via Natural or Artificial Opening 8 Via Natural or Artificial Opening Endoscopic	Ø Drainage Device 2 Monitoring Device Y Other Device	Z No Qualifier
Q Pleura	X External	Ø Drainage Device 2 Monitoring Device	Z No Qualifier
T Diaphragm	Ø Open 3 Percutaneous 4 Percutaneous Endoscopic 7 Via Natural or Artificial Opening 8 Via Natural or Artificial Opening Endoscopic	Ø Drainage Device 2 Monitoring Device 7 Autologous Tissue Substitute J Synthetic Substitute K Nonautologous Tissue Substitute M Diaphragmatic Pacemaker Lead Y Other Device	Z No Qualifier
T Diaphragm	X External	Ø Drainage Device 2 Monitoring Device 7 Autologous Tissue Substitute J Synthetic Substitute K Nonautologous Tissue Substitute M Diaphragmatic Pacemaker Lead	Z No Qualifier

Non-OR ØBWØ[3,4]YZ
Non-OR ØBWØ[7,8][2,3,D,Y]Z
Non-OR ØBWØX[Ø,2,3,7,C,D,J,K]Z
Non-OR ØBW1X[Ø,2,7,C,D,F,J,K]Z
Non-OR ØBW[K,L]3YZ
Non-OR ØBW[K,L]7[Ø,2,3,Y]Z
Non-OR ØBW[K,L]8[Ø,2,3]Z
Non-OR ØBW[K,L]X[Ø,2,3]Z
Non-OR ØBWQ[Ø,3,4,7,8][Ø,2]Z
Non-OR ØBWQ[Ø,3,7]YZ
Non-OR ØBWQX[Ø,2]Z
Non-OR ØBWT[3,7,8]YZ
Non-OR ØBWTX[Ø,2,7,J,K,M]Z

Ø Medical and Surgical
B Respiratory System
Y Transplantation Definition: Putting in or on all or a portion of a living body part taken from another individual or animal to physically take the place and/or function of all or a portion of a similar body part

Explanation: The native body part may or may not be taken out, and the transplanted body part may take over all or a portion of its function

Body Part Character 4	Approach Character 5	Device Character 6	Qualifier Character 7
C Upper Lung Lobe, Right LC D Middle Lung Lobe, Right LC F Lower Lung Lobe, Right LC G Upper Lung Lobe, Left LC H Lung Lingula LC J Lower Lung Lobe, Left LC K Lung, Right LC L Lung, Left LC M Lungs, Bilateral LC	Ø Open	Z No Device	Ø Allogeneic 1 Syngeneic 2 Zooplastic

LC ØBY[C,D,F,G,H,J,K,L,M]ØZ[Ø,1,2]

Mouth and Throat ØCØ–ØCX

Character Meanings

This Character Meaning table is provided as a guide to assist the user in the identification of character members that may be found in this section of code tables. It **SHOULD NOT** be used to build a PCS code.

Operation–Character 3		Body Part–Character 4		Approach–Character 5		Device–Character 6		Qualifier–Character 7	
Ø	Alteration	Ø	Upper Lip	Ø	Open	Ø	Drainage Device	Ø	Single
2	Change	1	Lower Lip	3	Percutaneous	1	Radioactive Element	1	Multiple
5	Destruction	2	Hard Palate	4	Percutaneous Endoscopic	5	External Fixation Device	2	All
7	Dilation	3	Soft Palate	7	Via Natural or Artificial Opening	7	Autologous Tissue Substitute	X	Diagnostic
9	Drainage	4	Buccal Mucosa	8	Via Natural or Artificial Opening Endoscopic	B	Intraluminal Device, Airway	Z	No Qualifier
B	Excision	5	Upper Gingiva	X	External	C	Extraluminal Device		
C	Extirpation	6	Lower Gingiva			D	Intraluminal Device		
D	Extraction	7	Tongue			J	Synthetic Substitute		
F	Fragmentation	8	Parotid Gland, Right			K	Nonautologous Tissue Substitute		
H	Insertion	9	Parotid Gland, Left			Y	Other Device		
J	Inspection	A	Salivary Gland			Z	No Device		
L	Occlusion	B	Parotid Duct, Right						
M	Reattachment	C	Parotid Duct, Left						
N	Release	D	Sublingual Gland, Right						
P	Removal	F	Sublingual Gland, Left						
Q	Repair	G	Submaxillary Gland, Right						
R	Replacement	H	Submaxillary Gland, Left						
S	Reposition	J	Minor Salivary Gland						
T	Resection	M	Pharynx						
U	Supplement	N	Uvula						
V	Restriction	P	Tonsils						
W	Revision	Q	Adenoids						
X	Transfer	R	Epiglottis						
		S	Larynx						
		T	Vocal Cord, Right						
		V	Vocal Cord, Left						
		W	Upper Tooth						
		X	Lower Tooth						
		Y	Mouth and Throat						

AHA Coding Clinic for table ØC9
2017, 2Q, 16 Incision and drainage of floor of mouth

AHA Coding Clinic for table ØCB
2017, 2Q, 16 Excision of floor of mouth
2016, 3Q, 28 Lingual tonsillectomy, tongue base excision and epiglottopexy
2016, 2Q, 19 Biopsy of the base of tongue
2014, 3Q, 21 Superficial parotidectomy

AHA Coding Clinic for table ØCC
2016, 2Q, 20 Sialendoscopy with stone removal

AHA Coding Clinic for table ØCQ
2017, 1Q, 20 Preparatory nasal adhesion repair before definitive cleft palate repair

AHA Coding Clinic for table ØCR
2014, 3Q, 25 Excision of soft palate with placement of surgical obturator
2014, 2Q, 5 Oasis acellular matrix graft
2014, 2Q, 6 Composite grafting (synthetic versus nonautologous tissue substitute)

AHA Coding Clinic for table ØCS
2016, 3Q, 28 Lingual tonsillectomy, tongue base excision and epiglottopexy

AHA Coding Clinic for table ØCT
2016, 2Q, 12 Resection of malignant neoplasm of infratemporal fossa
2014, 3Q, 21 Superficial parotidectomy
2014, 3Q, 23 Le Fort I osteotomy

Mouth and Throat

Salivary Glands

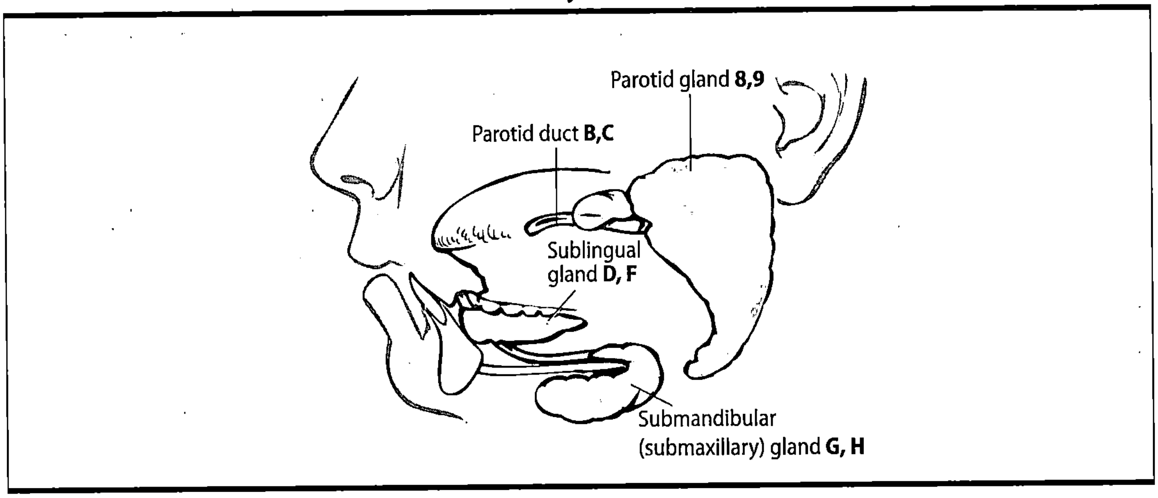

Oral Anatomy

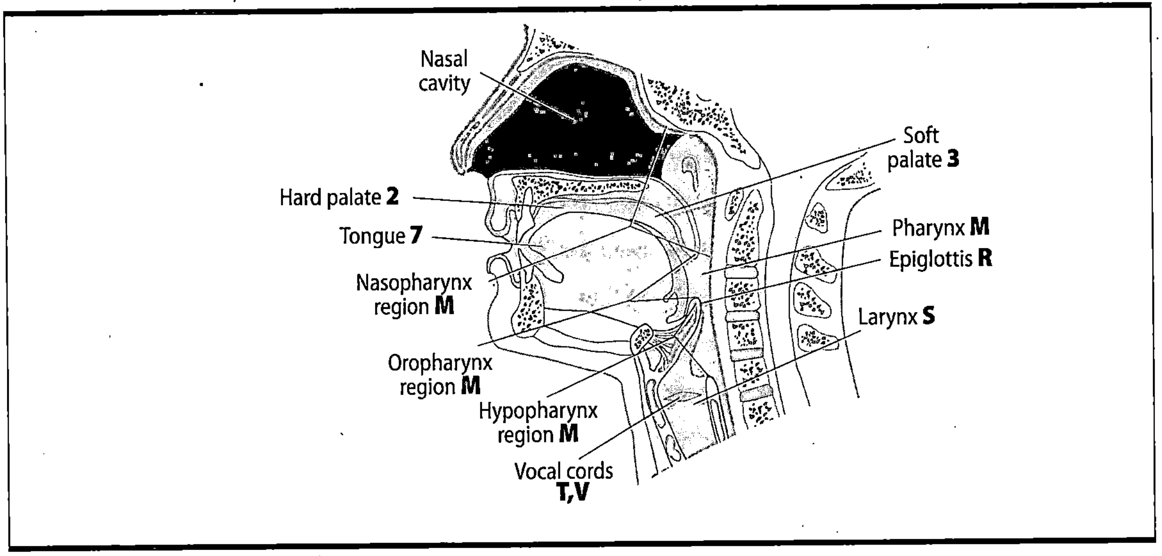

Mouth Frontal View (Upper)

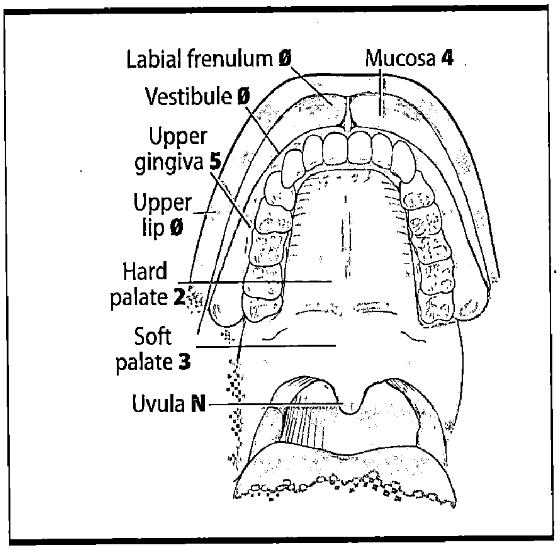

Mouth Frontal View (Lower)

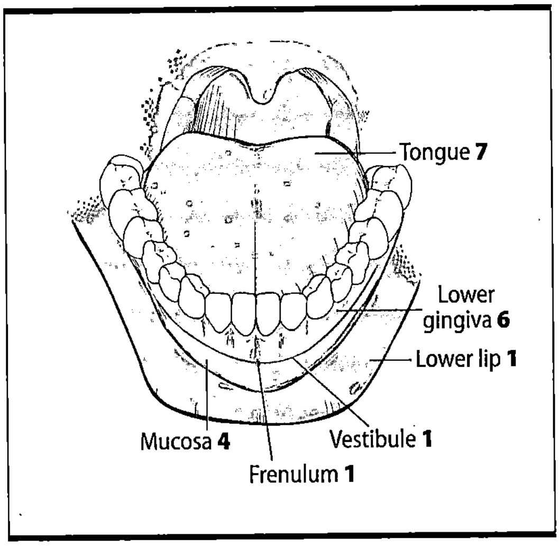

Ø Medical and Surgical
C Mouth and Throat
Ø Alteration Definition: Modifying the anatomic structure of a body part without affecting the function of the body part
Explanation: Principal purpose is to improve appearance

Body Part Character 4	Approach Character 5	Device Character 6	Qualifier Character 7
Ø Upper Lip Frenulum labii superioris Labial gland Vermilion border 1 Lower Lip Frenulum labii inferioris Labial gland Vermilion border	X External	7 Autologous Tissue Substitute J Synthetic Substitute K Nonautologous Tissue Substitute Z No Device	Z No Qualifier

Ø Medical and Surgical
C Mouth and Throat
2 Change Definition: Taking out or off a device from a body part and putting back an identical or similar device in or on the same body part without cutting or puncturing the skin or a mucous membrane
Explanation: All CHANGE procedures are coded using the approach EXTERNAL

Body Part Character 4	Approach Character 5	Device Character 6	Qualifier Character 7
A Salivary Gland S Larynx Aryepiglottic fold Arytenoid cartilage Corniculate cartilage Cuneiform cartilage False vocal cord Glottis Rima glottidis Thyroid cartilage Ventricular fold Y Mouth and Throat	X External	Ø Drainage Device Y Other Device	Z No Qualifier

Non-OR All body part, approach, device, and qualifier values

Ø Medical and Surgical
C Mouth and Throat
5 Destruction Definition: Physical eradication of all or a portion of a body part by the direct use of energy, force, or a destructive agent
Explanation: None of the body part is physically taken out

Body Part Character 4		Approach Character 5	Device Character 6	Qualifier Character 7
Ø Upper Lip Frenulum labii superioris Labial gland Vermilion border **1 Lower Lip** Frenulum labii inferioris Labial gland Vermilion border **2 Hard Palate** **3 Soft Palate** **4 Buccal Mucosa** Buccal gland Molar gland Palatine gland	**5 Upper Gingiva** **6 Lower Gingiva** **7 Tongue** Frenulum linguae **N Uvula** Palatine uvula **P Tonsils** Palatine tonsil **Q Adenoids** Pharyngeal tonsil	**Ø Open** **3 Percutaneous** **X External**	**Z No Device**	**Z No Qualifier**
8 Parotid Gland, Right **9 Parotid Gland, Left** **B Parotid Duct, Right** Stensen's duct **C Parotid Duct, Left** *See B Parotid Duct, Right* **D Sublingual Gland, Right**	**F Sublingual Gland, Left** **G Submaxillary Gland, Right** Submandibular gland **H Submaxillary Gland, Left** *See G Submaxillary Gland, Right* **J Minor Salivary Gland** Anterior lingual gland	**Ø Open** **3 Percutaneous**	**Z No Device**	**Z No Qualifier**
M Pharynx Base of tongue Hypopharynx Laryngopharynx Lingual tonsil Oropharynx Piriform recess (sinus) Tongue, base of **R Epiglottis** Glossoepiglottic fold	**S Larynx** Aryepiglottic fold Arytenoid cartilage Corniculate cartilage Cuneiform cartilage False vocal cord Glottis Rima glottidis Thyroid cartilage Ventricular fold **T Vocal Cord, Right** Vocal fold **V Vocal Cord, Left** *See T Vocal Cord, Right*	**Ø Open** **3 Percutaneous** **4 Percutaneous Endoscopic** **7 Via Natural or Artificial Opening** **8 Via Natural or Artificial Opening Endoscopic**	**Z No Device**	**Z No Qualifier**
W Upper Tooth **X Lower Tooth**		**Ø Open** **X External**	**Z No Device**	**Ø Single** **1 Multiple** **2 All**

Non-OR ØC5[5,6][Ø,3,X]ZZ
Non-OR ØC5[W,X][Ø,X]Z[Ø,1,2]

Ø Medical and Surgical
C Mouth and Throat
7 Dilation Definition: Expanding an orifice or the lumen of a tubular body part
Explanation: The orifice can be a natural orifice or an artificially created orifice. Accomplished by stretching a tubular body part using intraluminal pressure or by cutting part of the orifice or wall of the tubular body part.

Body Part Character 4	Approach Character 5	Device Character 6	Qualifier Character 7
B Parotid Duct, Right Stensen's duct **C Parotid Duct, Left** *See B Parotid Duct, Right*	**Ø Open** **3 Percutaneous** **7 Via Natural or Artificial Opening**	**D Intraluminal Device** **Z No Device**	**Z No Qualifier**
M Pharynx Base of tongue Hypopharynx Laryngopharynx Lingual tonsil Oropharynx Piriform recess (sinus) Tongue, base of	**7 Via Natural or Artificial Opening** **8 Via Natural or Artificial Opening Endoscopic**	**D Intraluminal Device** **Z No Device**	**Z No Qualifier**
S Larynx Aryepiglottic fold Arytenoid cartilage Corniculate cartilage Cuneiform cartilage False vocal cord Glottis Rima glottidis Thyroid cartilage Ventricular fold	**Ø Open** **3 Percutaneous** **4 Percutaneous Endoscopic** **7 Via Natural or Artificial Opening** **8 Via Natural or Artificial Opening Endoscopic**	**D Intraluminal Device** **Z No Device**	**Z No Qualifier**

Non-OR ØC7[B,C][Ø,3,7][D,Z]Z
Non-OR ØC7M[7,8][D,Z]Z

Ø Medical and Surgical
C Mouth and Throat
9 Drainage Definition: Taking or letting out fluids and/or gases from a body part
Explanation: The qualifier DIAGNOSTIC is used to identify drainage procedures that are biopsies

Body Part Character 4		Approach Character 5	Device Character 6	Qualifier Character 7
Ø Upper Lip Frenulum labii superioris Labial gland Vermilion border **1 Lower Lip** Frenulum labii inferioris Labial gland Vermilion border **2 Hard Palate** **3 Soft Palate** **4 Buccal Mucosa** Buccal gland Molar gland Palatine gland	**5 Upper Gingiva** **6 Lower Gingiva** **7 Tongue** Frenulum linguae **N Uvula** Palatine uvula **P Tonsils** Palatine tonsil **Q Adenoids** Pharyngeal tonsil	**Ø Open** **3 Percutaneous** **X External**	**Ø Drainage Device**	**Z No Qualifier**
Ø Upper Lip Frenulum labii superioris Labial gland Vermilion border **1 Lower Lip** Frenulum labii inferioris Labial gland Vermilion border **2 Hard Palate** **3 Soft Palate** **4 Buccal Mucosa** Buccal gland Molar gland Palatine gland	**5 Upper Gingiva** **6 Lower Gingiva** **7 Tongue** Frenulum linguae **N Uvula** Palatine uvula **P Tonsils** Palatine tonsil **Q Adenoids** Pharyngeal tonsil	**Ø Open** **3 Percutaneous** **X External**	**Z No Device**	**X Diagnostic** **Z No Qualifier**
8 Parotid Gland, Right **9 Parotid Gland, Left** **B Parotid Duct, Right** Stensen's duct **C Parotid Duct, Left** *See B Parotid Duct, Right* **D Sublingual Gland, Right**	**F Sublingual Gland, Left** **G Submaxillary Gland, Right** Submandibular gland **H Submaxillary Gland, Left** *See G Submaxillary Gland, Right* **J Minor Salivary Gland** Anterior lingual gland	**Ø Open** **3 Percutaneous**	**Ø Drainage Device**	**Z No Qualifier**
8 Parotid Gland, Right **9 Parotid Gland, Left** **B Parotid Duct, Right** Stensen's duct **C Parotid Duct, Left** *See B Parotid Duct, Right*	**D Sublingual Gland, Right** **F Sublingual Gland, Left** **G Submaxillary Gland, Right** Submandibular gland **H Submaxillary Gland, Left** *See G Submaxillary Gland, Right* **J Minor Salivary Gland** Anterior lingual gland	**Ø Open** **3 Percutaneous**	**Z No Device**	**X Diagnostic** **Z No Qualifier**
M Pharynx Base of tongue Hypopharynx Laryngopharynx Lingual tonsil Oropharynx Piriform recess (sinus) Tongue, base of **R Epiglottis** Glossoepiglottic fold	**S Larynx** Aryepiglottic fold Arytenoid cartilage Corniculate cartilage Cuneiform cartilage False vocal cord Glottis Rima glottidis Thyroid cartilage Ventricular fold **T Vocal Cord, Right** Vocal fold **V Vocal Cord, Left** *See T Vocal Cord, Right*	**Ø Open** **3 Percutaneous** **4 Percutaneous Endoscopic** **7 Via Natural or Artificial Opening** **8 Via Natural or Artificial Opening Endoscopic**	**Ø Drainage Device**	**Z No Qualifier**

ØC9 Continued on next page

Non-OR ØC9[Ø,1,2,3,4,7,N,P,Q]3ØZ
Non-OR ØC9[5,6][Ø,3,X]ØZ
Non-OR ØC9[Ø,1,4][Ø,3,X]ZX
Non-OR ØC9[Ø,1,2,3,4,7,N,P,Q]3ZZ
Non-OR ØC9[5,6][Ø,3,X]Z[X,Z]
Non-OR ØC97[3,X]ZX
Non-OR ØC9[8,9,B,C,D,F,G,H,J][Ø,3]ØZ
Non-OR ØC9[8,9,B,C,D,F,G,H,J]3ZX
Non-OR ØC9[8,9,B,C,D,F,G,H,J][Ø,3]ZZ
Non-OR ØC9[M,R,S,T,V]3ØZ

Mouth and Throat

ØC9 Continued

Ø Medical and Surgical
C Mouth and Throat
9 Drainage Definition: Taking or letting out fluids and/or gases from a body part
Explanation: The qualifier DIAGNOSTIC is used to identify drainage procedures that are biopsies

Body Part Character 4	Approach Character 5	Device Character 6	Qualifier Character 7
M Pharynx Base of tongue Hypopharynx Laryngopharynx Lingual tonsil Oropharynx Piriform recess (sinus) Tongue, base of **R** Epiglottis Glossoepiglottic fold **S** Larynx Aryepiglottic fold Arytenoid cartilage Corniculate cartilage Cuneiform cartilage False vocal cord Glottis Rima glottidis Thyroid cartilage Ventricular fold **T** Vocal Cord, Right Vocal fold **V** Vocal Cord, Left *See T Vocal Cord, Right*	**Ø** Open **3** Percutaneous **4** Percutaneous Endoscopic **7** Via Natural or Artificial Opening **8** Via Natural or Artificial Opening Endoscopic	**Z** No Device	**X** Diagnostic **Z** No Qualifier
W Upper Tooth **X** Lower Tooth	**Ø** Open **X** External	**Ø** Drainage Device **Z** No Device	**Ø** Single **1** Multiple **2** All

Non-OR ØC9M[Ø,3,4,7,8]ZX
Non-OR ØC9[M,R,S,T,V]3ZZ
Non-OR ØC9[R,S,T,V][3,4,7,8]ZX
Non-OR ØC9[W,X][Ø,X][Ø,Z][Ø,1,2]

Ø Medical and Surgical
C Mouth and Throat
B Excision Definition: Cutting out or off, without replacement, a portion of a body part
Explanation: The qualifier DIAGNOSTIC is used to identify excision procedures that are biopsies

Body Part Character 4	Approach Character 5	Device Character 6	Qualifier Character 7
Ø Upper Lip Frenulum labii superioris Labial gland Vermilion border **1** Lower Lip Frenulum labii inferioris Labial gland Vermilion border **2** Hard Palate **3** Soft Palate **4** Buccal Mucosa Buccal gland Molar gland Palatine gland **5** Upper Gingiva **6** Lower Gingiva **7** Tongue Frenulum linguae **N** Uvula Palatine uvula **P** Tonsils Palatine tonsil **Q** Adenoids Pharyngeal tonsil	**Ø** Open **3** Percutaneous **X** External	**Z** No Device	**X** Diagnostic **Z** No Qualifier
8 Parotid Gland, Right **9** Parotid Gland, Left **B** Parotid Duct, Right Stensen's duct **C** Parotid Duct, Left *See B Parotid Duct, Right* **D** Sublingual Gland, Right **F** Sublingual Gland, Left **G** Submaxillary Gland, Right Submandibular gland **H** Submaxillary Gland, Left *See G Submaxillary Gland, Right* **J** Minor Salivary Gland Anterior lingual gland	**Ø** Open **3** Percutaneous	**Z** No Device	**X** Diagnostic **Z** No Qualifier
M Pharynx Base of tongue Hypopharynx Laryngopharynx Lingual tonsil Oropharynx Piriform recess (sinus) Tongue, base of **R** Epiglottis Glossoepiglottic fold **S** Larynx Aryepiglottic fold Arytenoid cartilage Corniculate cartilage Cuneiform cartilage False vocal cord Glottis Rima glottidis Thyroid cartilage Ventricular fold **T** Vocal Cord, Right Vocal fold **V** Vocal Cord, Left *See T Vocal Cord, Right*	**Ø** Open **3** Percutaneous **4** Percutaneous Endoscopic **7** Via Natural or Artificial Opening **8** Via Natural or Artificial Opening Endoscopic	**Z** No Device	**X** Diagnostic **Z** No Qualifier
W Upper Tooth **X** Lower Tooth	**Ø** Open **X** External	**Z** No Device	**Ø** Single **1** Multiple **2** All

Non-OR ØCB[Ø,1,4][Ø,3,X]ZX
Non-OR ØCB[5,6][Ø,3,X]Z[X,Z]
Non-OR ØCB7[3,X]ZX
Non-OR ØCB[8,9,B,C,D,F,G,H,J]3ZX
Non-OR ØCBM[Ø,3,4,7,8]ZX
Non-OR ØCB[R,S,T,V][3,4,7,8]ZX
Non-OR ØCB[W,X][Ø,X]Z[Ø,1,2]

Ø Medical and Surgical
C Mouth and Throat
C Extirpation Definition: Taking or cutting out solid matter from a body part

Explanation: The solid matter may be an abnormal byproduct of a biological function or a foreign body; it may be imbedded in a body part or in the lumen of a tubular body part. The solid matter may or may not have been previously broken into pieces.

Body Part Character 4		Approach Character 5	Device Character 6	Qualifier Character 7
Ø Upper Lip Frenulum labii superioris Labial gland Vermilion border **1 Lower Lip** Frenulum labii inferioris Labial gland Vermilion border **2 Hard Palate** **3 Soft Palate** **4 Buccal Mucosa** Buccal gland Molar gland Palatine gland	**5 Upper Gingiva** **6 Lower Gingiva** **7 Tongue** Frenulum linguae **N Uvula** Palatine uvula **P Tonsils** Palatine tonsil **Q Adenoids** Pharyngeal tonsil	**Ø Open** **3 Percutaneous** **X External**	**Z No Device**	**Z No Qualifier**
8 Parotid Gland, Right **9 Parotid Gland, Left** **B Parotid Duct, Right** Stensen's duct **C Parotid Duct, Left** *See B Parotid Duct, Right* **D Sublingual Gland, Right**	**F Sublingual Gland, Left** **G Submaxillary Gland, Right** Submandibular gland **H Submaxillary Gland, Left** *See G Submaxillary Gland, Right* **J Minor Salivary Gland** Anterior lingual gland	**Ø Open** **3 Percutaneous**	**Z No Device**	**Z No Qualifier**
M Pharynx Base of tongue Hypopharynx Laryngopharynx Lingual tonsil Oropharynx Piriform recess (sinus) Tongue, base of **R Epiglottis** Glossoepiglottic fold	**S Larynx** Aryepiglottic fold Arytenoid cartilage Corniculate cartilage Cuneiform cartilage False vocal cord Glottis Rima glottidis Thyroid cartilage Ventricular fold **T Vocal Cord, Right** Vocal fold **V Vocal Cord, Left** *See T Vocal Cord, Right*	**Ø Open** **3 Percutaneous** **4 Percutaneous Endoscopic** **7 Via Natural or Artificial Opening** **8 Via Natural or Artificial Opening Endoscopic**	**Z No Device**	**Z No Qualifier**
W Upper Tooth **X Lower Tooth**		**Ø Open** **X External**	**Z No Device**	**Ø Single** **1 Multiple** **2 All**

Non-OR ØCC[Ø,1,2,3,4,7,N,P,Q]XZZ
Non-OR ØCC[5,6][Ø,3,X]ZZ
Non-OR ØCC[8,9,B,C,D,F,G,H,J][Ø,3]ZZ
Non-OR ØCC[M,S][7,8]ZZ
Non-OR ØCC[W,X][Ø,X]Z[Ø,1,2]

Ø Medical and Surgical
C Mouth and Throat
D Extraction Definition: Pulling or stripping out or off all or a portion of a body part by the use of force

Explanation: The qualifier DIAGNOSTIC is used to identify extraction procedures that are biopsies

Body Part Character 4	Approach Character 5	Device Character 6	Qualifier Character 7
T Vocal Cord, Right Vocal fold **V Vocal Cord, Left** *See T Vocal Cord, Right*	**Ø Open** **3 Percutaneous** **4 Percutaneous Endoscopic** **7 Via Natural or Artificial Opening** **8 Via Natural or Artificial Opening Endoscopic**	**Z No Device**	**Z No Qualifier**
W Upper Tooth **X Lower Tooth**	**X External**	**Z No Device**	**Ø Single** **1 Multiple** **2 All**

Non-OR ØCD[W,X]XZ[Ø,1,2]

Ø Medical and Surgical
C Mouth and Throat
F Fragmentation Definition: Breaking solid matter in a body part into pieces

Explanation: Physical force (e.g., manual, ultrasonic) applied directly or indirectly is used to break the solid matter into pieces. The solid matter may be an abnormal byproduct of a biological function or a foreign body. The pieces of solid matter are not taken out.

Body Part Character 4	Approach Character 5	Device Character 6	Qualifier Character 7
B Parotid Duct, Right NC Stensen's duct C Parotid Duct, Left NC *See B Parotid Duct, Right*	Ø Open 3 Percutaneous 7 Via Natural or Artificial Opening X External	Z No Device	Z No Qualifier

Non-OR All body part, approach, device, and qualifier values
NC ØCF[B,C]XZZ

Ø Medical and Surgical
C Mouth and Throat
H Insertion Definition: Putting in a nonbiological appliance that monitors, assists, performs, or prevents a physiological function but does not physically take the place of a body part

Explanation: None

Body Part Character 4	Approach Character 5	Device Character 6	Qualifier Character 7
7 Tongue Frenulum linguae	Ø Open 3 Percutaneous X External	1 Radioactive Element	Z No Qualifier
A Salivary Gland S Larynx Aryepiglottic fold Arytenoid cartilage Corniculate cartilage Cuneiform cartilage False vocal cord Glottis Rima glottidis Thyroid cartilage Ventricular fold	Ø Open 3 Percutaneous 7 Via Natural or Artificial Opening 8 Via Natural or Artificial Opening Endoscopic	Y Other Device	Z No Qualifier
Y Mouth and Throat	Ø Open 3 Percutaneous	Y Other Device	Z No Qualifier
Y Mouth and Throat	7 Via Natural or Artificial Opening 8 Via Natural or Artificial Opening Endoscopic	B Intraluminal Device, Airway Y Other Device	Z No Qualifier

Non-OR ØCH[A,S][3,7,8]YZ
Non-OR ØCHSØYZ
Non-OR ØCHY[Ø,3]YZ
Non-OR ØCHY[7,8][B,Y]Z

Ø Medical and Surgical
C Mouth and Throat
J Inspection Definition: Visually and/or manually exploring a body part

Explanation: Visual exploration may be performed with or without optical instrumentation. Manual exploration may be performed directly or through intervening body layers.

Body Part Character 4	Approach Character 5	Device Character 6	Qualifier Character 7
A Salivary Gland	Ø Open 3 Percutaneous X External	Z No Device	Z No Qualifier
S Larynx Aryepiglottic fold Arytenoid cartilage Corniculate cartilage Cuneiform cartilage False vocal cord Glottis Rima glottidis Thyroid cartilage Ventricular fold Y Mouth and Throat	Ø Open 3 Percutaneous 4 Percutaneous Endoscopic 7 Via Natural or Artificial Opening 8 Via Natural or Artificial Opening Endoscopic X External	Z No Device	Z No Qualifier

Non-OR All body part, approach, device, and qualifier values

Ø Medical and Surgical
C Mouth and Throat
L Occlusion Definition: Completely closing an orifice or the lumen of a tubular body part
Explanation: The orifice can be a natural orifice or an artificially created orifice

Body Part Character 4	Approach Character 5	Device Character 6	Qualifier Character 7
B Parotid Duct, Right Stensen's duct **C** Parotid Duct, Left *See B Parotid Duct, Right*	**Ø** Open **3** Percutaneous **4** Percutaneous Endoscopic	**C** Extraluminal Device **D** Intraluminal Device **Z** No Device	**Z** No Qualifier
B Parotid Duct, Right Stensen's duct **C** Parotid Duct, Left *See B Parotid Duct, Right*	**7** Via Natural or Artificial Opening **8** Via Natural or Artificial Opening Endoscopic	**D** Intraluminal Device **Z** No Device	**Z** No Qualifier

Ø Medical and Surgical
C Mouth and Throat
M Reattachment Definition: Putting back in or on all or a portion of a separated body part to its normal location or other suitable location
Explanation: Vascular circulation and nervous pathways may or may not be reestablished

Body Part Character 4	Approach Character 5	Device Character 6	Qualifier Character 7
Ø Upper Lip Frenulum labii superioris Labial gland Vermilion border **1** Lower Lip Frenulum labii inferioris Labial gland Vermilion border **3** Soft Palate **7** Tongue Frenulum linguae **N** Uvula Palatine uvula	**Ø** Open	**Z** No Device	**Z** No Qualifier
W Upper Tooth **X** Lower Tooth	**Ø** Open **X** External	**Z** No Device	**Ø** Single **1** Multiple **2** All

Non-OR ØCM[W,X][Ø,X]Z[Ø,1,2]

Mouth and Throat

Ø Medical and Surgical
C Mouth and Throat
N Release Definition: Freeing a body part from an abnormal physical constraint by cutting or by the use of force
Explanation: Some of the restraining tissue may be taken out but none of the body part is taken out

Body Part Character 4	Approach Character 5	Device Character 6	Qualifier Character 7
Ø Upper Lip Frenulum labii superioris Labial gland Vermilion border **1 Lower Lip** Frenulum labii inferioris Labial gland Vermilion border **2 Hard Palate** **3 Soft Palate** **4 Buccal Mucosa** Buccal gland Molar gland Palatine gland **5 Upper Gingiva** **6 Lower Gingiva** **7 Tongue** Frenulum linguae **N Uvula** Palatine uvula **P Tonsils** Palatine tonsil **Q Adenoids** Pharyngeal tonsil	**Ø Open** **3 Percutaneous** **X External**	**Z No Device**	**Z No Qualifier**
8 Parotid Gland, Right **9 Parotid Gland, Left** **B Parotid Duct, Right** Stensen's duct **C Parotid Duct, Left** *See B Parotid Duct, Right* **D Sublingual Gland, Right** **F Sublingual Gland, Left** **G Submaxillary Gland, Right** Submandibular gland **H Submaxillary Gland, Left** *See G Submaxillary Gland, Right* **J Minor Salivary Gland** Anterior lingual gland	**Ø Open** **3 Percutaneous**	**Z No Device**	**Z No Qualifier**
M Pharynx Base of tongue Hypopharynx Laryngopharynx Lingual tonsil Oropharynx Piriform recess (sinus) Tongue, base of **R Epiglottis** Glossoepiglottic fold **S Larynx** Aryepiglottic fold Arytenoid cartilage Corniculate cartilage Cuneiform cartilage False vocal cord Glottis Rima glottidis Thyroid cartilage Ventricular fold **T Vocal Cord, Right** Vocal fold **V Vocal Cord, Left** *See T Vocal Cord, Right*	**Ø Open** **3 Percutaneous** **4 Percutaneous Endoscopic** **7 Via Natural or Artificial Opening** **8 Via Natural or Artificial Opening Endoscopic**	**Z No Device**	**Z No Qualifier**
W Upper Tooth **X Lower Tooth**	**Ø Open** **X External**	**Z No Device**	**Ø Single** **1 Multiple** **2 All**

Non-OR ØCN[Ø,1,5,6,7][Ø,3,X]ZZ
Non-OR ØCN[W,X][Ø,X]Z[Ø,1,2]

Ø Medical and Surgical
C Mouth and Throat
P Removal Definition: Taking out or off a device from a body part

Explanation: If a device is taken out and a similar device put in without cutting or puncturing the skin or mucous membrane, the procedure is coded to the root operation CHANGE. Otherwise, the procedure for taking out a device is coded to the root operation REMOVAL.

Body Part Character 4	Approach Character 5	Device Character 6	Qualifier Character 7
A Salivary Gland	Ø Open 3 Percutaneous	Ø Drainage Device C Extraluminal Device Y Other Device	Z No Qualifier
A Salivary Gland	7 Via Natural or Artificial Opening 8 Via Natural or Artificial Opening Endoscopic	Y Other Device	Z No Qualifier
S Larynx Aryepiglottic fold Arytenoid cartilage Corniculate cartilage Cuneiform cartilage False vocal cord Glottis Rima glottidis Thyroid cartilage Ventricular fold	Ø Open 3 Percutaneous 7 Via Natural or Artificial Opening 8 Via Natural or Artificial Opening Endoscopic	Ø Drainage Device 7 Autologous Tissue Substitute D Intraluminal Device J Synthetic Substitute K Nonautologous Tissue Substitute Y Other Device	Z No Qualifier
S Larynx Aryepiglottic fold Arytenoid cartilage Corniculate cartilage Cuneiform cartilage False vocal cord Glottis Rima glottidis Thyroid cartilage Ventricular fold	X External	Ø Drainage Device 7 Autologous Tissue Substitute D Intraluminal Device J Synthetic Substitute K Nonautologous Tissue Substitute	Z No Qualifier
Y Mouth and Throat	Ø Open 3 Percutaneous 7 Via Natural or Artificial Opening 8 Via Natural or Artificial Opening Endoscopic	Ø Drainage Device 1 Radioactive Element 7 Autologous Tissue Substitute D Intraluminal Device J Synthetic Substitute K Nonautologous Tissue Substitute Y Other Device	Z No Qualifier
Y Mouth and Throat	X External	Ø Drainage Device 1 Radioactive Element 7 Autologous Tissue Substitute D Intraluminal Device J Synthetic Substitute K Nonautologous Tissue Substitute	Z No Qualifier

Non-OR ØCPA[Ø,3][Ø,C,Y]Z
Non-OR ØCPA[7,8]YZ
Non-OR ØCPS3YZ
Non-OR ØCPS[7,8][Ø,D,Y]Z
Non-OR ØCPSX[Ø,7,D,J,K]Z
Non-OR ØCPY3YZ
Non-OR ØCPY[7,8][Ø,D,Y]Z
Non-OR ØCPYX[Ø,1,7,D,J,K]Z

Ø Medical and Surgical
C Mouth and Throat
Q Repair Definition: Restoring, to the extent possible, a body part to its normal anatomic structure and function
Explanation: Used only when the method to accomplish the repair is not one of the other root operations

Body Part Character 4	Approach Character 5	Device Character 6	Qualifier Character 7
Ø Upper Lip Frenulum labii superioris Labial gland Vermilion border **1 Lower Lip** Frenulum labii inferioris Labial gland Vermilion border **2 Hard Palate** **3 Soft Palate** **4 Buccal Mucosa** Buccal gland Molar gland Palatine gland **5 Upper Gingiva** **6 Lower Gingiva** **7 Tongue** Frenulum linguae **N Uvula** Palatine uvula **P Tonsils** Palatine tonsil **Q Adenoids** Pharyngeal tonsil	**Ø Open** **3 Percutaneous** **X External**	**Z No Device**	**Z No Qualifier**
8 Parotid Gland, Right **9 Parotid Gland, Left** **B Parotid Duct, Right** Stensen's duct **C Parotid Duct, Left** *See B Parotid Duct, Right* **D Sublingual Gland, Right** **F Sublingual Gland, Left** **G Submaxillary Gland, Right** Submandibular gland **H Submaxillary Gland, Left** *See G Submaxillary Gland, Right* **J Minor Salivary Gland** Anterior lingual gland	**Ø Open** **3 Percutaneous**	**Z No Device**	**Z No Qualifier**
M Pharynx Base of tongue Hypopharynx Laryngopharynx Lingual tonsil Oropharynx Piriform recess (sinus) Tongue, base of **R Epiglottis** Glossoepiglottic fold **S Larynx** Aryepiglottic fold Arytenoid cartilage Corniculate cartilage Cuneiform cartilage False vocal cord Glottis Rima glottidis Thyroid cartilage Ventricular fold **T Vocal Cord, Right** Vocal fold **V Vocal Cord, Left** *See T Vocal Cord, Right*	**Ø Open** **3 Percutaneous** **4 Percutaneous Endoscopic** **7 Via Natural or Artificial Opening** **8 Via Natural or Artificial Opening Endoscopic**	**Z No Device**	**Z No Qualifier**
W Upper Tooth **X Lower Tooth**	**Ø Open** **X External**	**Z No Device**	**Ø Single** **1 Multiple** **2 All**

Non-OR ØCQ[Ø,1,4,7]XZZ
Non-OR ØCQ[5,6][Ø,3,X]ZZ
Non-OR ØCQ[W,X][Ø,X]Z[Ø,1,2]

Ø Medical and Surgical
C Mouth and Throat
R Replacement Definition: Putting in or on biological or synthetic material that physically takes the place and/or function of all or a portion of a body part

Explanation: The body part may have been taken out or replaced, or may be taken out, physically eradicated, or rendered nonfunctional during the REPLACEMENT procedure. A REMOVAL procedure is coded for taking out the device used in a previous replacement procedure.

Body Part Character 4	Approach Character 5	Device Character 6	Qualifier Character 7
Ø Upper Lip Frenulum labii superioris Labial gland Vermilion border **1 Lower Lip** Frenulum labii inferioris Labial gland Vermilion border **2 Hard Palate** **3 Soft Palate** **4 Buccal Mucosa** Buccal gland Molar gland Palatine gland **5 Upper Gingiva** **6 Lower Gingiva** **7 Tongue** Frenulum linguae **N Uvula** Palatine uvula	**Ø Open** **3 Percutaneous** **X External**	**7 Autologous Tissue Substitute** **J Synthetic Substitute** **K Nonautologous Tissue Substitute**	**Z No Qualifier**
B Parotid Duct, Right Stensen's duct **C Parotid Duct, Left** *See B Parotid Duct, Right*	**Ø Open** **3 Percutaneous**	**7 Autologous Tissue Substitute** **J Synthetic Substitute** **K Nonautologous Tissue Substitute**	**Z No Qualifier**
M Pharynx Base of tongue Hypopharynx Laryngopharynx Lingual tonsil Oropharynx Piriform recess (sinus) Tongue, base of **R Epiglottis** Glossoepiglottic fold **S Larynx** Aryepiglottic fold Arytenoid cartilage Corniculate cartilage Cuneiform cartilage False vocal cord Glottis Rima glottidis Thyroid cartilage Ventricular fold **T Vocal Cord, Right** Vocal fold **V Vocal Cord, Left** *See T Vocal Cord, Right*	**Ø Open** **7 Via Natural or Artificial Opening** **8 Via Natural or Artificial Opening Endoscopic**	**7 Autologous Tissue Substitute** **J Synthetic Substitute** **K Nonautologous Tissue Substitute**	**Z No Qualifier**
W Upper Tooth **X Lower Tooth**	**Ø Open** **X External**	**7 Autologous Tissue Substitute** **J Synthetic Substitute** **K Nonautologous Tissue Substitute**	**Ø Single** **1 Multiple** **2 All**

Non-OR ØCR[W,X][Ø,X][7,J,K][Ø,1,2]

Mouth and Throat
ØCR–ØCR

Mouth and Throat

Ø Medical and Surgical
C Mouth and Throat
S Reposition Definition: Moving to its normal location, or other suitable location, all or a portion of a body part

Explanation: The body part is moved to a new location from an abnormal location, or from a normal location where it is not functioning correctly. The body part may or may not be cut out or off to be moved to the new location.

Body Part Character 4	Approach Character 5	Device Character 6	Qualifier Character 7
Ø Upper Lip Frenulum labii superioris Labial gland Vermilion border **1 Lower Lip** Frenulum labii inferioris Labial gland Vermilion border **2 Hard Palate** **3 Soft Palate** **7 Tongue** Frenulum linguae **N Uvula** Palatine uvula	**Ø Open** **X External**	**Z No Device**	**Z No Qualifier**
B Parotid Duct, Right Stensen's duct **C Parotid Duct, Left** *See B Parotid Duct, Right*	**Ø Open** **3 Percutaneous**	**Z No Device**	**Z No Qualifier**
R Epiglottis Glossoepiglottic fold **T Vocal Cord, Right** Vocal fold **V Vocal Cord, Left** *See T Vocal Cord, Right*	**Ø Open** **7 Via Natural or Artificial Opening** **8 Via Natural or Artificial Opening Endoscopic**	**Z No Device**	**Z No Qualifier**
W Upper Tooth **X Lower Tooth**	**Ø Open** **X External**	**5 External Fixation Device** **Z No Device**	**Ø Single** **1 Multiple** **2 All**

Non-OR ØCS[W,X][Ø,X][5,Z][Ø,1,2]

Ø Medical and Surgical
C Mouth and Throat
T Resection Definition: Cutting out or off, without replacement, all of a body part
Explanation: None

Body Part Character 4	Approach Character 5	Device Character 6	Qualifier Character 7
Ø Upper Lip Frenulum labii superioris Labial gland Vermilion border **1 Lower Lip** Frenulum labii inferioris Labial gland Vermilion border **2 Hard Palate** **3 Soft Palate** **7 Tongue** Frenulum linguae **N Uvula** Palatine uvula **P Tonsils** Palatine tonsil **Q Adenoids** Pharyngeal tonsil	**Ø Open** **X External**	**Z No Device**	**Z No Qualifier**
8 Parotid Gland, Right **9 Parotid Gland, Left** **B Parotid Duct, Right** Stensen's duct **C Parotid Duct, Left** *See B Parotid Duct, Right* **D Sublingual Gland, Right** **F Sublingual Gland, Left** **G Submaxillary Gland, Right** Submandibular gland **H Submaxillary Gland, Left** *See G Submaxillary Gland, Right* **J Minor Salivary Gland** Anterior lingual gland	**Ø Open**	**Z No Device**	**Z No Qualifier**
M Pharynx Base of tongue Hypopharynx Laryngopharynx Lingual tonsil Oropharynx Piriform recess (sinus) Tongue, base of **R Epiglottis** Glossoepiglottic fold **S Larynx** Aryepiglottic fold Arytenoid cartilage Corniculate cartilage Cuneiform cartilage False vocal cord Glottis Rima glottidis Thyroid cartilage Ventricular fold **T Vocal Cord, Right** Vocal fold **V Vocal Cord, Left** *See T Vocal Cord, Right*	**Ø Open** **4 Percutaneous Endoscopic** **7 Via Natural or Artificial Opening** **8 Via Natural or Artificial Opening Endoscopic**	**Z No Device**	**Z No Qualifier**
W Upper Tooth **X Lower Tooth**	**Ø Open**	**Z No Device**	**Ø Single** **1 Multiple** **2 All**

Non-OR ØCT[W,X]ØZ[Ø,1,2]

Ø Medical and Surgical
C Mouth and Throat
U Supplement Definition: Putting in or on biological or synthetic material that physically reinforces and/or augments the function of a portion of a body part

Explanation: The biological material is non-living, or is living and from the same individual. The body part may have been previously replaced, and the SUPPLEMENT procedure is performed to physically reinforce and/or augment the function of the replaced body part.

Body Part Character 4	Approach Character 5	Device Character 6	Qualifier Character 7
Ø Upper Lip Frenulum labii superioris Labial gland Vermilion border **1 Lower Lip** Frenulum labii inferioris Labial gland Vermilion border **2 Hard Palate** **3 Soft Palate** **4 Buccal Mucosa** Buccal gland Molar gland Palatine gland **5 Upper Gingiva** **6 Lower Gingiva** **7 Tongue** Frenulum linguae **N Uvula** Palatine uvula	**Ø** Open **3** Percutaneous **X** External	**7** Autologous Tissue Substitute **J** Synthetic Substitute **K** Nonautologous Tissue Substitute	**Z** No Qualifier
M Pharynx Base of tongue Hypopharynx Laryngopharynx Lingual tonsil Oropharynx Piriform recess (sinus) Tongue, base of **R Epiglottis** Glossoepiglottic fold **S Larynx** Aryepiglottic fold Arytenoid cartilage Corniculate cartilage Cuneiform cartilage False vocal cord Glottis Rima glottidis Thyroid cartilage Ventricular fold **T Vocal Cord, Right** Vocal fold **V Vocal Cord, Left** *See T Vocal Cord, Right*	**Ø** Open **7** Via Natural or Artificial Opening **8** Via Natural or Artificial Opening Endoscopic	**7** Autologous Tissue Substitute **J** Synthetic Substitute **K** Nonautologous Tissue Substitute	**Z** No Qualifier

Non-OR ØCU2[Ø,3]JZ

Ø Medical and Surgical
C Mouth and Throat
V Restriction Definition: Partially closing an orifice or the lumen of a tubular body part

Explanation: The orifice can be a natural orifice or an artificially created orifice

Body Part Character 4	Approach Character 5	Device Character 6	Qualifier Character 7
B Parotid Duct, Right Stensen's duct **C Parotid Duct, Left** *See B Parotid Duct, Right*	**Ø** Open **3** Percutaneous	**C** Extraluminal Device **D** Intraluminal Device **Z** No Device	**Z** No Qualifier
B Parotid Duct, Right Stensen's duct **C Parotid Duct, Left** *See B Parotid Duct, Right*	**7** Via Natural or Artificial Opening **8** Via Natural or Artificial Opening Endoscopic	**D** Intraluminal Device **Z** No Device	**Z** No Qualifier

Ø Medical and Surgical
C Mouth and Throat
W Revision Definition: Correcting, to the extent possible, a portion of a malfunctioning device or the position of a displaced device

Explanation: Revision can include correcting a malfunctioning or displaced device by taking out or putting in components of the device such as a screw or pin

Body Part Character 4	Approach Character 5	Device Character 6	Qualifier Character 7
A Salivary Gland	**Ø** Open **3** Percutaneous	**Ø** Drainage Device **C** Extraluminal Device **Y** Other Device	**Z** No Qualifier
A Salivary Gland	**7** Via Natural or Artificial Opening **8** Via Natural or Artificial Opening Endoscopic	**Y** Other Device	**Z** No Qualifier
A Salivary Gland	**X** External	**Ø** Drainage Device **C** Extraluminal Device	**Z** No Qualifier
S Larynx Aryepiglottic fold Arytenoid cartilage Corniculate cartilage Cuneiform cartilage False vocal cord Glottis Rima glottidis Thyroid cartilage Ventricular fold	**Ø** Open **3** Percutaneous **7** Via Natural or Artificial Opening **8** Via Natural or Artificial Opening Endoscopic	**Ø** Drainage Device **7** Autologous Tissue Substitute **D** Intraluminal Device **J** Synthetic Substitute **K** Nonautologous Tissue Substitute **Y** Other Device	**Z** No Qualifier
S Larynx Aryepiglottic fold Arytenoid cartilage Corniculate cartilage Cuneiform cartilage False vocal cord Glottis Rima glottidis Thyroid cartilage Ventricular fold	**X** External	**Ø** Drainage Device **7** Autologous Tissue Substitute **D** Intraluminal Device **J** Synthetic Substitute **K** Nonautologous Tissue Substitute	**Z** No Qualifier
Y Mouth and Throat	**Ø** Open **3** Percutaneous **7** Via Natural or Artificial Opening **8** Via Natural or Artificial Opening Endoscopic	**Ø** Drainage Device **1** Radioactive Element **7** Autologous Tissue Substitute **D** Intraluminal Device **J** Synthetic Substitute **K** Nonautologous Tissue Substitute **Y** Other Device	**Z** No Qualifier
Y Mouth and Throat	**X** External	**Ø** Drainage Device **1** Radioactive Element **7** Autologous Tissue Substitute **D** Intraluminal Device **J** Synthetic Substitute **K** Nonautologous Tissue Substitute	**Z** No Qualifier

Non-OR ØCWA[Ø,3][Ø,C,Y]Z
Non-OR ØCWA[7,8]YZ
Non-OR ØCWAX[Ø,C]Z
Non-OR ØCWS[3,7,8]YZ
Non-OR ØCWSX[Ø,7,D,J,K]Z
Non-OR ØCWYØ7Z
Non-OR ØCWY[3,7,8]YZ
Non-OR ØCWYX[Ø,1,7,D,J,K]Z

Ø Medical and Surgical
C Mouth and Throat
X Transfer Definition: Moving, without taking out, all or a portion of a body part to another location to take over the function of all or a portion of a body part

Explanation: The body part transferred remains connected to its vascular and nervous supply

Body Part Character 4	Approach Character 5	Device Character 6	Qualifier Character 7
Ø Upper Lip Frenulum labii superioris Labial gland Vermilion border **1 Lower Lip** Frenulum labii inferioris Labial gland Vermilion border **3 Soft Palate** **4 Buccal Mucosa** Buccal gland Molar gland Palatine gland **5 Upper Gingiva** **6 Lower Gingiva** **7 Tongue** Frenulum linguae	**Ø Open** **X External**	**Z No Device**	**Z No Qualifier**

Gastrointestinal System ØD1–ØDY

Character Meanings

This Character Meaning table is provided as a guide to assist the user in the identification of character members that may be found in this section of code tables. It **SHOULD NOT** be used to build a PCS code.

Operation–Character 3	Body Part–Character 4	Approach–Character 5	Device–Character 6	Qualifier–Character 7
1 Bypass	Ø Upper Intestinal Tract	Ø Open	Ø Drainage Device	Ø Allogeneic
2 Change	1 Esophagus, Upper	3 Percutaneous	1 Radioactive Element	1 Syngeneic
5 Destruction	2 Esophagus, Middle	4 Percutaneous Endoscopic	2 Monitoring Device	2 Zooplastic
7 Dilation	3 Esophagus, Lower	7 Via Natural or Artificial Opening	3 Infusion Device	3 Vertical
8 Division	4 Esophagogastric Junction	8 Via Natural or Artificial Opening Endoscopic	7 Autologous Tissue Substitute	4 Cutaneous
9 Drainage	5 Esophagus	F Via Natural or Artificial Opening with Percutaneous Endoscopic Assistance	B Intraluminal Device, Airway	5 Esophagus
B Excision	6 Stomach	X External	C Extraluminal Device	6 Stomach
C Extirpation	7 Stomach, Pylorus		D Intraluminal Device	9 Duodenum
D Extraction	8 Small Intestine		J Synthetic Substitute	A Jejunum
F Fragmentation	9 Duodenum		K Nonautologous Tissue Substitute	B Ileum
H Insertion	A Jejunum		L Artificial Sphincter	H Cecum
J Inspection	B Ileum		M Stimulator Lead	K Ascending Colon
L Occlusion	C Ileocecal Valve		U Feeding Device	L Transverse Colon
M Reattachment	D Lower Intestinal Tract		Y Other Device	M Descending Colon
N Release	E Large Intestine		Z No Device	N Sigmoid Colon
P Removal	F Large Intestine, Right			P Rectum
Q Repair	G Large Intestine, Left			Q Anus
R Replacement	H Cecum			X Diagnostic
S Reposition	J Appendix			Z No Qualifier
T Resection	K Ascending Colon			
U Supplement	L Transverse Colon			
V Restriction	M Descending Colon			
W Revision	N Sigmoid Colon			
X Transfer	P Rectum			
Y Transplantation	Q Anus			
	R Anal Sphincter			
	U Omentum			
	V Mesentery			
	W Peritoneum			

AHA Coding Clinic for table ØD1
2017, 2Q, 17 Billroth II (distal gastrectomy and gastrojejunostomy)
2016, 2Q, 31 Laparoscopic biliopancreatic diversion with duodenal switch
2014, 4Q, 41 Abdominoperineal resection (APR) with flap closure of perineum and colostomy

AHA Coding Clinic for table ØD5
2017, 1Q, 34 Debulking of tumor and peritoneum ablation

AHA Coding Clinic for table ØD7
2017, 3Q, 23 Laparoscopic pyloromyotomy
2014, 4Q, 40 Dilation of gastrojejunostomy anastomosis stricture

AHA Coding Clinic for table ØD8
2017, 3Q, 22 Laparoscopic esophagomyotomy (Heller type) and Toupet fundoplication
2017, 3Q, 23 Laparoscopic pyloromyotomy

AHA Coding Clinic for table ØD9
2015, 2Q, 29 Insertion of nasogastric tube for drainage and feeding

AHA Coding Clinic for table ØDB
2017, 2Q, 17 Billroth II (distal gastrectomy and gastrojejunostomy)
2017, 1Q, 16 Hepatic flexure versus transverse colon
2016, 3Q, 3-7 Stoma creation & takedown procedures
2016, 2Q, 31 Laparoscopic biliopancreatic diversion with duodenal switch
2016, 1Q, 22 Perineal proctectomy
2016, 1Q, 24 Endoscopic brush biopsy of esophagus
2014, 4Q, 40 Abdominoperineal resection (APR) with flap closure of perineum and colostomy
2014, 3Q, 28 Ileostomy takedown and parastomal hernia repair
2014, 3Q, 32 Pyloric-sparing Whipple procedure

AHA Coding Clinic for table ØDD
2017, 4Q, 41-42 Extraction procedures

AHA Coding Clinic for table ØDH
2016, 3Q, 26 Insertion of gastrostomy tube
2013, 4Q, 117 Percutaneous endoscopic placement of gastrostomy tube

AHA Coding Clinic for table ØDJ
2017, 2Q, 15 Low anterior resection with sigmoidoscopy
2016, 2Q, 20 Capsule endoscopy of small intestine
2015, 3Q, 24 Esophagogastroduodenoscopy with epinephrine injection for control of bleeding

AHA Coding Clinic for table ØDL
2013, 4Q, 112 Endoscopic banding of esophageal varices

AHA Coding Clinic for table ØDN
2017, 4Q, 49-50 New and revised body part values - Repositioning of the intestine
2017, 1Q, 35 Lysis of omental and peritoneal adhesions
2015, 3Q, 15 Vascular ring surgery with release of esophagus and trachea
2015, 3Q, 16 Vascular ring surgery and double aortic arch

AHA Coding Clinic for table ØDQ
2018, 2Q, 25 Third and fourth degree obstetric lacerations
2018, 1Q, 11 Repair of internal hernia at Petersen space
2017, 3Q, 17 Posterior sagittal anorectoplasty
2016, 3Q, 3-7 Stoma creation & takedown procedures
2016, 3Q, 26 Insertion of gastrostomy tube
2016, 1Q, 7 Obstetrical perineal laceration repair
2016, 1Q, 8 Obstetrical perineal laceration repair
2014, 4Q, 20 Control of bleeding duodenal ulcer

AHA Coding Clinic for table ØDS
2017, 4Q, 49-50 New and revised body part values - Repositioning of the intestine
2017, 3Q, 9 Ileocolic intussusception reduction via air enema
2017, 3Q, 17 Posterior sagittal anorectoplasty
2016, 3Q, 3-5 Stoma creation & takedown procedures

AHA Coding Clinic for table ØDT
2017, 4Q, 49-50 New and revised body part values - Repositioning of the intestine
2014, 4Q, 40 Abdominoperineal resection (APR) with flap closure of perineum and colostomy
2014, 4Q, 42 Right colectomy with side-to-side functional end-to-end anastomosis
2014, 3Q, 6 Ileocecectomy including cecum, terminal ileum and appendix
2014, 3Q, 6 Right colectomy

AHA Coding Clinic for table ØDV
2017, 3Q, 22 Laparoscopic esophagomyotomy (Heller type) and Toupet fundoplication
2016, 2Q, 22 Esophageal lengthening Collis gastroplasty with Nissen fundoplication and hiatal hernia
2014, 3Q, 28 Laparoscopic Nissen fundoplication and diaphragmatic hernia repair

AHA Coding Clinic for table ØDW
2018, 1Q, 20 Adjustment of gastric band

AHA Coding Clinic for table ØDX
2017, 2Q, 18 Esophagectomy and esophagogastrectomy with cervical esophagogastrostomy
2016, 2Q, 22 Esophageal lengthening Collis gastroplasty with Nissen fundoplication and hiatal hernia
2015, 1Q, 28 Repair of bronchopleural fistula using omental pedicle graft

Upper Intestinal Tract (Ø) and Lower Intestinal Tract (D)

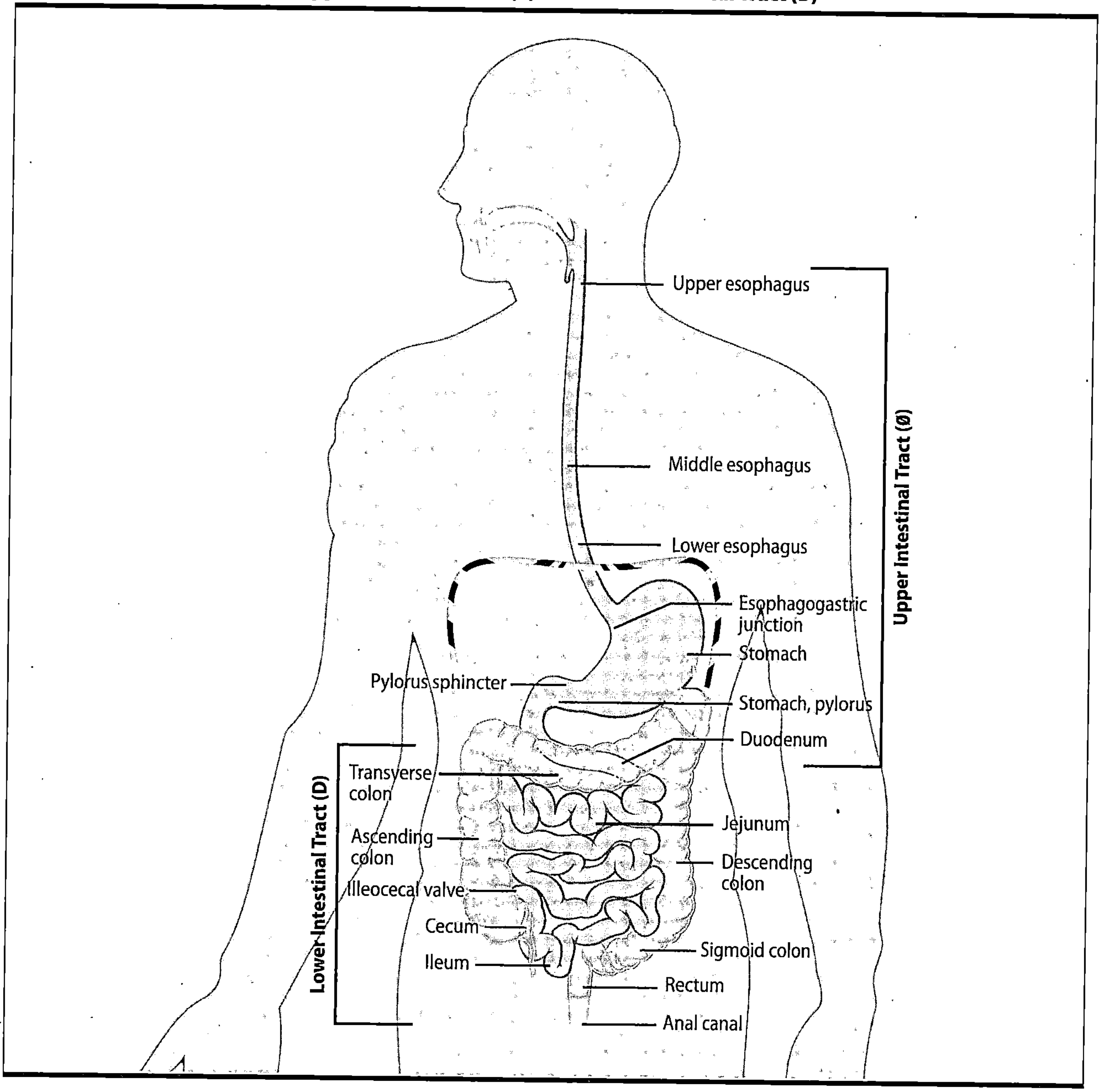

Upper Intestinal Tract

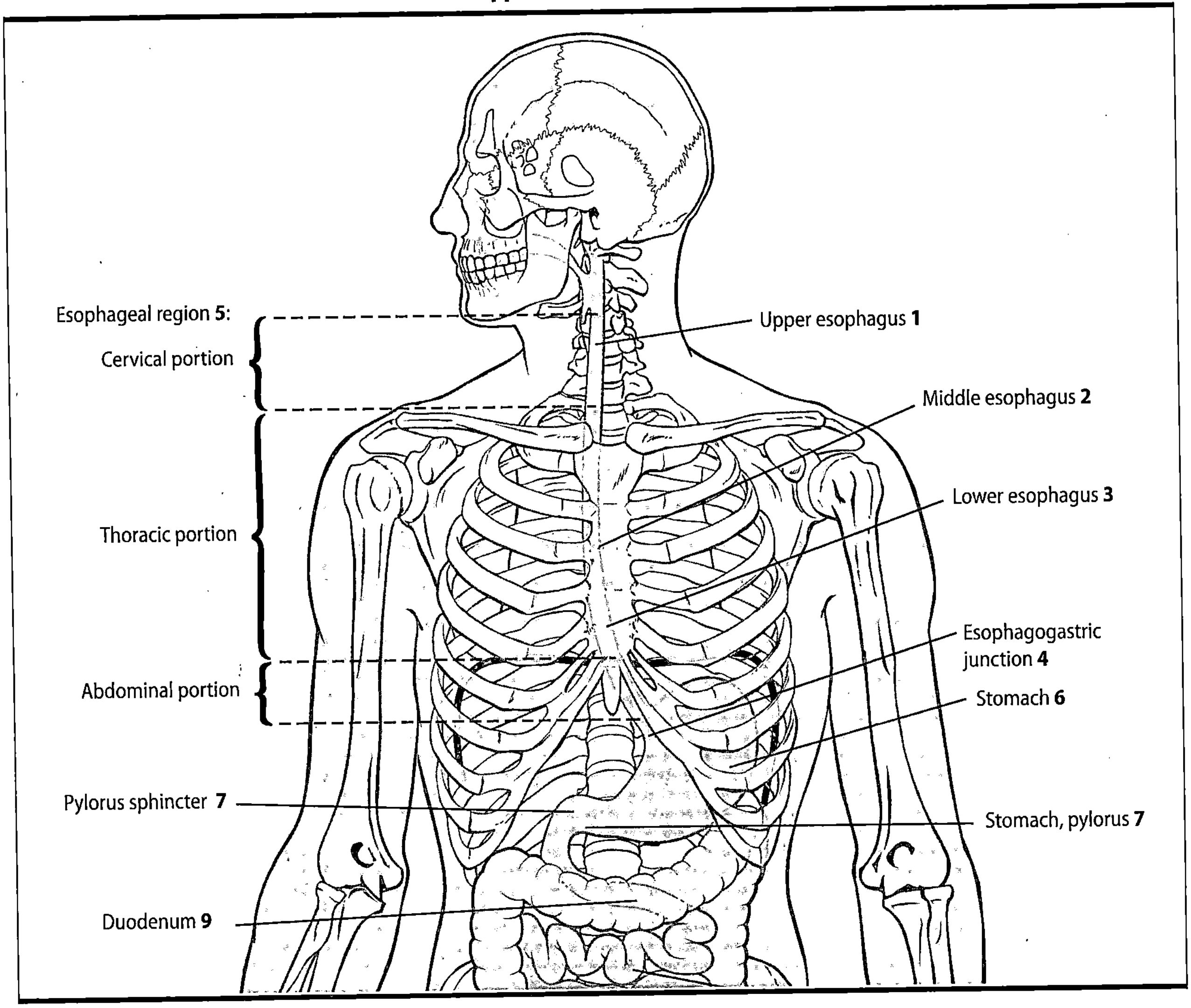

Lower Intestinal Tract (Jejunum Down to and Including Rectum/Anus)

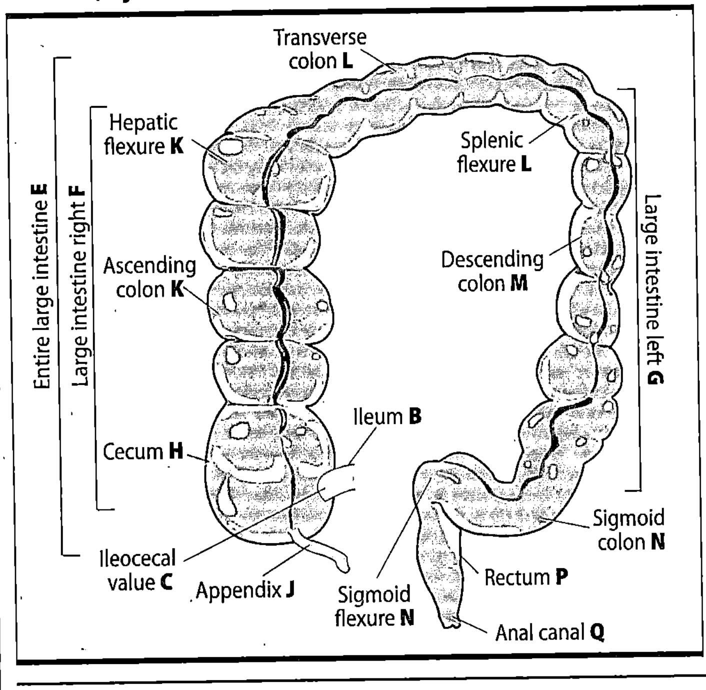

Rectum and Anus

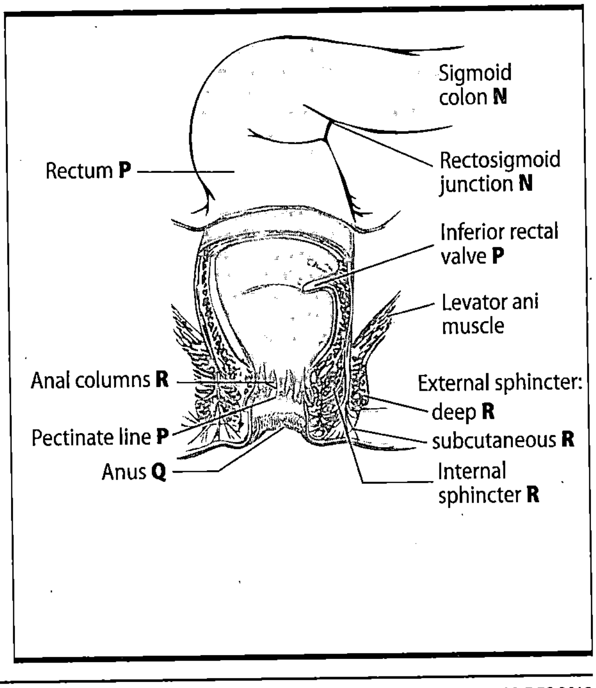

Ø Medical and Surgical
D Gastrointestinal System
1 Bypass Definition: Altering the route of passage of the contents of a tubular body part

Explanation: Rerouting contents of a body part to a downstream area of the normal route, to a similar route and body part, or to an abnormal route and dissimilar body part. Includes one or more anastomoses, with or without the use of a device.

Body Part Character 4	Approach Character 5	Device Character 6	Qualifier Character 7
1 Esophagus, Upper Cervical esophagus 2 Esophagus, Middle Thoracic esophagus 3 Esophagus, Lower Abdominal esophagus 5 Esophagus	Ø Open 4 Percutaneous Endoscopic 8 Via Natural or Artificial Opening Endoscopic	7 Autologous Tissue Substitute J Synthetic Substitute K Nonautologous Tissue Substitute Z No Device	4 Cutaneous 6 Stomach 9 Duodenum A Jejunum B Ileum
1 Esophagus, Upper Cervical esophagus 2 Esophagus, Middle Thoracic esophagus 3 Esophagus, Lower Abdominal esophagus 5 Esophagus	3 Percutaneous	J Synthetic Substitute	4 Cutaneous
6 Stomach 9 Duodenum	Ø Open 4 Percutaneous Endoscopic 8 Via Natural or Artificial Opening Endoscopic	7 Autologous Tissue Substitute J Synthetic Substitute K Nonautologous Tissue Substitute Z No Device	4 Cutaneous 9 Duodenum A Jejunum B Ileum L Transverse Colon
6 Stomach 9 Duodenum	3 Percutaneous	J Synthetic Substitute	4 Cutaneous
A Jejunum Duodenojejunal flexure	Ø Open 4 Percutaneous Endoscopic 8 Via Natural or Artificial Opening Endoscopic	7 Autologous Tissue Substitute J Synthetic Substitute K Nonautologous Tissue Substitute Z No Device	4 Cutaneous A Jejunum B Ileum H Cecum K Ascending Colon L Transverse Colon M Descending Colon N Sigmoid Colon P Rectum Q Anus
A Jejunum Duodenojejunal flexure	3 Percutaneous	J Synthetic Substitute	4 Cutaneous
B Ileum	Ø Open 4 Percutaneous Endoscopic 8 Via Natural or Artificial Opening Endoscopic	7 Autologous Tissue Substitute J Synthetic Substitute K Nonautologous Tissue Substitute Z No Device	4 Cutaneous B Ileum H Cecum K Ascending Colon L Transverse Colon M Descending Colon N Sigmoid Colon P Rectum Q Anus
B Ileum	3 Percutaneous	J Synthetic Substitute	4 Cutaneous
H Cecum	Ø Open 4 Percutaneous Endoscopic 8 Via Natural or Artificial Opening Endoscopic	7 Autologous Tissue Substitute J Synthetic Substitute K Nonautologous Tissue Substitute Z No Device	4 Cutaneous H Cecum K Ascending Colon L Transverse Colon M Descending Colon N Sigmoid Colon P Rectum
H Cecum	3 Percutaneous	J Synthetic Substitute	4 Cutaneous
K Ascending Colon	Ø Open 4 Percutaneous Endoscopic 8 Via Natural or Artificial Opening Endoscopic	7 Autologous Tissue Substitute J Synthetic Substitute K Nonautologous Tissue Substitute Z No Device	4 Cutaneous K Ascending Colon L Transverse Colon M Descending Colon N Sigmoid Colon P Rectum

ØD1 Continued on next page

Non-OR ØD16[Ø,4,8][7,J,K,Z]4
Non-OR ØD163J4
HAC ØD16[Ø,4,8][7,J,K,Z][9,A,B,L] when reported with PDx E66.Ø1 and SDx K68.11 or K95.Ø1 or K95.81 or T81.4XXA

Gastrointestinal System

ØD1 Continued

Ø Medical and Surgical
D Gastrointestinal System
1 Bypass Definition: Altering the route of passage of the contents of a tubular body part

Explanation: Rerouting contents of a body part to a downstream area of the normal route, to a similar route and body part, or to an abnormal route and dissimilar body part. Includes one or more anastomoses, with or without the use of a device.

Body Part Character 4	Approach Character 5	Device Character 6	Qualifier Character 7
K Ascending Colon	3 Percutaneous	J Synthetic Substitute	4 Cutaneous
L Transverse Colon Hepatic flexure Splenic flexure	Ø Open 4 Percutaneous Endoscopic 8 Via Natural or Artificial Opening Endoscopic	7 Autologous Tissue Substitute J Synthetic Substitute K Nonautologous Tissue Substitute Z No Device	4 Cutaneous L Transverse Colon M Descending Colon N Sigmoid Colon P Rectum
L Transverse Colon Hepatic flexure Splenic flexure	3 Percutaneous	J Synthetic Substitute	4 Cutaneous
M Descending Colon	Ø Open 4 Percutaneous Endoscopic 8 Via Natural or Artificial Opening Endoscopic	7 Autologous Tissue Substitute J Synthetic Substitute K Nonautologous Tissue Substitute Z No Device	4 Cutaneous M Descending Colon N Sigmoid Colon P Rectum
M Descending Colon	3 Percutaneous	J Synthetic Substitute	4 Cutaneous
N Sigmoid Colon Rectosigmoid junction Sigmoid flexure	Ø Open 4 Percutaneous Endoscopic 8 Via Natural or Artificial Opening Endoscopic	7 Autologous Tissue Substitute J Synthetic Substitute K Nonautologous Tissue Substitute Z No Device	4 Cutaneous N Sigmoid Colon P Rectum
N Sigmoid Colon Rectosigmoid junction Sigmoid flexure	3 Percutaneous	J Synthetic Substitute	4 Cutaneous

Ø Medical and Surgical
D Gastrointestinal System
2 Change Definition: Taking out or off a device from a body part and putting back an identical or similar device in or on the same body part without cutting or puncturing the skin or a mucous membrane

Explanation: All CHANGE procedures are coded using the approach EXTERNAL

Body Part Character 4	Approach Character 5	Device Character 6	Qualifier Character 7
Ø Upper Intestinal Tract D Lower Intestinal Tract	X External	Ø Drainage Device U Feeding Device Y Other Device	Z No Qualifier
U Omentum Gastrocolic ligament Gastrocolic omentum Gastrohepatic omentum Gastrophrenic ligament Gastrosplenic ligament Greater Omentum Hepatogastric ligament Lesser Omentum V Mesentery Mesoappendix Mesocolon W Peritoneum Epiploic foramen	X External	Ø Drainage Device Y Other Device	Z No Qualifier

Non-OR All body part, approach, device, and qualifier values

Ø Medical and Surgical
D Gastrointestinal System
5 Destruction Definition: Physical eradication of all or a portion of a body part by the direct use of energy, force, or a destructive agent
Explanation: None of the body part is physically taken out

Body Part Character 4	Approach Character 5	Device Character 6	Qualifier Character 7
1 Esophagus, Upper Cervical esophagus **2 Esophagus, Middle** Thoracic esophagus **3 Esophagus, Lower** Abdominal esophagus **4 Esophagogastric Junction** Cardia Cardioesophageal junction Gastroesophageal (GE) junction **5 Esophagus** **6 Stomach** **7 Stomach, Pylorus** Pyloric antrum Pyloric canal Pyloric sphincter **8 Small Intestine** **9 Duodenum** **A Jejunum** Duodenojejunal flexure **B Ileum** **C Ileocecal Valve** **E Large Intestine** **F Large Intestine, Right** **G Large Intestine, Left** **H Cecum** **J Appendix** Vermiform appendix **K Ascending Colon** **L Transverse Colon** Hepatic flexure Splenic flexure **M Descending Colon** **N Sigmoid Colon** Rectosigmoid junction Sigmoid flexure **P Rectum** Anorectal junction	**Ø Open** **3 Percutaneous** **4 Percutaneous Endoscopic** **7 Via Natural or Artificial Opening** **8 Via Natural or Artificial Opening Endoscopic**	**Z No Device**	**Z No Qualifier**
Q Anus Anal orifice	**Ø Open** **3 Percutaneous** **4 Percutaneous Endoscopic** **7 Via Natural or Artificial Opening** **8 Via Natural or Artificial Opening Endoscopic** **X External**	**Z No Device**	**Z No Qualifier**
R Anal Sphincter External anal sphincter Internal anal sphincter **U Omentum** Gastrocolic ligament Gastrocolic omentum Gastrohepatic omentum Gastrophrenic ligament Gastrosplenic ligament Greater Omentum Hepatogastric ligament Lesser Omentum **V Mesentery** Mesoappendix Mesocolon **W Peritoneum** Epiploic foramen	**Ø Open** **3 Percutaneous** **4 Percutaneous Endoscopic**	**Z No Device**	**Z No Qualifier**

Non-OR ØD5[1,2,3,4,5,6,7,9,E,F,G,H,K,L,M,N][4,8]ZZ
Non-OR ØD5P[Ø,3,4,7,8]ZZ
Non-OR ØD5Q[4,8]ZZ
Non-OR ØD5R4ZZ

Ø Medical and Surgical
D Gastrointestinal System
7 Dilation Definition: Expanding an orifice or the lumen of a tubular body part

Explanation: The orifice can be a natural orifice or an artificially created orifice. Accomplished by stretching a tubular body part using intraluminal pressure or by cutting part of the orifice or wall of the tubular body part.

Body Part Character 4	Approach Character 5	Device Character 6	Qualifier Character 7
1 Esophagus, Upper Cervical esophagus **2 Esophagus, Middle** Thoracic esophagus **3 Esophagus, Lower** Abdominal esophagus **4 Esophagogastric Junction** Cardia Cardioesophageal junction Gastroesophageal (GE) junction **5 Esophagus** **6 Stomach** **7 Stomach, Pylorus** Pyloric antrum Pyloric canal Pyloric sphincter **8 Small Intestine** **9 Duodenum** **A Jejunum** Duodenojejunal flexure **B Ileum** **C Ileocecal Valve** **E Large Intestine** **F Large Intestine, Right** **G Large Intestine, Left** **H Cecum** **K Ascending Colon** **L Transverse Colon** Hepatic flexure Splenic flexure **M Descending Colon** **N Sigmoid Colon** Rectosigmoid junction Sigmoid flexure **P Rectum** Anorectal junction **Q Anus** Anal orifice	**Ø Open** **3 Percutaneous** **4 Percutaneous Endoscopic** **7 Via Natural or Artificial Opening** **8 Via Natural or Artificial Opening Endoscopic**	**D Intraluminal Device** **Z No Device**	**Z No Qualifier**

Non-OR ØD7[1,2,3,4,5,6,8,9,A,B,C,E,F,G,H,K,L,M,N,P,Q][7,8][D,Z]Z
Non-OR ØD77[4,8]DZ
Non-OR ØD777[D,Z]Z
Non-OR ØD7[8,9,A,B,C,E,F,G,H,K,L,M,N][Ø,3,4]DZ

Ø Medical and Surgical
D Gastrointestinal System
8 Division Definition: Cutting into a body part, without draining fluids and/or gases from the body part, in order to separate or transect a body part

Explanation: All or a portion of the body part is separated into two or more portions

Body Part Character 4	Approach Character 5	Device Character 6	Qualifier Character 7
4 Esophagogastric Junction Cardia Cardioesophageal junction Gastroesophageal (GE) junction **7 Stomach, Pylorus** Pyloric antrum Pyloric canal Pyloric sphincter	**Ø Open** **3 Percutaneous** **4 Percutaneous Endoscopic** **7 Via Natural or Artificial Opening** **8 Via Natural or Artificial Opening Endoscopic**	**Z No Device**	**Z No Qualifier**
R Anal Sphincter External anal sphincter Internal anal sphincter	**Ø Open** **3 Percutaneous**	**Z No Device**	**Z No Qualifier**

Ø Medical and Surgical
D Gastrointestinal System
9 Drainage Definition: Taking or letting out fluids and/or gases from a body part
Explanation: The qualifier DIAGNOSTIC is used to identify drainage procedures that are biopsies

Body Part Character 4		Approach Character 5	Device Character 6	Qualifier Character 7
1 Esophagus, Upper Cervical esophagus **2 Esophagus, Middle** Thoracic esophagus **3 Esophagus, Lower** Abdominal esophagus **4 Esophagogastric Junction** Cardia Cardioesophageal junction Gastroesophageal (GE) junction **5 Esophagus** **6 Stomach** **7 Stomach, Pylorus** Pyloric antrum Pyloric canal Pyloric sphincter **8 Small Intestine** **9 Duodenum**	**A Jejunum** Duodenojejunal flexure **B Ileum** **C Ileocecal Valve** **E Large Intestine** **F Large Intestine, Right** **G Large Intestine, Left** **H Cecum** **J Appendix** Vermiform appendix **K Ascending Colon** **L Transverse Colon** Hepatic flexure Splenic flexure **M Descending Colon** **N Sigmoid Colon** Rectosigmoid junction Sigmoid flexure **P Rectum** Anorectal junction	**Ø Open** **3 Percutaneous** **4 Percutaneous Endoscopic** **7 Via Natural or Artificial Opening** **8 Via Natural or Artificial Opening Endoscopic**	**Ø Drainage Device**	**Z No Qualifier**
1 Esophagus, Upper Cervical esophagus **2 Esophagus, Middle** Thoracic esophagus **3 Esophagus, Lower** Abdominal esophagus **4 Esophagogastric Junction** Cardia Cardioesophageal junction Gastroesophageal (GE) junction **5 Esophagus** **6 Stomach** **7 Stomach, Pylorus** Pyloric antrum Pyloric canal Pyloric sphincter **8 Small Intestine** **9 Duodenum**	**A Jejunum** Duodenojejunal flexure **B Ileum** **C Ileocecal Valve** **E Large Intestine** **F Large Intestine, Right** **G Large Intestine, Left** **H Cecum** **J Appendix** Vermiform appendix **K Ascending Colon** **L Transverse Colon** Hepatic flexure Splenic flexure **M Descending Colon** **N Sigmoid Colon** Rectosigmoid junction Sigmoid flexure **P Rectum** Anorectal junction	**Ø Open** **3 Percutaneous** **4 Percutaneous Endoscopic** **7 Via Natural or Artificial Opening** **8 Via Natural or Artificial Opening Endoscopic**	**Z No Device**	**X Diagnostic** **Z No Qualifier**
Q Anus Anal orifice		**Ø Open** **3 Percutaneous** **4 Percutaneous Endoscopic** **7 Via Natural or Artificial Opening** **8 Via Natural or Artificial Opening Endoscopic** **X External**	**Ø Drainage Device**	**Z No Qualifier**
Q Anus Anal orifice		**Ø Open** **3 Percutaneous** **4 Percutaneous Endoscopic** **7 Via Natural or Artificial Opening** **8 Via Natural or Artificial Opening Endoscopic** **X External**	**Z No Device**	**X Diagnostic** **Z No Qualifier**

ØD9 Continued on next page

Non-OR ØD9[1,2,3,4,5,C,J]3ØZ
Non-OR ØD9[6,7,8,9,A,B,E,F,G,H,K,L,M,N,P][3,7,8]ØZ
Non-OR ØD9[1,2,3,4,5,6,7,8,9,A,B,C,E,F,G,H,K,L,M,N,P][3,4,7,8]ZX
Non-OR ØD9[1,2,3,4,5,6,7,8,9,A,B,C,E,F,G,H,J,K,L,M,N,P]3ZZ
Non-OR ØD9Q3ØZ
Non-OR ØD9Q[Ø,4,7,8,X]ZX
Non-OR ØD9Q3Z[X,Z]

Ø Medical and Surgical
D Gastrointestinal System
9 Drainage Definition: Taking or letting out fluids and/or gases from a body part
Explanation: The qualifier DIAGNOSTIC is used to identify drainage procedures that are biopsies

ØD9 Continued

Body Part Character 4	Approach Character 5	Device Character 6	Qualifier Character 7
R Anal Sphincter External anal sphincter Internal anal sphincter **U Omentum** Gastrocolic ligament Gastrocolic omentum Gastrohepatic omentum Gastrophrenic ligament Gastrosplenic ligament Greater Omentum Hepatogastric ligament Lesser Omentum **V Mesentery** Mesoappendix Mesocolon **W Peritoneum** Epiploic foramen	**Ø Open** **3 Percutaneous** **4 Percutaneous Endoscopic**	**Ø Drainage Device**	**Z No Qualifier**
R Anal Sphincter External anal sphincter Internal anal sphincter **U Omentum** Gastrocolic ligament Gastrocolic omentum Gastrohepatic omentum Gastrophrenic ligament Gastrosplenic ligament Greater Omentum Hepatogastric ligament Lesser Omentum **V Mesentery** Mesoappendix Mesocolon **W Peritoneum** Epiploic foramen	**Ø Open** **3 Percutaneous** **4 Percutaneous Endoscopic**	**Z No Device**	**X Diagnostic** **Z No Qualifier**

Non-OR ØD9R3ØZ
Non-OR ØD9[U,V,W][3,4]ØZ
Non-OR ØD9R[Ø,4]ZX
Non-OR ØD9[R,U,V,W]3Z[X,Z]
Non-OR ØD9[U,V,W]4ZZ

Ø Medical and Surgical
D Gastrointestinal System
B Excision Definition: Cutting out or off, without replacement, a portion of a body part
Explanation: The qualifier DIAGNOSTIC is used to identify excision procedures that are biopsies

Body Part Character 4	Approach Character 5	Device Character 6	Qualifier Character 7
1 Esophagus, Upper Cervical esophagus **2 Esophagus, Middle** Thoracic esophagus **3 Esophagus, Lower** Abdominal esophagus **4 Esophagogastric Junction** Cardia Cardioesophageal junction Gastroesophageal (GE) junction **5 Esophagus** **7 Stomach, Pylorus** Pyloric antrum Pyloric canal Pyloric sphincter **8 Small Intestine** **9 Duodenum** **A Jejunum** Duodenojejunal flexure **B Ileum** **C Ileocecal Valve** **E Large Intestine** **F Large Intestine, Right** **H Cecum** **J Appendix** Vermiform appendix **K Ascending Colon** **P Rectum** Anorectal junction	**Ø Open** **3 Percutaneous** **4 Percutaneous Endoscopic** **7 Via Natural or Artificial Opening** **8 Via Natural or Artificial Opening Endoscopic**	**Z No Device**	**X Diagnostic** **Z No Qualifier**
6 Stomach	**Ø Open** **3 Percutaneous** **4 Percutaneous Endoscopic** **7 Via Natural or Artificial Opening** **8 Via Natural or Artificial Opening Endoscopic**	**Z No Device**	**3 Vertical** **X Diagnostic** **Z No Qualifier**
G Large Intestine, Left **L Transverse Colon** Hepatic flexure Splenic flexure **M Descending Colon** **N Sigmoid Colon** Rectosigmoid junction Sigmoid flexure	**Ø Open** **3 Percutaneous** **4 Percutaneous Endoscopic** **7 Via Natural or Artificial Opening** **8 Via Natural or Artificial Opening Endoscopic**	**Z No Device**	**X Diagnostic** **Z No Qualifier**
G Large Intestine, Left **L Transverse Colon** Hepatic flexure Splenic flexure **M Descending Colon** **N Sigmoid Colon** Rectosigmoid junction Sigmoid flexure	**F Via Natural or Artificial Opening with Percutaneous Endoscopic Assistance**	**Z No Device**	**Z No Qualifier**
Q Anus Anal orifice	**Ø Open** **3 Percutaneous** **4 Percutaneous Endoscopic** **7 Via Natural or Artificial Opening** **8 Via Natural or Artificial Opening Endoscopic** **X External**	**Z No Device**	**X Diagnostic** **Z No Qualifier**
R Anal Sphincter External anal sphincter Internal anal sphincter **U Omentum** Gastrocolic ligament Gastrocolic omentum Gastrohepatic omentum Gastrophrenic ligament Gastrosplenic ligament Greater Omentum Hepatogastric ligament Lesser Omentum **V Mesentery** Mesoappendix Mesocolon **W Peritoneum** Epiploic foramen	**Ø Open** **3 Percutaneous** **4 Percutaneous Endoscopic**	**Z No Device**	**X Diagnostic** **Z No Qualifier**

Non-OR ØDB[1,2,3,4,5,7,8,9,A,B,C,E,F,H,K,P][3,4,7,8]ZX
Non-OR ØDB[1,2,3,5,7,9][4,8]ZZ
Non-OR ØDB[4,E,F,H,K,P]8ZZ
Non-OR ØDB6[3,4,7,8]ZX
Non-OR ØDB6[4,8]ZZ
Non-OR ØDB[G,L,M,N][3,4,7,8]ZX
Non-OR ØDB[G,L,M,N]8ZZ
Non-OR ØDBQ[Ø,3,4,7,8,X]ZX
Non-OR ØDBQ8ZZ
Non-OR ØDBR[Ø,3,4]ZX
Non-OR ØDB[U,V,W][3,4]ZX

Ø Medical and Surgical
D Gastrointestinal System
C Extirpation Definition: Taking or cutting out solid matter from a body part

Explanation: The solid matter may be an abnormal byproduct of a biological function or a foreign body; it may be imbedded in a body part or in the lumen of a tubular body part. The solid matter may or may not have been previously broken into pieces.

Body Part Character 4	Approach Character 5	Device Character 6	Qualifier Character 7
1 Esophagus, Upper Cervical esophagus **2 Esophagus, Middle** Thoracic esophagus **3 Esophagus, Lower** Abdominal esophagus **4 Esophagogastric Junction** Cardia Cardioesophageal junction Gastroesophageal (GE) junction **5 Esophagus** **6 Stomach** **7 Stomach, Pylorus** Pyloric antrum Pyloric canal Pyloric sphincter **8 Small Intestine** **9 Duodenum** **A Jejunum** Duodenojejunal flexure **B Ileum** **C Ileocecal Valve** **E Large Intestine** **F Large Intestine, Right** **G Large Intestine, Left** **H Cecum** **J Appendix** Vermiform appendix **K Ascending Colon** **L Transverse Colon** Hepatic flexure Splenic flexure **M Descending Colon** **N Sigmoid Colon** Rectosigmoid junction Sigmoid flexure **P Rectum** Anorectal junction	**Ø Open** **3 Percutaneous** **4 Percutaneous Endoscopic** **7 Via Natural or Artificial Opening** **8 Via Natural or Artificial Opening Endoscopic**	**Z No Device**	**Z No Qualifier**
Q Anus Anal orifice	**Ø Open** **3 Percutaneous** **4 Percutaneous Endoscopic** **7 Via Natural or Artificial Opening** **8 Via Natural or Artificial Opening Endoscopic** **X External**	**Z No Device**	**Z No Qualifier**
R Anal Sphincter External anal sphincter Internal anal sphincter **U Omentum** Gastrocolic ligament Gastrocolic omentum Gastrohepatic omentum Gastrophrenic ligament Gastrosplenic ligament Greater Omentum Hepatogastric ligament Lesser Omentum **V Mesentery** Mesoappendix Mesocolon **W Peritoneum** Epiploic foramen	**Ø Open** **3 Percutaneous** **4 Percutaneous Endoscopic**	**Z No Device**	**Z No Qualifier**

Non-OR ØDC[1,2,3,4,5,6,7,8,9,A,B,C,E,F,G,H,K,L,M,N,P][7,8]ZZ
Non-OR ØDCQ[7,8,X]ZZ

Ø Medical and Surgical
D Gastrointestinal System
D Extraction Definition: Pulling or stripping out or off all or a portion of a body part by the use of force
Explanation: The qualifier DIAGNOSTIC is used to identify extraction procedures that are biopsies

Body Part Character 4	Approach Character 5	Device Character 6	Qualifier Character 7
1 Esophagus, Upper Cervical esophagus **2 Esophagus, Middle** Thoracic esophagus **3 Esophagus, Lower** Abdominal esophagus **4 Esophagogastric Junction** Cardia, Cardioesophageal junction, Gastroesophageal (GE) junction **5 Esophagus** **6 Stomach** **7 Stomach, Pylorus** Pyloric antrum, Pyloric canal, Pyloric sphincter **8 Small Intestine** **9 Duodenum** **A Jejunum** Duodenojejunal flexure **B Ileum** **C Ileocecal Valve** **E Large Intestine** **F Large Intestine, Right** **G Large Intestine, Left** **H Cecum** **J Appendix** Vermiform appendix **K Ascending Colon** **L Transverse Colon** Hepatic flexure, Splenic flexure **M Descending Colon** **N Sigmoid Colon** Rectosigmoid junction, Sigmoid flexure **P Rectum** Anorectal junction	**3 Percutaneous** **4 Percutaneous Endoscopic** **8 Via Natural or Artificial Opening Endoscopic**	**Z No Device**	**X Diagnostic**
Q Anus Anal orifice	**3 Percutaneous** **4 Percutaneous Endoscopic** **8 Via Natural or Artificial Opening Endoscopic** **X External**	**Z No Device**	**X Diagnostic**

Non-OR ØDD[1,2,3,4,5,6,7,8,9,A,B,C,E,F,G,H,K,L,M,N,P][3,4,8]ZX
Non-OR ØDDQ[3,4,8,X]ZX

Ø Medical and Surgical
D Gastrointestinal System
F Fragmentation Definition: Breaking solid matter in a body part into pieces

Explanation: Physical force (e.g., manual, ultrasonic) applied directly or indirectly is used to break the solid matter into pieces. The solid matter may be an abnormal byproduct of a biological function or a foreign body. The pieces of solid matter are not taken out.

Body Part Character 4	Approach Character 5	Device Character 6	Qualifier Character 7
5 Esophagus NC 6 Stomach NC 8 Small Intestine NC 9 Duodenum NC A Jejunum NC Duodenojejunal flexure B Ileum NC E Large Intestine NC F Large Intestine, Right NC G Large Intestine, Left NC H Cecum NC J Appendix NC Vermiform appendix K Ascending Colon NC L Transverse Colon NC Hepatic flexure Splenic flexure M Descending Colon NC N Sigmoid Colon NC Rectosigmoid junction Sigmoid flexure P Rectum NC Anorectal junction Q Anus NC Anal orifice	Ø Open 3 Percutaneous 4 Percutaneous Endoscopic 7 Via Natural or Artificial Opening 8 Via Natural or Artificial Opening Endoscopic X External	Z No Device	Z No Qualifier

Non-OR ØDF[5,6,8,9,A,B,E,F,G,H,J,K,L,M,N,P,Q]XZZ
NC ØDF[5,6,8,9,A,B,E,F,G,H,J,K,L,M,N,P,Q]XZZ

Ø Medical and Surgical
D Gastrointestinal System
H Insertion Definition: Putting in a nonbiological appliance that monitors, assists, performs, or prevents a physiological function but does not physically take the place of a body part

Explanation: None

Body Part Character 4	Approach Character 5	Device Character 6	Qualifier Character 7
Ø Upper Intestinal Tract D Lower Intestinal Tract	Ø Open 3 Percutaneous 4 Percutaneous Endoscopic 7 Via Natural or Artificial Opening 8 Via Natural or Artificial Opening Endoscopic	Y Other Device	Z No Qualifier
5 Esophagus	Ø Open 3 Percutaneous 4 Percutaneous Endoscopic	1 Radioactive Element 2 Monitoring Device 3 Infusion Device D Intraluminal Device U Feeding Device Y Other Device	Z No Qualifier
5 Esophagus	7 Via Natural or Artificial Opening 8 Via Natural or Artificial Opening Endoscopic	1 Radioactive Element 2 Monitoring Device 3 Infusion Device B Intraluminal Device, Airway D Intraluminal Device U Feeding Device Y Other Device	Z No Qualifier
6 Stomach ⊞	Ø Open 3 Percutaneous 4 Percutaneous Endoscopic	2 Monitoring Device 3 Infusion Device D Intraluminal Device M Stimulator Lead U Feeding Device Y Other Device	Z No Qualifier
6 Stomach	7 Via Natural or Artificial Opening 8 Via Natural or Artificial Opening Endoscopic	2 Monitoring Device 3 Infusion Device D Intraluminal Device U Feeding Device Y Other Device	Z No Qualifier
8 Small Intestine 9 Duodenum A Jejunum Duodenojejunal flexure B Ileum	Ø Open 3 Percutaneous 4 Percutaneous Endoscopic 7 Via Natural or Artificial Opening 8 Via Natural or Artificial Opening Endoscopic	2 Monitoring Device 3 Infusion Device D Intraluminal Device U Feeding Device	Z No Qualifier
E Large Intestine	Ø Open 3 Percutaneous 4 Percutaneous Endoscopic 7 Via Natural or Artificial Opening 8 Via Natural or Artificial Opening Endoscopic	D Intraluminal Device	Z No Qualifier
P Rectum Anorectal junction	Ø Open 3 Percutaneous 4 Percutaneous Endoscopic 7 Via Natural or Artificial Opening 8 Via Natural or Artificial Opening Endoscopic	1 Radioactive Element D Intraluminal Device	Z No Qualifier
Q Anus Anal orifice	Ø Open 3 Percutaneous 4 Percutaneous Endoscopic	D Intraluminal Device L Artificial Sphincter	Z No Qualifier
Q Anus Anal orifice	7 Via Natural or Artificial Opening 8 Via Natural or Artificial Opening Endoscopic	D Intraluminal Device	Z No Qualifier
R Anal Sphincter External anal sphincter Internal anal sphincter	Ø Open 3 Percutaneous 4 Percutaneous Endoscopic	M Stimulator Lead	Z No Qualifier

Non-OR ØDH[Ø,D][Ø,3,4,7,8]YZ
Non-OR ØDH5[Ø,3,4][D,U]Z
Non-OR ØDH5[3,4]YZ
Non-OR ØDH5[7,8][2,3,B,D,U,Y]Z
Non-OR ØDH6[3,4][U,Y]Z
Non-OR ØDH6[7,8][2,3,D,U,Y]Z
Non-OR ØDH[8,9,A,B][Ø,3,4][D,U]Z
Non-OR ØDH[8,9,A,B][7,8][2,3,D,U]Z
Non-OR ØDHE[Ø,3,4,7,8]DZ
Non-OR ØDHP[Ø,3,4,7,8]DZ

See Appendix L for Procedure Combinations
⊞ ØDH6[Ø,3,4]MZ

Ø Medical and Surgical
D Gastrointestinal System
J Inspection Definition: Visually and/or manually exploring a body part

Explanation: Visual exploration may be performed with or without optical instrumentation. Manual exploration may be performed directly or through intervening body layers.

Body Part Character 4	Approach Character 5	Device Character 6	Qualifier Character 7
Ø Upper Intestinal Tract 6 Stomach D Lower Intestinal Tract	Ø Open 3 Percutaneous 4 Percutaneous Endoscopic 7 Via Natural or Artificial Opening 8 Via Natural or Artificial Opening Endoscopic X External	Z No Device	Z No Qualifier
U Omentum Gastrocolic ligament Gastrocolic omentum Gastrohepatic omentum Gastrophrenic ligament Gastrosplenic ligament Greater Omentum Hepatogastric ligament Lesser Omentum V Mesentery Mesoappendix Mesocolon W Peritoneum Epiploic foramen	Ø Open 3 Percutaneous 4 Percutaneous Endoscopic X External	Z No Device	Z No Qualifier

Non-OR ØDJ[Ø,6,D][3,7,8,X]ZZ
Non-OR ØDJ[U,V,W][3,X]ZZ

Ø Medical and Surgical
D Gastrointestinal System
L Occlusion Definition: Completely closing an orifice or the lumen of a tubular body part
Explanation: The orifice can be a natural orifice or an artificially created orifice

Body Part Character 4		Approach Character 5	Device Character 6	Qualifier Character 7
1 Esophagus, Upper Cervical esophagus **2 Esophagus, Middle** Thoracic esophagus **3 Esophagus, Lower** Abdominal esophagus **4 Esophagogastric Junction** Cardia; Cardioesophageal junction; Gastroesophageal (GE) junction **5 Esophagus** **6 Stomach** **7 Stomach, Pylorus** Pyloric antrum; Pyloric canal; Pyloric sphincter **8 Small Intestine**	**9 Duodenum** **A Jejunum** Duodenojejunal flexure **B Ileum** **C Ileocecal Valve** **E Large Intestine** **F Large Intestine, Right** **G Large Intestine, Left** **H Cecum** **K Ascending Colon** **L Transverse Colon** Hepatic flexure; Splenic flexure **M Descending Colon** **N Sigmoid Colon** Rectosigmoid junction; Sigmoid flexure **P Rectum** Anorectal junction	**Ø Open** **3 Percutaneous** **4 Percutaneous Endoscopic**	**C Extraluminal Device** **D Intraluminal Device** **Z No Device**	**Z No Qualifier**
1 Esophagus, Upper Cervical esophagus **2 Esophagus, Middle** Thoracic esophagus **3 Esophagus, Lower** Abdominal esophagus **4 Esophagogastric Junction** Cardia; Cardioesophageal junction; Gastroesophageal (GE) junction **5 Esophagus** **6 Stomach** **7 Stomach, Pylorus** Pyloric antrum; Pyloric canal; Pyloric sphincter **8 Small Intestine**	**9 Duodenum** **A Jejunum** Duodenojejunal flexure **B Ileum** **C Ileocecal Valve** **E Large Intestine** **F Large Intestine, Right** **G Large Intestine, Left** **H Cecum** **K Ascending Colon** **L Transverse Colon** Hepatic flexure; Splenic flexure **M Descending Colon** **N Sigmoid Colon** Rectosigmoid junction; Sigmoid flexure **P Rectum** Anorectal junction	**7 Via Natural or Artificial Opening** **8 Via Natural or Artificial Opening Endoscopic**	**D Intraluminal Device** **Z No Device**	**Z No Qualifier**
Q Anus Anal orifice		**Ø Open** **3 Percutaneous** **4 Percutaneous Endoscopic** **X External**	**C Extraluminal Device** **D Intraluminal Device** **Z No Device**	**Z No Qualifier**
Q Anus Anal orifice		**7 Via Natural or Artificial Opening** **8 Via Natural or Artificial Opening Endoscopic**	**D Intraluminal Device** **Z No Device**	**Z No Qualifier**

Non-OR ØDL[1,2,3,4,5][Ø,3,4][C,D,Z]Z
Non-OR ØDL[1,2,3,4,5][7,8][D,Z]Z

Ø Medical and Surgical
D Gastrointestinal System
M Reattachment Definition: Putting back in or on all or a portion of a separated body part to its normal location or other suitable location
Explanation: Vascular circulation and nervous pathways may or may not be reestablished

Body Part Character 4	Approach Character 5	Device Character 6	Qualifier Character 7
5 Esophagus 6 Stomach 8 Small Intestine 9 Duodenum A Jejunum Duodenojejunal flexure B Ileum E Large Intestine F Large Intestine, Right G Large Intestine, Left H Cecum K Ascending Colon L Transverse Colon Hepatic flexure Splenic flexure M Descending Colon N Sigmoid Colon Rectosigmoid junction Sigmoid flexure P Rectum Anorectal junction	Ø Open 4 Percutaneous Endoscopic	Z No Device	Z No Qualifier

Ø Medical and Surgical
D Gastrointestinal System
N Release Definition: Freeing a body part from an abnormal physical constraint by cutting or by the use of force
Explanation: Some of the restraining tissue may be taken out but none of the body part is taken out

Body Part Character 4	Body Part Character 4 (cont.)	Approach Character 5	Device Character 6	Qualifier Character 7
1 Esophagus, Upper Cervical esophagus 2 Esophagus, Middle Thoracic esophagus 3 Esophagus, Lower Abdominal esophagus 4 Esophagogastric Junction Cardia Cardioesophageal junction Gastroesophageal (GE) junction 5 Esophagus 6 Stomach 7 Stomach, Pylorus Pyloric antrum Pyloric canal Pyloric sphincter 8 Small Intestine 9 Duodenum	A Jejunum Duodenojejunal flexure B Ileum C Ileocecal Valve E Large Intestine F Large Intestine, Right G Large Intestine, Left H Cecum J Appendix Vermiform appendix K Ascending Colon L Transverse Colon Hepatic flexure Splenic flexure M Descending Colon N Sigmoid Colon Rectosigmoid junction Sigmoid flexure P Rectum Anorectal junction	Ø Open 3 Percutaneous 4 Percutaneous Endoscopic 7 Via Natural or Artificial Opening 8 Via Natural or Artificial Opening Endoscopic	Z No Device	Z No Qualifier
Q Anus Anal orifice		Ø Open 3 Percutaneous 4 Percutaneous Endoscopic 7 Via Natural or Artificial Opening 8 Via Natural or Artificial Opening Endoscopic X External	Z No Device	Z No Qualifier
R Anal Sphincter External anal sphincter Internal anal sphincter U Omentum Gastrocolic ligament Gastrocolic omentum Gastrohepatic omentum Gastrophrenic ligament Gastrosplenic ligament Greater Omentum Hepatogastric ligament Lesser Omentum V Mesentery Mesoappendix Mesocolon W Peritoneum Epiploic foramen		Ø Open 3 Percutaneous 4 Percutaneous Endoscopic	Z No Device	Z No Qualifier

Non-OR ØDN[8,9,A,B,E,F,G,H,K,L,M,N][7,8]ZZ

Ø Medical and Surgical
D Gastrointestinal System
P Removal Definition: Taking out or off a device from a body part

Explanation: If a device is taken out and a similar device put in without cutting or puncturing the skin or mucous membrane, the procedure is coded to the root operation CHANGE. Otherwise, the procedure for taking out a device is coded to the root operation REMOVAL.

Body Part Character 4	Approach Character 5	Device Character 6	Qualifier Character 7
Ø Upper Intestinal Tract D Lower Intestinal Tract	Ø Open 3 Percutaneous 4 Percutaneous Endoscopic 7 Via Natural or Artificial Opening 8 Via Natural or Artificial Opening Endoscopic	Ø Drainage Device 2 Monitoring Device 3 Infusion Device 7 Autologous Tissue Substitute C Extraluminal Device D Intraluminal Device J Synthetic Substitute K Nonautologous Tissue Substitute U Feeding Device Y Other Device	Z No Qualifier
Ø Upper Intestinal Tract D Lower Intestinal Tract	X External	Ø Drainage Device 2 Monitoring Device 3 Infusion Device D Intraluminal Device U Feeding Device	Z No Qualifier
5 Esophagus	Ø Open 3 Percutaneous 4 Percutaneous Endoscopic	1 Radioactive Element 2 Monitoring Device 3 Infusion Device U Feeding Device Y Other Device	Z No Qualifier
5 Esophagus	7 Via Natural or Artificial Opening 8 Via Natural or Artificial Opening Endoscopic	1 Radioactive Element D Intraluminal Device Y Other Device	Z No Qualifier
5 Esophagus	X External	1 Radioactive Element 2 Monitoring Device 3 Infusion Device D Intraluminal Device U Feeding Device	Z No Qualifier
6 Stomach	Ø Open 3 Percutaneous 4 Percutaneous Endoscopic	Ø Drainage Device 2 Monitoring Device 3 Infusion Device 7 Autologous Tissue Substitute C Extraluminal Device D Intraluminal Device J Synthetic Substitute K Nonautologous Tissue Substitute M Stimulator Lead U Feeding Device Y Other Device	Z No Qualifier
6 Stomach	7 Via Natural or Artificial Opening 8 Via Natural or Artificial Opening Endoscopic	Ø Drainage Device 2 Monitoring Device 3 Infusion Device 7 Autologous Tissue Substitute C Extraluminal Device D Intraluminal Device J Synthetic Substitute K Nonautologous Tissue Substitute U Feeding Device Y Other Device	Z No Qualifier
6 Stomach	X External	Ø Drainage Device 2 Monitoring Device 3 Infusion Device D Intraluminal Device U Feeding Device	Z No Qualifier

ØDP Continued on next page

Non-OR ØDP[Ø,D][3,4]YZ
Non-OR ØDP[Ø,D][7,8][Ø,2,3,D,U,Y]Z
Non-OR ØDP[Ø,D]X[Ø,2,3,D,U]Z
Non-OR ØDP5[3,4]YZ
Non-OR ØDP5[7,8][1,D,Y]Z
Non-OR ØDP5X[1,2,3,D,U]Z
Non-OR ØDP6[3,4]YZ
Non-OR ØDP6[7,8][Ø,2,3,D,U,Y]Z
Non-OR ØDP6X[Ø,2,3,D,U]Z

Ø Medical and Surgical
D Gastrointestinal System
P Removal Definition: Taking out or off a device from a body part

Explanation: If a device is taken out and a similar device put in without cutting or puncturing the skin or mucous membrane, the procedure is coded to the root operation CHANGE. Otherwise, the procedure for taking out a device is coded to the root operation REMOVAL.

ØDP Continued

Body Part Character 4	Approach Character 5	Device Character 6	Qualifier Character 7
P Rectum Anorectal junction	**Ø** Open **3** Percutaneous **4** Percutaneous Endoscopic **7** Via Natural or Artificial Opening **8** Via Natural or Artificial Opening Endoscopic **X** External	**1** Radioactive Element	**Z** No Qualifier
Q Anus Anal orifice	**Ø** Open **3** Percutaneous **4** Percutaneous Endoscopic **7** Via Natural or Artificial Opening **8** Via Natural or Artificial Opening Endoscopic	**L** Artificial Sphincter	**Z** No Qualifier
R Anal Sphincter External anal sphincter Internal anal sphincter	**Ø** Open **3** Percutaneous **4** Percutaneous Endoscopic	**M** Stimulator Lead	**Z** No Qualifier
U Omentum Gastrocolic ligament Gastrocolic omentum Gastrohepatic omentum Gastrophrenic ligament Gastrosplenic ligament Greater Omentum Hepatogastric ligament Lesser Omentum **V** Mesentery Mesoappendix Mesocolon **W** Peritoneum Epiploic foramen	**Ø** Open **3** Percutaneous **4** Percutaneous Endoscopic	**Ø** Drainage Device **1** Radioactive Element **7** Autologous Tissue Substitute **J** Synthetic Substitute **K** Nonautologous Tissue Substitute	**Z** No Qualifier

Non-OR ØDPP[7,8,X]1Z

Ø Medical and Surgical
D Gastrointestinal System
Q Repair Definition: Restoring, to the extent possible, a body part to its normal anatomic structure and function
Explanation: Used only when the method to accomplish the repair is not one of the other root operations

Body Part Character 4	Approach Character 5	Device Character 6	Qualifier Character 7
1 Esophagus, Upper Cervical esophagus **2 Esophagus, Middle** Thoracic esophagus **3 Esophagus, Lower** Abdominal esophagus **4 Esophagogastric Junction** Cardia Cardioesophageal junction Gastroesophageal (GE) junction **5 Esophagus** **6 Stomach** **7 Stomach, Pylorus** Pyloric antrum Pyloric canal Pyloric sphincter **8 Small Intestine** ⊞ **9 Duodenum** ⊞ **A Jejunum** ⊞ Duodenojejunal flexure **B Ileum** ⊞ **C Ileocecal Valve** **E Large Intestine** ⊞ **F Large Intestine, Right** ⊞ **G Large Intestine, Left** ⊞ **H Cecum** ⊞ **J Appendix** Vermiform appendix **K Ascending Colon** ⊞ **L Transverse Colon** ⊞ Hepatic flexure Splenic flexure **M Descending Colon** ⊞ **N Sigmoid Colon** ⊞ Rectosigmoid junction Sigmoid flexure **P Rectum** Anorectal junction	**Ø Open** **3 Percutaneous** **4 Percutaneous Endoscopic** **7 Via Natural or Artificial Opening** **8 Via Natural or Artificial Opening Endoscopic**	**Z No Device**	**Z No Qualifier**
Q Anus Anal orifice	**Ø Open** **3 Percutaneous** **4 Percutaneous Endoscopic** **7 Via Natural or Artificial Opening** **8 Via Natural or Artificial Opening Endoscopic** **X External**	**Z No Device**	**Z No Qualifier**
R Anal Sphincter External anal sphincter Internal anal sphincter **U Omentum** Gastrocolic ligament Gastrocolic omentum Gastrohepatic omentum Gastrophrenic ligament Gastrosplenic ligament Greater Omentum Hepatogastric ligament Lesser Omentum **V Mesentery** Mesoappendix Mesocolon **W Peritoneum** Epiploic foramen	**Ø Open** **3 Percutaneous** **4 Percutaneous Endoscopic**	**Z No Device**	**Z No Qualifier**

See Appendix L for Procedure Combinations
⊞ ØDQ[8,9,A,B,E,F,G,H,K,L,M,N]ØZZ

Ø Medical and Surgical
D Gastrointestinal System
R Replacement Definition: Putting in or on biological or synthetic material that physically takes the place and/or function of all or a portion of a body part

Explanation: The body part may have been taken out or replaced, or may be taken out, physically eradicated, or rendered nonfunctional during the REPLACEMENT procedure. A REMOVAL procedure is coded for taking out the device used in a previous replacement procedure.

Body Part Character 4	Approach Character 5	Device Character 6	Qualifier Character 7
5 Esophagus	Ø Open 4 Percutaneous Endoscopic 7 Via Natural or Artificial Opening 8 Via Natural or Artificial Opening Endoscopic	7 Autologous Tissue Substitute J Synthetic Substitute K Nonautologous Tissue Substitute	Z No Qualifier
R Anal Sphincter External anal sphincter Internal anal sphincter U Omentum Gastrocolic ligament Gastrocolic omentum Gastrohepatic omentum Gastrophrenic ligament Gastrosplenic ligament Greater Omentum Hepatogastric ligament Lesser Omentum V Mesentery Mesoappendix Mesocolon W Peritoneum Epiploic foramen	Ø Open 4 Percutaneous Endoscopic	7 Autologous Tissue Substitute J Synthetic Substitute K Nonautologous Tissue Substitute	Z No Qualifier

Ø Medical and Surgical
D Gastrointestinal System
S Reposition Definition: Moving to its normal location, or other suitable location, all or a portion of a body part

Explanation: The body part is moved to a new location from an abnormal location, or from a normal location where it is not functioning correctly. The body part may or may not be cut out or off to be moved to the new location.

Body Part Character 4	Approach Character 5	Device Character 6	Qualifier Character 7
5 Esophagus 6 Stomach 9 Duodenum A Jejunum Duodenojejunal flexure B Ileum H Cecum K Ascending Colon L Transverse Colon Hepatic flexure Splenic flexure M Descending Colon N Sigmoid Colon Rectosigmoid junction Sigmoid flexure P Rectum Anorectal junction Q Anus Anal orifice	Ø Open 4 Percutaneous Endoscopic 7 Via Natural or Artificial Opening 8 Via Natural or Artificial Opening Endoscopic X External	Z No Device	Z No Qualifier
8 Small Intestine E Large Intestine	Ø Open 4 Percutaneous Endoscopic 7 Via Natural or Artificial Opening 8 Via Natural or Artificial Opening Endoscopic	Z No Device	Z No Qualifier

Non-OR ØDS[5,6,9,A,B,H,K,L,M,N,P,Q]XZZ

Ø Medical and Surgical
D Gastrointestinal System
T Resection Definition: Cutting out or off, without replacement, all of a body part
Explanation: None

Body Part Character 4	Approach Character 5	Device Character 6	Qualifier Character 7
1 Esophagus, Upper Cervical esophagus **2 Esophagus, Middle** Thoracic esophagus **3 Esophagus, Lower** Abdominal esophagus **4 Esophagogastric Junction** Cardia; Cardioesophageal junction; Gastroesophageal (GE) junction **5 Esophagus** **6 Stomach** **7 Stomach, Pylorus** Pyloric antrum; Pyloric canal; Pyloric sphincter **8 Small Intestine** **9 Duodenum** ⊞ **A Jejunum** Duodenojejunal flexure **B Ileum** **C Ileocecal Valve** **E Large Intestine** **F Large Intestine, Right** **H Cecum** **J Appendix** Vermiform appendix **K Ascending Colon** **P Rectum** Anorectal junction **Q Anus** Anal orifice	**Ø Open** **4 Percutaneous Endoscopic** **7 Via Natural or Artificial Opening** **8 Via Natural or Artificial Opening Endoscopic**	**Z No Device**	**Z No Qualifier**
G Large Intestine, Left **L Transverse Colon** Hepatic flexure; Splenic flexure **M Descending Colon** **N Sigmoid Colon** Rectosigmoid junction; Sigmoid flexure	**Ø Open** **4 Percutaneous Endoscopic** **7 Via Natural or Artificial Opening** **8 Via Natural or Artificial Opening Endoscopic** **F Via Natural or Artificial Opening with Percutaneous Endoscopic Assistance**	**Z No Device**	**Z No Qualifier**
R Anal Sphincter External anal sphincter; Internal anal sphincter **U Omentum** Gastrocolic ligament; Gastrocolic omentum; Gastrohepatic omentum; Gastrophrenic ligament; Gastrosplenic ligament; Greater Omentum; Hepatogastric ligament; Lesser Omentum	**Ø Open** **4 Percutaneous Endoscopic**	**Z No Device**	**Z No Qualifier**

See Appendix L for Procedure Combinations
⊞ ØDT9ØZZ

Ø Medical and Surgical
D Gastrointestinal System
U Supplement Definition: Putting in or on biological or synthetic material that physically reinforces and/or augments the function of a portion of a body part

Explanation: The biological material is non-living, or is living and from the same individual. The body part may have been previously replaced, and the SUPPLEMENT procedure is performed to physically reinforce and/or augment the function of the replaced body part.

Body Part Character 4	Approach Character 5	Device Character 6	Qualifier Character 7
1 Esophagus, Upper Cervical esophagus **2 Esophagus, Middle** Thoracic esophagus **3 Esophagus, Lower** Abdominal esophagus **4 Esophagogastric Junction** Cardia Cardioesophageal junction Gastroesophageal (GE) junction **5 Esophagus** **6 Stomach** **7 Stomach, Pylorus** Pyloric antrum Pyloric canal Pyloric sphincter **8 Small Intestine** **9 Duodenum** **A Jejunum** Duodenojejunal flexure **B Ileum** **C Ileocecal Valve** **E Large Intestine** **F Large Intestine, Right** **G Large Intestine, Left** **H Cecum** **K Ascending Colon** **L Transverse Colon** Hepatic flexure Splenic flexure **M Descending Colon** **N Sigmoid Colon** Rectosigmoid junction Sigmoid flexure **P Rectum** Anorectal junction	**Ø Open** **4 Percutaneous Endoscopic** **7 Via Natural or Artificial Opening** **8 Via Natural or Artificial Opening Endoscopic**	**7 Autologous Tissue Substitute** **J Synthetic Substitute** **K Nonautologous Tissue Substitute**	**Z No Qualifier**
Q Anus Anal orifice	**Ø Open** **4 Percutaneous Endoscopic** **7 Via Natural or Artificial Opening** **8 Via Natural or Artificial Opening Endoscopic** **X External**	**7 Autologous Tissue Substitute** **J Synthetic Substitute** **K Nonautologous Tissue Substitute**	**Z No Qualifier**
R Anal Sphincter External anal sphincter Internal anal sphincter **U Omentum** Gastrocolic ligament Gastrocolic omentum Gastrohepatic omentum Gastrophrenic ligament Gastrosplenic ligament Greater Omentum Hepatogastric ligament Lesser Omentum **V Mesentery** Mesoappendix Mesocolon **W Peritoneum** Epiploic foramen	**Ø Open** **4 Percutaneous Endoscopic**	**7 Autologous Tissue Substitute** **J Synthetic Substitute** **K Nonautologous Tissue Substitute**	**Z No Qualifier**

Ø Medical and Surgical
D Gastrointestinal System
V Restriction Definition: Partially closing an orifice or the lumen of a tubular body part
Explanation: The orifice can be a natural orifice or an artificially created orifice

Body Part Character 4		Approach Character 5	Device Character 6	Qualifier Character 7
1 Esophagus, Upper Cervical esophagus **2 Esophagus, Middle** Thoracic esophagus **3 Esophagus, Lower** Abdominal esophagus **4 Esophagogastric Junction** Cardia, Cardioesophageal junction, Gastroesophageal (GE) junction **5 Esophagus** **6 Stomach** **7 Stomach, Pylorus** Pyloric antrum, Pyloric canal, Pyloric sphincter **8 Small Intestine**	**9 Duodenum** **A Jejunum** Duodenojejunal flexure **B Ileum** **C Ileocecal Valve** **E Large Intestine** **F Large Intestine, Right** **G Large Intestine, Left** **H Cecum** **K Ascending Colon** **L Transverse Colon** Hepatic flexure, Splenic flexure **M Descending Colon** **N Sigmoid Colon** Rectosigmoid junction, Sigmoid flexure **P Rectum** Anorectal junction	**Ø Open** **3 Percutaneous** **4 Percutaneous Endoscopic**	**C Extraluminal Device** **D Intraluminal Device** **Z No Device**	**Z No Qualifier**
1 Esophagus, Upper Cervical esophagus **2 Esophagus, Middle** Thoracic esophagus **3 Esophagus, Lower** Abdominal esophagus **4 Esophagogastric Junction** Cardia, Cardioesophageal junction, Gastroesophageal (GE) junction **5 Esophagus** **6 Stomach** NC **7 Stomach, Pylorus** Pyloric antrum, Pyloric canal, Pyloric sphincter **8 Small Intestine**	**9 Duodenum** **A Jejunum** Duodenojejunal flexure **B Ileum** **C Ileocecal Valve** **E Large Intestine** **F Large Intestine, Right** **G Large Intestine, Left** **H Cecum** **K Ascending Colon** **L Transverse Colon** Hepatic flexure, Splenic flexure **M Descending Colon** **N Sigmoid Colon** Rectosigmoid junction, Sigmoid flexure **P Rectum** Anorectal junction	**7 Via Natural or Artificial Opening** **8 Via Natural or Artificial Opening Endoscopic**	**D Intraluminal Device** **Z No Device**	**Z No Qualifier**
Q Anus Anal orifice		**Ø Open** **3 Percutaneous** **4 Percutaneous Endoscopic** **X External**	**C Extraluminal Device** **D Intraluminal Device** **Z No Device**	**Z No Qualifier**
Q Anus Anal orifice		**7 Via Natural or Artificial Opening** **8 Via Natural or Artificial Opening Endoscopic**	**D Intraluminal Device** **Z No Device**	**Z No Qualifier**

Non-OR ØDV6[7,8]DZ
HAC ØDV64CZ when reported with PDx E66.Ø1 and SDx K68.11 or K95.Ø1 or K95.81 or T81.4XXA
NC ØDV6[7,8]DZ

Ø Medical and Surgical
D Gastrointestinal System
W Revision Definition: Correcting, to the extent possible, a portion of a malfunctioning device or the position of a displaced device

Explanation: Revision can include correcting a malfunctioning or displaced device by taking out or putting in components of the device such as a screw or pin

Body Part Character 4	Approach Character 5	Device Character 6	Qualifier Character 7
Ø Upper Intestinal Tract D Lower Intestinal Tract	Ø Open 3 Percutaneous 4 Percutaneous Endoscopic 7 Via Natural or Artificial Opening 8 Via Natural or Artificial Opening Endoscopic	Ø Drainage Device 2 Monitoring Device 3 Infusion Device 7 Autologous Tissue Substitute C Extraluminal Device D Intraluminal Device J Synthetic Substitute K Nonautologous Tissue Substitute U Feeding Device Y Other Device	Z No Qualifier
Ø Upper Intestinal Tract D Lower Intestinal Tract	X External	Ø Drainage Device 2 Monitoring Device 3 Infusion Device 7 Autologous Tissue Substitute C Extraluminal Device D Intraluminal Device J Synthetic Substitute K Nonautologous Tissue Substitute U Feeding Device	Z No Qualifier
5 Esophagus	Ø Open 3 Percutaneous 4 Percutaneous Endoscopic	Y Other Device	Z No Qualifier
5 Esophagus	7 Via Natural or Artificial Opening 8 Via Natural or Artificial Opening Endoscopic	D Intraluminal Device Y Other Device	Z No Qualifier
5 Esophagus	X External	D Intraluminal Device	Z No Qualifier
6 Stomach	Ø Open 3 Percutaneous 4 Percutaneous Endoscopic	Ø Drainage Device 2 Monitoring Device 3 Infusion Device 7 Autologous Tissue Substitute C Extraluminal Device D Intraluminal Device J Synthetic Substitute K Nonautologous Tissue Substitute M Stimulator Lead U Feeding Device Y Other Device	Z No Qualifier
6 Stomach	7 Via Natural or Artificial Opening 8 Via Natural or Artificial Opening Endoscopic	Ø Drainage Device 2 Monitoring Device 3 Infusion Device 7 Autologous Tissue Substitute C Extraluminal Device D Intraluminal Device J Synthetic Substitute K Nonautologous Tissue Substitute U Feeding Device Y Other Device	Z No Qualifier
6 Stomach	X External	Ø Drainage Device 2 Monitoring Device 3 Infusion Device 7 Autologous Tissue Substitute C Extraluminal Device D Intraluminal Device J Synthetic Substitute K Nonautologous Tissue Substitute U Feeding Device	Z No Qualifier

ØDW Continued on next page

Non-OR ØDW[Ø,D][3,4,7,8]YZ
Non-OR ØDW[Ø,D]X[Ø,2,3,7,C,D,J,K,U]Z
Non-OR ØDW5[Ø,3,4]YZ
Non-OR ØDW5[7,8]YZ
Non-OR ØDW5XDZ
Non-OR ØDW6[3,4]YZ
Non-OR ØDW6[7,8]YZ
Non-OR ØDW6X[Ø,2,3,7,C,D,J,K,U]Z

Ø Medical and Surgical
D Gastrointestinal System
W Revision Definition: Correcting, to the extent possible, a portion of a malfunctioning device or the position of a displaced device

Explanation: Revision can include correcting a malfunctioning or displaced device by taking out or putting in components of the device such as a screw or pin

ØDW Continued

Body Part Character 4	Approach Character 5	Device Character 6	Qualifier Character 7
8 Small Intestine E Large Intestine	Ø Open 4 Percutaneous Endoscopic 7 Via Natural or Artificial Opening 8 Via Natural or Artificial Opening Endoscopic	7 Autologous Tissue Substitute J Synthetic Substitute K Nonautologous Tissue Substitute	Z No Qualifier
Q Anus Anal orifice	Ø Open 3 Percutaneous 4 Percutaneous Endoscopic 7 Via Natural or Artificial Opening 8 Via Natural or Artificial Opening Endoscopic	L Artificial Sphincter	Z No Qualifier
R Anal Sphincter External anal sphincter Internal anal sphincter	Ø Open 3 Percutaneous 4 Percutaneous Endoscopic	M Stimulator Lead	Z No Qualifier
U Omentum Gastrocolic ligament Gastrocolic omentum Gastrohepatic omentum Gastrophrenic ligament Gastrosplenic ligament Greater Omentum Hepatogastric ligament Lesser Omentum V Mesentery Mesoappendix Mesocolon W Peritoneum Epiploic foramen	Ø Open 3 Percutaneous 4 Percutaneous Endoscopic	Ø Drainage Device 7 Autologous Tissue Substitute J Synthetic Substitute K Nonautologous Tissue Substitute	Z No Qualifier

Non-OR ØDW[U,V,W][Ø,3,4]ØZ

Ø Medical and Surgical
D Gastrointestinal System
X Transfer Definition: Moving, without taking out, all or a portion of a body part to another location to take over the function of all or a portion of a body part

Explanation: The body part transferred remains connected to its vascular and nervous supply

Body Part Character 4	Approach Character 5	Device Character 6	Qualifier Character 7
6 Stomach 8 Small Intestine E Large Intestine	Ø Open 4 Percutaneous Endoscopic	Z No Device	5 Esophagus

Ø Medical and Surgical
D Gastrointestinal System
Y Transplantation Definition: Putting in or on all or a portion of a living body part taken from another individual or animal to physically take the place and/or function of all or a portion of a similar body part

Explanation: The native body part may or may not be taken out, and the transplanted body part may take over all or a portion of its function

Body Part Character 4	Approach Character 5	Device Character 6	Qualifier Character 7
5 Esophagus 6 Stomach 8 Small Intestine LC E Large Intestine LC	Ø Open	Z No Device	Ø Allogeneic 1 Syngeneic 2 Zooplastic

Non-OR ØDY5ØZ[Ø,1,2]
LC ØDY[8,E]ØZ[Ø,1,2]

Hepatobiliary System and Pancreas ØF1–ØFY

Character Meanings

This Character Meaning table is provided as a guide to assist the user in the identification of character members that may be found in this section of code tables. It **SHOULD NOT** be used to build a PCS code.

Operation–Character 3		Body Part–Character 4		Approach–Character 5		Device–Character 6		Qualifier–Character 7	
1	Bypass	Ø	Liver	Ø	Open	Ø	Drainage Device	Ø	Allogeneic
2	Change	1	Liver, Right Lobe	3	Percutaneous	1	Radioactive Element	1	Syngeneic
5	Destruction	2	Liver, Left Lobe	4	Percutaneous Endoscopic	2	Monitoring Device	2	Zooplastic
7	Dilation	4	Gallbladder	7	Via Natural or Artificial Opening	3	Infusion Device	3	Duodenum
8	Division	5	Hepatic Duct, Right	8	Via Natural or Artificial Opening Endoscopic	7	Autologous Tissue Substitute	4	Stomach
9	Drainage	6	Hepatic Duct, Left	X	External	C	Extraluminal Device	5	Hepatic Duct, Right
B	Excision	7	Hepatic Duct, Common			D	Intraluminal Device	6	Hepatic Duct, Left
C	Extirpation	8	Cystic Duct			J	Synthetic Substitute	7	Hepatic Duct, Caudate
D	Extraction	9	Common Bile Duct			K	Nonautologous Tissue Substitute		
F	Fragmentation	B	Hepatobiliary Duct			Y	Other Device	8	Cystic Duct
H	Insertion	C	Ampulla of Vater			Z	No Device	9	Common Bile Duct
J	Inspection	D	Pancreatic Duct					B	Small Intestine
L	Occlusion	F	Pancreatic Duct, Accessory					C	Large Intestine
M	Reattachment	G	Pancreas					F	Irreversible Electroporation
N	Release							X	Diagnostic
P	Removal							Z	No Qualifier
Q	Repair								
R	Replacement								
S	Reposition								
T	Resection								
U	Supplement								
V	Restriction								
W	Revision								
Y	Transplantation								

AHA Coding Clinic for table ØF7

2016, 3Q, 27 Endoscopic retrograde cholangiopancreatography with sphincterotomy and insertion of pancreatic stent
2016, 1Q, 25 Endoscopic retrograde cholangiopancreatography with brush biopsy of pancreatic and common bile ducts
2015, 1Q, 32 Percutaneous transhepatic biliary drainage catheter placement
2014, 3Q, 15 Drainage of pancreatic pseudocyst

AHA Coding Clinic for table ØF9

2015, 1Q, 32 Percutaneous transhepatic biliary drainage catheter placement
2014, 3Q, 15 Drainage of pancreatic pseudocyst

AHA Coding Clinic for table ØFB

2016, 3Q, 41 Open cholecystectomy with needle biopsy of liver
2016, 1Q, 23 Endoscopic ultrasound with aspiration biopsy of common hepatic duct
2016, 1Q, 25 Endoscopic retrograde cholangiopancreatography with brush biopsy of pancreatic and common bile ducts
2014, 3Q, 32 Pyloric-sparing Whipple procedure

AHA Coding Clinic for table ØFC

2016, 3Q, 27 Endoscopic retrograde cholangiopancreatography with sphincterotomy and insertion of pancreatic stent

AHA Coding Clinic for table ØFQ

2016, 3Q, 27 Revision of common bile duct anastomosis
2013, 4Q, 109 Separating conjoined twins

AHA Coding Clinic for table ØFT

2012, 4Q, 99 Domino liver transplant

AHA Coding Clinic for table ØFY

2014, 3Q, 13 Orthotopic liver transplant with end to side cavoplasty
2012, 4Q, 99 Domino liver transplant

Liver

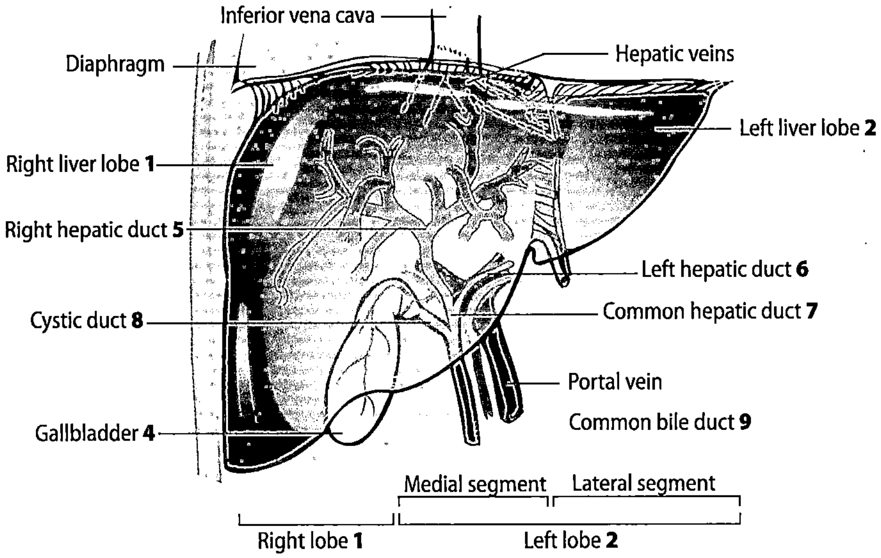

Pancreas

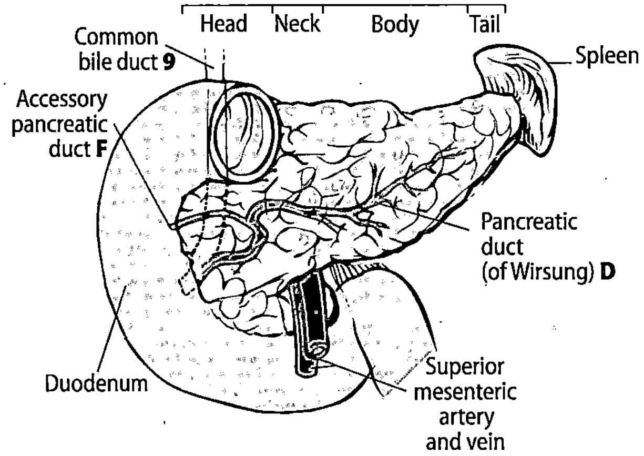

Gallbladder and Ducts

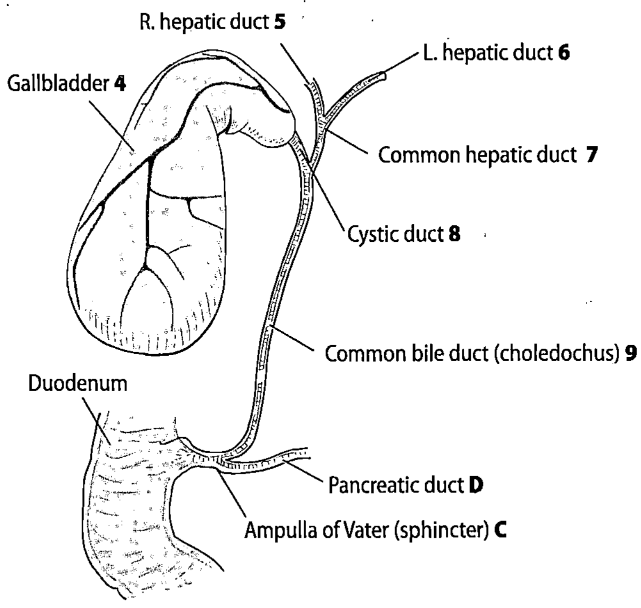

Ø Medical and Surgical
F Hepatobiliary System and Pancreas
1 Bypass Definition: Altering the route of passage of the contents of a tubular body part

Explanation: Rerouting contents of a body part to a downstream area of the normal route, to a similar route and body part, or to an abnormal route and dissimilar body part. Includes one or more anastomoses, with or without the use of a device.

Body Part Character 4	Approach Character 5	Device Character 6	Qualifier Character 7
4 Gallbladder 5 Hepatic Duct, Right 6 Hepatic Duct, Left 7 Hepatic Duct, Common 8 Cystic Duct 9 Common Bile Duct	Ø Open 4 Percutaneous Endoscopic	D Intraluminal Device Z No Device	3 Duodenum 4 Stomach 5 Hepatic Duct, Right 6 Hepatic Duct, Left 7 Hepatic Duct, Caudate 8 Cystic Duct 9 Common Bile Duct B Small Intestine
D Pancreatic Duct Duct of Wirsung F Pancreatic Duct, Accessory Duct of Santorini G Pancreas	Ø Open 4 Percutaneous Endoscopic	D Intraluminal Device Z No Device	3 Duodenum B Small Intestine C Large Intestine

Ø Medical and Surgical
F Hepatobiliary System and Pancreas
2 Change Definition: Taking out or off a device from a body part and putting back an identical or similar device in or on the same body part without cutting or puncturing the skin or a mucous membrane

Explanation: All CHANGE procedures are coded using the approach EXTERNAL

Body Part Character 4	Approach Character 5	Device Character 6	Qualifier Character 7
Ø Liver Quadrate lobe 4 Gallbladder B Hepatobiliary Duct D Pancreatic Duct Duct of Wirsung G Pancreas	X External	Ø Drainage Device Y Other Device	Z No Qualifier

Non-OR All body part, approach, device, and qualifier values

Ø Medical and Surgical
F Hepatobiliary System and Pancreas
5 Destruction Definition: Physical eradication of all or a portion of a body part by the direct use of energy, force, or a destructive agent

Explanation: None of the body part is physically taken out

Body Part Character 4	Approach Character 5	Device Character 6	Qualifier Character 7
Ø Liver Quadrate lobe 1 Liver, Right Lobe 2 Liver, Left Lobe	Ø Open 3 Percutaneous 4 Percutaneous Endoscopic	Z No Device	F Irreversible Electroporation Z No Qualifier
4 Gallbladder	Ø Open 3 Percutaneous 4 Percutaneous Endoscopic 8 Via Natural or Artificial Opening Endoscopic	Z No Device	Z No Qualifier
5 Hepatic Duct, Right 6 Hepatic Duct, Left 7 Hepatic Duct, Common 8 Cystic Duct 9 Common Bile Duct C Ampulla of Vater Duodenal ampulla Hepatopancreatic ampulla D Pancreatic Duct Duct of Wirsung F Pancreatic Duct, Accessory Duct of Santorini	Ø Open 3 Percutaneous 4 Percutaneous Endoscopic 7 Via Natural or Artificial Opening 8 Via Natural or Artificial Opening Endoscopic	Z No Device	Z No Qualifier
G Pancreas	Ø Open 3 Percutaneous 4 Percutaneous Endoscopic	Z No Device	F Irreversible Electroporation Z No Qualifier
G Pancreas	8 Via Natural or Artificial Opening Endoscopic	Z No Device	Z No Qualifier

Non-OR ØF5[5,6,7,8,9,C,D,F][4,8]ZZ
Non-OR ØF5G4ZZ
Non-OR ØF5G8ZZ

Ø Medical and Surgical
F Hepatobiliary System and Pancreas
7 Dilation Definition: Expanding an orifice or the lumen of a tubular body part

Explanation: The orifice can be a natural orifice or an artificially created orifice. Accomplished by stretching a tubular body part using intraluminal pressure or by cutting part of the orifice or wall of the tubular body part.

Body Part Character 4	Approach Character 5	Device Character 6	Qualifier Character 7
5 Hepatic Duct, Right 6 Hepatic Duct, Left 7 Hepatic Duct, Common 8 Cystic Duct 9 Common Bile Duct C Ampulla of Vater Duodenal ampulla Hepatopancreatic ampulla D Pancreatic Duct Duct of Wirsung F Pancreatic Duct, Accessory Duct of Santorini	Ø Open 3 Percutaneous 4 Percutaneous Endoscopic 7 Via Natural or Artificial Opening 8 Via Natural or Artificial Opening Endoscopic	D Intraluminal Device Z No Device	Z No Qualifier

Non-OR ØF7[5,6,7,8,9][3,4][D,Z]Z
Non-OR ØF7[5,6,7,8,9,D][7,8]DZ
Non-OR ØF7[5,6,7,8,9,C,D,F]8ZZ
Non-OR ØF7[D,F]4[D,Z]Z
Non-OR ØF7[C,F]8DZ

See Appendix L for Procedure Combinations
Combo-only ØF7[5,6,8,9,D][7,8]DZ

Ø Medical and Surgical
F Hepatobiliary System and Pancreas
8 Division Definition: Cutting into a body part, without draining fluids and/or gases from the body part, in order to separate or transect a body part

Explanation: All or a portion of the body part is separated into two or more portions

Body Part Character 4	Approach Character 5	Device Character 6	Qualifier Character 7
G Pancreas	Ø Open 3 Percutaneous 4 Percutaneous Endoscopic	Z No Device	Z No Qualifier

Ø Medical and Surgical
F Hepatobiliary System and Pancreas
9 Drainage Definition: Taking or letting out fluids and/or gases from a body part
Explanation: The qualifier DIAGNOSTIC is used to identify drainage procedures that are biopsies

Body Part Character 4	Approach Character 5	Device Character 6	Qualifier Character 7
Ø Liver Quadrate lobe **1** Liver, Right Lobe **2** Liver, Left Lobe	**Ø** Open **3** Percutaneous **4** Percutaneous Endoscopic	**Ø** Drainage Device	**Z** No Qualifier
Ø Liver Quadrate lobe **1** Liver, Right Lobe **2** Liver, Left Lobe	**Ø** Open **3** Percutaneous **4** Percutaneous Endoscopic	**Z** No Device	**X** Diagnostic **Z** No Qualifier
4 Gallbladder **G** Pancreas	**Ø** Open **3** Percutaneous **4** Percutaneous Endoscopic **8** Via Natural or Artificial Opening Endoscopic	**Ø** Drainage Device	**Z** No Qualifier
4 Gallbladder **G** Pancreas	**Ø** Open **3** Percutaneous **4** Percutaneous Endoscopic **8** Via Natural or Artificial Opening Endoscopic	**Z** No Device	**X** Diagnostic **Z** No Qualifier
5 Hepatic Duct, Right **6** Hepatic Duct, Left **7** Hepatic Duct, Common **8** Cystic Duct **9** Common Bile Duct **C** Ampulla of Vater Duodenal ampulla Hepatopancreatic ampulla **D** Pancreatic Duct Duct of Wirsung **F** Pancreatic Duct, Accessory Duct of Santorini	**Ø** Open **3** Percutaneous **4** Percutaneous Endoscopic **7** Via Natural or Artificial Opening **8** Via Natural or Artificial Opening Endoscopic	**Ø** Drainage Device	**Z** No Qualifier
5 Hepatic Duct, Right **6** Hepatic Duct, Left **7** Hepatic Duct, Common **8** Cystic Duct **9** Common Bile Duct **C** Ampulla of Vater Duodenal ampulla Hepatopancreatic ampulla **D** Pancreatic Duct Duct of Wirsung **F** Pancreatic Duct, Accessory Duct of Santorini	**Ø** Open **3** Percutaneous **4** Percutaneous Endoscopic **7** Via Natural or Artificial Opening **8** Via Natural or Artificial Opening Endoscopic	**Z** No Device	**X** Diagnostic **Z** No Qualifier

Non-OR ØF9[Ø,1,2][3,4]ØZ
Non-OR ØF9[Ø,1,2][3,4]Z[X,Z]
Non-OR ØF9[4,G]8ØZ
Non-OR ØF9G3ØZ
Non-OR ØF9[4,G]8Z[X,Z]
Non-OR ØF9G3Z[XZ]
Non-OR ØF9G4ZX
Non-OR ØF9[5,6,8][3,8]ØZ
Non-OR ØF97[3,4,7,8]ØZ
Non-OR ØF99[3,8]ØZ
Non-OR ØF9C[3,4,8]ØZ
Non-OR ØF9[D,F][3,8]ØZ
Non-OR ØF9[5,6,8,9,C,D,F]3Z[X,Z]
Non-OR ØF9[5,6,8,9,C,D,F][4,7,8]ZX
Non-OR ØF9[5,6,8,D,F]8ZZ
Non-OR ØF97[3,4,7,8]Z[X,Z]
Non-OR ØF99[4,7,8]ZZ
Non-OR ØF9C[4,8]ZZ

Ø Medical and Surgical
F Hepatobiliary System and Pancreas
B Excision Definition: Cutting out or off, without replacement, a portion of a body part
Explanation: The qualifier DIAGNOSTIC is used to identify excision procedures that are biopsies

Body Part Character 4	Approach Character 5	Device Character 6	Qualifier Character 7
Ø Liver Quadrate lobe 1 Liver, Right Lobe 2 Liver, Left Lobe	Ø Open 3 Percutaneous 4 Percutaneous Endoscopic	Z No Device	X Diagnostic Z No Qualifier
4 Gallbladder G Pancreas	Ø Open 3 Percutaneous 4 Percutaneous Endoscopic 8 Via Natural or Artificial Opening Endoscopic	Z No Device	X Diagnostic Z No Qualifier
5 Hepatic Duct, Right 6 Hepatic Duct, Left 7 Hepatic Duct, Common 8 Cystic Duct 9 Common Bile Duct C Ampulla of Vater Duodenal ampulla Hepatopancreatic ampulla D Pancreatic Duct Duct of Wirsung F Pancreatic Duct, Accessory Duct of Santorini	Ø Open 3 Percutaneous 4 Percutaneous Endoscopic 7 Via Natural or Artificial Opening 8 Via Natural or Artificial Opening Endoscopic	Z No Device	X Diagnostic Z No Qualifier

Non-OR ØFB[Ø,1,2]3ZX
Non-OR ØFB[4,G][3,4,8]ZX
Non-OR ØFB[5,6,7,8,9,C,D,F][3,4,7,8]ZX
Non-OR ØFB[5,6,7,8,9,C,D,F][4,8]ZZ

Ø Medical and Surgical
F Hepatobiliary System and Pancreas
C Extirpation Definition: Taking or cutting out solid matter from a body part
Explanation: The solid matter may be an abnormal byproduct of a biological function or a foreign body; it may be imbedded in a body part or in the lumen of a tubular body part. The solid matter may or may not have been previously broken into pieces.

Body Part Character 4	Approach Character 5	Device Character 6	Qualifier Character 7
Ø Liver Quadrate lobe 1 Liver, Right Lobe 2 Liver, Left Lobe	Ø Open 3 Percutaneous 4 Percutaneous Endoscopic	Z No Device	Z No Qualifier
4 Gallbladder G Pancreas	Ø Open 3 Percutaneous 4 Percutaneous Endoscopic 8 Via Natural or Artificial Opening Endoscopic	Z No Device	Z No Qualifier
5 Hepatic Duct, Right 6 Hepatic Duct, Left 7 Hepatic Duct, Common 8 Cystic Duct 9 Common Bile Duct C Ampulla of Vater Duodenal ampulla Hepatopancreatic ampulla D Pancreatic Duct Duct of Wirsung F Pancreatic Duct, Accessory Duct of Santorini	Ø Open 3 Percutaneous 4 Percutaneous Endoscopic 7 Via Natural or Artificial Opening 8 Via Natural or Artificial Opening Endoscopic	Z No Device	Z No Qualifier

Non-OR ØFC[5,6,7,8,9][3,4,7,8]ZZ
Non-OR ØFCC[4,8]ZZ
Non-OR ØFC[D,F][3,4,8]ZZ

Ø Medical and Surgical
F Hepatobiliary System and Pancreas
D Extraction Definition: Pulling or stripping out or off all or a portion of a body part by the use of force
Explanation: The qualifier DIAGNOSTIC is used to identify extraction procedures that are biopsies

Body Part Character 4	Approach Character 5	Device Character 6	Qualifier Character 7
Ø Liver Quadrate lobe **1** Liver, Right Lobe **2** Liver, Left Lobe	**3** Percutaneous **4** Percutaneous Endoscopic	**Z** No Device	**X** Diagnostic
4 Gallbladder **5** Hepatic Duct, Right **6** Hepatic Duct, Left **7** Hepatic Duct, Common **8** Cystic Duct **9** Common Bile Duct **C** Ampulla of Vater Duodenal ampulla Hepatopancreatic ampulla **D** Pancreatic Duct Duct of Wirsung **F** Pancreatic Duct, Accessory Duct of Santorini **G** Pancreas	**3** Percutaneous **4** Percutaneous Endoscopic **8** Via Natural or Artificial Opening Endoscopic	**Z** No Device	**X** Diagnostic

Ø Medical and Surgical
F Hepatobiliary System and Pancreas
F Fragmentation Definition: Breaking solid matter in a body part into pieces
Explanation: Physical force (e.g., manual, ultrasonic) applied directly or indirectly is used to break the solid matter into pieces. The solid matter may be an abnormal byproduct of a biological function or a foreign body. The pieces of solid matter are not taken out.

Body Part Character 4	Approach Character 5	Device Character 6	Qualifier Character 7
4 Gallbladder NC **5** Hepatic Duct, Right NC **6** Hepatic Duct, Left NC **7** Hepatic Duct, Common **8** Cystic Duct NC **9** Common Bile Duct NC **C** Ampulla of Vater NC Duodenal ampulla Hepatopancreatic ampulla **D** Pancreatic Duct NC Duct of Wirsung **F** Pancreatic Duct, Accessory NC Duct of Santorini	**Ø** Open **3** Percutaneous **4** Percutaneous Endoscopic **7** Via Natural or Artificial Opening **8** Via Natural or Artificial Opening Endoscopic **X** External	**Z** No Device	**Z** No Qualifier

Non-OR ØFF[4,5,6,7,8,9,C,D,F][8,X]ZZ
NC ØFF[4,5,6,8,9,C,D,F]XZZ

Ø Medical and Surgical
F Hepatobiliary System and Pancreas
H Insertion Definition: Putting in a nonbiological appliance that monitors, assists, performs, or prevents a physiological function but does not physically take the place of a body part
Explanation: None

Body Part Character 4	Approach Character 5	Device Character 6	Qualifier Character 7
Ø Liver Quadrate lobe **4** Gallbladder **G** Pancreas	**Ø** Open **3** Percutaneous **4** Percutaneous Endoscopic	**2** Monitoring Device **3** Infusion Device **Y** Other Device	**Z** No Qualifier
1 Liver, Right Lobe **2** Liver, Left Lobe	**Ø** Open **3** Percutaneous **4** Percutaneous Endoscopic	**2** Monitoring Device **3** Infusion Device	**Z** No Qualifier
B Hepatobiliary Duct **D** Pancreatic Duct Duct of Wirsung	**Ø** Open **3** Percutaneous **4** Percutaneous Endoscopic **7** Via Natural or Artificial Opening **8** Via Natural or Artificial Opening Endoscopic	**1** Radioactive Element **2** Monitoring Device **3** Infusion Device **D** Intraluminal Device **Y** Other Device	**Z** No Qualifier

Non-OR ØFH[Ø,4,G][Ø,3,4]3Z
Non-OR ØFH[Ø,4,G][3,4]YZ
Non-OR ØFH[1,2][Ø,3,4]3Z
Non-OR ØFH[B,D][Ø,3,4]3Z
Non-OR ØFH[B,D]4DZ
Non-OR ØFH[B,D][7,8][2,3]Z
Non-OR ØFH[B,D]8DZ
Non-OR ØFH[B,D][3,4,7,8]YZ

See Appendix L for Procedure Combinations
Combo-only ØFHB8DZ

Ø Medical and Surgical
F Hepatobiliary System and Pancreas
J Inspection Definition: Visually and/or manually exploring a body part

Explanation: Visual exploration may be performed with or without optical instrumentation. Manual exploration may be performed directly or through intervening body layers.

Body Part Character 4	Approach Character 5	Device Character 6	Qualifier Character 7
Ø Liver Quadrate lobe	Ø Open 3 Percutaneous 4 Percutaneous Endoscopic X External	Z No Device	Z No Qualifier
4 Gallbladder G Pancreas	Ø Open 3 Percutaneous 4 Percutaneous Endoscopic 8 Via Natural or Artificial Opening Endoscopic X External	Z No Device	Z No Qualifier
B Hepatobiliary Duct D Pancreatic Duct Duct of Wirsung	Ø Open 3 Percutaneous 4 Percutaneous Endoscopic 7 Via Natural or Artificial Opening 8 Via Natural or Artificial Opening Endoscopic	Z No Device	Z No Qualifier

Non-OR ØFJØ[3,X]ZZ
Non-OR ØFJ[4,G][3,8,X]ZZ
Non-OR ØFJ[B,D][3,7,8]ZZ

Ø Medical and Surgical
F Hepatobiliary System and Pancreas
L Occlusion Definition: Completely closing an orifice or the lumen of a tubular body part

Explanation: The orifice can be a natural orifice or an artificially created orifice

Body Part Character 4	Approach Character 5	Device Character 6	Qualifier Character 7
5 Hepatic Duct, Right 6 Hepatic Duct, Left 7 Hepatic Duct, Common 8 Cystic Duct 9 Common Bile Duct C Ampulla of Vater Duodenal ampulla Hepatopancreatic ampulla D Pancreatic Duct Duct of Wirsung F Pancreatic Duct, Accessory Duct of Santorini	Ø Open 3 Percutaneous 4 Percutaneous Endoscopic	C Extraluminal Device D Intraluminal Device Z No Device	Z No Qualifier
5 Hepatic Duct, Right 6 Hepatic Duct, Left 7 Hepatic Duct, Common 8 Cystic Duct 9 Common Bile Duct C Ampulla of Vater Duodenal ampulla Hepatopancreatic ampulla D Pancreatic Duct Duct of Wirsung F Pancreatic Duct, Accessory Duct of Santorini	7 Via Natural or Artificial Opening 8 Via Natural or Artificial Opening Endoscopic	D Intraluminal Device Z No Device	Z No Qualifier

Non-OR ØFL[5,6,7,8,9][3,4][C,D,Z]Z
Non-OR ØFL[5,6,7,8,9][7,8][D,Z]Z

Ø Medical and Surgical
F Hepatobiliary System and Pancreas
M Reattachment Definition: Putting back in or on all or a portion of a separated body part to its normal location or other suitable location
Explanation: Vascular circulation and nervous pathways may or may not be reestablished

Body Part Character 4	Approach Character 5	Device Character 6	Qualifier Character 7
Ø Liver Quadrate lobe 1 Liver, Right Lobe 2 Liver, Left Lobe 4 Gallbladder 5 Hepatic Duct, Right 6 Hepatic Duct, Left 7 Hepatic Duct, Common 8 Cystic Duct 9 Common Bile Duct C Ampulla of Vater Duodenal ampulla Hepatopancreatic ampulla D Pancreatic Duct Duct of Wirsung F Pancreatic Duct, Accessory Duct of Santorini G Pancreas	Ø Open 4 Percutaneous Endoscopic	Z No Device	Z No Qualifier

Non-OR ØFM[4,5,6,7,8,9]4ZZ

Ø Medical and Surgical
F Hepatobiliary System and Pancreas
N Release Definition: Freeing a body part from an abnormal physical constraint by cutting or by the use of force
Explanation: Some of the restraining tissue may be taken out but none of the body part is taken out

Body Part Character 4	Approach Character 5	Device Character 6	Qualifier Character 7
Ø Liver Quadrate lobe 1 Liver, Right Lobe 2 Liver, Left Lobe	Ø Open 3 Percutaneous 4 Percutaneous Endoscopic	Z No Device	Z No Qualifier
4 Gallbladder G Pancreas	Ø Open 3 Percutaneous 4 Percutaneous Endoscopic 8 Via Natural or Artificial Opening Endoscopic	Z No Device	Z No Qualifier
5 Hepatic Duct, Right 6 Hepatic Duct, Left 7 Hepatic Duct, Common 8 Cystic Duct 9 Common Bile Duct C Ampulla of Vater Duodenal ampulla Hepatopancreatic ampulla D Pancreatic Duct Duct of Wirsung F Pancreatic Duct, Accessory Duct of Santorini	Ø Open 3 Percutaneous 4 Percutaneous Endoscopic 7 Via Natural or Artificial Opening 8 Via Natural or Artificial Opening Endoscopic	Z No Device	Z No Qualifier

Ø Medical and Surgical
F Hepatobiliary System and Pancreas
P Removal Definition: Taking out or off a device from a body part

Explanation: If a device is taken out and a similar device put in without cutting or puncturing the skin or mucous membrane, the procedure is coded to the root operation CHANGE. Otherwise, the procedure for taking out a device is coded to the root operation REMOVAL.

Body Part Character 4	Approach Character 5	Device Character 6	Qualifier Character 7
Ø Liver Quadrate lobe	Ø Open 3 Percutaneous 4 Percutaneous Endoscopic	Ø Drainage Device 2 Monitoring Device 3 Infusion Device Y Other Device	Z No Qualifier
Ø Liver Quadrate lobe	X External	Ø Drainage Device 2 Monitoring Device 3 Infusion Device	Z No Qualifier
4 Gallbladder G Pancreas	Ø Open 3 Percutaneous 4 Percutaneous Endoscopic	Ø Drainage Device 2 Monitoring Device 3 Infusion Device D Intraluminal Device Y Other Device	Z No Qualifier
4 Gallbladder G Pancreas	X External	Ø Drainage Device 2 Monitoring Device 3 Infusion Device D Intraluminal Device	Z No Qualifier
B Hepatobiliary Duct D Pancreatic Duct Duct of Wirsung	Ø Open 3 Percutaneous 4 Percutaneous Endoscopic 7 Via Natural or Artificial Opening 8 Via Natural or Artificial Opening Endoscopic	Ø Drainage Device 1 Radioactive Element 2 Monitoring Device 3 Infusion Device 7 Autologous Tissue Substitute C Extraluminal Device D Intraluminal Device J Synthetic Substitute K Nonautologous Tissue Substitute Y Other Device	Z No Qualifier
B Hepatobiliary Duct D Pancreatic Duct Duct of Wirsung	X External	Ø Drainage Device 1 Radioactive Element 2 Monitoring Device 3 Infusion Device D Intraluminal Device	Z No Qualifier

Non-OR ØFPØ[3,4]YZ
Non-OR ØFPØX[Ø,2,3]Z
Non-OR ØFP[4,G][3,4]YZ
Non-OR ØFP4X[Ø,2,3,D]Z
Non-OR ØFPGX[Ø,2,3]Z
Non-OR ØFP[B,D][3,4]YZ
Non-OR ØFP[B,D][7,8][Ø,2,3,D,Y]Z
Non-OR ØFP[B,D]X[Ø,1,2,3,D]Z

See Appendix L for Procedure Combinations
Combo-only ØFP[B,D]XDZ

Ø Medical and Surgical
F Hepatobiliary System and Pancreas
Q Repair Definition: Restoring, to the extent possible, a body part to its normal anatomic structure and function
Explanation: Used only when the method to accomplish the repair is not one of the other root operations

Body Part Character 4	Approach Character 5	Device Character 6	Qualifier Character 7
Ø Liver Quadrate lobe 1 Liver, Right Lobe 2 Liver, Left Lobe	Ø Open 3 Percutaneous 4 Percutaneous Endoscopic	Z No Device	Z No Qualifier
4 Gallbladder G Pancreas	Ø Open 3 Percutaneous 4 Percutaneous Endoscopic 8 Via Natural or Artificial Opening Endoscopic	Z No Device	Z No Qualifier
5 Hepatic Duct, Right 6 Hepatic Duct, Left 7 Hepatic Duct, Common 8 Cystic Duct 9 Common Bile Duct C Ampulla of Vater Duodenal ampulla Hepatopancreatic ampulla D Pancreatic Duct Duct of Wirsung F Pancreatic Duct, Accessory Duct of Santorini	Ø Open 3 Percutaneous 4 Percutaneous Endoscopic 7 Via Natural or Artificial Opening 8 Via Natural or Artificial Opening Endoscopic	Z No Device	Z No Qualifier

Ø Medical and Surgical
F Hepatobiliary System and Pancreas
R Replacement Definition: Putting in or on biological or synthetic material that physically takes the place and/or function of all or a portion of a body part
Explanation: The body part may have been taken out or replaced, or may be taken out, physically eradicated, or rendered nonfunctional during the REPLACEMENT procedure. A REMOVAL procedure is coded for taking out the device used in a previous replacement procedure.

Body Part Character 4	Approach Character 5	Device Character 6	Qualifier Character 7
5 Hepatic Duct, Right 6 Hepatic Duct, Left 7 Hepatic Duct, Common 8 Cystic Duct 9 Common Bile Duct C Ampulla of Vater Duodenal ampulla Hepatopancreatic ampulla D Pancreatic Duct Duct of Wirsung F Pancreatic Duct, Accessory Duct of Santorini	Ø Open 4 Percutaneous Endoscopic 8 Via Natural or Artificial Opening Endoscopic	7 Autologous Tissue Substitute J Synthetic Substitute K Nonautologous Tissue Substitute	Z No Qualifier

Ø Medical and Surgical
F Hepatobiliary System and Pancreas
S Reposition Definition: Moving to its normal location, or other suitable location, all or a portion of a body part
Explanation: The body part is moved to a new location from an abnormal location, or from a normal location where it is not functioning correctly. The body part may or may not be cut out or off to be moved to the new location.

Body Part Character 4	Approach Character 5	Device Character 6	Qualifier Character 7
Ø Liver Quadrate lobe 4 Gallbladder 5 Hepatic Duct, Right 6 Hepatic Duct, Left 7 Hepatic Duct, Common 8 Cystic Duct 9 Common Bile Duct C Ampulla of Vater Duodenal ampulla Hepatopancreatic ampulla D Pancreatic Duct Duct of Wirsung F Pancreatic Duct, Accessory Duct of Santorini G Pancreas	Ø Open 4 Percutaneous Endoscopic	Z No Device	Z No Qualifier

Ø Medical and Surgical
F Hepatobiliary System and Pancreas
T Resection Definition: Cutting out or off, without replacement, all of a body part
Explanation: None

Body Part Character 4	Approach Character 5	Device Character 6	Qualifier Character 7
Ø Liver Quadrate lobe 1 Liver, Right Lobe 2 Liver, Left Lobe 4 Gallbladder G Pancreas ⊞	Ø Open 4 Percutaneous Endoscopic	Z No Device	Z No Qualifier
5 Hepatic Duct, Right 6 Hepatic Duct, Left 7 Hepatic Duct, Common 8 Cystic Duct 9 Common Bile Duct C Ampulla of Vater Duodenal ampulla Hepatopancreatic ampulla D Pancreatic Duct Duct of Wirsung F Pancreatic Duct, Accessory Duct of Santorini	Ø Open 4 Percutaneous Endoscopic 7 Via Natural or Artificial Opening 8 Via Natural or Artificial Opening Endoscopic	Z No Device	Z No Qualifier

Non-OR ØFT[D,F][4,8]ZZ

See Appendix L for Procedure Combinations
⊞ ØFTGØZZ

Ø Medical and Surgical
F Hepatobiliary System and Pancreas
U Supplement Definition: Putting in or on biological or synthetic material that physically reinforces and/or augments the function of a portion of a body part
Explanation: The biological material is non-living, or is living and from the same individual. The body part may have been previously replaced, and the SUPPLEMENT procedure is performed to physically reinforce and/or augment the function of the replaced body part.

Body Part Character 4	Approach Character 5	Device Character 6	Qualifier Character 7
5 Hepatic Duct, Right 6 Hepatic Duct, Left 7 Hepatic Duct, Common 8 Cystic Duct 9 Common Bile Duct C Ampulla of Vater Duodenal ampulla Hepatopancreatic ampulla D Pancreatic Duct Duct of Wirsung F Pancreatic Duct, Accessory Duct of Santorini	Ø Open 3 Percutaneous 4 Percutaneous Endoscopic 8 Via Natural or Artificial Opening Endoscopic	7 Autologous Tissue Substitute J Synthetic Substitute K Nonautologous Tissue Substitute	Z No Qualifier

Ø Medical and Surgical
F Hepatobiliary System and Pancreas
V Restriction Definition: Partially closing an orifice or the lumen of a tubular body part
Explanation: The orifice can be a natural orifice or an artificially created orifice

Body Part Character 4	Approach Character 5	Device Character 6	Qualifier Character 7
5 Hepatic Duct, Right **6** Hepatic Duct, Left **7** Hepatic Duct, Common **8** Cystic Duct **9** Common Bile Duct **C** Ampulla of Vater Duodenal ampulla Hepatopancreatic ampulla **D** Pancreatic Duct Duct of Wirsung **F** Pancreatic Duct, Accessory Duct of Santorini	**Ø** Open **3** Percutaneous **4** Percutaneous Endoscopic	**C** Extraluminal Device **D** Intraluminal Device **Z** No Device	**Z** No Qualifier
5 Hepatic Duct, Right **6** Hepatic Duct, Left **7** Hepatic Duct, Common **8** Cystic Duct **9** Common Bile Duct **C** Ampulla of Vater Duodenal ampulla Hepatopancreatic ampulla **D** Pancreatic Duct Duct of Wirsung **F** Pancreatic Duct, Accessory Duct of Santorini	**7** Via Natural or Artificial Opening **8** Via Natural or Artificial Opening Endoscopic	**D** Intraluminal Device **Z** No Device	**Z** No Qualifier

Non-OR ØFV[5,6,7,8,9][3,4][C,D,Z]Z
Non-OR ØFV[5,6,7,8,9][7,8][D,Z]Z

Ø Medical and Surgical
F Hepatobiliary System and Pancreas
W Revision Definition: Correcting, to the extent possible, a portion of a malfunctioning device or the position of a displaced device
Explanation: Revision can include correcting a malfunctioning or displaced device by taking out or putting in components of the device such as a screw or pin

Body Part Character 4	Approach Character 5	Device Character 6	Qualifier Character 7
Ø Liver Quadrate lobe	Ø Open 3 Percutaneous 4 Percutaneous Endoscopic	Ø Drainage Device 2 Monitoring Device 3 Infusion Device Y Other Device	Z No Qualifier
Ø Liver Quadrate lobe	X External	Ø Drainage Device 2 Monitoring Device 3 Infusion Device	Z No Qualifier
4 Gallbladder G Pancreas	Ø Open 3 Percutaneous 4 Percutaneous Endoscopic	Ø Drainage Device 2 Monitoring Device 3 Infusion Device D Intraluminal Device Y Other Device	Z No Qualifier
4 Gallbladder G Pancreas	X External	Ø Drainage Device 2 Monitoring Device 3 Infusion Device D Intraluminal Device	Z No Qualifier
B Hepatobiliary Duct D Pancreatic Duct Duct of Wirsung	Ø Open 3 Percutaneous 4 Percutaneous Endoscopic 7 Via Natural or Artificial Opening 8 Via Natural or Artificial Opening Endoscopic	Ø Drainage Device 2 Monitoring Device 3 Infusion Device 7 Autologous Tissue Substitute C Extraluminal Device D Intraluminal Device J Synthetic Substitute K Nonautologous Tissue Substitute Y Other Device	Z No Qualifier
B Hepatobiliary Duct D Pancreatic Duct Duct of Wirsung	X External	Ø Drainage Device 2 Monitoring Device 3 Infusion Device 7 Autologous Tissue Substitute C Extraluminal Device D Intraluminal Device J Synthetic Substitute K Nonautologous Tissue Substitute	Z No Qualifier

Non-OR ØFWØ[3,4]YZ
Non-OR ØFWØX[Ø,2,3]Z
Non-OR ØFW[4,G][3,4]YZ
Non-OR ØFW[4,G]X[Ø,2,3,D]Z
Non-OR ØFW[B,D][3,4,7,8]YZ
Non-OR ØFW[B,D]X[Ø,2,3,7,C,D,J,K]Z

Ø Medical and Surgical
F Hepatobiliary System and Pancreas
Y Transplantation Definition: Putting in or on all or a portion of a living body part taken from another individual or animal to physically take the place and/or function of all or a portion of a similar body part
Explanation: The native body part may or may not be taken out, and the transplanted body part may take over all or a portion of its function

Body Part Character 4	Approach Character 5	Device Character 6	Qualifier Character 7
Ø Liver LC Quadrate lobe G Pancreas ⊞ LC NC	Ø Open	Z No Device	Ø Allogeneic 1 Syngeneic 2 Zooplastic

LC ØFYØØZ[Ø,1,2]
LC ØFYGØZ[Ø,1]
NC ØFYGØZ2
NC ØFYGØZ[Ø,1] If reported alone without one of the following procedures ØTYØØZ[Ø,1,2], ØTY1ØZ[Ø,1,2] and without one of the following diagnoses E1Ø.1Ø-E1Ø.9, E89.1

See Appendix L for Procedure Combinations
⊞ ØFYGØZ[Ø,1,2]

Endocrine System ØG2–ØGW

Character Meanings

This Character Meaning table is provided as a guide to assist the user in the identification of character members that may be found in this section of code tables. It **SHOULD NOT** be used to build a PCS code.

Operation–Character 3	Body Part–Character 4	Approach–Character 5	Device–Character 6	Qualifier–Character 7
2 Change	Ø Pituitary Gland	Ø Open	Ø Drainage Device	X Diagnostic
5 Destruction	1 Pineal Body	3 Percutaneous	2 Monitoring Device	Z No Qualifier
8 Division	2 Adrenal Gland, Left	4 Percutaneous Endoscopic	3 Infusion Device	
9 Drainage	3 Adrenal Gland, Right	X External	Y Other Device	
B Excision	4 Adrenal Glands, Bilateral		Z No Device	
C Extirpation	5 Adrenal Gland			
H Insertion	6 Carotid Body, Left			
J Inspection	7 Carotid Body, Right			
M Reattachment	8 Carotid Bodies, Bilateral			
N Release	9 Para-aortic Body			
P Removal	B Coccygeal Glomus			
Q Repair	C Glomus Jugulare			
S Reposition	D Aortic Body			
T Resection	F Paraganglion Extremity			
W Revision	G Thyroid Gland Lobe, Left			
	H Thyroid Gland Lobe, Right			
	J Thyroid Gland Isthmus			
	K Thyroid Gland			
	L Superior Parathyroid Gland, Right			
	M Superior Parathyroid Gland, Left			
	N Inferior Parathyroid Gland, Right			
	P Inferior Parathyroid Gland, Left			
	Q Parathyroid Glands, Multiple			
	R Parathyroid Gland			
	S Endocrine Gland			

AHA Coding Clinic for table ØGB
2017, 2Q, 20 Near total thyroidectomy
2014, 3Q, 22 Transsphenoidal removal of pituitary tumor and fat graft placement

AHA Coding Clinic for table ØGT
2017, 2Q, 20 Near total thyroidectomy

Endocrine System

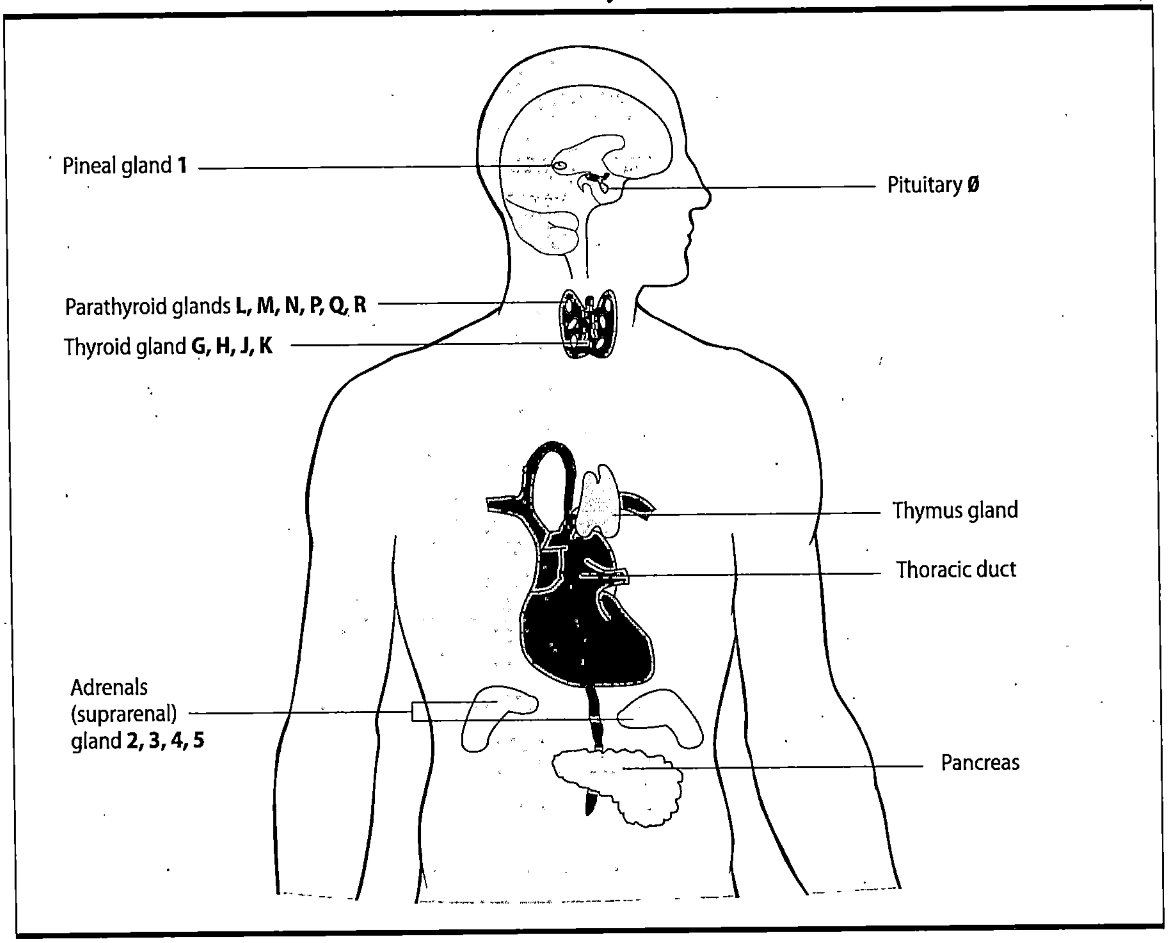

Left Adrenal Gland

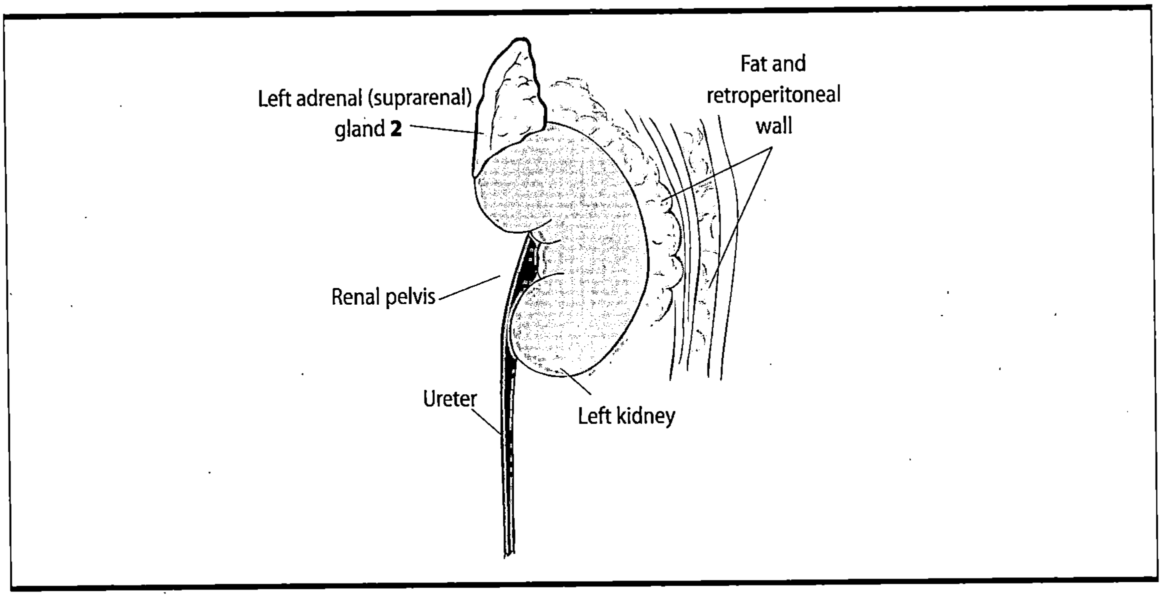

Thyroid

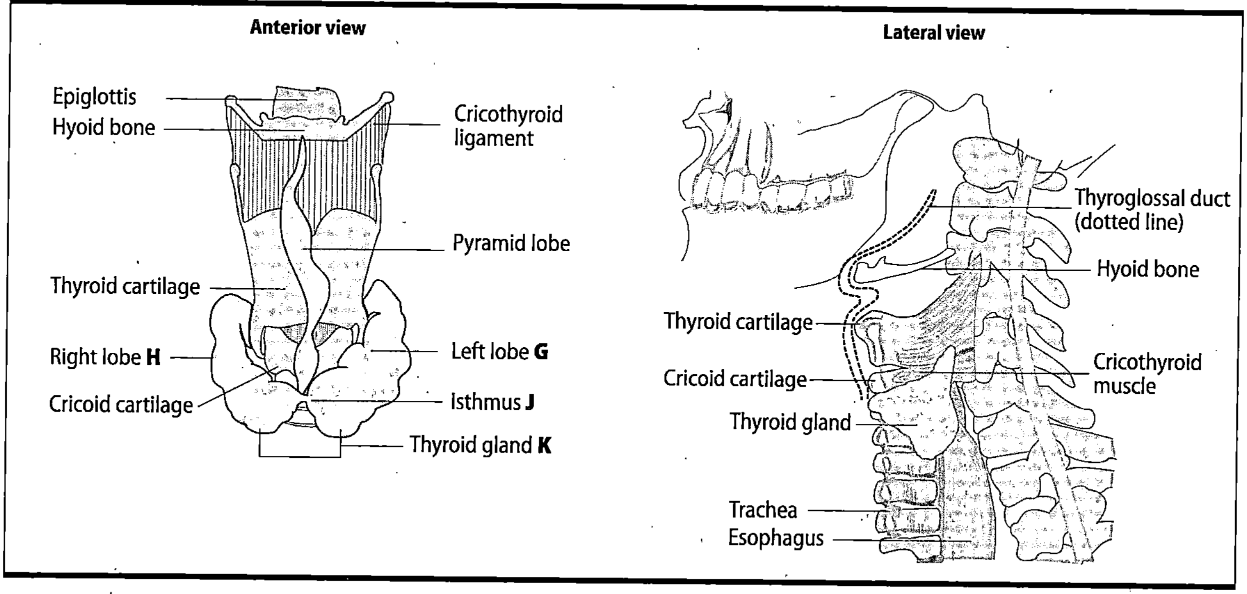
Anterior view
Epiglottis
Hyoid bone
Cricothyroid ligament
Pyramid lobe
Thyroid cartilage
Right lobe **H**
Left lobe **G**
Cricoid cartilage
Isthmus **J**
Thyroid gland **K**
Lateral view
Thyroglossal duct (dotted line)
Hyoid bone
Thyroid cartilage
Cricoid cartilage
Cricothyroid muscle
Thyroid gland
Trachea
Esophagus

Thyroid and Parathyroid Glands

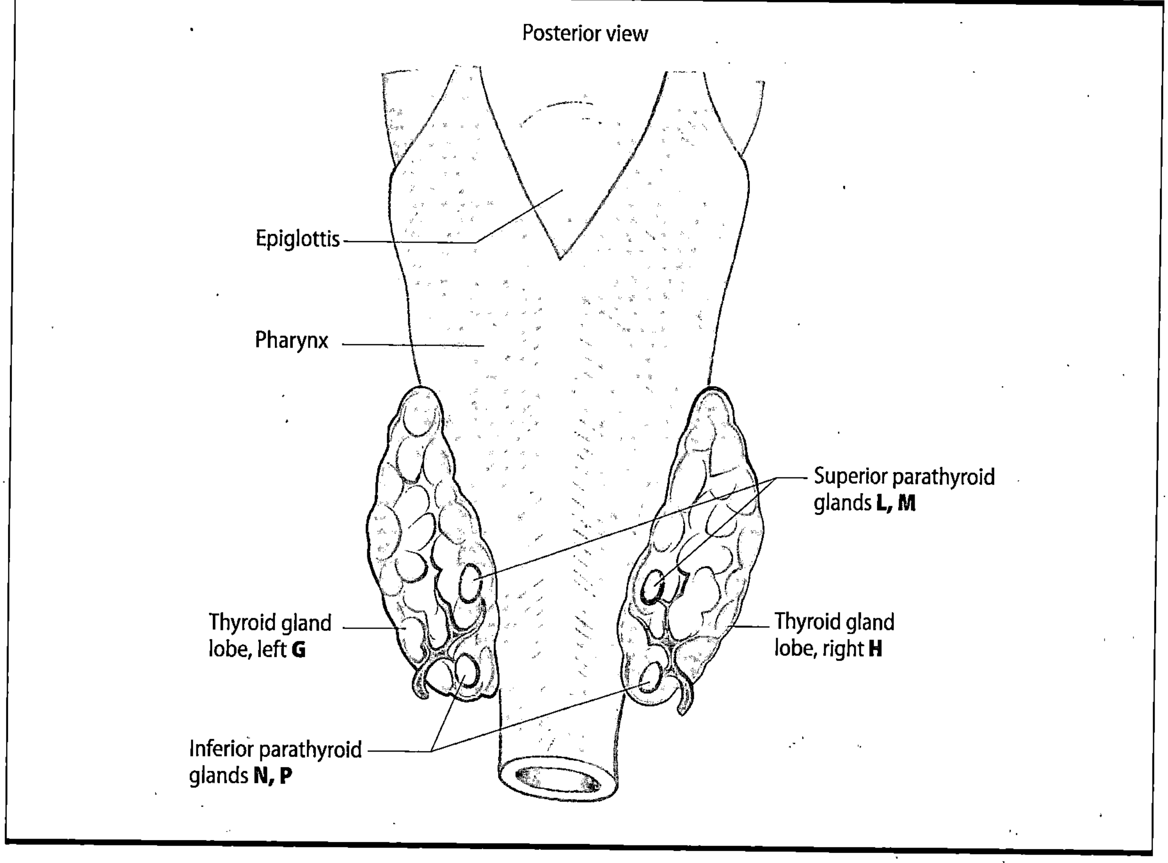
Posterior view
Epiglottis
Pharynx
Superior parathyroid glands **L, M**
Thyroid gland lobe, left **G**
Thyroid gland lobe, right **H**
Inferior parathyroid glands **N, P**

Ø Medical and Surgical
G Endocrine System
2 Change Definition: Taking out or off a device from a body part and putting back an identical or similar device in or on the same body part without cutting or puncturing the skin or a mucous membrane
Explanation: All CHANGE procedures are coded using the approach EXTERNAL

Body Part Character 4	Approach Character 5	Device Character 6	Qualifier Character 7
Ø Pituitary Gland Adenohypophysis Hypophysis Neurohypophysis **1** Pineal Body **5** Adrenal Gland Suprarenal gland **K** Thyroid Gland **R** Parathyroid Gland **S** Endocrine Gland	**X** External	**Ø** Drainage Device **Y** Other Device	**Z** No Qualifier

Non-OR All body part, approach, device, and qualifier values

Ø Medical and Surgical
G Endocrine System
5 Destruction Definition: Physical eradication of all or a portion of a body part by the direct use of energy, force, or a destructive agent
Explanation: None of the body part is physically taken out

Body Part Character 4	Approach Character 5	Device Character 6	Qualifier Character 7
Ø Pituitary Gland Adenohypophysis Hypophysis Neurohypophysis **1** Pineal Body **2** Adrenal Gland, Left Suprarenal gland **3** Adrenal Gland, Right *See 2 Adrenal Gland, Left* **4** Adrenal Glands, Bilateral *See 2 Adrenal Gland, Left* **6** Carotid Body, Left Carotid glomus **7** Carotid Body, Right *See 6 Carotid Body, Left* **8** Carotid Bodies, Bilateral *See 6 Carotid Body, Left* **9** Para-aortic Body **B** Coccygeal Glomus Coccygeal body **C** Glomus Jugulare Jugular body **D** Aortic Body **F** Paraganglion Extremity **G** Thyroid Gland Lobe, Left **H** Thyroid Gland Lobe, Right **K** Thyroid Gland **L** Superior Parathyroid Gland, Right **M** Superior Parathyroid Gland, Left **N** Inferior Parathyroid Gland, Right **P** Inferior Parathyroid Gland, Left **Q** Parathyroid Glands, Multiple **R** Parathyroid Gland	**Ø** Open **3** Percutaneous **4** Percutaneous Endoscopic	**Z** No Device	**Z** No Qualifier

Ø Medical and Surgical
G Endocrine System
8 Division Definition: Cutting into a body part, without draining fluids and/or gases from the body part, in order to separate or transect a body part
Explanation: All or a portion of the body part is separated into two or more portions

Body Part Character 4	Approach Character 5	Device Character 6	Qualifier Character 7
Ø Pituitary Gland Adenohypophysis Hypophysis Neurohypophysis **J** Thyroid Gland Isthmus	**Ø** Open **3** Percutaneous **4** Percutaneous Endoscopic	**Z** No Device	**Z** No Qualifier

Ø Medical and Surgical
G Endocrine System
9 Drainage Definition: Taking or letting out fluids and/or gases from a body part
Explanation: The qualifier DIAGNOSTIC is used to identify drainage procedures that are biopsies

Body Part Character 4	Approach Character 5	Device Character 6	Qualifier Character 7
Ø Pituitary Gland Adenohypophysis Hypophysis Neurohypophysis 1 Pineal Body 2 Adrenal Gland, Left Suprarenal gland 3 Adrenal Gland, Right *See 2 Adrenal Gland, Left* 4 Adrenal Glands, Bilateral *See 2 Adrenal Gland, Left* 6 Carotid Body, Left Carotid glomus 7 Carotid Body, Right *See 6 Carotid Body, Left* 8 Carotid Bodies, Bilateral *See 6 Carotid Body, Left* 9 Para-aortic Body B Coccygeal Glomus Coccygeal body C Glomus Jugulare Jugular body D Aortic Body F Paraganglion Extremity G Thyroid Gland Lobe, Left H Thyroid Gland Lobe, Right K Thyroid Gland L Superior Parathyroid Gland, Right M Superior Parathyroid Gland, Left N Inferior Parathyroid Gland, Right P Inferior Parathyroid Gland, Left Q Parathyroid Glands, Multiple R Parathyroid Gland	Ø Open 3 Percutaneous 4 Percutaneous Endoscopic	Ø Drainage Device	Z No Qualifier
Ø Pituitary Gland Adenohypophysis Hypophysis Neurohypophysis 1 Pineal Body 2 Adrenal Gland, Left Suprarenal gland 3 Adrenal Gland, Right *See 2 Adrenal Gland, Left* 4 Adrenal Glands, Bilateral *See 2 Adrenal Gland, Left* 6 Carotid Body, Left Carotid glomus 7 Carotid Body, Right *See 6 Carotid Body, Left* 8 Carotid Bodies, Bilateral *See 6 Carotid Body, Left* 9 Para-aortic Body B Coccygeal Glomus Coccygeal body C Glomus Jugulare Jugular body D Aortic Body F Paraganglion Extremity G Thyroid Gland Lobe, Left H Thyroid Gland Lobe, Right K Thyroid Gland L Superior Parathyroid Gland, Right M Superior Parathyroid Gland, Left N Inferior Parathyroid Gland, Right P Inferior Parathyroid Gland, Left Q Parathyroid Glands, Multiple R Parathyroid Gland	Ø Open 3 Percutaneous 4 Percutaneous Endoscopic	Z No Device	X Diagnostic Z No Qualifier

Non-OR ØG9[Ø,1,2,3,4,6,7,8,9,B,C,D,F,G,H,K,L,M,N,P,Q,R]3ØZ
Non-OR ØG9[G,H,K,L,M,N,P,Q,R]4ØZ
Non-OR ØG9[2,3,4,G,H,K][3,4]ZX
Non-OR ØG9[Ø,1,2,3,4,6,7,8,9,B,C,D,F,G,H,K,L,M,N,P,Q,R]3ZZ
Non-OR ØG9[G,H,K,L,M,N,P,Q,R]4ZZ

Ø Medical and Surgical
G Endocrine System
B Excision Definition: Cutting out or off, without replacement, a portion of a body part
Explanation: The qualifier DIAGNOSTIC is used to identify excision procedures that are biopsies

Body Part Character 4	Approach Character 5	Device Character 6	Qualifier Character 7
Ø Pituitary Gland Adenohypophysis Hypophysis Neurohypophysis **1** Pineal Body **2** Adrenal Gland, Left Suprarenal gland **3** Adrenal Gland, Right *See 2 Adrenal Gland, Left* **4** Adrenal Glands, Bilateral *See 2 Adrenal Gland, Left* **6** Carotid Body, Left Carotid glomus **7** Carotid Body, Right *See 6 Carotid Body, Left* **8** Carotid Bodies, Bilateral *See 6 Carotid Body, Left* **9** Para-aortic Body **B** Coccygeal Glomus Coccygeal body **C** Glomus Jugulare Jugular body **D** Aortic Body **F** Paraganglion Extremity **G** Thyroid Gland Lobe, Left **H** Thyroid Gland Lobe, Right **J** Thyroid Gland Isthmus **L** Superior Parathyroid Gland, Right **M** Superior Parathyroid Gland, Left **N** Inferior Parathyroid Gland, Right **P** Inferior Parathyroid Gland, Left **Q** Parathyroid Glands, Multiple **R** Parathyroid Gland	**Ø** Open **3** Percutaneous **4** Percutaneous Endoscopic	**Z** No Device	**X** Diagnostic **Z** No Qualifier

Non-OR ØGB[2,3,4,G,H,J][3,4]ZX

Ø Medical and Surgical
G Endocrine System
C Extirpation Definition: Taking or cutting out solid matter from a body part
Explanation: The solid matter may be an abnormal byproduct of a biological function or a foreign body; it may be imbedded in a body part or in the lumen of a tubular body part. The solid matter may or may not have been previously broken into pieces.

Body Part Character 4	Approach Character 5	Device Character 6	Qualifier Character 7
Ø Pituitary Gland Adenohypophysis Hypophysis Neurohypophysis **1** Pineal Body **2** Adrenal Gland, Left Suprarenal gland **3** Adrenal Gland, Right *See 2 Adrenal Gland, Left* **4** Adrenal Glands, Bilateral *See 2 Adrenal Gland, Left* **6** Carotid Body, Left Carotid glomus **7** Carotid Body, Right *See 6 Carotid Body, Left* **8** Carotid Bodies, Bilateral *See 6 Carotid Body, Left* **9** Para-aortic Body **B** Coccygeal Glomus Coccygeal body **C** Glomus Jugulare Jugular body **D** Aortic Body **F** Paraganglion Extremity **G** Thyroid Gland Lobe, Left **H** Thyroid Gland Lobe, Right **K** Thyroid Gland **L** Superior Parathyroid Gland, Right **M** Superior Parathyroid Gland, Left **N** Inferior Parathyroid Gland, Right **P** Inferior Parathyroid Gland, Left **Q** Parathyroid Glands, Multiple **R** Parathyroid Gland	**Ø** Open **3** Percutaneous **4** Percutaneous Endoscopic	**Z** No Device	**Z** No Qualifier

Ø Medical and Surgical
G Endocrine System
H Insertion Definition: Putting in a nonbiological appliance that monitors, assists, performs, or prevents a physiological function but does not physically take the place of a body part

Explanation: None

Body Part Character 4	Approach Character 5	Device Character 6	Qualifier Character 7
S Endocrine Gland	Ø Open 3 Percutaneous 4 Percutaneous Endoscopic	2 Monitoring Device 3 Infusion Device Y Other Device	Z No Qualifier

Non-OR ØGHS[3,4]YZ

Ø Medical and Surgical
G Endocrine System
J Inspection Definition: Visually and/or manually exploring a body part

Explanation: Visual exploration may be performed with or without optical instrumentation. Manual exploration may be performed directly or through intervening body layers.

Body Part Character 4	Approach Character 5	Device Character 6	Qualifier Character 7
Ø Pituitary Gland Adenohypophysis Hypophysis Neurohypophysis 1 Pineal Body 5 Adrenal Gland Suprarenal gland K Thyroid Gland R Parathyroid Gland S Endocrine Gland	Ø Open 3 Percutaneous 4 Percutaneous Endoscopic	Z No Device	Z No Qualifier

Non-OR ØGJ[Ø,1,5,K,R,S]3ZZ

Ø Medical and Surgical
G Endocrine System
M Reattachment Definition: Putting back in or on all or a portion of a separated body part to its normal location or other suitable location

Explanation: Vascular circulation and nervous pathways may or may not be reestablished

Body Part Character 4	Approach Character 5	Device Character 6	Qualifier Character 7
2 Adrenal Gland, Left Suprarenal gland 3 Adrenal Gland, Right *See 2 Adrenal Gland, Left* G Thyroid Gland Lobe, Left H Thyroid Gland Lobe, Right L Superior Parathyroid Gland, Right M Superior Parathyroid Gland, Left N Inferior Parathyroid Gland, Right P Inferior Parathyroid Gland, Left Q Parathyroid Glands, Multiple R Parathyroid Gland	Ø Open 4 Percutaneous Endoscopic	Z No Device	Z No Qualifier

Ø Medical and Surgical
G Endocrine System
N Release Definition: Freeing a body part from an abnormal physical constraint by cutting or by the use of force
Explanation: Some of the restraining tissue may be taken out but none of the body part is taken out

Body Part Character 4	Approach Character 5	Device Character 6	Qualifier Character 7
Ø Pituitary Gland Adenohypophysis Hypophysis Neurohypophysis 1 Pineal Body 2 Adrenal Gland, Left Suprarenal gland 3 Adrenal Gland, Right *See 2 Adrenal Gland, Left* 4 Adrenal Glands, Bilateral *See 2 Adrenal Gland, Left* 6 Carotid Body, Left Carotid glomus 7 Carotid Body, Right *See 6 Carotid Body, Left* 8 Carotid Bodies, Bilateral *See 6 Carotid Body, Left* 9 Para-aortic Body B Coccygeal Glomus Coccygeal body C Glomus Jugulare Jugular body D Aortic Body F Paraganglion Extremity G Thyroid Gland Lobe, Left H Thyroid Gland Lobe, Right K Thyroid Gland L Superior Parathyroid Gland, Right M Superior Parathyroid Gland, Left N Inferior Parathyroid Gland, Right P Inferior Parathyroid Gland, Left Q Parathyroid Glands, Multiple R Parathyroid Gland	Ø Open 3 Percutaneous 4 Percutaneous Endoscopic	Z No Device	Z No Qualifier

Non-OR ØGN[6,7,8,9,B,C,D,F][Ø,3,4]ZZ

Ø Medical and Surgical
G Endocrine System
P Removal Definition: Taking out or off a device from a body part
Explanation: If a device is taken out and a similar device put in without cutting or puncturing the skin or mucous membrane, the procedure is coded to the root operation CHANGE. Otherwise, the procedure for taking out a device is coded to the root operation REMOVAL.

Body Part Character 4	Approach Character 5	Device Character 6	Qualifier Character 7
Ø Pituitary Gland Adenohypophysis Hypophysis Neurohypophysis 1 Pineal Body 5 Adrenal Gland Suprarenal gland K Thyroid Gland R Parathyroid Gland	Ø Open 3 Percutaneous 4 Percutaneous Endoscopic X External	Ø Drainage Device	Z No Qualifier
S Endocrine Gland	Ø Open 3 Percutaneous 4 Percutaneous Endoscopic	Ø Drainage Device 2 Monitoring Device 3 Infusion Device Y Other Device	Z No Qualifier
S Endocrine Gland	X External	Ø Drainage Device 2 Monitoring Device 3 Infusion Device	Z No Qualifier

Non-OR ØGP[Ø,1,5,K,R]XØZ
Non-OR ØGPS[3,4]YZ
Non-OR ØGPSX[Ø,2,3]Z

Ø Medical and Surgical
G Endocrine System
Q Repair Definition: Restoring, to the extent possible, a body part to its normal anatomic structure and function

Explanation: Used only when the method to accomplish the repair is not one of the other root operations

Body Part Character 4	Approach Character 5	Device Character 6	Qualifier Character 7
Ø Pituitary Gland Adenohypophysis Hypophysis Neurohypophysis 1 Pineal Body 2 Adrenal Gland, Left Suprarenal gland 3 Adrenal Gland, Right *See 2 Adrenal Gland, Left* 4 Adrenal Glands, Bilateral *See 2 Adrenal Gland, Left* 6 Carotid Body, Left Carotid glomus 7 Carotid Body, Right *See 6 Carotid Body, Left* 8 Carotid Bodies, Bilateral *See 6 Carotid Body, Left* 9 Para-aortic Body B Coccygeal Glomus Coccygeal body C Glomus Jugulare Jugular body D Aortic Body F Paraganglion Extremity G Thyroid Gland Lobe, Left H Thyroid Gland Lobe, Right J Thyroid Gland Isthmus K Thyroid Gland L Superior Parathyroid Gland, Right M Superior Parathyroid Gland, Left N Inferior Parathyroid Gland, Right P Inferior Parathyroid Gland, Left Q Parathyroid Glands, Multiple R Parathyroid Gland	Ø Open 3 Percutaneous 4 Percutaneous Endoscopic	Z No Device	Z No Qualifier

Ø Medical and Surgical
G Endocrine System
S Reposition Definition: Moving to its normal location, or other suitable location, all or a portion of a body part

Explanation: The body part is moved to a new location from an abnormal location, or from a normal location where it is not functioning correctly. The body part may or may not be cut out or off to be moved to the new location.

Body Part Character 4	Approach Character 5	Device Character 6	Qualifier Character 7
2 Adrenal Gland, Left Suprarenal gland 3 Adrenal Gland, Right *See 2 Adrenal Gland, Left* G Thyroid Gland Lobe, Left H Thyroid Gland Lobe, Right L Superior Parathyroid Gland, Right M Superior Parathyroid Gland, Left N Inferior Parathyroid Gland, Right P Inferior Parathyroid Gland, Left Q Parathyroid Glands, Multiple R Parathyroid Gland	Ø Open 4 Percutaneous Endoscopic	Z No Device	Z No Qualifier

Ø Medical and Surgical
G Endocrine System
T Resection Definition: Cutting out or off, without replacement, all of a body part
Explanation: None

Body Part Character 4	Approach Character 5	Device Character 6	Qualifier Character 7
Ø Pituitary Gland Adenohypophysis Hypophysis Neurohypophysis **1** Pineal Body **2** Adrenal Gland, Left Suprarenal gland **3** Adrenal Gland, Right *See 2 Adrenal Gland, Left* **4** Adrenal Glands, Bilateral *See 2 Adrenal Gland, Left* **6** Carotid Body, Left Carotid glomus **7** Carotid Body, Right *See 6 Carotid Body, Left* **8** Carotid Bodies, Bilateral *See 6 Carotid Body, Left* **9** Para-aortic Body **B** Coccygeal Glomus Coccygeal body **C** Glomus Jugulare Jugular body **D** Aortic Body **F** Paraganglion Extremity **G** Thyroid Gland Lobe, Left **H** Thyroid Gland Lobe, Right **J** Thyroid Gland Isthmus **K** Thyroid Gland **L** Superior Parathyroid Gland, Right **M** Superior Parathyroid Gland, Left **N** Inferior Parathyroid Gland, Right **P** Inferior Parathyroid Gland, Left **Q** Parathyroid Glands, Multiple **R** Parathyroid Gland	**Ø** Open **4** Percutaneous Endoscopic	**Z** No Device	**Z** No Qualifier

Non-OR ØGT[6,7,8,9,B,C,D,F][Ø,4]ZZ

Ø Medical and Surgical
G Endocrine System
W Revision Definition: Correcting, to the extent possible, a portion of a malfunctioning device or the position of a displaced device
Explanation: Revision can include correcting a malfunctioning or displaced device by taking out or putting in components of the device such as a screw or pin

Body Part Character 4	Approach Character 5	Device Character 6	Qualifier Character 7
Ø Pituitary Gland Adenohypophysis Hypophysis Neurohypophysis **1** Pineal Body **5** Adrenal Gland Suprarenal gland **K** Thyroid Gland **R** Parathyroid Gland	**Ø** Open **3** Percutaneous **4** Percutaneous Endoscopic **X** External	**Ø** Drainage Device	**Z** No Qualifier
S Endocrine Gland	**Ø** Open **3** Percutaneous **4** Percutaneous Endoscopic	**Ø** Drainage Device **2** Monitoring Device **3** Infusion Device **Y** Other Device	**Z** No Qualifier
S Endocrine Gland	**X** External	**Ø** Drainage Device **2** Monitoring Device **3** Infusion Device	**Z** No Qualifier

Non-OR ØGW[Ø,1,5,K,R]XØZ
Non-OR ØGWS[3,4]YZ
Non-OR ØGWSX[Ø,2,3]Z

Skin and Breast ØHØ–ØHX

Character Meanings*

This Character Meaning table is provided as a guide to assist the user in the identification of character members that may be found in this section of code tables. It **SHOULD NOT** be used to build a PCS code.

Operation–Character 3	Body Part–Character 4	Approach–Character 5	Device–Character 6	Qualifier–Character 7
Ø Alteration	Ø Skin, Scalp	Ø Open	Ø Drainage Device	3 Full Thickness
2 Change	1 Skin, Face	3 Percutaneous	1 Radioactive Element	4 Partial Thickness
5 Destruction	2 Skin, Right Ear	7 Via Natural or Artificial Opening	7 Autologous Tissue Substitute	5 Latissimus Dorsi Myocutaneous Flap
8 Division	3 Skin, Left Ear	8 Via Natural or Artificial Opening Endoscopic	J Synthetic Substitute	6 Transverse Rectus Abdominis Myocutaneous Flap
9 Drainage	4 Skin, Neck	X External	K Nonautologous Tissue Substitute	7 Deep Inferior Epigastric Artery Perforator Flap
B Excision	5 Skin, Chest		N Tissue Expander	8 Superficial Inferior Epigastric Artery Flap
C Extirpation	6 Skin, Back		Y Other Device	9 Gluteal Artery Perforator Flap
D Extraction	7 Skin, Abdomen		Z No Device	D Multiple
H Insertion	8 Skin, Buttock			X Diagnostic
J Inspection	9 Skin, Perineum			Z No Qualifier
M Reattachment	A Skin, Inguinal			
N Release	B Skin, Right Upper Arm			
P Removal	C Skin, Left Upper Arm			
Q Repair	D Skin, Right Lower Arm			
R Replacement	E Skin, Left Lower Arm			
S Reposition	F Skin, Right Hand			
T Resection	G Skin, Left Hand			
U Supplement	H Skin, Right Upper Leg			
W Revision	J Skin, Left Upper Leg			
X Transfer	K Skin, Right Lower Leg			
	L Skin, Left Lower Leg			
	M Skin, Right Foot			
	N Skin, Left Foot			
	P Skin			
	Q Finger Nail			
	R Toe Nail			
	S Hair			
	T Breast, Right			
	U Breast, Left			
	V Breast, Bilateral			
	W Nipple, Right			
	X Nipple, Left			
	Y Supernumerary Breast			

* Includes skin and breast glands and ducts.

AHA Coding Clinic for table ØHB

2018, 1Q, 14 Excisional debridement of breast tissue and skin
2016, 3Q, 29 Closure of bilateral alveolar clefts
2015, 3Q, 3-8 Excisional and nonexcisional debridement

AHA Coding Clinic for table ØHD

2016, 1Q, 40 Nonexcisional debridement of skin and subcutaneous tissue
2015, 3Q, 3-8 Excisional and nonexcisional debridement

AHA Coding Clinic for table ØHH

2017, 4Q, 67 New qualifier values - Pedicle flap procedures
2014, 2Q, 12 Pedicle latissimus myocutaneous flap with placement of breast tissue expanders
2013, 4Q, 107 Breast tissue expander placement using acellular dermal matrix

AHA Coding Clinic for table ØHP

2016, 2Q, 27 Removal of nonviable transverse rectus abdominis myocutaneous (TRAM) flaps

AHA Coding Clinic for table ØHQ

2018, 2Q, 25 Third and fourth degree obstetric lacerations
2016, 1Q, 7 Obstetrical perineal laceration repair
2014, 4Q, 31 Delayed wound closure following fracture treatment

AHA Coding Clinic for table ØHR

2017, 1Q, 35 Epifix® allograft
2014, 3Q, 14 Application of TheraSkin® and excisional debridement

AHA Coding Clinic for table ØHT

2014, 4Q, 34 Skin-sparing mastectomy

Integumentary Anatomy

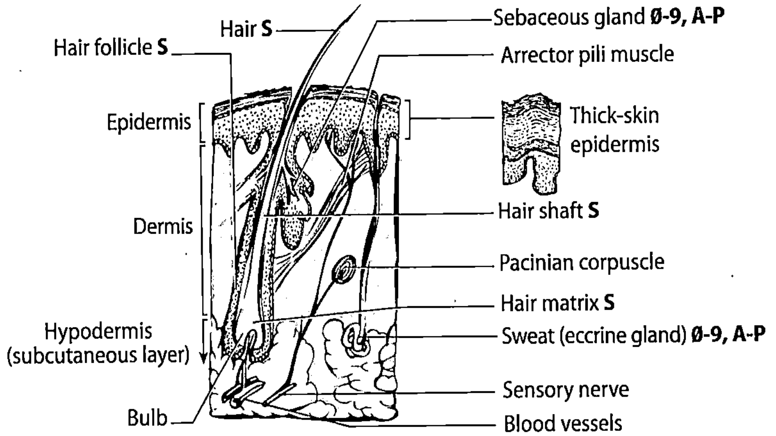

Nail Anatomy

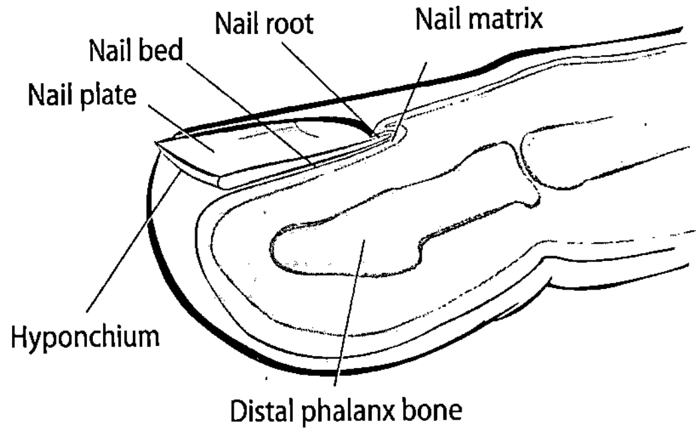

Breast

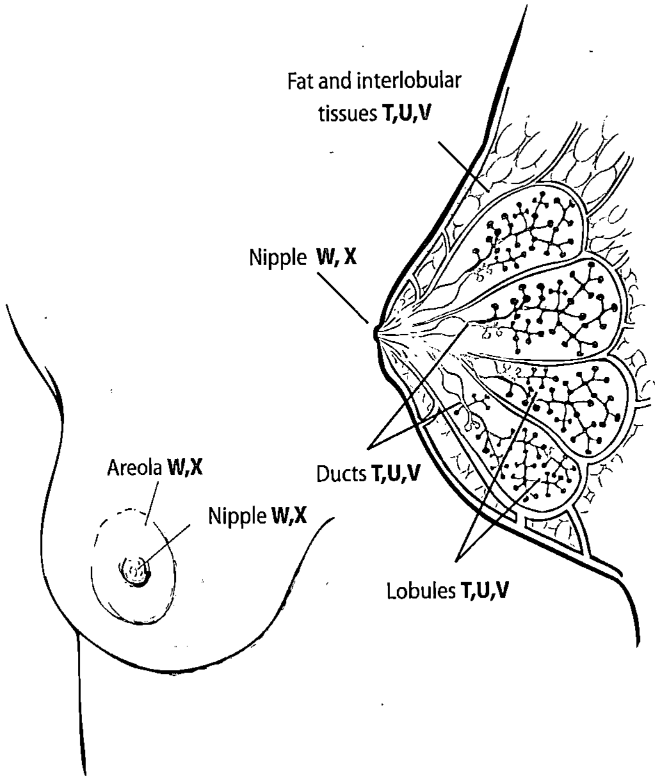

Ø Medical and Surgical
H Skin and Breast
Ø Alteration Definition: Modifying the anatomic structure of a body part without affecting the function of the body part
Explanation: Principal purpose is to improve appearance

Body Part Character 4	Approach Character 5	Device Character 6	Qualifier Character 7
T Breast, Right Mammary duct Mammary gland **U** Breast, Left *See T Breast, Right* **V** Breast, Bilateral *See T Breast, Right*	**Ø** Open **3** Percutaneous **X** External	**7** Autologous Tissue Substitute **J** Synthetic Substitute **K** Nonautologous Tissue Substitute **Z** No Device	**Z** No Qualifier

Non-OR ØHØ[T,U,V]3JZ

Ø Medical and Surgical
H Skin and Breast
2 Change Definition: Taking out or off a device from a body part and putting back an identical or similar device in or on the same body part without cutting or puncturing the skin or a mucous membrane
Explanation: All CHANGE procedures are coded using the approach EXTERNAL

Body Part Character 4	Approach Character 5	Device Character 6	Qualifier Character 7
P Skin Dermis Epidermis Sebaceous gland Sweat gland **T** Breast, Right Mammary duct Mammary gland **U** Breast, Left *See T Breast, Right*	**X** External	**Ø** Drainage Device **Y** Other Device	**Z** No Qualifier

Non-OR All body part, approach, device, and qualifier values

Ø Medical and Surgical
H Skin and Breast
5 Destruction Definition: Physical eradication of all or a portion of a body part by the direct use of energy, force, or a destructive agent
Explanation: None of the body part is physically taken out

Body Part Character 4	Approach Character 5	Device Character 6	Qualifier Character 7
Ø Skin, Scalp **1** Skin, Face **2** Skin, Right Ear **3** Skin, Left Ear **4** Skin, Neck **5** Skin, Chest **6** Skin, Back **7** Skin, Abdomen **8** Skin, Buttock **9** Skin, Perineum **A** Skin, Inguinal **B** Skin, Right Upper Arm **C** Skin, Left Upper Arm **D** Skin, Right Lower Arm **E** Skin, Left Lower Arm **F** Skin, Right Hand **G** Skin, Left Hand **H** Skin, Right Upper Leg **J** Skin, Left Upper Leg **K** Skin, Right Lower Leg **L** Skin, Left Lower Leg **M** Skin, Right Foot **N** Skin, Left Foot	**X** External	**Z** No Device	**D** Multiple **Z** No Qualifier
Q Finger Nail Nail bed Nail plate **R** Toe Nail *See Q Finger Nail*	**X** External	**Z** No Device	**Z** No Qualifier
T Breast, Right Mammary duct Mammary gland **U** Breast, Left *See T Breast, Right* **V** Breast, Bilateral *See T Breast, Right* **W** Nipple, Right Areola **X** Nipple, Left *See W Nipple, Right*	**Ø** Open **3** Percutaneous **7** Via Natural or Artificial Opening **8** Via Natural or Artificial Opening Endoscopic **X** External	**Z** No Device	**Z** No Qualifier

DRG Non-OR ØH5[Ø,1,4,5,6,7,8,9,A,B,C,D,E,F,G,H,J,K,L,M,N]XZ[D,Z]
DRG Non-OR ØH5[Q,R]XZZ
Non-OR ØH5[2,3]XZ[D,Z]

Ø Medical and Surgical
H Skin and Breast
8 Division Definition: Cutting into a body part, without draining fluids and/or gases from the body part, in order to separate or transect a body part
Explanation: All or a portion of the body part is separated into two or more portions

Body Part Character 4	Approach Character 5	Device Character 6	Qualifier Character 7
Ø Skin, Scalp 1 Skin, Face 2 Skin, Right Ear 3 Skin, Left Ear 4 Skin, Neck 5 Skin, Chest 6 Skin, Back 7 Skin, Abdomen 8 Skin, Buttock 9 Skin, Perineum A Skin, Inguinal B Skin, Right Upper Arm C Skin, Left Upper Arm D Skin, Right Lower Arm E Skin, Left Lower Arm F Skin, Right Hand G Skin, Left Hand H Skin, Right Upper Leg J Skin, Left Upper Leg K Skin, Right Lower Leg L Skin, Left Lower Leg M Skin, Right Foot N Skin, Left Foot	X External	Z No Device	Z No Qualifier

Non-OR All body part, approach, device, and qualifier values

Ø Medical and Surgical
H Skin and Breast
9 Drainage Definition: Taking or letting out fluids and/or gases from a body part
Explanation: The qualifier DIAGNOSTIC is used to identify drainage procedures that are biopsies

Body Part Character 4	Approach Character 5	Device Character 6	Qualifier Character 7
Ø Skin, Scalp 1 Skin, Face 2 Skin, Right Ear 3 Skin, Left Ear 4 Skin, Neck 5 Skin, Chest 6 Skin, Back 7 Skin, Abdomen 8 Skin, Buttock 9 Skin, Perineum A Skin, Inguinal B Skin, Right Upper Arm C Skin, Left Upper Arm D Skin, Right Lower Arm E Skin, Left Lower Arm F Skin, Right Hand G Skin, Left Hand H Skin, Right Upper Leg J Skin, Left Upper Leg K Skin, Right Lower Leg L Skin, Left Lower Leg M Skin, Right Foot N Skin, Left Foot Q Finger Nail Nail bed Nail plate R Toe Nail *See Q Finger Nail*	X External	Ø Drainage Device	Z No Qualifier
Ø Skin, Scalp 1 Skin, Face 2 Skin, Right Ear 3 Skin, Left Ear 4 Skin, Neck 5 Skin, Chest 6 Skin, Back 7 Skin, Abdomen 8 Skin, Buttock 9 Skin, Perineum A Skin, Inguinal B Skin, Right Upper Arm C Skin, Left Upper Arm D Skin, Right Lower Arm E Skin, Left Lower Arm F Skin, Right Hand G Skin, Left Hand H Skin, Right Upper Leg J Skin, Left Upper Leg K Skin, Right Lower Leg L Skin, Left Lower Leg M Skin, Right Foot N Skin, Left Foot Q Finger Nail Nail bed Nail plate R Toe Nail *See Q Finger Nail*	X External	Z No Device	X Diagnostic Z No Qualifier
T Breast, Right Mammary duct Mammary gland U Breast, Left *See T Breast, Right* V Breast, Bilateral *See T Breast, Right* W Nipple, Right Areola X Nipple, Left *See W Nipple, Right*	Ø Open 3 Percutaneous 7 Via Natural or Artificial Opening 8 Via Natural or Artificial Opening Endoscopic X External	Ø Drainage Device	Z No Qualifier
T Breast, Right Mammary duct Mammary gland U Breast, Left *See T Breast, Right* V Breast, Bilateral *See T Breast, Right* W Nipple, Right Areola X Nipple, Left *See W Nipple, Right*	Ø Open 3 Percutaneous 7 Via Natural or Artificial Opening 8 Via Natural or Artificial Opening Endoscopic X External	Z No Device	X Diagnostic Z No Qualifier

Non-OR ØH9[Ø,1,2,3,4,5,6,7,8,A,B,C,D,E,F,G,H,J,K,L,M,N,Q,R]XØZ
Non-OR ØH9[Ø,1,2,3,4,5,6,7,8,A,B,C,D,E,F,G,H,J,K,L,M,N,Q,R]XZ[X,Z]
Non-OR ØH99XZX
Non-OR ØH9[T,U,V,W,X][Ø,3,7,8,X]ØZ
Non-OR ØH9[T,U,V,W,X][3,7,8,X]Z[X,Z]
Non-OR ØH9[T,U,V,W,X]ØZZ

Ø Medical and Surgical
H Skin and Breast
B Excision Definition: Cutting out or off, without replacement, a portion of a body part
Explanation: The qualifier DIAGNOSTIC is used to identify excision procedures that are biopsies

Body Part Character 4	Approach Character 5	Device Character 6	Qualifier Character 7
Ø Skin, Scalp 1 Skin, Face 2 Skin, Right Ear 3 Skin, Left Ear 4 Skin, Neck 5 Skin, Chest 6 Skin, Back 7 Skin, Abdomen 8 Skin, Buttock 9 Skin, Perineum A Skin, Inguinal B Skin, Right Upper Arm C Skin, Left Upper Arm D Skin, Right Lower Arm E Skin, Left Lower Arm F Skin, Right Hand G Skin, Left Hand H Skin, Right Upper Leg J Skin, Left Upper Leg K Skin, Right Lower Leg L Skin, Left Lower Leg M Skin, Right Foot N Skin, Left Foot Q Finger Nail Nail bed Nail plate R Toe Nail *See Q Finger Nail*	X External	Z No Device	X Diagnostic Z No Qualifier
T Breast, Right Mammary duct Mammary gland U Breast, Left *See T Breast, Right* V Breast, Bilateral *See T Breast, Right* W Nipple, Right Areola X Nipple, Left *See W Nipple, Right* Y Supernumerary Breast	Ø Open 3 Percutaneous 7 Via Natural or Artificial Opening 8 Via Natural or Artificial Opening Endoscopic X External	Z No Device	X Diagnostic Z No Qualifier

DRG Non-OR ØHB9XZZ
Non-OR ØHB[Ø,1,2,3,4,5,6,7,8,A,B,C,D,E,F,G,H,J,K,L,M,N,Q,R]XZ[X,Z]
Non-OR ØHB9XZX
Non-OR ØHB[T,U,V,W,X,Y][3,7,8,X]ZX

Ø Medical and Surgical
H Skin and Breast
C Extirpation Definition: Taking or cutting out solid matter from a body part

Explanation: The solid matter may be an abnormal byproduct of a biological function or a foreign body; it may be imbedded in a body part or in the lumen of a tubular body part. The solid matter may or may not have been previously broken into pieces.

Body Part Character 4	Approach Character 5	Device Character 6	Qualifier Character 7
Ø Skin, Scalp 1 Skin, Face 2 Skin, Right Ear 3 Skin, Left Ear 4 Skin, Neck 5 Skin, Chest 6 Skin, Back 7 Skin, Abdomen 8 Skin, Buttock 9 Skin, Perineum A Skin, Inguinal B Skin, Right Upper Arm C Skin, Left Upper Arm D Skin, Right Lower Arm E Skin, Left Lower Arm F Skin, Right Hand G Skin, Left Hand H Skin, Right Upper Leg J Skin, Left Upper Leg K Skin, Right Lower Leg L Skin, Left Lower Leg M Skin, Right Foot N Skin, Left Foot Q Finger Nail Nail bed Nail plate R Toe Nail *See Q Finger Nail*	X External	Z No Device	Z No Qualifier
T Breast, Right Mammary duct Mammary gland U Breast, Left *See T Breast, Right* V Breast, Bilateral *See T Breast, Right* W Nipple, Right Areola X Nipple, Left *See W Nipple, Right*	Ø Open 3 Percutaneous 7 Via Natural or Artificial Opening 8 Via Natural or Artificial Opening Endoscopic X External	Z No Device	Z No Qualifier

Non-OR All body part, approach, device and qualifier values

Ø Medical and Surgical
H Skin and Breast
D Extraction Definition: Pulling or stripping out or off all or a portion of a body part by the use of force
Explanation: The qualifier DIAGNOSTIC is used to identify extraction procedures that are biopsies

Body Part Character 4	Approach Character 5	Device Character 6	Qualifier Character 7
Ø Skin, Scalp **1** Skin, Face **2** Skin, Right Ear **3** Skin, Left Ear **4** Skin, Neck **5** Skin, Chest **6** Skin, Back **7** Skin, Abdomen **8** Skin, Buttock **9** Skin, Perineum **A** Skin, Inguinal **B** Skin, Right Upper Arm **C** Skin, Left Upper Arm **D** Skin, Right Lower Arm **E** Skin, Left Lower Arm **F** Skin, Right Hand **G** Skin, Left Hand **H** Skin, Right Upper Leg **J** Skin, Left Upper Leg **K** Skin, Right Lower Leg **L** Skin, Left Lower Leg **M** Skin, Right Foot **N** Skin, Left Foot **Q** Finger Nail Nail bed Nail plate **R** Toe Nail *See Q Finger Nail* **S** Hair	**X** External	**Z** No Device	**Z** No Qualifier

Non-OR All body part, approach, device, and qualifier values

Ø Medical and Surgical
H Skin and Breast
H Insertion Definition: Putting in a nonbiological appliance that monitors, assists, performs, or prevents a physiological function but does not physically take the place of a body part
Explanation: None

Body Part Character 4	Approach Character 5	Device Character 6	Qualifier Character 7
P Skin	**X** External	**Y** Other Device	**Z** No Qualifier
T Breast, Right Mammary duct Mammary gland **U** Breast, Left *See T Breast, Right*	**Ø** Open **3** Percutaneous **7** Via Natural or Artificial Opening **8** Via Natural or Artificial Opening Endoscopic	**1** Radioactive Element **N** Tissue Expander **Y** Other Device	**Z** No Qualifier
T Breast, Right Mammary duct Mammary gland **U** Breast, Left *See T Breast, Right*	**X** External	**1** Radioactive Element	**Z** No Qualifier
V Breast, Bilateral *See T Breast, Right* **W** Nipple, Right Areola **X** Nipple, Left *See W Nipple, Right*	**Ø** Open **3** Percutaneous **7** Via Natural or Artificial Opening **8** Via Natural or Artificial Opening Endoscopic	**1** Radioactive Element **N** Tissue Expander	**Z** No Qualifier
V Breast, Bilateral *See T Breast, Right* **W** Nipple, Right Areola **X** Nipple, Left *See W Nipple, Right*	**X** External	**1** Radioactive Element	**Z** No Qualifier

Non-OR ØHHPXYZ
Non-OR ØHH[T,U][3,7,8]YZ

Ø Medical and Surgical
H Skin and Breast
J Inspection Definition: Visually and/or manually exploring a body part
Explanation: Visual exploration may be performed with or without optical instrumentation. Manual exploration may be performed directly or through intervening body layers.

Body Part Character 4	Approach Character 5	Device Character 6	Qualifier Character 7
P Skin Dermis Epidermis Sebaceous gland Sweat gland **Q** Finger Nail Nail bed Nail plate **R** Toe Nail *See Q Finger Nail*	**X** External	**Z** No Device	**Z** No Qualifier
T Breast, Right Mammary duct Mammary gland **U** Breast, Left *See T Breast, Right*	**Ø** Open **3** Percutaneous **7** Via Natural or Artificial Opening **8** Via Natural or Artificial Opening Endoscopic **X** External	**Z** No Device	**Z** No Qualifier

Non-OR All body part, approach, device and qualifier values

Ø Medical and Surgical
H Skin and Breast
M Reattachment Definition: Putting back in or on all or a portion of a separated body part to its normal location or other suitable location
Explanation: Vascular circulation and nervous pathways may or may not be reestablished

Body Part Character 4	Approach Character 5	Device Character 6	Qualifier Character 7
Ø Skin, Scalp **1** Skin, Face **2** Skin, Right Ear **3** Skin, Left Ear **4** Skin, Neck **5** Skin, Chest **6** Skin, Back **7** Skin, Abdomen **8** Skin, Buttock **9** Skin, Perineum **A** Skin, Inguinal **B** Skin, Right Upper Arm **C** Skin, Left Upper Arm **D** Skin, Right Lower Arm **E** Skin, Left Lower Arm **F** Skin, Right Hand **G** Skin, Left Hand **H** Skin, Right Upper Leg **J** Skin, Left Upper Leg **K** Skin, Right Lower Leg **L** Skin, Left Lower Leg **M** Skin, Right Foot **N** Skin, Left Foot **T** Breast, Right Mammary duct Mammary gland **U** Breast, Left *See T Breast, Right* **V** Breast, Bilateral *See T Breast, Right* **W** Nipple, Right Areola **X** Nipple, Left *See W Nipple, Right*	**X** External	**Z** No Device	**Z** No Qualifier

Non-OR ØHMØXZZ

Ø Medical and Surgical
H Skin and Breast
N Release Definition: Freeing a body part from an abnormal physical constraint by cutting or by the use of force
Explanation: Some of the restraining tissue may be taken out but none of the body part is taken out

Body Part Character 4	Approach Character 5	Device Character 6	Qualifier Character 7
Ø Skin, Scalp **1** Skin, Face **2** Skin, Right Ear **3** Skin, Left Ear **4** Skin, Neck **5** Skin, Chest **6** Skin, Back **7** Skin, Abdomen **8** Skin, Buttock **9** Skin, Perineum **A** Skin, Inguinal **B** Skin, Right Upper Arm **C** Skin, Left Upper Arm **D** Skin, Right Lower Arm **E** Skin, Left Lower Arm **F** Skin, Right Hand **G** Skin, Left Hand **H** Skin, Right Upper Leg **J** Skin, Left Upper Leg **K** Skin, Right Lower Leg **L** Skin, Left Lower Leg **M** Skin, Right Foot **N** Skin, Left Foot **Q** Finger Nail Nail bed Nail plate **R** Toe Nail *See Q Finger Nail*	**X** External	**Z** No Device	**Z** No Qualifier
T Breast, Right Mammary duct Mammary gland **U** Breast, Left *See T Breast, Right* **V** Breast, Bilateral *See T Breast, Right* **W** Nipple, Right Areola **X** Nipple, Left *See W Nipple, Right*	**Ø** Open **3** Percutaneous **7** Via Natural or Artificial Opening **8** Via Natural or Artificial Opening Endoscopic **X** External	**Z** No Device	**Z** No Qualifier

Skin and Breast

Ø Medical and Surgical
H Skin and Breast
P Removal Definition: Taking out or off a device from a body part

Explanation: If a device is taken out and a similar device put in without cutting or puncturing the skin or mucous membrane, the procedure is coded to the root operation CHANGE. Otherwise, the procedure for taking out a device is coded to the root operation REMOVAL.

Body Part Character 4	Approach Character 5	Device Character 6	Qualifier Character 7
P Skin Dermis Epidermis Sebaceous gland Sweat gland	**X** External	**Ø** Drainage Device **7** Autologous Tissue Substitute **J** Synthetic Substitute **K** Nonautologous Tissue Substitute **Y** Other Device	**Z** No Qualifier
Q Finger Nail Nail bed Nail plate **R** Toe Nail *See Q Finger Nail*	**X** External	**Ø** Drainage Device **7** Autologous Tissue Substitute **J** Synthetic Substitute **K** Nonautologous Tissue Substitute	**Z** No Qualifier
S Hair	**X** External	**7** Autologous Tissue Substitute **J** Synthetic Substitute **K** Nonautologous Tissue Substitute	**Z** No Qualifier
T Breast, Right Mammary duct Mammary gland **U** Breast, Left *See T Breast, Right*	**Ø** Open **3** Percutaneous **7** Via Natural or Artificial Opening **8** Via Natural or Artificial Opening Endoscopic	**Ø** Drainage Device **1** Radioactive Element **7** Autologous Tissue Substitute **J** Synthetic Substitute **K** Nonautologous Tissue Substitute **N** Tissue Expander **Y** Other Device	**Z** No Qualifier
T Breast, Right Mammary duct Mammary gland **U** Breast, Left *See T Breast, Right*	**X** External	**Ø** Drainage Device **1** Radioactive Element **7** Autologous Tissue Substitute **J** Synthetic Substitute **K** Nonautologous Tissue Substitute	**Z** No Qualifier

Non-OR ØHPPX[Ø,7,J,K,Y]Z
Non-OR ØHP[Q,R]X[Ø,7,J,K]Z
Non-OR ØHPSX[7,J,K]Z
Non-OR ØHP[T,U]Ø[Ø,1,7,K]Z
Non-OR ØHP[T,U]3[Ø,1,7,K,Y]Z
Non-OR ØHP[T,U][7,8][Ø,1,7,J,K,N,Y]Z
Non-OR ØHP[T,U]X[Ø,1,7,J,K]Z

Ø Medical and Surgical
H Skin and Breast
Q Repair Definition: Restoring, to the extent possible, a body part to its normal anatomic structure and function
Explanation: Used only when the method to accomplish the repair is not one of the other root operations

Body Part Character 4	Approach Character 5	Device Character 6	Qualifier Character 7
Ø Skin, Scalp **1** Skin, Face **2** Skin, Right Ear **3** Skin, Left Ear **4** Skin, Neck **5** Skin, Chest **6** Skin, Back **7** Skin, Abdomen **8** Skin, Buttock **9** Skin, Perineum **A** Skin, Inguinal **B** Skin, Right Upper Arm **C** Skin, Left Upper Arm **D** Skin, Right Lower Arm **E** Skin, Left Lower Arm **F** Skin, Right Hand **G** Skin, Left Hand **H** Skin, Right Upper Leg **J** Skin, Left Upper Leg **K** Skin, Right Lower Leg **L** Skin, Left Lower Leg **M** Skin, Right Foot **N** Skin, Left Foot **Q** Finger Nail Nail bed Nail plate **R** Toe Nail *See Q Finger Nail*	**X** External	**Z** No Device	**Z** No Qualifier
T Breast, Right Mammary duct Mammary gland **U** Breast, Left *See T Breast, Right* **V** Breast, Bilateral *See T Breast, Right* **W** Nipple, Right Areola **X** Nipple, Left *See W Nipple, Right* **Y** Supernumerary Breast	**Ø** Open **3** Percutaneous **7** Via Natural or Artificial Opening **8** Via Natural or Artificial Opening Endoscopic **X** External	**Z** No Device	**Z** No Qualifier

DRG Non-OR ØHQ9XZZ
Non-OR ØHQ[Ø,1,2,3,4,5,6,7,8,A,B,C,D,E,F,G,H,J,K,L,M,N]XZZ
Non-OR ØHQ[T,U,V,Y]XZZ

Ø Medical and Surgical
H Skin and Breast
R Replacement Definition: Putting in or on biological or synthetic material that physically takes the place and/or function of all or a portion of a body part

Explanation: The body part may have been taken out or replaced, or may be taken out, physically eradicated, or rendered nonfunctional during the REPLACEMENT procedure. A REMOVAL procedure is coded for taking out the device used in a previous replacement procedure.

Body Part Character 4	Approach Character 5	Device Character 6	Qualifier Character 7
Ø Skin, Scalp 1 Skin, Face 2 Skin, Right Ear 3 Skin, Left Ear 4 Skin, Neck 5 Skin, Chest 6 Skin, Back 7 Skin, Abdomen 8 Skin, Buttock 9 Skin, Perineum A Skin, Inguinal B Skin, Right Upper Arm C Skin, Left Upper Arm D Skin, Right Lower Arm E Skin, Left Lower Arm F Skin, Right Hand G Skin, Left Hand H Skin, Right Upper Leg J Skin, Left Upper Leg K Skin, Right Lower Leg L Skin, Left Lower Leg M Skin, Right Foot N Skin, Left Foot	X External	7 Autologous Tissue Substitute K Nonautologous Tissue Substitute	3 Full Thickness 4 Partial Thickness
Ø Skin, Scalp 1 Skin, Face 2 Skin, Right Ear 3 Skin, Left Ear 4 Skin, Neck 5 Skin, Chest 6 Skin, Back 7 Skin, Abdomen 8 Skin, Buttock 9 Skin, Perineum A Skin, Inguinal B Skin, Right Upper Arm C Skin, Left Upper Arm D Skin, Right Lower Arm E Skin, Left Lower Arm F Skin, Right Hand G Skin, Left Hand H Skin, Right Upper Leg J Skin, Left Upper Leg K Skin, Right Lower Leg L Skin, Left Lower Leg M Skin, Right Foot N Skin, Left Foot	X External	J Synthetic Substitute	3 Full Thickness 4 Partial Thickness Z No Qualifier
Q Finger Nail Nail bed Nail plate R Toe Nail *See Q Finger Nail* S Hair	X External	7 Autologous Tissue Substitute J Synthetic Substitute K Nonautologous Tissue Substitute	Z No Qualifier
T Breast, Right Mammary duct Mammary gland U Breast, Left *See T Breast, Right* V Breast, Bilateral *See T Breast, Right*	Ø Open	7 Autologous Tissue Substitute	5 Latissimus Dorsi Myocutaneous Flap 6 Transverse Rectus Abdominis Myocutaneous Flap 7 Deep Inferior Epigastric Artery Perforator Flap 8 Superficial Inferior Epigastric Artery Flap 9 Gluteal Artery Perforator Flap Z No Qualifier
T Breast, Right Mammary duct Mammary gland U Breast, Left *See T Breast, Right* V Breast, Bilateral *See T Breast, Right*	Ø Open	J Synthetic Substitute K Nonautologous Tissue Substitute	Z No Qualifier
T Breast, Right ⊞ Mammary duct Mammary gland U Breast, Left ⊞ *See T Breast, Right* V Breast, Bilateral ⊞ *See T Breast, Right*	3 Percutaneous X External	7 Autologous Tissue Substitute J Synthetic Substitute K Nonautologous Tissue Substitute	Z No Qualifier
W Nipple, Right Areola X Nipple, Left *See W Nipple, Right*	Ø Open 3 Percutaneous X External	7 Autologous Tissue Substitute J Synthetic Substitute K Nonautologous Tissue Substitute	Z No Qualifier

Non-OR ØHRSX7Z

See Appendix L for Procedure Combinations
⊞ ØHR[T,U,V]37Z

Ø Medical and Surgical
H Skin and Breast
S Reposition Definition: Moving to its normal location, or other suitable location, all or a portion of a body part

Explanation: The body part is moved to a new location from an abnormal location, or from a normal location where it is not functioning correctly. The body part may or may not be cut out or off to be moved to the new location.

Body Part Character 4	Approach Character 5	Device Character 6	Qualifier Character 7
S Hair **W** Nipple, Right Areola **X** Nipple, Left *See W Nipple, Right*	**X** External	**Z** No Device	**Z** No Qualifier
T Breast, Right Mammary duct Mammary gland **U** Breast, Left *See T Breast, Right* **V** Breast, Bilateral *See T Breast, Right*	**Ø** Open	**Z** No Device	**Z** No Qualifier

Non-OR ØHSSXZZ

Ø Medical and Surgical
H Skin and Breast
T Resection Definition: Cutting out or off, without replacement, all of a body part

Explanation: None

Body Part Character 4	Approach Character 5	Device Character 6	Qualifier Character 7
Q Finger Nail Nail bed Nail plate **R** Toe Nail *See Q Finger Nail* **W** Nipple, Right Areola **X** Nipple, Left *See W Nipple, Right*	**X** External	**Z** No Device	**Z** No Qualifier
T Breast, Right ⊞ Mammary duct Mammary gland **U** Breast, Left ⊞ *See T Breast, Right* **V** Breast, Bilateral ⊞ *See T Breast, Right* **Y** Supernumerary Breast	**Ø** Open	**Z** No Device	**Z** No Qualifier

Non-OR ØHT[Q,R]XZZ

See Appendix L for Procedure Combinations
⊞ ØHT[T,U,V]ØZZ

Ø Medical and Surgical
H Skin and Breast
U Supplement Definition: Putting in or on biological or synthetic material that physically reinforces and/or augments the function of a portion of a body part

Explanation: The biological material is non-living, or is living and from the same individual. The body part may have been previously replaced, and the SUPPLEMENT procedure is performed to physically reinforce and/or augment the function of the replaced body part.

Body Part Character 4	Approach Character 5	Device Character 6	Qualifier Character 7
T Breast, Right Mammary duct Mammary gland **U** Breast, Left *See T Breast, Right* **V** Breast, Bilateral *See T Breast, Right* **W** Nipple, Right Areola **X** Nipple, Left *See W Nipple, Right*	**Ø** Open **3** Percutaneous **7** Via Natural or Artificial Opening **8** Via Natural or Artificial Opening Endoscopic **X** External	**7** Autologous Tissue Substitute **J** Synthetic Substitute **K** Nonautologous Tissue Substitute	**Z** No Qualifier

Non-OR ØHU[T,U,V]3JZ

Ø Medical and Surgical
H Skin and Breast
W Revision Definition: Correcting, to the extent possible, a portion of a malfunctioning device or the position of a displaced device

Explanation: Revision can include correcting a malfunctioning or displaced device by taking out or putting in components of the device such as a screw or pin

Body Part Character 4	Approach Character 5	Device Character 6	Qualifier Character 7
P Skin Dermis Epidermis Sebaceous gland Sweat gland	**X** External	**Ø** Drainage Device **7** Autologous Tissue Substitute **J** Synthetic Substitute **K** Nonautologous Tissue Substitute **Y** Other Device	**Z** No Qualifier
Q Finger Nail Nail bed Nail plate **R** Toe Nail *See Q Finger Nail*	**X** External	**Ø** Drainage Device **7** Autologous Tissue Substitute **J** Synthetic Substitute **K** Nonautologous Tissue Substitute	**Z** No Qualifier
S Hair	**X** External	**7** Autologous Tissue Substitute **J** Synthetic Substitute **K** Nonautologous Tissue Substitute	**Z** No Qualifier
T Breast, Right Mammary duct Mammary gland **U** Breast, Left *See T Breast, Right*	**Ø** Open **3** Percutaneous **7** Via Natural or Artificial Opening **8** Via Natural or Artificial Opening Endoscopic	**Ø** Drainage Device **7** Autologous Tissue Substitute **J** Synthetic Substitute **K** Nonautologous Tissue Substitute **N** Tissue Expander **Y** Other Device	**Z** No Qualifier
T Breast, Right Mammary duct Mammary gland **U** Breast, Left *See T Breast, Right*	**X** External	**Ø** Drainage Device **7** Autologous Tissue Substitute **J** Synthetic Substitute **K** Nonautologous Tissue Substitute	**Z** No Qualifier

Non-OR ØHWPX[Ø,7,J,K,Y]Z
Non-OR ØHW[Q,R]X[Ø,7,J,K]Z
Non-OR ØHWSX[7,J,K]Z
Non-OR ØHW[T,U]Ø[Ø,7,K,N]Z
Non-OR ØHW[T,U]3[Ø,7,K,N,Y]Z
Non-OR ØHW[T,U][7,8][Ø,7,J,K,N,Y]Z
Non-OR ØHW[T,U]X[Ø,7,J,K]Z

Ø Medical and Surgical
H Skin and Breast
X Transfer Definition: Moving, without taking out, all or a portion of a body part to another location to take over the function of all or a portion of a body part

Explanation: The body part transferred remains connected to its vascular and nervous supply

Body Part Character 4	Approach Character 5	Device Character 6	Qualifier Character 7
Ø Skin, Scalp **1** Skin, Face **2** Skin, Right Ear **3** Skin, Left Ear **4** Skin, Neck **5** Skin, Chest **6** Skin, Back **7** Skin, Abdomen **8** Skin, Buttock **9** Skin, Perineum **A** Skin, Inguinal **B** Skin, Right Upper Arm **C** Skin, Left Upper Arm **D** Skin, Right Lower Arm **E** Skin, Left Lower Arm **F** Skin, Right Hand **G** Skin, Left Hand **H** Skin, Right Upper Leg **J** Skin, Left Upper Leg **K** Skin, Right Lower Leg **L** Skin, Left Lower Leg **M** Skin, Right Foot **N** Skin, Left Foot	**X** External	**Z** No Device	**Z** No Qualifier

Subcutaneous Tissue and Fascia ØJØ–ØJX

Character Meanings

This Character Meaning table is provided as a guide to assist the user in the identification of character members that may be found in this section of code tables. It **SHOULD NOT** be used to build a PCS code.

Operation–Character 3	Body Part–Character 4	Approach–Character 5	Device–Character 6	Qualifier–Character 7
Ø Alteration	Ø Subcutaneous Tissue and Fascia, Scalp	Ø Open	Ø Drainage Device OR Monitoring Device, Hemodynamic	B Skin and Subcutaneous Tissue
2 Change	1 Subcutaneous Tissue and Fascia, Face	3 Percutaneous	1 Radioactive Element	C Skin, Subcutaneous Tissue and Fascia
5 Destruction	4 Subcutaneous Tissue and Fascia, Right Neck	X External	2 Monitoring Device	X Diagnostic
8 Division	5 Subcutaneous Tissue and Fascia, Left Neck		3 Infusion Device	Z No Qualifier
9 Drainage	6 Subcutaneous Tissue and Fascia, Chest		4 Pacemaker, Single Chamber	
B Excision	7 Subcutaneous Tissue and Fascia, Back		5 Pacemaker, Single Chamber Rate Responsive	
C Extirpation	8 Subcutaneous Tissue and Fascia, Abdomen		6 Pacemaker, Dual Chamber	
D Extraction	9 Subcutaneous Tissue and Fascia, Buttock		7 Autologous Tissue Substitute OR Cardiac Resynchronization Pacemaker Pulse Generator	
H Insertion	B Subcutaneous Tissue and Fascia, Perineum		8 Defibrillator Generator	
J Inspection	C Subcutaneous Tissue and Fascia, Pelvic Region		9 Cardiac Resynchronization Defibrillator Pulse Generator	
N Release	D Subcutaneous Tissue and Fascia, Right Upper Arm		A Contractility Modulation Device	
P Removal	F Subcutaneous Tissue and Fascia, Left Upper Arm		B Stimulator Generator, Single Array	
Q Repair	G Subcutaneous Tissue and Fascia, Right Lower Arm		C Stimulator Generator, Single Array Rechargeable	
R Replacement	H Subcutaneous Tissue and Fascia, Left Lower Arm		D Stimulator Generator, Multiple Array	
U Supplement	J Subcutaneous Tissue and Fascia, Right Hand		E Stimulator Generator, Multiple Array Rechargeable	
W Revision	K Subcutaneous Tissue and Fascia, Left Hand		H Contraceptive Device	
X Transfer	L Subcutaneous Tissue and Fascia, Right Upper Leg		J Synthetic Substitute	
	M Subcutaneous Tissue and Fascia, Left Upper Leg		K Nonautologous Tissue Substitute	
	N Subcutaneous Tissue and Fascia, Right Lower Leg		M Stimulator Generator	
	P Subcutaneous Tissue and Fascia, Left Lower Leg		N Tissue Expander	
	Q Subcutaneous Tissue and Fascia, Right Foot		P Cardiac Rhythm Related Device	
	R Subcutaneous Tissue and Fascia, Left Foot		V Infusion Device, Pump	
	S Subcutaneous Tissue and Fascia, Head and Neck		W Vascular Access Device, Totally Implantable	
	T Subcutaneous Tissue and Fascia, Trunk		X Vascular Access Device, Tunneled	
	V Subcutaneous Tissue and Fascia, Upper Extremity		Y Other Device	
	W Subcutaneous Tissue and Fascia, Lower Extremity		Z No Device	

AHA Coding Clinic for table ØJ2

2017, 2Q, 26	Exchange of tunneled catheter

AHA Coding Clinic for table ØJ8

2017, 3Q, 11	Bilateral escharotomy of leg, thigh and foot

AHA Coding Clinic for table ØJ9

2015, 3Q, 23	Incision and drainage of multiple abscess cavities using vessel loop

AHA Coding Clinic for table ØJB

2018, 1Q, 7	Placement of fat graft following lumbar decompression surgery
2015, 3Q, 3-8	Excisional and nonexcisional debridement
2015, 2Q, 13	Transfer of free flap to reconstruct orbital defect
2015, 1Q, 29	Fistulectomy with placement of seton
2014, 4Q, 38	Abdominoplasty and abdominal wall plication for hernia repair
2014, 3Q, 22	Transsphenoidal removal of pituitary tumor and fat graft placement

AHA Coding Clinic for table ØJC

2017, 3Q, 22	Replacement of native skull bone flap

AHA Coding Clinic for table ØJD

2016, 3Q, 20	VersaJet™ nonexcisional debridement of leg muscle
2016, 3Q, 21	Nonexcisional debridement of infected lumbar wound
2016, 3Q, 21	Nonexcisional pulsed lavage debridement
2016, 3Q, 22	Debridement of bone and tendon using Tenex ultrasound device
2016, 1Q, 40	Nonexcisional debridement of skin and subcutaneous tissue
2015, 3Q, 3-8	Excisional and nonexcisional debridement
2015, 1Q, 23	Non-Excisional debridement with lavage of wound

AHA Coding Clinic for table ØJH

2017, 4Q, 63-64	Added and revised device values - Vascular access reservoir
2017, 2Q, 24	Tunneled catheter versus totally implantable catheter
2017, 2Q, 26	Exchange of tunneled catheter
2016, 4Q, 97-98	Phrenic neurostimulator
2016, 2Q, 14	Insertion of peritoneal totally implantable venous access device
2016, 2Q, 15	Removal and replacement of tunneled internal jugular catheter
2015, 4Q, 14	New Section X codes—New Technology procedures
2015, 4Q, 30-31	Vascular access devices
2015, 2Q, 33	Totally implantable central venous access device (Port-a-Cath)
2014, 3Q, 19	End of life replacement of Baclofen pump
2013, 4Q, 116	Device character for Port-A-Cath placement
2012, 4Q, 104	Placement of subcutaneous implantable cardioverter defibrillator

AHA Coding Clinic for table ØJN

2017, 3Q, 11	Bilateral escharotomy of leg, thigh and foot

AHA Coding Clinic for table ØJP

2016, 2Q, 15	Removal and replacement of tunneled internal jugular catheter
2015, 4Q, 31	Vascular access devices
2014, 3Q, 19	End of life replacement of Baclofen pump
2013, 4Q, 109	Separating conjoined twins
2012, 4Q, 104	Placement of subcutaneous implantable cardioverter defibrillator

AHA Coding Clinic for table ØJQ

2017, 3Q, 19	Anterior repair of cystocele
2014, 4Q, 44	Posterior colporrhaphy/rectocele repair

AHA Coding Clinic for table ØJR

2015, 2Q, 13	Transfer of free flap to reconstruct orbital defect

AHA Coding Clinic for table ØJU

2018, 2Q, 20	Prelaminated free flap graft using Alloderm™
2018, 1Q, 7	Placement of fat graft following lumbar decompression surgery

AHA Coding Clinic for table ØJW

2018, 1Q, 8	Ventricular peritoneal shunt ligation
2015, 4Q, 33	Externalization of peritoneal dialysis catheter
2015, 2Q, 9	Revision of ventriculoperitoneal (VP) shunt
2012, 4Q, 104	Placement of subcutaneous implantable cardioverter defibrillator

AHA Coding Clinic for table ØJX

2018, 1Q, 10	Complex wound closure using pericranial flap
2014, 3Q, 18	Placement of reverse sural fasciocutaneous pedicle flap
2013, 4Q, 109	Separating conjoined twins

Ø Medical and Surgical
J Subcutaneous Tissue and Fascia
Ø Alteration Definition: Modifying the anatomic structure of a body part without affecting the function of the body part
Explanation: Principal purpose is to improve appearance

Body Part Character 4	Approach Character 5	Device Character 6	Qualifier Character 7
1 Subcutaneous Tissue and Fascia, Face Masseteric fascia Orbital fascia **4 Subcutaneous Tissue and Fascia, Right Neck** Deep cervical fascia Pretracheal fascia Prevertebral fascia **5 Subcutaneous Tissue and Fascia, Left Neck** *See 4 Subcutaneous Tissue and Fascia, Right Neck* **6 Subcutaneous Tissue and Fascia, Chest** Pectoral fascia **7 Subcutaneous Tissue and Fascia, Back** **8 Subcutaneous Tissue and Fascia, Abdomen** **9 Subcutaneous Tissue and Fascia, Buttock** **D Subcutaneous Tissue and Fascia, Right Upper Arm** Axillary fascia Deltoid fascia Infraspinatus fascia Subscapular aponeurosis Supraspinatus fascia **F Subcutaneous Tissue and Fascia, Left Upper Arm** *See D Subcutaneous Tissue and Fascia, Right Upper Arm* **G Subcutaneous Tissue and Fascia, Right Lower Arm** Antebrachial fascia Bicipital aponeurosis **H Subcutaneous Tissue and Fascia, Left Lower Arm** *See G Subcutaneous Tissue and Fascia, Right Lower Arm* **L Subcutaneous Tissue and Fascia, Right Upper Leg** Crural fascia Fascia lata Iliac fascia Iliotibial tract (band) **M Subcutaneous Tissue and Fascia, Left Upper Leg** *See L Subcutaneous Tissue and Fascia, Right Upper Leg* **N Subcutaneous Tissue and Fascia, Right Lower Leg** **P Subcutaneous Tissue and Fascia, Left Lower Leg**	**Ø** Open **3** Percutaneous	**Z** No Device	**Z** No Qualifier

Ø Medical and Surgical
J Subcutaneous Tissue and Fascia
2 Change Definition: Taking out or off a device from a body part and putting back an identical or similar device in or on the same body part without cutting or puncturing the skin or a mucous membrane
Explanation: All CHANGE procedures are coded using the approach EXTERNAL

Body Part Character 4	Approach Character 5	Device Character 6	Qualifier Character 7
S Subcutaneous Tissue and Fascia, Head and Neck **T** Subcutaneous Tissue and Fascia, Trunk External oblique aponeurosis Transversalis fascia **V** Subcutaneous Tissue and Fascia, Upper Extremity **W** Subcutaneous Tissue and Fascia, Lower Extremity	**X** External	**Ø** Drainage Device **Y** Other Device	**Z** No Qualifier

Non-OR All body part, approach, device, and qualifier values

Ø Medical and Surgical
J Subcutaneous Tissue and Fascia
5 Destruction Definition: Physical eradication of all or a portion of a body part by the direct use of energy, force, or a destructive agent
Explanation: None of the body part is physically taken out

Body Part Character 4		Approach Character 5	Device Character 6	Qualifier Character 7
Ø Subcutaneous Tissue and Fascia, Scalp Galea aponeurotica **1** Subcutaneous Tissue and Fascia, Face Masseteric fascia Orbital fascia **4** Subcutaneous Tissue and Fascia, Right Neck Deep cervical fascia Pretracheal fascia Prevertebral fascia **5** Subcutaneous Tissue and Fascia, Left Neck *See 4 Subcutaneous Tissue and Fascia, Right Neck* **6** Subcutaneous Tissue and Fascia, Chest Pectoral fascia **7** Subcutaneous Tissue and Fascia, Back **8** Subcutaneous Tissue and Fascia, Abdomen **9** Subcutaneous Tissue and Fascia, Buttock **B** Subcutaneous Tissue and Fascia, Perineum **C** Subcutaneous Tissue and Fascia, Pelvic Region **D** Subcutaneous Tissue and Fascia, Right Upper Arm Axillary fascia Deltoid fascia Infraspinatus fascia Subscapular aponeurosis Supraspinatus fascia **F** Subcutaneous Tissue and Fascia, Left Upper Arm *See D Subcutaneous Tissue and Fascia, Right Upper Arm*	**G** Subcutaneous Tissue and Fascia, Right Lower Arm Antebrachial fascia Bicipital aponeurosis **H** Subcutaneous Tissue and Fascia, Left Lower Arm *See G Subcutaneous Tissue and Fascia, Right Lower Arm* **J** Subcutaneous Tissue and Fascia, Right Hand Palmar fascia (aponeurosis) **K** Subcutaneous Tissue and Fascia, Left Hand *See J Subcutaneous Tissue and Fascia, Right Hand* **L** Subcutaneous Tissue and Fascia, Right Upper Leg Crural fascia Fascia lata Iliac fascia Iliotibial tract (band) **M** Subcutaneous Tissue and Fascia, Left Upper Leg *See L Subcutaneous Tissue and Fascia, Right Upper Leg* **N** Subcutaneous Tissue and Fascia, Right Lower Leg **P** Subcutaneous Tissue and Fascia, Left Lower Leg **Q** Subcutaneous Tissue and Fascia, Right Foot Plantar fascia (aponeurosis) **R** Subcutaneous Tissue and Fascia, Left Foot *See Q Subcutaneous Tissue and Fascia, Right Foot*	**Ø** Open **3** Percutaneous	**Z** No Device	**Z** No Qualifier

DRG Non-OR All body part, approach, device, and qualifier values

Ø Medical and Surgical
J Subcutaneous Tissue and Fascia
8 Division Definition: Cutting into a body part, without draining fluids and/or gases from the body part, in order to separate or transect a body part
Explanation: All or a portion of the body part is separated into two or more portions

Body Part Character 4		Approach Character 5	Device Character 6	Qualifier Character 7
Ø Subcutaneous Tissue and Fascia, Scalp Galea aponeurotica **1 Subcutaneous Tissue and Fascia, Face** Masseteric fascia Orbital fascia **4 Subcutaneous Tissue and Fascia, Right Neck** Deep cervical fascia Pretracheal fascia Prevertebral fascia **5 Subcutaneous Tissue and Fascia, Left Neck** *See 4 Subcutaneous Tissue and Fascia, Right Neck* **6 Subcutaneous Tissue and Fascia, Chest** Pectoral fascia **7 Subcutaneous Tissue and Fascia, Back** **8 Subcutaneous Tissue and Fascia, Abdomen** **9 Subcutaneous Tissue and Fascia, Buttock** **B Subcutaneous Tissue and Fascia, Perineum** **C Subcutaneous Tissue and Fascia, Pelvic Region** **D Subcutaneous Tissue and Fascia, Right Upper Arm** Axillary fascia Deltoid fascia Infraspinatus fascia Subscapular aponeurosis Supraspinatus fascia **F Subcutaneous Tissue and Fascia, Left Upper Arm** *See D Subcutaneous Tissue and Fascia, Right Upper Arm* **G Subcutaneous Tissue and Fascia, Right Lower Arm** Antebrachial fascia Bicipital aponeurosis	**H Subcutaneous Tissue and Fascia, Left Lower Arm** *See G Subcutaneous Tissue and Fascia, Right Lower Arm* **J Subcutaneous Tissue and Fascia, Right Hand** Palmar fascia (aponeurosis) **K Subcutaneous Tissue and Fascia, Left Hand** *See J Subcutaneous Tissue and Fascia, Right Hand* **L Subcutaneous Tissue and Fascia, Right Upper Leg** Crural fascia Fascia lata Iliac fascia Iliotibial tract (band) **M Subcutaneous Tissue and Fascia, Left Upper Leg** *See L Subcutaneous Tissue and Fascia, Right Upper Leg* **N Subcutaneous Tissue and Fascia, Right Lower Leg** **P Subcutaneous Tissue and Fascia, Left Lower Leg** **Q Subcutaneous Tissue and Fascia, Right Foot** Plantar fascia (aponeurosis) **R Subcutaneous Tissue and Fascia, Left Foot** *See Q Subcutaneous Tissue and Fascia, Right Foot* **S Subcutaneous Tissue and Fascia, Head and Neck** **T Subcutaneous Tissue and Fascia, Trunk** External oblique aponeurosis Transversalis fascia **V Subcutaneous Tissue and Fascia, Upper Extremity** **W Subcutaneous Tissue and Fascia, Lower Extremity**	**Ø Open** **3 Percutaneous**	**Z No Device**	**Z No Qualifier**

Subcutaneous Tissue and Fascia
ØJ8–ØJ8

Ø Medical and Surgical
J Subcutaneous Tissue and Fascia
9 Drainage Definition: Taking or letting out fluids and/or gases from a body part
Explanation: The qualifier DIAGNOSTIC is used to identify drainage procedures that are biopsies

Body Part Character 4		Approach Character 5	Device Character 6	Qualifier Character 7
Ø Subcutaneous Tissue and Fascia, Scalp Galea aponeurotica **1 Subcutaneous Tissue and Fascia, Face** Masseteric fascia Orbital fascia **4 Subcutaneous Tissue and Fascia, Right Neck** Deep cervical fascia Pretracheal fascia Prevertebral fascia **5 Subcutaneous Tissue and Fascia, Left Neck** *See 4 Subcutaneous Tissue and Fascia, Right Neck* **6 Subcutaneous Tissue and Fascia, Chest** Pectoral fascia **7 Subcutaneous Tissue and Fascia, Back** **8 Subcutaneous Tissue and Fascia, Abdomen** **9 Subcutaneous Tissue and Fascia, Buttock** **B Subcutaneous Tissue and Fascia, Perineum** **C Subcutaneous Tissue and Fascia, Pelvic Region** **D Subcutaneous Tissue and Fascia, Right Upper Arm** Axillary fascia Deltoid fascia Infraspinatus fascia Subscapular aponeurosis Supraspinatus fascia **F Subcutaneous Tissue and Fascia, Left Upper Arm** *See D Subcutaneous Tissue and Fascia, Right Upper Arm*	**G Subcutaneous Tissue and Fascia, Right Lower Arm** Antebrachial fascia Bicipital aponeurosis **H Subcutaneous Tissue and Fascia, Left Lower Arm** *See G Subcutaneous Tissue and Fascia, Right Lower Arm* **J Subcutaneous Tissue and Fascia, Right Hand** Palmar fascia (aponeurosis) **K Subcutaneous Tissue and Fascia, Left Hand** *See J Subcutaneous Tissue and Fascia, Right Hand* **L Subcutaneous Tissue and Fascia, Right Upper Leg** Crural fascia Fascia lata Iliac fascia Iliotibial tract (band) **M Subcutaneous Tissue and Fascia, Left Upper Leg** *See L Subcutaneous Tissue and Fascia, Right Upper Leg* **N Subcutaneous Tissue and Fascia, Right Lower Leg** **P Subcutaneous Tissue and Fascia, Left Lower Leg** **Q Subcutaneous Tissue and Fascia, Right Foot** Plantar fascia (aponeurosis) **R Subcutaneous Tissue and Fascia, Left Foot** *See Q Subcutaneous Tissue and Fascia, Right Foot*	**Ø Open** **3 Percutaneous**	**Ø Drainage Device**	**Z No Qualifier**

ØJ9 Continued on next page

Non-OR ØJ9[Ø,1,4,5,6,7,8,9,B,C,D,F,G,H,J,K,L,M,N,P,Q,R][Ø,3]ØZ

Ø Medical and Surgical
J Subcutaneous Tissue and Fascia
9 Drainage Definition: Taking or letting out fluids and/or gases from a body part
Explanation: The qualifier DIAGNOSTIC is used to identify drainage procedures that are biopsies

ØJ9 Continued

Body Part Character 4		Approach Character 5	Device Character 6	Qualifier Character 7
Ø Subcutaneous Tissue and Fascia, Scalp Galea aponeurotica **1 Subcutaneous Tissue and Fascia, Face** Masseteric fascia Orbital fascia **4 Subcutaneous Tissue and Fascia, Right Neck** Deep cervical fascia Pretracheal fascia Prevertebral fascia **5 Subcutaneous Tissue and Fascia, Left Neck** *See 4 Subcutaneous Tissue and Fascia, Right Neck* **6 Subcutaneous Tissue and Fascia, Chest** Pectoral fascia **7 Subcutaneous Tissue and Fascia, Back** **8 Subcutaneous Tissue and Fascia, Abdomen** **9 Subcutaneous Tissue and Fascia, Buttock** **B Subcutaneous Tissue and Fascia, Perineum** **C Subcutaneous Tissue and Fascia, Pelvic Region** **D Subcutaneous Tissue and Fascia, Right Upper Arm** Axillary fascia Deltoid fascia Infraspinatus fascia Subscapular aponeurosis Supraspinatus fascia **F Subcutaneous Tissue and Fascia, Left Upper Arm** *See D Subcutaneous Tissue and Fascia, Right Upper Arm*	**G Subcutaneous Tissue and Fascia, Right Lower Arm** Antebrachial fascia Bicipital aponeurosis **H Subcutaneous Tissue and Fascia, Left Lower Arm** *See G Subcutaneous Tissue and Fascia, Right Lower Arm* **J Subcutaneous Tissue and Fascia, Right Hand** Palmar fascia (aponeurosis) **K Subcutaenous Tissue and Fascia, Left Hand** *See J Subcutaneous Tissue and Fascia, Right Hand* **L Subcutaneous Tissue and Fascia, Right Upper Leg** Crural fascia Fascia lata Iliac fascia Iliotibial tract (band) **M Subcutaneous Tissue and Fascia, Left Upper Leg** *See L Subcutaneous Tissue and Fascia, Right Upper Leg* **N Subcutaneous Tissue and Fascia, Right Lower Leg** **P Subcutaneous Tissue and Fascia, Left Lower Leg** **Q Subcutaneous Tissue and Fascia, Right Foot** Plantar fascia (aponeurosis) **R Subcutaneous Tissue and Fascia, Left Foot** *See Q Subcutaneous Tissue and Fascia, Right Foot*	Ø Open 3 Percutaneous	Z No Device	X Diagnostic Z No Qualifier

Non-OR ØJ9[Ø,1,4,5,6,7,8,9,B,C,D,F,G,H,J,K,L,M,N,P,Q,R][Ø,3]ZX
Non-OR ØJ9[Ø,1,4,5,6,7,8,9,B,C,D,F,G,H,J,K,L,M,N,P,Q,R]3ZZ

Ø Medical and Surgical
J Subcutaneous Tissue and Fascia
B Excision Definition: Cutting out or off, without replacement, a portion of a body part
Explanation: The qualifier DIAGNOSTIC is used to identify excision procedures that are biopsies

Body Part Character 4	Approach Character 5	Device Character 6	Qualifier Character 7
Ø Subcutaneous Tissue and Fascia, Scalp Galea aponeurotica **1** Subcutaneous Tissue and Fascia, Face Masseteric fascia Orbital fascia **4** Subcutaneous Tissue and Fascia, Right Neck Deep cervical fascia Pretracheal fascia Prevertebral fascia **5** Subcutaneous Tissue and Fascia, Left Neck *See 4 Subcutaneous Tissue and Fascia, Right Neck* **6** Subcutaneous Tissue and Fascia, Chest Pectoral fascia **7** Subcutaneous Tissue and Fascia, Back **8** Subcutaneous Tissue and Fascia, Abdomen **9** Subcutaneous Tissue and Fascia, Buttock **B** Subcutaneous Tissue and Fascia, Perineum **C** Subcutaneous Tissue and Fascia, Pelvic Region **D** Subcutaneous Tissue and Fascia, Right Upper Arm Axillary fascia Deltoid fascia Infraspinatus fascia Subscapular aponeurosis Supraspinatus fascia **F** Subcutaneous Tissue and Fascia, Left Upper Arm *See D Subcutaneous Tissue and Fascia, Right Upper Arm* **G** Subcutaneous Tissue and Fascia, Right Lower Arm Antebrachial fascia Bicipital aponeurosis **H** Subcutaneous Tissue and Fascia, Left Lower Arm *See G Subcutaneous Tissue and Fascia, Right Lower Arm* **J** Subcutaneous Tissue and Fascia, Right Hand Palmar fascia (aponeurosis) **K** Subcutaneous Tissue and Fascia, Left Hand *See J Subcutaneous Tissue and Fascia, Right Hand* **L** Subcutaneous Tissue and Fascia, Right Upper Leg Crural fascia Fascia lata Iliac fascia Iliotibial tract (band) **M** Subcutaneous Tissue and Fascia, Left Upper Leg *See L Subcutaneous Tissue and Fascia, Right Upper Leg* **N** Subcutaneous Tissue and Fascia, Right Lower Leg **P** Subcutaneous Tissue and Fascia, Left Lower Leg **Q** Subcutaneous Tissue and Fascia, Right Foot Plantar fascia (aponeurosis) **R** Subcutaneous Tissue and Fascia, Left Foot *See Q Subcutaneous Tissue and Fascia, Right Foot*	**Ø** Open **3** Percutaneous	**Z** No Device	**X** Diagnostic **Z** No Qualifier

DRG Non-OR ØJB[Ø,4,5,6,7,8,9,B,C,D,F,G,H,L,M,N,P,Q,R]3ZZ
Non-OR ØJB[Ø,1,4,5,6,7,8,9,B,C,D,F,G,H,J,K,L,M,N,P,Q,R][Ø,3]ZX

Ø Medical and Surgical
J Subcutaneous Tissue and Fascia
C Extirpation Definition: Taking or cutting out solid matter from a body part

Explanation: The solid matter may be an abnormal byproduct of a biological function or a foreign body; it may be imbedded in a body part or in the lumen of a tubular body part. The solid matter may or may not have been previously broken into pieces.

Body Part Character 4		Approach Character 5	Device Character 6	Qualifier Character 7
Ø Subcutaneous Tissue and Fascia, Scalp Galea aponeurotica **1** Subcutaneous Tissue and Fascia, Face Masseteric fascia Orbital fascia **4** Subcutaneous Tissue and Fascia, Right Neck Deep cervical fascia Pretracheal fascia Prevertebral fascia **5** Subcutaneous Tissue and Fascia, Left Neck *See 4 Subcutaneous Tissue and Fascia, Right Neck* **6** Subcutaneous Tissue and Fascia, Chest Pectoral fascia **7** Subcutaneous Tissue and Fascia, Back **8** Subcutaneous Tissue and Fascia, Abdomen **9** Subcutaneous Tissue and Fascia, Buttock **B** Subcutaneous Tissue and Fascia, Perineum **C** Subcutaneous Tissue and Fascia, Pelvic Region **D** Subcutaneous Tissue and Fascia, Right Upper Arm Axillary fascia Deltoid fascia Infraspinatus fascia Subscapular aponeurosis Supraspinatus fascia **F** Subcutaneous Tissue and Fascia, Left Upper Arm *See D Subcutaneous Tissue and Fascia, Right Upper Arm*	**G** Subcutaneous Tissue and Fascia, Right Lower Arm Antebrachial fascia Bicipital aponeurosis **H** Subcutaneous Tissue and Fascia, Left Lower Arm *See G Subcutaneous Tissue and Fascia, Right Lower Arm* **J** Subcutaneous Tissue and Fascia, Right Hand Palmar fascia (aponeurosis) **K** Subcutaneous Tissue and Fascia, Left Hand *See J Subcutaneous Tissue and Fascia, Right Hand* **L** Subcutaneous Tissue and Fascia, Right Upper Leg Crural fascia Fascia lata Iliac fascia Iliotibial tract (band) **M** Subcutaneous Tissue and Fascia, Left Upper Leg *See L Subcutaneous Tissue and Fascia, Right Upper Leg* **N** Subcutaneous Tissue and Fascia, Right Lower Leg **P** Subcutaneous Tissue and Fascia, Left Lower Leg **Q** Subcutaneous Tissue and Fascia, Right Foot Plantar fascia (aponeurosis) **R** Subcutaneous Tissue and Fascia, Left Foot *See Q Subcutaneous Tissue and Fascia, Right Foot*	**Ø** Open **3** Percutaneous	**Z** No Device	**Z** No Qualifier

Non-OR All body part, approach, device, and qualifier values

Ø Medical and Surgical
J Subcutaneous Tissue and Fascia
D Extraction Definition: Pulling or stripping out or off all or a portion of a body part by the use of force
Explanation: The qualifier DIAGNOSTIC is used to identify extraction procedures that are biopsies

Body Part Character 4	Approach Character 5	Device Character 6	Qualifier Character 7
Ø Subcutaneous Tissue and Fascia, Scalp Galea aponeurotica 1 Subcutaneous Tissue and Fascia, Face Masseteric fascia Orbital fascia 4 Subcutaneous Tissue and Fascia, Right Neck Deep cervical fascia Pretracheal fascia Prevertebral fascia 5 Subcutaneous Tissue and Fascia, Left Neck *See 4 Subcutaneous Tissue and Fascia, Right Neck* 6 Subcutaneous Tissue and Fascia, Chest Pectoral fascia 7 Subcutaneous Tissue and Fascia, Back 8 Subcutaneous Tissue and Fascia, Abdomen 9 Subcutaneous Tissue and Fascia, Buttock B Subcutaneous Tissue and Fascia, Perineum C Subcutaneous Tissue and Fascia, Pelvic Region D Subcutaneous Tissue and Fascia, Right Upper Arm Axillary fascia Deltoid fascia Infraspinatus fascia Subscapular aponeurosis Supraspinatus fascia F Subcutaneous Tissue and Fascia, Left Upper Arm *See D Subcutaneous Tissue and Fascia, Right Upper Arm* G Subcutaneous Tissue and Fascia, Right Lower Arm Antebrachial fascia Bicipital aponeurosis H Subcutaneous Tissue and Fascia, Left Lower Arm *See G Subcutaneous Tissue and Fascia, Right Lower Arm* J Subcutaneous Tissue and Fascia, Right Hand Palmar fascia (aponeurosis) K Subcutaneous Tissue and Fascia, Left Hand *See J Subcutaneous Tissue and Fascia, Right Hand* L Subcutaneous Tissue and Fascia, Right Upper Leg Crural fascia Fascia lata Iliac fascia Iliotibial tract (band) M Subcutaneous Tissue and Fascia, Left Upper Leg *See L Subcutaneous Tissue and Fascia, Right Upper Leg* N Subcutaneous Tissue and Fascia, Right Lower Leg P Subcutaneous Tissue and Fascia, Left Lower Leg Q Subcutaneous Tissue and Fascia, Right Foot Plantar fascia (aponeurosis) R Subcutaneous Tissue and Fascia, Left Foot *See Q Subcutaneous Tissue and Fascia, Right Foot*	Ø Open 3 Percutaneous	Z No Device	Z No Qualifier

Non-OR ØJD[Ø,1,4,5,B,C,D,F,G,H,J,K,N,P,Q,R]3ZZ

See Appendix L for Procedure Combinations
Combo-only ØJD[6,7,8,9,L,M]3ZZ

Ø Medical and Surgical
J Subcutaneous Tissue and Fascia
H Insertion Definition: Putting in a nonbiological appliance that monitors, assists, performs, or prevents a physiological function but does not physically take the place of a body part
Explanation: None

Body Part Character 4	Approach Character 5	Device Character 6	Qualifier Character 7
Ø Subcutaneous Tissue and Fascia, Scalp Galea aponeurotica 1 Subcutaneous Tissue and Fascia, Face Masseteric fascia Orbital fascia 4 Subcutaneous Tissue and Fascia, Right Neck Deep cervical fascia Pretracheal fascia Prevertebral fascia 5 Subcutaneous Tissue and Fascia, Left Neck *See 4 Subcutaneous Tissue and Fascia, Right Neck* 9 Subcutaneous Tissue and Fascia, Buttock B Subcutaneous Tissue and Fascia, Perineum C Subcutaneous Tissue and Fascia, Pelvic Region J Subcutaneous Tissue and Fascia, Right Hand Palmar fascia (aponeurosis) K Subcutaneous Tissue and Fascia, Left Hand *See J Subcutaneous Tissue and Fascia, Right Hand* Q Subcutaneous Tissue and Fascia, Right Foot Plantar fascia (aponeurosis) R Subcutaneous Tissue and Fascia, Left Foot *See Q Subcutaneous Tissue and Fascia, Right Foot*	Ø Open 3 Percutaneous	N Tissue Expander	Z No Qualifier

ØJH Continued on next page

Ø Medical and Surgical
J Subcutaneous Tissue and Fascia
H Insertion Definition: Putting in a nonbiological appliance that monitors, assists, performs, or prevents a physiological function but does not physically take the place of a body part
Explanation: None

ØJH Continued

Body Part Character 4	Approach Character 5	Device Character 6	Qualifier Character 7
6 Subcutaneous Tissue and Fascia, Chest ⊞ Pectoral fascia 8 Subcutaneous Tissue and Fascia, Abdomen ⊞ NC	Ø Open 3 Percutaneous	Ø Monitoring Device, Hemodynamic 2 Monitoring Device 4 Pacemaker, Single Chamber 5 Pacemaker, Single Chamber Rate Responsive 6 Pacemaker, Dual Chamber 7 Cardiac Resynchronization Pacemaker Pulse Generator 8 Defibrillator Generator 9 Cardiac Resynchronization Defibrillator Pulse Generator A Contractility Modulation Device B Stimulator Generator, Single Array C Stimulator Generator, Single Array Rechargeable D Stimulator Generator, Multiple Array E Stimulator Generator, Multiple Array Rechargeable H Contraceptive Device M Stimulator Generator N Tissue Expander P Cardiac Rhythm Related Device V Infusion Device, Pump W Vascular Access Device, Totally Implantable X Vascular Access Device, Tunneled	Z No Qualifier
7 Subcutaneous Tissue and Fascia, Back ⊞ NC	Ø Open 3 Percutaneous	B Stimulator Generator, Single Array C Stimulator Generator, Single Array Rechargeable D Stimulator Generator, Multiple Array E Stimulator Generator, Multiple Array Rechargeable M Stimulator Generator N Tissue Expander V Infusion Device, Pump	Z No Qualifier
D Subcutaneous Tissue and Fascia, Right Upper Arm Axillary fascia Deltoid fascia Infraspinatus fascia Subscapular aponeurosis Supraspinatus fascia F Subcutaneous Tissue and Fascia, Left Upper Arm *See D Subcutaneous Tissue and Fascia, Right Upper Arm* G Subcutaneous Tissue and Fascia, Right Lower Arm Antebrachial fascia Bicipital aponeurosis H Subcutaneous Tissue and Fascia, Left Lower Arm *See G Subcutaneous Tissue and Fascia, Right Lower Arm* L Subcutaneous Tissue and Fascia, Right Upper Leg Crural fascia Fascia lata Iliac fascia Iliotibial tract (band) M Subcutaneous Tissue and Fascia, Left Upper Leg *See L Subcutaneous Tissue and Fascia, Right Upper Leg* N Subcutaneous Tissue and Fascia, Right Lower Leg P Subcutaneous Tissue and Fascia, Left Lower Leg	Ø Open 3 Percutaneous	H Contraceptive Device N Tissue Expander V Infusion Device, Pump W Vascular Access Device, Totally Implantable X Vascular Access Device, Tunneled	Z No Qualifier
S Subcutaneous Tissue and Fascia, Head and Neck V Subcutaneous Tissue and Fascia, Upper Extremity W Subcutaneous Tissue and Fascia, Lower Extremity	Ø Open 3 Percutaneous	1 Radioactive Element 3 Infusion Device Y Other Device	Z No Qualifier
T Subcutaneous Tissue and Fascia, Trunk External oblique aponeurosis Transversalis fascia	Ø Open 3 Percutaneous	1 Radioactive Element 3 Infusion Device V Infusion Device, Pump Y Other Device	Z No Qualifier

DRG Non-OR ØJH6[Ø,3][4,5,6,H,W,X]Z
DRG Non-OR ØJH8[Ø,3][2,4,5,6,H,W,X]Z
DRG Non-OR ØJH[D,F,G,H,L,M][Ø,3][W,X]Z
DRG Non-OR ØJHNØ[W,X]Z
DRG Non-OR ØJHN3[H,W,X]Z
DRG Non-OR ØJHP[Ø,3][H,W,X]Z
Non-OR ØJH[D,F,G,H,L,M][Ø,3]HZ
Non-OR ØJHNØHZ
Non-OR ØJH[S,V,W]Ø3Z
Non-OR ØJH[S,V,W]3[3,Y]Z
Non-OR ØJHTØ3Z
Non-OR ØJHT3[3,Y]Z

HAC ØJH[6,8][Ø,3][4,5,6,7,8,9,P]Z when reported with SDx K68.11 or T81.4XXA or T82.6XXA or T82.7XXA
HAC ØJH63XZ when reported with SDx J95.811
NC ØJH8[Ø,3]MZ
NC ØJH7[Ø,3]MZ

See Appendix L for Procedure Combinations
⊞ ØJH[6,8][Ø,3][8,9,A,B,C,D,E]Z
⊞ ØJH7[Ø,3][B,C,D,E]Z

LC Limited Coverage NC Noncovered ⊞ Combination Member HAC associated procedure Combination Only DRG Non-OR Non-OR New/Revised in GREEN

Ø Medical and Surgical
J Subcutaneous Tissue and Fascia
J Inspection Definition: Visually and/or manually exploring a body part

Explanation: Visual exploration may be performed with or without optical instrumentation. Manual exploration may be performed directly or through intervening body layers.

Body Part Character 4	Approach Character 5	Device Character 6	Qualifier Character 7
S Subcutaneous Tissue and Fascia, Head and Neck **T** Subcutaneous Tissue and Fascia, Trunk External oblique aponeurosis Transversalis fascia **V** Subcutaneous Tissue and Fascia, Upper Extremity **W** Subcutaneous Tissue and Fascia, Lower Extremity	**Ø** Open **3** Percutaneous **X** External	**Z** No Device	**Z** No Qualifier

Non-OR All body part, approach, device, and qualifier values

Ø Medical and Surgical
J Subcutaneous Tissue and Fascia
N Release Definition: Freeing a body part from an abnormal physical constraint by cutting or by the use of force

Explanation: Some of the restraining tissue may be taken out but none of the body part is taken out

Body Part Character 4	Approach Character 5	Device Character 6	Qualifier Character 7
Ø Subcutaneous Tissue and Fascia, Scalp Galea aponeurotica **1** Subcutaneous Tissue and Fascia, Face Masseteric fascia Orbital fascia **4** Subcutaneous Tissue and Fascia, Right Neck Deep cervical fascia Pretracheal fascia Prevertebral fascia **5** Subcutaneous Tissue and Fascia, Left Neck *See 4 Subcutaneous Tissue and Fascia, Right Neck* **6** Subcutaneous Tissue and Fascia, Chest Pectoral fascia **7** Subcutaneous Tissue and Fascia, Back **8** Subcutaneous Tissue and Fascia, Abdomen **9** Subcutaneous Tissue and Fascia, Buttock **B** Subcutaneous Tissue and Fascia, Perineum **C** Subcutaneous Tissue and Fascia, Pelvic Region **D** Subcutaneous Tissue and Fascia, Right Upper Arm Axillary fascia Deltoid fascia Infraspinatus fascia Subscapular aponeurosis Supraspinatus fascia **F** Subcutaneous Tissue and Fascia, Left Upper Arm *See D Subcutaneous Tissue and Fascia, Right Upper Arm* **G** Subcutaneous Tissue and Fascia, Right Lower Arm Antebrachial fascia Bicipital aponeurosis **H** Subcutaneous Tissue and Fascia, Left Lower Arm *See G Subcutaneous Tissue and Fascia, Right Lower Arm* **J** Subcutaneous Tissue and Fascia, Right Hand Palmar fascia (aponeurosis) **K** Subcutaneous Tissue and Fascia, Left Hand *See J Subcutaneous Tissue and Fascia, Right Hand* **L** Subcutaneous Tissue and Fascia, Right Upper Leg Crural fascia Fascia lata Iliac fascia Iliotibial tract (band) **M** Subcutaneous Tissue and Fascia, Left Upper Leg *See L Subcutaneous Tissue and Fascia, Right Upper Leg* **N** Subcutaneous Tissue and Fascia, Right Lower Leg **P** Subcutaneous Tissue and Fascia, Left Lower Leg **Q** Subcutaneous Tissue and Fascia, Right Foot Plantar fascia (aponeurosis) **R** Subcutaneous Tissue and Fascia, Left Foot *See Q Subcutaneous Tissue and Fascia, Right Foot*	**Ø** Open **3** Percutaneous **X** External	**Z** No Device	**Z** No Qualifier

Non-OR ØJN[Ø,1,4,5,6,7,8,9,B,C,D,F,G,H,J,K,L,M,N,P,Q,R]XZZ

Ø Medical and Surgical
J Subcutaneous Tissue and Fascia
P Removal Definition: Taking out or off a device from a body part

Explanation: If a device is taken out and a similar device put in without cutting or puncturing the skin or mucous membrane, the procedure is coded to the root operation CHANGE. Otherwise, the procedure for taking out a device is coded to the root operation REMOVAL.

Body Part Character 4	Approach Character 5	Device Character 6	Qualifier Character 7
S Subcutaneous Tissue and Fascia, Head and Neck	Ø Open 3 Percutaneous	Ø Drainage Device 1 Radioactive Element 3 Infusion Device 7 Autologous Tissue Substitute J Synthetic Substitute K Nonautologous Tissue Substitute N Tissue Expander Y Other Device	Z No Qualifier
S Subcutaneous Tissue and Fascia, Head and Neck	X External	Ø Drainage Device 1 Radioactive Element 3 Infusion Device	Z No Qualifier
T Subcutaneous Tissue and Fascia, Trunk External oblique aponeurosis Transversalis fascia	Ø Open 3 Percutaneous	Ø Drainage Device 1 Radioactive Element 2 Monitoring Device 3 Infusion Device 7 Autologous Tissue Substitute H Contraceptive Device J Synthetic Substitute K Nonautologous Tissue Substitute M Stimulator Generator N Tissue Expander P Cardiac Rhythm Related Device V Infusion Device, Pump W Vascular Access Device, Totally Implantable X Vascular Access Device, Tunneled Y Other Device	Z No Qualifier
T Subcutaneous Tissue and Fascia, Trunk External oblique aponeurosis Transversalis fascia	X External	Ø Drainage Device 1 Radioactive Element 2 Monitoring Device 3 Infusion Device H Contraceptive Device V Infusion Device, Pump X Vascular Access Device, Tunneled	Z No Qualifier
V Subcutaneous Tissue and Fascia, Upper Extremity W Subcutaneous Tissue and Fascia, Lower Extremity	Ø Open 3 Percutaneous	Ø Drainage Device 1 Radioactive Element 3 Infusion Device 7 Autologous Tissue Substitute H Contraceptive Device J Synthetic Substitute K Nonautologous Tissue Substitute N Tissue Expander V Infusion Device, Pump W Vascular Access Device, Totally Implantable X Vascular Access Device, Tunneled Y Other Device	Z No Qualifier
V Subcutaneous Tissue and Fascia, Upper Extremity W Subcutaneous Tissue and Fascia, Lower Extremity	X External	Ø Drainage Device 1 Radioactive Element 3 Infusion Device H Contraceptive Device V Infusion Device, Pump X Vascular Access Device, Tunneled	Z No Qualifier

Non-OR ØJPS[Ø,3][Ø,1,3,7,J,K,N,Y]Z
Non-OR ØJPSX[Ø,1,3]Z
Non-OR ØJPT[Ø,3][Ø,1,2,3,7,H,J,K,M,N,V,W,X,Y]Z
Non-OR ØJPTX[Ø,1,2,3,H,V,X]Z
Non-OR ØJP[V,W][Ø,3][Ø,1,3,7,H,J,K,N,V,W,X,Y]Z
Non-OR ØJP[V,W]X[Ø,1,3,H,V,X]Z
HAC ØJPT[Ø,3]PZ when reported with SDx K68.11 or T81.4XXA or T82.6XXA or T82.7XXA

Ø Medical and Surgical
J Subcutaneous Tissue and Fascia
Q Repair Definition: Restoring, to the extent possible, a body part to its normal anatomic structure and function
Explanation: Used only when the method to accomplish the repair is not one of the other root operations

Body Part Character 4	Approach Character 5	Device Character 6	Qualifier Character 7
Ø Subcutaneous Tissue and Fascia, Scalp Galea aponeurotica **1** Subcutaneous Tissue and Fascia, Face Masseteric fascia Orbital fascia **4** Subcutaneous Tissue and Fascia, Right Neck Deep cervical fascia Pretracheal fascia Prevertebral fascia **5** Subcutaneous Tissue and Fascia, Left Neck *See 4 Subcutaneous Tissue and Fascia, Right Neck* **6** Subcutaneous Tissue and Fascia, Chest Pectoral fascia **7** Subcutaneous Tissue and Fascia, Back **8** Subcutaneous Tissue and Fascia, Abdomen **9** Subcutaneous Tissue and Fascia, Buttock **B** Subcutaneous Tissue and Fascia, Perineum **C** Subcutaneous Tissue and Fascia, Pelvic Region **D** Subcutaneous Tissue and Fascia, Right Upper Arm Axillary fascia Deltoid fascia Infraspinatus fascia Subscapular aponeurosis Supraspinatus fascia **F** Subcutaneous Tissue and Fascia, Left Upper Arm *See D Subcutaneous Tissue and Fascia, Right Upper Arm* **G** Subcutaneous Tissue and Fascia, Right Lower Arm Antebrachial fascia Bicipital aponeurosis **H** Subcutaneous Tissue and Fascia, Left Lower Arm *See G Subcutaneous Tissue and Fascia, Right Lower Arm* **J** Subcutaneous Tissue and Fascia, Right Hand Palmar fascia (aponeurosis) **K** Subcutaneous Tissue and Fascia, Left Hand *See J Subcutaneous Tissue and Fascia, Right Hand* **L** Subcutaneous Tissue and Fascia, Right Upper Leg Crural fascia Fascia lata Iliac fascia Iliotibial tract (band) **M** Subcutaneous Tissue and Fascia, Left Upper Leg *See L Subcutaneous Tissue and Fascia, Right Upper Leg* **N** Subcutaneous Tissue and Fascia, Right Lower Leg **P** Subcutaneous Tissue and Fascia, Left Lower Leg **Q** Subcutaneous Tissue and Fascia, Right Foot Plantar fascia (aponeurosis) **R** Subcutaneous Tissue and Fascia, Left Foot *See Q Subcutaneous Tissue and Fascia, Right Foot*	**Ø** Open **3** Percutaneous	**Z** No Device	**Z** No Qualifier

Non-OR ØJQ[Ø,1,4,5,6,7,8,9,B,C,D,F,G,H,J,K,L,M,N,P,Q,R]3ZZ

Ø Medical and Surgical
J Subcutaneous Tissue and Fascia
R Replacement Definition: Putting in or on biological or synthetic material that physically takes the place and/or function of all or a portion of a body part

Explanation: The body part may have been taken out or replaced, or may be taken out, physically eradicated, or rendered nonfunctional during the REPLACEMENT procedure. A REMOVAL procedure is coded for taking out the device used in a previous replacement procedure.

Body Part Character 4	Approach Character 5	Device Character 6	Qualifier Character 7
Ø Subcutaneous Tissue and Fascia, Scalp Galea aponeurotica **1 Subcutaneous Tissue and Fascia, Face** Masseteric fascia Orbital fascia **4 Subcutaneous Tissue and Fascia, Right Neck** Deep cervical fascia Pretracheal fascia Prevertebral fascia **5 Subcutaneous Tissue and Fascia, Left Neck** *See 4 Subcutaneous Tissue and Fascia, Right Neck* **6 Subcutaneous Tissue and Fascia, Chest** Pectoral fascia **7 Subcutaneous Tissue and Fascia, Back** **8 Subcutaneous Tissue and Fascia, Abdomen** **9 Subcutaneous Tissue and Fascia, Buttock** **B Subcutaneous Tissue and Fascia, Perineum** **C Subcutaneous Tissue and Fascia, Pelvic Region** **D Subcutaneous Tissue and Fascia, Right Upper Arm** Axillary fascia Deltoid fascia Infraspinatus fascia Subscapular aponeurosis Supraspinatus fascia **F Subcutaneous Tissue and Fascia, Left Upper Arm** *See D Subcutaneous Tissue and Fascia, Right Upper Arm* **G Subcutaneous Tissue and Fascia, Right Lower Arm** Antebrachial fascia Bicipital aponeurosis **H Subcutaneous Tissue and Fascia, Left Lower Arm** *See G Subcutaneous Tissue and Fascia, Right Lower Arm* **J Subcutaneous Tissue and Fascia, Right Hand** Palmar fascia (aponeurosis) **K Subcutaneous Tissue and Fascia, Left Hand** *See J Subcutaneous Tissue and Fascia, Right Hand* **L Subcutaneous Tissue and Fascia, Right Upper Leg** Crural fascia Fascia lata Iliac fascia Iliotibial tract (band) **M Subcutaneous Tissue and Fascia, Left Upper Leg** *See L Subcutaneous Tissue and Fascia, Right Upper Leg* **N Subcutaneous Tissue and Fascia, Right Lower Leg** **P Subcutaneous Tissue and Fascia, Left Lower Leg** **Q Subcutaneous Tissue and Fascia, Right Foot** Plantar fascia (aponeurosis) **R Subcutaneous Tissue and Fascia, Left Foot** *See Q Subcutaneous Tissue and Fascia, Right Foot*	**Ø Open** **3 Percutaneous**	**7 Autologous Tissue Substitute** **J Synthetic Substitute** **K Nonautologous Tissue Substitute**	**Z No Qualifier**

Subcutaneous Tissue and Fascia *(left margin)*

Ø Medical and Surgical
J Subcutaneous Tissue and Fascia
U Supplement: Definition: Putting in or on biological or synthetic material that physically reinforces and/or augments the function of a portion of a body part
Explanation: The biological material is non-living, or is living and from the same individual. The body part may have been previously replaced, and the SUPPLEMENT procedure is performed to physically reinforce and/or augment the function of the replaced body part.

Body Part Character 4		Approach Character 5	Device Character 6	Qualifier Character 7
Ø Subcutaneous Tissue and Fascia, Scalp Galea aponeurotica **1 Subcutaneous Tissue and Fascia, Face** Masseteric fascia Orbital fascia **4 Subcutaneous Tissue and Fascia, Right Neck** Deep cervical fascia Pretracheal fascia Prevertebral fascia **5 Subcutaneous Tissue and Fascia, Left Neck** *See 4 Subcutaneous Tissue and Fascia, Right Neck* **6 Subcutaneous Tissue and Fascia, Chest** Pectoral fascia **7 Subcutaneous Tissue and Fascia, Back** **8 Subcutaneous Tissue and Fascia, Abdomen** **9 Subcutaneous Tissue and Fascia, Buttock** **B Subcutaneous Tissue and Fascia, Perineum** **C Subcutaneous Tissue and Fascia, Pelvic Region** **D Subcutaneous Tissue and Fascia, Right Upper Arm** Axillary fascia Deltoid fascia Infraspinatus fascia Subscapular aponeurosis Supraspinatus fascia **F Subcutaneous Tissue and Fascia, Left Upper Arm** *See D Subcutaneous Tissue and Fascia, Right Upper Arm*	**G Subcutaneous Tissue and Fascia, Right Lower Arm** Antebrachial fascia Bicipital aponeurosis **H Subcutaneous Tissue and Fascia, Left Lower Arm** *See G Subcutaneous Tissue and Fascia, Right Lower Arm* **J Subcutaneous Tissue and Fascia, Right Hand** Palmar fascia (aponeurosis) **K Subcutaneous Tissue and Fascia, Left Hand** *See J Subcutaneous Tissue and Fascia, Right Hand* **L Subcutaneous Tissue and Fascia, Right Upper Leg** Crural fascia Fascia lata Iliac fascia Iliotibial tract (band) **M Subcutaneous Tissue and Fascia, Left Upper Leg** *See L Subcutaneous Tissue and Fascia, Right Upper Leg* **N Subcutaneous Tissue and Fascia, Right Lower Leg** **P Subcutaneous Tissue and Fascia, Left Lower Leg** **Q Subcutaneous Tissue and Fascia, Right Foot** Plantar fascia (aponeurosis) **R Subcutaneous Tissue and Fascia, Left Foot** *See Q Subcutaneous Tissue and Fascia, Right Foot*	**Ø Open** **3 Percutaneous**	**7 Autologous Tissue Substitute** **J Synthetic Substitute** **K Nonautologous Tissue Substitute**	**Z No Qualifier**

Ø Medical and Surgical
J Subcutaneous Tissue and Fascia
W Revision Definition: Correcting, to the extent possible, a portion of a malfunctioning device or the position of a displaced device

Explanation: Revision can include correcting a malfunctioning or displaced device by taking out or putting in components of the device such as a screw or pin

Body Part Character 4	Approach Character 5	Device Character 6	Qualifier Character 7
S Subcutaneous Tissue and Fascia, Head and Neck	Ø Open 3 Percutaneous	Ø Drainage Device 3 Infusion Device 7 Autologous Tissue Substitute J Synthetic Substitute K Nonautologous Tissue Substitute N Tissue Expander Y Other Device	Z No Qualifier
S Subcutaneous Tissue and Fascia, Head and Neck	X External	Ø Drainage Device 3 Infusion Device 7 Autologous Tissue Substitute J Synthetic Substitute K Nonautologous Tissue Substitute N Tissue Expander	Z No Qualifier
T Subcutaneous Tissue and Fascia, Trunk External oblique aponeurosis Transversalis fascia	Ø Open 3 Percutaneous	Ø Drainage Device 2 Monitoring Device 3 Infusion Device 7 Autologous Tissue Substitute H Contraceptive Device J Synthetic Substitute K Nonautologous Tissue Substitute M Stimulator Generator N Tissue Expander P Cardiac Rhythm Related Device V Infusion Device, Pump W Vascular Access Device, Totally Implantable X Vascular Access Device, Tunneled Y Other Device	Z No Qualifier
T Subcutaneous Tissue and Fascia, Trunk External oblique aponeurosis Transversalis fascia	X External	Ø Drainage Device 2 Monitoring Device 3 Infusion Device 7 Autologous Tissue Substitute H Contraceptive Device J Synthetic Substitute K Nonautologous Tissue Substitute M Stimulator Generator N Tissue Expander P Cardiac Rhythm Related Device V Infusion Device, Pump W Vascular Access Device, Totally Implantable X Vascular Access Device, Tunneled	Z No Qualifier
V Subcutaneous Tissue and Fascia, Upper Extremity W Subcutaneous Tissue and Fascia, Lower Extremity	Ø Open 3 Percutaneous	Ø Drainage Device 3 Infusion Device 7 Autologous Tissue Substitute H Contraceptive Device J Synthetic Substitute K Nonautologous Tissue Substitute N Tissue Expander V Infusion Device, Pump W Vascular Access Device, Totally Implantable X Vascular Access Device, Tunneled Y Other Device	Z No Qualifier
V Subcutaneous Tissue and Fascia, Upper Extremity W Subcutaneous Tissue and Fascia, Lower Extremity	X External	Ø Drainage Device 3 Infusion Device 7 Autologous Tissue Substitute H Contraceptive Device J Synthetic Substitute K Nonautologous Tissue Substitute N Tissue Expander V Infusion Device, Pump W Vascular Access Device, Totally Implantable X Vascular Access Device, Tunneled	Z No Qualifier

DRG Non-OR ØJWS[Ø,3][Ø,3,7,J,K,N,Y]Z
DRG Non-OR ØJWT[Ø,3][Ø,3,7,H,J,K,M,N,V,W,X]Z
DRG Non-OR ØJWTXMZ
DRG Non-OR ØJW[V,W][Ø,3][Ø,3,7,H,J,K,N,V,W,X,Y]Z
Non-OR ØJWSX[Ø,3,7,J,K,N]Z
Non-OR ØJWT3YZ
Non-OR ØJWTX[Ø,2,3,7,H,J,K,N,P,V,W,X]Z
Non-OR ØJW[V,W]X[Ø,3,7,H,J,K,N,V,W,X]Z

HAC ØJWT[Ø,3]PZ when reported with SDx K68.11 or T81.4XXA or T82.6XXA or T82.7XXA

Ø Medical and Surgical
J Subcutaneous Tissue and Fascia
X Transfer Definition: Moving, without taking out, all or a portion of a body part to another location to take over the function of all or a portion of a body part

Explanation: The body part transferred remains connected to its vascular and nervous supply

Body Part Character 4		Approach Character 5	Device Character 6	Qualifier Character 7
Ø Subcutaneous Tissue and Fascia, Scalp Galea aponeurotica **1 Subcutaneous Tissue and Fascia, Face** Masseteric fascia Orbital fascia **4 Subcutaneous Tissue and Fascia, Right Neck** Deep cervical fascia Pretracheal fascia Prevertebral fascia **5 Subcutaneous Tissue and Fascia, Left Neck** *See 4 Subcutaneous Tissue and Fascia, Right Neck* **6 Subcutaneous Tissue and Fascia, Chest** Pectoral fascia **7 Subcutaneous Tissue and Fascia, Back** **8 Subcutaneous Tissue and Fascia, Abdomen** **9 Subcutaneous Tissue and Fascia, Buttock** **B Subcutaneous Tissue and Fascia, Perineum** **C Subcutaneous Tissue and Fascia, Pelvic Region** **D Subcutaneous Tissue and Fascia, Right Upper Arm** Axillary fascia Deltoid fascia Infraspinatus fascia Subscapular aponeurosis Supraspinatus fascia **F Subcutaneous Tissue and Fascia, Left Upper Arm** *See D Subcutaneous Tissue and Fascia, Right Upper Arm*	**G Subcutaneous Tissue and Fascia, Right Lower Arm** Antebrachial fascia Bicipital aponeurosis **H Subcutaneous Tissue and Fascia, Left Lower Arm** *See G Subcutaneous Tissue and Fascia, Right Lower Arm* **J Subcutaneous Tissue and Fascia, Right Hand** Palmar fascia (aponeurosis) **K Subcutaneous Tissue and Fascia, Left Hand** *See J Subcutaneous Tissue and Fascia, Right Hand* **L Subcutaneous Tissue and Fascia, Right Upper Leg** Crural fascia Fascia lata Iliac fascia Iliotibial tract (band) **M Subcutaneous Tissue and Fascia, Left Upper Leg** *See L Subcutaneous Tissue and Fascia, Right Upper Leg* **N Subcutaneous Tissue and Fascia, Right Lower Leg** **P Subcutaneous Tissue and Fascia, Left Lower Leg** **Q Subcutaneous Tissue and Fascia, Right Foot** Plantar fascia (aponeurosis) **R Subcutaneous Tissue and Fascia, Left Foot** *See Q Subcutaneous Tissue and Fascia, Right Foot*	**Ø Open** **3 Percutaneous**	**Z No Device**	**B Skin and Subcutaneous Tissue** **C Skin, Subcutaneous Tissue and Fascia** **Z No Qualifier**

Muscles ØK2–ØKX

Character Meanings

This Character Meaning table is provided as a guide to assist the user in the identification of character members that may be found in this section of code tables. It **SHOULD NOT** be used to build a PCS code.

Operation–Character 3	Body Part–Character 4	Approach–Character 5	Device–Character 6	Qualifier–Character 7
2 Change	Ø Head Muscle	Ø Open	Ø Drainage Device	Ø Skin
5 Destruction	1 Facial Muscle	3 Percutaneous	7 Autologous Tissue Substitute	1 Subcutaneous Tissue
8 Division	2 Neck Muscle, Right	4 Percutaneous Endoscopic	J Synthetic Substitute	2 Skin and Subcutaneous Tissue
9 Drainage	3 Neck Muscle, Left	X External	K Nonautologous Tissue Substitute	5 Latissimus Dorsi Myocutaneous Flap
B Excision	4 Tongue, Palate, Pharynx Muscle		M Stimulator Lead	6 Transverse Rectus Abdominis Myocutaneous Flap
C Extirpation	5 Shoulder Muscle, Right		Y Other Device	7 Deep Inferior Epigastric Artery Perforator Flap
D Extraction	6 Shoulder Muscle, Left		Z No Device	8 Superficial Inferior Epigastric Artery Flap
H Insertion	7 Upper Arm Muscle, Right			9 Gluteal Artery Perforator Flap
J Inspection	8 Upper Arm Muscle, Left			X Diagnostic
M Reattachment	9 Lower Arm and Wrist Muscle, Right			Z No Qualifier
N Release	B Lower Arm and Wrist Muscle, Left			
P Removal	C Hand Muscle, Right			
Q Repair	D Hand Muscle, Left			
R Replacement	F Trunk Muscle, Right			
S Reposition	G Trunk Muscle, Left			
T Resection	H Thorax Muscle, Right			
U Supplement	J Thorax Muscle, Left			
W Revision	K Abdomen Muscle, Right			
X Transfer	L Abdomen Muscle, Left			
	M Perineum Muscle			
	N Hip Muscle, Right			
	P Hip Muscle, Left			
	Q Upper Leg Muscle, Right			
	R Upper Leg Muscle, Left			
	S Lower Leg Muscle, Right			
	T Lower Leg Muscle, Left			
	V Foot Muscle, Right			
	W Foot Muscle, Left			
	X Upper Muscle			
	Y Lower Muscle			

AHA Coding Clinic for table ØKB
2016, 3Q, 20 Excisional debridement of sacrum
2015, 3Q, 3-8 Excisional and nonexcisional debridement

AHA Coding Clinic for table ØKD
2017, 4Q, 41-42 Extraction procedures

AHA Coding Clinic for table ØKN
2017, 2Q, 12 Compartment syndrome and fasciotomy of foot
2017, 2Q, 13 Compartment syndrome and fasciotomy of leg
2015, 2Q, 22 Arthroscopic subacromial decompression
2014, 4Q, 39 Abdominal component release with placement of mesh for hernia repair

AHA Coding Clinic for table ØKQ
2018, 2Q, 25 Third and fourth degree obstetric lacerations
2016, 2Q, 34 Assisted vaginal delivery
2016, 1Q, 7 Obstetrical perineal laceration repair
2014, 4Q, 43 Second degree obstetric perineal laceration
2013, 4Q, 120 Repair of second degree perineum obstetric laceration

AHA Coding Clinic for table ØKS
2017, 1Q, 41 Manual reduction of hernia

AHA Coding Clinic for table ØKT
2016, 2Q, 12 Resection of malignant neoplasm of infratemporal fossa
2015, 1Q, 38 Abdominoperineal resection with flap closure of the perineum and colostomy

AHA Coding Clinic for table ØKX
2018, 2Q, 18 Transverse rectus abdominis myocutaneous (TRAM) delay
2017, 4Q, 67 New qualifier values - Pedicle flap procedures
2016, 3Q, 30 Resection of femur with interposition arthroplasty
2015, 3Q, 33 Cleft lip repair using Millard rotation advancement
2015, 2Q, 26 Pharyngeal flap to soft palate
2014, 4Q, 41 Abdominoperineal resection (APR) with flap closure of perineum and colostomy
2014, 2Q, 10 Transverse abdominomyocutaneous (TRAM) breast reconstruction
2014, 2Q, 12 Pedicle latissimus myocutaneous flap with placement of breast tissue expanders

Muscles

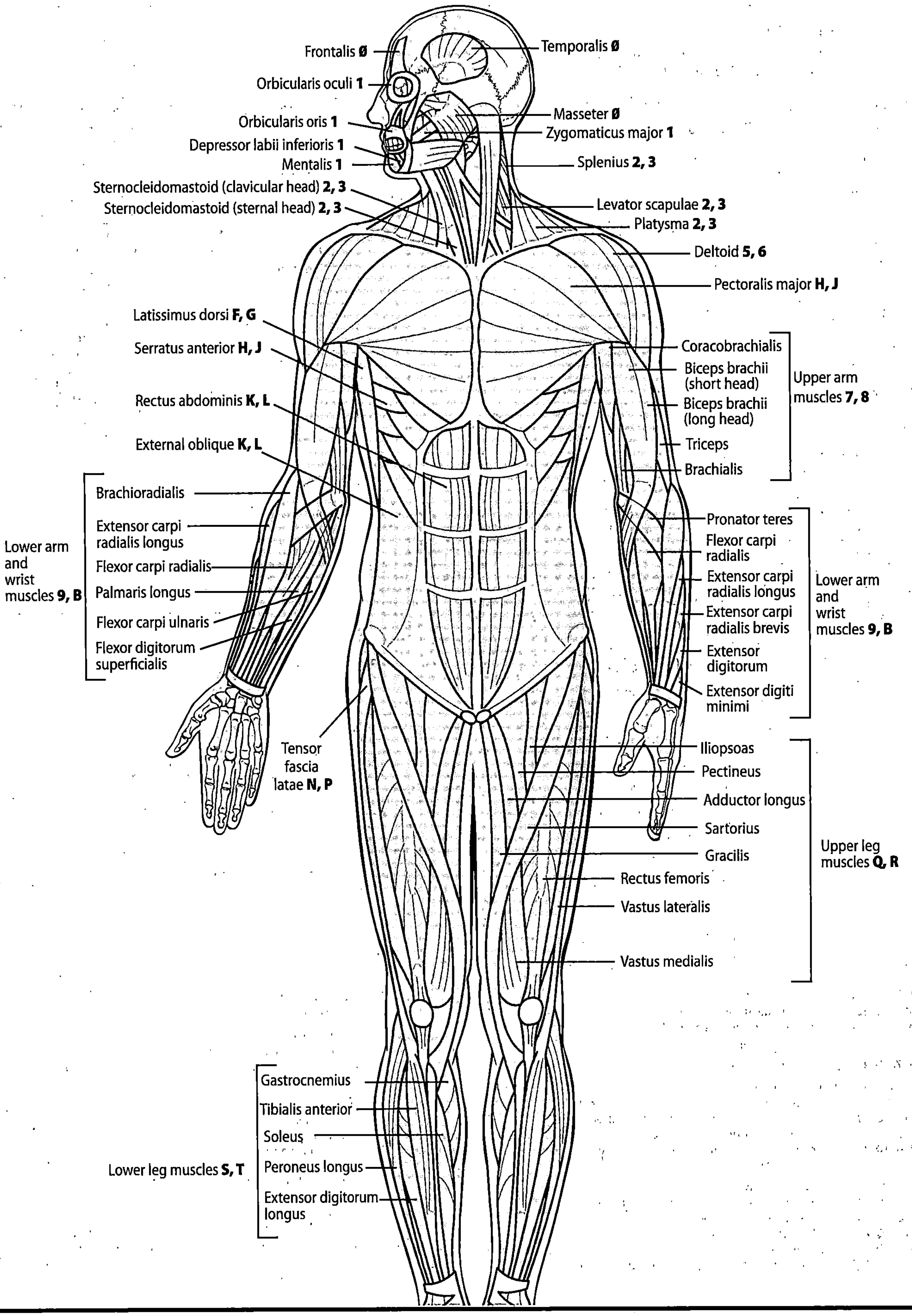
Frontalis Ø
Temporalis Ø
Orbicularis oculi 1
Orbicularis oris 1
Masseter Ø
Zygomaticus major 1
Depressor labii inferioris 1
Mentalis 1
Splenius 2, 3
Sternocleidomastoid (clavicular head) 2, 3
Sternocleidomastoid (sternal head) 2, 3
Levator scapulae 2, 3
Platysma 2, 3
Deltoid 5, 6
Pectoralis major H, J
Latissimus dorsi F, G
Serratus anterior H, J
Coracobrachialis
Biceps brachii (short head)
Biceps brachii (long head)
Triceps
Brachialis
Upper arm muscles 7, 8
Rectus abdominis K, L
External oblique K, L
Brachioradialis
Extensor carpi radialis longus
Flexor carpi radialis
Palmaris longus
Flexor carpi ulnaris
Flexor digitorum superficialis
Lower arm and wrist muscles 9, B
Pronator teres
Flexor carpi radialis
Extensor carpi radialis longus
Extensor carpi radialis brevis
Extensor digitorum
Extensor digiti minimi
Lower arm and wrist muscles 9, B
Tensor fascia latae N, P
Iliopsoas
Pectineus
Adductor longus
Sartorius
Gracilis
Rectus femoris
Vastus lateralis
Vastus medialis
Upper leg muscles Q, R
Gastrocnemius
Tibialis anterior
Soleus
Peroneus longus
Extensor digitorum longus
Lower leg muscles S, T

Ø   **Medical and Surgical**
K   **Muscles**
2   **Change**   Definition: Taking out or off a device from a body part and putting back an identical or similar device in or on the same body part without cutting or puncturing the skin or a mucous membrane
                 Explanation: All CHANGE procedures are coded using the approach EXTERNAL

Body Part Character 4	Approach Character 5	Device Character 6	Qualifier Character 7
X Upper Muscle **Y** Lower Muscle	**X** External	**Ø** Drainage Device **Y** Other Device	**Z** No Qualifier
Non-OR All body part, approach, device, and qualifier values			

Ø   **Medical and Surgical**
K   **Muscles**
5   **Destruction**   Definition: Physical eradication of all or a portion of a body part by the direct use of energy, force, or a destructive agent
                      Explanation: None of the body part is physically taken out

Body Part Character 4			Approach Character 5	Device Character 6	Qualifier Character 7

Ø   **Head Muscle**
    Auricularis muscle
    Masseter muscle
    Pterygoid muscle
    Splenius capitis muscle
    Temporalis muscle
    Temporoparietalis muscle
1   **Facial Muscle**
    Buccinator muscle
    Corrugator supercilii muscle
    Depressor anguli oris muscle
    Depressor labii inferioris muscle
    Depressor septi nasi muscle
    Depressor supercilii muscle
    Levator anguli oris muscle
    Levator labii superioris alaeque
       nasi muscle
    Levator labii superioris muscle
    Mentalis muscle
    Nasalis muscle
    Occipitofrontalis muscle
    Orbicularis oris muscle
    Procerus muscle
    Risorius muscle
    Zygomaticus muscle
2   **Neck Muscle, Right**
    Anterior vertebral muscle
    Arytenoid muscle
    Cricothyroid muscle
    Infrahyoid muscle
    Levator scapulae muscle
    Platysma muscle
    Scalene muscle
    Splenius cervicis muscle
    Sternocleidomastoid muscle
    Suprahyoid muscle
    Thyroarytenoid muscle
3   **Neck Muscle, Left**
    See 2 Neck Muscle, Right
4   **Tongue, Palate, Pharynx
    Muscle**
    Chondroglossus muscle
    Genioglossus muscle
    Hyoglossus muscle
    Inferior longitudinal muscle
    Levator veli palatini muscle
    Palatoglossal muscle
    Palatopharyngeal muscle
    Pharyngeal constrictor muscle
    Salpingopharyngeus muscle
    Styloglossus muscle
    Stylopharyngeus muscle
    Superior longitudinal muscle
    Tensor veli palatini muscle
5   **Shoulder Muscle, Right**
    Deltoid muscle
    Infraspinatus muscle
    Subscapularis muscle
    Supraspinatus muscle
    Teres major muscle
    Teres minor muscle
6   **Shoulder Muscle, Left**
    See 5 Shoulder Muscle, Right
	7 **Upper Arm Muscle, Right**
	    Biceps brachii muscle
	    Brachialis muscle
	    Coracobrachialis muscle
	    Triceps brachii muscle
	8 **Upper Arm Muscle, Left**
	    See 7 Upper Arm Muscle, Right
	9 **Lower Arm and Wrist Muscle,
	    Right**
	    Anatomical snuffbox
	    Brachioradialis muscle
	    Extensor carpi radialis muscle
	    Extensor carpi ulnaris muscle
	    Flexor carpi radialis muscle
	    Flexor carpi ulnaris muscle
	    Flexor pollicis longus muscle
	    Palmaris longus muscle
	    Pronator quadratus muscle
	    Pronator teres muscle
	B **Lower Arm and Wrist Muscle,
	    Left**
	    *See 9 Lower Arm and Wrist
	      Muscle, Right*
	C **Hand Muscle, Right**
	    Hypothenar muscle
	    Palmar interosseous muscle
	    Thenar muscle
	D **Hand Muscle, Left**
	    See C Hand Muscle, Right
	F **Trunk Muscle, Right**
	    Coccygeus muscle
	    Erector spinae muscle
	    Interspinalis muscle
	    Intertransversarius muscle
	    Latissimus dorsi muscle
	    Quadratus lumborum muscle
	    Rhomboid major muscle
	    Rhomboid minor muscle
	    Serratus posterior muscle
	    Transversospinalis muscle
	    Trapezius muscle
	G **Trunk Muscle, Left**
	    See F Trunk Muscle, Right
	H **Thorax Muscle, Right**
	    Intercostal muscle
	    Levatores costarum muscle
	    Pectoralis major muscle
	    Pectoralis minor muscle
	    Serratus anterior muscle
	    Subclavius muscle
	    Subcostal muscle
	    Transverse thoracis muscle
	J **Thorax Muscle, Left**
	    See H Thorax Muscle, Right
	K **Abdomen Muscle, Right**
	    External oblique muscle
	    Internal oblique muscle
	    Pyramidalis muscle
	    Rectus abdominis muscle
	    Transversus abdominis muscle
	L **Abdomen Muscle, Left**
	    See K Abdomen Muscle, Right
		M **Perineum Muscle**
		    Bulbospongiosus muscle
		    Cremaster muscle
		    Deep transverse perineal muscle
		    Ischiocavernosus muscle
		    Levator ani muscle
		    Superficial transverse perineal
		      muscle
		N **Hip Muscle, Right**
		    Gemellus muscle
		    Gluteus maximus muscle
		    Gluteus medius muscle
		    Gluteus minimus muscle
		    Iliacus muscle
		    Obturator muscle
		    Piriformis muscle
		    Psoas muscle
		    Quadratus femoris muscle
		    Tensor fasciae latae muscle
		P **Hip Muscle, Left**
		    See N Hip Muscle, Right
		Q **Upper Leg Muscle, Right**
		    Adductor brevis muscle
		    Adductor longus muscle
		    Adductor magnus muscle
		    Biceps femoris muscle
		    Gracilis muscle
		    Pectineus muscle
		    Quadriceps (femoris)
		    Rectus femoris muscle
		    Sartorius muscle
		    Semimembranosus muscle
		    Semitendinosus muscle
		    Vastus intermedius muscle
		    Vastus lateralis muscle
		    Vastus medialis muscle
		R **Upper Leg Muscle, Left**
		    See Q Upper Leg Muscle, Right
		S **Lower Leg Muscle, Right**
		    Extensor digitorum longus muscle
		    Extensor hallucis longus muscle
		    Fibularis brevis muscle
		    Fibularis longus muscle
		    Flexor digitorum longus muscle
		    Flexor hallucis longus muscle
		    Gastrocnemius muscle
		    Peroneus brevis muscle
		    Peroneus longus muscle
		    Popliteus muscle
		    Soleus muscle
		    Tibialis anterior muscle
		    Tibialis posterior muscle
		T **Lower Leg Muscle, Left**
		    See S Lower Leg Muscle, Right
		V **Foot Muscle, Right**
		    Abductor hallucis muscle
		    Adductor hallucis muscle
		    Extensor digitorum brevis muscle
		    Extensor hallucis brevis muscle
		    Flexor digitorum brevis muscle
		    Flexor hallucis brevis muscle
		    Quadratus plantae muscle
		W **Foot Muscle, Left**
		    See V Foot Muscle, Right
			Ø Open
			3 Percutaneous
			4 Percutaneous
			    Endoscopic
				Z No Device	**Z** No Qualifier

Ø Medical and Surgical
K Muscles
8 Division Definition: Cutting into a body part, without draining fluids and/or gases from the body part, in order to separate or transect a body part
Explanation: All or a portion of the body part is separated into two or more portions

Body Part Character 4	Approach Character 5	Device Character 6	Qualifier Character 7
Ø Head Muscle Auricularis muscle Masseter muscle Pterygoid muscle Splenius capitis muscle Temporalis muscle Temporoparietalis muscle **1 Facial Muscle** Buccinator muscle Corrugator supercilii muscle Depressor anguli oris muscle Depressor labii inferioris muscle Depressor septi nasi muscle Depressor supercilii muscle Levator anguli oris muscle Levator labii superioris alaeque nasi muscle Levator labii superioris muscle Mentalis muscle Nasalis muscle Occipitofrontalis muscle Orbicularis oris muscle Procerus muscle Risorius muscle Zygomaticus muscle **2 Neck Muscle, Right** Anterior vertebral muscle Arytenoid muscle Cricothyroid muscle Infrahyoid muscle Levator scapulae muscle Platysma muscle Scalene muscle Splenius cervicis muscle Sternocleidomastoid muscle Suprahyoid muscle Thyroarytenoid muscle **3 Neck Muscle, Left** *See 2 Neck Muscle, Right* **4 Tongue, Palate, Pharynx Muscle** Chondroglossus muscle Genioglossus muscle Hyoglossus muscle Inferior longitudinal muscle Levator veli palatini muscle Palatoglossal muscle Palatopharyngeal muscle Pharyngeal constrictor muscle Salpingopharyngeus muscle Styloglossus muscle Stylopharyngeus muscle Superior longitudinal muscle Tensor veli palatini muscle **5 Shoulder Muscle, Right** Deltoid muscle Infraspinatus muscle Subscapularis muscle Supraspinatus muscle Teres major muscle Teres minor muscle **6 Shoulder Muscle, Left** *See 5 Shoulder Muscle, Right* **7 Upper Arm Muscle, Right** Biceps brachii muscle Brachialis muscle Coracobrachialis muscle Triceps brachii muscle **8 Upper Arm Muscle, Left** *See 7 Upper Arm Muscle, Right* **9 Lower Arm and Wrist Muscle, Right** Anatomical snuffbox Brachioradialis muscle Extensor carpi radialis muscle Extensor carpi ulnaris muscle Flexor carpi radialis muscle Flexor carpi ulnaris muscle Flexor pollicis longus muscle Palmaris longus muscle Pronator quadratus muscle Pronator teres muscle **B Lower Arm and Wrist Muscle, Left** *See 9 Lower Arm and Wrist Muscle, Right* **C Hand Muscle, Right** Hypothenar muscle Palmar interosseous muscle Thenar muscle **D Hand Muscle, Left** *See C Hand Muscle, Right* **F Trunk Muscle, Right** Coccygeus muscle Erector spinae muscle Interspinalis muscle Intertransversarius muscle Latissimus dorsi muscle Quadratus lumborum muscle Rhomboid major muscle Rhomboid minor muscle Serratus posterior muscle Transversospinalis muscle Trapezius muscle **G Trunk Muscle, Left** *See F Trunk Muscle, Right* **H Thorax Muscle, Right** Intercostal muscle Levatores costarum muscle Pectoralis major muscle Pectoralis minor muscle Serratus anterior muscle Subclavius muscle Subcostal muscle Transverse thoracis muscle **J Thorax Muscle, Left** *See H Thorax Muscle, Right* **K Abdomen Muscle, Right** External oblique muscle Internal oblique muscle Pyramidalis muscle Rectus abdominis muscle Transversus abdominis muscle **L Abdomen Muscle, Left** *See K Abdomen Muscle, Right* **M Perineum Muscle** Bulbospongiosus muscle Cremaster muscle Deep transverse perineal muscle Ischiocavernosus muscle Levator ani muscle Superficial transverse perineal muscle **N Hip Muscle, Right** Gemellus muscle Gluteus maximus muscle Gluteus medius muscle Gluteus minimus muscle Iliacus muscle Obturator muscle Piriformis muscle Psoas muscle Quadratus femoris muscle Tensor fasciae latae muscle **P Hip Muscle, Left** *See N Hip Muscle, Right* **Q Upper Leg Muscle, Right** Adductor brevis muscle Adductor longus muscle Adductor magnus muscle Biceps femoris muscle Gracilis muscle Pectineus muscle Quadriceps (femoris) Rectus femoris muscle Sartorius muscle Semimembranosus muscle Semitendinosus muscle Vastus intermedius muscle Vastus lateralis muscle Vastus medialis muscle **R Upper Leg Muscle, Left** *See Q Upper Leg Muscle, Right* **S Lower Leg Muscle, Right** Extensor digitorum longus muscle Extensor hallucis longus muscle Fibularis brevis muscle Fibularis longus muscle Flexor digitorum longus muscle Flexor hallucis longus muscle Gastrocnemius muscle Peroneus brevis muscle Peroneus longus muscle Popliteus muscle Soleus muscle Tibialis anterior muscle Tibialis posterior muscle **T Lower Leg Muscle, Left** *See S Lower Leg Muscle, Right* **V Foot Muscle, Right** Abductor hallucis muscle Adductor hallucis muscle Extensor digitorum brevis muscle Extensor hallucis brevis muscle Flexor digitorum brevis muscle Flexor hallucis brevis muscle Quadratus plantae muscle **W Foot Muscle, Left** *See V Foot Muscle, Right*	**Ø Open** **3 Percutaneous** **4 Percutaneous Endoscopic**	**Z No Device**	**Z No Qualifier**

Ø Medical and Surgical
K Muscles
9 Drainage Definition: Taking or letting out fluids and/or gases from a body part

Explanation: The qualifier DIAGNOSTIC is used to identify drainage procedures that are biopsies

Body Part Character 4

- **Ø Head Muscle**
  Auriculariss muscle
  Masseter muscle
  Pterygoid muscle
  Splenius capitis muscle
  Temporalis muscle
  Temporoparietalis muscle
- **1 Facial Muscle**
  Buccinator muscle
  Corrugator supercilii muscle
  Depressor anguli oris muscle
  Depressor labii inferioris muscle
  Depressor septi nasi muscle
  Depressor supercilii muscle
  Levator anguli oris muscle
  Levator labii superioris alaeque nasi muscle
  Levator labii superioris muscle
  Mentalis muscle
  Nasalis muscle
  Occipitofrontalis muscle
  Orbicularis oris muscle
  Procerus muscle
  Risorius muscle
  Zygomaticus muscle
- **2 Neck Muscle, Right**
  Anterior vertebral muscle
  Arytenoid muscle
  Cricothyroid muscle
  Infrahyoid muscle
  Levator scapulae muscle
  Platysma muscle
  Scalene muscle
  Splenius cervicis muscle
  Sternocleidomastoid muscle
  Suprahyoid muscle
  Thyroarytenoid muscle
- **3 Neck Muscle, Left**
  See 2 Neck Muscle, Right
- **4 Tongue, Palate, Pharynx Muscle**
  Chondroglossus muscle
  Genioglossus muscle
  Hyoglossus muscle
  Inferior longitudinal muscle
  Levator veli palatini muscle
  Palatoglossal muscle
  Palatopharyngeal muscle
  Pharyngeal constrictor muscle
  Salpingopharyngeus muscle
  Styloglossus muscle
  Stylopharyngeus muscle
  Superior longitudinal muscle
  Tensor veli palatini muscle
- **5 Shoulder Muscle, Right**
  Deltoid muscle
  Infraspinatus muscle
  Subscapularis muscle
  Supraspinatus muscle
  Teres major muscle
  Teres minor muscle
- **6 Shoulder Muscle, Left**
  See 5 Shoulder Muscle, Right
- **7 Upper Arm Muscle, Right**
  Biceps brachii muscle
  Brachialis muscle
  Coracobrachialis muscle
  Triceps brachii muscle
- **8 Upper Arm Muscle, Left**
  See 7 Upper Arm Muscle, Right
- **9 Lower Arm and Wrist Muscle, Right**
  Anatomical snuffbox
  Brachioradialis muscle
  Extensor carpi radialis muscle
  Extensor carpi ulnaris muscle
  Flexor carpi radialis muscle
  Flexor carpi ulnaris muscle
  Flexor pollicis longus muscle
  Palmaris longus muscle
  Pronator quadratus muscle
  Pronator teres muscle
- **B Lower Arm and Wrist Muscle, Left**
  See 9 Lower Arm and Wrist Muscle, Right
- **C Hand Muscle, Right**
  Hypothenar muscle
  Palmar interosseous muscle
  Thenar muscle
- **D Hand Muscle, Left**
  See C Hand Muscle, Right
- **F Trunk Muscle, Right**
  Coccygeus muscle
  Erector spinae muscle
  Interspinalis muscle
  Intertransversarius muscle
  Latissimus dorsi muscle
  Quadratus lumborum muscle
  Rhomboid major muscle
  Rhomboid minor muscle
  Serratus posterior muscle
  Transversospinalis muscle
  Trapezius muscle
- **G Trunk Muscle, Left**
  See F Trunk Muscle, Right
- **H Thorax Muscle, Right**
  Intercostal muscle
  Levatores costarum muscle
  Pectoralis major muscle
  Pectoralis minor muscle
  Serratus anterior muscle
  Subclavius muscle
  Subcostal muscle
  Transverse thoracis muscle
- **J Thorax Muscle, Left**
  See H Thorax Muscle, Right
- **K Abdomen Muscle, Right**
  External oblique muscle
  Internal oblique muscle
  Pyramidalis muscle
  Rectus abdominis muscle
  Transversus abdominis muscle
- **L Abdomen Muscle, Left**
  See K Abdomen Muscle, Right
- **M Perineum Muscle**
  Bulbospongiosus muscle
  Cremaster muscle
  Deep transverse perineal muscle
  Ischiocavernosus muscle
  Levator ani muscle
  Superficial transverse perineal muscle
- **N Hip Muscle, Right**
  Gemellus muscle
  Gluteus maximus muscle
  Gluteus medius muscle
  Gluteus minimus muscle
  Iliacus muscle
  Obturator muscle
  Piriformis muscle
  Psoas muscle
  Quadratus femoris muscle
  Tensor fasciae latae muscle
- **P Hip Muscle, Left**
  See N Hip Muscle, Right
- **Q Upper Leg Muscle, Right**
  Adductor brevis muscle
  Adductor longus muscle
  Adductor magnus muscle
  Biceps femoris muscle
  Gracilis muscle
  Pectineus muscle
  Quadriceps (femoris)
  Rectus femoris muscle
  Sartorius muscle
  Semimembranosus muscle
  Semitendinosus muscle
  Vastus intermedius muscle
  Vastus lateralis muscle
  Vastus medialis muscle
- **R Upper Leg Muscle, Left**
  See Q Upper Leg Muscle, Right
- **S Lower Leg Muscle, Right**
  Extensor digitorum longus muscle
  Extensor hallucis longus muscle
  Fibularis brevis muscle
  Fibularis longus muscle
  Flexor digitorum longus muscle
  Flexor hallucis longus muscle
  Gastrocnemius muscle
  Peroneus brevis muscle
  Peroneus longus muscle
  Popliteus muscle
  Soleus muscle
  Tibialis anterior muscle
  Tibialis posterior muscle
- **T Lower Leg Muscle, Left**
  See S Lower Leg Muscle, Right
- **V Foot Muscle, Right**
  Abductor hallucis muscle
  Adductor hallucis muscle
  Extensor digitorum brevis muscle
  Extensor hallucis brevis muscle
  Flexor digitorum brevis muscle
  Flexor hallucis brevis muscle
  Quadratus plantae muscle
- **W Foot Muscle, Left**
  See V Foot Muscle, Right

Approach Character 5	Device Character 6	Qualifier Character 7
Ø Open 3 Percutaneous 4 Percutaneous Endoscopic	Ø Drainage Device	Z No Qualifier

Non-OR ØK9[Ø,1,2,3,4,5,6,7,8,9,B,C,D,F,G,H,J,K,L,M,N,P,Q,R,S,T,V,W]3ØZ

ØK9 Continued on next page

ØK9 Continued

Ø Medical and Surgical
K Muscles
9 Drainage Definition: Taking or letting out fluids and/or gases from a body part
Explanation: The qualifier DIAGNOSTIC is used to identify drainage procedures that are biopsies

Body Part Character 4	Approach Character 5	Device Character 6	Qualifier Character 7
Ø Head Muscle Auricularis muscle Masseter muscle Pterygoid muscle Splenius capitis muscle Temporalis muscle Temporoparietalis muscle **1 Facial Muscle** Buccinator muscle Corrugator supercilii muscle Depressor anguli oris muscle Depressor labii inferioris muscle Depressor septi nasi muscle Depressor supercilii muscle Levator anguli oris muscle Levator labii superioris alaeque nasi muscle Levator labii superioris muscle Mentalis muscle Nasalis muscle Occipitofrontalis muscle Orbicularis oris muscle Procerus muscle Risorius muscle Zygomaticus muscle **2 Neck Muscle, Right** Anterior vertebral muscle Arytenoid muscle Cricothyroid muscle Infrahyoid muscle Levator scapulae muscle Platysma muscle Scalene muscle Splenius cervicis muscle Sternocleidomastoid muscle Suprahyoid muscle Thyroarytenoid muscle **3 Neck Muscle, Left** *See 2 Neck Muscle, Right* **4 Tongue, Palate, Pharynx Muscle** Chondroglossus muscle Genioglossus muscle Hyoglossus muscle Inferior longitudinal muscle Levator veli palatini muscle Palatoglossal muscle Palatopharyngeal muscle Pharyngeal constrictor muscle Salpingopharyngeus muscle Styloglossus muscle Stylopharyngeus muscle Superior longitudinal muscle Tensor veli palatini muscle **5 Shoulder Muscle, Right** Deltoid muscle Infraspinatus muscle Subscapularis muscle Supraspinatus muscle Teres major muscle Teres minor muscle **6 Shoulder Muscle, Left** *See 5 Shoulder Muscle, Right* **7 Upper Arm Muscle, Right** Biceps brachii muscle Brachialis muscle Coracobrachialis muscle Triceps brachii muscle **8 Upper Arm Muscle, Left** *See 7 Upper Arm Muscle, Right* **9 Lower Arm and Wrist Muscle, Right** Anatomical snuffbox Brachioradialis muscle Extensor carpi radialis muscle Extensor carpi ulnaris muscle Flexor carpi radialis muscle Flexor carpi ulnaris muscle Flexor pollicis longus muscle Palmaris longus muscle Pronator quadratus muscle Pronator teres muscle **B Lower Arm and Wrist Muscle, Left** *See 9 Lower Arm and Wrist Muscle, Right* **C Hand Muscle, Right** Hypothenar muscle Palmar interosseous muscle Thenar muscle **D Hand Muscle, Left** *See C Hand Muscle, Right* **F Trunk Muscle, Right** Coccygeus muscle Erector spinae muscle Interspinalis muscle Intertransversarius muscle Latissimus dorsi muscle Quadratus lumborum muscle Rhomboid major muscle Rhomboid minor muscle Serratus posterior muscle Transversospinalis muscle Trapezius muscle **G Trunk Muscle, Left** *See F Trunk Muscle, Right* **H Thorax Muscle, Right** Intercostal muscle Levatores costarum muscle Pectoralis major muscle Pectoralis minor muscle Serratus anterior muscle Subclavius muscle Subcostal muscle Transverse thoracis muscle **J Thorax Muscle, Left** *See H Thorax Muscle, Right* **K Abdomen Muscle, Right** External oblique muscle Internal oblique muscle Pyramidalis muscle Rectus abdominis muscle Transversus abdominis muscle **L Abdomen Muscle, Left** *See K Abdomen Muscle, Right* **M Perineum Muscle** Bulbospongiosus muscle Cremaster muscle Deep transverse perineal muscle Ischiocavernosus muscle Levator ani muscle Superficial transverse perineal muscle **N Hip Muscle, Right** Gemellus muscle Gluteus maximus muscle Gluteus medius muscle Gluteus minimus muscle Iliacus muscle Obturator muscle Piriformis muscle Psoas muscle Quadratus femoris muscle Tensor fasciae latae muscle **P Hip Muscle, Left** *See N Hip Muscle, Right* **Q Upper Leg Muscle, Right** Adductor brevis muscle Adductor longus muscle Adductor magnus muscle Biceps femoris muscle Gracilis muscle Pectineus muscle Quadriceps (femoris) Rectus femoris muscle Sartorius muscle Semimembranosus muscle Semitendinosus muscle Vastus intermedius muscle Vastus lateralis muscle Vastus medialis muscle **R Upper Leg Muscle, Left** *See Q Upper Leg Muscle, Right* **S Lower Leg Muscle, Right** Extensor digitorum longus muscle Extensor hallucis longus muscle Fibularis brevis muscle Fibularis longus muscle Flexor digitorum longus muscle Flexor hallucis longus muscle Gastrocnemius muscle Peroneus brevis muscle Peroneus longus muscle Popliteus muscle Soleus muscle Tibialis anterior muscle Tibialis posterior muscle **T Lower Leg Muscle, Left** *See S Lower Leg Muscle, Right* **V Foot Muscle, Right** Abductor hallucis muscle Adductor hallucis muscle Extensor digitorum brevis muscle Extensor hallucis brevis muscle Flexor digitorum brevis muscle Flexor hallucis brevis muscle Quadratus plantae muscle **W Foot Muscle, Left** *See V Foot Muscle, Right*	Ø Open 3 Percutaneous 4 Percutaneous Endoscopic	Z No Device	X Diagnostic Z No Qualifier

Non-OR ØK9[Ø,1,2,3,4,5,6,7,8,9,B,F,G,H,J,K,L,M,N,P,Q,R,S,T,V,W]3ZZ
Non-OR ØK9[C,D][3,4]ZZ

Ø Medical and Surgical
K Muscles
B Excision Definition: Cutting out or off, without replacement, a portion of a body part
Explanation: The qualifier DIAGNOSTIC is used to identify excision procedures that are biopsies

Body Part Character 4	Approach Character 5	Device Character 6	Qualifier Character 7
Ø Head Muscle Auriculalis muscle Masseter muscle Pterygoid muscle Splenius capitis muscle Temporalis muscle Temporoparietalis muscle **1 Facial Muscle** Buccinator muscle Corrugator supercilii muscle Depressor anguli oris muscle Depressor labii inferioris muscle Depressor septi nasi muscle Depressor supercilii muscle Levator anguli oris muscle Levator labii superioris alaeque nasi muscle Levator labii superioris muscle Mentalis muscle Nasalis muscle Occipitofrontalis muscle Orbicularis oris muscle Procerus muscle Risorius muscle Zygomaticus muscle **2 Neck Muscle, Right** Anterior vertebral muscle Arytenoid muscle Cricothyroid muscle Infrahyoid muscle Levator scapulae muscle Platysma muscle Scalene muscle Splenius cervicis muscle Sternocleidomastoid muscle Suprahyoid muscle Thyroarytenoid muscle **3 Neck Muscle, Left** *See 2 Neck Muscle, Right* **4 Tongue, Palate, Pharynx Muscle** Chondroglossus muscle Genioglossus muscle Hyoglossus muscle Inferior longitudinal muscle Levator veli palatini muscle Palatoglossal muscle Palatopharyngeal muscle Pharyngeal constrictor muscle Salpingopharyngeus muscle Styloglossus muscle Stylopharyngeus muscle Superior longitudinal muscle Tensor veli palatini muscle **5 Shoulder Muscle, Right** Deltoid muscle Infraspinatus muscle Subscapularis muscle Supraspinatus muscle Teres major muscle Teres minor muscle **6 Shoulder Muscle, Left** *See 5 Shoulder Muscle, Right* **7 Upper Arm Muscle, Right** Biceps brachii muscle Brachialis muscle Coracobrachialis muscle Triceps brachii muscle **8 Upper Arm Muscle, Left** *See 7 Upper Arm Muscle, Right* **9 Lower Arm and Wrist Muscle, Right** Anatomical snuffbox Brachioradialis muscle Extensor carpi radialis muscle Extensor carpi ulnaris muscle Flexor carpi radialis muscle Flexor carpi ulnaris muscle Flexor pollicis longus muscle Palmaris longus muscle Pronator quadratus muscle Pronator teres muscle **B Lower Arm and Wrist Muscle, Left** *See 9 Lower Arm and Wrist Muscle, Right* **C Hand Muscle, Right** Hypothenar muscle Palmar interosseous muscle Thenar muscle **D Hand Muscle, Left** *See C Hand Muscle, Right* **F Trunk Muscle, Right** Coccygeus muscle Erector spinae muscle Interspinalis muscle Intertransversarius muscle Latissimus dorsi muscle Quadratus lumborum muscle Rhomboid major muscle Rhomboid minor muscle Serratus posterior muscle Transversospinalis muscle Trapezius muscle **G Trunk Muscle, Left** *See F Trunk Muscle, Right* **H Thorax Muscle, Right** Intercostal muscle Levatores costarum muscle Pectoralis major muscle Pectoralis minor muscle Serratus anterior muscle Subclavius muscle Subcostal muscle Transverse thoracis muscle **J Thorax Muscle, Left** *See H Thorax Muscle, Right* **K Abdomen Muscle, Right** External oblique muscle Internal oblique muscle Pyramidalis muscle Rectus abdominis muscle Transversus abdominis muscle **L Abdomen Muscle, Left** *See K Abdomen Muscle, Right* **M Perineum Muscle** Bulbospongiosus muscle Cremaster muscle Deep transverse perineal muscle Ischiocavernosus muscle Levator ani muscle Superficial transverse perineal muscle **N Hip Muscle, Right** Gemellus muscle Gluteus maximus muscle Gluteus medius muscle Gluteus minimus muscle Iliacus muscle Obturator muscle Piriformis muscle Psoas muscle Quadratus femoris muscle Tensor fasciae latae muscle **P Hip Muscle, Left** *See N Hip Muscle, Right* **Q Upper Leg Muscle, Right** Adductor brevis muscle Adductor longus muscle Adductor magnus muscle Biceps femoris muscle Gracilis muscle Pectineus muscle Quadriceps (femoris) Rectus femoris muscle Sartorius muscle Semimembranosus muscle Semitendinosus muscle Vastus intermedius muscle Vastus lateralis muscle Vastus medialis muscle **R Upper Leg Muscle, Left** *See Q Upper Leg Muscle, Right* **S Lower Leg Muscle, Right** Extensor digitorum longus muscle Extensor hallucis longus muscle Fibularis brevis muscle Fibularis longus muscle Flexor digitorum longus muscle Flexor hallucis longus muscle Gastrocnemius muscle Peroneus brevis muscle Peroneus longus muscle Popliteus muscle Soleus muscle Tibialis anterior muscle Tibialis posterior muscle **T Lower Leg Muscle, Left** *See S Lower Leg Muscle, Right* **V Foot Muscle, Right** Abductor hallucis muscle Adductor hallucis muscle Extensor digitorum brevis muscle Extensor hallucis brevis muscle Flexor digitorum brevis muscle Flexor hallucis brevis muscle Quadratus plantae muscle **W Foot Muscle, Left** *See V Foot Muscle, Right*	**Ø** Open **3** Percutaneous **4** Percutaneous Endoscopic	**Z** No Device	**X** Diagnostic **Z** No Qualifier

Ø Medical and Surgical
K Muscles
C Extirpation Definition: Taking or cutting out solid matter from a body part

Explanation: The solid matter may be an abnormal byproduct of a biological function or a foreign body; it may be imbedded in a body part or in the lumen of a tubular body part. The solid matter may or may not have been previously broken into pieces.

Body Part Character 4	Approach Character 5	Device Character 6	Qualifier Character 7
Ø Head Muscle Auricularis muscle Masseter muscle Pterygoid muscle Splenius capitis muscle Temporalis muscle Temporoparietalis muscle	**Ø Open**	**Z No Device**	**Z No Qualifier**
1 Facial Muscle Buccinator muscle Corrugator supercilii muscle Depressor anguli oris muscle Depressor labii inferioris muscle Depressor septi nasi muscle Depressor supercilii muscle Levator anguli oris muscle Levator labii superioris alaeque nasi muscle Levator labii superioris muscle Mentalis muscle Nasalis muscle Occipitofrontalis muscle Orbicularis oris muscle Procerus muscle Risorius muscle Zygomaticus muscle	**3 Percutaneous**		
2 Neck Muscle, Right Anterior vertebral muscle Arytenoid muscle Cricothyroid muscle Infrahyoid muscle Levator scapulae muscle Platysma muscle Scalene muscle Splenius cervicis muscle Sternocleidomastoid muscle Suprahyoid muscle Thyroarytenoid muscle	**4 Percutaneous Endoscopic**		
3 Neck Muscle, Left *See 2 Neck Muscle, Right*			
4 Tongue, Palate, Pharynx Muscle Chondroglossus muscle Genioglossus muscle Hyoglossus muscle Inferior longitudinal muscle Levator veli palatini muscle Palatoglossal muscle Palatopharyngeal muscle Pharyngeal constrictor muscle Salpingopharyngeus muscle Styloglossus muscle Stylopharyngeus muscle Superior longitudinal muscle Tensor veli palatini muscle			
5 Shoulder Muscle, Right Deltoid muscle Infraspinatus muscle Subscapularis muscle Supraspinatus muscle Teres major muscle Teres minor muscle			
6 Shoulder Muscle, Left *See 5 Shoulder Muscle, Right*			
7 Upper Arm Muscle, Right Biceps brachii muscle Brachialis muscle Coracobrachialis muscle Triceps brachii muscle			
8 Upper Arm Muscle, Left *See 7 Upper Arm Muscle, Right*			
9 Lower Arm and Wrist Muscle, Right Anatomical snuffbox Brachioradialis muscle Extensor carpi radialis muscle Extensor carpi ulnaris muscle Flexor carpi radialis muscle Flexor carpi ulnaris muscle Flexor pollicis longus muscle Palmaris longus muscle Pronator quadratus muscle Pronator teres muscle			
B Lower Arm and Wrist Muscle, Left *See 9 Lower Arm and Wrist Muscle, Right*			
C Hand Muscle, Right Hypothenar muscle Palmar interosseous muscle Thenar muscle			
D Hand Muscle, Left *See C Hand Muscle, Right*			
F Trunk Muscle, Right Coccygeus muscle Erector spinae muscle Interspinalis muscle Intertransversarius muscle Latissimus dorsi muscle Quadratus lumborum muscle Rhomboid major muscle Rhomboid minor muscle Serratus posterior muscle Transversospinalis muscle Trapezius muscle			
G Trunk Muscle, Left *See F Trunk Muscle, Right*			
H Thorax Muscle, Right Intercostal muscle Levatores costarum muscle Pectoralis major muscle Pectoralis minor muscle Serratus anterior muscle Subclavius muscle Subcostal muscle Transverse thoracis muscle			
J Thorax Muscle, Left *See H Thorax Muscle, Right*			
K Abdomen Muscle, Right External oblique muscle Internal oblique muscle Pyramidalis muscle Rectus abdominis muscle Transversus abdominis muscle			
L Abdomen Muscle, Left *See K Abdomen Muscle, Right*			
M Perineum Muscle Bulbospongiosus muscle Cremaster muscle Deep transverse perineal muscle Ischiocavernosus muscle Levator ani muscle Superficial transverse perineal muscle			
N Hip Muscle, Right Gemellus muscle Gluteus maximus muscle Gluteus medius muscle Gluteus minimus muscle Iliacus muscle Obturator muscle Piriformis muscle Psoas muscle Quadratus femoris muscle Tensor fasciae latae muscle			
P Hip Muscle, Left *See N Hip Muscle, Right*			
Q Upper Leg Muscle, Right Adductor brevis muscle Adductor longus muscle Adductor magnus muscle Biceps femoris muscle Gracilis muscle Pectineus muscle Quadriceps (femoris) Rectus femoris muscle Sartorius muscle Semimembranosus muscle Semitendinosus muscle Vastus intermedius muscle Vastus lateralis muscle Vastus medialis muscle			
R Upper Leg Muscle, Left *See Q Upper Leg Muscle, Right*			
S Lower Leg Muscle, Right Extensor digitorum longus muscle Extensor hallucis longus muscle Fibularis brevis muscle Fibularis longus muscle Flexor digitorum longus muscle Flexor hallucis longus muscle Gastrocnemius muscle Peroneus brevis muscle Peroneus longus muscle Popliteus muscle Soleus muscle Tibialis anterior muscle Tibialis posterior muscle			
T Lower Leg Muscle, Left *See S Lower Leg Muscle, Right*			
V Foot Muscle, Right Abductor hallucis muscle Adductor hallucis muscle Extensor digitorum brevis muscle Extensor hallucis brevis muscle Flexor digitorum brevis muscle Flexor hallucis brevis muscle Quadratus plantae muscle			
W Foot Muscle, Left *See V Foot Muscle, Right*			

Ø Medical and Surgical
K Muscles
D Extraction

Definition: Pulling or stripping out or off all or a portion of a body part by the use of force
Explanation: The qualifier DIAGNOSTIC is used to identify extraction procedures that are biopsies

Body Part Character 4	Approach Character 5	Device Character 6	Qualifier Character 7
Ø Head Muscle Auricularis muscle Masseter muscle Pterygoid muscle Splenius capitis muscle Temporalis muscle Temporoparietalis muscle **1 Facial Muscle** Buccinator muscle Corrugator supercilii muscle Depressor anguli oris muscle Depressor labii inferioris muscle Depressor septi nasi muscle Depressor supercilii muscle Levator anguli oris muscle Levator labii superioris alaeque nasi muscle Levator labii superioris muscle Mentalis muscle Nasalis muscle Occipitofrontalis muscle Orbicularis oris muscle Procerus muscle Risorius muscle Zygomaticus muscle **2 Neck Muscle, Right** Anterior vertebral muscle Arytenoid muscle Cricothyroid muscle Infrahyoid muscle Levator scapulae muscle Platysma muscle Scalene muscle Splenius cervicis muscle Sternocleidomastoid muscle Suprahyoid muscle Thyroarytenoid muscle **3 Neck Muscle, Left** *See 2 Neck Muscle, Right* **4 Tongue, Palate, Pharynx Muscle** Chondroglossus muscle Genioglossus muscle Hyoglossus muscle Inferior longitudinal muscle Levator veli palatini muscle Palatoglossal muscle Palatopharyngeal muscle Pharyngeal constrictor muscle Salpingopharyngeus muscle Styloglossus muscle Stylopharyngeus muscle Superior longitudinal muscle Tensor veli palatini muscle **5 Shoulder Muscle, Right** Deltoid muscle Infraspinatus muscle Subscapularis muscle Supraspinatus muscle Teres major muscle Teres minor muscle **6 Shoulder Muscle, Left** *See 5 Shoulder Muscle, Right* **7 Upper Arm Muscle, Right** Biceps brachii muscle Brachialis muscle Coracobrachialis muscle Triceps brachii muscle **8 Upper Arm Muscle, Left** *See 7 Upper Arm Muscle, Right* **9 Lower Arm and Wrist Muscle, Right** Anatomical snuffbox Brachioradialis muscle Extensor carpi radialis muscle Extensor carpi ulnaris muscle Flexor carpi radialis muscle Flexor carpi ulnaris muscle Flexor pollicis longus muscle Palmaris longus muscle Pronator quadratus muscle Pronator teres muscle **B Lower Arm and Wrist Muscle, Left** *See 9 Lower Arm and Wrist Muscle, Right* **C Hand Muscle, Right** Hypothenar muscle Palmar interosseous muscle Thenar muscle **D Hand Muscle, Left** *See C Hand Muscle, Right* **F Trunk Muscle, Right** Coccygeus muscle Erector spinae muscle Interspinalis muscle Intertransversarius muscle Latissimus dorsi muscle Quadratus lumborum muscle Rhomboid major muscle Rhomboid minor muscle Serratus posterior muscle Transversospinalis muscle Trapezius muscle **G Trunk Muscle, Left** *See F Trunk Muscle, Right* **H Thorax Muscle, Right** Intercostal muscle Levatores costarum muscle Pectoralis major muscle Pectoralis minor muscle Serratus anterior muscle Subclavius muscle Subcostal muscle Transverse thoracis muscle **J Thorax Muscle, Left** *See H Thorax Muscle, Right* **K Abdomen Muscle, Right** External oblique muscle Internal oblique muscle Pyramidalis muscle Rectus abdominis muscle Transversus abdominis muscle **L Abdomen Muscle, Left** *See K Abdomen Muscle, Right* **M Perineum Muscle** Bulbospongiosus muscle Cremaster muscle Deep transverse perineal muscle Ischiocavernosus muscle Levator ani muscle Superficial transverse perineal muscle **N Hip Muscle, Right** Gemellus muscle Gluteus maximus muscle Gluteus medius muscle Gluteus minimus muscle Iliacus muscle Obturator muscle Piriformis muscle Psoas muscle Quadratus femoris muscle Tensor fasciae latae muscle **P Hip Muscle, Left** *See N Hip Muscle, Right* **Q Upper Leg Muscle, Right** Adductor brevis muscle Adductor longus muscle Adductor magnus muscle Biceps femoris muscle Gracilis muscle Pectineus muscle Quadriceps (femoris) Rectus femoris muscle Sartorius muscle Semimembranosus muscle Semitendinosus muscle Vastus intermedius muscle Vastus lateralis muscle Vastus medialis muscle **R Upper Leg Muscle, Left** *See Q Upper Leg Muscle, Right* **S Lower Leg Muscle, Right** Extensor digitorum longus muscle Extensor hallucis longus muscle Fibularis brevis muscle Fibularis longus muscle Flexor digitorum longus muscle Flexor hallucis longus muscle Gastrocnemius muscle Peroneus brevis muscle Peroneus longus muscle Popliteus muscle Soleus muscle Tibialis anterior muscle Tibialis posterior muscle **T Lower Leg Muscle, Left** *See S Lower Leg Muscle, Right* **V Foot Muscle, Right** Abductor hallucis muscle Adductor hallucis muscle Extensor digitorum brevis muscle Extensor hallucis brevis muscle Flexor digitorum brevis muscle Flexor hallucis brevis muscle Quadratus plantae muscle **W Foot Muscle, Left** *See V Foot Muscle, Right*	**Ø** Open	**Z** No Device	**Z** No Qualifier

Ø Medical and Surgical
K Muscles
H Insertion Definition: Putting in a nonbiological appliance that monitors, assists, performs, or prevents a physiological function but does not physically take the place of a body part

Explanation: None

Body Part Character 4	Approach Character 5	Device Character 6	Qualifier Character 7
X Upper Muscle Y Lower Muscle	Ø Open 3 Percutaneous 4 Percutaneous Endoscopic	M Stimulator Lead Y Other Device	Z No Qualifier

Non-OR ØKH[X,Y][3,4]YZ

Ø Medical and Surgical
K Muscles
J Inspection Definition: Visually and/or manually exploring a body part

Explanation: Visual exploration may be performed with or without optical instrumentation. Manual exploration may be performed directly or through intervening body layers.

Body Part Character 4	Approach Character 5	Device Character 6	Qualifier Character 7
X Upper Muscle Y Lower Muscle	Ø Open 3 Percutaneous 4 Percutaneous Endoscopic X External	Z No Device	Z No Qualifier

Non-OR ØKJ[X,Y][3,X]ZZ

Ø Medical and Surgical
K Muscles
M Reattachment Definition: Putting back in or on all or a portion of a separated body part to its normal location or other suitable location
Explanation: Vascular circulation and nervous pathways may or may not be reestablished

Body Part Character 4	Approach Character 5	Device Character 6	Qualifier Character 7
Ø Head Muscle Auricularis muscle Masseter muscle Pterygoid muscle Splenius capitis muscle Temporalis muscle Temporoparietalis muscle	**Ø Open** **4 Percutaneous Endoscopic**	**Z No Device**	**Z No Qualifier**
1 Facial Muscle Buccinator muscle Corrugator supercilii muscle Depressor anguli oris muscle Depressor labii inferioris muscle Depressor septi nasi muscle Depressor supercilii muscle Levator anguli oris muscle Levator labii superioris alaeque nasi muscle Levator labii superioris muscle Mentalis muscle Nasalis muscle Occipitofrontalis muscle Orbicularis oris muscle Procerus muscle Risorius muscle Zygomaticus muscle			
2 Neck Muscle, Right Anterior vertebral muscle Arytenoid muscle Cricothyroid muscle Infrahyoid muscle Levator scapulae muscle Platysma muscle Scalene muscle Splenius cervicis muscle Sternocleidomastoid muscle Suprahyoid muscle Thyroarytenoid muscle			
3 Neck Muscle, Left *See 2 Neck Muscle, Right*			
4 Tongue, Palate, Pharynx Muscle Chondroglossus muscle Genioglossus muscle Hyoglossus muscle Inferior longitudinal muscle Levator veli palatini muscle Palatoglossal muscle Palatopharyngeal muscle Pharyngeal constrictor muscle Salpingopharyngeus muscle Styloglossus muscle Stylopharyngeus muscle Superior longitudinal muscle Tensor veli palatini muscle			
5 Shoulder Muscle, Right Deltoid muscle Infraspinatus muscle Subscapularis muscle Supraspinatus muscle Teres major muscle Teres minor muscle			
6 Shoulder Muscle, Left *See 5 Shoulder Muscle, Right*			
7 Upper Arm Muscle, Right Biceps brachii muscle Brachialis muscle Coracobrachialis muscle Triceps brachii muscle			
8 Upper Arm Muscle, Left *See 7 Upper Arm Muscle, Right*			
9 Lower Arm and Wrist Muscle, Right Anatomical snuffbox Brachioradialis muscle Extensor carpi radialis muscle Extensor carpi ulnaris muscle Flexor carpi radialis muscle Flexor carpi ulnaris muscle Flexor pollicis longus muscle Palmaris longus muscle Pronator quadratus muscle Pronator teres muscle			
B Lower Arm and Wrist Muscle, Left *See 9 Lower Arm and Wrist Muscle, Right*			
C Hand Muscle, Right Hypothenar muscle Palmar interosseous muscle Thenar muscle			
D Hand Muscle, Left *See C Hand Muscle, Right*			
F Trunk Muscle, Right Coccygeus muscle Erector spinae muscle Interspinalis muscle Intertransversarius muscle Latissimus dorsi muscle Quadratus lumborum muscle Rhomboid major muscle Rhomboid minor muscle Serratus posterior muscle Transversospinalis muscle Trapezius muscle			
G Trunk Muscle, Left *See F Trunk Muscle, Right*			
H Thorax Muscle, Right Intercostal muscle Levatores costarum muscle Pectoralis major muscle Pectoralis minor muscle Serratus anterior muscle Subclavius muscle Subcostal muscle Transverse thoracis muscle			
J Thorax Muscle, Left *See H Thorax Muscle, Right*			
K Abdomen Muscle, Right External oblique muscle Internal oblique muscle Pyramidalis muscle Rectus abdominis muscle Transversus abdominis muscle			
L Abdomen Muscle, Left *See K Abdomen Muscle, Right*			
M Perineum Muscle Bulbospongiosus muscle Cremaster muscle Deep transverse perineal muscle Ischiocavernosus muscle Levator ani muscle Superficial transverse perineal muscle			
N Hip Muscle, Right Gemellus muscle Gluteus maximus muscle Gluteus medius muscle Gluteus minimus muscle Iliacus muscle Obturator muscle Piriformis muscle Psoas muscle Quadratus femoris muscle Tensor fasciae latae muscle			
P Hip Muscle, Left *See N Hip Muscle, Right*			
Q Upper Leg Muscle, Right Adductor brevis muscle Adductor longus muscle Adductor magnus muscle Biceps femoris muscle Gracilis muscle Pectineus muscle Quadriceps (femoris) Rectus femoris muscle Sartorius muscle Semimembranosus muscle Semitendinosus muscle Vastus intermedius muscle Vastus lateralis muscle Vastus medialis muscle			
R Upper Leg Muscle, Left *See Q Upper Leg Muscle, Right*			
S Lower Leg Muscle, Right Extensor digitorum longus muscle Extensor hallucis longus muscle Fibularis brevis muscle Fibularis longus muscle Flexor digitorum longus muscle Flexor hallucis longus muscle Gastrocnemius muscle Peroneus brevis muscle Peroneus longus muscle Popliteus muscle Soleus muscle Tibialis anterior muscle Tibialis posterior muscle			
T Lower Leg Muscle, Left *See S Lower Leg Muscle, Right*			
V Foot Muscle, Right Abductor hallucis muscle Adductor hallucis muscle Extensor digitorum brevis muscle Extensor hallucis brevis muscle Flexor digitorum brevis muscle Flexor hallucis brevis muscle Quadratus plantae muscle			
W Foot Muscle, Left *See V Foot Muscle, Right*			

Ø Medical and Surgical
K Muscles
N Release Definition: Freeing a body part from an abnormal physical constraint by cutting or by the use of force
Explanation: Some of the restraining tissue may be taken out but none of the body part is taken out

Body Part Character 4	Approach Character 5	Device Character 6	Qualifier Character 7
Ø Head Muscle Auricularis muscle Masseter muscle Pterygoid muscle Splenius capitis muscle Temporalis muscle Temporoparietalis muscle **1 Facial Muscle** Buccinator muscle Corrugator supercilii muscle Depressor anguli oris muscle Depressor labii inferioris muscle Depressor septi nasi muscle Depressor supercilii muscle Levator anguli oris muscle Levator labii superioris alaeque nasi muscle Levator labii superioris muscle Mentalis muscle Nasalis muscle Occipitofrontalis muscle Orbicularis oris muscle Procerus muscle Risorius muscle Zygomaticus muscle **2 Neck Muscle, Right** Anterior vertebral muscle Arytenoid muscle Cricothyroid muscle Infrahyoid muscle Levator scapulae muscle Platysma muscle Scalene muscle Splenius cervicis muscle Sternocleidomastoid muscle Suprahyoid muscle Thyroarytenoid muscle **3 Neck Muscle, Left** *See 2 Neck Muscle, Right* **4 Tongue, Palate, Pharynx Muscle** Chondroglossus muscle Genioglossus muscle Hyoglossus muscle Inferior longitudinal muscle Levator veli palatini muscle Palatoglossal muscle Palatopharyngeal muscle Pharyngeal constrictor muscle Salpingopharyngeus muscle Styloglossus muscle Stylopharyngeus muscle Superior longitudinal muscle Tensor veli palatini muscle **5 Shoulder Muscle, Right** Deltoid muscle Infraspinatus muscle Subscapularis muscle Supraspinatus muscle Teres major muscle Teres minor muscle **6 Shoulder Muscle, Left** *See 5 Shoulder Muscle, Right* **7 Upper Arm Muscle, Right** Biceps brachii muscle Brachialis muscle Coracobrachialis muscle Triceps brachii muscle **8 Upper Arm Muscle, Left** *See 7 Upper Arm Muscle, Right* **9 Lower Arm and Wrist Muscle, Right** Anatomical snuffbox Brachioradialis muscle Extensor carpi radialis muscle Extensor carpi ulnaris muscle Flexor carpi radialis muscle Flexor carpi ulnaris muscle Flexor pollicis longus muscle Palmaris longus muscle Pronator quadratus muscle Pronator teres muscle **B Lower Arm and Wrist Muscle, Left** *See 9 Lower Arm and Wrist Muscle, Right* **C Hand Muscle, Right** Hypothenar muscle Palmar interosseous muscle Thenar muscle **D Hand Muscle, Left** *See C Hand Muscle, Right* **F Trunk Muscle, Right** Coccygeus muscle Erector spinae muscle Interspinalis muscle Intertransversarius muscle Latissimus dorsi muscle Quadratus lumborum muscle Rhomboid major muscle Rhomboid minor muscle Serratus posterior muscle Transversospinalis muscle Trapezius muscle **G Trunk Muscle, Left** *See F Trunk Muscle, Right* **H Thorax Muscle, Right** Intercostal muscle Levatores costarum muscle Pectoralis major muscle Pectoralis minor muscle Serratus anterior muscle Subclavius muscle Subcostal muscle Transverse thoracis muscle **J Thorax Muscle, Left** *See H Thorax Muscle, Right* **K Abdomen Muscle, Right** External oblique muscle Internal oblique muscle Pyramidalis muscle Rectus abdominis muscle Transversus abdominis muscle **L Abdomen Muscle, Left** *See K Abdomen Muscle, Right* **M Perineum Muscle** Bulbospongiosus muscle Cremaster muscle Deep transverse perineal muscle Ischiocavernosus muscle Levator ani muscle Superficial transverse perineal muscle **N Hip Muscle, Right** Gemellus muscle Gluteus maximus muscle Gluteus medius muscle Gluteus minimus muscle Iliacus muscle Obturator muscle Piriformis muscle Psoas muscle Quadratus femoris muscle Tensor fasciae latae muscle **P Hip Muscle, Left** *See N Hip Muscle, Right* **Q Upper Leg Muscle, Right** Adductor brevis muscle Adductor longus muscle Adductor magnus muscle Biceps femoris muscle Gracilis muscle Pectineus muscle Quadriceps (femoris) Rectus femoris muscle Sartorius muscle Semimembranosus muscle Semitendinosus muscle Vastus intermedius muscle Vastus lateralis muscle Vastus medialis muscle **R Upper Leg Muscle, Left** *See Q Upper Leg Muscle, Right* **S Lower Leg Muscle, Right** Extensor digitorum longus muscle Extensor hallucis longus muscle Fibularis brevis muscle Fibularis longus muscle Flexor digitorum longus muscle Flexor hallucis longus muscle Gastrocnemius muscle Peroneus brevis muscle Peroneus longus muscle Popliteus muscle Soleus muscle Tibialis anterior muscle Tibialis posterior muscle **T Lower Leg Muscle, Left** *See S Lower Leg Muscle, Right* **V Foot Muscle, Right** Abductor hallucis muscle Adductor hallucis muscle Extensor digitorum brevis muscle Extensor hallucis brevis muscle Flexor digitorum brevis muscle Flexor hallucis brevis muscle Quadratus plantae muscle **W Foot Muscle, Left** *See V Foot Muscle, Right*	**Ø Open** **3 Percutaneous** **4 Percutaneous Endoscopic** **X External**	**Z No Device**	**Z No Qualifier**

Non-OR ØKN[Ø,1,2,3,4,5,6,7,8,9,B,C,D,F,G,H,J,K,L,M,N,P,Q,R,S,T,V,W]XZZ

Ø Medical and Surgical
K Muscles
P Removal Definition: Taking out or off a device from a body part

Explanation: If a device is taken out and a similar device put in without cutting or puncturing the skin or mucous membrane, the procedure is coded to the root operation CHANGE. Otherwise, the procedure for taking out a device is coded to the root operation REMOVAL.

Body Part Character 4	Approach Character 5	Device Character 6	Qualifier Character 7
X Upper Muscle Y Lower Muscle	Ø Open 3 Percutaneous 4 Percutaneous Endoscopic	Ø Drainage Device 7 Autologous Tissue Substitute J Synthetic Substitute K Nonautologous Tissue Substitute M Stimulator Lead Y Other Device	Z No Qualifier
X Upper Muscle Y Lower Muscle	X External	Ø Drainage Device M Stimulator Lead	Z No Qualifier

Non-OR ØKP[X,Y][3,4]YZ
Non-OR ØKP[X,Y]X[Ø,M]Z

Ø Medical and Surgical
K Muscles
Q Repair Definition: Restoring, to the extent possible, a body part to its normal anatomic structure and function
Explanation: Used only when the method to accomplish the repair is not one of the other root operations

Body Part Character 4	Approach Character 5	Device Character 6	Qualifier Character 7
Ø Head Muscle Auricularis muscle Masseter muscle Pterygoid muscle Splenius capitis muscle Temporalis muscle Temporoparietalis muscle **1 Facial Muscle** Buccinator muscle Corrugator supercilii muscle Depressor anguli oris muscle Depressor labii inferioris muscle Depressor septi nasi muscle Depressor supercilii muscle Levator anguli oris muscle Levator labii superioris alaeque nasi muscle Levator labii superioris muscle Mentalis muscle Nasalis muscle Occipitofrontalis muscle Orbicularis oris muscle Procerus muscle Risorius muscle Zygomaticus muscle **2 Neck Muscle, Right** Anterior vertebral muscle Arytenoid muscle Cricothyroid muscle Infrahyoid muscle Levator scapulae muscle Platysma muscle Scalene muscle Splenius cervicis muscle Sternocleidomastoid muscle Suprahyoid muscle Thyroarytenoid muscle **3 Neck Muscle, Left** *See 2 Neck Muscle, Right* **4 Tongue, Palate, Pharynx Muscle** Chondroglossus muscle Genioglossus muscle Hyoglossus muscle Inferior longitudinal muscle Levator veli palatini muscle Palatoglossal muscle Palatopharyngeal muscle Pharyngeal constrictor muscle Salpingopharyngeus muscle Styloglossus muscle Stylopharyngeus muscle Superior longitudinal muscle Tensor veli palatini muscle **5 Shoulder Muscle, Right** Deltoid muscle Infraspinatus muscle Subscapularis muscle Supraspinatus muscle Teres major muscle Teres minor muscle **6 Shoulder Muscle, Left** *See 5 Shoulder Muscle, Right* **7 Upper Arm Muscle, Right** Biceps brachii muscle Brachialis muscle Coracobrachialis muscle Triceps brachii muscle **8 Upper Arm Muscle, Left** *See 7 Upper Arm Muscle, Right* **9 Lower Arm and Wrist Muscle, Right** Anatomical snuffbox Brachioradialis muscle Extensor carpi radialis muscle Extensor carpi ulnaris muscle Flexor carpi radialis muscle Flexor carpi ulnaris muscle Flexor pollicis longus muscle Palmaris longus muscle Pronator quadratus muscle Pronator teres muscle **B Lower Arm and Wrist Muscle, Left** *See 9 Lower Arm and Wrist Muscle, Right* **C Hand Muscle, Right** Hypothenar muscle Palmar interosseous muscle Thenar muscle **D Hand Muscle, Left** *See C Hand Muscle, Right* **F Trunk Muscle, Right** Coccygeus muscle Erector spinae muscle Interspinalis muscle Intertransversarius muscle Latissimus dorsi muscle Quadratus lumborum muscle Rhomboid major muscle Rhomboid minor muscle Serratus posterior muscle Transversospinalis muscle Trapezius muscle **G Trunk Muscle, Left** *See F Trunk Muscle, Right* **H Thorax Muscle, Right** Intercostal muscle Levatores costarum muscle Pectoralis major muscle Pectoralis minor muscle Serratus anterior muscle Subclavius muscle Subcostal muscle Transverse thoracis muscle **J Thorax Muscle, Left** *See H Thorax Muscle, Right* **K Abdomen Muscle, Right** External oblique muscle Internal oblique muscle Pyramidalis muscle Rectus abdominis muscle Transversus abdominis muscle **L Abdomen Muscle, Left** *See K Abdomen Muscle, Right* **M Perineum Muscle** Bulbospongiosus muscle Cremaster muscle Deep transverse perineal muscle Ischiocavernosus muscle Levator ani muscle Superficial transverse perineal muscle **N Hip Muscle, Right** Gemellus muscle Gluteus maximus muscle Gluteus medius muscle Gluteus minimus muscle Iliacus muscle Obturator muscle Piriformis muscle Psoas muscle Quadratus femoris muscle Tensor fasciae latae muscle **P Hip Muscle, Left** *See N Hip Muscle, Right* **Q Upper Leg Muscle, Right** Adductor brevis muscle Adductor longus muscle Adductor magnus muscle Biceps femoris muscle Gracilis muscle Pectineus muscle Quadriceps (femoris) Rectus femoris muscle Sartorius muscle Semimembranosus muscle Semitendinosus muscle Vastus intermedius muscle Vastus lateralis muscle Vastus medialis muscle **R Upper Leg Muscle, Left** *See Q Upper Leg Muscle, Right* **S Lower Leg Muscle, Right** Extensor digitorum longus muscle Extensor hallucis longus muscle Fibularis brevis muscle Fibularis longus muscle Flexor digitorum longus muscle Flexor hallucis longus muscle Gastrocnemius muscle Peroneus brevis muscle Peroneus longus muscle Popliteus muscle Soleus muscle Tibialis anterior muscle Tibialis posterior muscle **T Lower Leg Muscle, Left** *See S Lower Leg Muscle, Right* **V Foot Muscle, Right** Abductor hallucis muscle Adductor hallucis muscle Extensor digitorum brevis muscle Extensor hallucis brevis muscle Flexor digitorum brevis muscle Flexor hallucis brevis muscle Quadratus plantae muscle **W Foot Muscle, Left** *See V Foot Muscle, Right*	**Ø Open** **3 Percutaneous** **4 Percutaneous Endoscopic**	Z No Device	Z No Qualifier

Ø Medical and Surgical
K Muscles
R Replacement Definition: Putting in or on biological or synthetic material that physically takes the place and/or function of all or a portion of a body part

Explanation: The body part may have been taken out or replaced, or may be taken out, physically eradicated, or rendered nonfunctional during the REPLACEMENT procedure. A REMOVAL procedure is coded for taking out the device used in a previous replacement procedure.

Body Part Character 4	Approach Character 5	Device Character 6	Qualifier Character 7
Ø Head Muscle Auricularis muscle; Masseter muscle; Pterygoid muscle; Splenius capitis muscle; Temporalis muscle; Temporoparietalis muscle **1 Facial Muscle** Buccinator muscle; Corrugator supercilii muscle; Depressor anguli oris muscle; Depressor labii inferioris muscle; Depressor septi nasi muscle; Depressor supercilii muscle; Levator anguli oris muscle; Levator labii superioris alaeque nasi muscle; Levator labii superioris muscle; Mentalis muscle; Nasalis muscle; Occipitofrontalis muscle; Orbicularis oris muscle; Procerus muscle; Risorius muscle; Zygomaticus muscle **2 Neck Muscle, Right** Anterior vertebral muscle; Arytenoid muscle; Cricothyroid muscle; Infrahyoid muscle; Levator scapulae muscle; Platysma muscle; Scalene muscle; Splenius cervicis muscle; Sternocleidomastoid muscle; Suprahyoid muscle; Thyroarytenoid muscle **3 Neck Muscle, Left** *See 2 Neck Muscle, Right* **4 Tongue, Palate, Pharynx Muscle** Chondroglossus muscle; Genioglossus muscle; Hyoglossus muscle; Inferior longitudinal muscle; Levator veli palatini muscle; Palatoglossal muscle; Palatopharyngeal muscle; Pharyngeal constrictor muscle; Salpingopharyngeus muscle; Styloglossus muscle; Stylopharyngeus muscle; Superior longitudinal muscle; Tensor veli palatini muscle **5 Shoulder Muscle, Right** Deltoid muscle; Infraspinatus muscle; Subscapularis muscle; Supraspinatus muscle; Teres major muscle; Teres minor muscle **6 Shoulder Muscle, Left** *See 5 Shoulder Muscle, Right* **7 Upper Arm Muscle, Right** Biceps brachii muscle; Brachialis muscle; Coracobrachialis muscle; Triceps brachii muscle **8 Upper Arm Muscle, Left** *See 7 Upper Arm Muscle, Right* **9 Lower Arm and Wrist Muscle, Right** Anatomical snuffbox; Brachioradialis muscle; Extensor carpi radialis muscle; Extensor carpi ulnaris muscle; Flexor carpi radialis muscle; Flexor carpi ulnaris muscle; Flexor pollicis longus muscle; Palmaris longus muscle; Pronator quadratus muscle; Pronator teres muscle **B Lower Arm and Wrist Muscle, Left** *See 9 Lower Arm and Wrist Muscle, Right* **C Hand Muscle, Right** Hypothenar muscle; Palmar interosseous muscle; Thenar muscle **D Hand Muscle, Left** *See C Hand Muscle, Right* **F Trunk Muscle, Right** Coccygeus muscle; Erector spinae muscle; Interspinalis muscle; Intertransversarius muscle; Latissimus dorsi muscle; Quadratus lumborum muscle; Rhomboid major muscle; Rhomboid minor muscle; Serratus posterior muscle; Transversospinalis muscle; Trapezius muscle **G Trunk Muscle, Left** *See F Trunk Muscle, Right* **H Thorax Muscle, Right** Intercostal muscle; Levatores costarum muscle; Pectoralis major muscle; Pectoralis minor muscle; Serratus anterior muscle; Subclavius muscle; Subcostal muscle; Transverse thoracis muscle **J Thorax Muscle, Left** *See H Thorax Muscle, Right* **K Abdomen Muscle, Right** External oblique muscle; Internal oblique muscle; Pyramidalis muscle; Rectus abdominis muscle; Transversus abdominis muscle **L Abdomen Muscle, Left** *See K Abdomen Muscle, Right* **M Perineum Muscle** Bulbospongiosus muscle; Cremaster muscle; Deep transverse perineal muscle; Ischiocavernosus muscle; Levator ani muscle; Superficial transverse perineal muscle **N Hip Muscle, Right** Gemellus muscle; Gluteus maximus muscle; Gluteus medius muscle; Gluteus minimus muscle; Iliacus muscle; Obturator muscle; Piriformis muscle; Psoas muscle; Quadratus femoris muscle; Tensor fasciae latae muscle **P Hip Muscle, Left** *See N Hip Muscle, Right* **Q Upper Leg Muscle, Right** Adductor brevis muscle; Adductor longus muscle; Adductor magnus muscle; Biceps femoris muscle; Gracilis muscle; Pectineus muscle; Quadriceps (femoris); Rectus femoris muscle; Sartorius muscle; Semimembranosus muscle; Semitendinosus muscle; Vastus intermedius muscle; Vastus lateralis muscle; Vastus medialis muscle **R Upper Leg Muscle, Left** *See Q Upper Leg Muscle, Right* **S Lower Leg Muscle, Right** Extensor digitorum longus muscle; Extensor hallucis longus muscle; Fibularis brevis muscle; Fibularis longus muscle; Flexor digitorum longus muscle; Flexor hallucis longus muscle; Gastrocnemius muscle; Peroneus brevis muscle; Peroneus longus muscle; Popliteus muscle; Soleus muscle; Tibialis anterior muscle; Tibialis posterior muscle **T Lower Leg Muscle, Left** *See S Lower Leg Muscle, Right* **V Foot Muscle, Right** Abductor hallucis muscle; Adductor hallucis muscle; Extensor digitorum brevis muscle; Extensor hallucis brevis muscle; Flexor digitorum brevis muscle; Flexor hallucis brevis muscle; Quadratus plantae muscle **W Foot Muscle, Left** *See V Foot Muscle, Right*	**Ø Open** **4 Percutaneous Endoscopic**	**7 Autologous Tissue Substitute** **J Synthetic Substitute** **K Nonautologous Tissue Substitute**	**Z No Qualifier**

Muscles

Ø Medical and Surgical
K Muscles
S Reposition Definition: Moving to its normal location, or other suitable location, all or a portion of a body part

Explanation: The body part is moved to a new location from an abnormal location, or from a normal location where it is not functioning correctly. The body part may or may not be cut out or off to be moved to the new location.

Body Part Character 4	Approach Character 5	Device Character 6	Qualifier Character 7
Ø Head Muscle Auricularis muscle Masseter muscle Pterygoid muscle Splenius capitis muscle Temporalis muscle Temporoparietalis muscle **1 Facial Muscle** Buccinator muscle Corrugator supercilii muscle Depressor anguli oris muscle Depressor labii inferioris muscle Depressor septi nasi muscle Depressor supercilii muscle Levator anguli oris muscle Levator labii superioris alaeque nasi muscle Levator labii superioris muscle Mentalis muscle Nasalis muscle Occipitofrontalis muscle Orbicularis oris muscle Procerus muscle Risorius muscle Zygomaticus muscle **2 Neck Muscle, Right** Anterior vertebral muscle Arytenoid muscle Cricothyroid muscle Infrahyoid muscle Levator scapulae muscle Platysma muscle Scalene muscle Splenius cervicis muscle Sternocleidomastoid muscle Suprahyoid muscle Thyroarytenoid muscle **3 Neck Muscle, Left** *See 2 Neck Muscle, Right* **4 Tongue, Palate, Pharynx Muscle** Chondroglossus muscle Genioglossus muscle Hyoglossus muscle Inferior longitudinal muscle Levator veli palatini muscle Palatoglossal muscle Palatopharyngeal muscle Pharyngeal constrictor muscle Salpingopharyngeus muscle Styloglossus muscle Stylopharyngeus muscle Superior longitudinal muscle Tensor veli palatini muscle **5 Shoulder Muscle, Right** Deltoid muscle Infraspinatus muscle Subscapularis muscle Supraspinatus muscle Teres major muscle Teres minor muscle **6 Shoulder Muscle, Left** *See 5 Shoulder Muscle, Right* **7 Upper Arm Muscle, Right** Biceps brachii muscle Brachialis muscle Coracobrachialis muscle Triceps brachii muscle **8 Upper Arm Muscle, Left** *See 7 Upper Arm Muscle, Right* **9 Lower Arm and Wrist Muscle, Right** Anatomical snuffbox Brachioradialis muscle Extensor carpi radialis muscle Extensor carpi ulnaris muscle Flexor carpi radialis muscle Flexor carpi ulnaris muscle Flexor pollicis longus muscle Palmaris longus muscle Pronator quadratus muscle Pronator teres muscle **B Lower Arm and Wrist Muscle, Left** *See 9 Lower Arm and Wrist Muscle, Right* **C Hand Muscle, Right** Hypothenar muscle Palmar interosseous muscle Thenar muscle **D Hand Muscle, Left** *See C Hand Muscle, Right* **F Trunk Muscle, Right** Coccygeus muscle Erector spinae muscle Interspinalis muscle Intertransversarius muscle Latissimus dorsi muscle Quadratus lumborum muscle Rhomboid major muscle Rhomboid minor muscle Serratus posterior muscle Transversospinalis muscle Trapezius muscle **G Trunk Muscle, Left** *See F Trunk Muscle, Right* **H Thorax Muscle, Right** Intercostal muscle Levatores costarum muscle Pectoralis major muscle Pectoralis minor muscle Serratus anterior muscle Subclavius muscle Subcostal muscle Transverse thoracis muscle **J Thorax Muscle, Left** *See H Thorax Muscle, Right* **K Abdomen Muscle, Right** External oblique muscle Internal oblique muscle Pyramidalis muscle Rectus abdominis muscle Transversus abdominis muscle **L Abdomen Muscle, Left** *See K Abdomen Muscle, Right* **M Perineum Muscle** Bulbospongiosus muscle Cremaster muscle Deep transverse perineal muscle Ischiocavernosus muscle Levator ani muscle Superficial transverse perineal muscle **N Hip Muscle, Right** Gemellus muscle Gluteus maximus muscle Gluteus medius muscle Gluteus minimus muscle Iliacus muscle Obturator muscle Piriformis muscle Psoas muscle Quadratus femoris muscle Tensor fasciae latae muscle **P Hip Muscle, Left** *See N Hip Muscle, Right* **Q Upper Leg Muscle, Right** Adductor brevis muscle Adductor longus muscle Adductor magnus muscle Biceps femoris muscle Gracilis muscle Pectineus muscle Quadriceps (femoris) Rectus femoris muscle Sartorius muscle Semimembranosus muscle Semitendinosus muscle Vastus intermedius muscle Vastus lateralis muscle Vastus medialis muscle **R Upper Leg Muscle, Left** *See Q Upper Leg Muscle, Right* **S Lower Leg Muscle, Right** Extensor digitorum longus muscle Extensor hallucis longus muscle Fibularis brevis muscle Fibularis longus muscle Flexor digitorum longus muscle Flexor hallucis longus muscle Gastrocnemius muscle Peroneus brevis muscle Peroneus longus muscle Popliteus muscle Soleus muscle Tibialis anterior muscle Tibialis posterior muscle **T Lower Leg Muscle, Left** *See S Lower Leg Muscle, Right* **V Foot Muscle, Right** Abductor hallucis muscle Adductor hallucis muscle Extensor digitorum brevis muscle Extensor hallucis brevis muscle Flexor digitorum brevis muscle Flexor hallucis brevis muscle Quadratus plantae muscle **W Foot Muscle, Left** *See V Foot Muscle, Right*	**Ø Open** **4 Percutaneous Endoscopic**	**Z** No Device	**Z** No Qualifier

Ø Medical and Surgical
K Muscles
T Resection Definition: Cutting out or off, without replacement, all of a body part
Explanation: None

Body Part Character 4	Approach Character 5	Device Character 6	Qualifier Character 7
Ø Head Muscle Auricularis muscle Masseter muscle Pterygoid muscle Splenius capitis muscle Temporalis muscle Temporoparietalis muscle **1 Facial Muscle** Buccinator muscle Corrugator supercilii muscle Depressor anguli oris muscle Depressor labii inferioris muscle Depressor septi nasi muscle Depressor supercilii muscle Levator anguli oris muscle Levator labii superioris alaeque nasi muscle Levator labii superioris muscle Mentalis muscle Nasalis muscle Occipitofrontalis muscle Orbicularis oris muscle Procerus muscle Risorius muscle Zygomaticus muscle **2 Neck Muscle, Right** Anterior vertebral muscle Arytenoid muscle Cricothyroid muscle Infrahyoid muscle Levator scapulae muscle Platysma muscle Scalene muscle Splenius cervicis muscle Sternocleidomastoid muscle Suprahyoid muscle Thyroarytenoid muscle **3 Neck Muscle, Left** *See 2 Neck Muscle, Right* **4 Tongue, Palate, Pharynx Muscle** Chondroglossus muscle Genioglossus muscle Hyoglossus muscle Inferior longitudinal muscle Levator veli palatini muscle Palatoglossal muscle Palatopharyngeal muscle Pharyngeal constrictor muscle Salpingopharyngeus muscle Styloglossus muscle Stylopharyngeus muscle Superior longitudinal muscle Tensor veli palatini muscle **5 Shoulder Muscle, Right** Deltoid muscle Infraspinatus muscle Subscapularis muscle Supraspinatus muscle Teres major muscle Teres minor muscle **6 Shoulder Muscle, Left** *See 5 Shoulder Muscle, Right* **7 Upper Arm Muscle, Right** Biceps brachii muscle Brachialis muscle Coracobrachialis muscle Triceps brachii muscle **8 Upper Arm Muscle, Left** *See 7 Upper Arm Muscle, Right* **9 Lower Arm and Wrist Muscle, Right** Anatomical snuffbox Brachioradialis muscle Extensor carpi radialis muscle Extensor carpi ulnaris muscle Flexor carpi radialis muscle Flexor carpi ulnaris muscle Flexor pollicis longus muscle Palmaris longus muscle Pronator quadratus muscle Pronator teres muscle **B Lower Arm and Wrist Muscle, Left** *See 9 Lower Arm and Wrist Muscle, Right* **C Hand Muscle, Right** Hypothenar muscle Palmar interosseous muscle Thenar muscle **D Hand Muscle, Left** *See C Hand Muscle, Right* **F Trunk Muscle, Right** Coccygeus muscle Erector spinae muscle Interspinalis muscle Intertransversarius muscle Latissimus dorsi muscle Quadratus lumborum muscle Rhomboid major muscle Rhomboid minor muscle Serratus posterior muscle Transversospinalis muscle Trapezius muscle **G Trunk Muscle, Left** *See F Trunk Muscle, Right* **H Thorax Muscle, Right** ⊞ Intercostal muscle Levatores costarum muscle Pectoralis major muscle Pectoralis minor muscle Serratus anterior muscle Subclavius muscle Subcostal muscle Transverse thoracis muscle **J Thorax Muscle, Left** ⊞ *See H Thorax Muscle, Right* **K Abdomen Muscle, Right** External oblique muscle Internal oblique muscle Pyramidalis muscle Rectus abdominis muscle Transversus abdominis muscle **L Abdomen Muscle, Left** *See K Abdomen Muscle, Right* **M Perineum Muscle** Bulbospongiosus muscle Cremaster muscle Deep transverse perineal muscle Ischiocavernosus muscle Levator ani muscle Superficial transverse perineal muscle **N Hip Muscle, Right** Gemellus muscle Gluteus maximus muscle Gluteus medius muscle Gluteus minimus muscle Iliacus muscle Obturator muscle Piriformis muscle Psoas muscle Quadratus femoris muscle Tensor fasciae latae muscle **P Hip Muscle, Left** *See N Hip Muscle, Right* **Q Upper Leg Muscle, Right** Adductor brevis muscle Adductor longus muscle Adductor magnus muscle Biceps femoris muscle Gracilis muscle Pectineus muscle Quadriceps (femoris) Rectus femoris muscle Sartorius muscle Semimembranosus muscle Semitendinosus muscle Vastus intermedius muscle Vastus lateralis muscle Vastus medialis muscle **R Upper Leg Muscle, Left** *See Q Upper Leg Muscle, Right* **S Lower Leg Muscle, Right** Extensor digitorum longus muscle Extensor hallucis longus muscle Fibularis brevis muscle Fibularis longus muscle Flexor digitorum longus muscle Flexor hallucis longus muscle Gastrocnemius muscle Peroneus brevis muscle Peroneus longus muscle Popliteus muscle Soleus muscle Tibialis anterior muscle Tibialis posterior muscle **T Lower Leg Muscle, Left** *See S Lower Leg Muscle, Right* **V Foot Muscle, Right** Abductor hallucis muscle Adductor hallucis muscle Extensor digitorum brevis muscle Extensor hallucis brevis muscle Flexor digitorum brevis muscle Flexor hallucis brevis muscle Quadratus plantae muscle **W Foot Muscle, Left** *See V Foot Muscle, Right*	**Ø Open** **4 Percutaneous Endoscopic**	**Z No Device**	**Z No Qualifier**

See Appendix L for Procedure Combinations
⊞ ØKT[H,J]ØZZ

Ø Medical and Surgical
K Muscles
U Supplement Definition: Putting in or on biological or synthetic material that physically reinforces and/or augments the function of a portion of a body part

Explanation: The biological material is non-living, or is living and from the same individual. The body part may have been previously replaced, and the SUPPLEMENT procedure is performed to physically reinforce and/or augment the function of the replaced body part.

Body Part Character 4	Approach Character 5	Device Character 6	Qualifier Character 7
Ø Head Muscle Auricularis muscle Masseter muscle Pterygoid muscle Splenius capitis muscle Temporalis muscle Temporoparietalis muscle **1 Facial Muscle** Buccinator muscle Corrugator supercilii muscle Depressor anguli oris muscle Depressor labii inferioris muscle Depressor septi nasi muscle Depressor supercilii muscle Levator anguli oris muscle Levator labii superioris alaeque nasi muscle Levator labii superioris muscle Mentalis muscle Nasalis muscle Occipitofrontalis muscle Orbicularis oris muscle Procerus muscle Risorius muscle Zygomaticus muscle **2 Neck Muscle, Right** Anterior vertebral muscle Arytenoid muscle Cricothyroid muscle Infrahyoid muscle Levator scapulae muscle Platysma muscle Scalene muscle Splenius cervicis muscle Sternocleidomastoid muscle Suprahyoid muscle Thyroarytenoid muscle **3 Neck Muscle, Left** *See 2 Neck Muscle, Right* **4 Tongue, Palate, Pharynx Muscle** Chondroglossus muscle Genioglossus muscle Hyoglossus muscle Inferior longitudinal muscle Levator veli palatini muscle Palatoglossal muscle Palatopharyngeal muscle Pharyngeal constrictor muscle Salpingopharyngeus muscle Styloglossus muscle Stylopharyngeus muscle Superior longitudinal muscle Tensor veli palatini muscle **5 Shoulder Muscle, Right** Deltoid muscle Infraspinatus muscle Subscapularis muscle Supraspinatus muscle Teres major muscle Teres minor muscle **6 Shoulder Muscle, Left** *See 5 Shoulder Muscle, Right* **7 Upper Arm Muscle, Right** Biceps brachii muscle Brachialis muscle Coracobrachialis muscle Triceps brachii muscle **8 Upper Arm Muscle, Left** *See 7 Upper Arm Muscle, Right* **9 Lower Arm and Wrist Muscle, Right** Anatomical snuffbox Brachioradialis muscle Extensor carpi radialis muscle Extensor carpi ulnaris muscle Flexor carpi radialis muscle Flexor carpi ulnaris muscle Flexor pollicis longus muscle Palmaris longus muscle Pronator quadratus muscle Pronator teres muscle **B Lower Arm and Wrist Muscle, Left** *See 9 Lower Arm and Wrist Muscle, Right* **C Hand Muscle, Right** Hypothenar muscle Palmar interosseous muscle Thenar muscle **D Hand Muscle, Left** *See C Hand Muscle, Right* **F Trunk Muscle, Right** Coccygeus muscle Erector spinae muscle Interspinalis muscle Intertransversarius muscle Latissimus dorsi muscle Quadratus lumborum muscle Rhomboid major muscle Rhomboid minor muscle Serratus posterior muscle Transversospinalis muscle Trapezius muscle **G Trunk Muscle, Left** *See F Trunk Muscle, Right* **H Thorax Muscle, Right** Intercostal muscle Levatores costarum muscle Pectoralis major muscle Pectoralis minor muscle Serratus anterior muscle Subclavius muscle Subcostal muscle Transverse thoracis muscle **J Thorax Muscle, Left** *See H Thorax Muscle, Right* **K Abdomen Muscle, Right** External oblique muscle Internal oblique muscle Pyramidalis muscle Rectus abdominis muscle Transversus abdominis muscle **L Abdomen Muscle, Left** *See K Abdomen Muscle, Right* **M Perineum Muscle** Bulbospongiosus muscle Cremaster muscle Deep transverse perineal muscle Ischiocavernosus muscle Levator ani muscle Superficial transverse perineal muscle **N Hip Muscle, Right** Gemellus muscle Gluteus maximus muscle Gluteus medius muscle Gluteus minimus muscle Iliacus muscle Obturator muscle Piriformis muscle Psoas muscle Quadratus femoris muscle Tensor fasciae latae muscle **P Hip Muscle, Left** *See N Hip Muscle, Right* **Q Upper Leg Muscle, Right** Adductor brevis muscle Adductor longus muscle Adductor magnus muscle Biceps femoris muscle Gracilis muscle Pectineus muscle Quadriceps (femoris) Rectus femoris muscle Sartorius muscle Semimembranosus muscle Semitendinosus muscle Vastus intermedius muscle Vastus lateralis muscle Vastus medialis muscle **R Upper Leg Muscle, Left** *See Q Upper Leg Muscle, Right* **S Lower Leg Muscle, Right** Extensor digitorum longus muscle Extensor hallucis longus muscle Fibularis brevis muscle Fibularis longus muscle Flexor digitorum longus muscle Flexor hallucis longus muscle Gastrocnemius muscle Peroneus brevis muscle Peroneus longus muscle Popliteus muscle Soleus muscle Tibialis anterior muscle Tibialis posterior muscle **T Lower Leg Muscle, Left** *See S Lower Leg Muscle, Right* **V Foot Muscle, Right** Abductor hallucis muscle Adductor hallucis muscle Extensor digitorum brevis muscle Extensor hallucis brevis muscle Flexor digitorum brevis muscle Flexor hallucis brevis muscle Quadratus plantae muscle **W Foot Muscle, Left** *See V Foot Muscle, Right*	**Ø Open** **4 Percutaneous Endoscopic**	**7 Autologous Tissue Substitute** **J Synthetic Substitute** **K Nonautologous Tissue Substitute**	**Z No Qualifier**

Ø Medical and Surgical
K Muscles
W Revision Definition: Correcting, to the extent possible, a portion of a malfunctioning device or the position of a displaced device

Explanation: Revision can include correcting a malfunctioning or displaced device by taking out or putting in components of the device such as a screw or pin

Body Part Character 4	Approach Character 5	Device Character 6	Qualifier Character 7
X Upper Muscle Y Lower Muscle	Ø Open 3 Percutaneous 4 Percutaneous Endoscopic	Ø Drainage Device 7 Autologous Tissue Substitute J Synthetic Substitute K Nonautologous Tissue Substitute M Stimulator Lead Y Other Device	Z No Qualifier
X Upper Muscle Y Lower Muscle	X External	Ø Drainage Device 7 Autologous Tissue Substitute J Synthetic Substitute K Nonautologous Tissue Substitute M Stimulator Lead	Z No Qualifier

Non-OR ØKW[X,Y][3,4]YZ
Non-OR ØKW[X,Y]X[Ø,7,J,K,M]Z

Ø Medical and Surgical
K Muscles
X Transfer Definition: Moving, without taking out, all or a portion of a body part to another location to take over the function of all or a portion of a body part
Explanation: The body part transferred remains connected to its vascular and nervous supply

Body Part Character 4	Approach Character 5	Device Character 6	Qualifier Character 7
Ø Head Muscle Auricularis muscle Masseter muscle Pterygoid muscle Splenius capitis muscle Temporalis muscle Temporoparietalis muscle **1 Facial Muscle** Buccinator muscle Corrugator supercilii muscle Depressor anguli oris muscle Depressor labii inferioris muscle Depressor septi nasi muscle Depressor supercilii muscle Levator anguli oris muscle Levator labii superioris alaeque nasi muscle Levator labii superioris muscle Mentalis muscle Nasalis muscle Occipitofrontalis muscle Orbicularis oris muscle Procerus muscle Risorius muscle Zygomaticus muscle **2 Neck Muscle, Right** Anterior vertebral muscle Arytenoid muscle Cricothyroid muscle Infrahyoid muscle Levator scapulae muscle Platysma muscle Scalene muscle Splenius cervicis muscle Sternocleidomastoid muscle Suprahyoid muscle Thyroarytenoid muscle **3 Neck Muscle, Left** *See 2 Neck Muscle, Right* **4 Tongue, Palate, Pharynx Muscle** Chondroglossus muscle Genioglossus muscle Hyoglossus muscle Inferior longitudinal muscle Levator veli palatini muscle Palatoglossal muscle Palatopharyngeal muscle Pharyngeal constrictor muscle Salpingopharyngeus muscle Styloglossus muscle Stylopharyngeus muscle Superior longitudinal muscle Tensor veli palatini muscle **5 Shoulder Muscle, Right** Deltoid muscle Infraspinatus muscle Subscapularis muscle Supraspinatus muscle Teres major muscle Teres minor muscle **6 Shoulder Muscle, Left** *See 5 Shoulder Muscle, Right* **7 Upper Arm Muscle, Right** Biceps brachii muscle Brachialis muscle Coracobrachialis muscle Triceps brachii muscle **8 Upper Arm Muscle, Left** *See 7 Upper Arm Muscle, Right* **9 Lower Arm and Wrist Muscle, Right** Anatomical snuffbox Brachioradialis muscle Extensor carpi radialis muscle Extensor carpi ulnaris muscle Flexor carpi radialis muscle Flexor carpi ulnaris muscle Flexor pollicis longus muscle Palmaris longus muscle Pronator quadratus muscle Pronator teres muscle **B Lower Arm and Wrist Muscle, Left** *See 9 Lower Arm and Wrist Muscle, Right* **C Hand Muscle, Right** Hypothenar muscle Palmar interosseous muscle Thenar muscle **D Hand Muscle, Left** *See C Hand Muscle, Right* **H Thorax Muscle, Right** Intercostal muscle Levatores costarum muscle Pectoralis major muscle Pectoralis minor muscle Serratus anterior muscle Subclavius muscle Subcostal muscle Transverse thoracis muscle **J Thorax Muscle, Left** *See H Thorax Muscle, Right* **M Perineum Muscle** Bulbospongiosus muscle Cremaster muscle Deep transverse perineal muscle Ischiocavernosus muscle Levator ani muscle Superficial transverse perineal muscle **N Hip Muscle, Right** Gemellus muscle Gluteus maximus muscle Gluteus medius muscle Gluteus minimus muscle Iliacus muscle Obturator muscle Piriformis muscle Psoas muscle Quadratus femoris muscle Tensor fasciae latae muscle **P Hip Muscle, Left** *See N Hip Muscle, Right* **Q Upper Leg Muscle, Right** Adductor brevis muscle Adductor longus muscle Adductor magnus muscle Biceps femoris muscle Gracilis muscle Pectineus muscle Quadriceps (femoris) Rectus femoris muscle Sartorius muscle Semimembranosus muscle Semitendinosus muscle Vastus intermedius muscle Vastus lateralis muscle Vastus medialis muscle **R Upper Leg Muscle, Left** *See Q Upper Leg Muscle, Right* **S Lower Leg Muscle, Right** Extensor digitorum longus muscle Extensor hallucis longus muscle Fibularis brevis muscle Fibularis longus muscle Flexor digitorum longus muscle Flexor hallucis longus muscle Gastrocnemius muscle Peroneus brevis muscle Peroneus longus muscle Popliteus muscle Soleus muscle Tibialis anterior muscle Tibialis posterior muscle **T Lower Leg Muscle, Left** *See S Lower Leg Muscle, Right* **V Foot Muscle, Right** Abductor hallucis muscle Adductor hallucis muscle Extensor digitorum brevis muscle Extensor hallucis brevis muscle Flexor digitorum brevis muscle Flexor hallucis brevis muscle Quadratus plantae muscle **W Foot Muscle, Left** *See V Foot Muscle, Right*	Ø Open 4 Percutaneous Endoscopic	Z No Device	Ø Skin 1 Subcutaneous Tissue 2 Skin and Subcutaneous Tissue Z No Qualifier

ØKX Continued on next page

Ø Medical and Surgical
K Muscles
X Transfer Definition: Moving, without taking out, all or a portion of a body part to another location to take over the function of all or a portion of a body part
Explanation: The body part transferred remains connected to its vascular and nervous supply

ØKX Continued

Body Part Character 4	Approach Character 5	Device Character 6	Qualifier Character 7
F Trunk Muscle, Right Coccygeus muscle Erector spinae muscle Interspinalis muscle Intertransversarius muscle Latissimus dorsi muscle Quadratus lumborum muscle Rhomboid major muscle Rhomboid minor muscle Serratus posterior muscle Transversospinalis muscle Trapezius muscle **G Trunk Muscle, Left** *See F Trunk Muscle, Right*	**Ø Open** **4 Percutaneous Endoscopic**	**Z No Device**	**Ø Skin** **1 Subcutaneous Tissue** **2 Skin and Subcutaneous Tissue** **5 Latissimus Dorsi Myocutaneous Flap** **7 Deep Inferior Epigastric Artery Perforator Flap** **8 Superficial Inferior Epigastric Artery Flap** **9 Gluteal Artery Perforator Flap** **Z No Qualifier**
K Abdomen Muscle, Right External oblique muscle Internal oblique muscle Pyramidalis muscle Rectus abdominis muscle Transversus abdominis muscle **L Abdomen Muscle, Left** *See K Abdomen Muscle, Right*	**Ø Open** **4 Percutaneous Endoscopic**	**Z No Device**	**Ø Skin** **1 Subcutaneous Tissue** **2 Skin and Subcutaneous Tissue** **6 Transverse Rectus Abdominis Myocutaneous Flap** **Z No Qualifier**

Tendons ØL2–ØLX

Character Meanings*

This Character Meaning table is provided as a guide to assist the user in the identification of character members that may be found in this section of code tables. It **SHOULD NOT** be used to build a PCS code.

Operation–Character 3		Body Part–Character 4		Approach–Character 5		Device–Character 6		Qualifier–Character 7	
2	Change	Ø	Head and Neck Tendon	Ø	Open	Ø	Drainage Device	X	Diagnostic
5	Destruction	1	Shoulder Tendon, Right	3	Percutaneous	7	Autologous Tissue Substitute	Z	No Qualifier
8	Division	2	Shoulder Tendon, Left	4	Percutaneous Endoscopic	J	Synthetic Substitute		
9	Drainage	3	Upper Arm Tendon, Right	X	External	K	Nonautologous Tissue Substitute		
B	Excision	4	Upper Arm Tendon, Left			Y	Other Device		
C	Extirpation	5	Lower Arm and Wrist Tendon, Right			Z	No Device		
D	Extraction	6	Lower Arm and Wrist Tendon, Left						
H	Insertion	7	Hand Tendon, Right						
J	Inspection	8	Hand Tendon, Left						
M	Reattachment	9	Trunk Tendon, Right						
N	Release	B	Trunk Tendon, Left						
P	Removal	C	Thorax Tendon, Right						
Q	Repair	D	Thorax Tendon, Left						
R	Replacement	F	Abdomen Tendon, Right						
S	Reposition	G	Abdomen Tendon, Left						
T	Resection	H	Perineum Tendon						
U	Supplement	J	Hip Tendon, Right						
W	Revision	K	Hip Tendon, Left						
X	Transfer	L	Upper Leg Tendon, Right						
		M	Upper Leg Tendon, Left						
		N	Lower Leg Tendon, Right						
		P	Lower Leg Tendon, Left						
		Q	Knee Tendon, Right						
		R	Knee Tendon, Left						
		S	Ankle Tendon, Right						
		T	Ankle Tendon, Left						
		V	Foot Tendon, Right						
		W	Foot Tendon, Left						
		X	Upper Tendon						
		Y	Lower Tendon						

* Includes synovial membrane.

AHA Coding Clinic for table ØL8
2016, 3Q, 30 Resection of femur with interposition arthroplasty

AHA Coding Clinic for table ØLB
2017, 2Q, 21 Arthroscopic anterior cruciate ligament revision using autograft with anterolateral ligament reconstruction
2015, 3Q, 26 Thumb arthroplasty with resection of trapezium
2014, 3Q, 14 Application of TheraSkin® and excisional debridement
2014, 3Q, 18 Placement of reverse sural fasciocutaneous pedicle flap

AHA Coding Clinic for table ØLD
2017, 4Q, 41 Extraction procedures

AHA Coding Clinic for table ØLQ
2016, 3Q, 32 Rotator cuff repair, tenodesis, decompression, acromioplasty and coracoplasty
2015, 2Q, 11 Repair of patellar and quadriceps tendons with allograft
2013, 3Q, 20 Superior labrum anterior posterior (SLAP) repair and subacromial decompression

AHA Coding Clinic for table ØLS
2016, 3Q, 32 Rotator cuff repair, tenodesis, decompression, acromioplasty and coracoplasty
2015, 3Q, 14 Endoprosthetic replacement of humerus and tendon reattachment

AHA Coding Clinic for table ØLU
2015, 2Q, 11 Repair of patellar and quadriceps tendons with allograft

Foot Tendons

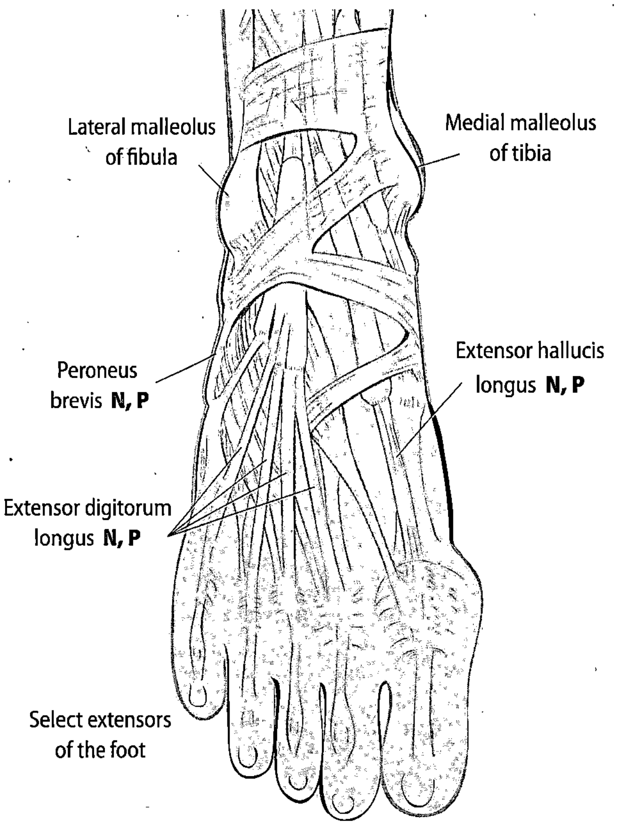

Shoulder Tendons

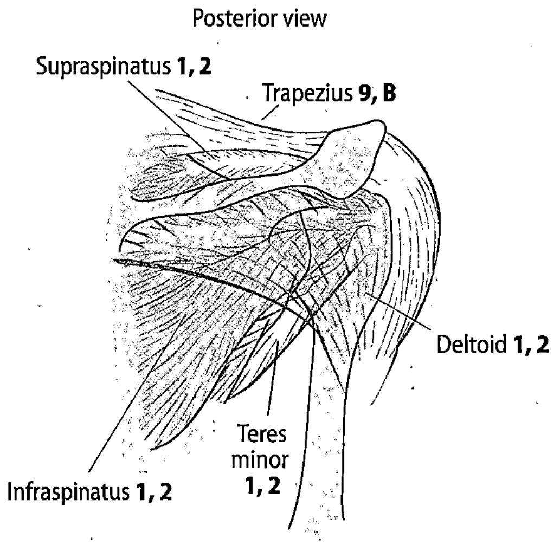

Tendons of Wrist and Hand

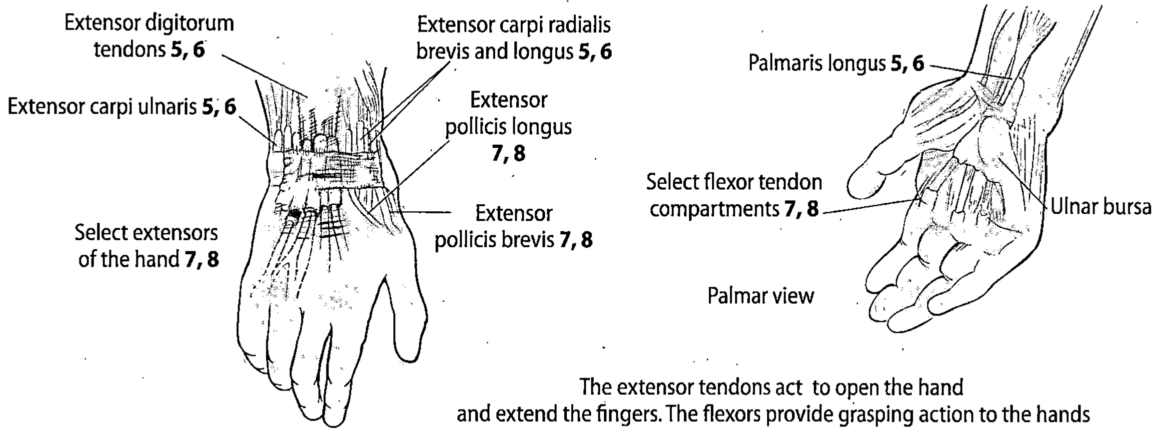

The extensor tendons act to open the hand and extend the fingers. The flexors provide grasping action to the hands

Leg Muscles and Tendons

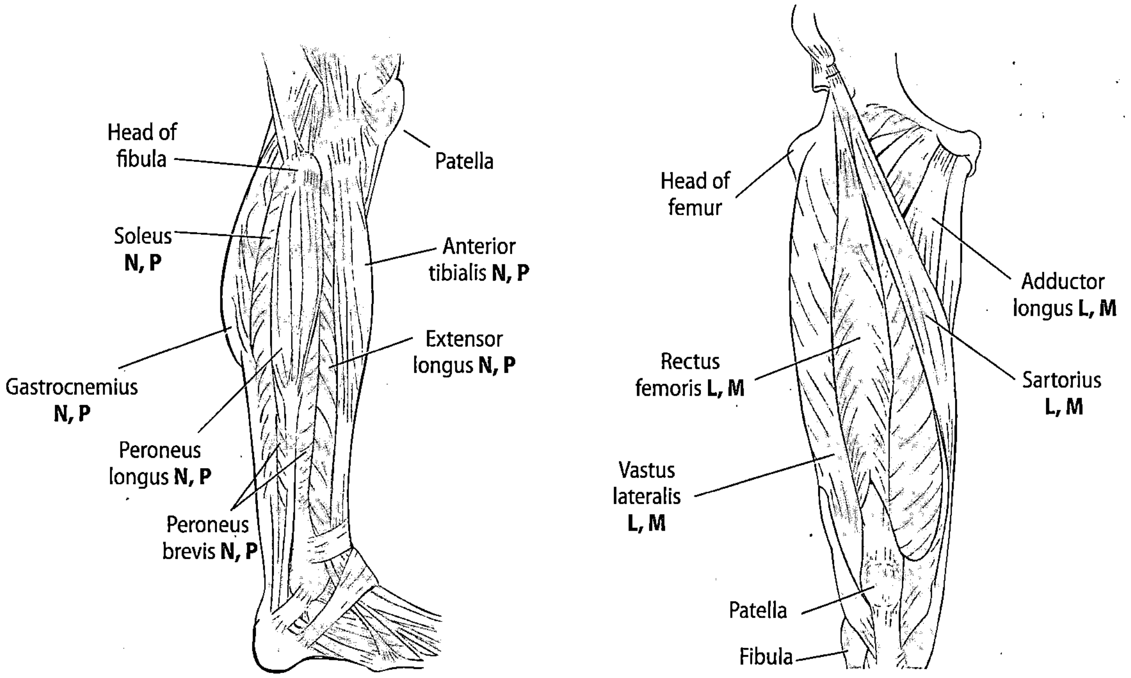

Ø Medical and Surgical
L Tendons
2 Change Definition: Taking out or off a device from a body part and putting back an identical or similar device in or on the same body part without cutting or puncturing the skin or a mucous membrane

Explanation: All CHANGE procedures are coded using the approach EXTERNAL

Body Part Character 4	Approach Character 5	Device Character 6	Qualifier Character 7
X Upper Tendon Y Lower Tendon	X External	Ø Drainage Device Y Other Device	Z No Qualifier

Non-OR All body part, approach, device, and qualifier values

Ø Medical and Surgical
L Tendons
5 Destruction Definition: Physical eradication of all or a portion of a body part by the direct use of energy, force, or a destructive agent

Explanation: None of the body part is physically taken out

Body Part Character 4	Approach Character 5	Device Character 6	Qualifier Character 7
Ø Head and Neck Tendon 1 Shoulder Tendon, Right 2 Shoulder Tendon, Left 3 Upper Arm Tendon, Right 4 Upper Arm Tendon, Left 5 Lower Arm and Wrist Tendon, Right 6 Lower Arm and Wrist Tendon, Left 7 Hand Tendon, Right 8 Hand Tendon, Left 9 Trunk Tendon, Right B Trunk Tendon, Left C Thorax Tendon, Right D Thorax Tendon, Left F Abdomen Tendon, Right G Abdomen Tendon, Left H Perineum Tendon J Hip Tendon, Right K Hip Tendon, Left L Upper Leg Tendon, Right M Upper Leg Tendon, Left N Lower Leg Tendon, Right Achilles tendon P Lower Leg Tendon, Left *See N Lower Leg Tendon, Right* Q Knee Tendon, Right Patellar tendon R Knee Tendon, Left *See Q Knee Tendon, Right* S Ankle Tendon, Right T Ankle Tendon, Left V Foot Tendon, Right W Foot Tendon, Left	Ø Open 3 Percutaneous 4 Percutaneous Endoscopic	Z No Device	Z No Qualifier

Ø Medical and Surgical
L Tendons
8 Division Definition: Cutting into a body part, without draining fluids and/or gases from the body part, in order to separate or transect a body part
Explanation: All or a portion of the body part is separated into two or more portions

Body Part Character 4	Approach Character 5	Device Character 6	Qualifier Character 7
Ø Head and Neck Tendon **1** Shoulder Tendon, Right **2** Shoulder Tendon, Left **3** Upper Arm Tendon, Right **4** Upper Arm Tendon, Left **5** Lower Arm and Wrist Tendon, Right **6** Lower Arm and Wrist Tendon, Left **7** Hand Tendon, Right **8** Hand Tendon, Left **9** Trunk Tendon, Right **B** Trunk Tendon, Left **C** Thorax Tendon, Right **D** Thorax Tendon, Left **F** Abdomen Tendon, Right **G** Abdomen Tendon, Left **H** Perineum Tendon **J** Hip Tendon, Right **K** Hip Tendon, Left **L** Upper Leg Tendon, Right **M** Upper Leg Tendon, Left **N** Lower Leg Tendon, Right Achilles tendon **P** Lower Leg Tendon, Left *See N Lower Leg Tendon, Right* **Q** Knee Tendon, Right Patellar tendon **R** Knee Tendon, Left *See Q Knee Tendon, Right* **S** Ankle Tendon, Right **T** Ankle Tendon, Left **V** Foot Tendon, Right **W** Foot Tendon, Left	**Ø** Open **3** Percutaneous **4** Percutaneous Endoscopic	**Z** No Device	**Z** No Qualifier

Ø Medical and Surgical
L Tendons
9 Drainage Definition: Taking or letting out fluids and/or gases from a body part
Explanation: The qualifier DIAGNOSTIC is used to identify drainage procedures that are biopsies

Body Part Character 4	Approach Character 5	Device Character 6	Qualifier Character 7
Ø Head and Neck Tendon **1** Shoulder Tendon, Right **2** Shoulder Tendon, Left **3** Upper Arm Tendon, Right **4** Upper Arm Tendon, Left **5** Lower Arm and Wrist Tendon, Right **6** Lower Arm and Wrist Tendon, Left **7** Hand Tendon, Right **8** Hand Tendon, Left **9** Trunk Tendon, Right **B** Trunk Tendon, Left **C** Thorax Tendon, Right **D** Thorax Tendon, Left **F** Abdomen Tendon, Right **G** Abdomen Tendon, Left **H** Perineum Tendon **J** Hip Tendon, Right **K** Hip Tendon, Left **L** Upper Leg Tendon, Right **M** Upper Leg Tendon, Left **N** Lower Leg Tendon, Right Achilles tendon **P** Lower Leg Tendon, Left *See N Lower Leg Tendon, Right* **Q** Knee Tendon, Right Patellar tendon **R** Knee Tendon, Left *See Q Knee Tendon, Right* **S** Ankle Tendon, Right **T** Ankle Tendon, Left **V** Foot Tendon, Right **W** Foot Tendon, Left	**Ø** Open **3** Percutaneous **4** Percutaneous Endoscopic	**Ø** Drainage Device	**Z** No Qualifier
Ø Head and Neck Tendon **1** Shoulder Tendon, Right **2** Shoulder Tendon, Left **3** Upper Arm Tendon, Right **4** Upper Arm Tendon, Left **5** Lower Arm and Wrist Tendon, Right **6** Lower Arm and Wrist Tendon, Left **7** Hand Tendon, Right **8** Hand Tendon, Left **9** Trunk Tendon, Right **B** Trunk Tendon, Left **C** Thorax Tendon, Right **D** Thorax Tendon, Left **F** Abdomen Tendon, Right **G** Abdomen Tendon, Left **H** Perineum Tendon **J** Hip Tendon, Right **K** Hip Tendon, Left **L** Upper Leg Tendon, Right **M** Upper Leg Tendon, Left **N** Lower Leg Tendon, Right Achilles tendon **P** Lower Leg Tendon, Left *See N Lower Leg Tendon, Right* **Q** Knee Tendon, Right Patellar tendon **R** Knee Tendon, Left *See Q Knee Tendon, Right* **S** Ankle Tendon, Right **T** Ankle Tendon, Left **V** Foot Tendon, Right **W** Foot Tendon, Left	**Ø** Open **3** Percutaneous **4** Percutaneous Endoscopic	**Z** No Device	**X** Diagnostic **Z** No Qualifier

Non-OR ØL9[Ø,1,2,3,4,5,6,7,8,9,B,C,D,F,G,H,J,K,L,M,N,P,Q,R,S,T,V,W]3ØZ
Non-OR ØL9[Ø,1,2,3,4,5,6,7,8,9,B,C,D,F,G,H,J,K,L,M,N,P,Q,R,S,T,V,W]3ZZ
Non-OR ØL9[7,8]4ZZ

Ø Medical and Surgical
L Tendons
B Excision Definition: Cutting out or off, without replacement, a portion of a body part
Explanation: The qualifier DIAGNOSTIC is used to identify excision procedures that are biopsies

Body Part Character 4	Approach Character 5	Device Character 6	Qualifier Character 7
Ø Head and Neck Tendon **1** Shoulder Tendon, Right **2** Shoulder Tendon, Left **3** Upper Arm Tendon, Right **4** Upper Arm Tendon, Left **5** Lower Arm and Wrist Tendon, Right **6** Lower Arm and Wrist Tendon, Left **7** Hand Tendon, Right **8** Hand Tendon, Left **9** Trunk Tendon, Right **B** Trunk Tendon, Left **C** Thorax Tendon, Right **D** Thorax Tendon, Left **F** Abdomen Tendon, Right **G** Abdomen Tendon, Left **H** Perineum Tendon **J** Hip Tendon, Right **K** Hip Tendon, Left **L** Upper Leg Tendon, Right **M** Upper Leg Tendon, Left **N** Lower Leg Tendon, Right Achilles tendon **P** Lower Leg Tendon, Left *See N Lower Leg Tendon, Right* **Q** Knee Tendon, Right Patellar tendon **R** Knee Tendon, Left *See Q Knee Tendon, Right* **S** Ankle Tendon, Right **T** Ankle Tendon, Left **V** Foot Tendon, Right **W** Foot Tendon, Left	**Ø** Open **3** Percutaneous **4** Percutaneous Endoscopic	**Z** No Device	**X** Diagnostic **Z** No Qualifier

Ø Medical and Surgical
L Tendons
C Extirpation Definition: Taking or cutting out solid matter from a body part

Explanation: The solid matter may be an abnormal byproduct of a biological function or a foreign body; it may be imbedded in a body part or in the lumen of a tubular body part. The solid matter may or may not have been previously broken into pieces.

Body Part Character 4	Approach Character 5	Device Character 6	Qualifier Character 7
Ø Head and Neck Tendon **1** Shoulder Tendon, Right **2** Shoulder Tendon, Left **3** Upper Arm Tendon, Right **4** Upper Arm Tendon, Left **5** Lower Arm and Wrist Tendon, Right **6** Lower Arm and Wrist Tendon, Left **7** Hand Tendon, Right **8** Hand Tendon, Left **9** Trunk Tendon, Right **B** Trunk Tendon, Left **C** Thorax Tendon, Right **D** Thorax Tendon, Left **F** Abdomen Tendon, Right **G** Abdomen Tendon, Left **H** Perineum Tendon **J** Hip Tendon, Right **K** Hip Tendon, Left **L** Upper Leg Tendon, Right **M** Upper Leg Tendon, Left **N** Lower Leg Tendon, Right Achilles tendon **P** Lower Leg Tendon, Left *See N Lower Leg Tendon, Right* **Q** Knee Tendon, Right Patellar tendon **R** Knee Tendon, Left *See Q Knee Tendon, Right* **S** Ankle Tendon, Right **T** Ankle Tendon, Left **V** Foot Tendon, Right **W** Foot Tendon, Left	**Ø** Open **3** Percutaneous **4** Percutaneous Endoscopic	**Z** No Device	**Z** No Qualifier

Ø Medical and Surgical
L Tendons
D Extraction Definition: Pulling or stripping out or off all or a portion of a body part by the use of force
Explanation: The qualifier DIAGNOSTIC is used to identify extraction procedures that are biopsies

Body Part Character 4	Approach Character 5	Device Character 6	Qualifier Character 7
Ø Head and Neck Tendon 1 Shoulder Tendon, Right 2 Shoulder Tendon, Left 3 Upper Arm Tendon, Right 4 Upper Arm Tendon, Left 5 Lower Arm and Wrist Tendon, Right 6 Lower Arm and Wrist Tendon, Left 7 Hand Tendon, Right 8 Hand Tendon, Left 9 Trunk Tendon, Right B Trunk Tendon, Left C Thorax Tendon, Right D Thorax Tendon, Left F Abdomen Tendon, Right G Abdomen Tendon, Left H Perineum Tendon J Hip Tendon, Right K Hip Tendon, Left L Upper Leg Tendon, Right M Upper Leg Tendon, Left N Lower Leg Tendon, Right Achilles tendon P Lower Leg Tendon, Left *See N Lower Leg Tendon, Right* Q Knee Tendon, Right Patellar tendon R Knee Tendon, Left *See Q Knee Tendon, Right* S Ankle Tendon, Right T Ankle Tendon, Left V Foot Tendon, Right W Foot Tendon, Left	Ø Open	Z No Device	Z No Qualifier

Ø Medical and Surgical
L Tendons
H Insertion Definition: Putting in a nonbiological appliance that monitors, assists, performs, or prevents a physiological function but does not physically take the place of a body part
Explanation: None

Body Part Character 4	Approach Character 5	Device Character 6	Qualifier Character 7
X Upper Tendon Y Lower Tendon	Ø Open 3 Percutaneous 4 Percutaneous Endoscopic	Y Other Device	Z No Qualifier

Non-OR ØLH[X,Y][3,4]YZ

Ø Medical and Surgical
L Tendons
J Inspection Definition: Visually and/or manually exploring a body part
Explanation: Visual exploration may be performed with or without optical instrumentation. Manual exploration may be performed directly or through intervening body layers.

Body Part Character 4	Approach Character 5	Device Character 6	Qualifier Character 7
X Upper Tendon Y Lower Tendon	Ø Open 3 Percutaneous 4 Percutaneous Endoscopic X External	Z No Device	Z No Qualifier

Non-OR ØLJ[X,Y][3,X]ZZ

Ø Medical and Surgical
L Tendons
M Reattachment Definition: Putting back in or on all or a portion of a separated body part to its normal location or other suitable location
Explanation: Vascular circulation and nervous pathways may or may not be reestablished

Body Part Character 4	Approach Character 5	Device Character 6	Qualifier Character 7
Ø Head and Neck Tendon 1 Shoulder Tendon, Right 2 Shoulder Tendon, Left 3 Upper Arm Tendon, Right 4 Upper Arm Tendon, Left 5 Lower Arm and Wrist Tendon, Right 6 Lower Arm and Wrist Tendon, Left 7 Hand Tendon, Right 8 Hand Tendon, Left 9 Trunk Tendon, Right B Trunk Tendon, Left C Thorax Tendon, Right D Thorax Tendon, Left F Abdomen Tendon, Right G Abdomen Tendon, Left H Perineum Tendon J Hip Tendon, Right K Hip Tendon, Left L Upper Leg Tendon, Right M Upper Leg Tendon, Left N Lower Leg Tendon, Right Achilles tendon P Lower Leg Tendon, Left *See N Lower Leg Tendon, Right* Q Knee Tendon, Right Patellar tendon R Knee Tendon, Left *See Q Knee Tendon, Right* S Ankle Tendon, Right T Ankle Tendon, Left V Foot Tendon, Right W Foot Tendon, Left	Ø Open 4 Percutaneous Endoscopic	Z No Device	Z No Qualifier

Ø Medical and Surgical
L Tendons
N Release Definition: Freeing a body part from an abnormal physical constraint by cutting or by the use of force
Explanation: Some of the restraining tissue may be taken out but none of the body part is taken out

Body Part Character 4	Approach Character 5	Device Character 6	Qualifier Character 7
Ø Head and Neck Tendon 1 Shoulder Tendon, Right 2 Shoulder Tendon, Left 3 Upper Arm Tendon, Right 4 Upper Arm Tendon, Left 5 Lower Arm and Wrist Tendon, Right 6 Lower Arm and Wrist Tendon, Left 7 Hand Tendon, Right 8 Hand Tendon, Left 9 Trunk Tendon, Right B Trunk Tendon, Left C Thorax Tendon, Right D Thorax Tendon, Left F Abdomen Tendon, Right G Abdomen Tendon, Left H Perineum Tendon J Hip Tendon, Right K Hip Tendon, Left L Upper Leg Tendon, Right M Upper Leg Tendon, Left N Lower Leg Tendon, Right Achilles tendon P Lower Leg Tendon, Left *See N Lower Leg Tendon, Right* Q Knee Tendon, Right Patellar tendon R Knee Tendon, Left *See Q Knee Tendon, Right* S Ankle Tendon, Right T Ankle Tendon, Left V Foot Tendon, Right W Foot Tendon, Left	Ø Open 3 Percutaneous 4 Percutaneous Endoscopic X External	Z No Device	Z No Qualifier

Non-OR ØLN[Ø,1,2,3,4,5,6,7,8,9,B,C,D,F,G,H,J,K,L,M,N,P,Q,R,S,T,V,W]XZZ

Ø Medical and Surgical
L Tendons
P Removal Definition: Taking out or off a device from a body part

Explanation: If a device is taken out and a similar device put in without cutting or puncturing the skin or mucous membrane, the procedure is coded to the root operation CHANGE. Otherwise, the procedure for taking out a device is coded to the root operation REMOVAL.

Body Part Character 4	Approach Character 5	Device Character 6	Qualifier Character 7
X Upper Tendon Y Lower Tendon	Ø Open 3 Percutaneous 4 Percutaneous Endoscopic	Ø Drainage Device 7 Autologous Tissue Substitute J Synthetic Substitute K Nonautologous Tissue Substitute Y Other Device	Z No Qualifier
X Upper Tendon Y Lower Tendon	X External	Ø Drainage Device	Z No Qualifier

Non-OR ØLP[X,Y]3ØZ
Non-OR ØLP[X,Y][3,4]YZ
Non-OR ØLP[X,Y]XØZ

Ø Medical and Surgical
L Tendons
Q Repair Definition: Restoring, to the extent possible, a body part to its normal anatomic structure and function

Explanation: Used only when the method to accomplish the repair is not one of the other root operations

Body Part Character 4	Approach Character 5	Device Character 6	Qualifier Character 7
Ø Head and Neck Tendon 1 Shoulder Tendon, Right 2 Shoulder Tendon, Left 3 Upper Arm Tendon, Right 4 Upper Arm Tendon, Left 5 Lower Arm and Wrist Tendon, Right 6 Lower Arm and Wrist Tendon, Left 7 Hand Tendon, Right 8 Hand Tendon, Left 9 Trunk Tendon, Right B Trunk Tendon, Left C Thorax Tendon, Right D Thorax Tendon, Left F Abdomen Tendon, Right G Abdomen Tendon, Left H Perineum Tendon J Hip Tendon, Right K Hip Tendon, Left L Upper Leg Tendon, Right M Upper Leg Tendon, Left N Lower Leg Tendon, Right Achilles tendon P Lower Leg Tendon, Left *See N Lower Leg Tendon, Right* Q Knee Tendon, Right Patellar tendon R Knee Tendon, Left *See Q Knee Tendon, Right* S Ankle Tendon, Right T Ankle Tendon, Left V Foot Tendon, Right W Foot Tendon, Left	Ø Open 3 Percutaneous 4 Percutaneous Endoscopic	Z No Device	Z No Qualifier

Ø Medical and Surgical
L Tendons
R Replacement Definition: Putting in or on biological or synthetic material that physically takes the place and/or function of all or a portion of a body part

Explanation: The body part may have been taken out or replaced, or may be taken out, physically eradicated, or rendered nonfunctional during the REPLACEMENT procedure. A REMOVAL procedure is coded for taking out the device used in a previous replacement procedure.

Body Part Character 4	Approach Character 5	Device Character 6	Qualifier Character 7
Ø Head and Neck Tendon 1 Shoulder Tendon, Right 2 Shoulder Tendon, Left 3 Upper Arm Tendon, Right 4 Upper Arm Tendon, Left 5 Lower Arm and Wrist Tendon, Right 6 Lower Arm and Wrist Tendon, Left 7 Hand Tendon, Right 8 Hand Tendon, Left 9 Trunk Tendon, Right B Trunk Tendon, Left C Thorax Tendon, Right D Thorax Tendon, Left F Abdomen Tendon, Right G Abdomen Tendon, Left H Perineum Tendon J Hip Tendon, Right K Hip Tendon, Left L Upper Leg Tendon, Right M Upper Leg Tendon, Left N Lower Leg Tendon, Right Achilles tendon P Lower Leg Tendon, Left *See N Lower Leg Tendon, Right* Q Knee Tendon, Right Patellar tendon R Knee Tendon, Left *See Q Knee Tendon, Right* S Ankle Tendon, Right T Ankle Tendon, Left V Foot Tendon, Right W Foot Tendon, Left	Ø Open 4 Percutaneous Endoscopic	7 Autologous Tissue Substitute J Synthetic Substitute K Nonautologous Tissue Substitute	Z No Qualifier

Ø Medical and Surgical
L Tendons
S Reposition Definition: Moving to its normal location, or other suitable location, all or a portion of a body part

Explanation: The body part is moved to a new location from an abnormal location, or from a normal location where it is not functioning correctly. The body part may or may not be cut out or off to be moved to the new location.

Body Part Character 4	Approach Character 5	Device Character 6	Qualifier Character 7
Ø Head and Neck Tendon 1 Shoulder Tendon, Right 2 Shoulder Tendon, Left 3 Upper Arm Tendon, Right 4 Upper Arm Tendon, Left 5 Lower Arm and Wrist Tendon, Right 6 Lower Arm and Wrist Tendon, Left 7 Hand Tendon, Right 8 Hand Tendon, Left 9 Trunk Tendon, Right B Trunk Tendon, Left C Thorax Tendon, Right D Thorax Tendon, Left F Abdomen Tendon, Right G Abdomen Tendon, Left H Perineum Tendon J Hip Tendon, Right K Hip Tendon, Left L Upper Leg Tendon, Right M Upper Leg Tendon, Left N Lower Leg Tendon, Right Achilles tendon P Lower Leg Tendon, Left *See N Lower Leg Tendon, Right* Q Knee Tendon, Right Patellar tendon R Knee Tendon, Left *See Q Knee Tendon, Right* S Ankle Tendon, Right T Ankle Tendon, Left V Foot Tendon, Right W Foot Tendon, Left	Ø Open 4 Percutaneous Endoscopic	Z No Device	Z No Qualifier

Ø Medical and Surgical
L Tendons
T Resection Definition: Cutting out or off, without replacement, all of a body part
Explanation: None

Body Part Character 4	Approach Character 5	Device Character 6	Qualifier Character 7
Ø Head and Neck Tendon 1 Shoulder Tendon, Right 2 Shoulder Tendon, Left 3 Upper Arm Tendon, Right 4 Upper Arm Tendon, Left 5 Lower Arm and Wrist Tendon, Right 6 Lower Arm and Wrist Tendon, Left 7 Hand Tendon, Right 8 Hand Tendon, Left 9 Trunk Tendon, Right B Trunk Tendon, Left C Thorax Tendon, Right D Thorax Tendon, Left F Abdomen Tendon, Right G Abdomen Tendon, Left H Perineum Tendon J Hip Tendon, Right K Hip Tendon, Left L Upper Leg Tendon, Right M Upper Leg Tendon, Left N Lower Leg Tendon, Right Achilles tendon P Lower Leg Tendon, Left *See N Lower Leg Tendon, Right* Q Knee Tendon, Right Patellar tendon R Knee Tendon, Left *See Q Knee Tendon, Right* S Ankle Tendon, Right T Ankle Tendon, Left V Foot Tendon, Right W Foot Tendon, Left	Ø Open 4 Percutaneous Endoscopic	Z No Device	Z No Qualifier

Ø Medical and Surgical
L Tendons
U Supplement Definition: Putting in or on biological or synthetic material that physically reinforces and/or augments the function of a portion of a body part
Explanation: The biological material is non-living, or is living and from the same individual. The body part may have been previously replaced, and the SUPPLEMENT procedure is performed to physically reinforce and/or augment the function of the replaced body part.

Body Part Character 4	Approach Character 5	Device Character 6	Qualifier Character 7
Ø Head and Neck Tendon 1 Shoulder Tendon, Right 2 Shoulder Tendon, Left 3 Upper Arm Tendon, Right 4 Upper Arm Tendon, Left 5 Lower Arm and Wrist Tendon, Right 6 Lower Arm and Wrist Tendon, Left 7 Hand Tendon, Right 8 Hand Tendon, Left 9 Trunk Tendon, Right B Trunk Tendon, Left C Thorax Tendon, Right D Thorax Tendon, Left F Abdomen Tendon, Right G Abdomen Tendon, Left H Perineum Tendon J Hip Tendon, Right K Hip Tendon, Left L Upper Leg Tendon, Right M Upper Leg Tendon, Left N Lower Leg Tendon, Right Achilles tendon P Lower Leg Tendon, Left *See N Lower Leg Tendon, Right* Q Knee Tendon, Right Patellar tendon R Knee Tendon, Left *See Q Knee Tendon, Right* S Ankle Tendon, Right T Ankle Tendon, Left V Foot Tendon, Right W Foot Tendon, Left	Ø Open 4 Percutaneous Endoscopic	7 Autologous Tissue Substitute J Synthetic Substitute K Nonautologous Tissue Substitute	Z No Qualifier

Ø Medical and Surgical
L Tendons
W Revision Definition: Correcting, to the extent possible, a portion of a malfunctioning device or the position of a displaced device
Explanation: Revision can include correcting a malfunctioning or displaced device by taking out or putting in components of the device such as a screw or pin

Body Part Character 4	Approach Character 5	Device Character 6	Qualifier Character 7
X Upper Tendon Y Lower Tendon	Ø Open 3 Percutaneous 4 Percutaneous Endoscopic	Ø Drainage Device 7 Autologous Tissue Substitute J Synthetic Substitute K Nonautologous Tissue Substitute Y Other Device	Z No Qualifier
X Upper Tendon Y Lower Tendon	X External	Ø Drainage Device 7 Autologous Tissue Substitute J Synthetic Substitute K Nonautologous Tissue Substitute	Z No Qualifier

Non-OR ØLW[X,Y][3,4]YZ
Non-OR ØLW[X,Y]X[Ø,7,J,K]Z

Ø Medical and Surgical
L Tendons
X Transfer Definition: Moving, without taking out, all or a portion of a body part to another location to take over the function of all or a portion of a body part
Explanation: The body part transferred remains connected to its vascular and nervous supply

Body Part Character 4	Approach Character 5	Device Character 6	Qualifier Character 7
Ø Head and Neck Tendon 1 Shoulder Tendon, Right 2 Shoulder Tendon, Left 3 Upper Arm Tendon, Right 4 Upper Arm Tendon, Left 5 Lower Arm and Wrist Tendon, Right 6 Lower Arm and Wrist Tendon, Left 7 Hand Tendon, Right 8 Hand Tendon, Left 9 Trunk Tendon, Right B Trunk Tendon, Left C Thorax Tendon, Right D Thorax Tendon, Left F Abdomen Tendon, Right G Abdomen Tendon, Left H Perineum Tendon J Hip Tendon, Right K Hip Tendon, Left L Upper Leg Tendon, Right M Upper Leg Tendon, Left N Lower Leg Tendon, Right Achilles tendon P Lower Leg Tendon, Left *See N Lower Leg Tendon, Right* Q Knee Tendon, Right Patellar tendon R Knee Tendon, Left *See Q Knee Tendon, Right* S Ankle Tendon, Right T Ankle Tendon, Left V Foot Tendon, Right W Foot Tendon, Left	Ø Open 4 Percutaneous Endoscopic	Z No Device	Z No Qualifier

Bursae and Ligaments ØM2–ØMX

Character Meanings*

This Character Meaning table is provided as a guide to assist the user in the identification of character members that may be found in this section of code tables. It **SHOULD NOT** be used to build a PCS code.

Operation–Character 3	Body Part–Character 4	Approach–Character 5	Device–Character 6	Qualifier–Character 7
2 Change	Ø Head and Neck Bursa and Ligament	Ø Open	Ø Drainage Device	X Diagnostic
5 Destruction	1 Shoulder Bursa and Ligament, Right	3 Percutaneous	7 Autologous Tissue Substitute	Z No Qualifier
8 Division	2 Shoulder Bursa and Ligament, Left	4 Percutaneous Endoscopic	J Synthetic Substitute	
9 Drainage	3 Elbow Bursa and Ligament, Right	X External	K Nonautologous Tissue Substitute	
B Excision	4 Elbow Bursa and Ligament, Left		Y Other Device	
C Extirpation	5 Wrist Bursa and Ligament, Right		Z No Device	
D Extraction	6 Wrist Bursa and Ligament, Left			
H Insertion	7 Hand Bursa and Ligament, Right			
J Inspection	8 Hand Bursa and Ligament, Left			
M Reattachment	9 Upper Extremity Bursa and Ligament, Right			
N Release	B Upper Extremity Bursa and Ligament, Left			
P Removal	C Upper Spine Bursa and Ligament			
Q Repair	D Lower Spine Bursa and Ligament			
R Replacement	F Sternum Bursa and Ligament			
S Reposition	G Rib(s) Bursa and Ligament			
T Resection	H Abdomen Bursa and Ligament, Right			
U Supplement	J Abdomen Bursa and Ligament, Left			
W Revision	K Perineum Bursa and Ligament			
X Transfer	L Hip Bursa and Ligament, Right			
	M Hip Bursa and Ligament, Left			
	N Knee Bursa and Ligament, Right			
	P Knee Bursa and Ligament, Left			
	Q Ankle Bursa and Ligament, Right			
	R Ankle Bursa and Ligament, Left			
	S Foot Bursa and Ligament, Right			
	T Foot Bursa and Ligament, Left			
	V Lower Extremity Bursa and Ligament, Right			
	W Lower Extremity Bursa and Ligament, Left			
	X Upper Bursa and Ligament			
	Y Lower Bursa and Ligament			

* Includes synovial membrane.

AHA Coding Clinic for table ØMM
2013, 3Q, 20 Superior labrum anterior posterior (SLAP) repair and subacromial decompression

AHA Coding Clinic for table ØMQ
2014, 3Q, 9 Interspinous ligamentoplasty

AHA Coding Clinic for table ØMT
2017, 2Q, 21 Arthroscopic anterior cruciate ligament revision using autograft with anterolateral ligament reconstruction

AHA Coding Clinic for table ØMU
2017, 2Q, 21 Arthroscopic anterior cruciate ligament revision using autograft with anterolateral ligament reconstruction

Shoulder Ligaments

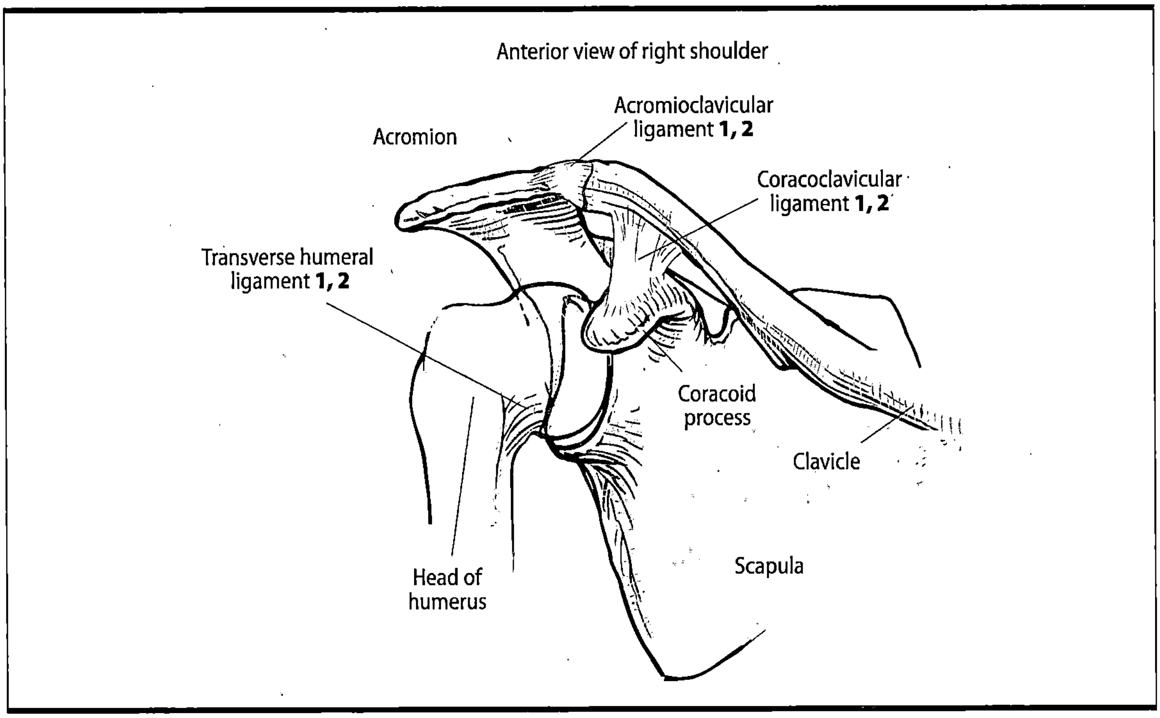

Knee Bursae

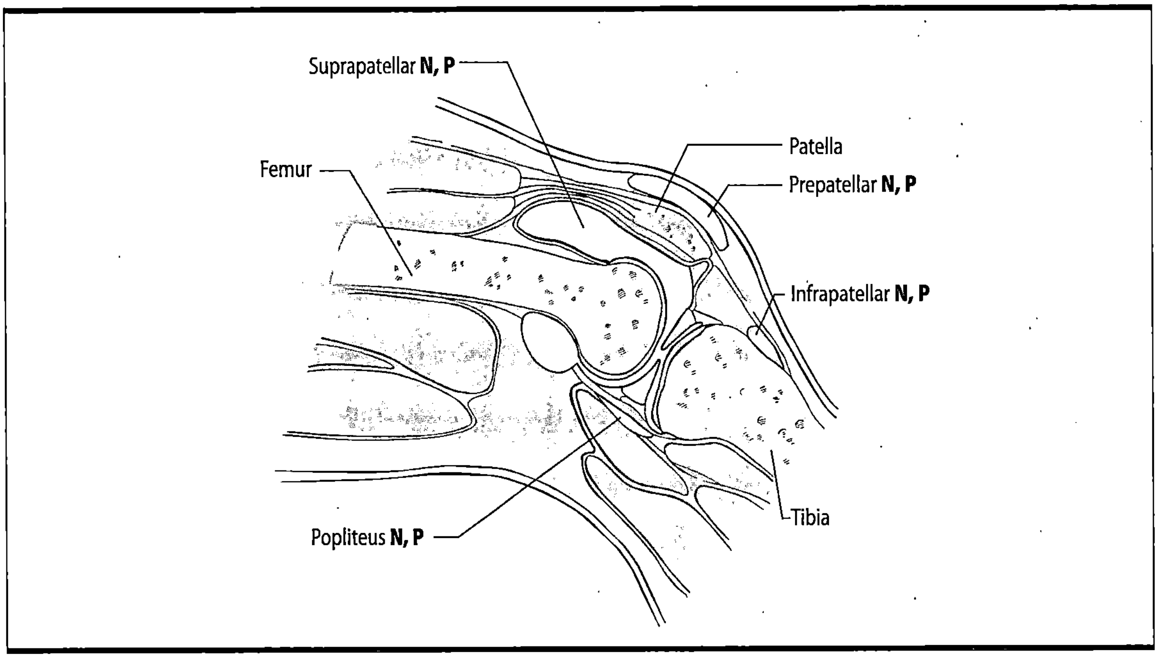

Knee Ligaments

Anterior view

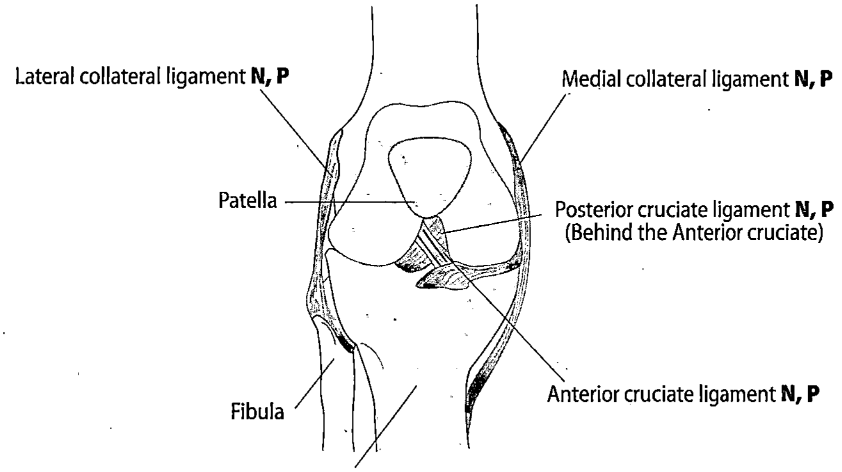

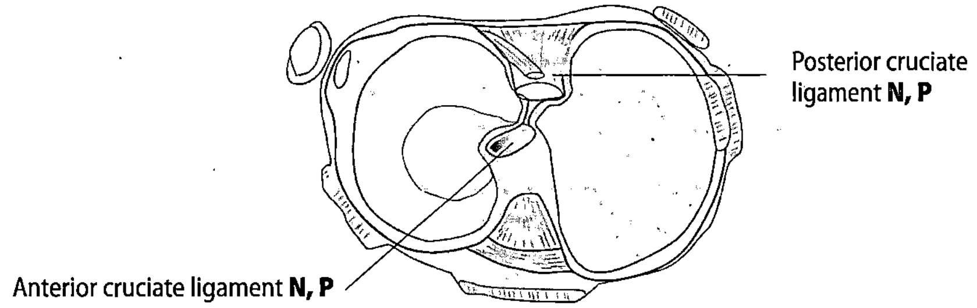

Wrist Ligaments

Palmar view

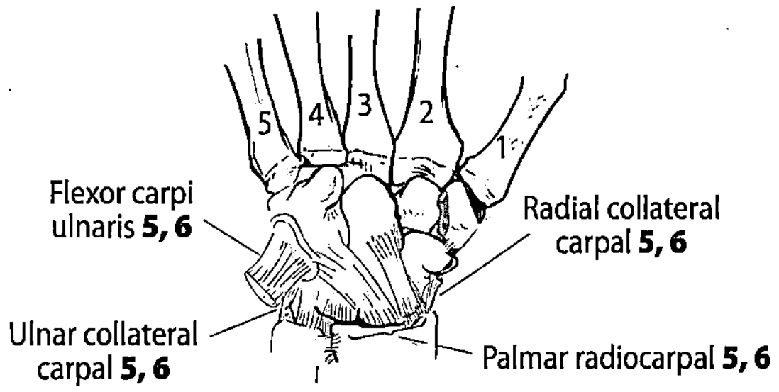

Dorsal view

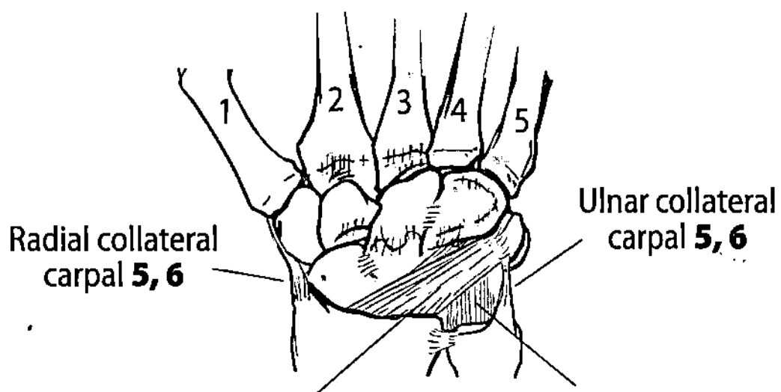

Ø Medical and Surgical
M Bursae and Ligaments
2 Change Definition: Taking out or off a device from a body part and putting back an identical or similar device in or on the same body part without cutting or puncturing the skin or a mucous membrane

Explanation: All CHANGE procedures are coded using the approach EXTERNAL

Body Part Character 4	Approach Character 5	Device Character 6	Qualifier Character 7
X Upper Bursa and Ligament Y Lower Bursa and Ligament	X External	Ø Drainage Device Y Other Device	Z No Qualifier

Non-OR All body part, approach, device, and qualifier values

Ø Medical and Surgical
M Bursae and Ligaments
5 Destruction Definition: Physical eradication of all or a portion of a body part by the direct use of energy, force, or a destructive agent

Explanation: None of the body part is physically taken out

Body Part Character 4	Approach Character 5	Device Character 6	Qualifier Character 7
Ø Head and Neck Bursa and Ligament Alar ligament of axis Cervical interspinous ligament Cervical intertransverse ligament Cervical ligamentum flavum Interspinous ligament, cervical Intertransverse ligament, cervical Lateral temporomandibular ligament Ligamentum flavum, cervical Sphenomandibular ligament Stylomandibular ligament Transverse ligament of atlas **1 Shoulder Bursa and Ligament, Right** Acromioclavicular ligament Coracoacromial ligament Coracoclavicular ligament Coracohumeral ligament Costoclavicular ligament Glenohumeral ligament Interclavicular ligament Sternoclavicular ligament Subacromial bursa Transverse humeral ligament Transverse scapular ligament **2 Shoulder Bursa and Ligament, Left** *See 1 Shoulder Bursa and Ligament, Right* **3 Elbow Bursa and Ligament, Right** Annular ligament Olecranon bursa Radial collateral ligament Ulnar collateral ligament **4 Elbow Bursa and Ligament, Left** *See 3 Elbow Bursa and Ligament, Right* **5 Wrist Bursa and Ligament, Right** Palmar ulnocarpal ligament Radial collateral carpal ligament Radiocarpal ligament Radioulnar ligament Ulnar collateral carpal ligament **6 Wrist Bursa and Ligament, Left** *See 5 Wrist Bursa and Ligament, Right* **7 Hand Bursa and Ligament, Right** Carpometacarpal ligament Intercarpal ligament Interphalangeal ligament Lunotriquetral ligament Metacarpal ligament Metacarpophalangeal ligament Pisohamate ligament Pisometacarpal ligament Scapholunate ligament Scaphotrapezium ligament **8 Hand Bursa and Ligament, Left** *See 7 Hand Bursa and Ligament, Right* **9 Upper Extremity Bursa and Ligament, Right** **B Upper Extremity Bursa and Ligament, Left** **C Upper Spine Bursa and Ligament** Interspinous ligament, thoracic Intertransverse ligament, thoracic Ligamentum flavum, thoracic Supraspinous ligament **D Lower Spine Bursa and Ligament** Iliolumbar ligament Interspinous ligament, lumbar Intertransverse ligament, lumbar Ligamentum flavum, lumbar Sacrococcygeal ligament Sacroiliac ligament Sacrospinous ligament Sacrotuberous ligament Supraspinous ligament **F Sternum Bursa and Ligament** Costoxiphoid ligament Sternocostal ligament **G Rib(s) Bursa and Ligament** Costotransverse ligament **H Abdomen Bursa and Ligament, Right** **J Abdomen Bursa and Ligament, Left** **K Perineum Bursa and Ligament** **L Hip Bursa and Ligament, Right** Iliofemoral ligament Ischiofemoral ligament Pubofemoral ligament Transverse acetabular ligament Trochanteric bursa **M Hip Bursa and Ligament, Left** *See L Hip Bursa and Ligament, Right* **N Knee Bursa and Ligament, Right** Anterior cruciate ligament (ACL) Lateral collateral ligament (LCL) Ligament of head of fibula Medial collateral ligament (MCL) Patellar ligament Popliteal ligament Posterior cruciate ligament (PCL) Prepatellar bursa **P Knee Bursa and Ligament, Left** *See N Knee Bursa and Ligament, Right* **Q Ankle Bursa and Ligament, Right** Calcaneofibular ligament Deltoid ligament Ligament of the lateral malleolus Talofibular ligament **R Ankle Bursa and Ligament, Left** *See Q Ankle Bursa and Ligament, Right* **S Foot Bursa and Ligament, Right** Calcaneocuboid ligament Cuneonavicular ligament Intercuneiform ligament Interphalangeal ligament Metatarsal ligament Metatarsophalangeal ligament Subtalar ligament Talocalcaneal ligament Talocalcaneonavicular ligament Tarsometatarsal ligament **T Foot Bursa and Ligament, Left** *See S Foot Bursa and Ligament, Right* **V Lower Extremity Bursa and Ligament, Right** **W Lower Extremity Bursa and Ligament, Left**	Ø Open 3 Percutaneous 4 Percutaneous Endoscopic	Z No Device	Z No Qualifier

Ø Medical and Surgical
M Bursae and Ligaments
8 Division Definition: Cutting into a body part, without draining fluids and/or gases from the body part, in order to separate or transect a body part
Explanation: All or a portion of the body part is separated into two or more portions

Body Part Character 4	Approach Character 5	Device Character 6	Qualifier Character 7
Ø Head and Neck Bursa and Ligament Alar ligament of axis Cervical interspinous ligament Cervical intertransverse ligament Cervical ligamentum flavum Interspinous ligament, cervical Intertransverse ligament, cervical Lateral temporomandibular ligament Ligamentum flavum, cervical Sphenomandibular ligament Stylomandibular ligament Transverse ligament of atlas **1 Shoulder Bursa and Ligament, Right** Acromioclavicular ligament Coracoacromial ligament Coracoclavicular ligament Coracohumeral ligament Costoclavicular ligament Glenohumeral ligament Interclavicular ligament Sternoclavicular ligament Subacromial bursa Transverse humeral ligament Transverse scapular ligament **2 Shoulder Bursa and Ligament, Left** *See 1 Shoulder Bursa and Ligament, Right* **3 Elbow Bursa and Ligament, Right** Annular ligament Olecranon bursa Radial collateral ligament Ulnar collateral ligament **4 Elbow Bursa and Ligament, Left** *See 3 Elbow Bursa and Ligament, Right* **5 Wrist Bursa and Ligament, Right** Palmar ulnocarpal ligament Radial collateral carpal ligament Radiocarpal ligament Radioulnar ligament Ulnar collateral carpal ligament **6 Wrist Bursa and Ligament, Left** *See 5 Wrist Bursa and Ligament, Right* **7 Hand Bursa and Ligament, Right** Carpometacarpal ligament Intercarpal ligament Interphalangeal ligament Lunotriquetral ligament Metacarpal ligament Metacarpophalangeal ligament Pisohamate ligament Pisometacarpal ligament Scapholunate ligament Scaphotrapezium ligament **8 Hand Bursa and Ligament, Left** *See 7 Hand Bursa and Ligament, Right* **9 Upper Extremity Bursa and Ligament, Right** **B Upper Extremity Bursa and Ligament, Left** **C Upper Spine Bursa and Ligament** Interspinous ligament, thoracic Intertransverse ligament, thoracic Ligamentum flavum, thoracic Supraspinous ligament **D Lower Spine Bursa and Ligament** Iliolumbar ligament Interspinous ligament, lumbar Intertransverse ligament, lumbar Ligamentum flavum, lumbar Sacrococcygeal ligament Sacroiliac ligament Sacrospinous ligament Sacrotuberous ligament Supraspinous ligament **F Sternum Bursa and Ligament** Costoxiphoid ligament Sternocostal ligament **G Rib(s) Bursa and Ligament** Costotransverse ligament **H Abdomen Bursa and Ligament, Right** **J Abdomen Bursa and Ligament, Left** **K Perineum Bursa and Ligament** **L Hip Bursa and Ligament, Right** Iliofemoral ligament Ischiofemoral ligament Pubofemoral ligament Transverse acetabular ligament Trochanteric bursa **M Hip Bursa and Ligament, Left** *See L Hip Bursa and Ligament, Right* **N Knee Bursa and Ligament, Right** Anterior cruciate ligament (ACL) Lateral collateral ligament (LCL) Ligament of head of fibula Medial collateral ligament (MCL) Patellar ligament Popliteal ligament Posterior cruciate ligament (PCL) Prepatellar bursa **P Knee Bursa and Ligament, Left** *See N Knee Bursa and Ligament, Right* **Q Ankle Bursa and Ligament, Right** Calcaneofibular ligament Deltoid ligament Ligament of the lateral malleolus Talofibular ligament **R Ankle Bursa and Ligament, Left** *See Q Ankle Bursa and Ligament, Right* **S Foot Bursa and Ligament, Right** Calcaneocuboid ligament Cuneonavicular ligament Intercuneiform ligament Interphalangeal ligament Metatarsal ligament Metatarsophalangeal ligament Subtalar ligament Talocalcaneal ligament Talocalcaneonavicular ligament Tarsometatarsal ligament **T Foot Bursa and Ligament, Left** *See S Foot Bursa and Ligament, Right* **V Lower Extremity Bursa and Ligament, Right** **W Lower Extremity Bursa and Ligament, Left**	Ø Open 3 Percutaneous 4 Percutaneous Endoscopic	Z No Device	Z No Qualifier

Ø Medical and Surgical
M Bursae and Ligaments
9 Drainage Definition: Taking or letting out fluids and/or gases from a body part
Explanation: The qualifier DIAGNOSTIC is used to identify drainage procedures that are biopsies

Body Part Character 4		Approach Character 5	Device Character 6	Qualifier Character 7
Ø Head and Neck Bursa and Ligament Alar ligament of axis Cervical interspinous ligament Cervical intertransverse ligament Cervical ligamentum flavum Interspinous ligament, cervical Intertransverse ligament, cervical Lateral temporomandibular ligament Ligamentum flavum, cervical Sphenomandibular ligament Stylomandibular ligament Transverse ligament of atlas **1 Shoulder Bursa and Ligament, Right** Acromioclavicular ligament Coracoacromial ligament Coracoclavicular ligament Coracohumeral ligament Costoclavicular ligament Glenohumeral ligament Interclavicular ligament Sternoclavicular ligament Subacromial bursa Transverse humeral ligament Transverse scapular ligament **2 Shoulder Bursa and Ligament, Left** *See 1 Shoulder Bursa and Ligament, Right* **3 Elbow Bursa and Ligament, Right** Annular ligament Olecranon bursa Radial collateral ligament Ulnar collateral ligament **4 Elbow Bursa and Ligament, Left** *See 3 Elbow Bursa and Ligament, Right* **5 Wrist Bursa and Ligament, Right** Palmar ulnocarpal ligament Radial collateral carpal ligament Radiocarpal ligament Radioulnar ligament Ulnar collateral carpal ligament **6 Wrist Bursa and Ligament, Left** *See 5 Wrist Bursa and Ligament, Right* **7 Hand Bursa and Ligament, Right** Carpometacarpal ligament Intercarpal ligament Interphalangeal ligament Lunotriquetral ligament Metacarpal ligament Metacarpophalangeal ligament Pisohamate ligament Pisometacarpal ligament Scapholunate ligament Scaphotrapezium ligament **8 Hand Bursa and Ligament, Left** *See 7 Hand Bursa and Ligament, Right* **9 Upper Extremity Bursa and Ligament, Right** **B Upper Extremity Bursa and Ligament, Left** **C Upper Spine Bursa and Ligament** Interspinous ligament, thoracic Intertransverse ligament, thoracic Ligamentum flavum, thoracic Supraspinous ligament	**D Lower Spine Bursa and Ligament** Iliolumbar ligament Interspinous ligament, lumbar Intertransverse ligament, lumbar Ligamentum flavum, lumbar Sacrococcygeal ligament Sacroiliac ligament Sacrospinous ligament Sacrotuberous ligament Supraspinous ligament **F Sternum Bursa and Ligament** Costoxiphoid ligament Sternocostal ligament **G Rib(s) Bursa and Ligament** Costotransverse ligament **H Abdomen Bursa and Ligament, Right** **J Abdomen Bursa and Ligament, Left** **K Perineum Bursa and Ligament** **L Hip Bursa and Ligament, Right** Iliofemoral ligament Ischiofemoral ligament Pubofemoral ligament Transverse acetabular ligament Trochanteric bursa **M Hip Bursa and Ligament, Left** *See L Hip Bursa and Ligament, Right* **N Knee Bursa and Ligament, Right** Anterior cruciate ligament (ACL) Lateral collateral ligament (LCL) Ligament of head of fibula Medial collateral ligament (MCL) Patellar ligament Popliteal ligament Posterior cruciate ligament (PCL) Prepatellar bursa **P Knee Bursa and Ligament, Left** *See N Knee Bursa and Ligament, Right* **Q Ankle Bursa and Ligament, Right** Calcaneofibular ligament Deltoid ligament Ligament of the lateral malleolus Talofibular ligament **R Ankle Bursa and Ligament, Left** *See Q Ankle Bursa and Ligament, Right* **S Foot Bursa and Ligament, Right** Calcaneocuboid ligament Cuneonavicular ligament Intercuneiform ligament Interphalangeal ligament Metatarsal ligament Metatarsophalangeal ligament Subtalar ligament Talocalcaneal ligament Talocalcaneonavicular ligament Tarsometatarsal ligament **T Foot Bursa and Ligament, Left** *See S Foot Bursa and Ligament, Right* **V Lower Extremity Bursa and Ligament, Right** **W Lower Extremity Bursa and Ligament, Left**	**Ø Open** **3 Percutaneous** **4 Percutaneous Endoscopic**	**Ø Drainage Device**	**Z No Qualifier**

ØM9 Continued on next page

Non-OR ØM9[Ø,1,2,3,4,5,6,7,8,9,B,C,D,F,G,H,J,K,L,M,N,P,Q,R,S,T,V,W]3ØZ
Non-OR ØM9[1,2,3,4,7,8,9,B,C,D,F,G,H,J,K,L,M,V,W]4ØZ

Ø Medical and Surgical
M Bursae and Ligaments
9 Drainage Definition: Taking or letting out fluids and/or gases from a body part
Explanation: The qualifier DIAGNOSTIC is used to identify drainage procedures that are biopsies

ØM9 Continued

Body Part Character 4	Approach Character 5	Device Character 6	Qualifier Character 7
Ø Head and Neck Bursa and Ligament Alar ligament of axis Cervical interspinous ligament Cervical intertransverse ligament Cervical ligamentum flavum Interspinous ligament, cervical Intertransverse ligament, cervical Lateral temporomandibular ligament Ligamentum flavum, cervical Sphenomandibular ligament Stylomandibular ligament Transverse ligament of atlas **1 Shoulder Bursa and Ligament, Right** Acromioclavicular ligament Coracoacromial ligament Coracoclavicular ligament Coracohumeral ligament Costoclavicular ligament Glenohumeral ligament Interclavicular ligament Sternoclavicular ligament Subacromial bursa Transverse humeral ligament Transverse scapular ligament **2 Shoulder Bursa and Ligament, Left** *See 1 Shoulder Bursa and Ligament, Right* **3 Elbow Bursa and Ligament, Right** Annular ligament Olecranon bursa Radial collateral ligament Ulnar collateral ligament **4 Elbow Bursa and Ligament, Left** *See 3 Elbow Bursa and Ligament, Right* **5 Wrist Bursa and Ligament, Right** Palmar ulnocarpal ligament Radial collateral carpal ligament Radiocarpal ligament Radioulnar ligament Ulnar collateral carpal ligament **6 Wrist Bursa and Ligament, Left** *See 5 Wrist Bursa and Ligament, Right* **7 Hand Bursa and Ligament, Right** Carpometacarpal ligament Intercarpal ligament Interphalangeal ligament Lunotriquetral ligament Metacarpal ligament Metacarpophalangeal ligament Pisohamate ligament Pisometacarpal ligament Scapholunate ligament Scaphotrapezium ligament **8 Hand Bursa and Ligament, Left** *See 7 Hand Bursa and Ligament, Right* **9 Upper Extremity Bursa and Ligament, Right** **B Upper Extremity Bursa and Ligament, Left** **C Upper Spine Bursa and Ligament** Interspinous ligament, thoracic Intertransverse ligament, thoracic Ligamentum flavum, thoracic Supraspinous ligament **D Lower Spine Bursa and Ligament** Iliolumbar ligament Interspinous ligament, lumbar Intertransverse ligament, lumbar Ligamentum flavum, lumbar Sacrococcygeal ligament Sacroiliac ligament Sacrospinous ligament Sacrotuberous ligament Supraspinous ligament **F Sternum Bursa and Ligament** Costoxiphoid ligament Sternocostal ligament **G Rib(s) Bursa and Ligament** Costotransverse ligament **H Abdomen Bursa and Ligament, Right** **J Abdomen Bursa and Ligament, Left** **K Perineum Bursa and Ligament** **L Hip Bursa and Ligament, Right** Iliofemoral ligament Ischiofemoral ligament Pubofemoral ligament Transverse acetabular ligament Trochanteric bursa **M Hip Bursa and Ligament, Left** *See L Hip Bursa and Ligament, Right* **N Knee Bursa and Ligament, Right** Anterior cruciate ligament (ACL) Lateral collateral ligament (LCL) Ligament of head of fibula Medial collateral ligament (MCL) Patellar ligament Popliteal ligament Posterior cruciate ligament (PCL) Prepatellar bursa **P Knee Bursa and Ligament, Left** *See N Knee Bursa and Ligament, Right* **Q Ankle Bursa and Ligament, Right** Calcaneofibular ligament Deltoid ligament Ligament of the lateral malleolus Talofibular ligament **R Ankle Bursa and Ligament, Left** *See Q Ankle Bursa and Ligament, Right* **S Foot Bursa and Ligament, Right** Calcaneocuboid ligament Cuneonavicular ligament Intercuneiform ligament Interphalangeal ligament Metatarsal ligament Metatarsophalangeal ligament Subtalar ligament Talocalcaneal ligament Talocalcaneonavicular ligament Tarsometatarsal ligament **T Foot Bursa and Ligament, Left** *See S Foot Bursa and Ligament, Right* **V Lower Extremity Bursa and Ligament, Right** **W Lower Extremity Bursa and Ligament, Left**	**Ø** Open **3** Percutaneous **4** Percutaneous Endoscopic	**Z** No Device	**X** Diagnostic **Z** No Qualifier

Non-OR ØM9[Ø,1,2,3,4,5,6,7,8,C,D,F,G,L,M,N,P,Q,R,S,T][Ø,3,4]ZX
Non-OR ØM9[Ø,1,2,3,4,5,6,7,8,9,B,C,D,F,G,H,J,K,L,M,N,P,Q,R,S,T,V,W]3ZZ
Non-OR ØM9[Ø,5,6,7,8,9,B,C,D,F,G,H,J,K,N,P,Q,R,S,T,V,W]4ZZ

Ø Medical and Surgical
M Bursae and Ligaments
B Excision Definition: Cutting out or off, without replacement, a portion of a body part

Explanation: The qualifier DIAGNOSTIC is used to identify excision procedures that are biopsies

Body Part Character 4	Approach Character 5	Device Character 6	Qualifier Character 7
Ø Head and Neck Bursa and Ligament Alar ligament of axis Cervical interspinous ligament Cervical intertransverse ligament Cervical ligamentum flavum Interspinous ligament, cervical Intertransverse ligament, cervical Lateral temporomandibular ligament Ligamentum flavum, cervical Sphenomandibular ligament Stylomandibular ligament Transverse ligament of atlas **1 Shoulder Bursa and Ligament, Right** Acromioclavicular ligament Coracoacromial ligament Coracoclavicular ligament Coracohumeral ligament Costoclavicular ligament Glenohumeral ligament Interclavicular ligament Sternoclavicular ligament Subacromial bursa Transverse humeral ligament Transverse scapular ligament **2 Shoulder Bursa and Ligament, Left** *See 1 Shoulder Bursa and Ligament, Right* **3 Elbow Bursa and Ligament, Right** Annular ligament Olecranon bursa Radial collateral ligament Ulnar collateral ligament **4 Elbow Bursa and Ligament, Left** *See 3 Elbow Bursa and Ligament, Right* **5 Wrist Bursa and Ligament, Right** Palmar ulnocarpal ligament Radial collateral carpal ligament Radiocarpal ligament Radioulnar ligament Ulnar collateral carpal ligament **6 Wrist Bursa and Ligament, Left** *See 5 Wrist Bursa and Ligament, Right* **7 Hand Bursa and Ligament, Right** Carpometacarpal ligament Intercarpal ligament Interphalangeal ligament Lunotriquetral ligament Metacarpal ligament Metacarpophalangeal ligament Pisohamate ligament Pisometacarpal ligament Scapholunate ligament Scaphotrapezium ligament **8 Hand Bursa and Ligament, Left** *See 7 Hand Bursa and Ligament, Right* **9 Upper Extremity Bursa and Ligament, Right** **B Upper Extremity Bursa and Ligament, Left** **C Upper Spine Bursa and Ligament** Interspinous ligament, thoracic Intertransverse ligament, thoracic Ligamentum flavum, thoracic Supraspinous ligament **D Lower Spine Bursa and Ligament** Iliolumbar ligament Interspinous ligament, lumbar Intertransverse ligament, lumbar Ligamentum flavum, lumbar Sacrococcygeal ligament Sacroiliac ligament Sacrospinous ligament Sacrotuberous ligament Supraspinous ligament **F Sternum Bursa and Ligament** Costoxiphoid ligament Sternocostal ligament **G Rib(s) Bursa and Ligament** Costotransverse ligament **H Abdomen Bursa and Ligament, Right** **J Abdomen Bursa and Ligament, Left** **K Perineum Bursa and Ligament** **L Hip Bursa and Ligament, Right** Iliofemoral ligament Ischiofemoral ligament Pubofemoral ligament Transverse acetabular ligament Trochanteric bursa **M Hip Bursa and Ligament, Left** *See L Hip Bursa and Ligament, Right* **N Knee Bursa and Ligament, Right** Anterior cruciate ligament (ACL) Lateral collateral ligament (LCL) Ligament of head of fibula Medial collateral ligament (MCL) Patellar ligament Popliteal ligament Posterior cruciate ligament (PCL) Prepatellar bursa **P Knee Bursa and Ligament, Left** *See N Knee Bursa and Ligament, Right* **Q Ankle Bursa and Ligament, Right** Calcaneofibular ligament Deltoid ligament Ligament of the lateral malleolus Talofibular ligament **R Ankle Bursa and Ligament, Left** *See Q Ankle Bursa and Ligament, Right* **S Foot Bursa and Ligament, Right** Calcaneocuboid ligament Cuneonavicular ligament Intercuneiform ligament Interphalangeal ligament Metatarsal ligament Metatarsophalangeal ligament Subtalar ligament Talocalcaneal ligament Talocalcaneonavicular ligament Tarsometatarsal ligament **T Foot Bursa and Ligament, Left** *See S Foot Bursa and Ligament, Right* **V Lower Extremity Bursa and Ligament, Right** **W Lower Extremity Bursa and Ligament, Left**	**Ø** Open **3** Percutaneous **4** Percutaneous Endoscopic	**Z** No Device	**X** Diagnostic **Z** No Qualifier

Non-OR ØMB[Ø,1,2,3,4,5,6,7,8,B,C,D,F,G,L,M,N,P,Q,R,S,T][Ø,3,4]ZX
Non-OR ØMB94ZX

Ø Medical and Surgical
M Bursae and Ligaments
C Extirpation Definition: Taking or cutting out solid matter from a body part

Explanation: The solid matter may be an abnormal byproduct of a biological function or a foreign body; it may be imbedded in a body part or in the lumen of a tubular body part. The solid matter may or may not have been previously broken into pieces.

Body Part Character 4	Approach Character 5	Device Character 6	Qualifier Character 7
Ø Head and Neck Bursa and Ligament Alar ligament of axis Cervical interspinous ligament Cervical intertransverse ligament Cervical ligamentum flavum Interspinous ligament, cervical Intertransverse ligament, cervical Lateral temporomandibular ligament Ligamentum flavum, cervical Sphenomandibular ligament Stylomandibular ligament Transverse ligament of atlas **1 Shoulder Bursa and Ligament, Right** Acromioclavicular ligament Coracoacromial ligament Coracoclavicular ligament Coracohumeral ligament Costoclavicular ligament Glenohumeral ligament Interclavicular ligament Sternoclavicular ligament Subacromial bursa Transverse humeral ligament Transverse scapular ligament **2 Shoulder Bursa and Ligament, Left** *See 1 Shoulder Bursa and Ligament, Right* **3 Elbow Bursa and Ligament, Right** Annular ligament Olecranon bursa Radial collateral ligament Ulnar collateral ligament **4 Elbow Bursa and Ligament, Left** *See 3 Elbow Bursa and Ligament, Right* **5 Wrist Bursa and Ligament, Right** Palmar ulnocarpal ligament Radial collateral carpal ligament Radiocarpal ligament Radioulnar ligament Ulnar collateral carpal ligament **6 Wrist Bursa and Ligament, Left** *See 5 Wrist Bursa and Ligament, Right* **7 Hand Bursa and Ligament, Right** Carpometacarpal ligament Intercarpal ligament Interphalangeal ligament Lunotriquetral ligament Metacarpal ligament Metacarpophalangeal ligament Pisohamate ligament Pisometacarpal ligament Scapholunate ligament Scaphotrapezium ligament **8 Hand Bursa and Ligament, Left** *See 7 Hand Bursa and Ligament, Right* **9 Upper Extremity Bursa and Ligament, Right** **B Upper Extremity Bursa and Ligament, Left** **C Upper Spine Bursa and Ligament** Interspinous ligament, thoracic Intertransverse ligament, thoracic Ligamentum flavum, thoracic Supraspinous ligament **D Lower Spine Bursa and Ligament** Iliolumbar ligament Interspinous ligament, lumbar Intertransverse ligament, lumbar Ligamentum flavum, lumbar Sacrococcygeal ligament Sacroiliac ligament Sacrospinous ligament Sacrotuberous ligament Supraspinous ligament **F Sternum Bursa and Ligament** Costoxiphoid ligament Sternocostal ligament **G Rib(s) Bursa and Ligament** Costotransverse ligament **H Abdomen Bursa and Ligament, Right** **J Abdomen Bursa and Ligament, Left** **K Perineum Bursa and Ligament** **L Hip Bursa and Ligament, Right** Iliofemoral ligament Ischiofemoral ligament Pubofemoral ligament Transverse acetabular ligament Trochanteric bursa **M Hip Bursa and Ligament, Left** *See L Hip Bursa and Ligament, Right* **N Knee Bursa and Ligament, Right** Anterior cruciate ligament (ACL) Lateral collateral ligament (LCL) Ligament of head of fibula Medial collateral ligament (MCL) Patellar ligament Popliteal ligament Posterior cruciate ligament (PCL) Prepatellar bursa **P Knee Bursa and Ligament, Left** *See N Knee Bursa and Ligament, Right* **Q Ankle Bursa and Ligament, Right** Calcaneofibular ligament Deltoid ligament Ligament of the lateral malleolus Talofibular ligament **R Ankle Bursa and Ligament, Left** *See Q Ankle Bursa and Ligament, Right* **S Foot Bursa and Ligament, Right** Calcaneocuboid ligament Cuneonavicular ligament Intercuneiform ligament Interphalangeal ligament Metatarsal ligament Metatarsophalangeal ligament Subtalar ligament Talocalcaneal ligament Talocalcaneonavicular ligament Tarsometatarsal ligament **T Foot Bursa and Ligament, Left** *See S Foot Bursa and Ligament, Right* **V Lower Extremity Bursa and Ligament, Right** **W Lower Extremity Bursa and Ligament, Left**	**Ø** Open **3** Percutaneous **4** Percutaneous Endoscopic	**Z** No Device	**Z** No Qualifier

Ø Medical and Surgical
M Bursae and Ligaments
D Extraction Definition: Pulling or stripping out or off all or a portion of a body part by the use of force
Explanation: The qualifier DIAGNOSTIC is used to identify extraction procedures that are biopsies

Body Part Character 4	Approach Character 5	Device Character 6	Qualifier Character 7
Ø Head and Neck Bursa and Ligament Alar ligament of axis Cervical interspinous ligament Cervical intertransverse ligament Cervical ligamentum flavum Interspinous ligament, cervical Intertransverse ligament, cervical Lateral temporomandibular ligament Ligamentum flavum, cervical Sphenomandibular ligament Stylomandibular ligament Transverse ligament of atlas **1 Shoulder Bursa and Ligament, Right** Acromioclavicular ligament Coracoacromial ligament Coracoclavicular ligament Coracohumeral ligament Costoclavicular ligament Glenohumeral ligament Interclavicular ligament Sternoclavicular ligament Subacromial bursa Transverse humeral ligament Transverse scapular ligament **2 Shoulder Bursa and Ligament, Left** *See 1 Shoulder Bursa and Ligament, Right* **3 Elbow Bursa and Ligament, Right** Annular ligament Olecranon bursa Radial collateral ligament Ulnar collateral ligament **4 Elbow Bursa and Ligament, Left** *See 3 Elbow Bursa and Ligament, Right* **5 Wrist Bursa and Ligament, Right** Palmar ulnocarpal ligament Radial collateral carpal ligament Radiocarpal ligament Radioulnar ligament Ulnar collateral carpal ligament **6 Wrist Bursa and Ligament, Left** *See 5 Wrist Bursa and Ligament, Right* **7 Hand Bursa and Ligament, Right** Carpometacarpal ligament Intercarpal ligament Interphalangeal ligament Lunotriquetral ligament Metacarpal ligament Metacarpophalangeal ligament Pisohamate ligament Pisometacarpal ligament Scapholunate ligament Scaphotrapezium ligament **8 Hand Bursa and Ligament, Left** *See 7 Hand Bursa and Ligament, Right* **9 Upper Extremity Bursa and Ligament, Right** **B Upper Extremity Bursa and Ligament, Left** **C Upper Spine Bursa and Ligament** Interspinous ligament, thoracic Intertransverse ligament, thoracic Ligamentum flavum, thoracic Supraspinous ligament **D Lower Spine Bursa and Ligament** Iliolumbar ligament Interspinous ligament, lumbar Intertransverse ligament, lumbar Ligamentum flavum, lumbar Sacrococcygeal ligament Sacroiliac ligament Sacrospinous ligament Sacrotuberous ligament Supraspinous ligament **F Sternum Bursa and Ligament** Costoxiphoid ligament Sternocostal ligament **G Rib(s) Bursa and Ligament** Costotransverse ligament **H Abdomen Bursa and Ligament, Right** **J Abdomen Bursa and Ligament, Left** **K Perineum Bursa and Ligament** **L Hip Bursa and Ligament, Right** Iliofemoral ligament Ischiofemoral ligament Pubofemoral ligament Transverse acetabular ligament Trochanteric bursa **M Hip Bursa and Ligament, Left** *See L Hip Bursa and Ligament, Right* **N Knee Bursa and Ligament, Right** Anterior cruciate ligament (ACL) Lateral collateral ligament (LCL) Ligament of head of fibula Medial collateral ligament (MCL) Patellar ligament Popliteal ligament Posterior cruciate ligament (PCL) Prepatellar bursa **P Knee Bursa and Ligament, Left** *See N Knee Bursa and Ligament, Right* **Q Ankle Bursa and Ligament, Right** Calcaneofibular ligament Deltoid ligament Ligament of the lateral malleolus Talofibular ligament **R Ankle Bursa and Ligament, Left** *See Q Ankle Bursa and Ligament, Right* **S Foot Bursa and Ligament, Right** Calcaneocuboid ligament Cuneonavicular ligament Intercuneiform ligament Interphalangeal ligament Metatarsal ligament Metatarsophalangeal ligament Subtalar ligament Talocalcaneal ligament Talocalcaneonavicular ligament Tarsometatarsal ligament **T Foot Bursa and Ligament, Left** *See S Foot Bursa and Ligament, Right* **V Lower Extremity Bursa and Ligament, Right** **W Lower Extremity Bursa and Ligament, Left**	**Ø** Open **3** Percutaneous **4** Percutaneous Endoscopic	**Z** No Device	**Z** No Qualifier

Ø Medical and Surgical
M Bursae and Ligaments
H Insertion Definition: Putting in a nonbiological appliance that monitors, assists, performs, or prevents a physiological function but does not physically take the place of a body part

Explanation: None

Body Part Character 4	Approach Character 5	Device Character 6	Qualifier Character 7
X Upper Bursa and Ligament Y Lower Bursa and Ligament	Ø Open 3 Percutaneous 4 Percutaneous Endoscopic	Y Other Device	Z No Qualifier

Non-OR ØMH[X,Y][3,4]YZ

Ø Medical and Surgical
M Bursae and Ligaments
J Inspection Definition: Visually and/or manually exploring a body part

Explanation: Visual exploration may be performed with or without optical instrumentation. Manual exploration may be performed directly or through intervening body layers.

Body Part Character 4	Approach Character 5	Device Character 6	Qualifier Character 7
X Upper Bursa and Ligament Y Lower Bursa and Ligament	Ø Open 3 Percutaneous 4 Percutaneous Endoscopic X External	Z No Device	Z No Qualifier

Non-OR ØMJ[X,Y][3,X]ZZ

Ø Medical and Surgical
M Bursae and Ligaments
M Reattachment Definition: Putting back in or on all or a portion of a separated body part to its normal location or other suitable location
Explanation: Vascular circulation and nervous pathways may or may not be reestablished

Body Part Character 4		Approach Character 5	Device Character 6	Qualifier Character 7
Ø Head and Neck Bursa and Ligament Alar ligament of axis Cervical interspinous ligament Cervical intertransverse ligament Cervical ligamentum flavum Interspinous ligament, cervical Intertransverse ligament, cervical Lateral temporomandibular ligament Ligamentum flavum, cervical Sphenomandibular ligament Stylomandibular ligament Transverse ligament of atlas **1 Shoulder Bursa and Ligament, Right** Acromioclavicular ligament Coracoacromial ligament Coracoclavicular ligament Coracohumeral ligament Costoclavicular ligament Glenohumeral ligament Interclavicular ligament Sternoclavicular ligament Subacromial bursa Transverse humeral ligament Transverse scapular ligament **2 Shoulder Bursa and Ligament, Left** *See 1 Shoulder Bursa and Ligament, Right* **3 Elbow Bursa and Ligament, Right** Annular ligament Olecranon bursa Radial collateral ligament Ulnar collateral ligament **4 Elbow Bursa and Ligament, Left** *See 3 Elbow Bursa and Ligament, Right* **5 Wrist Bursa and Ligament, Right** Palmar ulnocarpal ligament Radial collateral carpal ligament Radiocarpal ligament Radioulnar ligament Ulnar collateral carpal ligament **6 Wrist Bursa and Ligament, Left** *See 5 Wrist Bursa and Ligament, Right* **7 Hand Bursa and Ligament, Right** Carpometacarpal ligament Intercarpal ligament Interphalangeal ligament Lunotriquetral ligament Metacarpal ligament Metacarpophalangeal ligament Pisohamate ligament Pisometacarpal ligament Scapholunate ligament Scaphotrapezium ligament **8 Hand Bursa and Ligament, Left** *See 7 Hand Bursa and Ligament, Right* **9 Upper Extremity Bursa and Ligament, Right** **B Upper Extremity Bursa and Ligament, Left** **C Upper Spine Bursa and Ligament** Interspinous ligament, thoracic Intertransverse ligament, thoracic Ligamentum flavum, thoracic Supraspinous ligament	**D Lower Spine Bursa and Ligament** Iliolumbar ligament Interspinous ligament, lumbar Intertransverse ligament, lumbar Ligamentum flavum, lumbar Sacrococcygeal ligament Sacroiliac ligament Sacrospinous ligament Sacrotuberous ligament Supraspinous ligament **F Sternum Bursa and Ligament** Costoxiphoid ligament Sternocostal ligament **G Rib(s) Bursa and Ligament** Costotransverse ligament **H Abdomen Bursa and Ligament, Right** **J Abdomen Bursa and Ligament, Left** **K Perineum Bursa and Ligament** **L Hip Bursa and Ligament, Right** Iliofemoral ligament Ischiofemoral ligament Pubofemoral ligament Transverse acetabular ligament Trochanteric bursa **M Hip Bursa and Ligament, Left** *See L Hip Bursa and Ligament, Right* **N Knee Bursa and Ligament, Right** Anterior cruciate ligament (ACL) Lateral collateral ligament (LCL) Ligament of head of fibula Medial collateral ligament (MCL) Patellar ligament Popliteal ligament Posterior cruciate ligament (PCL) Prepatellar bursa **P Knee Bursa and Ligament, Left** *See N Knee Bursa and Ligament, Right* **Q Ankle Bursa and Ligament, Right** Calcaneofibular ligament Deltoid ligament Ligament of the lateral malleolus Talofibular ligament **R Ankle Bursa and Ligament, Left** *See Q Ankle Bursa and Ligament, Right* **S Foot Bursa and Ligament, Right** Calcaneocuboid ligament Cuneonavicular ligament Intercuneiform ligament Interphalangeal ligament Metatarsal ligament Metatarsophalangeal ligament Subtalar ligament Talocalcaneal ligament Talocalcaneonavicular ligament Tarsometatarsal ligament **T Foot Bursa and Ligament, Left** *See S Foot Bursa and Ligament, Right* **V Lower Extremity Bursa and Ligament, Right** **W Lower Extremity Bursa and Ligament, Left**	**Ø Open** **4 Percutaneous Endoscopic**	**Z No Device**	**Z No Qualifier**

Ø Medical and Surgical
M Bursae and Ligaments
N Release Definition: Freeing a body part from an abnormal physical constraint by cutting or by the use of force
Explanation: Some of the restraining tissue may be taken out but none of the body part is taken out

Body Part Character 4		Approach Character 5	Device Character 6	Qualifier Character 7
Ø Head and Neck Bursa and Ligament Alar ligament of axis Cervical interspinous ligament Cervical intertransverse ligament Cervical ligamentum flavum Interspinous ligament, cervical Intertransverse ligament, cervical Lateral temporomandibular ligament Ligamentum flavum, cervical Sphenomandibular ligament Stylomandibular ligament Transverse ligament of atlas **1 Shoulder Bursa and Ligament, Right** Acromioclavicular ligament Coracoacromial ligament Coracoclavicular ligament Coracohumeral ligament Costoclavicular ligament Glenohumeral ligament Interclavicular ligament Sternoclavicular ligament Subacromial bursa Transverse humeral ligament Transverse scapular ligament **2 Shoulder Bursa and Ligament, Left** *See 1 Shoulder Bursa and Ligament, Right* **3 Elbow Bursa and Ligament, Right** Annular ligament Olecranon bursa Radial collateral ligament Ulnar collateral ligament **4 Elbow Bursa and Ligament, Left** *See 3 Elbow Bursa and Ligament, Right* **5 Wrist Bursa and Ligament, Right** Palmar ulnocarpal ligament Radial collateral carpal ligament Radiocarpal ligament Radioulnar ligament Ulnar collateral carpal ligament **6 Wrist Bursa and Ligament, Left** *See 5 Wrist Bursa and Ligament, Right* **7 Hand Bursa and Ligament, Right** Carpometacarpal ligament Intercarpal ligament Interphalangeal ligament Lunotriquetral ligament Metacarpal ligament Metacarpophalangeal ligament Pisohamate ligament Pisometacarpal ligament Scapholunate ligament Scaphotrapezium ligament **8 Hand Bursa and Ligament, Left** *See 7 Hand Bursa and Ligament, Right* **9 Upper Extremity Bursa and Ligament, Right** **B Upper Extremity Bursa and Ligament, Left** **C Upper Spine Bursa and Ligament** Interspinous ligament, thoracic Intertransverse ligament, thoracic Ligamentum flavum, thoracic Supraspinous ligament	**D Lower Spine Bursa and Ligament** Iliolumbar ligament Interspinous ligament, lumbar Intertransverse ligament, lumbar Ligamentum flavum, lumbar Sacrococcygeal ligament Sacroiliac ligament Sacrospinous ligament Sacrotuberous ligament Supraspinous ligament **F Sternum Bursa and Ligament** Costoxiphoid ligament Sternocostal ligament **G Rib(s) Bursa and Ligament** Costotransverse ligament **H Abdomen Bursa and Ligament, Right** **J Abdomen Bursa and Ligament, Left** **K Perineum Bursa and Ligament** **L Hip Bursa and Ligament, Right** Iliofemoral ligament Ischiofemoral ligament Pubofemoral ligament Transverse acetabular ligament Trochanteric bursa **M Hip Bursa and Ligament, Left** *See L Hip Bursa and Ligament, Right* **N Knee Bursa and Ligament, Right** Anterior cruciate ligament (ACL) Lateral collateral ligament (LCL) Ligament of head of fibula Medial collateral ligament (MCL) Patellar ligament Popliteal ligament Posterior cruciate ligament (PCL) Prepatellar bursa **P Knee Bursa and Ligament, Left** *See N Knee Bursa and Ligament, Right* **Q Ankle Bursa and Ligament, Right** Calcaneofibular ligament Deltoid ligament Ligament of the lateral malleolus Talofibular ligament **R Ankle Bursa and Ligament, Left** *See Q Ankle Bursa and Ligament, Right* **S Foot Bursa and Ligament, Right** Calcaneocuboid ligament Cuneonavicular ligament Intercuneiform ligament Interphalangeal ligament Metatarsal ligament Metatarsophalangeal ligament Subtalar ligament Talocalcaneal ligament Talocalcaneonavicular ligament Tarsometatarsal ligament **T Foot Bursa and Ligament, Left** *See S Foot Bursa and Ligament, Right* **V Lower Extremity Bursa and Ligament, Right** **W Lower Extremity Bursa and Ligament, Left**	**Ø Open** **3 Percutaneous** **4 Percutaneous Endoscopic** **X External**	**Z No Device**	**Z No Qualifier**

Non-OR ØMN[Ø,1,2,3,4,5,6,7,8,9,B,C,D,F,G,H,J,K,L,M,N,P,Q,R,S,T,V,W]XZZ

Ø Medical and Surgical
M Bursae and Ligaments
P Removal Definition: Taking out or off a device from a body part

Explanation: If a device is taken out and a similar device put in without cutting or puncturing the skin or mucous membrane, the procedure is coded to the root operation CHANGE. Otherwise, the procedure for taking out a device is coded to the root operation REMOVAL.

Body Part Character 4	Approach Character 5	Device Character 6	Qualifier Character 7
X Upper Bursa and Ligament **Y** Lower Bursa and Ligament	**Ø** Open **3** Percutaneous **4** Percutaneous Endoscopic	**Ø** Drainage Device **7** Autologous Tissue Substitute **J** Synthetic Substitute **K** Nonautologous Tissue Substitute **Y** Other Device	**Z** No Qualifier
X Upper Bursa and Ligament **Y** Lower Bursa and Ligament	**X** External	**Ø** Drainage Device	**Z** No Qualifier

Non-OR ØMP[X,Y]3ØZ
Non-OR ØMP[X,Y][3,4]YZ
Non-OR ØMP[X,Y]XØZ

Ø Medical and Surgical
M Bursae and Ligaments
Q Repair Definition: Restoring, to the extent possible, a body part to its normal anatomic structure and function
Explanation: Used only when the method to accomplish the repair is not one of the other root operations

Body Part Character 4	Approach Character 5	Device Character 6	Qualifier Character 7
Ø Head and Neck Bursa and Ligament Alar ligament of axis Cervical interspinous ligament Cervical intertransverse ligament Cervical ligamentum flavum Interspinous ligament, cervical Intertransverse ligament, cervical Lateral temporomandibular ligament Ligamentum flavum, cervical Sphenomandibular ligament Stylomandibular ligament Transverse ligament of atlas **1 Shoulder Bursa and Ligament, Right** Acromioclavicular ligament Coracoacromial ligament Coracoclavicular ligament Coracohumeral ligament Costoclavicular ligament Glenohumeral ligament Interclavicular ligament Sternoclavicular ligament Subacromial bursa Transverse humeral ligament Transverse scapular ligament **2 Shoulder Bursa and Ligament, Left** *See 1 Shoulder Bursa and Ligament, Right* **3 Elbow Bursa and Ligament, Right** Annular ligament Olecranon bursa Radial collateral ligament Ulnar collateral ligament **4 Elbow Bursa and Ligament, Left** *See 3 Elbow Bursa and Ligament, Right* **5 Wrist Bursa and Ligament, Right** Palmar ulnocarpal ligament Radial collateral carpal ligament Radiocarpal ligament Radioulnar ligament Ulnar collateral carpal ligament **6 Wrist Bursa and Ligament, Left** *See 5 Wrist Bursa and Ligament, Right* **7 Hand Bursa and Ligament, Right** Carpometacarpal ligament Intercarpal ligament Interphalangeal ligament Lunotriquetral ligament Metacarpal ligament Metacarpophalangeal ligament Pisohamate ligament Pisometacarpal ligament Scapholunate ligament Scaphotrapezium ligament **8 Hand Bursa and Ligament, Left** *See 7 Hand Bursa and Ligament, Right* **9 Upper Extremity Bursa and Ligament, Right** **B Upper Extremity Bursa and Ligament, Left** **C Upper Spine Bursa and Ligament** Interspinous ligament, thoracic Intertransverse ligament, thoracic Ligamentum flavum, thoracic Supraspinous ligament **D Lower Spine Bursa and Ligament** Iliolumbar ligament Interspinous ligament, lumbar Intertransverse ligament, lumbar Ligamentum flavum, lumbar Sacrococcygeal ligament Sacroiliac ligament Sacrospinous ligament Sacrotuberous ligament Supraspinous ligament **F Sternum Bursa and Ligament** Costoxiphoid ligament Sternocostal ligament **G Rib(s) Bursa and Ligament** Costotransverse ligament **H Abdomen Bursa and Ligament, Right** **J Abdomen Bursa and Ligament, Left** **K Perineum Bursa and Ligament** **L Hip Bursa and Ligament, Right** Iliofemoral ligament Ischiofemoral ligament Pubofemoral ligament Transverse acetabular ligament Trochanteric bursa **M Hip Bursa and Ligament, Left** *See L Hip Bursa and Ligament, Right* **N Knee Bursa and Ligament, Right** Anterior cruciate ligament (ACL) Lateral collateral ligament (LCL) Ligament of head of fibula Medial collateral ligament (MCL) Patellar ligament Popliteal ligament Posterior cruciate ligament (PCL) Prepatellar bursa **P Knee Bursa and Ligament, Left** *See N Knee Bursa and Ligament, Right* **Q Ankle Bursa and Ligament, Right** Calcaneofibular ligament Deltoid ligament Ligament of the lateral malleolus Talofibular ligament **R Ankle Bursa and Ligament, Left** *See Q Ankle Bursa and Ligament, Right* **S Foot Bursa and Ligament, Right** Calcaneocuboid ligament Cuneonavicular ligament Intercuneiform ligament Interphalangeal ligament Metatarsal ligament Metatarsophalangeal ligament Subtalar ligament Talocalcaneal ligament Talocalcaneonavicular ligament Tarsometatarsal ligament **T Foot Bursa and Ligament, Left** *See S Foot Bursa and Ligament, Right* **V Lower Extremity Bursa and Ligament, Right** **W Lower Extremity Bursa and Ligament, Left**	**Ø Open** **3 Percutaneous** **4 Percutaneous Endoscopic**	**Z No Device**	**Z No Qualifier**

Ø Medical and Surgical
M Bursae and Ligaments
R Replacement Definition: Putting in or on biological or synthetic material that physically takes the place and/or function of all or a portion of a body part

Explanation: The body part may have been taken out or replaced, or may be taken out, physically eradicated, or rendered nonfunctional during the REPLACEMENT procedure. A REMOVAL procedure is coded for taking out the device used in a previous replacement procedure.

Body Part Character 4	Approach Character 5	Device Character 6	Qualifier Character 7
Ø Head and Neck Bursa and Ligament Alar ligament of axis Cervical interspinous ligament Cervical intertransverse ligament Cervical ligamentum flavum Interspinous ligament, cervical Intertransverse ligament, cervical Lateral temporomandibular ligament Ligamentum flavum, cervical Sphenomandibular ligament Stylomandibular ligament Transverse ligament of atlas **1 Shoulder Bursa and Ligament, Right** Acromioclavicular ligament Coracoacromial ligament Coracoclavicular ligament Coracohumeral ligament Costoclavicular ligament Glenohumeral ligament Interclavicular ligament Sternoclavicular ligament Subacromial bursa Transverse humeral ligament Transverse scapular ligament **2 Shoulder Bursa and Ligament, Left** *See 1 Shoulder Bursa and Ligament, Right* **3 Elbow Bursa and Ligament, Right** Annular ligament Olecranon bursa Radial collateral ligament Ulnar collateral ligament **4 Elbow Bursa and Ligament, Left** *See 3 Elbow Bursa and Ligament, Right* **5 Wrist Bursa and Ligament, Right** Palmar ulnocarpal ligament Radial collateral carpal ligament Radiocarpal ligament Radioulnar ligament Ulnar collateral carpal ligament **6 Wrist Bursa and Ligament, Left** *See 5 Wrist Bursa and Ligament, Right* **7 Hand Bursa and Ligament, Right** Carpometacarpal ligament Intercarpal ligament Interphalangeal ligament Lunotriquetral ligament Metacarpal ligament Metacarpophalangeal ligament Pisohamate ligament Pisometacarpal ligament Scapholunate ligament Scaphotrapezium ligament **8 Hand Bursa and Ligament, Left** *See 7 Hand Bursa and Ligament, Right* **9 Upper Extremity Bursa and Ligament, Right** **B Upper Extremity Bursa and Ligament, Left** **C Upper Spine Bursa and Ligament** Interspinous ligament, thoracic Intertransverse ligament, thoracic Ligamentum flavum, thoracic Supraspinous ligament **D Lower Spine Bursa and Ligament** Iliolumbar ligament Interspinous ligament, lumbar Intertransverse ligament, lumbar Ligamentum flavum, lumbar Sacrococcygeal ligament Sacroiliac ligament Sacrospinous ligament Sacrotuberous ligament Supraspinous ligament **F Sternum Bursa and Ligament** Costoxiphoid ligament Sternocostal ligament **G Rib(s) Bursa and Ligament** Costotransverse ligament **H Abdomen Bursa and Ligament, Right** **J Abdomen Bursa and Ligament, Left** **K Perineum Bursa and Ligament** **L Hip Bursa and Ligament, Right** Iliofemoral ligament Ischiofemoral ligament Pubofemoral ligament Transverse acetabular ligament Trochanteric bursa **M Hip Bursa and Ligament, Left** *See L Hip Bursa and Ligament, Right* **N Knee Bursa and Ligament, Right** Anterior cruciate ligament (ACL) Lateral collateral ligament (LCL) Ligament of head of fibula Medial collateral ligament (MCL) Patellar ligament Popliteal ligament Posterior cruciate ligament (PCL) Prepatellar bursa **P Knee Bursa and Ligament, Left** *See N Knee Bursa and Ligament, Right* **Q Ankle Bursa and Ligament, Right** Calcaneofibular ligament Deltoid ligament Ligament of the lateral malleolus Talofibular ligament **R Ankle Bursa and Ligament, Left** *See Q Ankle Bursa and Ligament, Right* **S Foot Bursa and Ligament, Right** Calcaneocuboid ligament Cuneonavicular ligament Intercuneiform ligament Interphalangeal ligament Metatarsal ligament Metatarsophalangeal ligament Subtalar ligament Talocalcaneal ligament Talocalcaneonavicular ligament Tarsometatarsal ligament **T Foot Bursa and Ligament, Left** *See S Foot Bursa and Ligament, Right* **V Lower Extremity Bursa and Ligament, Right** **W Lower Extremity Bursa and Ligament, Left**	**Ø Open** **4 Percutaneous Endoscopic**	**7 Autologous Tissue Substitute** **J Synthetic Substitute** **K Nonautologous Tissue Substitute**	**Z No Qualifier**

Ø Medical and Surgical
M Bursae and Ligaments
S Reposition Definition: Moving to its normal location, or other suitable location, all or a portion of a body part

Explanation: The body part is moved to a new location from an abnormal location, or from a normal location where it is not functioning correctly. The body part may or may not be cut out or off to be moved to the new location.

Body Part Character 4		Approach Character 5	Device Character 6	Qualifier Character 7
Ø Head and Neck Bursa and Ligament Alar ligament of axis Cervical interspinous ligament Cervical intertransverse ligament Cervical ligamentum flavum Interspinous ligament, cervical Intertransverse ligament, cervical Lateral temporomandibular ligament Ligamentum flavum, cervical Sphenomandibular ligament Stylomandibular ligament Transverse ligament of atlas **1 Shoulder Bursa and Ligament, Right** Acromioclavicular ligament Coracoacromial ligament Coracoclavicular ligament Coracohumeral ligament Costoclavicular ligament Glenohumeral ligament Interclavicular ligament Sternoclavicular ligament Subacromial bursa Transverse humeral ligament Transverse scapular ligament **2 Shoulder Bursa and Ligament, Left** *See 1 Shoulder Bursa and Ligament, Right* **3 Elbow Bursa and Ligament, Right** Annular ligament Olecranon bursa Radial collateral ligament Ulnar collateral ligament **4 Elbow Bursa and Ligament, Left** *See 3 Elbow Bursa and Ligament, Right* **5 Wrist Bursa and Ligament, Right** Palmar ulnocarpal ligament Radial collateral carpal ligament Radiocarpal ligament Radioulnar ligament Ulnar collateral carpal ligament **6 Wrist Bursa and Ligament, Left** *See 5 Wrist Bursa and Ligament, Right* **7 Hand Bursa and Ligament, Right** Carpometacarpal ligament Intercarpal ligament Interphalangeal ligament Lunotriquetral ligament Metacarpal ligament Metacarpophalangeal ligament Pisohamate ligament Pisometacarpal ligament Scapholunate ligament Scaphotrapezium ligament **8 Hand Bursa and Ligament, Left** *See 7 Hand Bursa and Ligament, Right* **9 Upper Extremity Bursa and Ligament, Right** **B Upper Extremity Bursa and Ligament, Left** **C Upper Spine Bursa and Ligament** Interspinous ligament, thoracic Intertransverse ligament, thoracic Ligamentum flavum, thoracic Supraspinous ligament	**D Lower Spine Bursa and Ligament** Iliolumbar ligament Interspinous ligament, lumbar Intertransverse ligament, lumbar Ligamentum flavum, lumbar Sacrococcygeal ligament Sacroiliac ligament Sacrospinous ligament Sacrotuberous ligament Supraspinous ligament **F Sternum Bursa and Ligament** Costoxiphoid ligament Sternocostal ligament **G Rib(s) Bursa and Ligament** Costotransverse ligament **H Abdomen Bursa and Ligament, Right** **J Abdomen Bursa and Ligament, Left** **K Perineum Bursa and Ligament** **L Hip Bursa and Ligament, Right** Iliofemoral ligament Ischiofemoral ligament Pubofemoral ligament Transverse acetabular ligament Trochanteric bursa **M Hip Bursa and Ligament, Left** *See L Hip Bursa and Ligament, Right* **N Knee Bursa and Ligament, Right** Anterior cruciate ligament (ACL) Lateral collateral ligament (LCL) Ligament of head of fibula Medial collateral ligament (MCL) Patellar ligament Popliteal ligament Posterior cruciate ligament (PCL) Prepatellar bursa **P Knee Bursa and Ligament, Left** *See N Knee Bursa and Ligament, Right* **Q Ankle Bursa and Ligament, Right** Calcaneofibular ligament Deltoid ligament Ligament of the lateral malleolus Talofibular ligament **R Ankle Bursa and Ligament, Left** *See Q Ankle Bursa and Ligament, Right* **S Foot Bursa and Ligament, Right** Calcaneocuboid ligament Cuneonavicular ligament Intercuneiform ligament Interphalangeal ligament Metatarsal ligament Metatarsophalangeal ligament Subtalar ligament Talocalcaneal ligament Talocalcaneonavicular ligament Tarsometatarsal ligament **T Foot Bursa and Ligament, Left** *See S Foot Bursa and Ligament, Right* **V Lower Extremity Bursa and Ligament, Right** **W Lower Extremity Bursa and Ligament, Left**	Ø Open 4 Percutaneous Endoscopic	Z No Device	Z No Qualifier

Ø Medical and Surgical
M Bursae and Ligaments
T Resection Definition: Cutting out or off, without replacement, all of a body part
Explanation: None

Body Part Character 4	Approach Character 5	Device Character 6	Qualifier Character 7
Ø Head and Neck Bursa and Ligament Alar ligament of axis Cervical interspinous ligament Cervical intertransverse ligament Cervical ligamentum flavum Interspinous ligament, cervical Intertransverse ligament, cervical Lateral temporomandibular ligament Ligamentum flavum, cervical Sphenomandibular ligament Stylomandibular ligament Transverse ligament of atlas **1 Shoulder Bursa and Ligament, Right** Acromioclavicular ligament Coracoacromial ligament Coracoclavicular ligament Coracohumeral ligament Costoclavicular ligament Glenohumeral ligament Interclavicular ligament Sternoclavicular ligament Subacromial bursa Transverse humeral ligament Transverse scapular ligament **2 Shoulder Bursa and Ligament, Left** *See 1 Shoulder Bursa and Ligament, Right* **3 Elbow Bursa and Ligament, Right** Annular ligament Olecranon bursa Radial collateral ligament Ulnar collateral ligament **4 Elbow Bursa and Ligament, Left** *See 3 Elbow Bursa and Ligament, Right* **5 Wrist Bursa and Ligament, Right** Palmar ulnocarpal ligament Radial collateral carpal ligament Radiocarpal ligament Radioulnar ligament Ulnar collateral carpal ligament **6 Wrist Bursa and Ligament, Left** *See 5 Wrist Bursa and Ligament, Right* **7 Hand Bursa and Ligament, Right** Carpometacarpal ligament Intercarpal ligament Interphalangeal ligament Lunotriquetral ligament Metacarpal ligament Metacarpophalangeal ligament Pisohamate ligament Pisometacarpal ligament Scapholunate ligament Scaphotrapezium ligament **8 Hand Bursa and Ligament, Left** *See 7 Hand Bursa and Ligament, Right* **9 Upper Extremity Bursa and Ligament, Right** **B Upper Extremity Bursa and Ligament, Left** **C Upper Spine Bursa and Ligament** Interspinous ligament, thoracic Intertransverse ligament, thoracic Ligamentum flavum, thoracic Supraspinous ligament **D Lower Spine Bursa and Ligament** Iliolumbar ligament Interspinous ligament, lumbar Intertransverse ligament, lumbar Ligamentum flavum, lumbar Sacrococcygeal ligament Sacroiliac ligament Sacrospinous ligament Sacrotuberous ligament Supraspinous ligament **F Sternum Bursa and Ligament** Costoxiphoid ligament Sternocostal ligament **G Rib(s) Bursa and Ligament** Costotransverse ligament **H Abdomen Bursa and Ligament, Right** **J Abdomen Bursa and Ligament, Left** **K Perineum Bursa and Ligament** **L Hip Bursa and Ligament, Right** Iliofemoral ligament Ischiofemoral ligament Pubofemoral ligament Transverse acetabular ligament Trochanteric bursa **M Hip Bursa and Ligament, Left** *See L Hip Bursa and Ligament, Right* **N Knee Bursa and Ligament, Right** Anterior cruciate ligament (ACL) Lateral collateral ligament (LCL) Ligament of head of fibula Medial collateral ligament (MCL) Patellar ligament Popliteal ligament Posterior cruciate ligament (PCL) Prepatellar bursa **P Knee Bursa and Ligament, Left** *See N Knee Bursa and Ligament, Right* **Q Ankle Bursa and Ligament, Right** Calcaneofibular ligament Deltoid ligament Ligament of the lateral malleolus Talofibular ligament **R Ankle Bursa and Ligament, Left** *See Q Ankle Bursa and Ligament, Right* **S Foot Bursa and Ligament, Right** Calcaneocuboid ligament Cuneonavicular ligament Intercuneiform ligament Interphalangeal ligament Metatarsal ligament Metatarsophalangeal ligament Subtalar ligament Talocalcaneal ligament Talocalcaneonavicular ligament Tarsometatarsal ligament **T Foot Bursa and Ligament, Left** *See S Foot Bursa and Ligament, Right* **V Lower Extremity Bursa and Ligament, Right** **W Lower Extremity Bursa and Ligament, Left**	**Ø Open** **4 Percutaneous Endoscopic**	**Z No Device**	**Z No Qualifier**

Ø Medical and Surgical
M Bursae and Ligaments
U Supplement Definition: Putting in or on biological or synthetic material that physically reinforces and/or augments the function of a portion of a body part

Explanation: The biological material is non-living, or is living and from the same individual. The body part may have been previously replaced, and the SUPPLEMENT procedure is performed to physically reinforce and/or augment the function of the replaced body part.

Body Part Character 4	Approach Character 5	Device Character 6	Qualifier Character 7
Ø Head and Neck Bursa and Ligament Alar ligament of axis Cervical interspinous ligament Cervical intertransverse ligament Cervical ligamentum flavum Interspinous ligament, cervical Intertransverse ligament, cervical Lateral temporomandibular ligament Ligamentum flavum, cervical Sphenomandibular ligament Stylomandibular ligament Transverse ligament of atlas **1 Shoulder Bursa and Ligament, Right** Acromioclavicular ligament Coracoacromial ligament Coracoclavicular ligament Coracohumeral ligament Costoclavicular ligament Glenohumeral ligament Interclavicular ligament Sternoclavicular ligament Subacromial bursa Transverse humeral ligament Transverse scapular ligament **2 Shoulder Bursa and Ligament, Left** *See 1 Shoulder Bursa and Ligament, Right* **3 Elbow Bursa and Ligament, Right** Annular ligament Olecranon bursa Radial collateral ligament Ulnar collateral ligament **4 Elbow Bursa and Ligament, Left** *See 3 Elbow Bursa and Ligament, Right* **5 Wrist Bursa and Ligament, Right** Palmar ulnocarpal ligament Radial collateral carpal ligament Radiocarpal ligament Radioulnar ligament Ulnar collateral carpal ligament **6 Wrist Bursa and Ligament, Left** *See 5 Wrist Bursa and Ligament, Right* **7 Hand Bursa and Ligament, Right** Carpometacarpal ligament Intercarpal ligament Interphalangeal ligament Lunotriquetral ligament Metacarpal ligament Metacarpophalangeal ligament Pisohamate ligament Pisometacarpal ligament Scapholunate ligament Scaphotrapezium ligament **8 Hand Bursa and Ligament, Left** *See 7 Hand Bursa and Ligament, Right* **9 Upper Extremity Bursa and Ligament, Right** **B Upper Extremity Bursa and Ligament, Left** **C Upper Spine Bursa and Ligament** Interspinous ligament, thoracic Intertransverse ligament, thoracic Ligamentum flavum, thoracic Supraspinous ligament **D Lower Spine Bursa and Ligament** Iliolumbar ligament Interspinous ligament, lumbar Intertransverse ligament, lumbar Ligamentum flavum, lumbar Sacrococcygeal ligament Sacroiliac ligament Sacrospinous ligament Sacrotuberous ligament Supraspinous ligament **F Sternum Bursa and Ligament** Costoxiphoid ligament Sternocostal ligament **G Rib(s) Bursa and Ligament** Costotransverse ligament **H Abdomen Bursa and Ligament, Right** **J Abdomen Bursa and Ligament, Left** **K Perineum Bursa and Ligament** **L Hip Bursa and Ligament, Right** Iliofemoral ligament Ischiofemoral ligament Pubofemoral ligament Transverse acetabular ligament Trochanteric bursa **M Hip Bursa and Ligament, Left** *See L Hip Bursa and Ligament, Right* **N Knee Bursa and Ligament, Right** Anterior cruciate ligament (ACL) Lateral collateral ligament (LCL) Ligament of head of fibula Medial collateral ligament (MCL) Patellar ligament Popliteal ligament Posterior cruciate ligament (PCL) Prepatellar bursa **P Knee Bursa and Ligament, Left** *See N Knee Bursa and Ligament, Right* **Q Ankle Bursa and Ligament, Right** Calcaneofibular ligament Deltoid ligament Ligament of the lateral malleolus Talofibular ligament **R Ankle Bursa and Ligament, Left** *See Q Ankle Bursa and Ligament, Right* **S Foot Bursa and Ligament, Right** Calcaneocuboid ligament Cuneonavicular ligament Intercuneiform ligament Interphalangeal ligament Metatarsal ligament Metatarsophalangeal ligament Subtalar ligament Talocalcaneal ligament Talocalcaneonavicular ligament Tarsometatarsal ligament **T Foot Bursa and Ligament, Left** *See S Foot Bursa and Ligament, Right* **V Lower Extremity Bursa and Ligament, Right** **W Lower Extremity Bursa and Ligament, Left**	**Ø** Open **4** Percutaneous Endoscopic	**7** Autologous Tissue Substitute **J** Synthetic Substitute **K** Nonautologous Tissue Substitute	**Z** No Qualifier

Bursae and Ligaments

Ø Medical and Surgical
M Bursae and Ligaments
W Revision Definition: Correcting, to the extent possible, a portion of a malfunctioning device or the position of a displaced device

Explanation: Revision can include correcting a malfunctioning or displaced device by taking out or putting in components of the device such as a screw or pin

Body Part Character 4	Approach Character 5	Device Character 6	Qualifier Character 7
X Upper Bursa and Ligament Y Lower Bursa and Ligament	Ø Open 3 Percutaneous 4 Percutaneous Endoscopic	Ø Drainage Device 7 Autologous Tissue Substitute J Synthetic Substitute K Nonautologous Tissue Substitute Y Other Device	Z No Qualifier
X Upper Bursa and Ligament Y Lower Bursa and Ligament	X External	Ø Drainage Device 7 Autologous Tissue Substitute J Synthetic Substitute K Nonautologous Tissue Substitute	Z No Qualifier

Non-OR ØMW[X,Y][3,4]YZ
Non-OR ØMW[X,Y]X[Ø,7,J,K]Z

Ø Medical and Surgical
M Bursae and Ligaments
X Transfer Definition: Moving, without taking out, all or a portion of a body part to another location to take over the function of all or a portion of a body part
Explanation: The body part transferred remains connected to its vascular and nervous supply

Body Part Character 4	Approach Character 5	Device Character 6	Qualifier Character 7
Ø Head and Neck Bursa and Ligament Alar ligament of axis Cervical interspinous ligament Cervical intertransverse ligament Cervical ligamentum flavum Interspinous ligament, cervical Intertransverse ligament, cervical Lateral temporomandibular ligament Ligamentum flavum, cervical Sphenomandibular ligament Stylomandibular ligament Transverse ligament of atlas **1 Shoulder Bursa and Ligament, Right** Acromioclavicular ligament Coracoacromial ligament Coracoclavicular ligament Coracohumeral ligament Costoclavicular ligament Glenohumeral ligament Interclavicular ligament Sternoclavicular ligament Subacromial bursa Transverse humeral ligament Transverse scapular ligament **2 Shoulder Bursa and Ligament, Left** *See 1 Shoulder Bursa and Ligament, Right* **3 Elbow Bursa and Ligament, Right** Annular ligament Olecranon bursa Radial collateral ligament Ulnar collateral ligament **4 Elbow Bursa and Ligament, Left** *See 3 Elbow Bursa and Ligament, Right* **5 Wrist Bursa and Ligament, Right** Palmar ulnocarpal ligament Radial collateral carpal ligament Radiocarpal ligament Radioulnar ligament Ulnar collateral carpal ligament **6 Wrist Bursa and Ligament, Left** *See 5 Wrist Bursa and Ligament, Right* **7 Hand Bursa and Ligament, Right** Carpometacarpal ligament Intercarpal ligament Interphalangeal ligament Lunotriquetral ligament Metacarpal ligament Metacarpophalangeal ligament Pisohamate ligament Pisometacarpal ligament Scapholunate ligament Scaphotrapezium ligament **8 Hand Bursa and Ligament, Left** *See 7 Hand Bursa and Ligament, Right* **9 Upper Extremity Bursa and Ligament, Right** **B Upper Extremity Bursa and Ligament, Left** **C Upper Spine Bursa and Ligament** Interspinous ligament, thoracic Intertransverse ligament, thoracic Ligamentum flavum, thoracic Supraspinous ligament **D Lower Spine Bursa and Ligament** Iliolumbar ligament Interspinous ligament, lumbar Intertransverse ligament, lumbar Ligamentum flavum, lumbar Sacrococcygeal ligament Sacroiliac ligament Sacrospinous ligament Sacrotuberous ligament Supraspinous ligament **F Sternum Bursa and Ligament** Costoxiphoid ligament Sternocostal ligament **G Rib(s) Bursa and Ligament** Costotransverse ligament **H Abdomen Bursa and Ligament, Right** **J Abdomen Bursa and Ligament, Left** **K Perineum Bursa and Ligament** **L Hip Bursa and Ligament, Right** Iliofemoral ligament Ischiofemoral ligament Pubofemoral ligament Transverse acetabular ligament Trochanteric bursa **M Hip Bursa and Ligament, Left** *See L Hip Bursa and Ligament, Right* **N Knee Bursa and Ligament, Right** Anterior cruciate ligament (ACL) Lateral collateral ligament (LCL) Ligament of head of fibula Medial collateral ligament (MCL) Patellar ligament Popliteal ligament Posterior cruciate ligament (PCL) Prepatellar bursa **P Knee Bursa and Ligament, Left** *See N Knee Bursa and Ligament, Right* **Q Ankle Bursa and Ligament, Right** Calcaneofibular ligament Deltoid ligament Ligament of the lateral malleolus Talofibular ligament **R Ankle Bursa and Ligament, Left** *See Q Ankle Bursa and Ligament, Right* **S Foot Bursa and Ligament, Right** Calcaneocuboid ligament Cuneonavicular ligament Intercuneiform ligament Interphalangeal ligament Metatarsal ligament Metatarsophalangeal ligament Subtalar ligament Talocalcaneal ligament Talocalcaneonavicular ligament Tarsometatarsal ligament **T Foot Bursa and Ligament, Left** *See S Foot Bursa and Ligament, Right* **V Lower Extremity Bursa and Ligament, Right** **W Lower Extremity Bursa and Ligament, Left**	**Ø Open** **4 Percutaneous Endoscopic**	**Z No Device**	**Z No Qualifier**

Head and Facial Bones ØN2–ØNW

Character Meanings

This Character Meaning table is provided as a guide to assist the user in the identification of character members that may be found in this section of code tables. It **SHOULD NOT** be used to build a PCS code.

Operation–Character 3	Body Part–Character 4	Approach–Character 5	Device–Character 6	Qualifier–Character 7
2 Change	Ø Skull	Ø Open	Ø Drainage Device	X Diagnostic
5 Destruction	1 Frontal Bone	3 Percutaneous	4 Internal Fixation Device	Z No Qualifier
8 Division	3 Parietal Bone, Right	4 Percutaneous Endoscopic	5 External Fixation Device	
9 Drainage	4 Parietal Bone, Left	X External	7 Autologous Tissue Substitute	
B Excision	5 Temporal Bone, Right		J Synthetic Substitute	
C Extirpation	6 Temporal Bone, Left		K Nonautologous Tissue Substitute	
D Extraction	7 Occipital Bone		M Bone Growth Stimulator	
H Insertion	B Nasal Bone		N Neurostimulator Generator	
J Inspection	C Sphenoid Bone		S Hearing Device	
N Release	F Ethmoid Bone, Right		Y Other Device	
P Removal	G Ethmoid Bone, Left		Z No Device	
Q Repair	H Lacrimal Bone, Right			
R Replacement	J Lacrimal Bone, Left			
S Reposition	K Palatine Bone, Right			
T Resection	L Palatine Bone, Left			
U Supplement	M Zygomatic Bone, Right			
W Revision	N Zygomatic Bone, Left			
	P Orbit, Right			
	Q Orbit, Left			
	R Maxilla			
	T Mandible, Right			
	V Mandible, Left			
	W Facial Bone			
	X Hyoid Bone			

AHA Coding Clinic for table ØNB
2017, 1Q, 20 Preparatory nasal adhesion repair before definitive cleft palate repair
2015, 3Q, 3-8 Excisional and nonexcisional debridement
2015, 2Q, 12 Orbital exenteration

AHA Coding Clinic for table ØND
2017, 4Q, 41 Extraction procedures

AHA Coding Clinic for table ØNH
2015, 3Q, 13 Nonexcisional debridement of cranial wound with removal and replacement of hardware

AHA Coding Clinic for table ØNP
2015, 3Q, 13 Nonexcisional debridement of cranial wound with removal and replacement of hardware

AHA Coding Clinic for table ØNQ
2016, 3Q, 29 Closure of bilateral alveolar clefts

AHA Coding Clinic for table ØNR
2017, 3Q, 17 Resection of schwannoma and placement of DuraGen and Lorenz cranial plating system
2017, 3Q, 22 Replacement of native skull bone flap
2017, 1Q, 23 Reconstruction of mandible using titanium and bone
2014, 3Q, 7 Hemi-cranioplasty for repair of cranial defect

AHA Coding Clinic for table ØNS
2017, 3Q, 22 Replacement of native skull bone flap
2017, 1Q, 20 Preparatory nasal adhesion repair before definitive cleft palate repair
2016, 2Q, 30 Clipping (occlusion) of cerebral artery, decompressive craniectomy and storage of bone flap in abdominal wall
2015, 3Q, 17 Craniosynostosis with cranial vault reconstruction
2015, 3Q, 27 Moyamoya disease and hemispheric pial synagiosis with craniotomy
2014, 3Q, 23 Le Fort I osteotomy
2013, 3Q, 24 Distraction osteogenesis
2013, 3Q, 25 Fracture of frontal bone with repair and coagulation for hemostasis

AHA Coding Clinic for table ØNU
2016, 3Q, 29 Closure of bilateral alveolar clefts
2013, 3Q, 24 Distraction osteogenesis

Head and Facial Bones

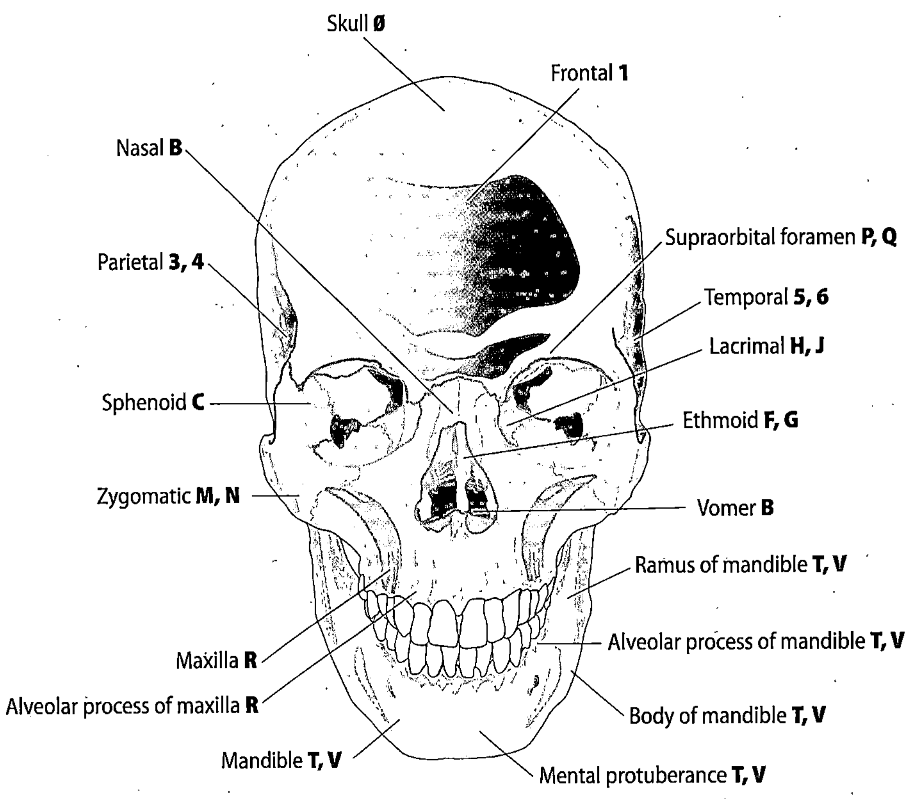

Skull Bones

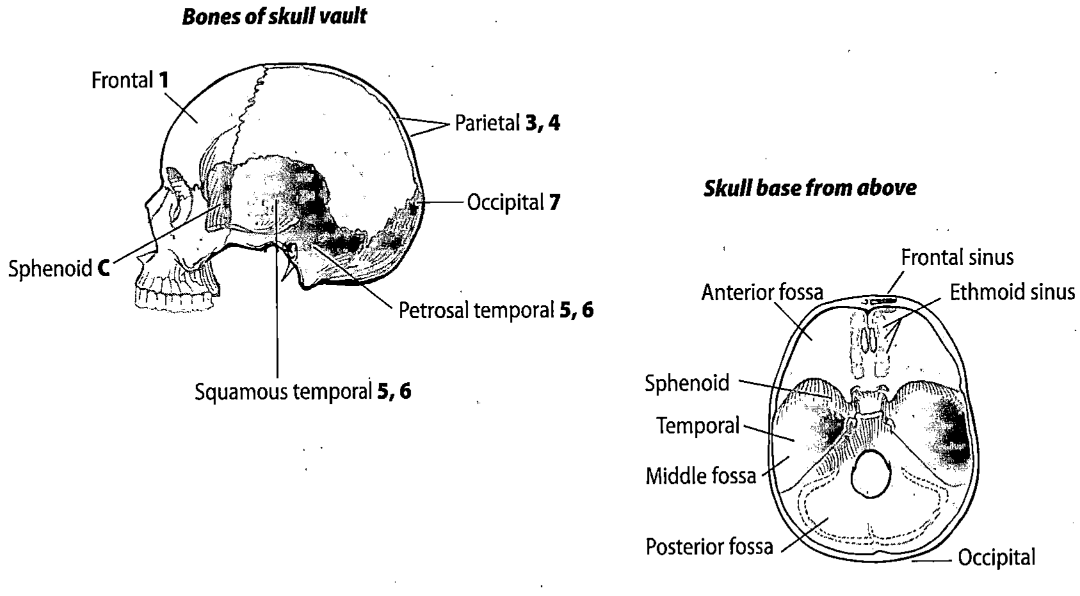

Ø Medical and Surgical
N Head and Facial Bones
2 Change Definition: Taking out or off a device from a body part and putting back an identical or similar device in or on the same body part without cutting or puncturing the skin or a mucous membrane
Explanation: All CHANGE procedures are coded using the approach EXTERNAL

Body Part Character 4	Approach Character 5	Device Character 6	Qualifier Character 7
Ø Skull **B** Nasal Bone Vomer of nasal septum **W** Facial Bone	**X** External	**Ø** Drainage Device **Y** Other Device	**Z** No Qualifier

Non-OR All body part, approach, device, and qualifier values

Ø Medical and Surgical
N Head and Facial Bones
5 Destruction Definition: Physical eradication of all or a portion of a body part by the direct use of energy, force, or a destructive agent
Explanation: None of the body part is physically taken out

Body Part Character 4	Approach Character 5	Device Character 6	Qualifier Character 7
Ø Skull **1** Frontal Bone Zygomatic process of frontal bone **3** Parietal Bone, Right **4** Parietal Bone, Left **5** Temporal Bone, Right Mastoid process Petrous part of temporal bone Tympanic part of temporal bone Zygomatic process of temporal bone **6** Temporal Bone, Left *See 5 Temporal Bone, Right* **7** Occipital Bone Foramen magnum **B** Nasal Bone Vomer of nasal septum **C** Sphenoid Bone Greater wing Lesser wing Optic foramen Pterygoid process Sella turcica **F** Ethmoid Bone, Right Cribriform plate **G** Ethmoid Bone, Left *See F Ethmoid Bone, Right* **H** Lacrimal Bone, Right **J** Lacrimal Bone, Left **K** Palatine Bone, Right **L** Palatine Bone, Left **M** Zygomatic Bone, Right **N** Zygomatic Bone, Left **P** Orbit, Right Bony orbit Orbital portion of ethmoid bone Orbital portion of frontal bone Orbital portion of lacrimal bone Orbital portion of maxilla Orbital portion of palatine bone Orbital portion of sphenoid bone Orbital portion of zygomatic bone **Q** Orbit, Left *See P Orbit, Right* **R** Maxilla Alveolar process of maxilla **T** Mandible, Right Alveolar process of mandible Condyloid process Mandibular notch Mental foramen **V** Mandible, Left *See T Mandible, Right* **X** Hyoid Bone	**Ø** Open **3** Percutaneous **4** Percutaneous Endoscopic	**Z** No Device	**Z** No Qualifier

Ø Medical and Surgical
N Head and Facial Bones
8 Division Definition: Cutting into a body part, without draining fluids and/or gases from the body part, in order to separate or transect a body part
Explanation: All or a portion of the body part is separated into two or more portions

Body Part Character 4	Approach Character 5	Device Character 6	Qualifier Character 7
Ø Skull **1 Frontal Bone** Zygomatic process of frontal bone **3 Parietal Bone, Right** **4 Parietal Bone, Left** **5 Temporal Bone, Right** Mastoid process Petrous part of temporal bone Tympanic part of temporal bone Zygomatic process of temporal bone **6 Temporal Bone, Left** *See 5 Temporal Bone, Right* **7 Occipital Bone** Foramen magnum **B Nasal Bone** Vomer of nasal septum **C Sphenoid Bone** Greater wing Lesser wing Optic foramen Pterygoid process Sella turcica **F Ethmoid Bone, Right** Cribriform plate **G Ethmoid Bone, Left** *See F Ethmoid Bone, Right* **H Lacrimal Bone, Right** **J Lacrimal Bone, Left** **K Palatine Bone, Right** **L Palatine Bone, Left** **M Zygomatic Bone, Right** **N Zygomatic Bone, Left** **P Orbit, Right** Bony orbit Orbital portion of ethmoid bone Orbital portion of frontal bone Orbital portion of lacrimal bone Orbital portion of maxilla Orbital portion of palatine bone Orbital portion of sphenoid bone Orbital portion of zygomatic bone **Q Orbit, Left** *See P Orbit, Right* **R Maxilla** Alveolar process of maxilla **T Mandible, Right** Alveolar process of mandible Condyloid process Mandibular notch Mental foramen **V Mandible, Left** *See T Mandible, Right* **X Hyoid Bone**	**Ø Open** **3 Percutaneous** **4 Percutaneous Endoscopic**	**Z No Device**	**Z No Qualifier**

Non-OR ØN8B[Ø,3,4]ZZ

Ø Medical and Surgical
N Head and Facial Bones
9 Drainage Definition: Taking or letting out fluids and/or gases from a body part
Explanation: The qualifier DIAGNOSTIC is used to identify drainage procedures that are biopsies

Body Part Character 4	Approach Character 5	Device Character 6	Qualifier Character 7
Ø Skull 1 Frontal Bone Zygomatic process of frontal bone 3 Parietal Bone, Right 4 Parietal Bone, Left 5 Temporal Bone, Right Mastoid process Petrous part of temporal bone Tympanic part of temporal bone Zygomatic process of temporal bone 6 Temporal Bone, Left *See 5 Temporal Bone, Right* 7 Occipital Bone Foramen magnum B Nasal Bone Vomer of nasal septum C Sphenoid Bone Greater wing Lesser wing Optic foramen Pterygoid process Sella turcica F Ethmoid Bone, Right Cribriform plate G Ethmoid Bone, Left *See F Ethmoid Bone, Right* H Lacrimal Bone, Right J Lacrimal Bone, Left K Palatine Bone, Right L Palatine Bone, Left M Zygomatic Bone, Right N Zygomatic Bone, Left P Orbit, Right Bony orbit Orbital portion of ethmoid bone Orbital portion of frontal bone Orbital portion of lacrimal bone Orbital portion of maxilla Orbital portion of palatine bone Orbital portion of sphenoid bone Orbital portion of zygomatic bone Q Orbit, Left *See P Orbit, Right* R Maxilla Alveolar process of maxilla T Mandible, Right Alveolar process of mandible Condyloid process Mandibular notch Mental foramen V Mandible, Left *See T Mandible, Right* X Hyoid Bone	Ø Open 3 Percutaneous 4 Percutaneous Endoscopic	Ø Drainage Device	Z No Qualifier

ØN9 Continued on next page

Non-OR ØN9[Ø,1,3,4,5,6,7,C,F,G,H,J,K,L,M,N,P,Q,X]3ØZ
Non-OR ØN9[B,R,T,V][Ø,3,4]ØZ

ØN9 Continued

Ø Medical and Surgical
N Head and Facial Bones
9 Drainage Definition: Taking or letting out fluids and/or gases from a body part
Explanation: The qualifier DIAGNOSTIC is used to identify drainage procedures that are biopsies

Body Part Character 4	Approach Character 5	Device Character 6	Qualifier Character 7
Ø Skull 1 Frontal Bone Zygomatic process of frontal bone 3 Parietal Bone, Right 4 Parietal Bone, Left 5 Temporal Bone, Right Mastoid process Petrous part of temporal bone Tympanic part of temporal bone Zygomatic process of temporal bone 6 Temporal Bone, Left *See 5 Temporal Bone, Right* 7 Occipital Bone Foramen magnum B Nasal Bone Vomer of nasal septum C Sphenoid Bone Greater wing Lesser wing Optic foramen Pterygoid process Sella turcica F Ethmoid Bone, Right Cribriform plate G Ethmoid Bone, Left *See F Ethmoid Bone, Right* H Lacrimal Bone, Right J Lacrimal Bone, Left K Palatine Bone, Right L Palatine Bone, Left M Zygomatic Bone, Right N Zygomatic Bone, Left P Orbit, Right Bony orbit Orbital portion of ethmoid bone Orbital portion of frontal bone Orbital portion of lacrimal bone Orbital portion of maxilla Orbital portion of palatine bone Orbital portion of sphenoid bone Orbital portion of zygomatic bone Q Orbit, Left *See P Orbit, Right* R Maxilla Alveolar process of maxilla T Mandible, Right Alveolar process of mandible Condyloid process Mandibular notch Mental foramen V Mandible, Left *See T Mandible, Right* X Hyoid Bone	Ø Open 3 Percutaneous 4 Percutaneous Endoscopic	Z No Device	X Diagnostic Z No Qualifier

Non-OR ØN9[Ø,1,3,4,5,6,7,C,F,G,H,J,K,L,M,N,P,Q,X]3ZZ
Non-OR ØN9B[Ø,3,4]Z[X,Z]
Non-OR ØN9[R,T,V][Ø,3,4]ZZ

Ø Medical and Surgical
N Head and Facial Bones
B Excision Definition: Cutting out or off, without replacement, a portion of a body part
Explanation: The qualifier DIAGNOSTIC is used to identify excision procedures that are biopsies

Body Part Character 4	Approach Character 5	Device Character 6	Qualifier Character 7
Ø Skull **1 Frontal Bone** Zygomatic process of frontal bone **3 Parietal Bone, Right** **4 Parietal Bone, Left** **5 Temporal Bone, Right** Mastoid process Petrous part of temporal bone Tympanic part of temporal bone Zygomatic process of temporal bone **6 Temporal Bone, Left** *See 5 Temporal Bone, Right* **7 Occipital Bone** Foramen magnum **B Nasal Bone** Vomer of nasal septum **C Sphenoid Bone** Greater wing Lesser wing Optic foramen Pterygoid process Sella turcica **F Ethmoid Bone, Right** Cribriform plate **G Ethmoid Bone, Left** *See F Ethmoid Bone, Right* **H Lacrimal Bone, Right** **J Lacrimal Bone, Left** **K Palatine Bone, Right** **L Palatine Bone, Left** **M Zygomatic Bone, Right** **N Zygomatic Bone, Left** **P Orbit, Right** Bony orbit Orbital portion of ethmoid bone Orbital portion of frontal bone Orbital portion of lacrimal bone Orbital portion of maxilla Orbital portion of palatine bone Orbital portion of sphenoid bone Orbital portion of zygomatic bone **Q Orbit, Left** *See P Orbit, Right* **R Maxilla** Alveolar process of maxilla **T Mandible, Right** Alveolar process of mandible Condyloid process Mandibular notch Mental foramen **V Mandible, Left** *See T Mandible, Right* **X Hyoid Bone**	**Ø Open** **3 Percutaneous** **4 Percutaneous Endoscopic**	**Z No Device**	**X Diagnostic** **Z No Qualifier**

Non-OR ØNB[B,R,T,V][Ø,3,4]ZX

Ø Medical and Surgical
N Head and Facial Bones
C Extirpation Definition: Taking or cutting out solid matter from a body part

Explanation: The solid matter may be an abnormal byproduct of a biological function or a foreign body; it may be imbedded in a body part or in the lumen of a tubular body part. The solid matter may or may not have been previously broken into pieces.

Body Part Character 4	Approach Character 5	Device Character 6	Qualifier Character 7
1 Frontal Bone Zygomatic process of frontal bone **3 Parietal Bone, Right** **4 Parietal Bone, Left** **5 Temporal Bone, Right** Mastoid process Petrous part of temporal bone Tympanic part of temporal bone Zygomatic process of temporal bone **6 Temporal Bone, Left** *See 5 Temporal Bone, Right* **7 Occipital Bone** Foramen magnum **B Nasal Bone** Vomer of nasal septum **C Sphenoid Bone** Greater wing Lesser wing Optic foramen Pterygoid process Sella turcica **F Ethmoid Bone, Right** Cribriform plate **G Ethmoid Bone, Left** *See F Ethmoid Bone, Right* **H Lacrimal Bone, Right** **J Lacrimal Bone, Left** **K Palatine Bone, Right** **L Palatine Bone, Left** **M Zygomatic Bone, Right** **N Zygomatic Bone, Left** **P Orbit, Right** Bony orbit Orbital portion of ethmoid bone Orbital portion of frontal bone Orbital portion of lacrimal bone Orbital portion of maxilla Orbital portion of palatine bone Orbital portion of sphenoid bone Orbital portion of zygomatic bone **Q Orbit, Left** *See P Orbit, Right* **R Maxilla** Alveolar process of maxilla **T Mandible, Right** Alveolar process of mandible Condyloid process Mandibular notch Mental foramen **V Mandible, Left** *See T Mandible, Right* **X Hyoid Bone**	**Ø Open** **3 Percutaneous** **4 Percutaneous Endoscopic**	**Z No Device**	**Z No Qualifier**

Non-OR ØNC[B,R,T,V][Ø,3,4]ZZ

Ø Medical and Surgical
N Head and Facial Bones
D Extraction Definition: Pulling or stripping out or off all or a portion of a body part by the use of force
Explanation: The qualifier DIAGNOSTIC is used to identify extraction procedures that are biopsies

Body Part Character 4	Approach Character 5	Device Character 6	Qualifier Character 7
Ø Skull **1 Frontal Bone** Zygomatic process of frontal bone **3 Parietal Bone, Right** **4 Parietal Bone, Left** **5 Temporal Bone, Right** Mastoid process Petrous part of temporal bone Tympanic part of temporal bone Zygomatic process of temporal bone **6 Temporal Bone, Left** *See 5 Temporal Bone, Right* **7 Occipital Bone** Foramen magnum **B Nasal Bone** Vomer of nasal septum **C Sphenoid Bone** Greater wing Lesser wing Optic foramen Pterygoid process Sella turcica **F Ethmoid Bone, Right** Cribriform plate **G Ethmoid Bone, Left** *See F Ethmoid Bone, Right* **H Lacrimal Bone, Right** **J Lacrimal Bone, Left** **K Palatine Bone, Right** **L Palatine Bone, Left** **M Zygomatic Bone, Right** **N Zygomatic Bone, Left** **P Orbit, Right** Bony orbit Orbital portion of ethmoid bone Orbital portion of frontal bone Orbital portion of lacrimal bone Orbital portion of maxilla Orbital portion of palatine bone Orbital portion of sphenoid bone Orbital portion of zygomatic bone **Q Orbit, Left** *See P Orbit, Right* **R Maxilla** Alveolar process of maxilla **T Mandible, Right** Alveolar process of mandible Condyloid process Mandibular notch Mental foramen **V Mandible, Left** *See T Mandible, Right* **X Hyoid Bone**	**Ø Open**	**Z No Device**	**Z No Qualifier**

Ø Medical and Surgical
N Head and Facial Bones
H Insertion Definition: Putting in a nonbiological appliance that monitors, assists, performs, or prevents a physiological function but does not physically take the place of a body part
Explanation: None

Body Part Character 4	Approach Character 5	Device Character 6	Qualifier Character 7
Ø Skull ⊞	**Ø Open**	**4 Internal Fixation Device** **5 External Fixation Device** **M Bone Growth Stimulator** **N Neurostimulator Generator**	**Z No Qualifier**
Ø Skull	**3 Percutaneous** **4 Percutaneous Endoscopic**	**4 Internal Fixation Device** **5 External Fixation Device** **M Bone Growth Stimulator**	**Z No Qualifier**
1 Frontal Bone Zygomatic process of frontal bone **3 Parietal Bone, Right** **4 Parietal Bone, Left** **7 Occipital Bone** Foramen magnum **C Sphenoid Bone** Greater wing Lesser wing Optic foramen Pterygoid process Sella turcica **F Ethmoid Bone, Right** Cribriform plate **G Ethmoid Bone, Left** *See F Ethmoid Bone, Right* **H Lacrimal Bone, Right** **J Lacrimal Bone, Left** **K Palatine Bone, Right** **L Palatine Bone, Left** **M Zygomatic Bone, Right** **N Zygomatic Bone, Left** **P Orbit, Right** Bony orbit Orbital portion of ethmoid bone Orbital portion of frontal bone Orbital portion of lacrimal bone Orbital portion of maxilla Orbital portion of palatine bone Orbital portion of sphenoid bone Orbital portion of zygomatic bone **Q Orbit, Left** *See P Orbit, Right* **X Hyoid Bone**	**Ø Open** **3 Percutaneous** **4 Percutaneous Endoscopic**	**4 Internal Fixation Device**	**Z No Qualifier**
5 Temporal Bone, Right Mastoid process Petrous part of temporal bone Tympanic part of temporal bone Zygomatic process of temporal bone **6 Temporal Bone, Left** *See 5 Temporal Bone, Right*	**Ø Open** **3 Percutaneous** **4 Percutaneous Endoscopic**	**4 Internal Fixation Device** **S Hearing Device**	**Z No Qualifier**
B Nasal Bone Vomer of nasal septum	**Ø Open** **3 Percutaneous** **4 Percutaneous Endoscopic**	**4 Internal Fixation Device** **M Bone Growth Stimulator**	**Z No Qualifier**
R Maxilla Alveolar process of maxilla **T Mandible, Right** Alveolar process of mandible Condyloid process Mandibular notch Mental foramen **V Mandible, Left** *See T Mandible, Right*	**Ø Open** **3 Percutaneous** **4 Percutaneous Endoscopic**	**4 Internal Fixation Device** **5 External Fixation Device**	**Z No Qualifier**
W Facial Bone	**Ø Open** **3 Percutaneous** **4 Percutaneous Endoscopic**	**M Bone Growth Stimulator**	**Z No Qualifier**

Non-OR ØNHØØ5Z
Non-OR ØNHØ[3,4]5Z
Non-OR ØNHB[Ø,3,4][4,M]Z

See Appendix L for Procedure Combinations
⊞ ØNHØØNZ

Ø Medical and Surgical
N Head and Facial Bones
J Inspection Definition: Visually and/or manually exploring a body part

Explanation: Visual exploration may be performed with or without optical instrumentation. Manual exploration may be performed directly or through intervening body layers.

Body Part Character 4	Approach Character 5	Device Character 6	Qualifier Character 7
Ø Skull B Nasal Bone Vomer of nasal septum W Facial Bone	Ø Open 3 Percutaneous 4 Percutaneous Endoscopic X External	Z No Device	Z No Qualifier

Non-OR ØNJ[Ø,B,W][3,X]ZZ

Ø Medical and Surgical
N Head and Facial Bones
N Release Definition: Freeing a body part from an abnormal physical constraint by cutting or by the use of force

Explanation: Some of the restraining tissue may be taken out but none of the body part is taken out

Body Part Character 4	Approach Character 5	Device Character 6	Qualifier Character 7
1 Frontal Bone Zygomatic process of frontal bone 3 Parietal Bone, Right 4 Parietal Bone, Left 5 Temporal Bone, Right Mastoid process Petrous part of temporal bone Tympanic part of temporal bone Zygomatic process of temporal bone 6 Temporal Bone, Left *See 5 Temporal Bone, Right* 7 Occipital Bone Foramen magnum B Nasal Bone Vomer of nasal septum C Sphenoid Bone Greater wing Lesser wing Optic foramen Pterygoid process Sella turcica F Ethmoid Bone, Right Cribriform plate G Ethmoid Bone, Left *See F Ethmoid Bone, Right* H Lacrimal Bone, Right J Lacrimal Bone, Left K Palatine Bone, Right L Palatine Bone, Left M Zygomatic Bone, Right N Zygomatic Bone, Left P Orbit, Right Bony orbit Orbital portion of ethmoid bone Orbital portion of frontal bone Orbital portion of lacrimal bone Orbital portion of maxilla Orbital portion of palatine bone Orbital portion of sphenoid bone Orbital portion of zygomatic bone Q Orbit, Left *See P Orbit, Right* R Maxilla Alveolar process of maxilla T Mandible, Right Alveolar process of mandible Condyloid process Mandibular notch Mental foramen V Mandible, Left *See T Mandible, Right* X Hyoid Bone	Ø Open 3 Percutaneous 4 Percutaneous Endoscopic	Z No Device	Z No Qualifier

Non-OR ØNNB[Ø,3,4]ZZ

Ø Medical and Surgical
N Head and Facial Bones
P Removal Definition: Taking out or off a device from a body part

Explanation: If a device is taken out and a similar device put in without cutting or puncturing the skin or mucous membrane, the procedure is coded to the root operation CHANGE. Otherwise, the procedure for taking out a device is coded to the root operation REMOVAL.

Body Part Character 4	Approach Character 5	Device Character 6	Qualifier Character 7
Ø Skull	**Ø** Open	**Ø** Drainage Device **4** Internal Fixation Device **5** External Fixation Device **7** Autologous Tissue Substitute **J** Synthetic Substitute **K** Nonautologous Tissue Substitute **M** Bone Growth Stimulator **N** Neurostimulator Generator **S** Hearing Device	**Z** No Qualifier
Ø Skull	**3** Percutaneous **4** Percutaneous Endoscopic	**Ø** Drainage Device **4** Internal Fixation Device **5** External Fixation Device **7** Autologous Tissue Substitute **J** Synthetic Substitute **K** Nonautologous Tissue Substitute **M** Bone Growth Stimulator **S** Hearing Device	**Z** No Qualifier
Ø Skull	**X** External	**Ø** Drainage Device **4** Internal Fixation Device **5** External Fixation Device **M** Bone Growth Stimulator **S** Hearing Device	**Z** No Qualifier
B Nasal Bone Vomer of nasal septum **W** Facial Bone	**Ø** Open **3** Percutaneous **4** Percutaneous Endoscopic	**Ø** Drainage Device **4** Internal Fixation Device **7** Autologous Tissue Substitute **J** Synthetic Substitute **K** Nonautologous Tissue Substitute **M** Bone Growth Stimulator	**Z** No Qualifier
B Nasal Bone Vomer of nasal septum **W** Facial Bone	**X** External	**Ø** Drainage Device **4** Internal Fixation Device **M** Bone Growth Stimulator	**Z** No Qualifier

Non-OR ØNPØ[3,4]5Z
Non-OR ØNPØX[Ø,5]Z
Non-OR ØNPB[Ø,3,4][Ø,4,7,J,K,M]Z
Non-OR ØNPBX[Ø,4,M]Z
Non-OR ØNPWX[Ø,M]Z

Ø Medical and Surgical
N Head and Facial Bones
Q Repair Definition: Restoring, to the extent possible, a body part to its normal anatomic structure and function
Explanation: Used only when the method to accomplish the repair is not one of the other root operations

Body Part Character 4	Approach Character 5	Device Character 6	Qualifier Character 7
Ø Skull **1** Frontal Bone Zygomatic process of frontal bone **3** Parietal Bone, Right **4** Parietal Bone, Left **5** Temporal Bone, Right Mastoid process Petrous part of temporal bone Tympanic part of temporal bone Zygomatic process of temporal bone **6** Temporal Bone, Left *See 5 Temporal Bone, Right* **7** Occipital Bone Foramen magnum **B** Nasal Bone Vomer of nasal septum **C** Sphenoid Bone Greater wing Lesser wing Optic foramen Pterygoid process Sella turcica **F** Ethmoid Bone, Right Cribriform plate **G** Ethmoid Bone, Left *See F Ethmoid Bone, Right* **H** Lacrimal Bone, Right **J** Lacrimal Bone, Left **K** Palatine Bone, Right **L** Palatine Bone, Left **M** Zygomatic Bone, Right **N** Zygomatic Bone, Left **P** Orbit, Right Bony orbit Orbital portion of ethmoid bone Orbital portion of frontal bone Orbital portion of lacrimal bone Orbital portion of maxilla Orbital portion of palatine bone Orbital portion of sphenoid bone Orbital portion of zygomatic bone **Q** Orbit, Left *See P Orbit, Right* **R** Maxilla Alveolar process of maxilla **T** Mandible, Right Alveolar process of mandible Condyloid process Mandibular notch Mental foramen **V** Mandible, Left *See T Mandible, Right* **X** Hyoid Bone	**Ø** Open **3** Percutaneous **4** Percutaneous Endoscopic **X** External	**Z** No Device	**Z** No Qualifier

Non-OR ØNQ[Ø,1,3,4,5,6,7,B,C,F,G,H,J,K,L,M,N,P,Q,R,T,V,X]XZZ

Ø Medical and Surgical
N Head and Facial Bones
R Replacement Definition: Putting in or on biological or synthetic material that physically takes the place and/or function of all or a portion of a body part

Explanation: The body part may have been taken out or replaced, or may be taken out, physically eradicated, or rendered nonfunctional during the REPLACEMENT procedure. A REMOVAL procedure is coded for taking out the device used in a previous replacement procedure.

Body Part Character 4	Approach Character 5	Device Character 6	Qualifier Character 7
Ø Skull **1 Frontal Bone** Zygomatic process of frontal bone **3 Parietal Bone, Right** **4 Parietal Bone, Left** **5 Temporal Bone, Right** Mastoid process Petrous part of temporal bone Tympanic part of temporal bone Zygomatic process of temporal bone **6 Temporal Bone, Left** *See 5 Temporal Bone, Right* **7 Occipital Bone** Foramen magnum **B Nasal Bone** Vomer of nasal septum **C Sphenoid Bone** Greater wing Lesser wing Optic foramen Pterygoid process Sella turcica **F Ethmoid Bone, Right** Cribriform plate **G Ethmoid Bone, Left** *See F Ethmoid Bone, Right* **H Lacrimal Bone, Right** **J Lacrimal Bone, Left** **K Palatine Bone, Right** **L Palatine Bone, Left** **M Zygomatic Bone, Right** **N Zygomatic Bone, Left** **P Orbit, Right** Bony orbit Orbital portion of ethmoid bone Orbital portion of frontal bone Orbital portion of lacrimal bone Orbital portion of maxilla Orbital portion of palatine bone Orbital portion of sphenoid bone Orbital portion of zygomatic bone **Q Orbit, Left** *See P Orbit, Right* **R Maxilla** Alveolar process of maxilla **T Mandible, Right** Alveolar process of mandible Condyloid process Mandibular notch Mental foramen **V Mandible, Left** *See T Mandible, Right* **X Hyoid Bone**	**Ø Open** **3 Percutaneous** **4 Percutaneous Endoscopic**	**7 Autologous Tissue Substitute** **J Synthetic Substitute** **K Nonautologous Tissue Substitute**	**Z No Qualifier**

Ø Medical and Surgical
N Head and Facial Bones
S Reposition Definition: Moving to its normal location, or other suitable location, all or a portion of a body part

Explanation: The body part is moved to a new location from an abnormal location, or from a normal location where it is not functioning correctly. The body part may or may not be cut out or off to be moved to the new location.

Body Part Character 4	Approach Character 5	Device Character 6	Qualifier Character 7
Ø Skull **R Maxilla** Alveolar process of maxilla **T Mandible, Right** Alveolar process of mandible Condyloid process Mandibular notch Mental foramen **V Mandible, Left** *See T Mandible, Right*	**Ø Open** **3 Percutaneous** **4 Percutaneous Endoscopic**	**4 Internal Fixation Device** **5 External Fixation Device** **Z No Device**	**Z No Qualifier**
Ø Skull **R Maxilla** Alveolar process of maxilla **T Mandible, Right** Alveolar process of mandible Condyloid process Mandibular notch Mental foramen **V Mandible, Left** *See T Mandible, Right*	**X External**	**Z No Device**	**Z No Qualifier**
1 Frontal Bone Zygomatic process of frontal bone **3 Parietal Bone, Right** **4 Parietal Bone, Left** **5 Temporal Bone, Right** Mastoid process Petrous part of temporal bone Tympanic part of temporal bone Zygomatic process of temporal bone **6 Temporal Bone, Left** *See 5 Temporal Bone, Right* **7 Occipital Bone** Foramen magnum **B Nasal Bone** Vomer of nasal septum **C Sphenoid Bone** Greater wing Lesser wing Optic foramen Pterygoid process Sella turcica **F Ethmoid Bone, Right** Cribriform plate **G Ethmoid Bone, Left** *See F Ethmoid Bone, Right* **H Lacrimal Bone, Right** **J Lacrimal Bone, Left** **K Palatine Bone, Right** **L Palatine Bone, Left** **M Zygomatic Bone, Right** **N Zygomatic Bone, Left** **P Orbit, Right** Bony orbit Orbital portion of ethmoid bone Orbital portion of frontal bone Orbital portion of lacrimal bone Orbital portion of maxilla Orbital portion of palatine bone Orbital portion of sphenoid bone Orbital portion of zygomatic bone **Q Orbit, Left** *See P Orbit, Right* **X Hyoid Bone**	**Ø Open** **3 Percutaneous** **4 Percutaneous Endoscopic**	**4 Internal Fixation Device** **Z No Device**	**Z No Qualifier**

ØNS Continued on next page

Non-OR ØNS[R,T,V][3,4][4,5,Z]Z
Non-OR ØNS[Ø,R,T,V]XZZ
Non-OR ØNS[B,C,F,G,H,J,K,L,M,N,P,Q,X][3,4][4,Z]Z

Ø Medical and Surgical
N Head and Facial Bones
S Reposition Definition: Moving to its normal location, or other suitable location, all or a portion of a body part

Explanation: The body part is moved to a new location from an abnormal location, or from a normal location where it is not functioning correctly. The body part may or may not be cut out or off to be moved to the new location.

ØNS Continued

Body Part Character 4	Approach Character 5	Device Character 6	Qualifier Character 7
1 Frontal Bone Zygomatic process of frontal bone **3 Parietal Bone, Right** **4 Parietal Bone, Left** **5 Temporal Bone, Right** Mastoid process Petrous part of temporal bone Tympanic part of temporal bone Zygomatic process of temporal bone **6 Temporal Bone, Left** *See 5 Temporal Bone, Right* **7 Occipital Bone** Foramen magnum **B Nasal Bone** Vomer of nasal septum **C Sphenoid Bone** Greater wing Lesser wing Optic foramen Pterygoid process Sella turcica **F Ethmoid Bone, Right** Cribriform plate **G Ethmoid Bone, Left** *See F Ethmoid Bone, Right* **H Lacrimal Bone, Right** **J Lacrimal Bone, Left** **K Palatine Bone, Right** **L Palatine Bone, Left** **M Zygomatic Bone, Right** **N Zygomatic Bone, Left** **P Orbit, Right** Bony orbit Orbital portion of ethmoid bone Orbital portion of frontal bone Orbital portion of lacrimal bone Orbital portion of maxilla Orbital portion of palatine bone Orbital portion of sphenoid bone Orbital portion of zygomatic bone **Q Orbit, Left** *See P Orbit, Right* **X Hyoid Bone**	**X External**	**Z No Device**	**Z No Qualifier**

Non-OR ØNS[1,3,4,5,6,7,B,C,F,G,H,J,K,L,M,N,P,Q,X]XZZ

Ø Medical and Surgical
N Head and Facial Bones
T Resection Definition: Cutting out or off, without replacement, all of a body part
Explanation: None

Body Part Character 4	Approach Character 5	Device Character 6	Qualifier Character 7
1 Frontal Bone Zygomatic process of frontal bone **3 Parietal Bone, Right** **4 Parietal Bone, Left** **5 Temporal Bone, Right** Mastoid process Petrous part of temporal bone Tympanic part of temporal bone Zygomatic process of temporal bone **6 Temporal Bone, Left** *See 5 Temporal Bone, Right* **7 Occipital Bone** Foramen magnum **B Nasal Bone** Vomer of nasal septum **C Sphenoid Bone** Greater wing Lesser wing Optic foramen Pterygoid process Sella turcica **F Ethmoid Bone, Right** Cribriform plate **G Ethmoid Bone, Left** *See F Ethmoid Bone, Right* **H Lacrimal Bone, Right** **J Lacrimal Bone, Left** **K Palatine Bone, Right** **L Palatine Bone, Left** **M Zygomatic Bone, Right** **N Zygomatic Bone, Left** **P Orbit, Right** Bony orbit Orbital portion of ethmoid bone Orbital portion of frontal bone Orbital portion of lacrimal bone Orbital portion of maxilla Orbital portion of palatine bone Orbital portion of sphenoid bone Orbital portion of zygomatic bone **Q Orbit, Left** *See P Orbit, Right* **R Maxilla** Alveolar process of maxilla **T Mandible, Right** Alveolar process of mandible Condyloid process Mandibular notch Mental foramen **V Mandible, Left** *See T Mandible, Right* **X Hyoid Bone**	**Ø Open**	**Z No Device**	**Z No Qualifier**

Ø Medical and Surgical
N Head and Facial Bones
U Supplement Definition: Putting in or on biological or synthetic material that physically reinforces and/or augments the function of a portion of a body part

Explanation: The biological material is non-living, or is living and from the same individual. The body part may have been previously replaced, and the SUPPLEMENT procedure is performed to physically reinforce and/or augment the function of the replaced body part.

Body Part Character 4	Approach Character 5	Device Character 6	Qualifier Character 7
Ø Skull **1 Frontal Bone** Zygomatic process of frontal bone **3 Parietal Bone, Right** **4 Parietal Bone, Left** **5 Temporal Bone, Right** Mastoid process Petrous part of temporal bone Tympanic part of temporal bone Zygomatic process of temporal bone **6 Temporal Bone, Left** *See 5 Temporal Bone, Right* **7 Occipital Bone** Foramen magnum **B Nasal Bone** Vomer of nasal septum **C Sphenoid Bone** Greater wing Lesser wing Optic foramen Pterygoid process Sella turcica **F Ethmoid Bone, Right** Cribriform plate **G Ethmoid Bone, Left** *See F Ethmoid Bone, Right* **H Lacrimal Bone, Right** **J Lacrimal Bone, Left** **K Palatine Bone, Right** **L Palatine Bone, Left** **M Zygomatic Bone, Right** **N Zygomatic Bone, Left** **P Orbit, Right** Bony orbit Orbital portion of ethmoid bone Orbital portion of frontal bone Orbital portion of lacrimal bone Orbital portion of maxilla Orbital portion of palatine bone Orbital portion of sphenoid bone Orbital portion of zygomatic bone **Q Orbit, Left** *See P Orbit, Right* **R Maxilla** Alveolar process of maxilla **T Mandible, Right** Alveolar process of mandible Condyloid process Mandibular notch Mental foramen **V Mandible, Left** *See T Mandible, Right* **X Hyoid Bone**	**Ø Open** **3 Percutaneous** **4 Percutaneous Endoscopic**	**7 Autologous Tissue Substitute** **J Synthetic Substitute** **K Nonautologous Tissue Substitute**	**Z No Qualifier**

Ø Medical and Surgical
N Head and Facial Bones
W Revision Definition: Correcting, to the extent possible, a portion of a malfunctioning device or the position of a displaced device

Explanation: Revision can include correcting a malfunctioning or displaced device by taking out or putting in components of the device such as a screw or pin

Body Part Character 4	Approach Character 5	Device Character 6	Qualifier Character 7
Ø Skull	**Ø** Open	**Ø** Drainage Device **4** Internal Fixation Device **5** External Fixation Device **7** Autologous Tissue Substitute **J** Synthetic Substitute **K** Nonautologous Tissue Substitute **M** Bone Growth Stimulator **N** Neurostimulator Generator **S** Hearing Device	**Z** No Qualifier
Ø Skull	**3** Percutaneous **4** Percutaneous Endoscopic **X** External	**Ø** Drainage Device **4** Internal Fixation Device **5** External Fixation Device **7** Autologous Tissue Substitute **J** Synthetic Substitute **K** Nonautologous Tissue Substitute **M** Bone Growth Stimulator **S** Hearing Device	**Z** No Qualifier
B Nasal Bone Vomer of nasal septum **W** Facial Bone	**Ø** Open **3** Percutaneous **4** Percutaneous Endoscopic **X** External	**Ø** Drainage Device **4** Internal Fixation Device **7** Autologous Tissue Substitute **J** Synthetic Substitute **K** Nonautologous Tissue Substitute **M** Bone Growth Stimulator	**Z** No Qualifier

Non-OR ØNWØX[Ø,4,5,7,J,K,M,S]Z
Non-OR ØNWB[Ø,3,4,X][Ø,4,7,J,K,M]Z
Non-OR ØNWWX[Ø,4,7,J,K,M]Z

Upper Bones ØP2–ØPW

Character Meanings

This Character Meaning table is provided as a guide to assist the user in the identification of character members that may be found in this section of code tables. It **SHOULD NOT** be used to build a PCS code.

Operation–Character 3	Body Part–Character 4	Approach–Character 5	Device–Character 6	Qualifier–Character 7
2 Change	Ø Sternum	Ø Open	Ø Drainage Device OR Internal Fixation Device, Rigid Plate	X Diagnostic
5 Destruction	1 Ribs, 1 to 2	3 Percutaneous	4 Internal Fixation Device	Z No Qualifier
8 Division	2 Ribs, 3 or more	4 Percutaneous Endoscopic	5 External Fixation Device	
9 Drainage	3 Cervical Vertebra	X External	6 Internal Fixation Device, Intramedullary	
B Excision	4 Thoracic Vertebra		7 Autologous Tissue Substitute	
C Extirpation	5 Scapula, Right		8 External Fixation Device, Limb Lengthening	
D Extraction	6 Scapula, Left		B External Fixation Device, Monoplanar	
H Insertion	7 Glenoid Cavity, Right		C External Fixation Device, Ring	
J Inspection	8 Glenoid Cavity, Left		D External Fixation Device, Hybrid	
N Release	9 Clavicle, Right		J Synthetic Substitute	
P Removal	B Clavicle, Left		K Nonautologous Tissue Substitute	
Q Repair	C Humeral Head, Right		M Bone Growth Stimulator	
R Replacement	D Humeral Head, Left		Y Other Device	
S Reposition	F Humeral Shaft, Right		Z No Device	
T Resection	G Humeral Shaft, Left			
U Supplement	H Radius, Right			
W Revision	J Radius, Left			
	K Ulna, Right			
	L Ulna, Left			
	M Carpal, Right			
	N Carpal, Left			
	P Metacarpal, Right			
	Q Metacarpal, Left			
	R Thumb Phalanx, Right			
	S Thumb Phalanx, Left			
	T Finger Phalanx, Right			
	V Finger Phalanx, Left			
	Y Upper Bone			

AHA Coding Clinic for table ØPB

2015, 3Q, 3-8 Excisional and nonexcisional debridement
2015, 2Q, 34 Decompressive laminectomy
2013, 4Q, 109 Separating conjoined twins
2013, 4Q, 116 Spinal decompression
2013, 3Q, 20 Superior labrum anterior posterior (SLAP) repair and subacromialdecompression
2012, 4Q, 101 Rib resection with reconstruction of anterior chest wall
2012, 2Q, 19 Multiple decompressive cervical laminectomies

AHA Coding Clinic for table ØPD

2017, 4Q, 41 Extraction procedures

AHA Coding Clinic for table ØPH

2017, 2Q, 20 Exchange of intramedullary antibiotic impregnated spacer
2016, 4Q, 117 Placement of magnetic growth rods
2014, 4Q, 28 Removal and replacement of displaced growing rods

AHA Coding Clinic for table ØPP

2017, 2Q, 20 Exchange of intramedullary antibiotic impregnated spacer
2016, 4Q, 117 Placement of magnetic growth rods
2014, 4Q, 28 Removal and replacement of displaced growing rods

AHA Coding Clinic for table ØPS

2017, 4Q, 53 New and revised body part values - Ribs
2016, 1Q, 21 Elongation derotation flexion casting
2015, 4Q, 33 Ravitch operation
2015, 2Q, 35 Application of tongs to reduce and stabilize cervical fracture
2014, 4Q, 26 Placement of vertical expandable prosthetic titanium rib (VEPTR)
2014, 4Q, 32 Open reduction internal fixation of fracture with debridement
2014, 3Q, 33 Radial fracture treatment with open reduction internal fixation, and release of carpal ligament

AHA Coding Clinic for table ØPT

2015, 3Q, 26 Thumb arthroplasty with resection of trapezium

AHA Coding Clinic for table ØPU

2015, 2Q, 20 Cervical laminoplasty
2013, 4Q, 109 Separating conjoined twins

AHA Coding Clinic for table ØPW

2014, 4Q, 26 Adjustment of VEPTR lengthening mechanism
2014, 4Q, 27 Bilateral lengthening of growing rods

Upper Bones

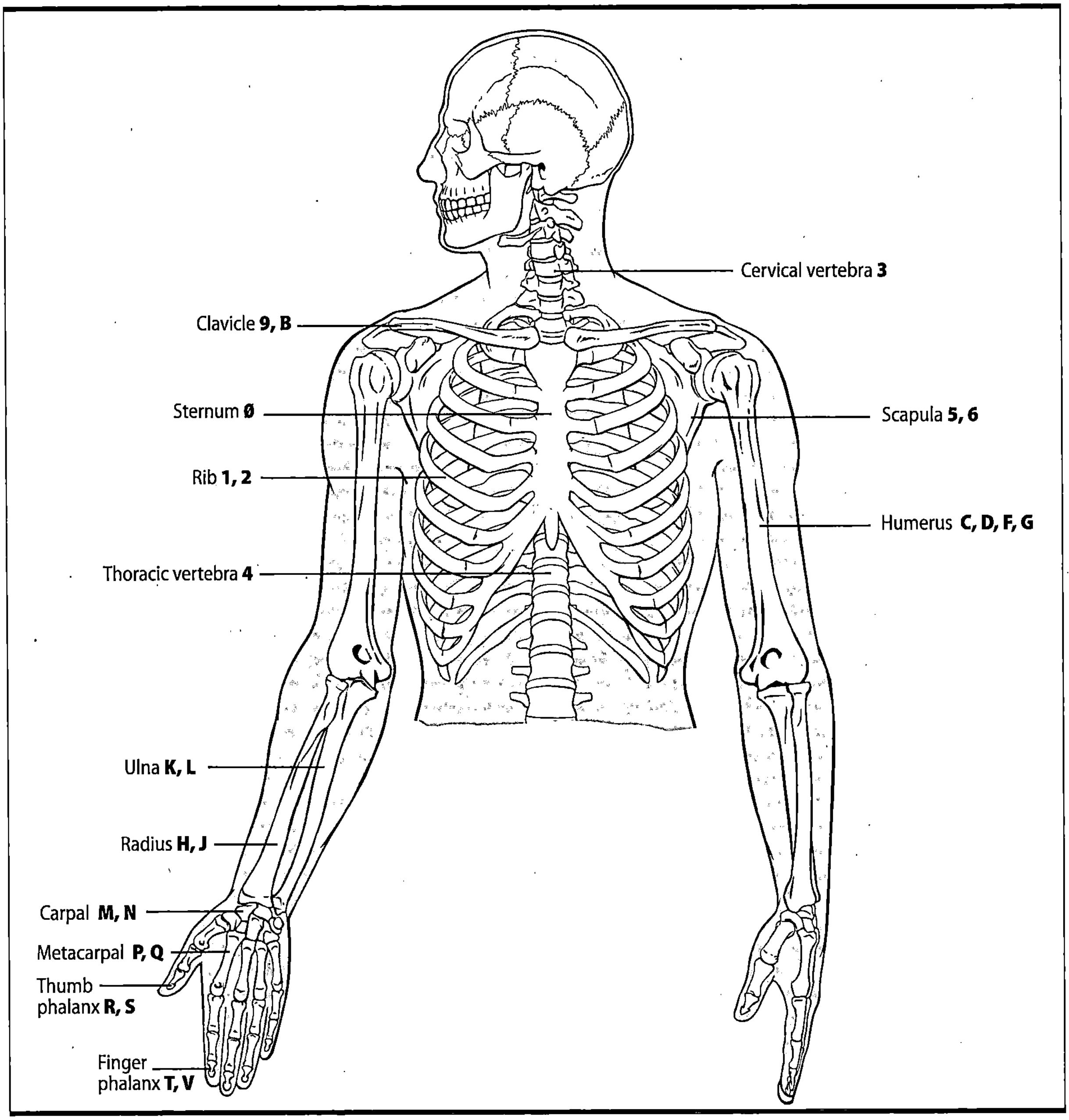
Cervical vertebra **3**
Clavicle **9, B**
Sternum **Ø**
Scapula **5, 6**
Rib **1, 2**
Humerus **C, D, F, G**
Thoracic vertebra **4**
Ulna **K, L**
Radius **H, J**
Carpal **M, N**
Metacarpal **P, Q**
Thumb phalanx **R, S**
Finger phalanx **T, V**

Humerus and Scapula

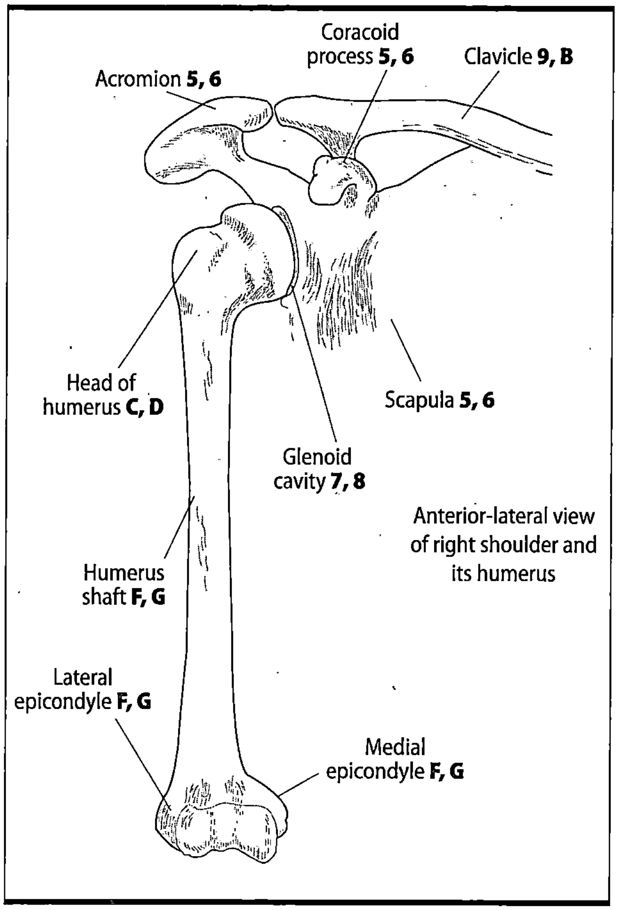
Coracoid process 5, 6
Clavicle 9, B
Acromion 5, 6
Head of humerus C, D
Scapula 5, 6
Glenoid cavity 7, 8
Anterior-lateral view of right shoulder and its humerus
Humerus shaft F, G
Lateral epicondyle F, G
Medial epicondyle F, G

Radius and Ulna

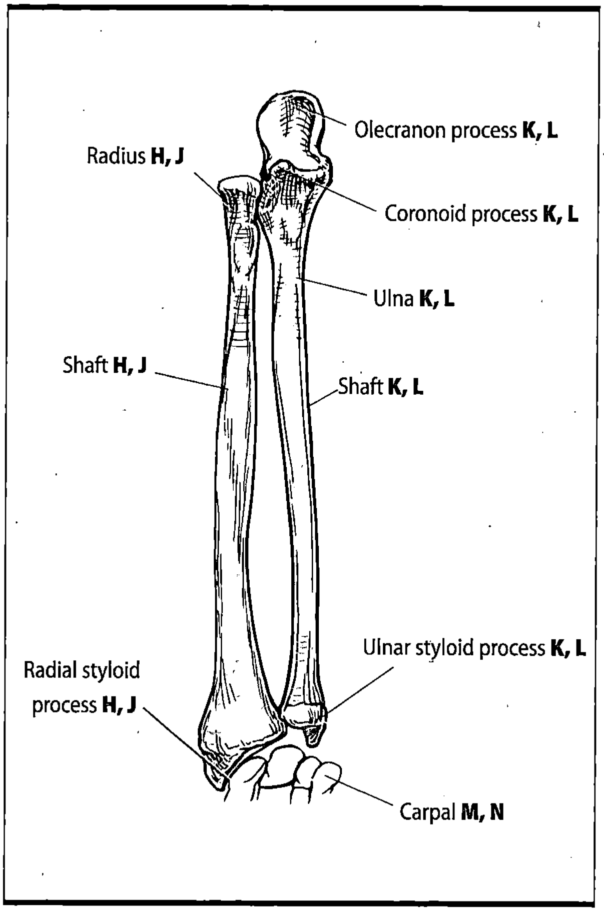
Olecranon process K, L
Radius H, J
Coronoid process K, L
Ulna K, L
Shaft H, J
Shaft K, L
Ulnar styloid process K, L
Radial styloid process H, J
Carpal M, N

Hand

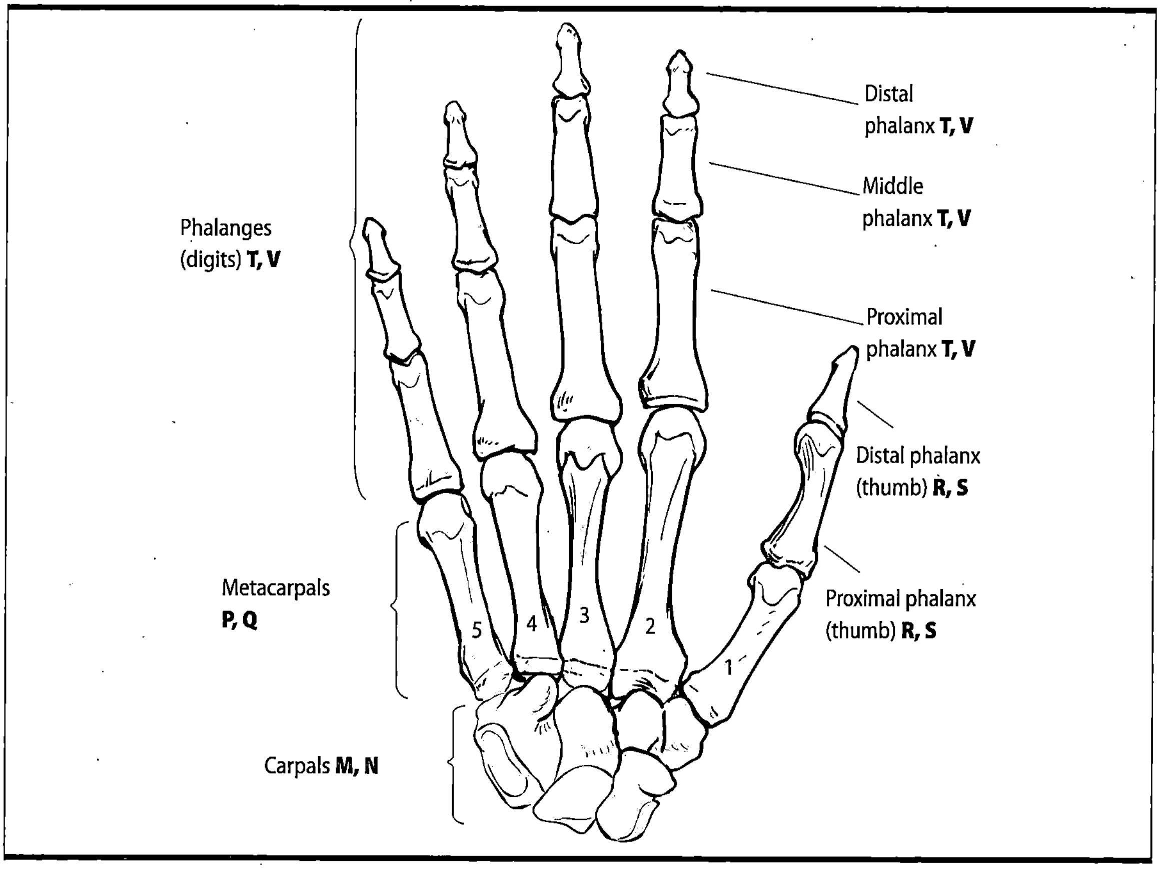
Distal phalanx T, V
Middle phalanx T, V
Phalanges (digits) T, V
Proximal phalanx T, V
Distal phalanx (thumb) R, S
Metacarpals P, Q
5
4
3
2
1
Proximal phalanx (thumb) R, S
Carpals M, N

Ø Medical and Surgical
P Upper Bones
2 Change Definition: Taking out or off a device from a body part and putting back an identical or similar device in or on the same body part without cutting or puncturing the skin or a mucous membrane

Explanation: All CHANGE procedures are coded using the approach EXTERNAL

Body Part Character 4	Approach Character 5	Device Character 6	Qualifier Character 7
Y Upper Bone	X External	Ø Drainage Device Y Other Device	Z No Qualifier

Non-OR All body part, approach, device, and qualifier values

Ø Medical and Surgical
P Upper Bones
5 Destruction Definition: Physical eradication of all or a portion of a body part by the direct use of energy, force, or a destructive agent

Explanation: None of the body part is physically taken out

Body Part Character 4	Approach Character 5	Device Character 6	Qualifier Character 7
Ø Sternum Manubrium Suprasternal notch Xiphoid process **1 Ribs, 1 to 2** **2 Ribs, 3 or More** **3 Cervical Vertebra** Dens Odontoid process Spinous process Transverse foramen Transverse process Vertebral arch Vertebral body Vertebral foramen Vertebral lamina Vertebral pedicle **4 Thoracic Vertebra** Spinous process Transverse process Vertebral arch Vertebral body Vertebral foramen Vertebral lamina Vertebral pedicle **5 Scapula, Right** Acromion (process) Coracoid process **6 Scapula, Left** *See 5 Scapula, Right* **7 Glenoid Cavity, Right** Glenoid fossa (of scapula) **8 Glenoid Cavity, Left** *See 7 Glenoid Cavity, Right* **9 Clavicle, Right** **B Clavicle, Left** **C Humeral Head, Right** Greater tuberosity Lesser tuberosity Neck of humerus (anatomical)(surgical) **D Humeral Head, Left** *See C Humeral Head, Right* **F Humeral Shaft, Right** Distal humerus Humerus, distal Lateral epicondyle of humerus Medial epicondyle of humerus **G Humeral Shaft, Left** *See F Humeral Shaft, Right* **H Radius, Right** Ulnar notch **J Radius, Left** *See H Radius, Right* **K Ulna, Right** Olecranon process Radial notch **L Ulna, Left** *See K Ulna, Right* **M Carpal, Right** Capitate bone Hamate bone Lunate bone Pisiform bone Scaphoid bone Trapezium bone Trapezoid bone Triquetral bone **N Carpal, Left** *See M Carpal, Right* **P Metacarpal, Right** **Q Metacarpal, Left** **R Thumb Phalanx, Right** **S Thumb Phalanx, Left** **T Finger Phalanx, Right** **V Finger Phalanx, Left**	Ø Open 3 Percutaneous 4 Percutaneous Endoscopic	Z No Device	Z No Qualifier

Ø Medical and Surgical
P Upper Bones
8 Division Definition: Cutting into a body part, without draining fluids and/or gases from the body part, in order to separate or transect a body part
Explanation: All or a portion of the body part is separated into two or more portions

Body Part Character 4		Approach Character 5	Device Character 6	Qualifier Character 7
Ø Sternum Manubrium Suprasternal notch Xiphoid process **1 Ribs, 1 to 2** **2 Ribs, 3 or More** **3 Cervical Vertebra** Dens Odontoid process Spinous process Transverse foramen Transverse process Vertebral arch Vertebral body Vertebral foramen Vertebral lamina Vertebral pedicle **4 Thoracic Vertebra** Spinous process Transverse process Vertebral arch Vertebral body Vertebral foramen Vertebral lamina Vertebral pedicle **5 Scapula, Right** Acromion (process) Coracoid process **6 Scapula, Left** *See 5 Scapula, Right* **7 Glenoid Cavity, Right** Glenoid fossa (of scapula) **8 Glenoid Cavity, Left** *See 7 Glenoid Cavity, Right* **9 Clavicle, Right** **B Clavicle, Left** **C Humeral Head, Right** Greater tuberosity Lesser tuberosity Neck of humerus (anatomical)(surgical) **D Humeral Head, Left** *See C Humeral Head, Right*	**F Humeral Shaft, Right** Distal humerus Humerus, distal Lateral epicondyle of humerus Medial epicondyle of humerus **G Humeral Shaft, Left** *See F Humeral Shaft, Right* **H Radius, Right** Ulnar notch **J Radius, Left** *See H Radius, Right* **K Ulna, Right** Olecranon process Radial notch **L Ulna, Left** *See K Ulna, Right* **M Carpal, Right** Capitate bone Hamate bone Lunate bone Pisiform bone Scaphoid bone Trapezium bone Trapezoid bone Triquetral bone **N Carpal, Left** *See M Carpal, Right* **P Metacarpal, Right** **Q Metacarpal, Left** **R Thumb Phalanx, Right** **S Thumb Phalanx, Left** **T Finger Phalanx, Right** **V Finger Phalanx, Left**	**Ø Open** **3 Percutaneous** **4 Percutaneous Endoscopic**	**Z No Device**	**Z No Qualifier**

Ø Medical and Surgical
P Upper Bones
9 Drainage Definition: Taking or letting out fluids and/or gases from a body part
Explanation: The qualifier DIAGNOSTIC is used to identify drainage procedures that are biopsies

Body Part Character 4	Approach Character 5	Device Character 6	Qualifier Character 7
Ø Sternum Manubrium Suprasternal notch Xiphoid process **1 Ribs, 1 to 2** **2 Ribs, 3 or More** **3 Cervical Vertebra** Dens Odontoid process Spinous process Transverse foramen Transverse process Vertebral arch Vertebral body Vertebral foramen Vertebral lamina Vertebral pedicle **4 Thoracic Vertebra** Spinous process Transverse process Vertebral arch Vertebral body Vertebral foramen Vertebral lamina Vertebral pedicle **5 Scapula, Right** Acromion (process) Coracoid process **6 Scapula, Left** *See 5 Scapula, Right* **7 Glenoid Cavity, Right** Glenoid fossa (of scapula) **8 Glenoid Cavity, Left** *See 7 Glenoid Cavity, Right* **9 Clavicle, Right** **B Clavicle, Left** **C Humeral Head, Right** Greater tuberosity Lesser tuberosity Neck of humerus (anatomical)(surgical) **D Humeral Head, Left** *See C Humeral Head, Right* **F Humeral Shaft, Right** Distal humerus Humerus, distal Lateral epicondyle of humerus Medial epicondyle of humerus **G Humeral Shaft, Left** *See F Humeral Shaft, Right* **H Radius, Right** Ulnar notch **J Radius, Left** *See H Radius, Right* **K Ulna, Right** Olecranon process Radial notch **L Ulna, Left** *See K Ulna, Right* **M Carpal, Right** Capitate bone Hamate bone Lunate bone Pisiform bone Scaphoid bone Trapezium bone Trapezoid bone Triquetral bone **N Carpal, Left** *See M Carpal, Right* **P Metacarpal, Right** **Q Metacarpal, Left** **R Thumb Phalanx, Right** **S Thumb Phalanx, Left** **T Finger Phalanx, Right** **V Finger Phalanx, Left**	**Ø Open** **3 Percutaneous** **4 Percutaneous Endoscopic**	**Ø Drainage Device**	**Z No Qualifier**

ØP9 Continued on next page

Non-OR ØP9[Ø,1,2,3,4,5,6,7,8,9,B,C,D,F,G,H,J,K,L,M,N,P,Q,R,S,T,V]3ØZ

Ø Medical and Surgical
P Upper Bones
9 Drainage Definition: Taking or letting out fluids and/or gases from a body part
Explanation: The qualifier DIAGNOSTIC is used to identify drainage procedures that are biopsies

ØP9 Continued

Body Part Character 4	Approach Character 5	Device Character 6	Qualifier Character 7
Ø Sternum Manubrium Suprasternal notch Xiphoid process **1 Ribs, 1 to 2** **2 Ribs, 3 or More** **3 Cervical Vertebra** Dens Odontoid process Spinous process Transverse foramen Transverse process Vertebral arch Vertebral body Vertebral foramen Vertebral lamina Vertebral pedicle **4 Thoracic Vertebra** Spinous process Transverse process Vertebral arch Vertebral body Vertebral foramen Vertebral lamina Vertebral pedicle **5 Scapula, Right** Acromion (process) Coracoid process **6 Scapula, Left** *See 5 Scapula, Right* **7 Glenoid Cavity, Right** Glenoid fossa (of scapula) **8 Glenoid Cavity, Left** *See 7 Glenoid Cavity, Right* **9 Clavicle, Right** **B Clavicle, Left** **C Humeral Head, Right** Greater tuberosity Lesser tuberosity Neck of humerus (anatomical)(surgical) **D Humeral Head, Left** *See C Humeral Head, Right* **F Humeral Shaft, Right** Distal humerus Humerus, distal Lateral epicondyle of humerus Medial epicondyle of humerus **G Humeral Shaft, Left** *See F Humeral Shaft, Right* **H Radius, Right** Ulnar notch **J Radius, Left** *See H Radius, Right* **K Ulna, Right** Olecranon process Radial notch **L Ulna, Left** *See K Ulna, Right* **M Carpal, Right** Capitate bone Hamate bone Lunate bone Pisiform bone Scaphoid bone Trapezium bone Trapezoid bone Triquetral bone **N Carpal, Left** *See M Carpal, Right* **P Metacarpal, Right** **Q Metacarpal, Left** **R Thumb Phalanx, Right** **S Thumb Phalanx, Left** **T Finger Phalanx, Right** **V Finger Phalanx, Left**	**Ø Open** **3 Percutaneous** **4 Percutaneous Endoscopic**	**Z No Device**	**X Diagnostic** **Z No Qualifier**

Non-OR ØP9[Ø,1,2,3,4,5,6,7,8,9,B,C,D,F,G,H,J,K,L,M,N,P,Q,R,S,T,V]3ZZ

Ø Medical and Surgical
P Upper Bones
B Excision Definition: Cutting out or off, without replacement, a portion of a body part
Explanation: The qualifier DIAGNOSTIC is used to identify excision procedures that are biopsies

Body Part Character 4		Approach Character 5	Device Character 6	Qualifier Character 7
Ø Sternum Manubrium Suprasternal notch Xiphoid process **1 Ribs, 1 to 2** **2 Ribs, 3 or More** **3 Cervical Vertebra** Dens Odontoid process Spinous process Transverse foramen Transverse process Vertebral arch Vertebral body Vertebral foramen Vertebral lamina Vertebral pedicle **4 Thoracic Vertebra** Spinous process Transverse process Vertebral arch Vertebral body Vertebral foramen Vertebral lamina Vertebral pedicle **5 Scapula, Right** Acromion (process) Coracoid process **6 Scapula, Left** *See 5 Scapula, Right* **7 Glenoid Cavity, Right** Glenoid fossa (of scapula) **8 Glenoid Cavity, Left** *See 7 Glenoid Cavity, Right* **9 Clavicle, Right** **B Clavicle, Left** **C Humeral Head, Right** Greater tuberosity Lesser tuberosity Neck of humerus (anatomical)(surgical) **D Humeral Head, Left** *See C Humeral Head, Right*	**F Humeral Shaft, Right** Distal humerus Humerus, distal Lateral epicondyle of humerus Medial epicondyle of humerus **G Humeral Shaft, Left** *See F Humeral Shaft, Right* **H Radius, Right** Ulnar notch **J Radius, Left** *See H Radius, Right* **K Ulna, Right** Olecranon process Radial notch **L Ulna, Left** *See K Ulna, Right* **M Carpal, Right** Capitate bone Hamate bone Lunate bone Pisiform bone Scaphoid bone Trapezium bone Trapezoid bone Triquetral bone **N Carpal, Left** *See M Carpal, Right* **P Metacarpal, Right** **Q Metacarpal, Left** **R Thumb Phalanx, Right** **S Thumb Phalanx, Left** **T Finger Phalanx, Right** **V Finger Phalanx, Left**	**Ø Open** **3 Percutaneous** **4 Percutaneous Endoscopic**	**Z No Device**	**X Diagnostic** **Z No Qualifier**

Ø Medical and Surgical
P Upper Bones
C Extirpation Definition: Taking or cutting out solid matter from a body part

Explanation: The solid matter may be an abnormal byproduct of a biological function or a foreign body; it may be imbedded in a body part or in the lumen of a tubular body part. The solid matter may or may not have been previously broken into pieces.

Body Part Character 4		Approach Character 5	Device Character 6	Qualifier Character 7
Ø Sternum Manubrium Suprasternal notch Xiphoid process **1 Ribs, 1 to 2** **2 Ribs, 3 or More** **3 Cervical Vertebra** Dens Odontoid process Spinous process Transverse foramen Transverse process Vertebral arch Vertebral body Vertebral foramen Vertebral lamina Vertebral pedicle **4 Thoracic Vertebra** Spinous process Transverse process Vertebral arch Vertebral body Vertebral foramen Vertebral lamina Vertebral pedicle **5 Scapula, Right** Acromion (process) Coracoid process **6 Scapula, Left** *See 5 Scapula, Right* **7 Glenoid Cavity, Right** Glenoid fossa (of scapula) **8 Glenoid Cavity, Left** *See 7 Glenoid Cavity, Right* **9 Clavicle, Right** **B Clavicle, Left** **C Humeral Head, Right** Greater tuberosity Lesser tuberosity Neck of humerus (anatomical)(surgical) **D Humeral Head, Left** *See C Humeral Head, Right*	**F Humeral Shaft, Right** Distal humerus Humerus, distal Lateral epicondyle of humerus Medial epicondyle of humerus **G Humeral Shaft, Left** *See F Humeral Shaft, Right* **H Radius, Right** Ulnar notch **J Radius, Left** *See H Radius, Right* **K Ulna, Right** Olecranon process Radial notch **L Ulna, Left** *See K Ulna, Right* **M Carpal, Right** Capitate bone Hamate bone Lunate bone Pisiform bone Scaphoid bone Trapezium bone Trapezoid bone Triquetral bone **N Carpal, Left** *See M Carpal, Right* **P Metacarpal, Right** **Q Metacarpal, Left** **R Thumb Phalanx, Right** **S Thumb Phalanx, Left** **T Finger Phalanx, Right** **V Finger Phalanx, Left**	**Ø** Open **3** Percutaneous **4** Percutaneous Endoscopic	**Z** No Device	**Z** No Qualifier

Ø Medical and Surgical
P Upper Bones
D Extraction Definition: Pulling or stripping out or off all or a portion of a body part by the use of force
Explanation: The qualifier DIAGNOSTIC is used to identify extraction procedures that are biopsies

Body Part Character 4		Approach Character 5	Device Character 6	Qualifier Character 7
Ø Sternum Manubrium Suprasternal notch Xiphoid process **1 Ribs, 1 to 2** **2 Ribs, 3 or More** **3 Cervical Vertebra** Dens Odontoid process Spinous process Transverse foramen Transverse process Vertebral arch Vertebral body Vertebral foramen Vertebral lamina Vertebral pedicle **4 Thoracic Vertebra** Spinous process Transverse process Vertebral arch Vertebral body Vertebral foramen Vertebral lamina Vertebral pedicle **5 Scapula, Right** Acromion (process) Coracoid process **6 Scapula, Left** *See 5 Scapula, Right* **7 Glenoid Cavity, Right** Glenoid fossa (of scapula) **8 Glenoid Cavity, Left** *See 7 Glenoid Cavity, Right* **9 Clavicle, Right** **B Clavicle, Left** **C Humeral Head, Right** Greater tuberosity Lesser tuberosity Neck of humerus (anatomical)(surgical) **D Humeral Head, Left** *See C Humeral Head, Right*	**F Humeral Shaft, Right** Distal humerus Humerus, distal Lateral epicondyle of humerus Medial epicondyle of humerus **G Humeral Shaft, Left** *See F Humeral Shaft, Right* **H Radius, Right** Ulnar notch **J Radius, Left** *See H Radius, Right* **K Ulna, Right** Olecranon process Radial notch **L Ulna, Left** *See K Ulna, Right* **M Carpal, Right** Capitate bone Hamate bone Lunate bone Pisiform bone Scaphoid bone Trapezium bone Trapezoid bone Triquetral bone **N Carpal, Left** *See M Carpal, Right* **P Metacarpal, Right** **Q Metacarpal, Left** **R Thumb Phalanx, Right** **S Thumb Phalanx, Left** **T Finger Phalanx, Right** **V Finger Phalanx, Left**	Ø Open	Z No Device	Z No Qualifier

Ø Medical and Surgical
P Upper Bones
H Insertion Definition: Putting in a nonbiological appliance that monitors, assists, performs, or prevents a physiological function but does not physically take the place of a body part
Explanation: None

Body Part Character 4		Approach Character 5	Device Character 6	Qualifier Character 7
Ø Sternum Manubrium Suprasternal notch Xiphoid process		**Ø Open** **3 Percutaneous** **4 Percutaneous Endoscopic**	**Ø Internal Fixation Device, Rigid Plate** **4 Internal Fixation Device**	**Z No Qualifier**
1 Ribs, 1 to 2 **2 Ribs, 3 or More** **3 Cervical Vertebra** Dens Odontoid process Spinous process Transverse foramen Transverse process Vertebral arch Vertebral body Vertebral foramen Vertebral lamina Vertebral pedicle **4 Thoracic Vertebra** Spinous process Transverse process Vertebral arch Vertebral body Vertebral foramen Vertebral lamina Vertebral pedicle	**5 Scapula, Right** Acromion (process) Coracoid process **6 Scapula, Left** *See 5 Scapula, Right* **7 Glenoid Cavity, Right** Glenoid fossa (of scapula) **8 Glenoid Cavity, Left** *See 7 Glenoid Cavity, Right* **9 Clavicle, Right** **B Clavicle, Left**	**Ø Open** **3 Percutaneous** **4 Percutaneous Endoscopic**	**4 Internal Fixation Device**	**Z No Qualifier**
C Humeral Head, Right Greater tuberosity Lesser tuberosity Neck of humerus (anatomical)(surgical) **D Humeral Head, Left** *See C Humeral Head, Right* **F Humeral Shaft, Right** Distal humerus Humerus, distal Lateral epicondyle of humerus Medial epicondyle of humerus	**G Humeral Shaft, Left** *See F Humeral Shaft, Right* **H Radius, Right** Ulnar notch **J Radius, Left** *See H Radius, Right* **K Ulna, Right** Olecranon process Radial notch **L Ulna, Left** *See K Ulna, Right*	**Ø Open** **3 Percutaneous** **4 Percutaneous Endoscopic**	**4 Internal Fixation Device** **5 External Fixation Device** **6 Internal Fixation Device, Intramedullary** **8 External Fixation Device, Limb Lengthening** **B External Fixation Device, Monoplanar** **C External Fixation Device, Ring** **D External Fixation Device, Hybrid**	**Z No Qualifier**
M Carpal, Right Capitate bone Hamate bone Lunate bone Pisiform bone Scaphoid bone Trapezium bone Trapezoid bone Triquetral bone **N Carpal, Left** *See M Carpal, Right*	**P Metacarpal, Right** **Q Metacarpal, Left** **R Thumb Phalanx, Right** **S Thumb Phalanx, Left** **T Finger Phalanx, Right** **V Finger Phalanx, Left**	**Ø Open** **3 Percutaneous** **4 Percutaneous Endoscopic**	**4 Internal Fixation Device** **5 External Fixation Device**	**Z No Qualifier**
Y Upper Bone		**Ø Open** **3 Percutaneous** **4 Percutaneous Endoscopic**	**M Bone Growth Stimulator**	**Z No Qualifier**

Non-OR ØPH[C,D,F,G,H,J,K,L][Ø,3,4]8Z

Ø Medical and Surgical
P Upper Bones
J Inspection Definition: Visually and/or manually exploring a body part

Explanation: Visual exploration may be performed with or without optical instrumentation. Manual exploration may be performed directly or through intervening body layers.

Body Part Character 4	Approach Character 5	Device Character 6	Qualifier Character 7
Y Upper Bone	Ø Open 3 Percutaneous 4 Percutaneous Endoscopic X External	Z No Device	Z No Qualifier

Non-OR ØPJY[3,X]ZZ

Ø Medical and Surgical
P Upper Bones
N Release Definition: Freeing a body part from an abnormal physical constraint by cutting or by the use of force

Explanation: Some of the restraining tissue may be taken out but none of the body part is taken out

Body Part Character 4		Approach Character 5	Device Character 6	Qualifier Character 7
Ø Sternum Manubrium Suprasternal notch Xiphoid process **1 Ribs, 1 to 2** **2 Ribs, 3 or More** **3 Cervical Vertebra** Dens Odontoid process Spinous process Transverse foramen Transverse process Vertebral arch Vertebral body Vertebral foramen Vertebral lamina Vertebral pedicle **4 Thoracic Vertebra** Spinous process Transverse process Vertebral arch Vertebral body Vertebral foramen Vertebral lamina Vertebral pedicle **5 Scapula, Right** Acromion (process) Coracoid process **6 Scapula, Left** *See 5 Scapula, Right* **7 Glenoid Cavity, Right** Glenoid fossa (of scapula) **8 Glenoid Cavity, Left** *See 7 Glenoid Cavity, Right* **9 Clavicle, Right** **B Clavicle, Left** **C Humeral Head, Right** Greater tuberosity Lesser tuberosity Neck of humerus (anatomical) (surgical) **D Humeral Head, Left** *See C Humeral Head, Right*	**F Humeral Shaft, Right** Distal humerus Humerus, distal Lateral epicondyle of humerus Medial epicondyle of humerus **G Humeral Shaft, Left** *See F Humeral Shaft, Right* **H Radius, Right** Ulnar notch **J Radius, Left** *See H Radius, Right* **K Ulna, Right** Olecranon process Radial notch **L Ulna, Left** *See K Ulna, Right* **M Carpal, Right** Capitate bone Hamate bone Lunate bone Pisiform bone Scaphoid bone Trapezium bone Trapezoid bone Triquetral bone **N Carpal, Left** *See M Carpal, Right* **P Metacarpal, Right** **Q Metacarpal, Left** **R Thumb Phalanx, Right** **S Thumb Phalanx, Left** **T Finger Phalanx, Right** **V Finger Phalanx, Left**	Ø Open 3 Percutaneous 4 Percutaneous Endoscopic	Z No Device	Z No Qualifier

Ø Medical and Surgical
P Upper Bones
P Removal Definition: Taking out or off a device from a body part

Explanation: If a device is taken out and a similar device put in without cutting or puncturing the skin or mucous membrane, the procedure is coded to the root operation CHANGE. Otherwise, the procedure for taking out a device is coded to the root operation REMOVAL.

Body Part Character 4	Approach Character 5	Device Character 6	Qualifier Character 7
Ø Sternum Manubrium Suprasternal notch Xiphoid process **1 Ribs, 1 to 2** **2 Ribs, 3 or More** **3 Cervical Vertebra** Dens Odontoid process Spinous process Transverse foramen Transverse process Vertebral arch Vertebral body Vertebral foramen Vertebral lamina Vertebral pedicle **4 Thoracic Vertebra** Spinous process Transverse process Vertebral arch Vertebral body Vertebral foramen Vertebral lamina Vertebral pedicle **5 Scapula, Right** Acromion (process) Coracoid process **6 Scapula, Left** *See 5 Scapula, Right* **7 Glenoid Cavity, Right** Glenoid fossa (of scapula) **8 Glenoid Cavity, Left** *See 7 Glenoid Cavity, Right* **9 Clavicle, Right** **B Clavicle, Left**	Ø Open 3 Percutaneous 4 Percutaneous Endoscopic	4 Internal Fixation Device 7 Autologous Tissue Substitute J Synthetic Substitute K Nonautologous Tissue Substitute	Z No Qualifier
Ø Sternum Manubrium Suprasternal notch Xiphoid process **1 Ribs, 1 to 2** **2 Ribs, 3 or More** **3 Cervical Vertebra** Dens Odontoid process Spinous process Transverse foramen Transverse process Vertebral arch Vertebral body Vertebral foramen Vertebral lamina Vertebral pedicle **4 Thoracic Vertebra** Spinous process Transverse process Vertebral arch Vertebral body Vertebral foramen Vertebral lamina Vertebral pedicle **5 Scapula, Right** Acromion (process) Coracoid process **6 Scapula, Left** *See 5 Scapula, Right* **7 Glenoid Cavity, Right** Glenoid fossa (of scapula) **8 Glenoid Cavity, Left** *See 7 Glenoid Cavity, Right* **9 Clavicle, Right** **B Clavicle, Left**	X External	4 Internal Fixation Device	Z No Qualifier
C Humeral Head, Right Greater tuberosity Lesser tuberosity Neck of humerus (anatomical) (surgical) **D Humeral Head, Left** *See C Humeral Head, Right* **F Humeral Shaft, Right** Distal humerus Humerus, distal Lateral epicondyle of humerus Medial epicondyle of humerus **G Humeral Shaft, Left** *See F Humeral Shaft, Right* **H Radius, Right** Ulnar notch **J Radius, Left** *See H Radius, Right* **K Ulna, Right** Olecranon process Radial notch **L Ulna, Left** *See K Ulna, Right* **M Carpal, Right** Capitate bone Hamate bone Lunate bone Pisiform bone Scaphoid bone Trapezium bone Trapezoid bone Triquetral bone **N Carpal, Left** *See M Carpal, Right* **P Metacarpal, Right** **Q Metacarpal, Left** **R Thumb Phalanx, Right** **S Thumb Phalanx, Left** **T Finger Phalanx, Right** **V Finger Phalanx, Left**	Ø Open 3 Percutaneous 4 Percutaneous Endoscopic	4 Internal Fixation Device 5 External Fixation Device 7 Autologous Tissue Substitute J Synthetic Substitute K Nonautologous Tissue Substitute	Z No Qualifier

ØPP Continued on next page

Non-OR ØPP[Ø,1,2,3,4,5,6,7,8,9,B]X4Z

ØPP Continued

Ø Medical and Surgical
P Upper Bones
P Removal Definition: Taking out or off a device from a body part

Explanation: If a device is taken out and a similar device put in without cutting or puncturing the skin or mucous membrane, the procedure is coded to the root operation CHANGE. Otherwise, the procedure for taking out a device is coded to the root operation REMOVAL.

Body Part Character 4	Approach Character 5	Device Character 6	Qualifier Character 7
C Humeral Head, Right Greater tuberosity Lesser tuberosity Neck of humerus (anatomical) (surgical) **D Humeral Head, Left** *See C Humeral Head, Right* **F Humeral Shaft, Right** Distal humerus Humerus, distal Lateral epicondyle of humerus Medial epicondyle of humerus **G Humeral Shaft, Left** *See F Humeral Shaft, Right* **H Radius, Right** Ulnar notch **J Radius, Left** *See H Radius, Right* **K Ulna, Right** Olecranon process Radial notch **L Ulna, Left** *See K Ulna, Right* **M Carpal, Right** Capitate bone Hamate bone Lunate bone Pisiform bone Scaphoid bone Trapezium bone Trapezoid bone Triquetral bone **N Carpal, Left** *See M Carpal, Right* **P Metacarpal, Right** **Q Metacarpal, Left** **R Thumb Phalanx, Right** **S Thumb Phalanx, Left** **T Finger Phalanx, Right** **V Finger Phalanx, Left**	**X External**	**4 Internal Fixation Device** **5 External Fixation Device**	**Z No Qualifier**
Y Upper Bone	**Ø Open** **3 Percutaneous** **4 Percutaneous Endoscopic** **X External**	**Ø Drainage Device** **M Bone Growth Stimulator**	**Z No Qualifier**

Non-OR ØPP[C,D,F,G,H,J,K,L,M,N,P,Q,R,S,T,V]X[4,5]Z
Non-OR ØPPY3ØZ
Non-OR ØPPYX[Ø,M]Z

Ø Medical and Surgical
P Upper Bones
Q Repair Definition: Restoring, to the extent possible, a body part to its normal anatomic structure and function
Explanation: Used only when the method to accomplish the repair is not one of the other root operations

Body Part Character 4	Approach Character 5	Device Character 6	Qualifier Character 7
Ø Sternum Manubrium Suprasternal notch Xiphoid process **1 Ribs, 1 to 2** **2 Ribs, 3 or More** **3 Cervical Vertebra** Dens Odontoid process Spinous process Transverse foramen Transverse process Vertebral arch Vertebral body Vertebral foramen Vertebral lamina Vertebral pedicle **4 Thoracic Vertebra** Spinous process Transverse process Vertebral arch Vertebral body Vertebral foramen Vertebral lamina Vertebral pedicle **5 Scapula, Right** Acromion (process) Coracoid process **6 Scapula, Left** *See 5 Scapula, Right* **7 Glenoid Cavity, Right** Glenoid fossa (of scapula) **8 Glenoid Cavity, Left** *See 7 Glenoid Cavity, Right* **9 Clavicle, Right** **B Clavicle, Left** **C Humeral Head, Right** Greater tuberosity Lesser tuberosity Neck of humerus (anatomical)(surgical) **D Humeral Head, Left** *See C Humeral Head, Right* **F Humeral Shaft, Right** Distal humerus Humerus, distal Lateral epicondyle of humerus Medial epicondyle of humerus **G Humeral Shaft, Left** *See F Humeral Shaft, Right* **H Radius, Right** Ulnar notch **J Radius, Left** *See H Radius, Right* **K Ulna, Right** Olecranon process Radial notch **L Ulna, Left** *See K Ulna, Right* **M Carpal, Right** Capitate bone Hamate bone Lunate bone Pisiform bone Scaphoid bone Trapezium bone Trapezoid bone Triquetral bone **N Carpal, Left** *See M Carpal, Right* **P Metacarpal, Right** **Q Metacarpal, Left** **R Thumb Phalanx, Right** **S Thumb Phalanx, Left** **T Finger Phalanx, Right** **V Finger Phalanx, Left**	**Ø Open** **3 Percutaneous** **4 Percutaneous Endoscopic** **X External**	**Z No Device**	**Z No Qualifier**

Non-OR ØPQ[Ø,1,2,3,4,5,6,7,8,9,B,C,D,F,G,H,J,K,L,M,N,P,Q,R,S,T,V]XZZ

Ø Medical and Surgical
P Upper Bones
R Replacement Definition: Putting in or on biological or synthetic material that physically takes the place and/or function of all or a portion of a body part

Explanation: The body part may have been taken out or replaced, or may be taken out, physically eradicated, or rendered nonfunctional during the REPLACEMENT procedure. A REMOVAL procedure is coded for taking out the device used in a previous replacement procedure.

Body Part Character 4		Approach Character 5	Device Character 6	Qualifier Character 7
Ø Sternum Manubrium Suprasternal notch Xiphoid process **1 Ribs, 1 to 2** **2 Ribs, 3 or More** **3 Cervical Vertebra** Dens Odontoid process Spinous process Transverse foramen Transverse process Vertebral arch Vertebral body Vertebral foramen Vertebral lamina Vertebral pedicle **4 Thoracic Vertebra** Spinous process Transverse process Vertebral arch Vertebral body Vertebral foramen Vertebral lamina Vertebral pedicle **5 Scapula, Right** Acromion (process) Coracoid process **6 Scapula, Left** *See 5 Scapula, Right* **7 Glenoid Cavity, Right** Glenoid fossa (of scapula) **8 Glenoid Cavity, Left** *See 7 Glenoid Cavity, Right* **9 Clavicle, Right** **B Clavicle, Left** **C Humeral Head, Right** Greater tuberosity Lesser tuberosity Neck of humerus (anatomical)(surgical) **D Humeral Head, Left** *See C Humeral Head, Right*	**F Humeral Shaft, Right** Distal humerus Humerus, distal Lateral epicondyle of humerus Medial epicondyle of humerus **G Humeral Shaft, Left** *See F Humeral Shaft, Right* **H Radius, Right** Ulnar notch **J Radius, Left** *See H Radius, Right* **K Ulna, Right** Olecranon process Radial notch **L Ulna, Left** *See K Ulna, Right* **M Carpal, Right** Capitate bone Hamate bone Lunate bone Pisiform bone Scaphoid bone Trapezium bone Trapezoid bone Triquetral bone **N Carpal, Left** *See M Carpal, Right* **P Metacarpal, Right** **Q Metacarpal, Left** **R Thumb Phalanx, Right** **S Thumb Phalanx, Left** **T Finger Phalanx, Right** **V Finger Phalanx, Left**	**Ø Open** **3 Percutaneous** **4 Percutaneous Endoscopic**	**7 Autologous Tissue Substitute** **J Synthetic Substitute** **K Nonautologous Tissue Substitute**	**Z No Qualifier**

Ø Medical and Surgical
P Upper Bones
S Reposition Definition: Moving to its normal location, or other suitable location, all or a portion of a body part

Explanation: The body part is moved to a new location from an abnormal location, or from a normal location where it is not functioning correctly. The body part may or may not be cut out or off to be moved to the new location.

Body Part Character 4	Approach Character 5	Device Character 6	Qualifier Character 7
Ø Sternum Manubrium Suprasternal notch Xiphoid process	Ø Open 3 Percutaneous 4 Percutaneous Endoscopic	Ø Internal Fixation Device, Rigid Plate 4 Internal Fixation Device Z No Device	Z No Qualifier
Ø Sternum Manubrium Suprasternal notch Xiphoid process	X External	Z No Device	Z No Qualifier
1 Ribs, 1 to 2 2 Ribs, 3 or More 3 Cervical Vertebra ⊞ Dens Odontoid process Spinous process Transverse foramen Transverse process Vertebral arch Vertebral body Vertebral foramen Vertebral lamina Vertebral pedicle 4 Thoracic Vertebra ⊞ Spinous process Transverse process Vertebral arch Vertebral body Vertebral foramen Vertebral lamina Vertebral pedicle 5 Scapula, Right Acromion (process) Coracoid process 6 Scapula, Left *See 5 Scapula, Right* 7 Glenoid Cavity, Right Glenoid fossa (of scapula) 8 Glenoid Cavity, Left *See 7 Glenoid Cavity, Right* 9 Clavicle, Right B Clavicle, Left	Ø Open 3 Percutaneous 4 Percutaneous Endoscopic	4 Internal Fixation Device Z No Device	Z No Qualifier
1 Ribs, 1 to 2 2 Ribs, 3 or More 3 Cervical Vertebra Dens Odontoid process Spinous process Transverse foramen Transverse process Vertebral arch Vertebral body Vertebral foramen Vertebral lamina Vertebral pedicle 4 Thoracic Vertebra Spinous process Transverse process Vertebral arch Vertebral body Vertebral foramen Vertebral lamina Vertebral pedicle 5 Scapula, Right Acromion (process) Coracoid process 6 Scapula, Left *See 5 Scapula, Right* 7 Glenoid Cavity, Right Glenoid fossa (of scapula) 8 Glenoid Cavity, Left *See 7 Glenoid Cavity, Right* 9 Clavicle, Right B Clavicle, Left	X External	Z No Device	Z No Qualifier
C Humeral Head, Right Greater tuberosity Lesser tuberosity Neck of humerus (anatomical)(surgical) D Humeral Head, Left *See C Humeral Head, Right* F Humeral Shaft, Right Distal humerus Humerus, distal Lateral epicondyle of humerus Medial epicondyle of humerus G Humeral Shaft, Left *See F Humeral Shaft, Right* H Radius, Right Ulnar notch J Radius, Left *See H Radius, Right* K Ulna, Right Olecranon process Radial notch L Ulna, Left *See K Ulna, Right*	Ø Open 3 Percutaneous 4 Percutaneous Endoscopic	4 Internal Fixation Device 5 External Fixation Device 6 Internal Fixation Device, Intramedullary B External Fixation Device, Monoplanar C External Fixation Device, Ring D External Fixation Device, Hybrid Z No Device	Z No Qualifier

ØPS Continued on next page

Non-OR ØPSØ[3,4]ZZ
Non-OR ØPSØXZZ
Non-OR ØPS[1,2,5,6,7,8,9,B][3,4]ZZ
Non-OR ØPS[1,2,3,4,5,6,7,8,9,B]XZZ
Non-OR ØPS[C,D,F,G,H,J,K,L][3,4]ZZ

See Appendix L for Procedure Combinations
⊞ ØPS[3,4]3ZZ

ØPS Continued

Ø Medical and Surgical
P Upper Bones
S Reposition

Definition: Moving to its normal location, or other suitable location, all or a portion of a body part

Explanation: The body part is moved to a new location from an abnormal location, or from a normal location where it is not functioning correctly. The body part may or may not be cut out or off to be moved to the new location.

Body Part Character 4	Approach Character 5	Device Character 6	Qualifier Character 7
C Humeral Head, Right Greater tuberosity Lesser tuberosity Neck of humerus (anatomical)(surgical) **D Humeral Head, Left** *See C Humeral Head, Right* **F Humeral Shaft, Right** Distal humerus Humerus, distal Lateral epicondyle of humerus Medial epicondyle of humerus **G Humeral Shaft, Left** *See F Humeral Shaft, Right* **H Radius, Right** Ulnar notch **J Radius, Left** *See H Radius, Right* **K Ulna, Right** Olecranon process Radial notch **L Ulna, Left** *See K Ulna, Right*	**X** External	**Z** No Device	**Z** No Qualifier
M Carpal, Right Capitate bone Hamate bone Lunate bone Pisiform bone Scaphoid bone Trapezium bone Trapezoid bone Triquetral bone **N Carpal, Left** *See M Carpal, Right* **P Metacarpal, Right** **Q Metacarpal, Left** **R Thumb Phalanx, Right** **S Thumb Phalanx, Left** **T Finger Phalanx, Right** **V Finger Phalanx, Left**	**Ø** Open **3** Percutaneous **4** Percutaneous Endoscopic	**4** Internal Fixation Device **5** External Fixation Device **Z** No Device	**Z** No Qualifier
M Carpal, Right Capitate bone Hamate bone Lunate bone Pisiform bone Scaphoid bone Trapezium bone Trapezoid bone Triquetral bone **N Carpal, Left** *See M Carpal, Right* **P Metacarpal, Right** **Q Metacarpal, Left** **R Thumb Phalanx, Right** **S Thumb Phalanx, Left** **T Finger Phalanx, Right** **V Finger Phalanx, Left**	**X** External	**Z** No Device	**Z** No Qualifier

Non-OR ØPS[C,D,F,G,H,J,K,L]XZZ
Non-OR ØPS[M,N,P,Q,R,S,T,V][3,4]ZZ
Non-OR ØPS[M,N,P,Q,R,S,T,V]XZZ

Ø Medical and Surgical
P Upper Bones
T Resection

Definition: Cutting out or off, without replacement, all of a body part

Explanation: None

Body Part Character 4	Approach Character 5	Device Character 6	Qualifier Character 7
Ø Sternum Manubrium Suprasternal notch Xiphoid process **1 Ribs, 1 to 2** **2 Ribs, 3 or More** **5 Scapula, Right** Acromion (process) Coracoid process **6 Scapula, Left** *See 5 Scapula, Right* **7 Glenoid Cavity, Right** Glenoid fossa (of scapula) **8 Glenoid Cavity, Left** *See 7 Glenoid Cavity, Right* **9 Clavicle, Right** **B Clavicle, Left** **C Humeral Head, Right** Greater tuberosity Lesser tuberosity Neck of humerus (anatomical) (surgical) **D Humeral Head, Left** *See C Humeral Head, Right* **F Humeral Shaft, Right** Distal humerus Humerus, distal Lateral epicondyle of humerus Medial epicondyle of humerus **G Humeral Shaft, Left** *See F Humeral Shaft, Right* **H Radius, Right** Ulnar notch **J Radius, Left** *See H Radius, Right* **K Ulna, Right** Olecranon process Radial notch **L Ulna, Left** *See K Ulna, Right* **M Carpal, Right** Capitate bone Hamate bone Lunate bone Pisiform bone Scaphoid bone Trapezium bone Trapezoid bone Triquetral bone **N Carpal, Left** *See M Carpal, Right* **P Metacarpal, Right** **Q Metacarpal, Left** **R Thumb Phalanx, Right** **S Thumb Phalanx, Left** **T Finger Phalanx, Right** **V Finger Phalanx, Left**	**Ø** Open	**Z** No Device	**Z** No Qualifier

Upper Bones
ØPS–ØPT

Ø Medical and Surgical
P Upper Bones
U Supplement Definition: Putting in or on biological or synthetic material that physically reinforces and/or augments the function of a portion of a body part

Explanation: The biological material is non-living, or is living and from the same individual. The body part may have been previously replaced, and the SUPPLEMENT procedure is performed to physically reinforce and/or augment the function of the replaced body part.

Body Part Character 4		Approach Character 5	Device Character 6	Qualifier Character 7
Ø Sternum Manubrium Suprasternal notch Xiphoid process **1 Ribs, 1 to 2** **2 Ribs, 3 or More** **3 Cervical Vertebra** ⊞ Dens Odontoid process Spinous process Transverse foramen Transverse process Vertebral arch Vertebral body Vertebral foramen Vertebral lamina Vertebral pedicle **4 Thoracic Vertebra** ⊞ Spinous process Transverse process Vertebral arch Vertebral body Vertebral foramen Vertebral lamina Vertebral pedicle **5 Scapula, Right** Acromion (process) Coracoid process **6 Scapula, Left** *See 5 Scapula, Right* **7 Glenoid Cavity, Right** Glenoid fossa (of scapula) **8 Glenoid Cavity, Left** *See 7 Glenoid Cavity, Right* **9 Clavicle, Right** **B Clavicle, Left** **C Humeral Head, Right** Greater tuberosity Lesser tuberosity Neck of humerus (anatomical) (surgical)	**D Humeral Head, Left** *See C Humeral Head, Right* **F Humeral Shaft, Right** Distal humerus Humerus, distal Lateral epicondyle of humerus Medial epicondyle of humerus **G Humeral Shaft, Left** *See F Humeral Shaft, Right* **H Radius, Right** Ulnar notch **J Radius, Left** *See H Radius, Right* **K Ulna, Right** Olecranon process Radial notch **L Ulna, Left** *See K Ulna, Right* **M Carpal, Right** Capitate bone Hamate bone Lunate bone Pisiform bone Scaphoid bone Trapezium bone Trapezoid bone Triquetral bone **N Carpal, Left** *See M Carpal, Right* **P Metacarpal, Right** **Q Metacarpal, Left** **R Thumb Phalanx, Right** **S Thumb Phalanx, Left** **T Finger Phalanx, Right** **V Finger Phalanx, Left**	**Ø Open** **3 Percutaneous** **4 Percutaneous Endoscopic**	**7 Autologous Tissue Substitute** **J Synthetic Substitute** **K Nonautologous Tissue Substitute**	**Z No Qualifier**

See Appendix L for Procedure Combinations
⊞ ØPU[3,4]3JZ

Ø Medical and Surgical
P Upper Bones
W Revision Definition: Correcting, to the extent possible, a portion of a malfunctioning device or the position of a displaced device
Explanation: Revision can include correcting a malfunctioning or displaced device by taking out or putting in components of the device such as a screw or pin

Body Part Character 4		Approach Character 5	Device Character 6	Qualifier Character 7
Ø Sternum Manubrium Suprasternal notch Xiphoid process **1 Ribs, 1 to 2** **2 Ribs, 3 or More** **3 Cervical Vertebra** Dens Odontoid process Spinous process Transverse foramen Transverse process Vertebral arch Vertebral body Vertebral foramen Vertebral lamina Vertebral pedicle **4 Thoracic Vertebra** Spinous process Transverse process Vertebral arch Vertebral body Vertebral foramen Vertebral lamina Vertebral pedicle	**5 Scapula, Right** Acromion (process) Coracoid process **6 Scapula, Left** *See 5 Scapula, Right* **7 Glenoid Cavity, Right** Glenoid fossa (of scapula) **8 Glenoid Cavity, Left** *See 7 Glenoid Cavity, Right* **9 Clavicle, Right** **B Clavicle, Left**	**Ø Open** **3 Percutaneous** **4 Percutaneous Endoscopic** **X External**	**4 Internal Fixation Device** **7 Autologous Tissue Substitute** **J Synthetic Substitute** **K Nonautologous Tissue Substitute**	**Z No Qualifier**
C Humeral Head, Right Greater tuberosity Lesser tuberosity Neck of humerus (anatomical)(surgical) **D Humeral Head, Left** *See C Humeral Head, Right* **F Humeral Shaft, Right** Distal humerus Humerus, distal Lateral epicondyle of humerus Medial epicondyle of humerus **G Humeral Shaft, Left** *See F Humeral Shaft, Right* **H Radius, Right** Ulnar notch **J Radius, Left** *See H Radius, Right* **K Ulna, Right** Olecranon process Radial notch	**L Ulna, Left** *See K Ulna, Right* **M Carpal, Right** Capitate bone Hamate bone Lunate bone Pisiform bone Scaphoid bone Trapezium bone Trapezoid bone Triquetral bone **N Carpal, Left** *See M Carpal, Right* **P Metacarpal, Right** **Q Metacarpal, Left** **R Thumb Phalanx, Right** **S Thumb Phalanx, Left** **T Finger Phalanx, Right** **V Finger Phalanx, Left**	**Ø Open** **3 Percutaneous** **4 Percutaneous Endoscopic** **X External**	**4 Internal Fixation Device** **5 External Fixation Device** **7 Autologous Tissue Substitute** **J Synthetic Substitute** **K Nonautologous Tissue Substitute**	**Z No Qualifier**
Y Upper Bone		**Ø Open** **3 Percutaneous** **4 Percutaneous Endoscopic** **X External**	**Ø Drainage Device** **M Bone Growth Stimulator**	**Z No Qualifier**

Non-OR ØPW[Ø,1,2,3,4,5,6,7,8,9,B]X[4,7,J,K]Z
Non-OR ØPW[C,D,F,G,H,J,K,L,M,N,P,Q,R,S,T,V]X[4,5,7,J,K]Z
Non-OR ØPWYX[Ø,M]Z

Lower Bones ØQ2–ØQW

Character Meanings

This Character Meaning table is provided as a guide to assist the user in the identification of character members that may be found in this section of code tables. It **SHOULD NOT** be used to build a PCS code.

Operation–Character 3	Body Part–Character 4	Approach–Character 5	Device–Character 6	Qualifier–Character 7
2 Change	Ø Lumbar Vertebra	Ø Open	Ø Drainage Device	2 Sesamoid Bone(s) 1st Toe
5 Destruction	1 Sacrum	3 Percutaneous	4 Internal Fixation Device	X Diagnostic
8 Division	2 Pelvic Bone, Right	4 Percutaneous Endoscopic	5 External Fixation Device	Z No Qualifier
9 Drainage	3 Pelvic Bone, Left	X External	6 Internal Fixation Device, Intramedullary	
B Excision	4 Acetabulum, Right		7 Autologous Tissue Substitute	
C Extirpation	5 Acetabulum, Left		8 External Fixation Device, Limb Lengthening	
D Extraction	6 Upper Femur, Right		B External Fixation Device, Monoplanar	
H Insertion	7 Upper Femur, Left		C External Fixation Device, Ring	
J Inspection	8 Femoral Shaft, Right		D External Fixation Device, Hybrid	
N Release	9 Femoral Shaft, Left		J Synthetic Substitute	
P Removal	B Lower Femur, Right		K Nonautologous Tissue Substitute	
Q Repair	C Lower Femur, Left		M Bone Growth Stimulator	
R Replacement	D Patella, Right		Y Other Device	
S Reposition	F Patella, Left		Z No Device	
T Resection	G Tibia, Right			
U Supplement	H Tibia, Left			
W Revision	J Fibula, Right			
	K Fibula, Left			
	L Tarsal, Right			
	M Tarsal, Left			
	N Metatarsal, Right			
	P Metatarsal, Left			
	Q Toe Phalanx, Right			
	R Toe Phalanx, Left			
	S Coccyx			
	Y Lower Bone			

AHA Coding Clinic for table ØQ8

2018, 1Q, 25	Periacetabular osteotomy for repair of congenital hip dysplasia
2016, 2Q, 31	Periacetabular ostectomy for repair of congenital hip dysplasia

AHA Coding Clinic for table ØQB

2017, 1Q, 23	Reconstruction of mandible using titanium and bone
2016, 3Q, 30	Resection of femur with interposition arthroplasty
2015, 3Q, 3-8	Excisional and nonexcisional debridement
2015, 3Q, 26	Femoral head resection
2015, 2Q, 34	Decompressive laminectomy
2014, 4Q, 25	Femoroacetabular impingement and labral tear with repair
2014, 2Q, 6	Posterior lumbar fusion with discectomy
2013, 4Q, 116	Spinal decompression
2013, 2Q, 39	Ankle fusion, osteotomy, and removal of hardware
2012, 2Q, 19	Multiple decompressive cervical laminectomies

AHA Coding Clinic for table ØQD

2017, 4Q, 41	Extraction procedures

AHA Coding Clinic for table ØQH

2017, 1Q, 21	Staged scoliosis surgery with iliac fixation and spinal fusion
2016, 3Q, 34	Tibial/fibula epiphysiodesis

AHA Coding Clinic for table ØQP

2017, 4Q, 74-75	Magnetic growth rods
2015, 2Q, 6	Planned implant break

AHA Coding Clinic for table ØQQ

2018, 1Q, 15	Pubic symphysis fusion
2014, 3Q, 24	Repair of lipomyelomeningocele and tethered cord

AHA Coding Clinic for table ØQR

2017, 1Q, 22	Total knee replacement and patellar component
2016, 3Q, 30	Resection of femur with interposition arthroplasty

AHA Coding Clinic for table ØQS

2018, 1Q, 13	Bilateral cuboid osteotomy for repair of congenital talipes equinovarus
2018, 1Q, 25	Periacetabular osteotomy for repair of congenital hip dysplasia
2016, 3Q, 34	Tibial/fibula epiphysiodesis
2014, 4Q, 29	Rotational osteosynthesis
2014, 4Q, 31	Reposition of femur for correction of valgus and recurvatum deformities

AHA Coding Clinic for table ØQT

2017, 1Q, 22	Chopart amputation of foot
2016, 3Q, 30	Resection of femur with interposition arthroplasty
2015, 3Q, 26	Femoral head resection
2014, 4Q, 29	Rotational osteosynthesis

AHA Coding Clinic for table ØQU

2015, 3Q, 18	Total hip replacement with acetabular reconstruction
2014, 4Q, 31	Reposition of femur for correction of valgus and recurvatum deformities
2014, 2Q, 12	Percutaneous vertebroplasty using cement
2013, 2Q, 35	Use of bone void filler in grafting

AHA Coding Clinic for table ØQW

2017, 4Q, 74-75	Magnetic growth rods

Lower Bones

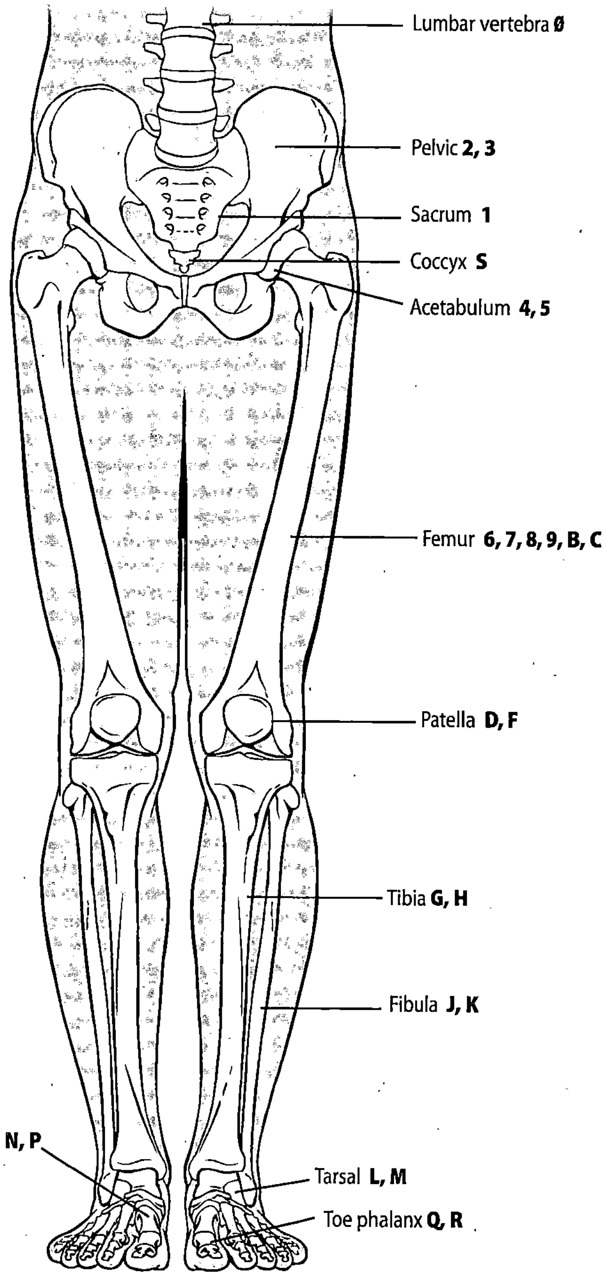
Lumbar vertebra Ø
Pelvic 2, 3
Sacrum 1
Coccyx S
Acetabulum 4, 5
Femur 6, 7, 8, 9, B, C
Patella D, F
Tibia G, H
Fibula J, K
Metatarsal N, P
Tarsal L, M
Toe phalanx Q, R

Hip Bone Anatomy

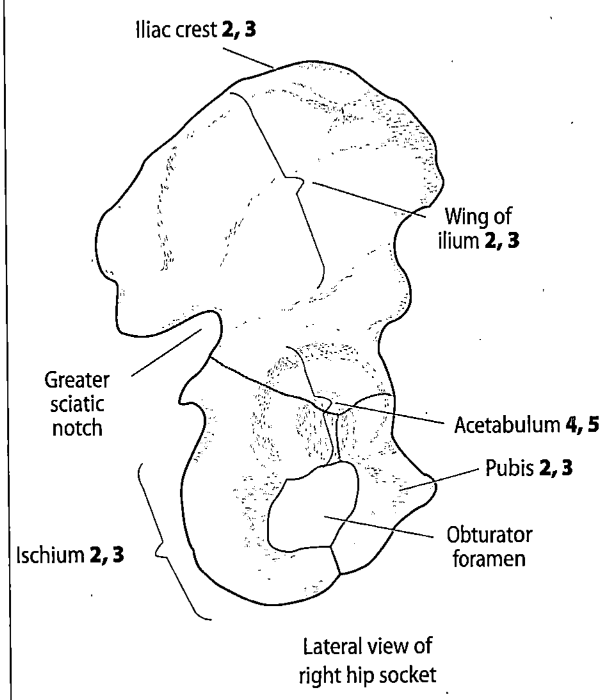
Iliac crest 2, 3
Wing of ilium 2, 3
Greater sciatic notch
Acetabulum 4, 5
Pubis 2, 3
Obturator foramen
Ischium 2, 3
Lateral view of right hip socket

Pelvic and Lower Extremity Bones

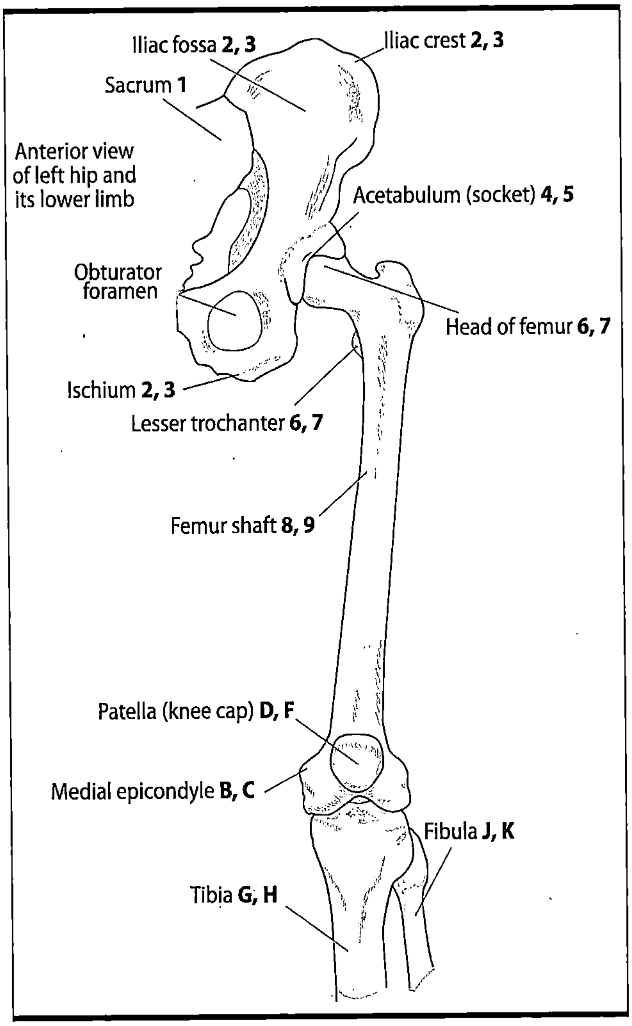
Iliac fossa 2, 3
Iliac crest 2, 3
Sacrum 1
Anterior view of left hip and its lower limb
Acetabulum (socket) 4, 5
Obturator foramen
Head of femur 6, 7
Ischium 2, 3
Lesser trochanter 6, 7
Femur shaft 8, 9
Patella (knee cap) D, F
Medial epicondyle B, C
Fibula J, K
Tibia G, H

Foot Bones

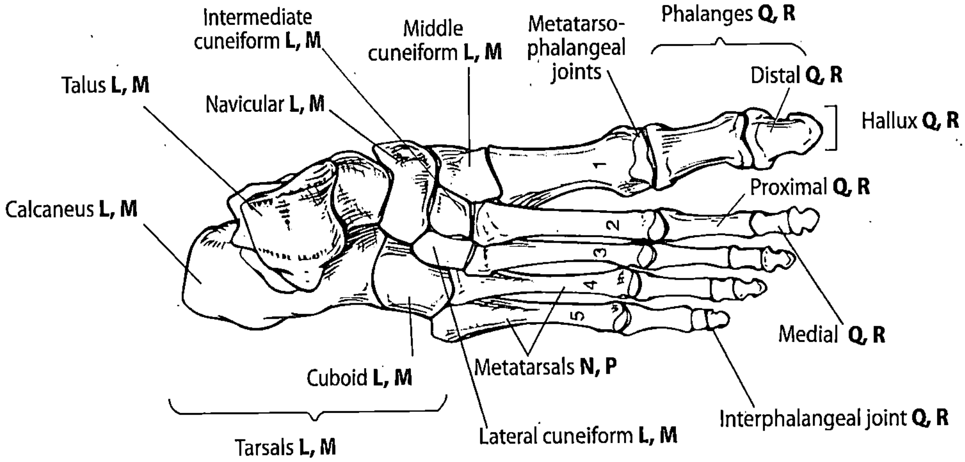
Intermediate cuneiform L, M
Middle cuneiform L, M
Metatarso-phalangeal joints
Phalanges Q, R
Talus L, M
Navicular L, M
Distal Q, R
Hallux Q, R
Calcaneus L, M
Proximal Q, R
1
2
3
4
5
Medial Q, R
Cuboid L, M
Metatarsals N, P
Interphalangeal joint Q, R
Tarsals L, M
Lateral cuneiform L, M

Ø Medical and Surgical
Q Lower Bones
2 Change Definition: Taking out or off a device from a body part and putting back an identical or similar device in or on the same body part without cutting or puncturing the skin or a mucous membrane

Explanation: All CHANGE procedures are coded using the approach EXTERNAL

Body Part Character 4	Approach Character 5	Device Character 6	Qualifier Character 7
Y Lower Bone	X External	Ø Drainage Device Y Other Device	Z No Qualifier

Non-OR All body part, approach, device, and qualifier values

Ø Medical and Surgical
Q Lower Bones
5 Destruction Definition: Physical eradication of all or a portion of a body part by the direct use of energy, force, or a destructive agent

Explanation: None of the body part is physically taken out

Body Part Character 4	Approach Character 5	Device Character 6	Qualifier Character 7
Ø Lumbar Vertebra Spinous process Transverse process Vertebral arch Vertebral body Vertebral foramen Vertebral lamina Vertebral pedicle **1 Sacrum** **2 Pelvic Bone, Right** Iliac crest Ilium Ischium Pubis **3 Pelvic Bone, Left** *See 2 Pelvic Bone, Right* **4 Acetabulum, Right** **5 Acetabulum, Left** **6 Upper Femur, Right** Femoral head Greater trochanter Lesser trochanter Neck of femur **7 Upper Femur, Left** *See 6 Upper Femur, Right* **8 Femoral Shaft, Right** Body of femur **9 Femoral Shaft, Left** *See 8 Femoral Shaft, Right* **B Lower Femur, Right** Lateral condyle of femur Lateral epicondyle of femur Medial condyle of femur Medial epicondyle of femur **C Lower Femur, Left** *See B Lower Femur, Right* **D Patella, Right** **F Patella, Left** **G Tibia, Right** Lateral condyle of tibia Medial condyle of tibia Medial malleolus **H Tibia, Left** *See G Tibia, Right* **J Fibula, Right** Body of fibula Head of fibula Lateral malleolus **K Fibula, Left** *See J Fibula, Right* **L Tarsal, Right** Calcaneus Cuboid bone Intermediate cuneiform bone Lateral cuneiform bone Medial cuneiform bone Navicular bone Talus bone **M Tarsal, Left** *See L Tarsal, Right* **N Metatarsal, Right** **P Metatarsal, Left** **Q Toe Phalanx, Right** **R Toe Phalanx, Left** **S Coccyx**	Ø Open 3 Percutaneous 4 Percutaneous Endoscopic	Z No Device	Z No Qualifier

Ø Medical and Surgical
Q Lower Bones
8 Division Definition: Cutting into a body part, without draining fluids and/or gases from the body part, in order to separate or transect a body part
Explanation: All or a portion of the body part is separated into two or more portions

Body Part Character 4	Approach Character 5	Device Character 6	Qualifier Character 7
Ø Lumbar Vertebra Spinous process Transverse process Vertebral arch Vertebral body Vertebral foramen Vertebral lamina Vertebral pedicle **1 Sacrum** **2 Pelvic Bone, Right** Iliac crest Ilium Ischium Pubis **3 Pelvic Bone, Left** *See 2 Pelvic Bone, Right* **4 Acetabulum, Right** **5 Acetabulum, Left** **6 Upper Femur, Right** Femoral head Greater trochanter Lesser trochanter Neck of femur **7 Upper Femur, Left** *See 6 Upper Femur, Right* **8 Femoral Shaft, Right** Body of femur **9 Femoral Shaft, Left** *See 8 Femoral Shaft, Right* **B Lower Femur, Right** Lateral condyle of femur Lateral epicondyle of femur Medial condyle of femur Medial epicondyle of femur **C Lower Femur, Left** *See B Lower Femur, Right* **D Patella, Right** **F Patella, Left** **G Tibia, Right** Lateral condyle of tibia Medial condyle of tibia Medial malleolus **H Tibia, Left** *See G Tibia, Right* **J Fibula, Right** Body of fibula Head of fibula Lateral malleolus **K Fibula, Left** *See J Fibula, Right* **L Tarsal, Right** Calcaneus Cuboid bone Intermediate cuneiform bone Lateral cuneiform bone Medial cuneiform bone Navicular bone Talus bone **M Tarsal, Left** *See L Tarsal, Right* **N Metatarsal, Right** **P Metatarsal, Left** **Q Toe Phalanx, Right** **R Toe Phalanx, Left** **S Coccyx**	**Ø Open** **3 Percutaneous** **4 Percutaneous Endoscopic**	**Z No Device**	**Z No Qualifier**

Ø Medical and Surgical
Q Lower Bones
9 Drainage Definition: Taking or letting out fluids and/or gases from a body part
Explanation: The qualifier DIAGNOSTIC is used to identify drainage procedures that are biopsies

Body Part Character 4		Approach Character 5	Device Character 6	Qualifier Character 7
Ø Lumbar Vertebra Spinous process Transverse process Vertebral arch Vertebral body Vertebral foramen Vertebral lamina Vertebral pedicle **1 Sacrum** **2 Pelvic Bone, Right** Iliac crest Ilium Ischium Pubis **3 Pelvic Bone, Left** *See 2 Pelvic Bone, Right* **4 Acetabulum, Right** **5 Acetabulum, Left** **6 Upper Femur, Right** Femoral head Greater trochanter Lesser trochanter Neck of femur **7 Upper Femur, Left** *See 6 Upper Femur, Right* **8 Femoral Shaft, Right** Body of femur **9 Femoral Shaft, Left** *See 8 Femoral Shaft, Right* **B Lower Femur, Right** Lateral condyle of femur Lateral epicondyle of femur Medial condyle of femur Medial epicondyle of femur	**C Lower Femur, Left** *See B Lower Femur, Right* **D Patella, Right** **F Patella, Left** **G Tibia, Right** Lateral condyle of tibia Medial condyle of tibia Medial malleolus **H Tibia, Left** *See G Tibia, Right* **J Fibula, Right** Body of fibula Head of fibula Lateral malleolus **K Fibula, Left** *See J Fibula, Right* **L Tarsal, Right** Calcaneus Cuboid bone Intermediate cuneiform bone Lateral cuneiform bone Medial cuneiform bone Navicular bone Talus bone **M Tarsal, Left** *See L Tarsal, Right* **N Metatarsal, Right** **P Metatarsal, Left** **Q Toe Phalanx, Right** **R Toe Phalanx, Left** **S Coccyx**	**Ø Open** **3 Percutaneous** **4 Percutaneous Endoscopic**	**Ø Drainage Device**	**Z No Qualifier**
Ø Lumbar Vertebra Spinous process Transverse process Vertebral arch Vertebral body Vertebral foramen Vertebral lamina Vertebral pedicle **1 Sacrum** **2 Pelvic Bone, Right** Iliac crest Ilium Ischium Pubis **3 Pelvic Bone, Left** *See 2 Pelvic Bone, Right* **4 Acetabulum, Right** **5 Acetabulum, Left** **6 Upper Femur, Right** Femoral head Greater trochanter Lesser trochanter Neck of femur **7 Upper Femur, Left** *See 6 Upper Femur, Right* **8 Femoral Shaft, Right** Body of femur **9 Femoral Shaft, Left** *See 8 Femoral Shaft, Right* **B Lower Femur, Right** Lateral condyle of femur Lateral epicondyle of femur Medial condyle of femur Medial epicondyle of femur	**C Lower Femur, Left** *See B Lower Femur, Right* **D Patella, Right** **F Patella, Left** **G Tibia, Right** Lateral condyle of tibia Medial condyle of tibia Medial malleolus **H Tibia, Left** *See G Tibia, Right* **J Fibula, Right** Body of fibula Head of fibula Lateral malleolus **K Fibula, Left** *See J Fibula, Right* **L Tarsal, Right** Calcaneus Cuboid bone Intermediate cuneiform bone Lateral cuneiform bone Medial cuneiform bone Navicular bone Talus bone **M Tarsal, Left** *See L Tarsal, Right* **N Metatarsal, Right** **P Metatarsal, Left** **Q Toe Phalanx, Right** **R Toe Phalanx, Left** **S Coccyx**	**Ø Open** **3 Percutaneous** **4 Percutaneous Endoscopic**	**Z No Device**	**X Diagnostic** **Z No Qualifier**

Non-OR ØQ9[Ø,1,2,3,4,5,6,7,8,9,B,C,D,F,G,H,J,K,L,M,P,Q,R,S]3ØZ
Non-OR ØQ9[Ø,1,2,3,4,5,6,7,8,9,B,C,D,F,G,H,J,K,L,M,P,Q,R,S]3ZZ

Ø Medical and Surgical
Q Lower Bones
B Excision **Definition: Cutting out or off, without replacement, a portion of a body part**
Explanation: The qualifier DIAGNOSTIC is used to identify excision procedures that are biopsies

Body Part Character 4	Approach Character 5	Device Character 6	Qualifier Character 7
Ø Lumbar Vertebra Spinous process Transverse process Vertebral arch Vertebral body Vertebral foramen Vertebral lamina Vertebral pedicle **1 Sacrum** **2 Pelvic Bone, Right** Iliac crest Ilium Ischium Pubis **3 Pelvic Bone, Left** *See 2 Pelvic Bone, Right* **4 Acetabulum, Right** **5 Acetabulum, Left** **6 Upper Femur, Right** Femoral head Greater trochanter Lesser trochanter Neck of femur **7 Upper Femur, Left** *See 6 Upper Femur, Right* **8 Femoral Shaft, Right** Body of femur **9 Femoral Shaft, Left** *See 8 Femoral Shaft, Right* **B Lower Femur, Right** Lateral condyle of femur Lateral epicondyle of femur Medial condyle of femur Medial epicondyle of femur **C Lower Femur, Left** *See B Lower Femur, Right* **D Patella, Right** **F Patella, Left** **G Tibia, Right** Lateral condyle of tibia Medial condyle of tibia Medial malleolus **H Tibia, Left** *See G Tibia, Right* **J Fibula, Right** Body of fibula Head of fibula Lateral malleolus **K Fibula, Left** *See J Fibula, Right* **L Tarsal, Right** Calcaneus Cuboid bone Intermediate cuneiform bone Lateral cuneiform bone Medial cuneiform bone Navicular bone Talus bone **M Tarsal, Left** *See L Tarsal, Right* **N Metatarsal, Right** **P Metatarsal, Left** **Q Toe Phalanx, Right** **R Toe Phalanx, Left** **S Coccyx**	**Ø Open** **3 Percutaneous** **4 Percutaneous Endoscopic**	**Z No Device**	**X Diagnostic** **Z No Qualifier**

Ø Medical and Surgical
Q Lower Bones
C Extirpation Definition: Taking or cutting out solid matter from a body part

Explanation: The solid matter may be an abnormal byproduct of a biological function or a foreign body; it may be imbedded in a body part or in the lumen of a tubular body part. The solid matter may or may not have been previously broken into pieces.

Body Part Character 4		Approach Character 5	Device Character 6	Qualifier Character 7
Ø Lumbar Vertebra Spinous process Transverse process Vertebral arch Vertebral body Vertebral foramen Vertebral lamina Vertebral pedicle **1 Sacrum** **2 Pelvic Bone, Right** Iliac crest Ilium Ischium Pubis **3 Pelvic Bone, Left** *See 2 Pelvic Bone, Right* **4 Acetabulum, Right** **5 Acetabulum, Left** **6 Upper Femur, Right** Femoral head Greater trochanter Lesser trochanter Neck of femur **7 Upper Femur, Left** *See 6 Upper Femur, Right* **8 Femoral Shaft, Right** Body of femur **9 Femoral Shaft, Left** *See 8 Femoral Shaft, Right* **B Lower Femur, Right** Lateral condyle of femur Lateral epicondyle of femur Medial condyle of femur Medial epicondyle of femur	**C Lower Femur, Left** *See B Lower Femur, Right* **D Patella, Right** **F Patella, Left** **G Tibia, Right** Lateral condyle of tibia Medial condyle of tibia Medial malleolus **H Tibia, Left** *See G Tibia, Right* **J Fibula, Right** Body of fibula Head of fibula Lateral malleolus **K Fibula, Left** *See J Fibula, Right* **L Tarsal, Right** Calcaneus Cuboid bone Intermediate cuneiform bone Lateral cuneiform bone Medial cuneiform bone Navicular bone Talus bone **M Tarsal, Left** *See L Tarsal, Right* **N Metatarsal, Right** **P Metatarsal, Left** **Q Toe Phalanx, Right** **R Toe Phalanx, Left** **S Coccyx**	**Ø** Open **3** Percutaneous **4** Percutaneous Endoscopic	**Z** No Device	**Z** No Qualifier

Ø Medical and Surgical
Q Lower Bones
D Extraction Definition: Pulling or stripping out or off all or a portion of a body part by the use of force

Explanation: The qualifier DIAGNOSTIC is used to identify extraction procedures that are biopsies

Body Part Character 4		Approach Character 5	Device Character 6	Qualifier Character 7
Ø Lumbar Vertebra Spinous process Transverse process Vertebral arch Vertebral body Vertebral foramen Vertebral lamina Vertebral pedicle **1 Sacrum** **2 Pelvic Bone, Right** Iliac crest Ilium Ischium Pubis **3 Pelvic Bone, Left** *See 2 Pelvic Bone, Right* **4 Acetabulum, Right** **5 Acetabulum, Left** **6 Upper Femur, Right** Femoral head Greater trochanter Lesser trochanter Neck of femur **7 Upper Femur, Left** *See 6 Upper Femur, Right* **8 Femoral Shaft, Right** Body of femur **9 Femoral Shaft, Left** *See 8 Femoral Shaft, Right* **B Lower Femur, Right** Lateral condyle of femur Lateral epicondyle of femur Medial condyle of femur Medial epicondyle of femur	**C Lower Femur, Left** *See B Lower Femur, Right* **D Patella, Right** **F Patella, Left** **G Tibia, Right** Lateral condyle of tibia Medial condyle of tibia Medial malleolus **H Tibia, Left** *See G Tibia, Right* **J Fibula, Right** Body of fibula Head of fibula Lateral malleolus **K Fibula, Left** *See J Fibula, Right* **L Tarsal, Right** Calcaneus Cuboid bone Intermediate cuneiform bone Lateral cuneiform bone Medial cuneiform bone Navicular bone Talus bone **M Tarsal, Left** *See L Tarsal, Right* **N Metatarsal, Right** **P Metatarsal, Left** **Q Toe Phalanx, Right** **R Toe Phalanx, Left** **S Coccyx**	**Ø** Open	**Z** No Device	**Z** No Qualifier

Ø Medical and Surgical
Q Lower Bones
H Insertion Definition: Putting in a nonbiological appliance that monitors, assists, performs, or prevents a physiological function but does not physically take the place of a body part

Explanation: None

Body Part Character 4		Approach Character 5	Device Character 6	Qualifier Character 7
Ø Lumbar Vertebra Spinous process Transverse process Vertebral arch Vertebral body Vertebral foramen Vertebral lamina Vertebral pedicle **1 Sacrum** **2 Pelvic Bone, Right** Iliac crest Ilium Ischium Pubis **3 Pelvic Bone, Left** *See 2 Pelvic Bone, Right* **4 Acetabulum, Right** **5 Acetabulum, Left**	**D Patella, Right** **F Patella, Left** **L Tarsal, Right** Calcaneus Cuboid bone Intermediate cuneiform bone Lateral cuneiform bone Medial cuneiform bone Navicular bone Talus bone **M Tarsal, Left** *See L Tarsal, Right* **N Metatarsal, Right** **P Metatarsal, Left** **Q Toe Phalanx, Right** **R Toe Phalanx, Left** **S Coccyx**	**Ø Open** **3 Percutaneous** **4 Percutaneous Endoscopic**	**4 Internal Fixation Device** **5 External Fixation Device**	**Z No Qualifier**
6 Upper Femur, Right Femoral head Greater trochanter Lesser trochanter Neck of femur **7 Upper Femur, Left** *See 6 Upper Femur, Right* **8 Femoral Shaft, Right** Body of femur **9 Femoral Shaft, Left** *See 8 Femoral Shaft, Right* **B Lower Femur, Right** Lateral condyle of femur Lateral epicondyle of femur Medial condyle of femur Medial epicondyle of femur	**C Lower Femur, Left** *See B Lower Femur, Right* **G Tibia, Right** Lateral condyle of tibia Medial condyle of tibia Medial malleolus **H Tibia, Left** *See G Tibia, Right* **J Fibula, Right** Body of fibula Head of fibula Lateral malleolus **K Fibula, Left** *See J Fibula, Right*	**Ø Open** **3 Percutaneous** **4 Percutaneous Endoscopic**	**4 Internal Fixation Device** **5 External Fixation Device** **6 Internal Fixation Device, Intramedullary** **8 External Fixation Device, Limb Lengthening** **B External Fixation Device, Monoplanar** **C External Fixation Device, Ring** **D External Fixation Device, Hybrid**	**Z No Qualifier**
Y Lower Bone		**Ø Open** **3 Percutaneous** **4 Percutaneous Endoscopic**	**M Bone Growth Stimulator**	**Z No Qualifier**

Non-OR ØQH[6,7,8,9,B,C,G,H,J,K][Ø,3,4]8Z

Ø Medical and Surgical
Q Lower Bones
J Inspection Definition: Visually and/or manually exploring a body part

Explanation: Visual exploration may be performed with or without optical instrumentation. Manual exploration may be performed directly or through intervening body layers.

Body Part Character 4	Approach Character 5	Device Character 6	Qualifier Character 7
Y Lower Bone	**Ø Open** **3 Percutaneous** **4 Percutaneous Endoscopic** **X External**	**Z No Device**	**Z No Qualifier**

Non-OR ØQJY[3,X]ZZ

Ø Medical and Surgical
Q Lower Bones
N Release Definition: Freeing a body part from an abnormal physical constraint by cutting or by the use of force
Explanation: Some of the restraining tissue may be taken out but none of the body part is taken out

Body Part Character 4		Approach Character 5	Device Character 6	Qualifier Character 7
Ø Lumbar Vertebra Spinous process Transverse process Vertebral arch Vertebral body Vertebral foramen Vertebral lamina Vertebral pedicle **1 Sacrum** **2 Pelvic Bone, Right** Iliac crest Ilium Ischium Pubis **3 Pelvic Bone, Left** *See 2 Pelvic Bone, Right* **4 Acetabulum, Right** **5 Acetabulum, Left** **6 Upper Femur, Right** Femoral head Greater trochanter Lesser trochanter Neck of femur **7 Upper Femur, Left** *See 6 Upper Femur, Right* **8 Femoral Shaft, Right** Body of femur **9 Femoral Shaft, Left** *See 8 Femoral Shaft, Right* **B Lower Femur, Right** Lateral condyle of femur Lateral epicondyle of femur Medial condyle of femur Medial epicondyle of femur	**C Lower Femur, Left** *See B Lower Femur, Right* **D Patella, Right** **F Patella, Left** **G Tibia, Right** Lateral condyle of tibia Medial condyle of tibia Medial malleolus **H Tibia, Left** *See G Tibia, Right* **J Fibula, Right** Body of fibula Head of fibula Lateral malleolus **K Fibula, Left** *See J Fibula, Right* **L Tarsal, Right** Calcaneus Cuboid bone Intermediate cuneiform bone Lateral cuneiform bone Medial cuneiform bone Navicular bone Talus bone **M Tarsal, Left** *See L Tarsal, Right* **N Metatarsal, Right** **P Metatarsal, Left** **Q Toe Phalanx, Right** **R Toe Phalanx, Left** **S Coccyx**	Ø Open 3 Percutaneous 4 Percutaneous Endoscopic	Z No Device	Z No Qualifier

Ø Medical and Surgical
Q Lower Bones
P Removal Definition: Taking out or off a device from a body part
Explanation: If a device is taken out and a similar device put in without cutting or puncturing the skin or mucous membrane, the procedure is coded to the root operation CHANGE. Otherwise, the procedure for taking out a device is coded to the root operation REMOVAL.

Body Part Character 4	Approach Character 5	Device Character 6	Qualifier Character 7
Ø Lumbar Vertebra Spinous process Transverse process Vertebral arch Vertebral body Vertebral foramen Vertebral lamina Vertebral pedicle **1 Sacrum** **4 Acetabulum, Right** **5 Acetabulum, Left** **S Coccyx**	Ø Open 3 Percutaneous 4 Percutaneous Endoscopic	4 Internal Fixation Device 7 Autologous Tissue Substitute J Synthetic Substitute K Nonautologous Tissue Substitute	Z No Qualifier
Ø Lumbar Vertebra Spinous process Transverse process Vertebral arch Vertebral body Vertebral foramen Vertebral lamina Vertebral pedicle **1 Sacrum** **4 Acetabulum, Right** **5 Acetabulum, Left** **S Coccyx**	X External	4 Internal Fixation Device	Z No Qualifier

ØQP Continued on next page

Non-OR ØQP[Ø,1,4,5,S]X4Z

ØQP Continued

Ø Medical and Surgical
Q Lower Bones
P Removal Definition: Taking out or off a device from a body part

Explanation: If a device is taken out and a similar device put in without cutting or puncturing the skin or mucous membrane, the procedure is coded to the root operation CHANGE. Otherwise, the procedure for taking out a device is coded to the root operation REMOVAL.

Body Part Character 4		Approach Character 5	Device Character 6	Qualifier Character 7
2 Pelvic Bone, Right Iliac crest Ilium Ischium Pubis **3 Pelvic Bone, Left** *See 2 Pelvic Bone, Right* **6 Upper Femur, Right** Femoral head Greater trochanter Lesser trochanter Neck of femur **7 Upper Femur, Left** *See 6 Upper Femur, Right* **8 Femoral Shaft, Right** Body of femur **9 Femoral Shaft, Left** *See 8 Femoral Shaft, Right* **B Lower Femur, Right** Lateral condyle of femur Lateral epicondyle of femur Medial condyle of femur Medial epicondyle of femur **C Lower Femur, Left** *See B Lower Femur, Right* **D Patella, Right** **F Patella, Left**	**G Tibia, Right** Lateral condyle of tibia Medial condyle of tibia Medial malleolus **H Tibia, Left** *See G Tibia, Right* **J Fibula, Right** Body of fibula Head of fibula Lateral malleolus **K Fibula, Left** *See J Fibula, Right* **L Tarsal, Right** Calcaneus Cuboid bone Intermediate cuneiform bone Lateral cuneiform bone Medial cuneiform bone Navicular bone Talus bone **M Tarsal, Left** *See L Tarsal, Right* **N Metatarsal, Right** **P Metatarsal, Left** **Q Toe Phalanx, Right** **R Toe Phalanx, Left**	**Ø Open** **3 Percutaneous** **4 Percutaneous Endoscopic**	**4 Internal Fixation Device** **5 External Fixation Device** **7 Autologous Tissue Substitute** **J Synthetic Substitute** **K Nonautologous Tissue Substitute**	**Z No Qualifier**
2 Pelvic Bone, Right Iliac crest Ilium Ischium Pubis **3 Pelvic Bone, Left** *See 2 Pelvic Bone, Right* **6 Upper Femur, Right** Femoral head Greater trochanter Lesser trochanter Neck of femur **7 Upper Femur, Left** *See 6 Upper Femur, Right* **8 Femoral Shaft, Right** Body of femur **9 Femoral Shaft, Left** *See 8 Femoral Shaft, Right* **B Lower Femur, Right** Lateral condyle of femur Lateral epicondyle of femur Medial condyle of femur Medial epicondyle of femur **C Lower Femur, Left** *See B Lower Femur, Right* **D Patella, Right** **F Patella, Left**	**G Tibia, Right** Lateral condyle of tibia Medial condyle of tibia Medial malleolus **H Tibia, Left** *See G Tibia, Right* **J Fibula, Right** Body of fibula Head of fibula Lateral malleolus **K Fibula, Left** *See J Fibula, Right* **L Tarsal, Right** Calcaneus Cuboid bone Intermediate cuneiform bone Lateral cuneiform bone Medial cuneiform bone Navicular bone Talus bone **M Tarsal, Left** *See L Tarsal, Right* **N Metatarsal, Right** **P Metatarsal, Left** **Q Toe Phalanx, Right** **R Toe Phalanx, Left**	**X External**	**4 Internal Fixation Device** **5 External Fixation Device**	**Z No Qualifier**
Y Lower Bone		**Ø Open** **3 Percutaneous** **4 Percutaneous Endoscopic** **X External**	**Ø Drainage Device** **M Bone Growth Stimulator**	**Z No Qualifier**

Non-OR ØQP[2,3,6,7,8,9,B,C,D,F,G,H,J,K,L,M,N,P,Q,R]X[4,5]Z
Non-OR ØQPY3ØZ
Non-OR ØQPYX[Ø,M]Z

Ø Medical and Surgical
Q Lower Bones
Q Repair Definition: Restoring, to the extent possible, a body part to its normal anatomic structure and function
Explanation: Used only when the method to accomplish the repair is not one of the other root operations

Body Part Character 4	Approach Character 5	Device Character 6	Qualifier Character 7
Ø Lumbar Vertebra Spinous process Transverse process Vertebral arch Vertebral body Vertebral foramen Vertebral lamina Vertebral pedicle **1 Sacrum** **2 Pelvic Bone, Right** Iliac crest Ilium Ischium Pubis **3 Pelvic Bone, Left** *See 2 Pelvic Bone, Right* **4 Acetabulum, Right** **5 Acetabulum, Left** **6 Upper Femur, Right** Femoral head Greater trochanter Lesser trochanter Neck of femur **7 Upper Femur, Left** *See 6 Upper Femur, Right* **8 Femoral Shaft, Right** Body of femur **9 Femoral Shaft, Left** *See 8 Femoral Shaft, Right* **B Lower Femur, Right** Lateral condyle of femur Lateral epicondyle of femur Medial condyle of femur Medial epicondyle of femur **C Lower Femur, Left** *See B Lower Femur, Right* **D Patella, Right** **F Patella, Left** **G Tibia, Right** Lateral condyle of tibia Medial condyle of tibia Medial malleolus **H Tibia, Left** *See G Tibia, Right* **J Fibula, Right** Body of fibula Head of fibula Lateral malleolus **K Fibula, Left** *See J Fibula, Right* **L Tarsal, Right** Calcaneus Cuboid bone Intermediate cuneiform bone Lateral cuneiform bone Medial cuneiform bone Navicular bone Talus bone **M Tarsal, Left** *See L Tarsal, Right* **N Metatarsal, Right** **P Metatarsal, Left** **Q Toe Phalanx, Right** **R Toe Phalanx, Left** **S Coccyx**	**Ø Open** **3 Percutaneous** **4 Percutaneous Endoscopic** **X External**	**Z No Device**	**Z No Qualifier**

Non-OR ØQQ[Ø,1,2,3,4,5,6,7,8,9,B,C,D,F,G,H,J,K,L,M,N,P,Q,R,S]XZZ

Ø Medical and Surgical
Q Lower Bones
R Replacement Definition: Putting in or on biological or synthetic material that physically takes the place and/or function of all or a portion of a body part

Explanation: The body part may have been taken out or replaced, or may be taken out, physically eradicated, or rendered nonfunctional during the REPLACEMENT procedure. A REMOVAL procedure is coded for taking out the device used in a previous replacement procedure.

Body Part Character 4	Approach Character 5	Device Character 6	Qualifier Character 7
Ø Lumbar Vertebra Spinous process Transverse process Vertebral arch Vertebral body Vertebral foramen Vertebral lamina Vertebral pedicle **1 Sacrum** **2 Pelvic Bone, Right** Iliac crest Ilium Ischium Pubis **3 Pelvic Bone, Left** *See 2 Pelvic Bone, Right* **4 Acetabulum, Right** **5 Acetabulum, Left** **6 Upper Femur, Right** Femoral head Greater trochanter Lesser trochanter Neck of femur **7 Upper Femur, Left** *See 6 Upper Femur, Right* **8 Femoral Shaft, Right** Body of femur **9 Femoral Shaft, Left** *See 8 Femoral Shaft, Right* **B Lower Femur, Right** Lateral condyle of femur Lateral epicondyle of femur Medial condyle of femur Medial epicondyle of femur **C Lower Femur, Left** *See B Lower Femur, Right* **D Patella, Right** **F Patella, Left** **G Tibia, Right** Lateral condyle of tibia Medial condyle of tibia Medial malleolus **H Tibia, Left** *See G Tibia, Right* **J Fibula, Right** Body of fibula Head of fibula Lateral malleolus **K Fibula, Left** *See J Fibula, Right* **L Tarsal, Right** Calcaneus Cuboid bone Intermediate cuneiform bone Lateral cuneiform bone Medial cuneiform bone Navicular bone Talus bone **M Tarsal, Left** *See L Tarsal, Right* **N Metatarsal, Right** **P Metatarsal, Left** **Q Toe Phalanx, Right** **R Toe Phalanx, Left** **S Coccyx**	**Ø Open** **3 Percutaneous** **4 Percutaneous Endoscopic**	**7 Autologous Tissue Substitute** **J Synthetic Substitute** **K Nonautologous Tissue Substitute**	**Z No Qualifier**

Ø Medical and Surgical
Q Lower Bones
S Reposition Definition: Moving to its normal location, or other suitable location, all or a portion of a body part

Explanation: The body part is moved to a new location from an abnormal location, or from a normal location where it is not functioning correctly. The body part may or may not be cut out or off to be moved to the new location.

Body Part Character 4	Approach Character 5	Device Character 6	Qualifier Character 7
Ø Lumbar Vertebra ⊞ Spinous process Transverse process Vertebral arch Vertebral body Vertebral foramen Vertebral lamina Vertebral pedicle 1 Sacrum ⊞ 4 Acetabulum, Right 5 Acetabulum, Left S Coccyx ⊞	Ø Open 3 Percutaneous 4 Percutaneous Endoscopic	4 Internal Fixation Device Z No Device	Z No Qualifier
Ø Lumbar Vertebra Spinous process Transverse process Vertebral arch Vertebral body Vertebral foramen Vertebral lamina Vertebral pedicle 1 Sacrum 4 Acetabulum, Right 5 Acetabulum, Left S Coccyx	X External	Z No Device	Z No Qualifier
2 Pelvic Bone, Right Iliac crest Ilium Ischium Pubis 3 Pelvic Bone, Left *See 2 Pelvic Bone, Right* D Patella, Right F Patella, Left L Tarsal, Right Calcaneus Cuboid bone Intermediate cuneiform bone Lateral cuneiform bone Medial cuneiform bone Navicular bone Talus bone M Tarsal, Left *See L Tarsal, Right* Q Toe Phalanx, Right R Toe Phalanx, Left	Ø Open 3 Percutaneous 4 Percutaneous Endoscopic	4 Internal Fixation Device 5 External Fixation Device Z No Device	Z No Qualifier
2 Pelvic Bone, Right Iliac crest Ilium Ischium Pubis 3 Pelvic Bone, Left *See 2 Pelvic Bone, Right* D Patella, Right F Patella, Left L Tarsal, Right Calcaneus Cuboid bone Intermediate cuneiform bone Lateral cuneiform bone Medial cuneiform bone Navicular bone Talus bone M Tarsal, Left *See L Tarsal, Right* Q Toe Phalanx, Right R Toe Phalanx, Left	X External	Z No Device	Z No Qualifier

ØQS Continued on next page

Non-OR ØQS[4,5][3,4]ZZ
Non-OR ØQS[Ø,1,4,5,S]XZZ
Non-OR ØQS[2,3,D,F,L,M,Q,R][3,4]ZZ
Non-OR ØQS[2,3,D,F,L,M,Q,R]XZZ

See Appendix L for Procedure Combinations
⊞ ØQS[Ø,1,S]3ZZ

ØQS Continued

Ø Medical and Surgical
Q Lower Bones
S Reposition Definition: Moving to its normal location, or other suitable location, all or a portion of a body part

Explanation: The body part is moved to a new location from an abnormal location, or from a normal location where it is not functioning correctly. The body part may or may not be cut out or off to be moved to the new location.

Body Part Character 4	Approach Character 5	Device Character 6	Qualifier Character 7
6 Upper Femur, Right Femoral head Greater trochanter Lesser trochanter Neck of femur **7 Upper Femur, Left** *See 6 Upper Femur, Right* **8 Femoral Shaft, Right** Body of femur **9 Femoral Shaft, Left** *See 8 Femoral Shaft, Right* **B Lower Femur, Right** Lateral condyle of femur Lateral epicondyle of femur Medial condyle of femur Medial epicondyle of femur **C Lower Femur, Left** *See B Lower Femur, Right* **G Tibia, Right** Lateral condyle of tibia Medial condyle of tibia Medial malleolus **H Tibia, Left** *See G Tibia, Right* **J Fibula, Right** Body of fibula Head of fibula Lateral malleolus **K Fibula, Left** *See J Fibula, Right*	**Ø Open** **3 Percutaneous** **4 Percutaneous Endoscopic**	**4 Internal Fixation Device** **5 External Fixation Device** **6 Internal Fixation Device, Intramedullary** **B External Fixation Device, Monoplanar** **C External Fixation Device, Ring** **D External Fixation Device, Hybrid** **Z No Device**	**Z No Qualifier**
6 Upper Femur, Right Femoral head Greater trochanter Lesser trochanter Neck of femur **7 Upper Femur, Left** *See 6 Upper Femur, Right* **8 Femoral Shaft, Right** Body of femur **9 Femoral Shaft, Left** *See 8 Femoral Shaft, Right* **B Lower Femur, Right** Lateral condyle of femur Lateral epicondyle of femur Medial condyle of femur Medial epicondyle of femur **C Lower Femur, Left** *See B Lower Femur, Right* **G Tibia, Right** Lateral condyle of tibia Medial condyle of tibia Medial malleolus **H Tibia, Left** *See G Tibia, Right* **J Fibula, Right** Body of fibula Head of fibula Lateral malleolus **K Fibula, Left** *See J Fibula, Right*	**X External**	**Z No Device**	**Z No Qualifier**
N Metatarsal, Right **P Metatarsal, Left**	**Ø Open** **3 Percutaneous** **4 Percutaneous Endoscopic**	**4 Internal Fixation Device** **5 External Fixation Device** **Z No Device**	**2 Sesamoid Bone(s) 1st Toe** **Z No Qualifier**
N Metatarsal, Right **P Metatarsal, Left**	**X External**	**Z No Device**	**2 Sesamoid Bone(s) 1st Toe** **Z No Qualifier**

Non-OR ØQS[6,7,8,9,B,C,G,H,J,K][3,4]ZZ
Non-OR ØQS[6,7,8,9,B,C,G,H,J,K]XZZ
Non-OR ØQS[N,P][3,4]Z[2,Z]
Non-OR ØQS[N,P]XZ[2,Z]

Ø Medical and Surgical
Q Lower Bones
T Resection Definition: Cutting out or off, without replacement, all of a body part
Explanation: None

Body Part Character 4	Body Part Character 4	Approach Character 5	Device Character 6	Qualifier Character 7
2 Pelvic Bone, Right Iliac crest Ilium Ischium Pubis **3 Pelvic Bone, Left** *See 2 Pelvic Bone, Right* **4 Acetabulum, Right** **5 Acetabulum, Left** **6 Upper Femur, Right** Femoral head Greater trochanter Lesser trochanter Neck of femur **7 Upper Femur, Left** *See 6 Upper Femur, Right* **8 Femoral Shaft, Right** Body of femur **9 Femoral Shaft, Left** *See 8 Femoral Shaft, Right* **B Lower Femur, Right** Lateral condyle of femur Lateral epicondyle of femur Medial condyle of femur Medial epicondyle of femur **C Lower Femur, Left** *See B Lower Femur, Right* **D Patella, Right**	**F Patella, Left** **G Tibia, Right** Lateral condyle of tibia Medial condyle of tibia Medial malleolus **H Tibia, Left** *See G Tibia, Right* **J Fibula, Right** Body of fibula Head of fibula Lateral malleolus **K Fibula, Left** *See J Fibula, Right* **L Tarsal, Right** Calcaneus Cuboid bone Intermediate cuneiform bone Lateral cuneiform bone Medial cuneiform bone Navicular bone Talus bone **M Tarsal, Left** *See L Tarsal, Right* **N Metatarsal, Right** **P Metatarsal, Left** **Q Toe Phalanx, Right** **R Toe Phalanx, Left** **S Coccyx**	**Ø Open**	**Z No Device**	**Z No Qualifier**

Ø Medical and Surgical
Q Lower Bones
U Supplement Definition: Putting in or on biological or synthetic material that physically reinforces and/or augments the function of a portion of a body part
Explanation: The biological material is non-living, or is living and from the same individual. The body part may have been previously replaced, and the SUPPLEMENT procedure is performed to physically reinforce and/or augment the function of the replaced body part.

Body Part Character 4	Body Part Character 4	Approach Character 5	Device Character 6	Qualifier Character 7
Ø Lumbar Vertebra ⊞ Spinous process Transverse process Vertebral arch Vertebral body Vertebral foramen Vertebral lamina Vertebral pedicle **1 Sacrum** ⊞ **2 Pelvic Bone, Right** Iliac crest Ilium Ischium Pubis **3 Pelvic Bone, Left** *See 2 Pelvic Bone, Right* **4 Acetabulum, Right** **5 Acetabulum, Left** **6 Upper Femur, Right** Femoral head Greater trochanter Lesser trochanter Neck of femur **7 Upper Femur, Left** *See 6 Upper Femur, Right* **8 Femoral Shaft, Right** Body of femur **9 Femoral Shaft, Left** *See 8 Femoral Shaft, Right* **B Lower Femur, Right** Lateral condyle of femur Lateral epicondyle of femur Medial condyle of femur Medial epicondyle of femur	**C Lower Femur, Left** *See B Lower Femur, Right* **D Patella, Right** **F Patella, Left** **G Tibia, Right** Lateral condyle of tibia Medial condyle of tibia Medial malleolus **H Tibia, Left** *See G Tibia, Right* **J Fibula, Right** Body of fibula Head of fibula Lateral malleolus **K Fibula, Left** *See J Fibula, Right* **L Tarsal, Right** Calcaneus Cuboid bone Intermediate cuneiform bone Lateral cuneiform bone Medial cuneiform bone Navicular bone Talus bone **M Tarsal, Left** *See L Tarsal, Right* **N Metatarsal, Right** **P Metatarsal, Left** **Q Toe Phalanx, Right** **R Toe Phalanx, Left** **S Coccyx** ⊞	**Ø Open** **3 Percutaneous** **4 Percutaneous Endoscopic**	**7 Autologous Tissue Substitute** **J Synthetic Substitute** **K Nonautologous Tissue Substitute**	**Z No Qualifier**

See Appendix L for Procedure Combinations
⊞ ØQU[Ø,1,S]3JZ

Ø Medical and Surgical
Q Lower Bones
W Revision Definition: Correcting, to the extent possible, a portion of a malfunctioning device or the position of a displaced device
Explanation: Revision can include correcting a malfunctioning or displaced device by taking out or putting in components of the device such as a screw or pin

Body Part Character 4	Approach Character 5	Device Character 6	Qualifier Character 7
Ø Lumbar Vertebra Spinous process Transverse process Vertebral arch Vertebral body Vertebral foramen Vertebral lamina Vertebral pedicle **1 Sacrum** **4 Acetabulum, Right** **5 Acetabulum, Left** **S Coccyx**	**Ø Open** **3 Percutaneous** **4 Percutaneous Endoscopic** **X External**	**4 Internal Fixation Device** **7 Autologous Tissue Substitute** **J Synthetic Substitute** **K Nonautologous Tissue Substitute**	**Z No Qualifier**
2 Pelvic Bone, Right Iliac crest Ilium Ischium Pubis **3 Pelvic Bone, Left** *See 2 Pelvic Bone, Right* **6 Upper Femur, Right** Femoral head Greater trochanter Lesser trochanter Neck of femur **7 Upper Femur, Left** *See 6 Upper Femur, Right* **8 Femoral Shaft, Right** Body of femur **9 Femoral Shaft, Left** *See 8 Femoral Shaft, Right* **B Lower Femur, Right** Lateral condyle of femur Lateral epicondyle of femur Medial condyle of femur Medial epicondyle of femur **C Lower Femur, Left** *See B Lower Femur, Right* **D Patella, Right** **F Patella, Left** **G Tibia, Right** Lateral condyle of tibia Medial condyle of tibia Medial malleolus **H Tibia, Left** *See G Tibia, Right* **J Fibula, Right** Body of fibula Head of fibula Lateral malleolus **K Fibula, Left** *See J Fibula, Right* **L Tarsal, Right** Calcaneus Cuboid bone Intermediate cuneiform bone Lateral cuneiform bone Medial cuneiform bone Navicular bone Talus bone **M Tarsal, Left** *See L Tarsal, Right* **N Metatarsal, Right** **P Metatarsal, Left** **Q Toe Phalanx, Right** **R Toe Phalanx, Left**	**Ø Open** **3 Percutaneous** **4 Percutaneous Endoscopic** **X External**	**4 Internal Fixation Device** **5 External Fixation Device** **7 Autologous Tissue Substitute** **J Synthetic Substitute** **K Nonautologous Tissue Substitute**	**Z No Qualifier**
Y Lower Bone	**Ø Open** **3 Percutaneous** **4 Percutaneous Endoscopic** **X External**	**Ø Drainage Device** **M Bone Growth Stimulator**	**Z No Qualifier**

Non-OR ØQW[Ø,1,4,5,S]X[4,7,J,K]Z
Non-OR ØQW[2,3,6,7,8,9,B,C,D,F,G,H,J,K,L,M,N,P,Q,R]X[4,5,7,J,K]Z
Non-OR ØQWYX[Ø,M]Z

Upper Joints ØR2–ØRW

Character Meanings*

This Character Meaning table is provided as a guide to assist the user in the identification of character members that may be found in this section of code tables. It **SHOULD NOT** be used to build a PCS code.

Operation–Character 3	Body Part–Character 4	Approach–Character 5	Device–Character 6	Qualifier–Character 7
2 Change	Ø Occipital-cervical Joint	Ø Open	Ø Drainage Device OR Synthetic Substitute, Reverse Ball and Socket	Ø Anterior Approach, Anterior Column
5 Destruction	1 Cervical Vertebral Joint	3 Percutaneous	3 Infusion Device	1 Posterior Approach, Posterior Column
9 Drainage	2 Cervical Vertebral Joint, 2 or more	4 Percutaneous Endoscopic	4 Internal Fixation Device	6 Humeral Surface
B Excision	3 Cervical Vertebral Disc	X External	5 External Fixation Device	7 Glenoid Surface
C Extirpation	4 Cervicothoracic Vertebral Joint		7 Autologous Tissue Substitute	J Posterior Approach, Anterior Column
G Fusion	5 Cervicothoracic Vertebral Disc		8 Spacer	X Diagnostic
H Insertion	6 Thoracic Vertebral Joint		A Interbody Fusion Device	Z No Qualifier
J Inspection	7 Thoracic Vertebral Joint, 2 to 7		B Spinal Stabilization Device, Interspinous Process	
N Release	8 Thoracic Vertebral Joint, 8 or more		C Spinal Stabilization Device, Pedicle-Based	
P Removal	9 Thoracic Vertebral Disc		D Spinal Stabilization Device, Facet Replacement	
Q Repair	A Thoracolumbar Vertebral Joint		J Synthetic Substitute	
R Replacement	B Thoracolumbar Vertebral Disc		K Nonautologous Tissue Substitute	
S Reposition	C Temporomandibular Joint, Right		Y Other Device	
T Resection	D Temporomandibular Joint, Left		Z No Device	
U Supplement	E Sternoclavicular Joint, Right			
W Revision	F Sternoclavicular Joint, Left			
	G Acromioclavicular Joint, Right			
	H Acromioclavicular Joint, Left			
	J Shoulder Joint, Right			
	K Shoulder Joint, Left			
	L Elbow Joint, Right			
	M Elbow Joint, Left			
	N Wrist Joint, Right			
	P Wrist Joint, Left			
	Q Carpal Joint, Right			
	R Carpal Joint, Left			
	S Carpometacarpal Joint, Right			
	T Carpometacarpal Joint, Left			
	U Metacarpophalangeal Joint, Right			
	V Metacarpophalangeal Joint, Left			
	W Finger Phalangeal Joint, Right			
	X Finger Phalangeal Joint, Left			
	Y Upper Joint			

* Includes synovial membrane.

AHA Coding Clinic for table ØRG
2018, 1Q, 22 Spinal fusion procedures without bone graft
2017, 4Q, 62 Added and revised device values - Nerve substitutes
2017, 4Q, 76 Radiolucent porous interbody fusion device
2017, 2Q, 23 Decompression of spinal cord and placement of instrumentation
2014, 3Q, 30 Spinal fusion and fixation instrumentation
2014, 2Q, 7 Anterior cervical thoracic fusion with total discectomy
2013, 1Q, 21-23 Spinal fusion of thoracic and lumbar vertebrae
2013, 1Q, 29 Cervical and thoracic spinal fusion

AHA Coding Clinic for table ØRH
2017, 2Q, 23 Decompression of spinal cord and placement of instrumentation
2016, 3Q, 32 Rotator cuff repair, tenodesis, decompression, acromioplasty and coracoplasty

AHA Coding Clinic for table ØRN
2016, 3Q, 32 Rotator cuff repair, tenodesis, decompression, acromioplasty and coracoplasty
2015, 2Q, 22 Arthroscopic subacromial decompression
2015, 2Q, 23 Arthroscopic release of shoulder joint

AHA Coding Clinic for table ØRP
2017, 4Q, 107 Total ankle replacement versus revision

AHA Coding Clinic for table ØRQ
2016, 1Q, 30 Thermal capsulorrhapy of shoulder

AHA Coding Clinic for table ØRR
2017, 4Q, 107 Total ankle replacement versus revision
2015, 3Q, 14 Endoprosthetic replacement of humerus and tendon reattachment
2015, 1Q, 27 Reverse total shoulder arthroplasty

AHA Coding Clinic for table ØRS
2015, 2Q, 35 Application of tongs to reduce and stabilize cervical fracture
2014, 4Q, 32 Open reduction internal fixation of fracture with debridement
2014, 3Q, 33 Radial fracture treatment with open reduction internal fixation, and release of carpal ligament
2013, 2Q, 39 Application of cervical tongs for reduction of cervical fracture

AHA Coding Clinic for table ØRT
2014, 2Q, 7 Anterior cervical thoracic fusion with total discectomy

AHA Coding Clinic for table ØRU
2015, 3Q, 26 Thumb arthroplasty with resection of trapezium

AHA Coding Clinic for table ØRW
2017, 4Q, 107 Total ankle replacement versus revision

Upper Joints

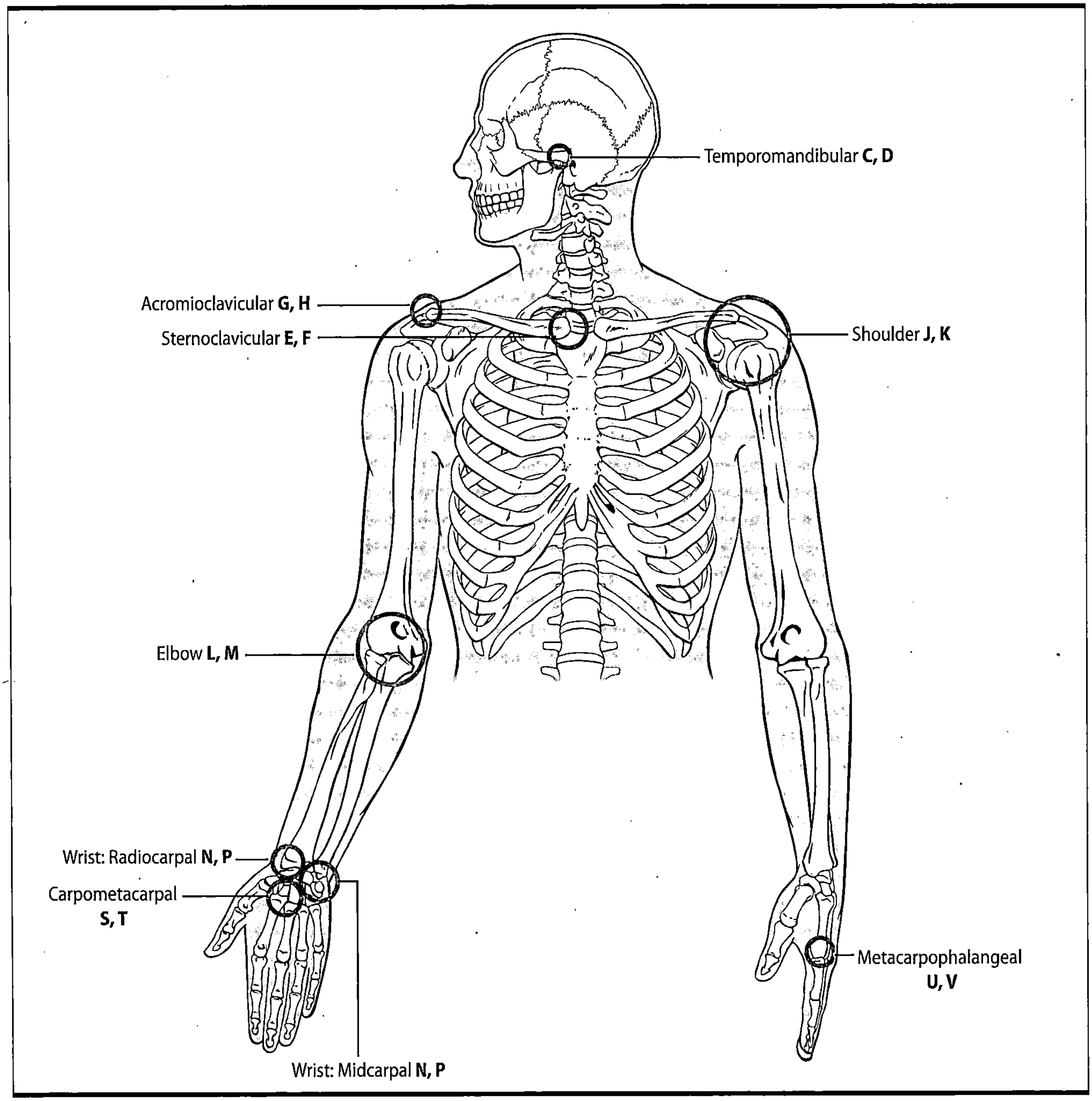

Hand Joints

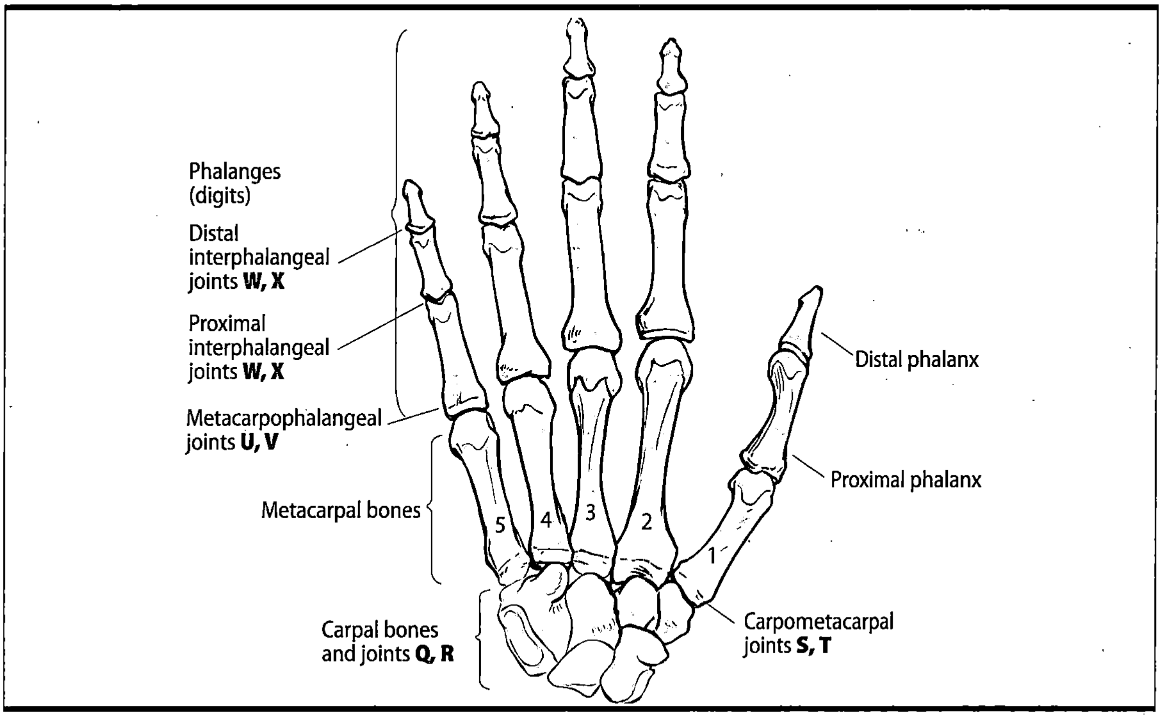
Phalanges (digits)
Distal interphalangeal joints **W, X**
Proximal interphalangeal joints **W, X**
Metacarpophalangeal joints **U, V**
Metacarpal bones
Carpal bones and joints **Q, R**
Distal phalanx
Proximal phalanx
Carpometacarpal joints **S, T**
5
4
3
2
1

Shoulder Joints

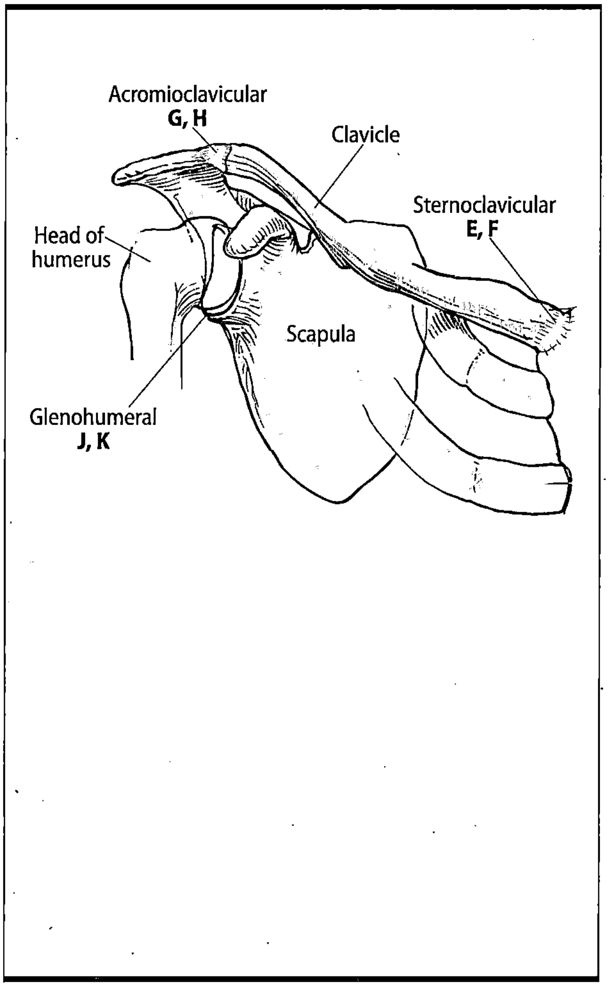
Acromioclavicular **G, H**
Clavicle
Sternoclavicular **E, F**
Head of humerus
Scapula
Glenohumeral **J, K**

Upper Vertebral Joints

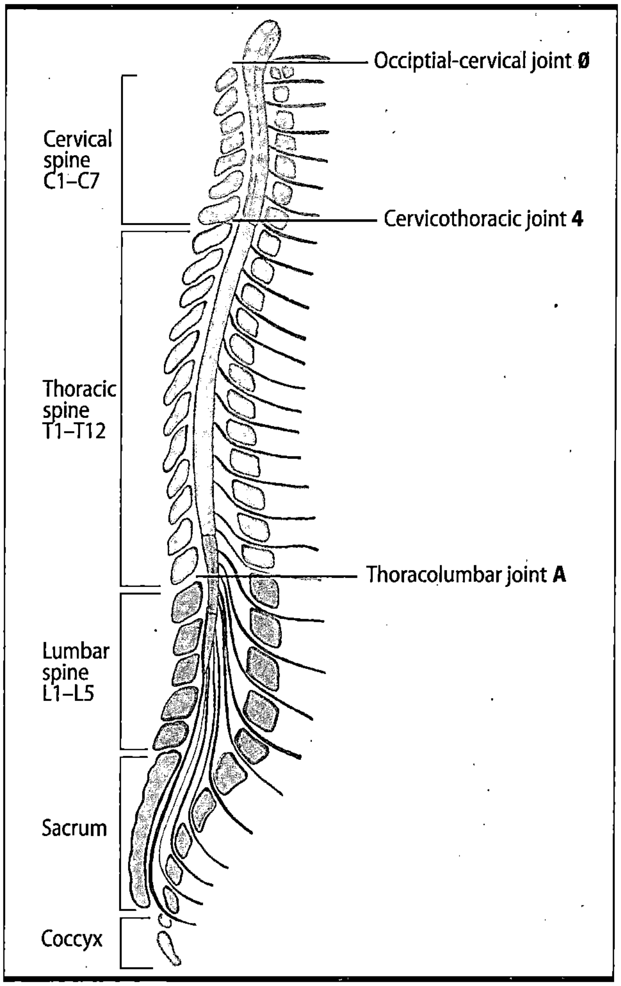
Occiptial-cervical joint **Ø**
Cervical spine C1–C7
Cervicothoracic joint **4**
Thoracic spine T1–T12
Thoracolumbar joint **A**
Lumbar spine L1–L5
Sacrum
Coccyx

Ø Medical and Surgical
R Upper Joints
2 Change Definition: Taking out or off a device from a body part and putting back an identical or similar device in or on the same body part without cutting or puncturing the skin or a mucous membrane

Explanation: All CHANGE procedures are coded using the approach EXTERNAL

Body Part Character 4	Approach Character 5	Device Character 6	Qualifier Character 7
Y Upper Joint	X External	Ø Drainage Device Y Other Device	Z No Qualifier

Non-OR All body part, approach, device, and qualifier values

Ø Medical and Surgical
R Upper Joints
5 Destruction Definition: Physical eradication of all or a portion of a body part by the direct use of energy, force, or a destructive agent

Explanation: None of the body part is physically taken out

Body Part Character 4	Approach Character 5	Device Character 6	Qualifier Character 7
Ø Occipital-cervical Joint 1 Cervical Vertebral Joint Atlantoaxial joint Cervical facet joint 3 Cervical Vertebral Disc 4 Cervicothoracic Vertebral Joint Cervicothoracic facet joint 5 Cervicothoracic Vertebral Disc 6 Thoracic Vertebral Joint Costotransverse joint Costovertebral joint Thoracic facet joint 9 Thoracic Vertebral Disc A Thoracolumbar Vertebral Joint Thoracolumbar facet joint B Thoracolumbar Vertebral Disc C Temporomandibular Joint, Right D Temporomandibular Joint, Left E Sternoclavicular Joint, Right F Sternoclavicular Joint, Left G Acromioclavicular Joint, Right H Acromioclavicular Joint, Left J Shoulder Joint, Right Glenohumeral joint Glenoid ligament (labrum) K Shoulder Joint, Left *See J Shoulder Joint, Right* L Elbow Joint, Right Distal humerus, involving joint Humeroradial joint Humeroulnar joint Proximal radioulnar joint M Elbow Joint, Left *See L Elbow Joint, Right* N Wrist Joint, Right Distal radioulnar joint Radiocarpal joint P Wrist Joint, Left *See N Wrist Joint, Right* Q Carpal Joint, Right Intercarpal joint Midcarpal joint R Carpal Joint, Left *See Q Carpal Joint, Right* S Carpometacarpal Joint, Right T Carpometacarpal Joint, Left U Metacarpophalangeal Joint, Right V Metacarpophalangeal Joint, Left W Finger Phalangeal Joint, Right Interphalangeal (IP) joint X Finger Phalangeal Joint, Left *See W Finger Phalangeal Joint, Right*	Ø Open 3 Percutaneous 4 Percutaneous Endoscopic	Z No Device	Z No Qualifier

Non-OR ØR5[3,5,9,B][3,4]ZZ

Ø Medical and Surgical
R Upper Joints
9 Drainage Definition: Taking or letting out fluids and/or gases from a body part
Explanation: The qualifier DIAGNOSTIC is used to identify drainage procedures that are biopsies

Body Part Character 4	Approach Character 5	Device Character 6	Qualifier Character 7
Ø Occipital-cervical Joint **1 Cervical Vertebral Joint** Atlantoaxial joint Cervical facet joint **3 Cervical Vertebral Disc** **4 Cervicothoracic Vertebral Joint** Cervicothoracic facet joint **5 Cervicothoracic Vertebral Disc** **6 Thoracic Vertebral Joint** Costotransverse joint Costovertebral joint Thoracic facet joint **9 Thoracic Vertebral Disc** **A Thoracolumbar Vertebral Joint** Thoracolumbar facet joint **B Thoracolumbar Vertebral Disc** **C Temporomandibular Joint, Right** **D Temporomandibular Joint, Left** **E Sternoclavicular Joint, Right** **F Sternoclavicular Joint, Left** **G Acromioclavicular Joint, Right** **H Acromioclavicular Joint, Left** **J Shoulder Joint, Right** Glenohumeral joint Glenoid ligament (labrum) **K Shoulder Joint, Left** *See J Shoulder Joint, Right* **L Elbow Joint, Right** Distal humerus, involving joint Humeroradial joint Humeroulnar joint Proximal radioulnar joint **M Elbow Joint, Left** *See L Elbow Joint, Right* **N Wrist Joint, Right** Distal radioulnar joint Radiocarpal joint **P Wrist Joint, Left** *See N Wrist Joint, Right* **Q Carpal Joint, Right** Intercarpal joint Midcarpal joint **R Carpal Joint, Left** *See Q Carpal Joint, Right* **S Carpometacarpal Joint, Right** **T Carpometacarpal Joint, Left** **U Metacarpophalangeal Joint, Right** **V Metacarpophalangeal Joint, Left** **W Finger Phalangeal Joint, Right** Interphalangeal (IP) joint **X Finger Phalangeal Joint, Left** *See W Finger Phalangeal Joint, Right*	**Ø Open** **3 Percutaneous** **4 Percutaneous Endoscopic**	**Ø Drainage Device**	**Z No Qualifier**
Ø Occipital-cervical Joint **1 Cervical Vertebral Joint** Atlantoaxial joint Cervical facet joint **3 Cervical Vertebral Disc** **4 Cervicothoracic Vertebral Joint** Cervicothoracic facet joint **5 Cervicothoracic Vertebral Disc** **6 Thoracic Vertebral Joint** Costotransverse joint Costovertebral joint Thoracic facet joint **9 Thoracic Vertebral Disc** **A Thoracolumbar Vertebral Joint** Thoracolumbar facet joint **B Thoracolumbar Vertebral Disc** **C Temporomandibular Joint, Right** **D Temporomandibular Joint, Left** **E Sternoclavicular Joint, Right** **F Sternoclavicular Joint, Left** **G Acromioclavicular Joint, Right** **H Acromioclavicular Joint, Left** **J Shoulder Joint, Right** Glenohumeral joint Glenoid ligament (labrum) **K Shoulder Joint, Left** *See J Shoulder Joint, Right* **L Elbow Joint, Right** Distal humerus, involving joint Humeroradial joint Humeroulnar joint Proximal radioulnar joint **M Elbow Joint, Left** *See L Elbow Joint, Right* **N Wrist Joint, Right** Distal radioulnar joint Radiocarpal joint **P Wrist Joint, Left** *See N Wrist Joint, Right* **Q Carpal Joint, Right** Intercarpal joint Midcarpal joint **R Carpal Joint, Left** *See Q Carpal Joint, Right* **S Carpometacarpal Joint, Right** **T Carpometacarpal Joint, Left** **U Metacarpophalangeal Joint, Right** **V Metacarpophalangeal Joint, Left** **W Finger Phalangeal Joint, Right** Interphalangeal (IP) joint **X Finger Phalangeal Joint, Left** *See W Finger Phalangeal Joint, Right*	**Ø Open** **3 Percutaneous** **4 Percutaneous Endoscopic**	**Z No Device**	**X Diagnostic** **Z No Qualifier**

Non-OR ØR9[Ø,1,3,4,5,6,9,A,B,E,F,G,H,J,K,L,M,N,P,Q,R,S,T,U,V,W,X][3,4]ØZ
Non-OR ØR9[C,D]3ØZ
Non-OR ØR9[Ø,1,3,4,5,6,9,A,B,E,F,G,H,J,K,L,M,N,P,Q,R,S,T,U,V,W,X][Ø,3,4]ZX
Non-OR ØR9[Ø,1,3,4,5,6,9,A,B,E,F,G,H,J,K,L,M,N,P,Q,R,S,T,U,V,W,X][3,4]ZZ
Non-OR ØR9[C,D]3ZZ

Upper Joints

ØRB–ØRB

Ø Medical and Surgical
R Upper Joints
B Excision Definition: Cutting out or off, without replacement, a portion of a body part
Explanation: The qualifier DIAGNOSTIC is used to identify excision procedures that are biopsies

Body Part Character 4	Approach Character 5	Device Character 6	Qualifier Character 7
Ø Occipital-cervical Joint **1** Cervical Vertebral Joint Atlantoaxial joint Cervical facet joint **3** Cervical Vertebral Disc **4** Cervicothoracic Vertebral Joint Cervicothoracic facet joint **5** Cervicothoracic Vertebral Disc **6** Thoracic Vertebral Joint Costotransverse joint Costovertebral joint Thoracic facet joint **9** Thoracic Vertebral Disc **A** Thoracolumbar Vertebral Joint Thoracolumbar facet joint **B** Thoracolumbar Vertebral Disc **C** Temporomandibular Joint, Right **D** Temporomandibular Joint, Left **E** Sternoclavicular Joint, Right **F** Sternoclavicular Joint, Left **G** Acromioclavicular Joint, Right **H** Acromioclavicular Joint, Left **J** Shoulder Joint, Right Glenohumeral joint Glenoid ligament (labrum) **K** Shoulder Joint, Left *See J Shoulder Joint, Right* **L** Elbow Joint, Right Distal humerus, involving joint Humeroradial joint Humeroulnar joint Proximal radioulnar joint **M** Elbow Joint, Left *See L Elbow Joint, Right* **N** Wrist Joint, Right Distal radioulnar joint Radiocarpal joint **P** Wrist Joint, Left *See N Wrist Joint, Right* **Q** Carpal Joint, Right Intercarpal joint Midcarpal joint **R** Carpal Joint, Left *See Q Carpal Joint, Right* **S** Carpometacarpal Joint, Right **T** Carpometacarpal Joint, Left **U** Metacarpophalangeal Joint, Right **V** Metacarpophalangeal Joint, Left **W** Finger Phalangeal Joint, Right Interphalangeal (IP) joint **X** Finger Phalangeal Joint, Left *See W Finger Phalangeal Joint, Right*	**Ø** Open **3** Percutaneous **4** Percutaneous Endoscopic	**Z** No Device	**X** Diagnostic **Z** No Qualifier

Non-OR ØRB[Ø,1,3,4,5,6,9,A,B,E,F,G,H,J,K,L,M,N,P,Q,R,S,T,U,V,W,X][Ø,3,4]ZX

Ø Medical and Surgical
R Upper Joints
C Extirpation Definition: Taking or cutting out solid matter from a body part

Explanation: The solid matter may be an abnormal byproduct of a biological function or a foreign body; it may be imbedded in a body part or in the lumen of a tubular body part. The solid matter may or may not have been previously broken into pieces.

Body Part Character 4	Approach Character 5	Device Character 6	Qualifier Character 7
Ø Occipital-cervical Joint **1 Cervical Vertebral Joint** Atlantoaxial joint Cervical facet joint **3 Cervical Vertebral Disc** **4 Cervicothoracic Vertebral Joint** Cervicothoracic facet joint **5 Cervicothoracic Vertebral Disc** **6 Thoracic Vertebral Joint** Costotransverse joint Costovertebral joint Thoracic facet joint **9 Thoracic Vertebral Disc** **A Thoracolumbar Vertebral Joint** Thoracolumbar facet joint **B Thoracolumbar Vertebral Disc** **C Temporomandibular Joint, Right** **D Temporomandibular Joint, Left** **E Sternoclavicular Joint, Right** **F Sternoclavicular Joint, Left** **G Acromioclavicular Joint, Right** **H Acromioclavicular Joint, Left** **J Shoulder Joint, Right** Glenohumeral joint Glenoid ligament (labrum) **K Shoulder Joint, Left** *See J Shoulder Joint, Right* **L Elbow Joint, Right** Distal humerus, involving joint Humeroradial joint Humeroulnar joint Proximal radioulnar joint **M Elbow Joint, Left** *See L Elbow Joint, Right* **N Wrist Joint, Right** Distal radioulnar joint Radiocarpal joint **P Wrist Joint, Left** *See N Wrist Joint, Right* **Q Carpal Joint, Right** Intercarpal joint Midcarpal joint **R Carpal Joint, Left** *See Q Carpal Joint, Right* **S Carpometacarpal Joint, Right** **T Carpometacarpal Joint, Left** **U Metacarpophalangeal Joint, Right** **V Metacarpophalangeal Joint, Left** **W Finger Phalangeal Joint, Right** Interphalangeal (IP) joint **X Finger Phalangeal Joint, Left** *See W Finger Phalangeal Joint, Right*	**Ø Open** **3 Percutaneous** **4 Percutaneous Endoscopic**	**Z No Device**	**Z No Qualifier**

Ø Medical and Surgical
R Upper Joints
G Fusion Definition: Joining together portions of an articular body part rendering the articular body part immobile
Explanation: The body part is joined together by fixation device, bone graft, or other means

Body Part Character 4	Approach Character 5	Device Character 6	Qualifier Character 7
Ø Occipital-cervical Joint **1 Cervical Vertebral Joint** Atlantoaxial joint Cervical facet joint **2 Cervical Vertebral Joints, 2 or more** Cervical facet joint **4 Cervicothoracic Vertebral Joint** Cervicothoracic facet joint **6 Thoracic Vertebral Joint** Costotransverse joint Costovertebral joint Thoracic facet joint **7 Thoracic Vertebral Joints, 2 to 7** ⊞ **8 Thoracic Vertebral Joints, 8 or more** **A Thoracolumbar Vertebral Joint** Thoracolumbar facet joint	**Ø Open** **3 Percutaneous** **4 Percutaneous Endoscopic**	**7 Autologous Tissue Substitute** **J Synthetic Substitute** **K Nonautologous Tissue Substitute**	**Ø Anterior Approach, Anterior Column** **1 Posterior Approach, Posterior Column** **J Posterior Approach, Anterior Column**
Ø Occipital-cervical Joint **1 Cervical Vertebral Joint** Atlantoaxial joint Cervical facet joint **2 Cervical Vertebral Joints, 2 or more** Cervical facet joint **4 Cervicothoracic Vertebral Joint** Cervicothoracic facet joint **6 Thoracic Vertebral Joint** Costotransverse joint Costovertebral joint Thoracic facet joint **7 Thoracic Vertebral Joints, 2 to 7** ⊞ **8 Thoracic Vertebral Joints, 8 or more** **A Thoracolumbar Vertebral Joint** Thoracolumbar facet joint	**Ø Open** **3 Percutaneous** **4 Percutaneous Endoscopic**	**A Interbody Fusion Device**	**Ø Anterior Approach, Anterior Column** **J Posterior Approach, Anterior Column**
C Temporomandibular Joint, Right **D Temporomandibular Joint, Left** **E Sternoclavicular Joint, Right** **F Sternoclavicular Joint, Left** **G Acromioclavicular Joint, Right** **H Acromioclavicular Joint, Left** **J Shoulder Joint, Right** Glenohumeral joint Glenoid ligament (labrum) **K Shoulder Joint, Left** *See J Shoulder Joint, Right*	**Ø Open** **3 Percutaneous** **4 Percutaneous Endoscopic**	**4 Internal Fixation Device** **7 Autologous Tissue Substitute** **J Synthetic Substitute** **K Nonautologous Tissue Substitute**	**Z No Qualifier**
L Elbow Joint, Right Distal humerus, involving joint Humeroradial joint Humeroulnar joint Proximal radioulnar joint **M Elbow Joint, Left** *See L Elbow Joint, Right* **N Wrist Joint, Right** Distal radioulnar joint Radiocarpal joint **P Wrist Joint, Left** *See N Wrist Joint, Right* **Q Carpal Joint, Right** Intercarpal joint Midcarpal joint **R Carpal Joint, Left** *See Q Carpal Joint, Right* **S Carpometacarpal Joint, Right** **T Carpometacarpal Joint, Left** **U Metacarpophalangeal Joint, Right** **V Metacarpophalangeal Joint, Left** **W Finger Phalangeal Joint, Right** Interphalangeal (IP) joint **X Finger Phalangeal Joint, Left** *See W Finger Phalangeal Joint, Right*	**Ø Open** **3 Percutaneous** **4 Percutaneous Endoscopic**	**4 Internal Fixation Device** **5 External Fixation Device** **7 Autologous Tissue Substitute** **J Synthetic Substitute** **K Nonautologous Tissue Substitute**	**Z No Qualifier**

HAC ØRG[Ø,1,2,4,6,7,8,A][Ø,3,4][7,J,K][Ø,1,J] when reported with SDx K68.11 or T81.4XXA or T84.6Ø-T84.619, T84.63-T84.7 with 7th character A

HAC ØRG[Ø,1,2,4,6,7,8,A][Ø,3,4]A[Ø,J] when reported with SDx K68.11 or T81.4XXA or T84.6Ø-T84.619, T84.63-T84.7 with 7th character A

HAC ØRG[E,F,G,H,J,K][Ø,3,4][4,7,J,K]Z when reported with SDx K68.11 or T81.4XXA or T84.6Ø-T84.619, T84.63-T84.7 with 7th character A

HAC ØRG[L,M][Ø,3,4][4,5,7,J,K]Z when reported with SDx K68.11 or T81.4XXA or T84.6Ø-T84.619, T84.63-T84.7 with 7th character A

See Appendix L for Procedure Combinations

⊞ ØRG7[Ø,3,4][7,J,K][Ø,1,J]

⊞ ØRG7[Ø,3,4]A[Ø,J]

Ø Medical and Surgical
R Upper Joints
H Insertion Definition: Putting in a nonbiological appliance that monitors, assists, performs, or prevents a physiological function but does not physically take the place of a body part

Explanation: None

Body Part Character 4	Approach Character 5	Device Character 6	Qualifier Character 7
Ø Occipital-cervical Joint **1** Cervical Vertebral Joint Atlantoaxial joint Cervical facet joint **4** Cervicothoracic Vertebral Joint Cervicothoracic facet joint **6** Thoracic Vertebral Joint Costotransverse joint Costovertebral joint Thoracic facet joint **A** Thoracolumbar Vertebral Joint Thoracolumbar facet joint	**Ø** Open **3** Percutaneous **4** Percutaneous Endoscopic	**3** Infusion Device **4** Internal Fixation Device **8** Spacer **B** Spinal Stabilization Device, Interspinous Process **C** Spinal Stabilization Device, Pedicle-Based **D** Spinal Stabilization Device, Facet Replacement	**Z** No Qualifier
3 Cervical Vertebral Disc **5** Cervicothoracic Vertebral Disc **9** Thoracic Vertebral Disc **B** Thoracolumbar Vertebral Disc	**Ø** Open **3** Percutaneous **4** Percutaneous Endoscopic	**3** Infusion Device	**Z** No Qualifier
C Temporomandibular Joint, Right **D** Temporomandibular Joint, Left **E** Sternoclavicular Joint, Right **F** Sternoclavicular Joint, Left **G** Acromioclavicular Joint, Right **H** Acromioclavicular Joint, Left **J** Shoulder Joint, Right Glenohumeral joint Glenoid ligament (labrum) **K** Shoulder Joint, Left *See J Shoulder Joint, Right*	**Ø** Open **3** Percutaneous **4** Percutaneous Endoscopic	**3** Infusion Device **4** Internal Fixation Device **8** Spacer	**Z** No Qualifier
L Elbow Joint, Right Distal humerus, involving joint Humeroradial joint Humeroulnar joint Proximal radioulnar joint **M** Elbow Joint, Left *See L Elbow Joint, Right* **N** Wrist Joint, Right Distal radioulnar joint Radiocarpal joint **P** Wrist Joint, Left *See N Wrist Joint, Right* **Q** Carpal Joint, Right Intercarpal joint Midcarpal joint **R** Carpal Joint, Left *See Q Carpal Joint, Right* **S** Carpometacarpal Joint, Right **T** Carpometacarpal Joint, Left **U** Metacarpophalangeal Joint, Right **V** Metacarpophalangeal Joint, Left **W** Finger Phalangeal Joint, Right Interphalangeal (IP) joint **X** Finger Phalangeal Joint, Left *See W Finger Phalangeal Joint, Right*	**Ø** Open **3** Percutaneous **4** Percutaneous Endoscopic	**3** Infusion Device **4** Internal Fixation Device **5** External Fixation Device **8** Spacer	**Z** No Qualifier

Non-OR ØRH[Ø,1,4,6,A][Ø,3,4][3,8]Z
Non-OR ØRH[3,5,9,B][Ø,3,4]3Z
Non-OR ØRH[C,D][Ø,4]8Z
Non-OR ØRH[C,D]3[3,8]Z
Non-OR ØRH[E,F,G,H,J,K][Ø,3,4][3,8]Z
Non-OR ØRH[L,M,N,P,Q,R,S,T,U,V,W,X][Ø,3,4][3,8]Z

Ø Medical and Surgical
R Upper Joints
J Inspection Definition: Visually and/or manually exploring a body part

Explanation: Visual exploration may be performed with or without optical instrumentation. Manual exploration may be performed directly or through intervening body layers.

Body Part Character 4	Approach Character 5	Device Character 6	Qualifier Character 7
Ø Occipital-cervical Joint 1 Cervical Vertebral Joint Atlantoaxial joint Cervical facet joint 3 Cervical Vertebral Disc 4 Cervicothoracic Vertebral Joint Cervicothoracic facet joint 5 Cervicothoracic Vertebral Disc 6 Thoracic Vertebral Joint Costotransverse joint Costovertebral joint Thoracic facet joint 9 Thoracic Vertebral Disc A Thoracolumbar Vertebral Joint Thoracolumbar facet joint B Thoracolumbar Vertebral Disc C Temporomandibular Joint, Right D Temporomandibular Joint, Left E Sternoclavicular Joint, Right F Sternoclavicular Joint, Left G Acromioclavicular Joint, Right H Acromioclavicular Joint, Left J Shoulder Joint, Right Glenohumeral joint Glenoid ligament (labrum) K Shoulder Joint, Left *See J Shoulder Joint, Right* L Elbow Joint, Right Distal humerus, involving joint Humeroradial joint Humeroulnar joint Proximal radioulnar joint M Elbow Joint, Left *See L Elbow Joint, Right* N Wrist Joint, Right Distal radioulnar joint Radiocarpal joint P Wrist Joint, Left *See N Wrist Joint, Right* Q Carpal Joint, Right Intercarpal joint Midcarpal joint R Carpal Joint, Left *See Q Carpal Joint, Right* S Carpometacarpal Joint, Right T Carpometacarpal Joint, Left U Metacarpophalangeal Joint, Right V Metacarpophalangeal Joint, Left W Finger Phalangeal Joint, Right Interphalangeal (IP) joint X Finger Phalangeal Joint, Left *See W Finger Phalangeal Joint, Right*	Ø Open 3 Percutaneous 4 Percutaneous Endoscopic X External	Z No Device	Z No Qualifier

Non-OR ØRJ[Ø,1,3,4,5,6,9,A,B,C,D,E,F,G,H,J,K,L,M,N,P,Q,R,S,T,U,V,W,X][3,X]ZZ

Ø Medical and Surgical
R Upper Joints
N Release Definition: Freeing a body part from an abnormal physical constraint by cutting or by the use of force
Explanation: Some of the restraining tissue may be taken out but none of the body part is taken out

Body Part Character 4	Approach Character 5	Device Character 6	Qualifier Character 7
Ø Occipital-cervical Joint **1** Cervical Vertebral Joint Atlantoaxial joint Cervical facet joint **3** Cervical Vertebral Disc **4** Cervicothoracic Vertebral Joint Cervicothoracic facet joint **5** Cervicothoracic Vertebral Disc **6** Thoracic Vertebral Joint Costotransverse joint Costovertebral joint Thoracic facet joint **9** Thoracic Vertebral Disc **A** Thoracolumbar Vertebral Joint Thoracolumbar facet joint **B** Thoracolumbar Vertebral Disc **C** Temporomandibular Joint, Right **D** Temporomandibular Joint, Left **E** Sternoclavicular Joint, Right **F** Sternoclavicular Joint, Left **G** Acromioclavicular Joint, Right **H** Acromioclavicular Joint, Left **J** Shoulder Joint, Right Glenohumeral joint Glenoid ligament (labrum) **K** Shoulder Joint, Left *See J Shoulder Joint, Right* **L** Elbow Joint, Right Distal humerus, involving joint Humeroradial joint Humeroulnar joint Proximal radioulnar joint **M** Elbow Joint, Left *See L Elbow Joint, Right* **N** Wrist Joint, Right Distal radioulnar joint Radiocarpal joint **P** Wrist Joint, Left *See N Wrist Joint, Right* **Q** Carpal Joint, Right Intercarpal joint Midcarpal joint **R** Carpal Joint, Left *See Q Carpal Joint, Right* **S** Carpometacarpal Joint, Right **T** Carpometacarpal Joint, Left **U** Metacarpophalangeal Joint, Right **V** Metacarpophalangeal Joint, Left **W** Finger Phalangeal Joint, Right Interphalangeal (IP) joint **X** Finger Phalangeal Joint, Left *See W Finger Phalangeal Joint, Right*	**Ø** Open **3** Percutaneous **4** Percutaneous Endoscopic **X** External	**Z** No Device	**Z** No Qualifier

Non-OR ØRN[Ø,1,3,4,5,6,9,A,B,C,D,E,F,G,H,J,K,L,M,N,P,Q,R,S,T,U,V,W,X]XZZ

Ø Medical and Surgical
R Upper Joints
P Removal Definition: Taking out or off a device from a body part

Explanation: If a device is taken out and a similar device put in without cutting or puncturing the skin or mucous membrane, the procedure is coded to the root operation CHANGE. Otherwise, the procedure for taking out the device is coded to the root operation REMOVAL.

Body Part Character 4	Approach Character 5	Device Character 6	Qualifier Character 7
Ø Occipital-cervical Joint **1** Cervical Vertebral Joint Atlantoaxial joint Cervical facet joint **4** Cervicothoracic Vertebral Joint Cervicothoracic facet joint **6** Thoracic Vertebral Joint Costotransverse joint Costovertebral joint Thoracic facet joint **A** Thoracolumbar Vertebral Joint Thoracolumbar facet joint	**Ø** Open **3** Percutaneous **4** Percutaneous Endoscopic	**Ø** Drainage Device **3** Infusion Device **4** Internal Fixation Device **7** Autologous Tissue Substitute **8** Spacer **A** Interbody Fusion Device **J** Synthetic Substitute **K** Nonautologous Tissue Substitute	**Z** No Qualifier
Ø Occipital-cervical Joint **1** Cervical Vertebral Joint Atlantoaxial joint Cervical facet joint **4** Cervicothoracic Vertebral Joint Cervicothoracic facet joint **6** Thoracic Vertebral Joint Costotransverse joint Costovertebral joint Thoracic facet joint **A** Thoracolumbar Vertebral Joint Thoracolumbar facet joint	**X** External	**Ø** Drainage Device **3** Infusion Device **4** Internal Fixation Device	**Z** No Qualifier
3 Cervical Vertebral Disc **5** Cervicothoracic Vertebral Disc **9** Thoracic Vertebral Disc **B** Thoracolumbar Vertebral Disc	**Ø** Open **3** Percutaneous **4** Percutaneous Endoscopic	**Ø** Drainage Device **3** Infusion Device **7** Autologous Tissue Substitute **J** Synthetic Substitute **K** Nonautologous Tissue Substitute	**Z** No Qualifier
3 Cervical Vertebral Disc **5** Cervicothoracic Vertebral Disc **9** Thoracic Vertebral Disc **B** Thoracolumbar Vertebral Disc	**X** External	**Ø** Drainage Device **3** Infusion Device	**Z** No Qualifier
C Temporomandibular Joint, Right **D** Temporomandibular Joint, Left **E** Sternoclavicular Joint, Right **F** Sternoclavicular Joint, Left **G** Acromioclavicular Joint, Right **H** Acromioclavicular Joint, Left **J** Shoulder Joint, Right Glenohumeral joint Glenoid ligament (labrum) **K** Shoulder Joint, Left *See J Shoulder Joint, Right*	**Ø** Open **3** Percutaneous **4** Percutaneous Endoscopic	**Ø** Drainage Device **3** Infusion Device **4** Internal Fixation Device **7** Autologous Tissue Substitute **8** Spacer **J** Synthetic Substitute **K** Nonautologous Tissue Substitute	**Z** No Qualifier
C Temporomandibular Joint, Right **D** Temporomandibular Joint, Left **E** Sternoclavicular Joint, Right **F** Sternoclavicular Joint, Left **G** Acromioclavicular Joint, Right **H** Acromioclavicular Joint, Left **J** Shoulder Joint, Right Glenohumeral joint Glenoid ligament (labrum) **K** Shoulder Joint, Left *See J Shoulder Joint, Right*	**X** External	**Ø** Drainage Device **3** Infusion Device **4** Internal Fixation Device	**Z** No Qualifier

ØRP Continued on next page

Non-OR ØRP[Ø,1,4,6,A]3[Ø,3,8]Z
Non-OR ØRP[Ø,1,4,6,A][Ø,4]8Z
Non-OR ØRP[Ø,1,4,6,A]X[Ø,3,4]Z
Non-OR ØRP[3,5,9,B]3[Ø,3]Z
Non-OR ØRP[3,5,9,B]X[Ø,3]Z
Non-OR ØRP[C,D,E,F,G,H,J,K]3[Ø,3,8]Z
Non-OR ØRP[C,D,E,F,G,H,J,K][Ø,4]8Z
Non-OR ØRP[C,D]X[Ø,3]Z
Non-OR ØRP[E,F,G,H,J,K]X[Ø,3,4]Z

Ø Medical and Surgical
R Upper Joints
P Removal Definition: Taking out or off a device from a body part

Explanation: If a device is taken out and a similar device put in without cutting or puncturing the skin or mucous membrane, the procedure is coded to the root operation CHANGE. Otherwise, the procedure for taking out the device is coded to the root operation REMOVAL.

ØRP Continued

Body Part Character 4	Approach Character 5	Device Character 6	Qualifier Character 7
L Elbow Joint, Right Distal humerus, involving joint Humeroradial joint Humeroulnar joint Proximal radioulnar joint **M** Elbow Joint, Left *See L Elbow Joint, Right* **N** Wrist Joint, Right Distal radioulnar joint Radiocarpal joint **P** Wrist Joint, Left *See N Wrist Joint, Right* **Q** Carpal Joint, Right Intercarpal joint Midcarpal joint **R** Carpal Joint, Left *See Q Carpal Joint, Right* **S** Carpometacarpal Joint, Right **T** Carpometacarpal Joint, Left **U** Metacarpophalangeal Joint, Right **V** Metacarpophalangeal Joint, Left **W** Finger Phalangeal Joint, Right Interphalangeal (IP) joint **X** Finger Phalangeal Joint, Left *See W Finger Phalangeal Joint, Right*	**Ø** Open **3** Percutaneous **4** Percutaneous Endoscopic	**Ø** Drainage Device **3** Infusion Device **4** Internal Fixation Device **5** External Fixation Device **7** Autologous Tissue Substitute **8** Spacer **J** Synthetic Substitute **K** Nonautologous Tissue Substitute	**Z** No Qualifier
L Elbow Joint, Right Distal humerus, involving joint Humeroradial joint Humeroulnar joint Proximal radioulnar joint **M** Elbow Joint, Left *See L Elbow Joint, Right* **N** Wrist Joint, Right Distal radioulnar joint Radiocarpal joint **P** Wrist Joint, Left *See N Wrist Joint, Right* **Q** Carpal Joint, Right Intercarpal joint Midcarpal joint **R** Carpal Joint, Left *See Q Carpal Joint, Right* **S** Carpometacarpal Joint, Right **T** Carpometacarpal Joint, Left **U** Metacarpophalangeal Joint, Right **V** Metacarpophalangeal Joint, Left **W** Finger Phalangeal Joint, Right Interphalangeal (IP) joint **X** Finger Phalangeal Joint, Left *See W Finger Phalangeal Joint, Right*	**X** External	**Ø** Drainage Device **3** Infusion Device **4** Internal Fixation Device **5** External Fixation Device	**Z** No Qualifier

Non-OR ØRP[L,M,N,P,Q,R,S,T,U,V,W,X]3[Ø,3,8]Z
Non-OR ØRP[L,M,N,P,Q,R,S,T,U,V,W,X][Ø,4]8Z
Non-OR ØRP[L,M,N,P,Q,R,S,T,U,V,W,X]X[Ø,3,4,5]Z

Ø Medical and Surgical
R Upper Joints
Q Repair Definition: Restoring, to the extent possible, a body part to its normal anatomic structure and function
Explanation: Used only when the method to accomplish the repair is not one of the other root operations

Body Part Character 4	Approach Character 5	Device Character 6	Qualifier Character 7
Ø Occipital-cervical Joint **1** Cervical Vertebral Joint Atlantoaxial joint Cervical facet joint **3** Cervical Vertebral Disc **4** Cervicothoracic Vertebral Joint Cervicothoracic facet joint **5** Cervicothoracic Vertebral Disc **6** Thoracic Vertebral Joint Costotransverse joint Costovertebral joint Thoracic facet joint **9** Thoracic Vertebral Disc **A** Thoracolumbar Vertebral Joint Thoracolumbar facet joint **B** Thoracolumbar Vertebral Disc **C** Temporomandibular Joint, Right **D** Temporomandibular Joint, Left **E** Sternoclavicular Joint, Right **F** Sternoclavicular Joint, Left **G** Acromioclavicular Joint, Right **H** Acromioclavicular Joint, Left **J** Shoulder Joint, Right Glenohumeral joint Glenoid ligament (labrum) **K** Shoulder Joint, Left *See J Shoulder Joint, Right* **L** Elbow Joint, Right Distal humerus, involving joint Humeroradial joint Humeroulnar joint Proximal radioulnar joint **M** Elbow Joint, Left *See L Elbow Joint, Right* **N** Wrist Joint, Right Distal radioulnar joint Radiocarpal joint **P** Wrist Joint, Left *See N Wrist Joint, Right* **Q** Carpal Joint, Right Intercarpal joint Midcarpal joint **R** Carpal Joint, Left *See Q Carpal Joint, Right* **S** Carpometacarpal Joint, Right **T** Carpometacarpal Joint, Left **U** Metacarpophalangeal Joint, Right **V** Metacarpophalangeal Joint, Left **W** Finger Phalangeal Joint, Right Interphalangeal (IP) joint **X** Finger Phalangeal Joint, Left *See W Finger Phalangeal Joint, Right*	**Ø** Open **3** Percutaneous **4** Percutaneous Endoscopic **X** External	**Z** No Device	**Z** No Qualifier

Non-OR ØRQ[Ø,1,3,4,5,6,9,A,B,C,D,E,F,G,H,J,K,L,M,N,P,Q,R,S,T,U,V,W,X]XZZ
HAC ØRQ[E,F,G,H,J,K,L,M][Ø,3,4,X]ZZ when reported with SDx K68.11 or T81.4XXA or T84.6Ø-T84.619, T84.63-T84.7 with 7th character A

Ø Medical and Surgical
R Upper Joints
R Replacement Definition: Putting in or on biological or synthetic material that physically takes the place and/or function of all or a portion of a body part
Explanation: The body part may have been taken out or replaced, or may be taken out, physically eradicated, or rendered nonfunctional during the REPLACEMENT procedure. A REMOVAL procedure is coded for taking out the device used in a previous replacement procedure.

Body Part Character 4	Approach Character 5	Device Character 6	Qualifier Character 7
Ø Occipital-cervical Joint **1 Cervical Vertebral Joint** Atlantoaxial joint Cervical facet joint **3 Cervical Vertebral Disc** **4 Cervicothoracic Vertebral Joint** Cervicothoracic facet joint **5 Cervicothoracic Vertebral Disc** **6 Thoracic Vertebral Joint** Costotransverse joint Costovertebral joint Thoracic facet joint **9 Thoracic Vertebral Disc** **A Thoracolumbar Vertebral Joint** Thoracolumbar facet joint **B Thoracolumbar Vertebral Disc** **C Temporomandibular Joint, Right** **D Temporomandibular Joint, Left** **E Sternoclavicular Joint, Right** **F Sternoclavicular Joint, Left** **G Acromioclavicular Joint, Right** **H Acromioclavicular Joint, Left** **L Elbow Joint, Right** Distal humerus, involving joint Humeroradial joint Humeroulnar joint Proximal radioulnar joint **M Elbow Joint, Left** *See L Elbow Joint, Right* **N Wrist Joint, Right** Distal radioulnar joint Radiocarpal joint **P Wrist Joint, Left** *See N Wrist Joint, Right* **Q Carpal Joint, Right** Intercarpal joint Midcarpal joint **R Carpal Joint, Left** *See Q Carpal Joint, Right* **S Carpometacarpal Joint, Right** **T Carpometacarpal Joint, Left** **U Metacarpophalangeal Joint, Right** **V Metacarpophalangeal Joint, Left** **W Finger Phalangeal Joint, Right** Interphalangeal (IP) joint **X Finger Phalangeal Joint, Left** *See W Finger Phalangeal Joint, Right*	**Ø Open**	**7 Autologous Tissue Substitute** **J Synthetic Substitute** **K Nonautologous Tissue Substitute**	**Z No Qualifier**
J Shoulder Joint, Right Glenohumeral joint Glenoid ligament (labrum) **K Shoulder Joint, Left** *See J Shoulder Joint, Right*	**Ø Open**	**Ø Synthetic Substitute, Reverse Ball and Socket** **7 Autologous Tissue Substitute** **K Nonautologous Tissue Substitute**	**Z No Qualifier**
J Shoulder Joint, Right Glenohumeral joint Glenoid ligament (labrum) **K Shoulder Joint, Left** *See J Shoulder Joint, Right*	**Ø Open**	**J Synthetic Substitute**	**6 Humeral Surface** **7 Glenoid Surface** **Z No Qualifier**

Upper Joints ØRS–ØRS

Ø Medical and Surgical
R Upper Joints
S Reposition Definition: Moving to its normal location, or other suitable location, all or a portion of a body part

Explanation: The body part is moved to a new location from an abnormal location, or from a normal location where it is not functioning correctly. The body part may or may not be cut out or off to be moved to the new location.

Body Part Character 4	Approach Character 5	Device Character 6	Qualifier Character 7
Ø Occipital-cervical Joint **1** Cervical Vertebral Joint Atlantoaxial joint Cervical facet joint **4** Cervicothoracic Vertebral Joint Cervicothoracic facet joint **6** Thoracic Vertebral Joint Costotransverse joint Costovertebral joint Thoracic facet joint **A** Thoracolumbar Vertebral Joint Thoracolumbar facet joint **C** Temporomandibular Joint, Right **D** Temporomandibular Joint, Left **E** Sternoclavicular Joint, Right **F** Sternoclavicular Joint, Left **G** Acromioclavicular Joint, Right **H** Acromioclavicular Joint, Left **J** Shoulder Joint, Right Glenohumeral joint Glenoid ligament (labrum) **K** Shoulder Joint, Left *See J Shoulder Joint, Right*	**Ø** Open **3** Percutaneous **4** Percutaneous Endoscopic **X** External	**4** Internal Fixation Device **Z** No Device	**Z** No Qualifier
L Elbow Joint, Right Distal humerus, involving joint Humeroradial joint Humeroulnar joint Proximal radioulnar joint **M** Elbow Joint, Left *See L Elbow Joint, Right* **N** Wrist Joint, Right Distal radioulnar joint Radiocarpal joint **P** Wrist Joint, Left *See N Wrist Joint, Right* **Q** Carpal Joint, Right Intercarpal joint Midcarpal joint **R** Carpal Joint, Left *See Q Carpal Joint, Right* **S** Carpometacarpal Joint, Right **T** Carpometacarpal Joint, Left **U** Metacarpophalangeal Joint, Right **V** Metacarpophalangeal Joint, Left **W** Finger Phalangeal Joint, Right Interphalangeal (IP) joint **X** Finger Phalangeal Joint, Left *See W Finger Phalangeal Joint, Right*	**Ø** Open **3** Percutaneous **4** Percutaneous Endoscopic **X** External	**4** Internal Fixation Device **5** External Fixation Device **Z** No Device	**Z** No Qualifier

Non-OR ØRS[Ø,1,4,6,A,C,D,E,F,G,H,J,K][3,4,X][4,Z]Z
Non-OR ØRS[L,M,N,P,Q,R,S,T,U,V,W,X][3,4,X][4,5,Z]Z

Ø Medical and Surgical
R Upper Joints
T Resection Definition: Cutting out or off, without replacement, all of a body part
Explanation: None

Body Part Character 4		Approach Character 5	Device Character 6	Qualifier Character 7
3 Cervical Vertebral Disc **4 Cervicothoracic Vertebral Joint** Cervicothoracic facet joint **5 Cervicothoracic Vertebral Disc** **9 Thoracic Vertebral Disc** **B Thoracolumbar Vertebral Disc** **C Temporomandibular Joint, Right** **D Temporomandibular Joint, Left** **E Sternoclavicular Joint, Right** **F Sternoclavicular Joint, Left** **G Acromioclavicular Joint, Right** **H Acromioclavicular Joint, Left** **J Shoulder Joint, Right** Glenohumeral joint Glenoid ligament (labrum) **K Shoulder Joint, Left** *See J Shoulder Joint, Right* **L Elbow Joint, Right** Distal humerus, involving joint Humeroradial joint Humeroulnar joint Proximal radioulnar joint	**M Elbow Joint, Left** *See L Elbow Joint, Right* **N Wrist Joint, Right** Distal radioulnar joint Radiocarpal joint **P Wrist Joint, Left** *See N Wrist Joint, Right* **Q Carpal Joint, Right** Intercarpal joint Midcarpal joint **R Carpal Joint, Left** *See Q Carpal Joint, Right* **S Carpometacarpal Joint, Right** **T Carpometacarpal Joint, Left** **U Metacarpophalangeal Joint, Right** **V Metacarpophalangeal Joint, Left** **W Finger Phalangeal Joint, Right** Interphalangeal (IP) joint **X Finger Phalangeal Joint, Left** *See W Finger Phalangeal Joint, Right*	**Ø Open**	**Z No Device**	**Z No Qualifier**

Ø Medical and Surgical
R Upper Joints
U Supplement Definition: Putting in or on biological or synthetic material that physically reinforces and/or augments the function of a portion of a body part
Explanation: The biological material is non-living, or is living and from the same individual. The body part may have been previously replaced, and the SUPPLEMENT procedure is performed to physically reinforce and/or augment the function of the replaced body part.

Body Part Character 4		Approach Character 5	Device Character 6	Qualifier Character 7
Ø Occipital-cervical Joint **1 Cervical Vertebral Joint** Atlantoaxial joint Cervical facet joint **3 Cervical Vertebral Disc** **4 Cervicothoracic Vertebral Joint** Cervicothoracic facet joint **5 Cervicothoracic Vertebral Disc** **6 Thoracic Vertebral Joint** Costotransverse joint Costovertebral joint Thoracic facet joint **9 Thoracic Vertebral Disc** **A Thoracolumbar Vertebral Joint** Thoracolumbar facet joint **B Thoracolumbar Vertebral Disc** **C Temporomandibular Joint, Right** **D Temporomandibular Joint, Left** **E Sternoclavicular Joint, Right** **F Sternoclavicular Joint, Left** **G Acromioclavicular Joint, Right** **H Acromioclavicular Joint, Left** **J Shoulder Joint, Right** Glenohumeral joint Glenoid ligament (labrum) **K Shoulder Joint, Left** *See J Shoulder Joint, Right*	**L Elbow Joint, Right** Distal humerus, involving joint Humeroradial joint Humeroulnar joint Proximal radioulnar joint **M Elbow Joint, Left** *See L Elbow Joint, Right* **N Wrist Joint, Right** Distal radioulnar joint Radiocarpal joint **P Wrist Joint, Left** *See N Wrist Joint, Right* **Q Carpal Joint, Right** Intercarpal joint Midcarpal joint **R Carpal Joint, Left** *See Q Carpal Joint, Right* **S Carpometacarpal Joint, Right** **T Carpometacarpal Joint, Left** **U Metacarpophalangeal Joint, Right** **V Metacarpophalangeal Joint, Left** **W Finger Phalangeal Joint, Right** Interphalangeal (IP) joint **X Finger Phalangeal Joint, Left** *See W Finger Phalangeal Joint, Right*	**Ø Open** **3 Percutaneous** **4 Percutaneous Endoscopic**	**7 Autologous Tissue Substitute** **J Synthetic Substitute** **K Nonautologous Tissue Substitute**	**Z No Qualifier**

HAC ØRU[E,F,G,H,J,K,L,M][Ø,3,4][7,J,K]Z when reported with SDx K68.11 or T81.4XXA or T84.6Ø-T84.619, T84.63-T84.7 with 7th character A

Ø Medical and Surgical
R Upper Joints
W Revision Definition: Correcting, to the extent possible, a portion of a malfunctioning device or the position of a displaced device

Explanation: Revision can include correcting a malfunctioning or displaced device by taking out or putting in components of the device such as a screw or pin

Body Part Character 4	Approach Character 5	Device Character 6	Qualifier Character 7
Ø Occipital-cervical Joint **1** Cervical Vertebral Joint Atlantoaxial joint Cervical facet joint **4** Cervicothoracic Vertebral Joint Cervicothoracic facet joint **6** Thoracic Vertebral Joint Costotransverse joint Costovertebral joint Thoracic facet joint **A** Thoracolumbar Vertebral Joint Thoracolumbar facet joint	**Ø** Open **3** Percutaneous **4** Percutaneous Endoscopic **X** External	**Ø** Drainage Device **3** Infusion Device **4** Internal Fixation Device **7** Autologous Tissue Substitute **8** Spacer **A** Interbody Fusion Device **J** Synthetic Substitute **K** Nonautologous Tissue Substitute	**Z** No Qualifier
3 Cervical Vertebral Disc **5** Cervicothoracic Vertebral Disc **9** Thoracic Vertebral Disc **B** Thoracolumbar Vertebral Disc	**Ø** Open **3** Percutaneous **4** Percutaneous Endoscopic **X** External	**Ø** Drainage Device **3** Infusion Device **7** Autologous Tissue Substitute **J** Synthetic Substitute **K** Nonautologous Tissue Substitute	**Z** No Qualifier
C Temporomandibular Joint, Right **D** Temporomandibular Joint, Left **E** Sternoclavicular Joint, Right **F** Sternoclavicular Joint, Left **G** Acromioclavicular Joint, Right **H** Acromioclavicular Joint, Left **J** Shoulder Joint, Right Glenohumeral joint Glenoid ligament (labrum) **K** Shoulder Joint, Left *See J Shoulder Joint, Right*	**Ø** Open **3** Percutaneous **4** Percutaneous Endoscopic **X** External	**Ø** Drainage Device **3** Infusion Device **4** Internal Fixation Device **7** Autologous Tissue Substitute **8** Spacer **J** Synthetic Substitute **K** Nonautologous Tissue Substitute	**Z** No Qualifier
L Elbow Joint, Right Distal humerus, involving joint Humeroradial joint Humeroulnar joint Proximal radioulnar joint **M** Elbow Joint, Left *See L Elbow Joint, Right* **N** Wrist Joint, Right Distal radioulnar joint Radiocarpal joint **P** Wrist Joint, Left *See N Wrist Joint, Right* **Q** Carpal Joint, Right Intercarpal joint Midcarpal joint **R** Carpal Joint, Left *See Q Carpal Joint, Right* **S** Carpometacarpal Joint, Right **T** Carpometacarpal Joint, Left **U** Metacarpophalangeal Joint, Right **V** Metacarpophalangeal Joint, Left **W** Finger Phalangeal Joint, Right Interphalangeal (IP) joint **X** Finger Phalangeal Joint, Left *See W Finger Phalangeal Joint, Right*	**Ø** Open **3** Percutaneous **4** Percutaneous Endoscopic **X** External	**Ø** Drainage Device **3** Infusion Device **4** Internal Fixation Device **5** External Fixation Device **7** Autologous Tissue Substitute **8** Spacer **J** Synthetic Substitute **K** Nonautologous Tissue Substitute	**Z** No Qualifier

Non-OR ØRW[Ø,1,4,6,A]X[Ø,3,4,7,8,A,J,K]Z
Non-OR ØRW[3,5,9,B]X[Ø,3,7,J,K]Z
Non-OR ØRW[C,D,E,F,G,H,J,K]X[Ø,3,4,7,8,J,K]Z
Non-OR ØRW[L,M,N,P,Q,R,S,T,U,V,W,X]X[Ø,3,4,5,7,8,J,K]Z

Lower Joints ØS2–ØSW

Character Meanings*

This Character Meaning table is provided as a guide to assist the user in the identification of character members that may be found in this section of code tables. It **SHOULD NOT** be used to build a PCS code.

Operation–Character 3	Body Part–Character 4	Approach–Character 5	Device–Character 6	Qualifier–Character 7
2 Change	Ø Lumbar Vertebral Joint	Ø Open	Ø Drainage Device OR Synthetic Substitute, Polyethylene	Ø Anterior Approach, Anterior Column
5 Destruction	1 Lumbar Vertebral Joint, 2 or more	3 Percutaneous	1 Synthetic Substitute, Metal	1 Posterior Approach, Posterior Column
9 Drainage	2 Lumbar Vertebral Disc	4 Percutaneous Endoscopic	2 Synthetic Substitute, Metal on Polyethylene	9 Cemented
B Excision	3 Lumbosacral Joint	X External	3 Infusion Device OR Synthetic Substitute, Ceramic	A Uncemented
C Extirpation	4 Lumbosacral Disc		4 Internal Fixation Device OR Synthetic Substitute, Ceramic on Polyethylene	C Patellar Surface
G Fusion	5 Sacrococcygeal Joint		5 External Fixation Device	J Posterior Approach, Anterior Column
H Insertion	6 Coccygeal Joint		6 Synthetic Substitute, Oxidized Zirconium on Polyethylene	X Diagnostic
J Inspection	7 Sacroiliac Joint, Right		7 Autologous Tissue Substitute	Z No Qualifier
N Release	8 Sacroiliac Joint, Left		8 Spacer	
P Removal	9 Hip Joint, Right		9 Liner	
	A Hip Joint, Acetabular Surface, Right		A Interbody Fusion Device	
Q Repair	B Hip Joint, Left		B Resurfacing Device OR Spinal Stabilization Device, Interspinous Process	
R Replacement	C Knee Joint, Right		C Spinal Stabilization Device, Pedicle-Based	
S Reposition	D Knee Joint, Left		D Spinal Stabilization Device, Facet Replacement	
T Resection	E Hip Joint, Acetabular Surface, Left		E Articulating Spacer	
U Supplement	F Ankle Joint, Right		J Synthetic Substitute	
W Revision	G Ankle Joint, Left		K Nonautologous Tissue Substitute	
	H Tarsal Joint, Right		L Synthetic Substitute, Unicondylar Medial	
	J Tarsal Joint, Left		M Synthetic Substitute, Unicondylar Lateral	
	K Tarsometatarsal Joint, Right		N Synthetic Substitute, Patellofemoral	
	L Tarsometatarsal Joint, Left		Y Other Device	
	M Metatarsal-Phalangeal Joint, Right		Z No Device	
	N Metatarsal-Phalangeal Joint, Left			
	P Toe Phalangeal Joint, Right			
	Q Toe Phalangeal Joint, Left			
	R Hip Joint, Femoral Surface, Right			
	S Hip Joint, Femoral Surface, Left			
	T Knee Joint, Femoral Surface, Right			
	U Knee Joint, Femoral Surface, Left			
	V Knee Joint, Tibial Surface, Right			
	W Knee Joint, Tibial Surface, Left			
	Y Lower Joint			

* Includes synovial membrane.

AHA Coding Clinic for table ØS9

2018, 2Q, 17	Arthroscopic drainage of knee and nonexcisional debridement
2017, 1Q, 50	Dry aspiration of ankle joint

AHA Coding Clinic for table ØSB

2017, 4Q, 76	Radiolucent porous interbody fusion device
2016, 2Q, 16	Decompressive laminectomy/foraminotomy and lumbar discectomy
2016, 1Q, 20	Metatarsophalangeal joint resection arthroplasty
2015, 1Q, 34	Arthroscopic meniscectomy with debridement and abrasion chondroplasty
2014, 2Q, 6	Posterior lumbar fusion with discectomy

AHA Coding Clinic for table ØSG

2018, 1Q, 22	Spinal fusion procedures without bone graft
2017, 4Q, 76	Radiolucent porous interbody fusion device
2017, 2Q, 23	Decompression of spinal cord and placement of instrumentation
2014, 3Q, 30	Spinal fusion and fixation instrumentation
2014, 3Q, 36	Lumbar interbody fusion of two vertebral levels
2014, 2Q, 6	Posterior lumbar fusion with discectomy
2013, 3Q, 25	36Ø-degree spinal fusion
2013, 2Q, 39	Ankle fusion, osteotomy, and removal of hardware
2013, 1Q, 21-23	Spinal fusion of thoracic and lumbar vertebrae

AHA Coding Clinic for table ØSH

2017, 2Q, 23	Decompression of spinal cord and placement of instrumentation

AHA Coding Clinic for table ØSJ

2017, 1Q, 50	Dry aspiration of ankle joint

AHA Coding Clinic for table ØSP

2018, 2Q, 16	Exchange of tibial polyethylene component with stabilizing insert (tibial tray)
2017, 4Q, 107	Total ankle replacement versus revision
2016, 4Q, 110-112	Removal and revision of hip and knee devices
2015, 2Q, 18	Total knee revision
2015, 2Q, 19	Revision of femoral head and acetabular liner
2013, 2Q, 39	Ankle fusion, osteotomy, and removal of hardware

AHA Coding Clinic for table ØSQ

2014, 4Q, 25	Femoroacetabular impingement and labral tear with repair

AHA Coding Clinic for table ØSR

2018, 2Q, 16	Exchange of tibial polyethylene component with stabilizing insert (tibial tray)
2017, 4Q, 38-39	Oxidized zirconium on polyethylene bearing surface
2017, 4Q, 107	Total ankle replacement versus revision
2017, 1Q, 22	Total knee replacement and patellar component
2016, 4Q, 110-111	Partial (unicondylar) knee replacement
2016, 4Q, 111-112	Removal and revision of hip and knee devices
2016, 3Q, 35	Use of cemented versus uncemented qualifier for joint replacement
2015, 3Q, 18	Total hip replacement with acetabular reconstruction
2015, 2Q, 18	Total knee revision
2015, 2Q, 19	Revision of femoral head and acetabular liner

AHA Coding Clinic for table ØSS

2016, 2Q, 31	Periacetabular ostectomy for repair of congenital hip dysplasia

AHA Coding Clinic for table ØST

2016, 1Q, 20	Metatarsophalangeal joint resection arthroplasty
2014, 4Q, 29	Rotational osteosynthesis

AHA Coding Clinic for table ØSU

2018, 2Q, 16	Exchange of tibial polyethylene component with stabilizing insert (tibial tray)
2016, 4Q, 111	Removal and revision of hip and knee devices
2015, 2Q, 19	Revision of femoral head and acetabular liner

AHA Coding Clinic for table ØSW

2017, 4Q, 107	Total ankle replacement versus revision
2016, 4Q, 110-112	Removal and revision of hip and knee devices
2015, 2Q, 18	Total knee revision
2015, 2Q, 19	Revision of femoral head and acetabular liner

Lower Joints

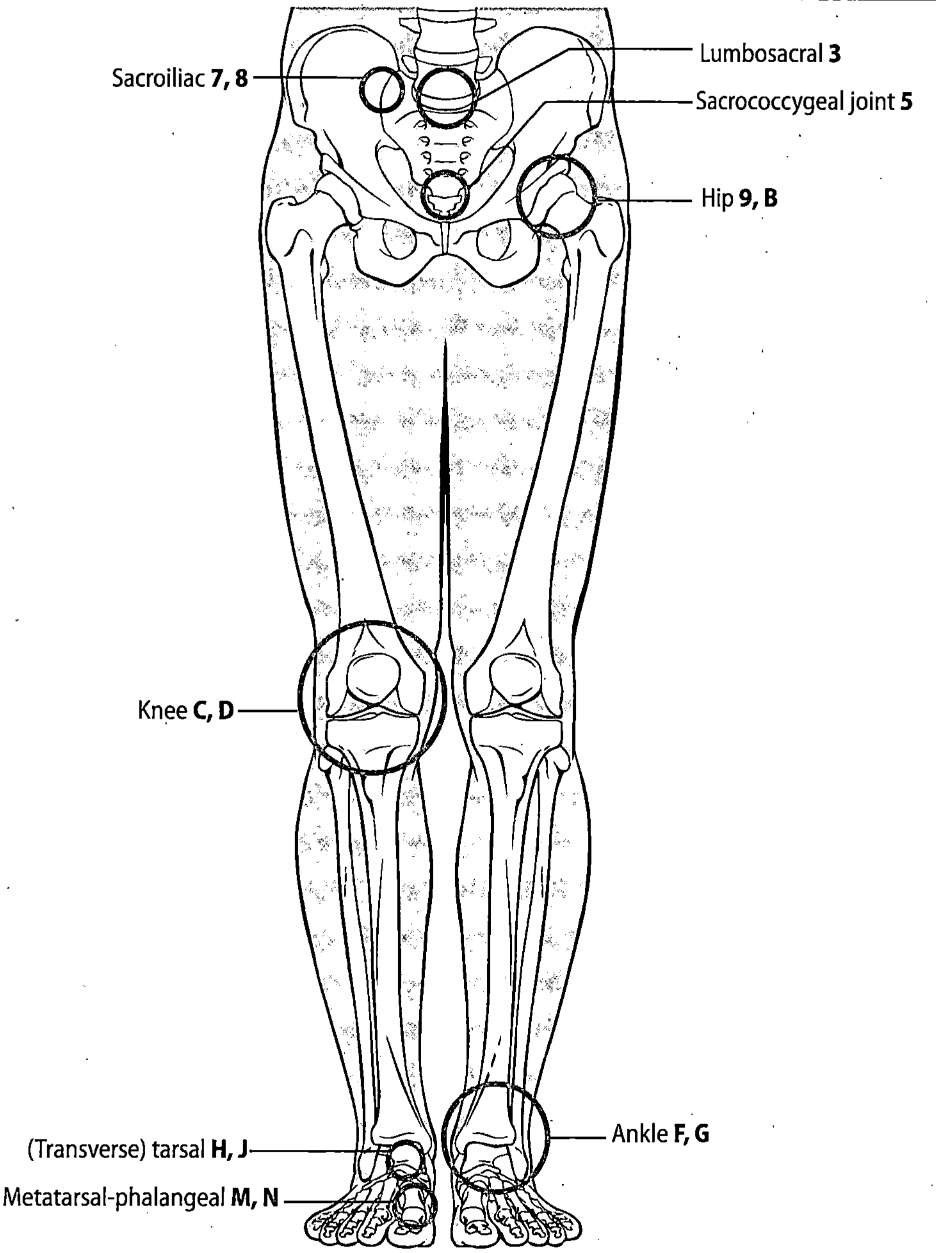
Sacroiliac 7, 8
Lumbosacral 3
Sacrococcygeal joint 5
Hip 9, B
Knee C, D
(Transverse) tarsal H, J
Metatarsal-phalangeal M, N
Ankle F, G

Hip Joint

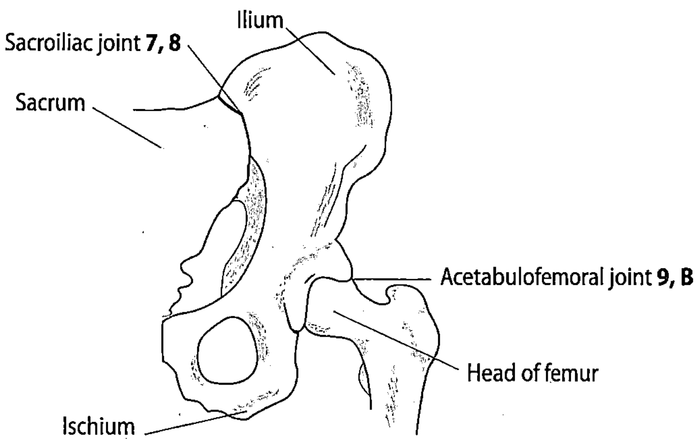
Ilium
Sacroiliac joint 7, 8
Sacrum
Acetabulofemoral joint 9, B
Head of femur
Ischium

Knee Joint

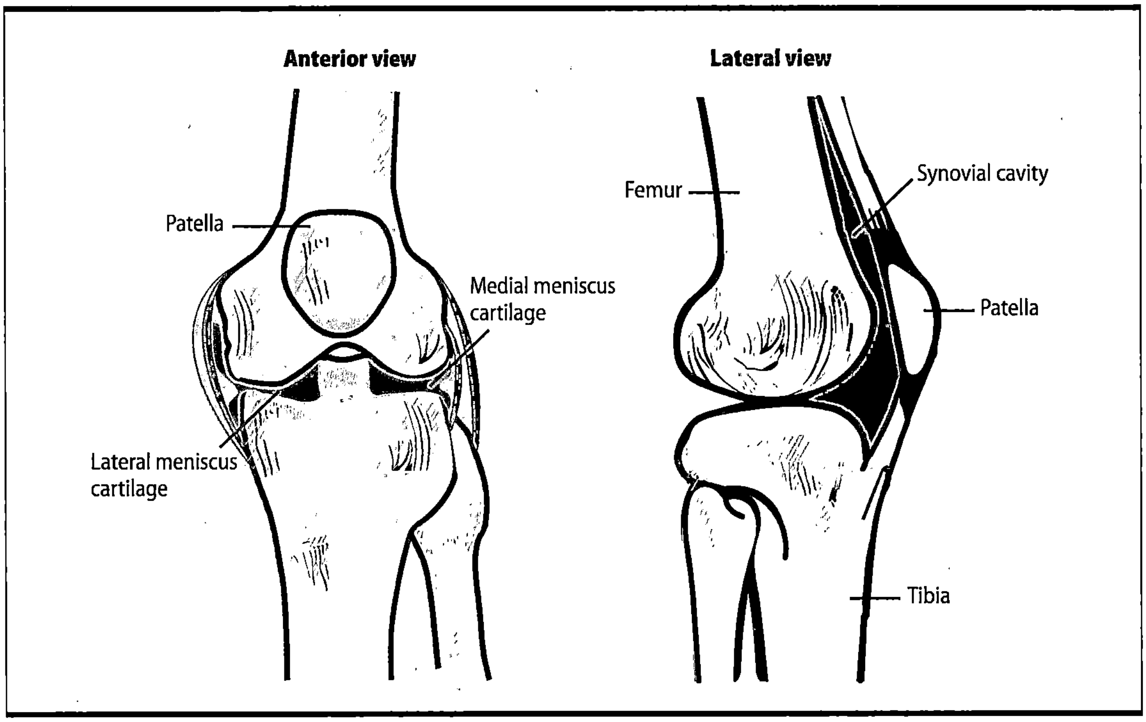
Anterior view
Patella
Medial meniscus cartilage
Lateral meniscus cartilage
Lateral view
Femur
Synovial cavity
Patella
Tibia

Foot Joints

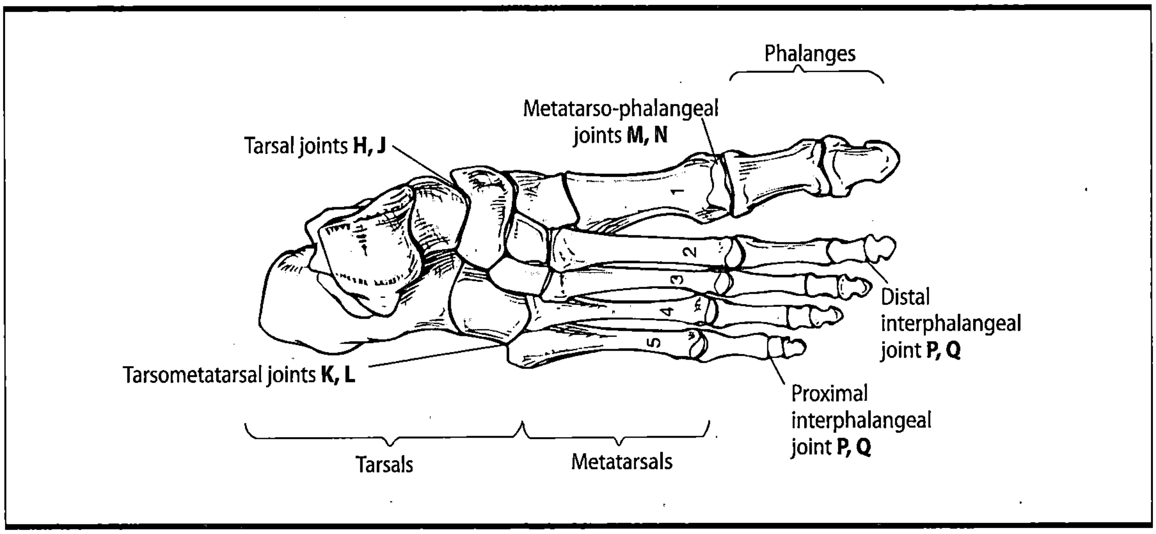
Phalanges
Metatarso-phalangeal joints **M, N**
Tarsal joints **H, J**
1
2
3
4
5
Distal interphalangeal joint **P, Q**
Tarsometatarsal joints **K, L**
Proximal interphalangeal joint **P, Q**
Tarsals
Metatarsals

Ø Medical and Surgical
S Lower Joints
2 Change Definition: Taking out or off a device from a body part and putting back an identical or similar device in or on the same body part without cutting or puncturing the skin or a mucous membrane

Explanation: All CHANGE procedures are coded using the approach EXTERNAL

Body Part Character 4	Approach Character 5	Device Character 6	Qualifier Character 7
Y Lower Joint	X External	Ø Drainage Device Y Other Device	Z No Qualifier

Non-OR All body part, approach, device, and qualifier values

Ø Medical and Surgical
S Lower Joints
5 Destruction Definition: Physical eradication of all or a portion of a body part by the direct use of energy, force, or a destructive agent

Explanation: None of the body part is physically taken out

Body Part Character 4	Approach Character 5	Device Character 6	Qualifier Character 7
Ø Lumbar Vertebral Joint Lumbar facet joint **2 Lumbar Vertebral Disc** **3 Lumbosacral Joint** Lumbosacral facet joint **4 Lumbosacral Disc** **5 Sacrococcygeal Joint** Sacrococcygeal symphysis **6 Coccygeal Joint** **7 Sacroiliac Joint, Right** **8 Sacroiliac Joint, Left** **9 Hip Joint, Right** Acetabulofemoral joint **B Hip Joint, Left** *See 9 Hip Joint, Right* **C Knee Joint, Right** Femoropatellar joint Femorotibial joint Lateral meniscus Medial meniscus Patellofemoral joint Tibiofemoral joint **D Knee Joint, Left** *See C Knee Joint, Right* **F Ankle Joint, Right** Inferior tibiofibular joint Talocrural joint **G Ankle Joint, Left** *See F Ankle Joint, Right* **H Tarsal Joint, Right** Calcaneocuboid joint Cuboideonavicular joint Cuneonavicular joint Intercuneiform joint Subtalar (talocalcaneal) joint Talocalcaneal (subtalar) joint Talocalcaneonavicular joint **J Tarsal Joint, Left** *See H Tarsal Joint, Right* **K Tarsometatarsal Joint, Right** **L Tarsometatarsal Joint, Left** **M Metatarsal-Phalangeal Joint, Right** Metatarsophalangeal (MTP) joint **N Metatarsal-Phalangeal Joint, Left** *See M Metatarsal-Phalangeal Joint, Right* **P Toe Phalangeal Joint, Right** Interphalangeal (IP) joint **Q Toe Phalangeal Joint, Left** *See P Toe Phalangeal Joint, Right*	Ø Open 3 Percutaneous 4 Percutaneous Endoscopic	Z No Device	Z No Qualifier

Ø Medical and Surgical
S Lower Joints
9 Drainage Definition: Taking or letting out fluids and/or gases from a body part
Explanation: The qualifier DIAGNOSTIC is used to identify drainage procedures that are biopsies

Body Part Character 4		Approach Character 5	Device Character 6	Qualifier Character 7
Ø Lumbar Vertebral Joint Lumbar facet joint **2** Lumbar Vertebral Disc **3** Lumbosacral Joint Lumbosacral facet joint **4** Lumbosacral Disc **5** Sacrococcygeal Joint Sacrococcygeal symphysis **6** Coccygeal Joint **7** Sacroiliac Joint, Right **8** Sacroiliac Joint, Left **9** Hip Joint, Right Acetabulofemoral joint **B** Hip Joint, Left *See 9 Hip Joint, Right* **C** Knee Joint, Right Femoropatellar joint Femorotibial joint Lateral meniscus Medial meniscus Patellofemoral joint Tibiofemoral joint **D** Knee Joint, Left *See C Knee Joint, Right* **F** Ankle Joint, Right Inferior tibiofibular joint Talocrural joint **G** Ankle Joint, Left *See F Ankle Joint, Right*	**H** Tarsal Joint, Right Calcaneocuboid joint Cuboideonavicular joint Cuneonavicular joint Intercuneiform joint Subtalar (talocalcaneal) joint Talocalcaneal (subtalar) joint Talocalcaneonavicular joint **J** Tarsal Joint, Left *See H Tarsal Joint, Right* **K** Tarsometatarsal Joint, Right **L** Tarsometatarsal Joint, Left **M** Metatarsal-Phalangeal Joint, Right Metatarsophalangeal (MTP) joint **N** Metatarsal-Phalangeal Joint, Left *See M Metatarsal-Phalangeal Joint, Right* **P** Toe Phalangeal Joint, Right Interphalangeal (IP) joint **Q** Toe Phalangeal Joint, Left *See P Toe Phalangeal Joint, Right*	**Ø** Open **3** Percutaneous **4** Percutaneous Endoscopic	**Ø** Drainage Device	**Z** No Qualifier
Ø Lumbar Vertebral Joint Lumbar facet joint **2** Lumbar Vertebral Disc **3** Lumbosacral Joint Lumbosacral facet joint **4** Lumbosacral Disc **5** Sacrococcygeal Joint Sacrococcygeal symphysis **6** Coccygeal Joint **7** Sacroiliac Joint, Right **8** Sacroiliac Joint, Left **9** Hip Joint, Right Acetabulofemoral joint **B** Hip Joint, Left *See 9 Hip Joint, Right* **C** Knee Joint, Right Femoropatellar joint Femorotibial joint Lateral meniscus Medial meniscus Patellofemoral joint Tibiofemoral joint **D** Knee Joint, Left *See C Knee Joint, Right* **F** Ankle Joint, Right Inferior tibiofibular joint Talocrural joint **G** Ankle Joint, Left *See F Ankle Joint, Right*	**H** Tarsal Joint, Right Calcaneocuboid joint Cuboideonavicular joint Cuneonavicular joint Intercuneiform joint Subtalar (talocalcaneal) joint Talocalcaneal (subtalar) joint Talocalcaneonavicular joint **J** Tarsal Joint, Left *See H Tarsal Joint, Right* **K** Tarsometatarsal Joint, Right **L** Tarsometatarsal Joint, Left **M** Metatarsal-Phalangeal Joint, Right Metatarsophalangeal (MTP) joint **N** Metatarsal-Phalangeal Joint, Left *See M Metatarsal-Phalangeal Joint, Right* **P** Toe Phalangeal Joint, Right Interphalangeal (IP) joint **Q** Toe Phalangeal Joint, Left *See P Toe Phalangeal Joint, Right*	**Ø** Open **3** Percutaneous **4** Percutaneous Endoscopic	**Z** No Device	**X** Diagnostic **Z** No Qualifier

Non-OR ØS9[Ø,2,3,4,5,6,7,8,9,B,C,D,F,G,H,J,K,L,M,N,P,Q][3,4]ØZ
Non-OR ØS9[Ø,2,3,4,5,6,7,8,9,B,C,D,F,G,H,J,K,L,M,N,P,Q][Ø,3,4]ZX
Non-OR ØS9[Ø,2,3,4,5,6,7,8,9,B,C,D,F,G,H,J,K,L,M,N,P,Q][3,4]ZZ

Ø Medical and Surgical
S Lower Joints
B Excision Definition: Cutting out or off, without replacement, a portion of a body part
Explanation: The qualifier DIAGNOSTIC is used to identify excision procedures that are biopsies

Body Part Character 4		Approach Character 5	Device Character 6	Qualifier Character 7
Ø Lumbar Vertebral Joint Lumbar facet joint 2 Lumbar Vertebral Disc 3 Lumbosacral Joint Lumbosacral facet joint 4 Lumbosacral Disc 5 Sacrococcygeal Joint Sacrococcygeal symphysis 6 Coccygeal Joint 7 Sacroiliac Joint, Right 8 Sacroiliac Joint, Left 9 Hip Joint, Right Acetabulofemoral joint B Hip Joint, Left *See 9 Hip Joint, Right* C Knee Joint, Right Femoropatellar joint Femorotibial joint Lateral meniscus Medial meniscus Patellofemoral joint Tibiofemoral joint D Knee Joint, Left *See C Knee Joint, Right* F Ankle Joint, Right Inferior tibiofibular joint Talocrural joint G Ankle Joint, Left *See F Ankle Joint, Right*	H Tarsal Joint, Right Calcaneocuboid joint Cuboideonavicular joint Cuneonavicular joint Intercuneiform joint Subtalar (talocalcaneal) joint Talocalcaneal (subtalar) joint Talocalcaneonavicular joint J Tarsal Joint, Left *See H Tarsal Joint, Right* K Tarsometatarsal Joint, Right L Tarsometatarsal Joint, Left M Metatarsal-Phalangeal Joint, Right Metatarsophalangeal (MTP) joint N Metatarsal-Phalangeal Joint, Left *See M Metatarsal-Phalangeal Joint, Right* P Toe Phalangeal Joint, Right Interphalangeal (IP) joint Q Toe Phalangeal Joint, Left *See P Toe Phalangeal Joint, Right*	Ø Open 3 Percutaneous 4 Percutaneous Endoscopic	Z No Device	X Diagnostic Z No Qualifier

Non-OR ØSB[Ø,2,3,4,5,6,7,8,9,B,C,D,F,G,H,J,K,L,M,N,P,Q][Ø,3,4]ZX

Ø Medical and Surgical
S Lower Joints
C Extirpation Definition: Taking or cutting out solid matter from a body part
Explanation: The solid matter may be an abnormal byproduct of a biological function or a foreign body; it may be imbedded in a body part or in the lumen of a tubular body part. The solid matter may or may not have been previously broken into pieces.

Body Part Character 4		Approach Character 5	Device Character 6	Qualifier Character 7
Ø Lumbar Vertebral Joint Lumbar facet joint 2 Lumbar Vertebral Disc 3 Lumbosacral Joint Lumbosacral facet joint 4 Lumbosacral Disc 5 Sacrococcygeal Joint Sacrococcygeal symphysis 6 Coccygeal Joint 7 Sacroiliac Joint, Right 8 Sacroiliac Joint, Left 9 Hip Joint, Right Acetabulofemoral joint B Hip Joint, Left *See 9 Hip Joint, Right* C Knee Joint, Right Femoropatellar joint Femorotibial joint Lateral meniscus Medial meniscus Patellofemoral joint Tibiofemoral joint D Knee Joint, Left *See C Knee Joint, Right* F Ankle Joint, Right Inferior tibiofibular joint Talocrural joint G Ankle Joint, Left *See F Ankle Joint, Right*	H Tarsal Joint, Right Calcaneocuboid joint Cuboideonavicular joint Cuneonavicular joint Intercuneiform joint Subtalar (talocalcaneal) joint Talocalcaneal (subtalar) joint Talocalcaneonavicular joint J Tarsal Joint, Left *See H Tarsal Joint, Right* K Tarsometatarsal Joint, Right L Tarsometatarsal Joint, Left M Metatarsal-Phalangeal Joint, Right Metatarsophalangeal (MTP) joint N Metatarsal-Phalangeal Joint, Left *See M Metatarsal-Phalangeal Joint, Right* P Toe Phalangeal Joint, Right Interphalangeal (IP) joint Q Toe Phalangeal Joint, Left *See P Toe Phalangeal Joint, Right*	Ø Open 3 Percutaneous 4 Percutaneous Endoscopic	Z No Device	Z No Qualifier

Ø Medical and Surgical
S Lower Joints
G Fusion Definition: Joining together portions of an articular body part rendering the articular body part immobile
Explanation: The body part is joined together by fixation device, bone graft, or other means

Body Part Character 4	Approach Character 5	Device Character 6	Qualifier Character 7
Ø Lumbar Vertebral Joint Lumbar facet joint **1 Lumbar Vertebral Joints, 2 or more** ⊞ **3 Lumbosacral Joint** Lumbosacral facet joint	**Ø Open** **3 Percutaneous** **4 Percutaneous Endoscopic**	**7 Autologous Tissue Substitute** **J Synthetic Substitute** **K Nonautologous Tissue Substitute**	**Ø Anterior Approach, Anterior Column** **1 Posterior Approach, Posterior Column** **J Posterior Approach, Anterior Column**
Ø Lumbar Vertebral Joint Lumbar facet joint **1 Lumbar Vertebral Joints, 2 or more** ⊞ **3 Lumbosacral Joint** Lumbosacral facet joint	**Ø Open** **3 Percutaneous** **4 Percutaneous Endoscopic**	**A Interbody Fusion Device**	**Ø Anterior Approach, Anterior Column** **J Posterior Approach, Anterior Column**
5 Sacrococcygeal Joint Sacrococcygeal symphysis **6 Coccygeal Joint** **7 Sacroiliac Joint, Right** **8 Sacroiliac Joint, Left**	**Ø Open** **3 Percutaneous** **4 Percutaneous Endoscopic**	**4 Internal Fixation Device** **7 Autologous Tissue Substitute** **J Synthetic Substitute** **K Nonautologous Tissue Substitute**	**Z No Qualifier**
9 Hip Joint, Right Acetabulofemoral joint **B Hip Joint, Left** *See 9 Hip Joint, Right* **C Knee Joint, Right** Femoropatellar joint Femorotibial joint Lateral meniscus Medial meniscus Patellofemoral joint Tibiofemoral joint **D Knee Joint, Left** *See C Knee Joint, Right* **F Ankle Joint, Right** Inferior tibiofibular joint Talocrural joint **G Ankle Joint, Left** *See F Ankle Joint, Right* **H Tarsal Joint, Right** Calcaneocuboid joint Cuboideonavicular joint Cuneonavicular joint Intercuneiform joint Subtalar (talocalcaneal) joint Talocalcaneal (subtalar) joint Talocalcaneonavicular joint **J Tarsal Joint, Left** *See H Tarsal Joint, Right* **K Tarsometatarsal Joint, Right** **L Tarsometatarsal Joint, Left** **M Metatarsal-Phalangeal Joint, Right** Metatarsophalangeal (MTP) joint **N Metatarsal-Phalangeal Joint, Left** *See M Metatarsal-Phalangeal Joint, Right* **P Toe Phalangeal Joint, Right** Interphalangeal (IP) joint **Q Toe Phalangeal Joint, Left** *See P Toe Phalangeal Joint, Right*	**Ø Open** **3 Percutaneous** **4 Percutaneous Endoscopic**	**4 Internal Fixation Device** **5 External Fixation Device** **7 Autologous Tissue Substitute** **J Synthetic Substitute** **K Nonautologous Tissue Substitute**	**Z No Qualifier**

HAC ØSG[Ø,1,3][Ø,3,4][7,J,K][Ø,1,J] when reported with SDx K68.11 or T81.4XXA or T84.6Ø-T84.619, T84.63-T84.7 with 7th character A
HAC ØSG[Ø,1,3][Ø,3,4]A[Ø,J] when reported with SDx K68.11 or T81.4XXA or T84.6Ø-T84.619, T84.63-T84.7 with 7th character A
HAC ØSG[7,8][Ø,3,4][4,7,J,K]Z when reported with SDx K68.11 or T81.4XXA or T84.6Ø-T84.619, T84.63-T84.7 with 7th character A

See Appendix L for Procedure Combinations
⊞ ØSG1[Ø,3,4][7,J,K][Ø,1,J]
⊞ ØSG1[Ø,3,4]A[Ø,J]

Ø Medical and Surgical
S Lower Joints
H Insertion Definition: Putting in a nonbiological appliance that monitors, assists, performs, or prevents a physiological function but does not physically take the place of a body part

Explanation: None

Body Part Character 4	Approach Character 5	Device Character 6	Qualifier Character 7
Ø Lumbar Vertebral Joint Lumbar facet joint 3 Lumbosacral Joint Lumbosacral facet joint	Ø Open 3 Percutaneous 4 Percutaneous Endoscopic	3 Infusion Device 4 Internal Fixation Device 8 Spacer B Spinal Stabilization Device, Interspinous Process C Spinal Stabilization Device, Pedicle-Based D Spinal Stabilization Device, Facet Replacement	Z No Qualifier
2 Lumbar Vertebral Disc 4 Lumbosacral Disc	Ø Open 3 Percutaneous 4 Percutaneous Endoscopic	3 Infusion Device 8 Spacer	Z No Qualifier
5 Sacrococcygeal Joint Sacrococcygeal symphysis 6 Coccygeal Joint 7 Sacroiliac Joint, Right 8 Sacroiliac Joint, Left	Ø Open 3 Percutaneous 4 Percutaneous Endoscopic	3 Infusion Device 4 Internal Fixation Device 8 Spacer	Z No Qualifier
9 Hip Joint, Right Acetabulofemoral joint B Hip Joint, Left *See 9 Hip Joint, Right* C Knee Joint, Right Femoropatellar joint Femorotibial joint Lateral meniscus Medial meniscus Patellofemoral joint Tibiofemoral joint D Knee Joint, Left *See C Knee Joint, Right* F Ankle Joint, Right Inferior tibiofibular joint Talocrural joint G Ankle Joint, Left *See F Ankle Joint, Right* H Tarsal Joint, Right Calcaneocuboid joint Cuboideonavicular joint Cuneonavicular joint Intercuneiform joint Subtalar (talocalcaneal) joint Talocalcaneal (subtalar) joint Talocalcaneonavicular joint J Tarsal Joint, Left *See H Tarsal Joint, Right* K Tarsometatarsal Joint, Right L Tarsometatarsal Joint, Left M Metatarsal-Phalangeal Joint, Right Metatarsophalangeal (MTP) joint N Metatarsal-Phalangeal Joint, Left *See M Metatarsal-Phalangeal Joint, Right* P Toe Phalangeal Joint, Right Interphalangeal (IP) joint Q Toe Phalangeal Joint, Left *See P Toe Phalangeal Joint, Right*	Ø Open 3 Percutaneous 4 Percutaneous Endoscopic	3 Infusion Device 4 Internal Fixation Device 5 External Fixation Device 8 Spacer	Z No Qualifier

Non-OR ØSH[Ø,3][Ø,3,4][3,8]Z
Non-OR ØSH[2,4][Ø,3,4][3,8]Z
Non-OR ØSH[5,6,7,8][Ø,3,4][3,8]Z
Non-OR ØSH[9,B,C,D,F,G,H,J,K,L,M,N,P,Q][Ø,3,4][3,8]Z

Lower Joints
ØSH–ØSH

Ø Medical and Surgical
S Lower Joints
J Inspection Definition: Visually and/or manually exploring a body part

Explanation: Visual exploration may be performed with or without optical instrumentation. Manual exploration may be performed directly or through intervening body layers.

Body Part Character 4		Approach Character 5	Device Character 6	Qualifier Character 7
Ø Lumbar Vertebral Joint Lumbar facet joint **2 Lumbar Vertebral Disc** **3 Lumbosacral Joint** Lumbosacral facet joint **4 Lumbosacral Disc** **5 Sacrococcygeal Joint** Sacrococcygeal symphysis **6 Coccygeal Joint** **7 Sacroiliac Joint, Right** **8 Sacroiliac Joint, Left** **9 Hip Joint, Right** Acetabulofemoral joint **B Hip Joint, Left** *See 9 Hip Joint, Right* **C Knee Joint, Right** Femoropatellar joint Femorotibial joint Lateral meniscus Medial meniscus Patellofemoral joint Tibiofemoral joint **D Knee Joint, Left** *See C Knee Joint, Right* **F Ankle Joint, Right** Inferior tibiofibular joint Talocrural joint **G Ankle Joint, Left** *See F Ankle Joint, Right*	**H Tarsal Joint, Right** Calcaneocuboid joint Cuboideonavicular joint Cuneonavicular joint Intercuneiform joint Subtalar (talocalcaneal) joint Talocalcaneal (subtalar) joint Talocalcaneonavicular joint **J Tarsal Joint, Left** *See H Tarsal Joint, Right* **K Tarsometatarsal Joint, Right** **L Tarsometatarsal Joint, Left** **M Metatarsal-Phalangeal Joint, Right** Metatarsophalangeal (MTP) joint **N Metatarsal-Phalangeal Joint, Left** *See M Metatarsal-Phalangeal Joint, Right* **P Toe Phalangeal Joint, Right** Interphalangeal (IP) joint **Q Toe Phalangeal Joint, Left** *See P Toe Phalangeal Joint, Right*	**Ø Open** **3 Percutaneous** **4 Percutaneous Endoscopic** **X External**	**Z No Device**	**Z No Qualifier**

Non-OR ØSJ[Ø,2,3,4,5,6,7,8,9,B,C,D,F,G,H,J,K,L,M,N,P,Q][3,X]ZZ

Ø Medical and Surgical
S Lower Joints
N Release Definition: Freeing a body part from an abnormal physical constraint by cutting or by the use of force

Explanation: Some of the restraining tissue may be taken out but none of the body part is taken out

Body Part Character 4		Approach Character 5	Device Character 6	Qualifier Character 7
Ø Lumbar Vertebral Joint Lumbar facet joint **2 Lumbar Vertebral Disc** **3 Lumbosacral Joint** Lumbosacral facet joint **4 Lumbosacral Disc** **5 Sacrococcygeal Joint** Sacrococcygeal symphysis **6 Coccygeal Joint** **7 Sacroiliac Joint, Right** **8 Sacroiliac Joint, Left** **9 Hip Joint, Right** Acetabulofemoral joint **B Hip Joint, Left** *See 9 Hip Joint, Right* **C Knee Joint, Right** Femoropatellar joint Femorotibial joint Lateral meniscus Medial meniscus Patellofemoral joint Tibiofemoral joint **D Knee Joint, Left** *See C Knee Joint, Right* **F Ankle Joint, Right** Inferior tibiofibular joint Talocrural joint **G Ankle Joint, Left** *See F Ankle Joint, Right*	**H Tarsal Joint, Right** Calcaneocuboid joint Cuboideonavicular joint Cuneonavicular joint Intercuneiform joint Subtalar (talocalcaneal) joint Talocalcaneal (subtalar) joint Talocalcaneonavicular joint **J Tarsal Joint, Left** *See H Tarsal Joint, Right* **K Tarsometatarsal Joint, Right** **L Tarsometatarsal Joint, Left** **M Metatarsal-Phalangeal Joint, Right** Metatarsophalangeal (MTP) joint **N Metatarsal-Phalangeal Joint, Left** *See M Metatarsal-Phalangeal Joint, Right* **P Toe Phalangeal Joint, Right** Interphalangeal (IP) joint **Q Toe Phalangeal Joint, Left** *See P Toe Phalangeal Joint, Right*	**Ø Open** **3 Percutaneous** **4 Percutaneous Endoscopic** **X External**	**Z No Device**	**Z No Qualifier**

Non-OR ØSN[Ø,2,3,4,5,6,7,8,9,B,C,D,F,G,H,J,K,L,M,N,P,Q]XZZ

Ø Medical and Surgical
S Lower Joints
P Removal Definition: Taking out or off a device from a body part

Explanation: If a device is taken out and a similar device put in without cutting or puncturing the skin or mucous membrane, the procedure is coded to the root operation CHANGE. Otherwise, the procedure for taking out the device is coded to the root operation REMOVAL.

Body Part Character 4	Approach Character 5	Device Character 6	Qualifier Character 7
Ø Lumbar Vertebral Joint Lumbar facet joint 3 Lumbosacral Joint Lumbosacral facet joint	Ø Open 3 Percutaneous 4 Percutaneous Endoscopic	Ø Drainage Device 3 Infusion Device 4 Internal Fixation Device 7 Autologous Tissue Substitute 8 Spacer A Interbody Fusion Device J Synthetic Substitute K Nonautologous Tissue Substitute	Z No Qualifier
Ø Lumbar Vertebral Joint Lumbar facet joint 3 Lumbosacral Joint Lumbosacral facet joint	X External	Ø Drainage Device 3 Infusion Device 4 Internal Fixation Device	Z No Qualifier
2 Lumbar Vertebral Disc 4 Lumbosacral Disc	Ø Open 3 Percutaneous 4 Percutaneous Endoscopic	Ø Drainage Device 3 Infusion Device 7 Autologous Tissue Substitute J Synthetic Substitute K Nonautologous Tissue Substitute	Z No Qualifier
2 Lumbar Vertebral Disc 4 Lumbosacral Disc	X External	Ø Drainage Device 3 Infusion Device	Z No Qualifier
5 Sacrococcygeal Joint Sacrococcygeal symphysis 6 Coccygeal Joint 7 Sacroiliac Joint, Right 8 Sacroiliac Joint, Left	Ø Open 3 Percutaneous 4 Percutaneous Endoscopic	Ø Drainage Device 3 Infusion Device 4 Internal Fixation Device 7 Autologous Tissue Substitute 8 Spacer J Synthetic Substitute K Nonautologous Tissue Substitute	Z No Qualifier
5 Sacrococcygeal Joint Sacrococcygeal symphysis 6 Coccygeal Joint 7 Sacroiliac Joint, Right 8 Sacroiliac Joint, Left	X External	Ø Drainage Device 3 Infusion Device 4 Internal Fixation Device	Z No Qualifier
9 Hip Joint, Right ⊞ Acetabulofemoral joint B Hip Joint, Left ⊞ *See 9 Hip Joint, Right*	Ø Open	Ø Drainage Device 3 Infusion Device 4 Internal Fixation Device 5 External Fixation Device 7 Autologous Tissue Substitute 8 Spacer 9 Liner B Resurfacing Device E Articulating Spacer J Synthetic Substitute K Nonautologous Tissue Substitute	Z No Qualifier
9 Hip Joint, Right ⊞ Acetabulofemoral joint B Hip Joint, Left ⊞ *See 9 Hip Joint, Right*	3 Percutaneous 4 Percutaneous Endoscopic	Ø Drainage Device 3 Infusion Device 4 Internal Fixation Device 5 External Fixation Device 7 Autologous Tissue Substitute 8 Spacer J Synthetic Substitute K Nonautologous Tissue Substitute	Z No Qualifier
9 Hip Joint, Right Acetabulofemoral joint B Hip Joint, Left *See 9 Hip Joint, Right*	X External	Ø Drainage Device 3 Infusion Device 4 Internal Fixation Device 5 External Fixation Device	Z No Qualifier

ØSP Continued on next page

Non-OR ØSP[Ø,3][Ø,3,4]8Z
Non-OR ØSP[Ø,3]3[Ø,3]Z
Non-OR ØSP[Ø,3]X[Ø,3,4]Z
Non-OR ØSP[2,4]3[Ø,3]Z
Non-OR ØSP[2,4]X[Ø,3]Z
Non-OR ØSP[5,6,7,8][Ø,3,4]8Z
Non-OR ØSP[5,6,7,8]3[Ø,3]Z
Non-OR ØSP[5,6,7,8]X[Ø,3,4]Z
Non-OR ØSP[9,B]3[Ø,3,8]Z
Non-OR ØSP[9,B]X[Ø,3,4,5]Z

See Appendix L for Procedure Combinations
Combo-only ØSP[9,B]Ø8Z
Combo-only ØSP[9,B]48Z
⊞ ØSP[9,B]Ø[9,B,J]Z
⊞ ØSP[9,B]4JZ

ØSP Continued

Ø Medical and Surgical
S Lower Joints
P Removal Definition: Taking out or off a device from a body part

Explanation: If a device is taken out and a similar device put in without cutting or puncturing the skin or mucous membrane, the procedure is coded to the root operation CHANGE. Otherwise, the procedure for taking out the device is coded to the root operation REMOVAL.

Body Part Character 4	Approach Character 5	Device Character 6	Qualifier Character 7
A Hip Joint, Acetabular Surface, Right ⊞ **E** Hip Joint, Acetabular Surface, Left ⊞ **R** Hip Joint, Femoral Surface, Right ⊞ **S** Hip Joint, Femoral Surface, Left ⊞ **T** Knee Joint, Femoral Surface, Right ⊞ Femoropatellar joint Patellofemoral joint **U** Knee Joint, Femoral Surface, Left ⊞ *See T Knee Joint, Femoral Surface, Right* **V** Knee Joint, Tibial Surface, Right ⊞ Femorotibial joint Tibiofemoral joint **W** Knee Joint, Tibial Surface, Left ⊞ *See V Knee Joint, Tibial Surface, Right*	**Ø** Open **3** Percutaneous **4** Percutaneous Endoscopic	**J** Synthetic Substitute	**Z** No Qualifier
C Knee Joint, Right ⊞ Femoropatellar joint Femorotibial joint Lateral meniscus Medial meniscus Patellofemoral joint Tibiofemoral joint **D** Knee Joint, Left ⊞ *See C Knee Joint, Right*	**Ø** Open	**Ø** Drainage Device **3** Infusion Device **4** Internal Fixation Device **5** External Fixation Device **7** Autologous Tissue Substitute **8** Spacer **9** Liner **E** Articulating Spacer **K** Nonautologous Tissue Substitute **L** Synthetic Substitute, Unicondylar Medial **M** Synthetic Substitute, Unicondylar Lateral **N** Synthetic Substitute, Patellofemoral	**Z** No Qualifier
C Knee Joint, Right ⊞ Femoropatellar joint Femorotibial joint Lateral meniscus Medial meniscus Patellofemoral joint Tibiofemoral joint **D** Knee Joint, Left ⊞ *See C Knee Joint, Right*	**Ø** Open	**J** Synthetic Substitute	**C** Patellar Surface **Z** No Qualifier
C Knee Joint, Right Femoropatellar joint Femorotibial joint Lateral meniscus Medial meniscus Patellofemoral joint Tibiofemoral joint **D** Knee Joint, Left *See C Knee Joint, Right*	**3** Percutaneous **4** Percutaneous Endoscopic	**Ø** Drainage Device **3** Infusion Device **4** Internal Fixation Device **5** External Fixation Device **7** Autologous Tissue Substitute **8** Spacer **K** Nonautologous Tissue Substitute **L** Synthetic Substitute, Unicondylar Medial **M** Synthetic Substitute, Unicondylar Lateral **N** Synthetic Substitute, Patellofemoral	**Z** No Qualifier
C Knee Joint, Right ⊞ Femoropatellar joint Femorotibial joint Lateral meniscus Medial meniscus Patellofemoral joint Tibiofemoral joint **D** Knee Joint, Left ⊞ *See C Knee Joint, Right*	**3** Percutaneous **4** Percutaneous Endoscopic	**J** Synthetic Substitute	**C** Patellar Surface **Z** No Qualifier

ØSP Continued on next page

Non-OR ØSP[C,D]3[Ø,3]Z

See Appendix L for Procedure Combinations

Combo-only ØSP[C,D]Ø8Z
Combo-only ØSP[C,D][3,4]8Z
⊞ ØSP[A,E,R,S,T,U,V,W][Ø,4]JZ
⊞ ØSP[C,D]Ø9Z
⊞ ØSP[C,D]ØJ[C,Z]
⊞ ØSP[C,D]4J[C,Z]

Ø Medical and Surgical
S Lower Joints
P Removal Definition: Taking out or off a device from a body part

Explanation: If a device is taken out and a similar device put in without cutting or puncturing the skin or mucous membrane, the procedure is coded to the root operation CHANGE. Otherwise, the procedure for taking out the device is coded to the root operation REMOVAL.

ØSP Continued

Body Part Character 4	Approach Character 5	Device Character 6	Qualifier Character 7
C Knee Joint, Right Femoropatellar joint Femorotibial joint Lateral meniscus Medial meniscus Patellofemoral joint Tibiofemoral joint **D Knee Joint, Left** *See C Knee Joint, Right*	X External	Ø Drainage Device 3 Infusion Device 4 Internal Fixation Device 5 External Fixation Device	Z No Qualifier
F Ankle Joint, Right Inferior tibiofibular joint Talocrural joint **G Ankle Joint, Left** *See F Ankle Joint, Right* **H Tarsal Joint, Right** Calcaneocuboid joint Cuboideonavicular joint Cuneonavicular joint Intercuneiform joint Subtalar (talocalcaneal) joint Talocalcaneal (subtalar) joint Talocalcaneonavicular joint **J Tarsal Joint, Left** *See H Tarsal Joint, Right* **K Tarsometatarsal Joint, Right** **L Tarsometatarsal Joint, Left** **M Metatarsal-Phalangeal Joint, Right** Metatarsophalangeal (MTP) joint **N Metatarsal-Phalangeal Joint, Left** *See M Metatarsal-Phalangeal Joint, Right* **P Toe Phalangeal Joint, Right** Interphalangeal (IP) joint **Q Toe Phalangeal Joint, Left** *See P Toe Phalangeal Joint, Right*	Ø Open 3 Percutaneous 4 Percutaneous Endoscopic	Ø Drainage Device 3 Infusion Device 4 Internal Fixation Device 5 External Fixation Device 7 Autologous Tissue Substitute 8 Spacer J Synthetic Substitute K Nonautologous Tissue Substitute	Z No Qualifier
F Ankle Joint, Right Inferior tibiofibular joint Talocrural joint **G Ankle Joint, Left** *See F Ankle Joint, Right* **H Tarsal Joint, Right** Calcaneocuboid joint Cuboideonavicular joint Cuneonavicular joint Intercuneiform joint Subtalar (talocalcaneal) joint Talocalcaneal (subtalar) joint Talocalcaneonavicular joint **J Tarsal Joint, Left** *See H Tarsal Joint, Right* **K Tarsometatarsal Joint, Right** **L Tarsometatarsal Joint, Left** **M Metatarsal-Phalangeal Joint, Right** Metatarsophalangeal (MTP) joint **N Metatarsal-Phalangeal Joint, Left** *See M Metatarsal-Phalangeal Joint, Right* **P Toe Phalangeal Joint, Right** Interphalangeal (IP) joint **Q Toe Phalangeal Joint, Left** *See P Toe Phalangeal Joint, Right*	X External	Ø Drainage Device 3 Infusion Device 4 Internal Fixation Device 5 External Fixation Device	Z No Qualifier

Non-OR ØSP[C,D]X[Ø,3,4,5]Z
Non-OR ØSP[F,G,H,J,K,L,M,N,P,Q]3[Ø,3,8]Z
Non-OR ØSP[F,G,H,J,K,L,M,N,P,Q][Ø,4]8Z
Non-OR ØSP[F,G,H,J,K,L,M,N,P,Q]X[Ø,3,4,5]Z

Ø Medical and Surgical
S Lower Joints
Q Repair Definition: Restoring, to the extent possible, a body part to its normal anatomic structure and function
Explanation: Used only when the method to accomplish the repair is not one of the other root operations

Body Part Character 4	Approach Character 5	Device Character 6	Qualifier Character 7
Ø Lumbar Vertebral Joint Lumbar facet joint **2 Lumbar Vertebral Disc** **3 Lumbosacral Joint** Lumbosacral facet joint **4 Lumbosacral Disc** **5 Sacrococcygeal Joint** Sacrococcygeal symphysis **6 Coccygeal Joint** **7 Sacroiliac Joint, Right** **8 Sacroiliac Joint, Left** **9 Hip Joint, Right** Acetabulofemoral joint **B Hip Joint, Left** *See 9 Hip Joint, Right* **C Knee Joint, Right** Femoropatellar joint Femorotibial joint Lateral meniscus Medial meniscus Patellofemoral joint Tibiofemoral joint **D Knee Joint, Left** *See C Knee Joint, Right* **F Ankle Joint, Right** Inferior tibiofibular joint Talocrural joint **G Ankle Joint, Left** *See F Ankle Joint, Right* **H Tarsal Joint, Right** Calcaneocuboid joint Cuboideonavicular joint Cuneonavicular joint Intercuneiform joint Subtalar (talocalcaneal) joint Talocalcaneal (subtalar) joint Talocalcaneonavicular joint **J Tarsal Joint, Left** *See H Tarsal Joint, Right* **K Tarsometatarsal Joint, Right** **L Tarsometatarsal Joint, Left** **M Metatarsal-Phalangeal Joint, Right** Metatarsophalangeal (MTP) joint **N Metatarsal-Phalangeal Joint, Left** *See M Metatarsal-Phalangeal Joint, Right* **P Toe Phalangeal Joint, Right** Interphalangeal (IP) joint **Q Toe Phalangeal Joint, Left** *See P Toe Phalangeal Joint, Right*	**Ø Open** **3 Percutaneous** **4 Percutaneous Endoscopic** **X External**	**Z No Device**	**Z No Qualifier**

Non-OR ØSQ[Ø,2,3,4,5,6,7,8,9,B,C,D,F,G,H,J,K,L,M,N,P,Q]XZZ

Ø Medical and Surgical
S Lower Joints
R Replacement Definition: Putting in or on biological or synthetic material that physically takes the place and/or function of all or a portion of a body part

Explanation: The body part may have been taken out or replaced, or may be taken out, physically eradicated, or rendered nonfunctional during the REPLACEMENT procedure. A REMOVAL procedure is coded for taking out the device used in a previous replacement procedure.

Body Part Character 4	Approach Character 5	Device Character 6	Qualifier Character 7
Ø Lumbar Vertebral Joint Lumbar facet joint **2 Lumbar Vertebral Disc** NC **3 Lumbosacral Joint** Lumbosacral facet joint **4 Lumbosacral Disc** NC **5 Sacrococcygeal Joint** Sacrococcygeal symphysis **6 Coccygeal Joint** **7 Sacroiliac Joint, Right** **8 Sacroiliac Joint, Left** **H Tarsal Joint, Right** Calcaneocuboid joint Cuboideonavicular joint Cuneonavicular joint Intercuneiform joint Subtalar (talocalcaneal) joint Talocalcaneal (subtalar) joint Talocalcaneonavicular joint **J Tarsal Joint, Left** *See H Tarsal Joint, Right* **K Tarsometatarsal Joint, Right** **L Tarsometatarsal Joint, Left** **M Metatarsal-Phalangeal Joint, Right** Metatarsophalangeal (MTP) joint **N Metatarsal-Phalangeal Joint, Left** *See M Metatarsal-Phalangeal Joint, Right* **P Toe Phalangeal Joint, Right** Interphalangeal (IP) joint **Q Toe Phalangeal Joint, Left** *See P Toe Phalangeal Joint, Right*	Ø Open	7 Autologous Tissue Substitute J Synthetic Substitute K Nonautologous Tissue Substitute	Z No Qualifier
9 Hip Joint, Right ⊞ Acetabulofemoral joint **B Hip Joint, Left** ⊞ *See 9 Hip Joint, Right*	Ø Open	1 Synthetic Substitute, Metal 2 Synthetic Substitute, Metal on Polyethylene 3 Synthetic Substitute, Ceramic 4 Synthetic Substitute, Ceramic on Polyethylene 6 Synthetic Substitute, Oxidized Zirconium on Polyethylene J Synthetic Substitute	9 Cemented A Uncemented Z No Qualifier
9 Hip Joint, Right Acetabulofemoral joint **B Hip Joint, Left** *See 9 Hip Joint, Right*	Ø Open	7 Autologous Tissue Substitute E Articulating Spacer K Nonautologous Tissue Substitute	Z No Qualifier
A Hip Joint, Acetabular Surface, Right ⊞ **E Hip Joint, Acetabular Surface, Left** ⊞	Ø Open	Ø Synthetic Substitute, Polyethylene 1 Synthetic Substitute, Metal 3 Synthetic Substitute, Ceramic J Synthetic Substitute	9 Cemented A Uncemented Z No Qualifier
A Hip Joint, Acetabular Surface, Right **E Hip Joint, Acetabular Surface, Left**	Ø Open	7 Autologous Tissue Substitute K Nonautologous Tissue Substitute	Z No Qualifier

ØSR Continued on next page

HAC ØSR[9,B]Ø[1,2,3,4,6,J][9,A,Z] when reported with SDx of I26.Ø2-I26.Ø9, I26.92-I26.99, or I82.4Ø1-I82.4Z9
HAC ØSR[9,B]Ø[7,K]Z when reported with SDx of I26.Ø2-I26.Ø9, I26.92-I26.99, or I82.4Ø1-I82.4Z9
HAC ØSR[A,E]Ø[Ø,1,3,J][9,A,Z] when reported with SDx of I26.Ø2-I26.Ø9, I26.92-I26.99, or I82.4Ø1-I82.4Z9
HAC ØSR[A,E]Ø[7,K]Z when reported with SDx of I26.Ø2-I26.Ø9, I26.92-I26.99, or I82.4Ø1-I82.4Z9
NC ØSR[2,4]ØJZ when beneficiary age is over 6Ø

See Appendix L for Procedure Combinations
⊞ ØSR[9,B]Ø[1,2,3,4,6,J][9,A,Z]
⊞ ØSR[A,E]Ø[Ø,1,3,J][9,A,Z]

ØSR Continued

Ø Medical and Surgical
S Lower Joints
R Replacement Definition: Putting in or on biological or synthetic material that physically takes the place and/or function of all or a portion of a body part

Explanation: The body part may have been taken out or replaced, or may be taken out, physically eradicated, or rendered nonfunctional during the REPLACEMENT procedure. A REMOVAL procedure is coded for taking out the device used in a previous replacement procedure.

Body Part Character 4	Approach Character 5	Device Character 6	Qualifier Character 7
C Knee Joint, Right Femoropatellar joint Femorotibial joint Lateral meniscus Medial meniscus Patellofemoral joint Tibiofemoral joint **D Knee Joint, Left** *See C Knee Joint, Right*	**Ø Open**	**6 Synthetic Substitute, Oxidized Zirconium on Polyethylene** **J Synthetic Substitute** **L Synthetic Substitute, Unicondylar Medial** **M Synthetic Substitute, Unicondylar Lateral** **N Synthetic Substitute, Patellofemoral**	**9 Cemented** **A Uncemented** **Z No Qualifier**
C Knee Joint, Right ⊞ Femoropatellar joint Femorotibial joint Lateral meniscus Medial meniscus Patellofemoral joint Tibiofemoral joint **D Knee Joint, Left** ⊞ *See C Knee Joint, Right*	**Ø Open**	**7 Autologous Tissue Substitute** **E Articulating Spacer** **K Nonautologous Tissue Substitute**	**Z No Qualifier**
F Ankle Joint, Right Inferior tibiofibular joint Talocrural joint **G Ankle Joint, Left** *See F Ankle Joint, Right* **T Knee Joint, Femoral Surface, Right** Femoropatellar joint Patellofemoral joint **U Knee Joint, Femoral Surface, Left** *See T Knee Joint, Femoral Surface, Right* **V Knee Joint, Tibial Surface, Right** Femorotibial joint Tibiofemoral joint **W Knee Joint, Tibial Surface, Left** *See V Knee Joint, Tibial Surface, Right*	**Ø Open**	**7 Autologous Tissue Substitute** **K Nonautologous Tissue Substitute**	**Z No Qualifier**
F Ankle Joint, Right Inferior tibiofibular joint Talocrural joint **G Ankle Joint, Left** *See F Ankle Joint, Right* **T Knee Joint, Femoral Surface, Right** ⊞ Femoropatellar joint Patellofemoral joint **U Knee Joint, Femoral Surface, Left** ⊞ *See T Knee Joint, Femoral Surface, Right* **V Knee Joint, Tibial Surface, Right** ⊞ Femorotibial joint Tibiofemoral joint **W Knee Joint, Tibial Surface, Left** ⊞ *See V Knee Joint, Tibial Surface, Right*	**Ø Open**	**J Synthetic Substitute**	**9 Cemented** **A Uncemented** **Z No Qualifier**
R Hip Joint, Femoral Surface, Right ⊞ **S Hip Joint, Femoral Surface, Left** ⊞	**Ø Open**	**1 Synthetic Substitute, Metal** **3 Synthetic Substitute, Ceramic** **J Synthetic Substitute**	**9 Cemented** **A Uncemented** **Z No Qualifier**
R Hip Joint, Femoral Surface, Right **S Hip Joint, Femoral Surface, Left**	**Ø Open**	**7 Autologous Tissue Substitute** **K Nonautologous Tissue Substitute**	**Z No Qualifier**

HAC ØSR[C,D]Ø[6,J][9,A,Z] when reported with SDx of I26.Ø2-I26.Ø9, I26.92-I26.99 or I82.4Ø1-I82.4Z9
HAC ØSR[C,D]Ø[7,K]Z when reported with SDx of I26.Ø2-I26.Ø9, I26.92-I26.99 or I82.4Ø1-I82.4Z9
HAC ØSR[T,U,V,W]Ø[7,K]Z when reported with SDx of I26.Ø2-I26.Ø9, I26.92-I26.99 or I82.4Ø1-I82.4Z9
HAC ØSR[T,U,V,W]ØJ[9,A,Z] when reported with SDx of I26.Ø2-I26.Ø9, I26.92-I26.99 or I82.4Ø1-I82.4Z9
HAC ØSR[R,S]Ø[1,3,J][9,A,Z] when reported with SDx of I26.Ø2-I26.Ø9, I26.92-I26.99, or I82.4Ø1-I82.4Z9
HAC ØSR[R,S]Ø[7,K]Z when reported with SDx of I26.Ø2-I26.Ø9, I26.92-I26.99, or I82.4Ø1-I82.4Z9

See Appendix L for Procedure Combinations
⊞ ØSR[C,D]Ø[6,J][9,A,Z]
⊞ ØSR[T,U,V,W]ØJ[9,A,Z]
⊞ ØSR[R,S]Ø[1,3,J][9,A,Z]

Ø Medical and Surgical
S Lower Joints
S Reposition Definition: Moving to its normal location, or other suitable location, all or a portion of a body part

Explanation: The body part is moved to a new location from an abnormal location, or from a normal location where it is not functioning correctly. The body part may or may not be cut out or off to be moved to the new location.

Body Part Character 4	Approach Character 5	Device Character 6	Qualifier Character 7
Ø Lumbar Vertebral Joint Lumbar facet joint **3 Lumbosacral Joint** Lumbosacral facet joint **5 Sacrococcygeal Joint** Sacrococcygeal symphysis **6 Coccygeal Joint** **7 Sacroiliac Joint, Right** **8 Sacroiliac Joint, Left**	Ø Open 3 Percutaneous 4 Percutaneous Endoscopic X External	4 Internal Fixation Device Z No Device	Z No Qualifier
9 Hip Joint, Right Acetabulofemoral joint **B Hip Joint, Left** *See 9 Hip Joint, Right* **C Knee Joint, Right** Femoropatellar joint; Femorotibial joint; Lateral meniscus; Medial meniscus; Patellofemoral joint; Tibiofemoral joint **D Knee Joint, Left** *See C Knee Joint, Right* **F Ankle Joint, Right** Inferior tibiofibular joint; Talocrural joint **G Ankle Joint, Left** *See F Ankle Joint, Right* **H Tarsal Joint, Right** Calcaneocuboid joint; Cuboideonavicular joint; Cuneonavicular joint; Intercuneiform joint; Subtalar (talocalcaneal) joint; Talocalcaneal (subtalar) joint; Talocalcaneonavicular joint **J Tarsal Joint, Left** *See H Tarsal Joint, Right* **K Tarsometatarsal Joint, Right** **L Tarsometatarsal Joint, Left** **M Metatarsal-Phalangeal Joint, Right** Metatarsophalangeal (MTP) joint **N Metatarsal-Phalangeal Joint, Left** *See M Metatarsal-Phalangeal Joint, Right* **P Toe Phalangeal Joint, Right** Interphalangeal (IP) joint **Q Toe Phalangeal Joint, Left** *See P Toe Phalangeal Joint, Right*	Ø Open 3 Percutaneous 4 Percutaneous Endoscopic X External	4 Internal Fixation Device 5 External Fixation Device Z No Device	Z No Qualifier

Non-OR ØSS[Ø,3,5,6,7,8][3,4,X][4,Z]Z
Non-OR ØSS[9,B,C,D,F,G,H,J,K,L,M,N,P,Q][3,4,X][4,5,Z]Z

Ø Medical and Surgical
S Lower Joints
T Resection Definition: Cutting out or off, without replacement, all of a body part

Explanation: None

Body Part Character 4	Approach Character 5	Device Character 6	Qualifier Character 7
2 Lumbar Vertebral Disc **4 Lumbosacral Disc** **5 Sacrococcygeal Joint** Sacrococcygeal symphysis **6 Coccygeal Joint** **7 Sacroiliac Joint, Right** **8 Sacroiliac Joint, Left** **9 Hip Joint, Right** Acetabulofemoral joint **B Hip Joint, Left** *See 9 Hip Joint, Right* **C Knee Joint, Right** Femoropatellar joint; Femorotibial joint; Lateral meniscus; Medial meniscus; Patellofemoral joint; Tibiofemoral joint **D Knee Joint, Left** *See C Knee Joint, Right* **F Ankle Joint, Right** Inferior tibiofibular joint; Talocrural joint **G Ankle Joint, Left** *See F Ankle Joint, Right* **H Tarsal Joint, Right** Calcaneocuboid joint; Cuboideonavicular joint; Cuneonavicular joint; Intercuneiform joint; Subtalar (talocalcaneal) joint; Talocalcaneal (subtalar) joint; Talocalcaneonavicular joint **J Tarsal Joint, Left** *See H Tarsal Joint, Right* **K Tarsometatarsal Joint, Right** **L Tarsometatarsal Joint, Left** **M Metatarsal-Phalangeal Joint, Right** Metatarsophalangeal (MTP) joint **N Metatarsal-Phalangeal Joint, Left** *See M Metatarsal-Phalangeal Joint, Right* **P Toe Phalangeal Joint, Right** Interphalangeal (IP) joint **Q Toe Phalangeal Joint, Left** *See P Toe Phalangeal Joint, Right*	Ø Open	Z No Device	Z No Qualifier

Ø Medical and Surgical
S Lower Joints
U Supplement Definition: Putting in or on biological or synthetic material that physically reinforces and/or augments the function of a portion of a body part
Explanation: The biological material is non-living, or is living and from the same individual. The body part may have been previously replaced, and the SUPPLEMENT procedure is performed to physically reinforce and/or augment the function of the replaced body part.

Body Part Character 4	Approach Character 5	Device Character 6	Qualifier Character 7
Ø Lumbar Vertebral Joint Lumbar facet joint **2 Lumbar Vertebral Disc** **3 Lumbosacral Joint** Lumbosacral facet joint **4 Lumbosacral Disc** **5 Sacrococcygeal Joint** Sacrococcygeal symphysis **6 Coccygeal Joint** **7 Sacroiliac Joint, Right** **8 Sacroiliac Joint, Left** **F Ankle Joint, Right** Inferior tibiofibular joint Talocrural joint **G Ankle Joint, Left** *See F Ankle Joint, Right* **H Tarsal Joint, Right** Calcaneocuboid joint Cuboideonavicular joint Cuneonavicular joint Intercuneiform joint Subtalar (talocalcaneal) joint Talocalcaneal (subtalar) joint Talocalcaneonavicular joint **J Tarsal Joint, Left** *See H Tarsal Joint, Right* **K Tarsometatarsal Joint, Right** **L Tarsometatarsal Joint, Left** **M Metatarsal-Phalangeal Joint, Right** Metatarsophalangeal (MTP) joint **N Metatarsal-Phalangeal Joint, Left** *See M Metatarsal-Phalangeal Joint, Right* **P Toe Phalangeal Joint, Right** Interphalangeal (IP) joint **Q Toe Phalangeal Joint, Left** *See P Toe Phalangeal Joint, Right*	**Ø Open** **3 Percutaneous** **4 Percutaneous Endoscopic**	**7 Autologous Tissue Substitute** **J Synthetic Substitute** **K Nonautologous Tissue Substitute**	**Z No Qualifier**
9 Hip Joint, Right ⊞ Acetabulofemoral joint **B Hip Joint, Left** ⊞ *See 9 Hip Joint, Right*	**Ø Open**	**7 Autologous Tissue Substitute** **9 Liner** **B Resurfacing Device** **J Synthetic Substitute** **K Nonautologous Tissue Substitute**	**Z No Qualifier**
9 Hip Joint, Right Acetabulofemoral joint **B Hip Joint, Left** *See 9 Hip Joint, Right*	**3 Percutaneous** **4 Percutaneous Endoscopic**	**7 Autologous Tissue Substitute** **J Synthetic Substitute** **K Nonautologous Tissue Substitute**	**Z No Qualifier**
A Hip Joint, Acetabular Surface, Right ⊞ **E Hip Joint, Acetabular Surface, Left** ⊞ **R Hip Joint, Femoral Surface, Right** ⊞ **S Hip Joint, Femoral Surface, Left** ⊞	**Ø Open**	**9 Liner** **B Resurfacing Device**	**Z No Qualifier**
C Knee Joint, Right Femoropatellar joint Femorotibial joint Lateral meniscus Medial meniscus Patellofemoral joint Tibiofemoral joint **D Knee Joint, Left** *See C Knee Joint, Right*	**Ø Open**	**7 Autologous Tissue Substitute** **J Synthetic Substitute** **K Nonautologous Tissue Substitute**	**Z No Qualifier**
C Knee Joint, Right Femoropatellar joint Femorotibial joint Lateral meniscus Medial meniscus Patellofemoral joint Tibiofemoral joint **D Knee Joint, Left** *See C Knee Joint, Right*	**Ø Open**	**9 Liner**	**C Patellar Surface** **Z No Qualifier**

ØSU Continued on next page

HAC ØSU[9,B]ØBZ when reported with SDx of I26.Ø2-I26.Ø9, I26.92-I26.99, or I82.4Ø1-I82.4Z9
HAC ØSU[A,E,R,S]ØBZ when reported with SDx of I26.Ø2-I26.Ø9, I26.92-I26.99, or I82.4Ø1-I82.4Z9

See Appendix L for Procedure Combinations
⊞ ØSU[9,B]Ø9Z
⊞ ØSU[A,E,R,S]Ø9Z

Ø Medical and Surgical
S Lower Joints
U Supplement Definition: Putting in or on biological or synthetic material that physically reinforces and/or augments the function of a portion of a body part
Explanation: The biological material is non-living, or is living and from the same individual. The body part may have been previously replaced, and the SUPPLEMENT procedure is performed to physically reinforce and/or augment the function of the replaced body part.

ØSU Continued

Body Part Character 4	Approach Character 5	Device Character 6	Qualifier Character 7
C Knee Joint, Right Femoropatellar joint Femorotibial joint Lateral meniscus Medial meniscus Patellofemoral joint Tibiofemoral joint **D Knee Joint, Left** *See C Knee Joint, Right*	**3 Percutaneous** **4 Percutaneous Endoscopic**	**7 Autologous Tissue Substitute** **J Synthetic Substitute** **K Nonautologous Tissue Substitute**	**Z No Qualifier**
T Knee Joint, Femoral Surface, Right Femoropatellar joint Patellofemoral joint **U Knee Joint, Femoral Surface, Left** *See T Knee Joint, Femoral Surface, Right* **V Knee Joint, Tibial Surface, Right** ⊞ Femorotibial joint Tibiofemoral joint **W Knee Joint, Tibial Surface, Left** ⊞ *See V Knee Joint, Tibial Surface, Right*	**Ø Open**	**9 Liner**	**Z No Qualifier**

See Appendix L for Procedure Combinations
⊞ ØSU[V,W]Ø9Z

Ø Medical and Surgical
S Lower Joints
W Revision Definition: Correcting, to the extent possible, a portion of a malfunctioning device or the position of a displaced device
Explanation: Revision can include correcting a malfunctioning or displaced device by taking out or putting in components of the device such as a screw or pin

Body Part Character 4	Approach Character 5	Device Character 6	Qualifier Character 7
Ø Lumbar Vertebral Joint Lumbar facet joint **3** Lumbosacral Joint Lumbosacral facet joint	**Ø** Open **3** Percutaneous **4** Percutaneous Endoscopic **X** External	**Ø** Drainage Device **3** Infusion Device **4** Internal Fixation Device **7** Autologous Tissue Substitute **8** Spacer **A** Interbody Fusion Device **J** Synthetic Substitute **K** Nonautologous Tissue Substitute	**Z** No Qualifier
2 Lumbar Vertebral Disc **4** Lumbosacral Disc	**Ø** Open **3** Percutaneous **4** Percutaneous Endoscopic **X** External	**Ø** Drainage Device **3** Infusion Device **7** Autologous Tissue Substitute **J** Synthetic Substitute **K** Nonautologous Tissue Substitute	**Z** No Qualifier
5 Sacrococcygeal Joint Sacrococcygeal symphysis **6** Coccygeal Joint **7** Sacroiliac Joint, Right **8** Sacroiliac Joint, Left	**Ø** Open **3** Percutaneous **4** Percutaneous Endoscopic **X** External	**Ø** Drainage Device **3** Infusion Device **4** Internal Fixation Device **7** Autologous Tissue Substitute **8** Spacer **J** Synthetic Substitute **K** Nonautologous Tissue Substitute	**Z** No Qualifier
9 Hip Joint, Right Acetabulofemoral joint **B** Hip Joint, Left *See 9 Hip Joint, Right*	**Ø** Open	**Ø** Drainage Device **3** Infusion Device **4** Internal Fixation Device **5** External Fixation Device **7** Autologous Tissue Substitute **8** Spacer **9** Liner **B** Resurfacing Device **J** Synthetic Substitute **K** Nonautologous Tissue Substitute	**Z** No Qualifier
9 Hip Joint, Right Acetabulofemoral joint **B** Hip Joint, Left *See 9 Hip Joint, Right*	**3** Percutaneous **4** Percutaneous Endoscopic **X** External	**Ø** Drainage Device **3** Infusion Device **4** Internal Fixation Device **5** External Fixation Device **7** Autologous Tissue Substitute **8** Spacer **J** Synthetic Substitute **K** Nonautologous Tissue Substitute	**Z** No Qualifier
A Hip Joint, Acetabular Surface, Right **E** Hip Joint, Acetabular Surface, Left **R** Hip Joint, Femoral Surface, Right **S** Hip Joint, Femoral Surface, Left **T** Knee Joint, Femoral Surface, Right Femoropatellar joint Patellofemoral joint **U** Knee Joint, Femoral Surface, Left *See T Knee Joint, Femoral Surface, Right* **V** Knee Joint, Tibial Surface, Right Femorotibial joint Tibiofemoral joint **W** Knee Joint, Tibial Surface, Left *See V Knee Joint, Tibial Surface, Right*	**Ø** Open **3** Percutaneous **4** Percutaneous Endoscopic **X** External	**J** Synthetic Substitute	**Z** No Qualifier
C Knee Joint, Right Femoropatellar joint Femorotibial joint Lateral meniscus Medial meniscus Patellofemoral joint Tibiofemoral joint **D** Knee Joint, Left *See C Knee Joint, Right*	**Ø** Open	**Ø** Drainage Device **3** Infusion Device **4** Internal Fixation Device **5** External Fixation Device **7** Autologous Tissue Substitute **8** Spacer **9** Liner **K** Nonautologous Tissue Substitute	**Z** No Qualifier

ØSW Continued on next page

Non-OR ØSW[Ø,3]X[Ø,3,4,7,8,A,J,K]Z
Non-OR ØSW[2,4]X[Ø,3,7,J,K]Z
Non-OR ØSW[5,6,7,8]X[Ø,3,4,7,8,J,K]Z
Non-OR ØSW[9,B]X[Ø,3,4,5,7,8,J,K]Z
Non-OR ØSW[A,E,R,S,T,U,V,W]XJZ

Ø Medical and Surgical
S Lower Joints
W Revision

ØSW Continued

Definition: Correcting, to the extent possible, a portion of a malfunctioning device or the position of a displaced device

Explanation: Revision can include correcting a malfunctioning or displaced device by taking out or putting in components of the device such as a screw or pin

Body Part Character 4	Approach Character 5	Device Character 6	Qualifier Character 7
C Knee Joint, Right Femoropatellar joint Femorotibial joint Lateral meniscus Medial meniscus Patellofemoral joint Tibiofemoral joint **D** Knee Joint, Left *See C Knee Joint, Right*	**Ø** Open	**J** Synthetic Substitute	**C** Patellar Surface **Z** No Qualifier
C Knee Joint, Right Femoropatellar joint Femorotibial joint Lateral meniscus Medial meniscus Patellofemoral joint Tibiofemoral joint **D** Knee Joint, Left *See C Knee Joint, Right*	**3** Percutaneous **4** Percutaneous Endoscopic **X** External	**Ø** Drainage Device **3** Infusion Device **4** Internal Fixation Device **5** External Fixation Device **7** Autologous Tissue Substitute **8** Spacer **K** Nonautologous Tissue Substitute	**Z** No Qualifier
C Knee Joint, Right Femoropatellar joint Femorotibial joint Lateral meniscus Medial meniscus Patellofemoral joint Tibiofemoral joint **D** Knee Joint, Left *See C Knee Joint, Right*	**3** Percutaneous **4** Percutaneous Endoscopic **X** External	**J** Synthetic Substitute	**C** Patellar Surface **Z** No Qualifier
F Ankle Joint, Right Inferior tibiofibular joint Talocrural joint **G** Ankle Joint, Left *See F Ankle Joint, Right* **H** Tarsal Joint, Right Calcaneocuboid joint Cuboideonavicular joint Cuneonavicular joint Intercuneiform joint Subtalar (talocalcaneal) joint Talocalcaneal (subtalar) joint Talocalcaneonavicular joint **J** Tarsal Joint, Left *See H Tarsal Joint, Right* **K** Tarsometatarsal Joint, Right **L** Tarsometatarsal Joint, Left **M** Metatarsal-Phalangeal Joint, Right Metatarsophalangeal (MTP) joint **N** Metatarsal-Phalangeal Joint, Left *See M Metatarsal-Phalangeal Joint, Right* **P** Toe Phalangeal Joint, Right Interphalangeal (IP) joint **Q** Toe Phalangeal Joint, Left *See P Toe Phalangeal Joint, Right*	**Ø** Open **3** Percutaneous **4** Percutaneous Endoscopic **X** External	**Ø** Drainage Device **3** Infusion Device **4** Internal Fixation Device **5** External Fixation Device **7** Autologous Tissue Substitute **8** Spacer **J** Synthetic Substitute **K** Nonautologous Tissue Substitute	**Z** No Qualifier

Non-OR ØSW[C,D]X[Ø,3,4,5,7,8,K]Z
Non-OR ØSW[C,D]XJ[C,Z]
Non-OR ØSW[F,G,H,J,K,L,M,N,P,Q]X[Ø,3,4,5,7,8,J,K]Z

Urinary System ØT1–ØTY

Character Meanings

This Character Meaning table is provided as a guide to assist the user in the identification of character members that may be found in this section of code tables. It **SHOULD NOT** be used to build a PCS code.

Operation–Character 3	Body Part–Character 4	Approach–Character 5	Device–Character 6	Qualifier–Character 7
1 Bypass	Ø Kidney, Right	Ø Open	Ø Drainage Device	Ø Allogeneic
2 Change	1 Kidney, Left	3 Percutaneous	2 Monitoring Device	1 Syngeneic
5 Destruction	2 Kidneys, Bilateral	4 Percutaneous Endoscopic	3 Infusion Device	2 Zooplastic
7 Dilation	3 Kidney Pelvis, Right	7 Via Natural or Artificial Opening	7 Autologous Tissue Substitute	3 Kidney Pelvis, Right
8 Division	4 Kidney Pelvis, Left	8 Via Natural or Artificial Opening Endoscopic	C Extraluminal Device	4 Kidney Pelvis, Left
9 Drainage	5 Kidney	X External	D Intraluminal Device	6 Ureter, Right
B Excision	6 Ureter, Right		J Synthetic Substitute	7 Ureter, Left
C Extirpation	7 Ureter, Left		K Nonautologous Tissue Substitute	8 Colon
D Extraction	8 Ureters, Bilateral		L Artificial Sphincter	9 Colocutaneous
F Fragmentation	9 Ureter		M Stimulator Lead	A Ileum
H Insertion	B Bladder		Y Other Device	B Bladder
J Inspection	C Bladder Neck		Z No Device	C Ileocutaneous
L Occlusion	D Urethra			D Cutaneous
M Reattachment				X Diagnostic
N Release				Z No Qualifier
P Removal				
Q Repair				
R Replacement				
S Reposition				
T Resection				
U Supplement				
V Restriction				
W Revision				
Y Transplantation				

AHA Coding Clinic for table ØT1
2017, 3Q, 20 Creation of Indiana pouch
2017, 3Q, 21 Augmentation cystoplasty with Indiana pouch and continent urinary diversion
2017, 1Q, 37 Perineal urethrostomy
2015, 3Q, 34 Redo urinary diversion surgery via left ureteral reimplantation

AHA Coding Clinic for table ØT7
2017, 4Q, 111 Exchange of ureteral stent
2016, 2Q, 27 Exchange of ureteral stents
2015, 2Q, 8 Urinary calculi fragmentation and evacuation
2013, 4Q, 123 Urolift® procedure

AHA Coding Clinic for table ØT9
2017, 3Q, 19 Ureteral stent placement for urinary leakage
2017, 3Q, 20 Creation of Indiana pouch
2017, 3Q, 21 Augmentation cystoplasty with Indiana pouch and continent urinary diversion

AHA Coding Clinic for table ØTB
2016, 1Q, 19 Biopsy of neobladder malignancy
2015, 3Q, 34 Excision of Mitrofanoff polyp
2014, 2Q, 8 Ileoscopy with excision of polyp of ileal loop urinary diversion

AHA Coding Clinic for table ØTC
2016, 3Q, 23 Ureteral stone migrating into bladder
2015, 2Q, 7 Urinary calculi fragmentation and evacuation
2015, 2Q, 8 Urinary calculi fragmentation and evacuation
2013, 4Q, 122 Laser lithotripsy with removal of fragments

AHA Coding Clinic for table ØTF
2015, 2Q, 7 Urinary calculi fragmentation and evacuation
2013, 4Q, 122 Extracorporeal shock wave lithotripsy
2013, 4Q, 122 Laser lithotripsy with removal of fragments

AHA Coding Clinic for table ØTP
2017, 4Q, 111 Exchange of ureteral stent
2016, 2Q, 27 Exchange of ureteral stents

AHA Coding Clinic for table ØTQ
2018, 2Q, 27 Dismembered pyeloplasty
2017, 1Q, 37 Perineal urethrostomy

AHA Coding Clinic for table ØTR
2017, 3Q, 20 Creation of Indiana pouch

AHA Coding Clinic for table ØTS
2018, 2Q, 27 Dismembered pyeloplasty
2017, 1Q, 36 Dismembered pyeloplasty
2016, 1Q, 15 Pubovaginal sling placement

AHA Coding Clinic for table ØTT
2014, 3Q, 16 Hand-assisted laparoscopy nephroureterectomy

AHA Coding Clinic for table ØTU
2017, 3Q, 21 Augmentation cystoplasty with Indiana pouch and continent urinary diversion

AHA Coding Clinic for table ØTV
2015, 2Q, 11 Cystourethroscopic Deflux® injection

Urinary System

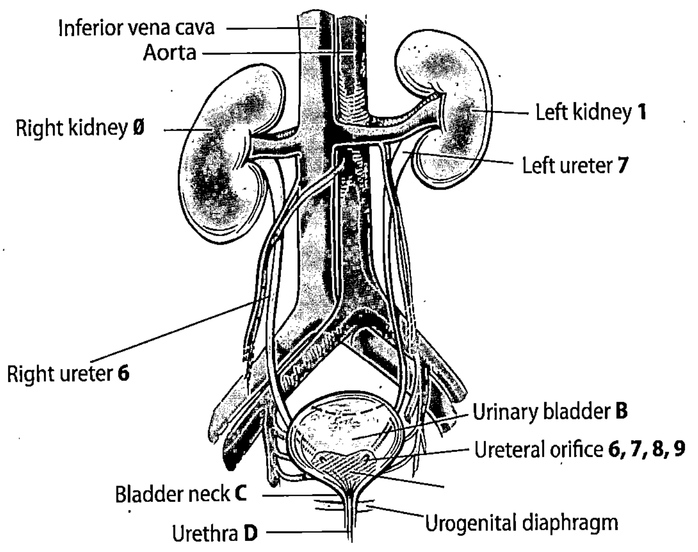

Kidney

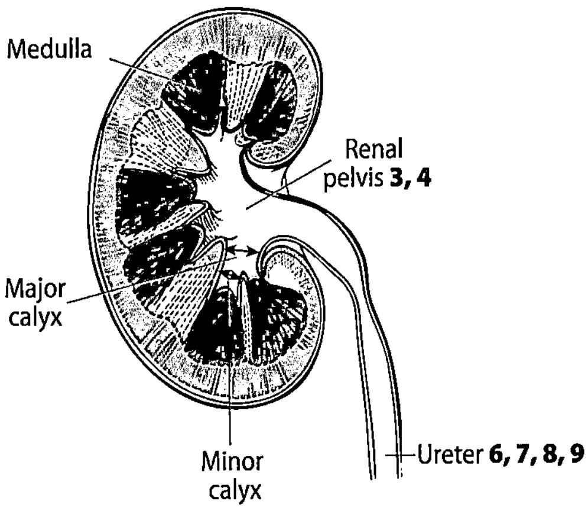

Cutaway detail of normal right kidney and ureter

Bladder

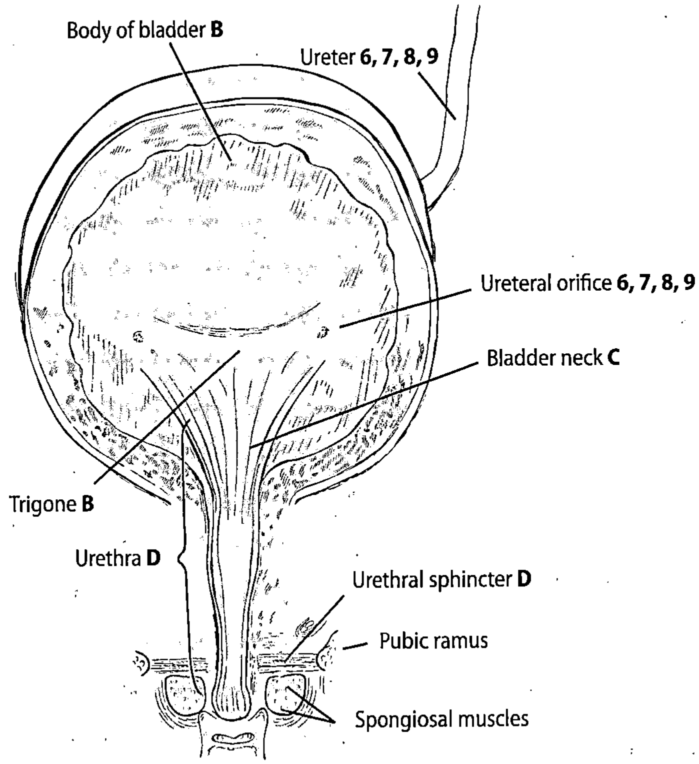

Ø Medical and Surgical
T Urinary System
1 Bypass Definition: Altering the route of passage of the contents of a tubular body part

Explanation: Rerouting contents of a body part to a downstream area of the normal route, to a similar route and body part, or to an abnormal route and dissimilar body part. Includes one or more anastomoses, with or without the use of a device.

Body Part Character 4	Approach Character 5	Device Character 6	Qualifier Character 7
3 Kidney Pelvis, Right Ureteropelvic junction (UPJ) **4 Kidney Pelvis, Left** *See 3 Kidney Pelvis, Right*	**Ø Open** **4 Percutaneous Endoscopic**	**7 Autologous Tissue Substitute** **J Synthetic Substitute** **K Nonautologous Tissue Substitute** **Z No Device**	**3 Kidney Pelvis, Right** **4 Kidney Pelvis, Left** **6 Ureter, Right** **7 Ureter, Left** **8 Colon** **9 Colocutaneous** **A Ileum** **B Bladder** **C Ileocutaneous** **D Cutaneous**
3 Kidney Pelvis, Right Ureteropelvic junction (UPJ) **4 Kidney Pelvis, Left** *See 3 Kidney Pelvis, Right*	**3 Percutaneous**	**J Synthetic Substitute**	**D Cutaneous**
6 Ureter, Right Ureteral orifice Ureterovesical orifice **7 Ureter, Left** *See 6 Ureter, Right* **8 Ureters, Bilateral** *See 6 Ureter, Right*	**Ø Open** **4 Percutaneous Endoscopic**	**7 Autologous Tissue Substitute** **J Synthetic Substitute** **K Nonautologous Tissue Substitute** **Z No Device**	**6 Ureter, Right** **7 Ureter, Left** **8 Colon** **9 Colocutaneous** **A Ileum** **B Bladder** **C Ileocutaneous** **D Cutaneous**
6 Ureter, Right Ureteral orifice Ureterovesical orifice **7 Ureter, Left** *See 6 Ureter, Right* **8 Ureters, Bilateral** *See 6 Ureter, Right*	**3 Percutaneous**	**J Synthetic Substitute**	**D Cutaneous**
B Bladder Trigone of bladder	**Ø Open** **4 Percutaneous Endoscopic**	**7 Autologous Tissue Substitute** **J Synthetic Substitute** **K Nonautologous Tissue Substitute** **Z No Device**	**9 Colocutaneous** **C Ileocutaneous** **D Cutaneous**
B Bladder Trigone of bladder	**3 Percutaneous**	**J Synthetic Substitute**	**D Cutaneous**

Ø Medical and Surgical
T Urinary System
2 Change Definition: Taking out or off a device from a body part and putting back an identical or similar device in or on the same body part without cutting or puncturing the skin or a mucous membrane

Explanation: All CHANGE procedures are coded using the approach EXTERNAL

Body Part Character 4	Approach Character 5	Device Character 6	Qualifier Character 7
5 Kidney Renal calyx Renal capsule Renal cortex Renal segment **9 Ureter** Ureteral orifice Ureterovesical orifice **B Bladder** Trigone of bladder **D Urethra** Bulbourethral (Cowper's) gland Cowper's (bulbourethral) gland External urethral sphincter Internal urethral sphincter Membranous urethra Penile urethra Prostatic urethra	**X External**	**Ø Drainage Device** **Y Other Device**	**Z No Qualifier**

Non-OR All body part, approach, device, and qualifier values

Ø Medical and Surgical
T Urinary System
5 Destruction Definition: Physical eradication of all or a portion of a body part by the direct use of energy, force, or a destructive agent
Explanation: None of the body part is physically taken out

Body Part Character 4	Approach Character 5	Device Character 6	Qualifier Character 7
Ø Kidney, Right Renal calyx Renal capsule Renal cortex Renal segment **1 Kidney, Left** *See Ø Kidney, Right* **3 Kidney Pelvis, Right** Ureteropelvic junction (UPJ) **4 Kidney Pelvis, Left** *See 3 Kidney Pelvis, Right* **6 Ureter, Right** Ureteral orifice Ureterovesical orifice **7 Ureter, Left** *See 6 Ureter, Right* **B Bladder** Trigone of bladder **C Bladder Neck**	**Ø Open** **3 Percutaneous** **4 Percutaneous Endoscopic** **7 Via Natural or Artificial Opening** **8 Via Natural or Artificial Opening Endoscopic**	**Z No Device**	**Z No Qualifier**
D Urethra Bulbourethral (Cowper's) gland Cowper's (bulbourethral) gland External urethral sphincter Internal urethral sphincter Membranous urethra Penile urethra Prostatic urethra	**Ø Open** **3 Percutaneous** **4 Percutaneous Endoscopic** **7 Via Natural or Artificial Opening** **8 Via Natural or Artificial Opening Endoscopic** **X External**	**Z No Device**	**Z No Qualifier**

Non-OR ØT5D[Ø,3,4,7,8,X]ZZ

Ø Medical and Surgical
T Urinary System
7 Dilation Definition: Expanding an orifice or the lumen of a tubular body part
Explanation: The orifice can be a natural orifice or an artificially created orifice. Accomplished by stretching a tubular body part using intraluminal pressure or by cutting part of the orifice or wall of the tubular body part.

Body Part Character 4	Approach Character 5	Device Character 6	Qualifier Character 7
3 Kidney Pelvis, Right Ureteropelvic junction (UPJ) **4 Kidney Pelvis, Left** *See 3 Kidney Pelvis, Right* **6 Ureter, Right** Ureteral orifice Ureterovesical orifice **7 Ureter, Left** *See 6 Ureter, Right* **8 Ureters, Bilateral** *See 6 Ureter, Right* **B Bladder** Trigone of bladder **C Bladder Neck** **D Urethra** Bulbourethral (Cowper's) gland Cowper's (bulbourethral) gland External urethral sphincter Internal urethral sphincter Membranous urethra Penile urethra Prostatic urethra	**Ø Open** **3 Percutaneous** **4 Percutaneous Endoscopic** **7 Via Natural or Artificial Opening** **8 Via Natural or Artificial Opening Endoscopic**	**D Intraluminal Device** **Z No Device**	**Z No Qualifier**

Non-OR ØT7[6,7][Ø,3,4,7,8]DZ
Non-OR ØT7[6,7][7,8]ZZ
Non-OR ØT7[8,D][Ø,3,4]DZ
Non-OR ØT7[8,B,D][7,8][D,Z]Z
Non-OR ØT7C[Ø,3,4,7,8][D,Z]Z

Ø Medical and Surgical
T Urinary System
8 Division Definition: Cutting into a body part, without draining fluids and/or gases from the body part, in order to separate or transect a body part
Explanation: All or a portion of the body part is separated into two or more portions

Body Part Character 4	Approach Character 5	Device Character 6	Qualifier Character 7
2 Kidneys, Bilateral Renal calyx Renal capsule Renal cortex Renal segment **C Bladder Neck**	**Ø Open** **3 Percutaneous** **4 Percutaneous Endoscopic**	**Z No Device**	**Z No Qualifier**

Ø Medical and Surgical
T Urinary System
9 Drainage Definition: Taking or letting out fluids and/or gases from a body part
Explanation: The qualifier DIAGNOSTIC is used to identify drainage procedures that are biopsies

Body Part Character 4	Approach Character 5	Device Character 6	Qualifier Character 7
Ø Kidney, Right Renal calyx Renal capsule Renal cortex Renal segment **1 Kidney, Left** *See Ø Kidney, Right* **3 Kidney Pelvis, Right** Ureteropelvic junction (UPJ) **4 Kidney Pelvis, Left** *See 3 Kidney Pelvis, Right* **6 Ureter, Right** Ureteral orifice Ureterovesical orifice **7 Ureter, Left** *See 6 Ureter, Right* **8 Ureters, Bilateral** *See 6 Ureter, Right* **B Bladder** Trigone of bladder **C Bladder Neck**	**Ø Open** **3 Percutaneous** **4 Percutaneous Endoscopic** **7 Via Natural or Artificial Opening** **8 Via Natural or Artificial Opening Endoscopic**	**Ø Drainage Device**	**Z No Qualifier**
Ø Kidney, Right Renal calyx Renal capsule Renal cortex Renal segment **1 Kidney, Left** *See Ø Kidney, Right* **3 Kidney Pelvis, Right** Ureteropelvic junction (UPJ) **4 Kidney Pelvis, Left** *See 3 Kidney Pelvis, Right* **6 Ureter, Right** Ureteral orifice Ureterovesical orifice **7 Ureter, Left** *See 6 Ureter, Right* **8 Ureters, Bilateral** *See 6 Ureter, Right* **B Bladder** Trigone of bladder **C Bladder Neck**	**Ø Open** **3 Percutaneous** **4 Percutaneous Endoscopic** **7 Via Natural or Artificial Opening** **8 Via Natural or Artificial Opening Endoscopic**	**Z No Device**	**X Diagnostic** **Z No Qualifier**
D Urethra Bulbourethral (Cowper's) gland Cowper's (bulbourethral) gland External urethral sphincter Internal urethral sphincter Membranous urethra Penile urethra Prostatic urethra	**Ø Open** **3 Percutaneous** **4 Percutaneous Endoscopic** **7 Via Natural or Artificial Opening** **8 Via Natural or Artificial Opening Endoscopic** **X External**	**Ø Drainage Device**	**Z No Qualifier**
D Urethra Bulbourethral (Cowper's) gland Cowper's (bulbourethral) gland External urethral sphincter Internal urethral sphincter Membranous urethra Penile urethra Prostatic urethra	**Ø Open** **3 Percutaneous** **4 Percutaneous Endoscopic** **7 Via Natural or Artificial Opening** **8 Via Natural or Artificial Opening Endoscopic** **X External**	**Z No Device**	**X Diagnostic** **Z No Qualifier**

Non-OR ØT9[Ø,1,3,4]3ØZ
Non-OR ØT9[6,7,8][Ø,3,4,7,8]ØZ
Non-OR ØT9[B,C][3,4,7,8]ØZ
Non-OR ØT9[Ø,1,3,4,6,7,8][3,4,7,8]ZX
Non-OR ØT9[Ø,1,3,4][3,4]ZZ
Non-OR ØT9[6,7,8]3ZZ
Non-OR ØT9[B,C][3,4,7,8]ZZ
Non-OR ØT9D3ØZ
Non-OR ØT9D[Ø,3,4,7,8,X]ZX
Non-OR ØT9D3ZZ

Urinary System

Ø Medical and Surgical
T Urinary System
B Excision Definition: Cutting out or off, without replacement, a portion of a body part
Explanation: The qualifier DIAGNOSTIC is used to identify excision procedures that are biopsies

Body Part Character 4	Approach Character 5	Device Character 6	Qualifier Character 7
Ø Kidney, Right Renal calyx Renal capsule Renal cortex Renal segment **1 Kidney, Left** *See Ø Kidney, Right* **3 Kidney Pelvis, Right** Ureteropelvic junction (UPJ) **4 Kidney Pelvis, Left** *See 3 Kidney Pelvis, Right* **6 Ureter, Right** Ureteral orifice Ureterovesical orifice **7 Ureter, Left** *See 6 Ureter, Right* **B Bladder** Trigone of bladder **C Bladder Neck**	**Ø Open** **3 Percutaneous** **4 Percutaneous Endoscopic** **7 Via Natural or Artificial Opening** **8 Via Natural or Artificial Opening Endoscopic**	**Z No Device**	**X Diagnostic** **Z No Qualifier**
D Urethra Bulbourethral (Cowper's) gland Cowper's (bulbourethral) gland External urethral sphincter Internal urethral sphincter Membranous urethra Penile urethra Prostatic urethra	**Ø Open** **3 Percutaneous** **4 Percutaneous Endoscopic** **7 Via Natural or Artificial Opening** **8 Via Natural or Artificial Opening Endoscopic** **X External**	**Z No Device**	**X Diagnostic** **Z No Qualifier**

Non-OR ØTB[Ø,1,3,4,6,7][3,4,7,8]ZX
Non-OR ØTBD[Ø,3,4,7,8,X]ZX

Ø Medical and Surgical
T Urinary System
C Extirpation Definition: Taking or cutting out solid matter from a body part
Explanation: The solid matter may be an abnormal byproduct of a biological function or a foreign body; it may be imbedded in a body part or in the lumen of a tubular body part. The solid matter may or may not have been previously broken into pieces.

Body Part Character 4	Approach Character 5	Device Character 6	Qualifier Character 7
Ø Kidney, Right Renal calyx Renal capsule Renal cortex Renal segment **1 Kidney, Left** *See Ø Kidney, Right* **3 Kidney Pelvis, Right** Ureteropelvic junction (UPJ) **4 Kidney Pelvis, Left** *See 3 Kidney Pelvis, Right* **6 Ureter, Right** Ureteral orifice Ureterovesical orifice **7 Ureter, Left** *See 6 Ureter, Right* **B Bladder** Trigone of bladder **C Bladder Neck**	**Ø Open** **3 Percutaneous** **4 Percutaneous Endoscopic** **7 Via Natural or Artificial Opening** **8 Via Natural or Artificial Opening Endoscopic**	**Z No Device**	**Z No Qualifier**
D Urethra Bulbourethral (Cowper's) gland Cowper's (bulbourethral) gland External urethral sphincter Internal urethral sphincter Membranous urethra Penile urethra Prostatic urethra	**Ø Open** **3 Percutaneous** **4 Percutaneous Endoscopic** **7 Via Natural or Artificial Opening** **8 Via Natural or Artificial Opening Endoscopic** **X External**	**Z No Device**	**Z No Qualifier**

Non-OR ØTC[B,C][7,8]ZZ
Non-OR ØTCD[7,8,X]ZZ

ØTB–ØTC

Ø Medical and Surgical
T Urinary System
D Extraction Definition: Pulling or stripping out or off all or a portion of a body part by the use of force
Explanation: The qualifier DIAGNOSTIC is used to identify extraction procedures that are biopsies

Body Part Character 4	Approach Character 5	Device Character 6	Qualifier Character 7
Ø Kidney, Right Renal calyx Renal capsule Renal cortex Renal segment **1 Kidney, Left** *See Ø Kidney, Right*	**Ø Open** **3 Percutaneous** **4 Percutaneous Endoscopic**	**Z No Device**	**Z No Qualifier**

Ø Medical and Surgical
T Urinary System
F Fragmentation Definition: Breaking solid matter in a body part into pieces
Explanation: Physical force (e.g., manual, ultrasonic) applied directly or indirectly is used to break the solid matter into pieces. The solid matter may be an abnormal byproduct of a biological function or a foreign body. The pieces of solid matter are not taken out.

Body Part Character 4	Approach Character 5	Device Character 6	Qualifier Character 7
3 Kidney Pelvis, Right Ureteropelvic junction (UPJ) **4 Kidney Pelvis, Left** *See 3 Kidney Pelvis, Right* **6 Ureter, Right** Ureteral orifice Ureterovesical orifice **7 Ureter, Left** *See 6 Ureter, Right* **B Bladder** Trigone of bladder **C Bladder Neck** **D Urethra** NC Bulbourethral (Cowper's) gland Cowper's (bulbourethral) gland External urethral sphincter Internal urethral sphincter Membranous urethra Penile urethra Prostatic urethra	**Ø Open** **3 Percutaneous** **4 Percutaneous Endoscopic** **7 Via Natural or Artificial Opening** **8 Via Natural or Artificial Opening Endoscopic** **X External**	**Z No Device**	**Z No Qualifier**

DRG Non-OR ØTF[3,4,6,7,B,C]XZZ
Non-OR ØTF[3,4][Ø,7,8]ZZ
Non-OR ØTF[6,7,B,C][Ø,3,4,7,8]ZZ
Non-OR ØTFD[Ø,3,4,7,8,X]ZZ
NC ØTFDXZZ

Ø Medical and Surgical
T Urinary System
H Insertion Definition: Putting in a nonbiological appliance that monitors, assists, performs, or prevents a physiological function but does not physically take the place of a body part

Explanation: None

Body Part Character 4	Approach Character 5	Device Character 6	Qualifier Character 7
5 Kidney Renal calyx Renal capsule Renal cortex Renal segment	**Ø Open** **3 Percutaneous** **4 Percutaneous Endoscopic** **7 Via Natural or Artificial Opening** **8 Via Natural or Artificial Opening Endoscopic**	**2 Monitoring Device** **3 Infusion Device** **Y Other Device**	**Z No Qualifier**
9 Ureter Ureteral orifice Ureterovesical orifice	**Ø Open** **3 Percutaneous** **4 Percutaneous Endoscopic** **7 Via Natural or Artificial Opening** **8 Via Natural or Artificial Opening Endoscopic**	**2 Monitoring Device** **3 Infusion Device** **M Stimulator Lead** **Y Other Device**	**Z No Qualifier**
B Bladder NC Trigone of bladder	**Ø Open** **3 Percutaneous** **4 Percutaneous Endoscopic** **7 Via Natural or Artificial Opening** **8 Via Natural or Artificial Opening Endoscopic**	**2 Monitoring Device** **3 Infusion Device** **L Artificial Sphincter** **M Stimulator Lead** **Y Other Device**	**Z No Qualifier**
C Bladder Neck	**Ø Open** **3 Percutaneous** **4 Percutaneous Endoscopic** **7 Via Natural or Artificial Opening** **8 Via Natural or Artificial Opening Endoscopic**	**L Artificial Sphincter**	**Z No Qualifier**
D Urethra Bulbourethral (Cowper's) gland Cowper's (bulbourethral) gland External urethral sphincter Internal urethral sphincter Membranous urethra Penile urethra Prostatic urethra	**Ø Open** **3 Percutaneous** **4 Percutaneous Endoscopic** **7 Via Natural or Artificial Opening** **8 Via Natural or Artificial Opening Endoscopic**	**2 Monitoring Device** **3 Infusion Device** **L Artificial Sphincter** **Y Other Device**	**Z No Qualifier**
D Urethra Bulbourethral (Cowper's) gland Cowper's (bulbourethral) gland External urethral sphincter Internal urethral sphincter Membranous urethra Penile urethra Prostatic urethra	**X External**	**2 Monitoring Device** **3 Infusion Device** **L Artificial Sphincter**	**Z No Qualifier**

Non-OR ØTH5Ø3Z
Non-OR ØTH5[3,4][3,Y]Z
Non-OR ØTH57[2,3,Y]Z
Non-OR ØTH58[2,3]Z
Non-OR ØTH9Ø3Z
Non-OR ØTH9[3,4][3,Y]Z
Non-OR ØTH97[2,3,Y]Z
Non-OR ØTH98[2,3]Z
Non-OR ØTHBØ3Z
Non-OR ØTHB[3,4][3,Y]Z
Non-OR ØTHB7[2,3,Y]Z
Non-OR ØTHB8[2,3]Z
Non-OR ØTHDØ3Z
Non-OR ØTHD[3,4][3,Y]Z
Non-OR ØTHD[7,8][2,3,Y]Z
Non-OR ØTHDX3Z
NC ØTHB[Ø,3,4,7,8]MZ

Ø Medical and Surgical
T Urinary System
J Inspection Definition: Visually and/or manually exploring a body part

Explanation: Visual exploration may be performed with or without optical instrumentation. Manual exploration may be performed directly or through intervening body layers.

Body Part Character 4	Approach Character 5	Device Character 6	Qualifier Character 7
5 Kidney Renal calyx Renal capsule Renal cortex Renal segment **9** Ureter Ureteral orifice Ureterovesical orifice **B** Bladder Trigone of bladder **D** Urethra Bulbourethral (Cowper's) gland Cowper's (bulbourethral) gland External urethral sphincter Internal urethral sphincter Membranous urethra Penile urethra Prostatic urethra	**Ø** Open **3** Percutaneous **4** Percutaneous Endoscopic **7** Via Natural or Artificial Opening **8** Via Natural or Artificial Opening Endoscopic **X** External	**Z** No Device	**Z** No Qualifier

Non-OR ØTJ[5,9,D][3,4,7,8,X]ZZ
Non-OR ØTJB[3,7,8,X]ZZ

Ø Medical and Surgical
T Urinary System
L Occlusion Definition: Completely closing an orifice or the lumen of a tubular body part

Explanation: The orifice can be a natural orifice or an artificially created orifice

Body Part Character 4	Approach Character 5	Device Character 6	Qualifier Character 7
3 Kidney Pelvis, Right Ureteropelvic junction (UPJ) **4** Kidney Pelvis, Left *See 3 Kidney Pelvis, Right* **6** Ureter, Right Ureteral orifice Ureterovesical orifice **7** Ureter, Left *See 6 Ureter, Right* **B** Bladder Trigone of bladder **C** Bladder Neck	**Ø** Open **3** Percutaneous **4** Percutaneous Endoscopic	**C** Extraluminal Device **D** Intraluminal Device **Z** No Device	**Z** No Qualifier
3 Kidney Pelvis, Right Ureteropelvic junction (UPJ) **4** Kidney Pelvis, Left *See 3 Kidney Pelvis, Right* **6** Ureter, Right Ureteral orifice Ureterovesical orifice **7** Ureter, Left *See 6 Ureter, Right* **B** Bladder Trigone of bladder **C** Bladder Neck	**7** Via Natural or Artificial Opening **8** Via Natural or Artificial Opening Endoscopic	**D** Intraluminal Device **Z** No Device	**Z** No Qualifier
D Urethra Bulbourethral (Cowper's) gland Cowper's (bulbourethral) gland External urethral sphincter Internal urethral sphincter Membranous urethra Penile urethra Prostatic urethra	**Ø** Open **3** Percutaneous **4** Percutaneous Endoscopic **X** External	**C** Extraluminal Device **D** Intraluminal Device **Z** No Device	**Z** No Qualifier
D Urethra Bulbourethral (Cowper's) gland Cowper's (bulbourethral) gland External urethral sphincter Internal urethral sphincter Membranous urethra Penile urethra Prostatic urethra	**7** Via Natural or Artificial Opening **8** Via Natural or Artificial Opening Endoscopic	**D** Intraluminal Device **Z** No Device	**Z** No Qualifier

Ø Medical and Surgical
T Urinary System
M Reattachment Definition: Putting back in or on all or a portion of a separated body part to its normal location or other suitable location
Explanation: Vascular circulation and nervous pathways may or may not be reestablished

Body Part Character 4	Approach Character 5	Device Character 6	Qualifier Character 7
Ø Kidney, Right Renal calyx Renal capsule Renal cortex Renal segment **1 Kidney, Left** *See Ø Kidney, Right* **2 Kidneys, Bilateral** *See Ø Kidney, Right* **3 Kidney Pelvis, Right** Ureteropelvic junction (UPJ) **4 Kidney Pelvis, Left** *See 3 Kidney Pelvis, Right* **6 Ureter, Right** Ureteral orifice Ureterovesical orifice **7 Ureter, Left** *See 6 Ureter, Right* **8 Ureters, Bilateral** *See 6 Ureter, Right* **B Bladder** Trigone of bladder **C Bladder Neck** **D Urethra** Bulbourethral (Cowper's) gland Cowper's (bulbourethral) gland External urethral sphincter Internal urethral sphincter Membranous urethra Penile urethra Prostatic urethra	**Ø Open** **4 Percutaneous Endoscopic**	**Z No Device**	**Z No Qualifier**

Ø Medical and Surgical
T Urinary System
N Release Definition: Freeing a body part from an abnormal physical constraint by cutting or by the use of force
Explanation: Some of the restraining tissue may be taken out but none of the body part is taken out

Body Part Character 4	Approach Character 5	Device Character 6	Qualifier Character 7
Ø Kidney, Right Renal calyx Renal capsule Renal cortex Renal segment **1 Kidney, Left** *See Ø Kidney, Right* **3 Kidney Pelvis, Right** Ureteropelvic junction (UPJ) **4 Kidney Pelvis, Left** *See 3 Kidney Pelvis, Right* **6 Ureter, Right** Ureteral orifice Ureterovesical orifice **7 Ureter, Left** *See 6 Ureter, Right* **B Bladder** Trigone of bladder **C Bladder Neck**	**Ø Open** **3 Percutaneous** **4 Percutaneous Endoscopic** **7 Via Natural or Artificial Opening** **8 Via Natural or Artificial Opening Endoscopic**	**Z No Device**	**Z No Qualifier**
D Urethra Bulbourethral (Cowper's) gland Cowper's (bulbourethral) gland External urethral sphincter Internal urethral sphincter Membranous urethra Penile urethra Prostatic urethra	**Ø Open** **3 Percutaneous** **4 Percutaneous Endoscopic** **7 Via Natural or Artificial Opening** **8 Via Natural or Artificial Opening Endoscopic** **X External**	**Z No Device**	**Z No Qualifier**

Ø Medical and Surgical
T Urinary System
P Removal Definition: Taking out or off a device from a body part

Explanation: If a device is taken out and a similar device put in without cutting or puncturing the skin or mucous membrane, the procedure is coded to the root operation CHANGE. Otherwise, the procedure for taking out the device is coded to the root operation REMOVAL.

Body Part Character 4	Approach Character 5	Device Character 6	Qualifier Character 7
5 Kidney Renal calyx Renal capsule Renal cortex Renal segment	Ø Open 3 Percutaneous 4 Percutaneous Endoscopic 7 Via Natural or Artificial Opening 8 Via Natural or Artificial Opening Endoscopic	Ø Drainage Device 2 Monitoring Device 3 Infusion Device 7 Autologous Tissue Substitute C Extraluminal Device D Intraluminal Device J Synthetic Substitute K Nonautologous Tissue Substitute Y Other Device	Z No Qualifier
5 Kidney Renal calyx Renal capsule Renal cortex Renal segment	X External	Ø Drainage Device 2 Monitoring Device 3 Infusion Device D Intraluminal Device	Z No Qualifier
9 Ureter Ureteral orifice Ureterovesical orifice	Ø Open 3 Percutaneous 4 Percutaneous Endoscopic 7 Via Natural or Artificial Opening 8 Via Natural or Artificial Opening Endoscopic	Ø Drainage Device 2 Monitoring Device 3 Infusion Device 7 Autologous Tissue Substitute C Extraluminal Device D Intraluminal Device J Synthetic Substitute K Nonautologous Tissue Substitute M Stimulator Lead Y Other Device	Z No Qualifier
9 Ureter Ureteral orifice Ureterovesical orifice	X External	Ø Drainage Device 2 Monitoring Device 3 Infusion Device D Intraluminal Device M Stimulator Lead	Z No Qualifier
B Bladder NC Trigone of bladder	Ø Open 3 Percutaneous 4 Percutaneous Endoscopic 7 Via Natural or Artificial Opening 8 Via Natural or Artificial Opening Endoscopic	Ø Drainage Device 2 Monitoring Device 3 Infusion Device 7 Autologous Tissue Substitute C Extraluminal Device D Intraluminal Device J Synthetic Substitute K Nonautologous Tissue Substitute L Artificial Sphincter M Stimulator Lead Y Other Device	Z No Qualifier
B Bladder Trigone of bladder	X External	Ø Drainage Device 2 Monitoring Device 3 Infusion Device D Intraluminal Device L Artificial Sphincter M Stimulator Lead	Z No Qualifier
D Urethra Bulbourethral (Cowper's) gland Cowper's (bulbourethral) gland External urethral sphincter Internal urethral sphincter Membranous urethra Penile urethra Prostatic urethra	Ø Open 3 Percutaneous 4 Percutaneous Endoscopic 7 Via Natural or Artificial Opening 8 Via Natural or Artificial Opening Endoscopic	Ø Drainage Device 2 Monitoring Device 3 Infusion Device 7 Autologous Tissue Substitute C Extraluminal Device D Intraluminal Device J Synthetic Substitute K Nonautologous Tissue Substitute L Artificial Sphincter Y Other Device	Z No Qualifier
D Urethra Bulbourethral (Cowper's) gland Cowper's (bulbourethral) gland External urethral sphincter Internal urethral sphincter Membranous urethra Penile urethra Prostatic urethra	X External	Ø Drainage Device 2 Monitoring Device 3 Infusion Device D Intraluminal Device L Artificial Sphincter	Z No Qualifier

Non-OR ØTP5[3,4,7]YZ
Non-OR ØTP5[7,8][Ø,2,3,D]Z
Non-OR ØTP5X[Ø,2,3,D]Z
Non-OR ØTP9[3,4,7]YZ
Non-OR ØTP9[7,8][Ø,2,3,D]Z
Non-OR ØTP9X[Ø,2,3,D]Z
Non-OR ØTPB[3,4,7]YZ
Non-OR ØTPB[7,8][Ø,2,3,D]Z
Non-OR ØTPBX[Ø,2,3,D,L]Z
Non-OR ØTPD[3,4]YZ
Non-OR ØTPD[7,8][Ø,2,3,D,Y]Z
Non-OR ØTPDX[Ø,2,3,D]Z
NC ØTPB[Ø,3,4,7,8]MZ

Ø Medical and Surgical
T Urinary System
Q Repair Definition: Restoring, to the extent possible, a body part to its normal anatomic structure and function
Explanation: Used only when the method to accomplish the repair is not one of the other root operations

Body Part Character 4	Approach Character 5	Device Character 6	Qualifier Character 7
Ø Kidney, Right Renal calyx Renal capsule Renal cortex Renal segment **1 Kidney, Left** *See Ø Kidney, Right* **3 Kidney Pelvis, Right** Ureteropelvic junction (UPJ) **4 Kidney Pelvis, Left** *See 3 Kidney Pelvis, Right* **6 Ureter, Right** Ureteral orifice Ureterovesical orifice **7 Ureter, Left** *See 6 Ureter, Right* **B Bladder** ⊞ Trigone of bladder **C Bladder Neck**	**Ø Open** **3 Percutaneous** **4 Percutaneous Endoscopic** **7 Via Natural or Artificial Opening** **8 Via Natural or Artificial Opening Endoscopic**	**Z No Device**	**Z No Qualifier**
D Urethra Bulbourethral (Cowper's) gland Cowper's (bulbourethral) gland External urethral sphincter Internal urethral sphincter Membranous urethra Penile urethra Prostatic urethra	**Ø Open** **3 Percutaneous** **4 Percutaneous Endoscopic** **7 Via Natural or Artificial Opening** **8 Via Natural or Artificial Opening Endoscopic** **X External**	**Z No Device**	**Z No Qualifier**

See Appendix L for Procedure Combinations
⊞ ØTQB[Ø,3,4]ZZ

Ø Medical and Surgical
T Urinary System
R Replacement Definition: Putting in or on biological or synthetic material that physically takes the place and/or function of all or a portion of a body part
Explanation: The body part may have been taken out or replaced, or may be taken out, physically eradicated, or rendered nonfunctional during the REPLACEMENT procedure. A REMOVAL procedure is coded for taking out the device used in a previous replacement procedure.

Body Part Character 4	Approach Character 5	Device Character 6	Qualifier Character 7
3 Kidney Pelvis, Right Ureteropelvic junction (UPJ) **4 Kidney Pelvis, Left** *See 3 Kidney Pelvis, Right* **6 Ureter, Right** Ureteral orifice Ureterovesical orifice **7 Ureter, Left** *See 6 Ureter, Right* **B Bladder** Trigone of bladder **C Bladder Neck**	**Ø Open** **4 Percutaneous Endoscopic** **7 Via Natural or Artificial Opening** **8 Via Natural or Artificial Opening Endoscopic**	**7 Autologous Tissue Substitute** **J Synthetic Substitute** **K Nonautologous Tissue Substitute**	**Z No Qualifier**
D Urethra Bulbourethral (Cowper's) gland Cowper's (bulbourethral) gland External urethral sphincter Internal urethral sphincter Membranous urethra Penile urethra Prostatic urethra	**Ø Open** **4 Percutaneous Endoscopic** **7 Via Natural or Artificial Opening** **8 Via Natural or Artificial Opening Endoscopic** **X External**	**7 Autologous Tissue Substitute** **J Synthetic Substitute** **K Nonautologous Tissue Substitute**	**Z No Qualifier**

Ø Medical and Surgical
T Urinary System
S Reposition Definition: Moving to its normal location, or other suitable location, all or a portion of a body part

Explanation: The body part is moved to a new location from an abnormal location, or from a normal location where it is not functioning correctly. The body part may or may not be cut out or off to be moved to the new location.

Body Part Character 4	Approach Character 5	Device Character 6	Qualifier Character 7
Ø Kidney, Right Renal calyx Renal capsule Renal cortex Renal segment **1 Kidney, Left** *See Ø Kidney, Right* **2 Kidneys, Bilateral** *See Ø Kidney, Right* **3 Kidney Pelvis, Right** Ureteropelvic junction (UPJ) **4 Kidney Pelvis, Left** *See 3 Kidney Pelvis, Right* **6 Ureter, Right** Ureteral orifice Ureterovesical orifice **7 Ureter, Left** *See 6 Ureter, Right* **8 Ureters, Bilateral** *See 6 Ureter, Right* **B Bladder** Trigone of bladder **C Bladder Neck** **D Urethra** Bulbourethral (Cowper's) gland Cowper's (bulbourethral) gland External urethral sphincter Internal urethral sphincter Membranous urethra Penile urethra Prostatic urethra	**Ø** Open **4** Percutaneous Endoscopic	**Z** No Device	**Z** No Qualifier

Ø Medical and Surgical
T Urinary System
T Resection Definition: Cutting out or off, without replacement, all of a body part

Explanation: None

Body Part Character 4	Approach Character 5	Device Character 6	Qualifier Character 7
Ø Kidney, Right Renal calyx Renal capsule Renal cortex Renal segment **1 Kidney, Left** *See Ø Kidney, Right* **2 Kidneys, Bilateral** *See Ø Kidney, Right*	**Ø** Open **4** Percutaneous Endoscopic	**Z** No Device	**Z** No Qualifier
3 Kidney Pelvis, Right Ureteropelvic junction (UPJ) **4 Kidney Pelvis, Left** *See 3 Kidney Pelvis, Right* **6 Ureter, Right** Ureteral orifice Ureterovesical orifice **7 Ureter, Left** *See 6 Ureter, Right* **B Bladder** ⊞ Trigone of bladder **C Bladder Neck** **D Urethra** Bulbourethral (Cowper's) gland Cowper's (bulbourethral) gland External urethral sphincter Internal urethral sphincter Membranous urethra Penile urethra Prostatic urethra	**Ø** Open **4** Percutaneous Endoscopic **7** Via Natural or Artificial Opening **8** Via Natural or Artificial Opening Endoscopic	**Z** No Device	**Z** No Qualifier

Non-OR ØTTD[4,7,8]ZZ

See Appendix L for Procedure Combinations
Combo-only ØTTDØZZ
⊞ ØTTBØZZ

Ø Medical and Surgical
T Urinary System
U Supplement Definition: Putting in or on biological or synthetic material that physically reinforces and/or augments the function of a portion of a body part

Explanation: The biological material is non-living, or is living and from the same individual. The body part may have been previously replaced, and the SUPPLEMENT procedure is performed to physically reinforce and/or augment the function of the replaced body part.

Body Part Character 4	Approach Character 5	Device Character 6	Qualifier Character 7
3 Kidney Pelvis, Right Ureteropelvic junction (UPJ) 4 Kidney Pelvis, Left *See 3 Kidney Pelvis, Right* 6 Ureter, Right Ureteral orifice Ureterovesical orifice 7 Ureter, Left *See 6 Ureter, Right* B Bladder Trigone of bladder C Bladder Neck	Ø Open 4 Percutaneous Endoscopic 7 Via Natural or Artificial Opening 8 Via Natural or Artificial Opening Endoscopic	7 Autologous Tissue Substitute J Synthetic Substitute K Nonautologous Tissue Substitute	Z No Qualifier
D Urethra Bulbourethral (Cowper's) gland Cowper's (bulbourethral) gland External urethral sphincter Internal urethral sphincter Membranous urethra Penile urethra Prostatic urethra	Ø Open 4 Percutaneous Endoscopic 7 Via Natural or Artificial Opening 8 Via Natural or Artificial Opening Endoscopic X External	7 Autologous Tissue Substitute J Synthetic Substitute K Nonautologous Tissue Substitute	Z No Qualifier

Ø Medical and Surgical
T Urinary System
V Restriction Definition: Partially closing an orifice or the lumen of a tubular body part

Explanation: The orifice can be a natural orifice or an artificially created orifice

Body Part Character 4	Approach Character 5	Device Character 6	Qualifier Character 7
3 Kidney Pelvis, Right Ureteropelvic junction (UPJ) 4 Kidney Pelvis, Left *See 3 Kidney Pelvis, Right* 6 Ureter, Right Ureteral orifice Ureterovesical orifice 7 Ureter, Left *See 6 Ureter, Right* B Bladder Trigone of bladder C Bladder Neck	Ø Open 3 Percutaneous 4 Percutaneous Endoscopic	C Extraluminal Device D Intraluminal Device Z No Device	Z No Qualifier
3 Kidney Pelvis, Right Ureteropelvic junction (UPJ) 4 Kidney Pelvis, Left *See 3 Kidney Pelvis, Right* 6 Ureter, Right Ureteral orifice Ureterovesical orifice 7 Ureter, Left *See 6 Ureter, Right* B Bladder Trigone of bladder C Bladder Neck	7 Via Natural or Artificial Opening 8 Via Natural or Artificial Opening Endoscopic	D Intraluminal Device Z No Device	Z No Qualifier
D Urethra Bulbourethral (Cowper's) gland Cowper's (bulbourethral) gland External urethral sphincter Internal urethral sphincter Membranous urethra Penile urethra Prostatic urethra	Ø Open 3 Percutaneous 4 Percutaneous Endoscopic	C Extraluminal Device D Intraluminal Device Z No Device	Z No Qualifier
D Urethra Bulbourethral (Cowper's) gland Cowper's (bulbourethral) gland External urethral sphincter Internal urethral sphincter Membranous urethra Penile urethra Prostatic urethra	7 Via Natural or Artificial Opening 8 Via Natural or Artificial Opening Endoscopic	D Intraluminal Device Z No Device	Z No Qualifier
D Urethra Bulbourethral (Cowper's) gland Cowper's (bulbourethral) gland External urethral sphincter Internal urethral sphincter Membranous urethra Penile urethra Prostatic urethra	X External	Z No Device	Z No Qualifier

LC Limited Coverage NC Noncovered ⊞ Combination Member HAC associated procedure Combination Only DRG Non-OR Non-OR New/Revised in GREEN

Ø Medical and Surgical
T Urinary System
W Revision

Definition: Correcting, to the extent possible, a portion of a malfunctioning device or the position of a displaced device

Explanation: Revision can include correcting a malfunctioning or displaced device by taking out or putting in components of the device such as a screw or pin

Body Part Character 4	Approach Character 5	Device Character 6	Qualifier Character 7
5 Kidney Renal calyx Renal capsule Renal cortex Renal segment	**Ø** Open **3** Percutaneous **4** Percutaneous Endoscopic **7** Via Natural or Artificial Opening **8** Via Natural or Artificial Opening Endoscopic	**Ø** Drainage Device **2** Monitoring Device **3** Infusion Device **7** Autologous Tissue Substitute **C** Extraluminal Device **D** Intraluminal Device **J** Synthetic Substitute **K** Nonautologous Tissue Substitute **Y** Other Device	**Z** No Qualifier
5 Kidney Renal calyx Renal capsule Renal cortex Renal segment	**X** External	**Ø** Drainage Device **2** Monitoring Device **3** Infusion Device **7** Autologous Tissue Substitute **C** Extraluminal Device **D** Intraluminal Device **J** Synthetic Substitute **K** Nonautologous Tissue Substitute	**Z** No Qualifier
9 Ureter Ureteral orifice Ureterovesical orifice	**Ø** Open **3** Percutaneous **4** Percutaneous Endoscopic **7** Via Natural or Artificial Opening **8** Via Natural or Artificial Opening Endoscopic	**Ø** Drainage Device **2** Monitoring Device **3** Infusion Device **7** Autologous Tissue Substitute **C** Extraluminal Device **D** Intraluminal Device **J** Synthetic Substitute **K** Nonautologous Tissue Substitute **M** Stimulator Lead **Y** Other Device	**Z** No Qualifier
9 Ureter Ureteral orifice Ureterovesical orifice	**X** External	**Ø** Drainage Device **2** Monitoring Device **3** Infusion Device **7** Autologous Tissue Substitute **C** Extraluminal Device **D** Intraluminal Device **J** Synthetic Substitute **K** Nonautologous Tissue Substitute **M** Stimulator Lead	**Z** No Qualifier
B Bladder Trigone of bladder	**Ø** Open **3** Percutaneous **4** Percutaneous Endoscopic **7** Via Natural or Artificial Opening **8** Via Natural or Artificial Opening Endoscopic	**Ø** Drainage Device **2** Monitoring Device **3** Infusion Device **7** Autologous Tissue Substitute **C** Extraluminal Device **D** Intraluminal Device **J** Synthetic Substitute **K** Nonautologous Tissue Substitute **L** Artificial Sphincter **M** Stimulator Lead **Y** Other Device	**Z** No Qualifier
B Bladder Trigone of bladder	**X** External	**Ø** Drainage Device **2** Monitoring Device **3** Infusion Device **7** Autologous Tissue Substitute **C** Extraluminal Device **D** Intraluminal Device **J** Synthetic Substitute **K** Nonautologous Tissue Substitute **L** Artificial Sphincter **M** Stimulator Lead	**Z** No Qualifier

ØTW Continued on next page

Non-OR ØTW5[3,4,7]YZ
Non-OR ØTW5X[Ø,2,3,7,C,D,J,K]Z
Non-OR ØTW9[3,4,7]YZ
Non-OR ØTW9X[Ø,2,3,7,C,D,J,K,M]Z
Non-OR ØTWB[3,4,7]YZ
Non-OR ØTWBX[Ø,2,3,7,C,D,J,K,L,M]Z

Urinary System

Ø Medical and Surgical
T Urinary System
W Revision Definition: Correcting, to the extent possible, a portion of a malfunctioning device or the position of a displaced device

Explanation: Revision can include correcting a malfunctioning or displaced device by taking out or putting in components of the device such as a screw or pin

ØTW Continued

Body Part Character 4	Approach Character 5	Device Character 6	Qualifier Character 7
D Urethra Bulbourethral (Cowper's) gland Cowper's (bulbourethral) gland External urethral sphincter Internal urethral sphincter Membranous urethra Penile urethra Prostatic urethra	**Ø** Open **3** Percutaneous **4** Percutaneous Endoscopic **7** Via Natural or Artificial Opening **8** Via Natural or Artificial Opening Endoscopic	**Ø** Drainage Device **2** Monitoring Device **3** Infusion Device **7** Autologous Tissue Substitute **C** Extraluminal Device **D** Intraluminal Device **J** Synthetic Substitute **K** Nonautologous Tissue Substitute **L** Artificial Sphincter **Y** Other Device	**Z** No Qualifier
D Urethra Bulbourethral (Cowper's) gland Cowper's (bulbourethral) gland External urethral sphincter Internal urethral sphincter Membranous urethra Penile urethra Prostatic urethra	**X** External	**Ø** Drainage Device **2** Monitoring Device **3** Infusion Device **7** Autologous Tissue Substitute **C** Extraluminal Device **D** Intraluminal Device **J** Synthetic Substitute **K** Nonautologous Tissue Substitute **L** Artificial Sphincter	**Z** No Qualifier

Non-OR ØTWD[3,4,7,8]YZ
Non-OR ØTWDX[Ø,2,3,7,C,D,J,K,L]Z

Ø Medical and Surgical
T Urinary System
Y Transplantation Definition: Putting in or on all or a portion of a living body part taken from another individual or animal to physically take the place and/or function of all or a portion of a similar body part

Explanation: The native body part may or may not be taken out, and the transplanted body part may take over all or a portion of its function

Body Part Character 4	Approach Character 5	Device Character 6	Qualifier Character 7
Ø Kidney, Right ⊞ LC Renal calyx Renal capsule Renal cortex Renal segment **1** Kidney, Left ⊞ LC *See Ø Kidney, Right*	**Ø** Open	**Z** No Device	**Ø** Allogeneic **1** Syngeneic **2** Zooplastic

LC ØTY[Ø,1]ØZ[Ø,1,2]

See Appendix L for Procedure Combinations
⊞ ØTY[Ø,1]ØZ[Ø,1,2]

Female Reproductive System ØU1–ØUY

Character Meanings

This Character Meaning table is provided as a guide to assist the user in the identification of character members that may be found in this section of code tables. It **SHOULD NOT** be used to build a PCS code.

Operation–Character 3	Body Part–Character 4	Approach–Character 5	Device–Character 6	Qualifier–Character 7
1 Bypass	Ø Ovary, Right	Ø Open	Ø Drainage Device	Ø Allogeneic
2 Change	1 Ovary, Left	3 Percutaneous	1 Radioactive Element	1 Syngeneic
5 Destruction	2 Ovaries, Bilateral	4 Percutaneous Endoscopic	3 Infusion Device	2 Zooplastic
7 Dilation	3 Ovary	7 Via Natural or Artificial Opening	7 Autologous Tissue Substitute	5 Fallopian Tube, Right
8 Division	4 Uterine Supporting Structure	8 Via Natural or Artificial Opening Endoscopic	C Extraluminal Device	6 Fallopian Tube, Left
9 Drainage	5 Fallopian Tube, Right	F Via Natural or Artificial Opening With Percutaneous Endoscopic Assistance	D Intraluminal Device	9 Uterus
B Excision	6 Fallopian Tube, Left	X External	G Intraluminal Device, Pessary	L Supracervical
C Extirpation	7 Fallopian Tubes, Bilateral		H Contraceptive Device	X Diagnostic
D Extraction	8 Fallopian Tube		J Synthetic Substitute	Z No Qualifier
F Fragmentation	9 Uterus		K Nonautologous Tissue Substitute	
H Insertion	B Endometrium		Y Other Device	
J Inspection	C Cervix		Z No Device	
L Occlusion	D Uterus and Cervix			
M Reattachment	F Cul-de-sac			
N Release	G Vagina			
P Removal	H Vagina and Cul-de-sac			
Q Repair	J Clitoris			
S Reposition	K Hymen			
T Resection	L Vestibular Gland			
U Supplement	M Vulva			
V Restriction	N Ova			
W Revision				
Y Transplantation				

AHA Coding Clinic for table ØU5
2015, 3Q, 31 Tubal ligation for sterilization

AHA Coding Clinic for table ØU9
2016, 4Q, 58 Longitudinal vaginal septum

AHA Coding Clinic for table ØUB
2018, 1Q, 23 Tubal ligation procedure
2015, 3Q, 31 Laparoscopic partial salpingectomy for ectopic pregnancy
2015, 3Q, 31 Tubal ligation for sterilization
2014, 4Q, 16 Excision of multiple uterine fibroids
2014, 3Q, 12 Excision of skin tag from labia majora

AHA Coding Clinic for table ØUC
2015, 3Q, 30 Removal of cervical cerclage
2013, 2Q, 38 Evacuation of clot post-partum

AHA Coding Clinic for table ØUH
2018, 1Q, 25 Intrauterine brachytherapy & placement of tandems & ovoids
2013, 2Q, 34 Placement of intrauterine device via open approach

AHA Coding Clinic for table ØUJ
2015, 1Q, 33 Robotic-assisted laparoscopic hysterectomy converted to open procedure

AHA Coding Clinic for table ØUL
2018, 1Q, 23 Tubal ligation procedure
2015, 3Q, 31 Tubal ligation for sterilization

AHA Coding Clinic for table ØUQ
2014, 4Q, 18 Obstetrical periurethral laceration
2013, 4Q, 120 Repair of clitoral obstetric laceration

AHA Coding Clinic for table ØUS
2016, 1Q, 9 Anteversion of retroverted pregnant uterus

AHA Coding Clinic for table ØUT
2017, 4Q, 68 New qualifier values - Supracervical hysterectomy
2015, 1Q, 33 Robotic-assisted laparoscopic hysterectomy converted to open procedure
2013, 3Q, 28 Total hysterectomy
2013, 1Q, 24 Excision versus Resection of remaining ovarian remnant following previous excision

AHA Coding Clinic for table ØUV
2015, 3Q, 30 Insertion of cervical cerclage

Female Reproductive System

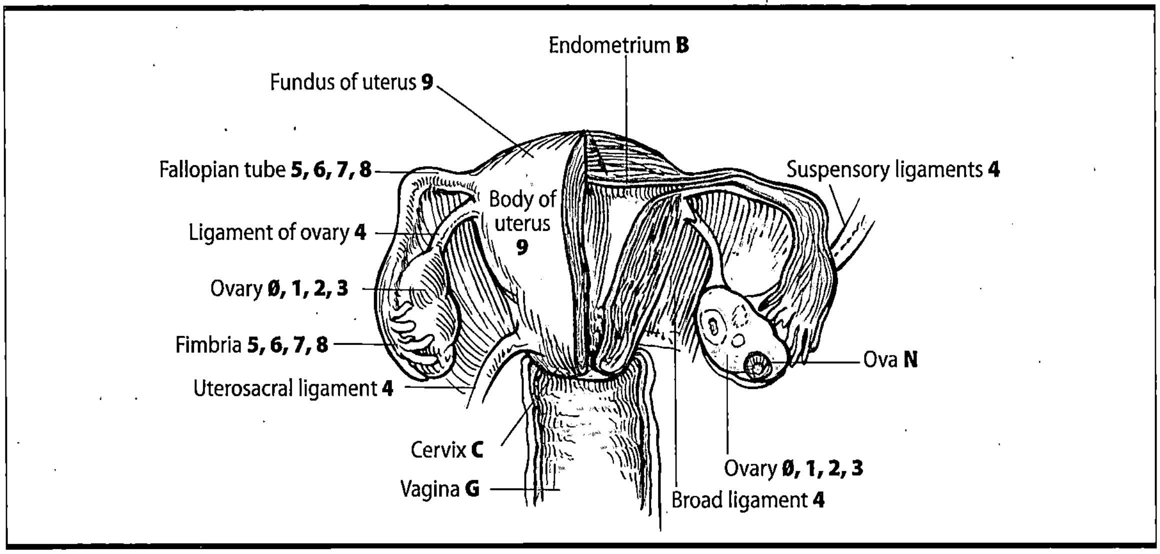

Female Internal/External Structures

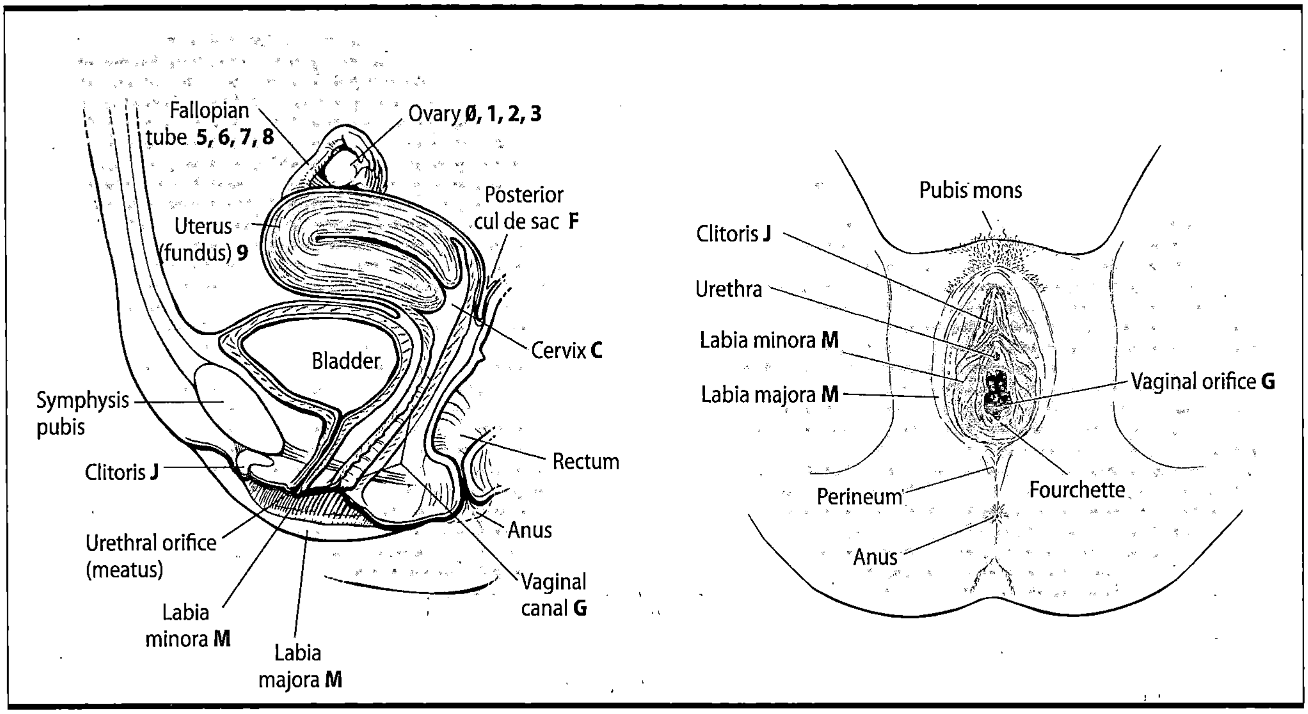

Ø Medical and Surgical
U Female Reproductive System
1 Bypass Definition: Altering the route of passage of the contents of a tubular body part

Explanation: Rerouting contents of a body part to a downstream area of the normal route, to a similar route and body part, or to an abnormal route and dissimilar body part. Includes one or more anastomoses, with or without the use of a device.

Body Part Character 4	Approach Character 5	Device Character 6	Qualifier Character 7
5 Fallopian Tube, Right ♀ Oviduct Salpinx Uterine tube 6 Fallopian Tube, Left ♀ *See 5 Fallopian Tube, Right*	Ø Open 4 Percutaneous Endoscopic	7 Autologous Tissue Substitute J Synthetic Substitute K Nonautologous Tissue Substitute Z No Device	5 Fallopian Tube, Right 6 Fallopian Tube, Left 9 Uterus

♀ All body part, approach, device, and qualifier values

Ø Medical and Surgical
U Female Reproductive System
2 Change Definition: Taking out or off a device from a body part and putting back an identical or similar device in or on the same body part without cutting or puncturing the skin or a mucous membrane

Explanation: All CHANGE procedures are coded using the approach EXTERNAL

Body Part Character 4	Approach Character 5	Device Character 6	Qualifier Character 7
3 Ovary ♀ 8 Fallopian Tube ♀ M Vulva ♀ Labia majora Labia minora	X External	Ø Drainage Device Y Other Device	Z No Qualifier
D Uterus and Cervix ♀	X External	Ø Drainage Device H Contraceptive Device Y Other Device	Z No Qualifier
H Vagina and Cul-de-sac ♀	X External	Ø Drainage Device G Intraluminal Device, Pessary Y Other Device	Z No Qualifier

Non-OR All body part, approach, device, and qualifier values ♀ All body part, approach, device, and qualifier values

Ø Medical and Surgical
U Female Reproductive System
5 Destruction Definition: Physical eradication of all or a portion of a body part by the direct use of energy, force, or a destructive agent
Explanation: None of the body part is physically taken out

Body Part Character 4	Approach Character 5	Device Character 6	Qualifier Character 7
Ø Ovary, Right ♀ **1 Ovary, Left** ♀ **2 Ovaries, Bilateral** ♀ **4 Uterine Supporting Structure** ♀ Broad ligament Infundibulopelvic ligament Ovarian ligament Round ligament of uterus	**Ø Open** **3 Percutaneous** **4 Percutaneous Endoscopic** **8 Via Natural or Artificial Opening Endoscopic**	**Z No Device**	**Z No Qualifier**
5 Fallopian Tube, Right ♀ Oviduct Salpinx Uterine tube **6 Fallopian Tube, Left** ♀ *See 5 Fallopian Tube, Right* **7 Fallopian Tubes, Bilateral** NC ♀ **9 Uterus** ♀ Fundus uteri Myometrium Perimetrium Uterine cornu **B Endometrium** ♀ **C Cervix** ♀ **F Cul-de-sac** ♀	**Ø Open** **3 Percutaneous** **4 Percutaneous Endoscopic** **7 Via Natural or Artificial Opening** **8 Via Natural or Artificial Opening Endoscopic**	**Z No Device**	**Z No Qualifier**
G Vagina ♀ **K Hymen** ♀	**Ø Open** **3 Percutaneous** **4 Percutaneous Endoscopic** **7 Via Natural or Artificial Opening** **8 Via Natural or Artificial Opening Endoscopic** **X External**	**Z No Device**	**Z No Qualifier**
J Clitoris ♀ **L Vestibular Gland** ♀ Bartholin's (greater vestibular) gland Greater vestibular (Bartholin's) gland Paraurethral (Skene's) gland Skene's (paraurethral) gland **M Vulva** ♀ Labia majora Labia minora	**Ø Open** **X External**	**Z No Device**	**Z No Qualifier**

NC ØU57[Ø,3,4,7,8]ZZ with principal or secondary diagnosis of Z3Ø.2 ♀ All body part, approach, device, and qualifier values

Ø Medical and Surgical
U Female Reproductive System
7 Dilation Definition: Expanding an orifice or the lumen of a tubular body part

Explanation: The orifice can be a natural orifice or an artificially created orifice. Accomplished by stretching a tubular body part using intraluminal pressure or by cutting part of the orifice or wall of the tubular body part.

Body Part Character 4	Approach Character 5	Device Character 6	Qualifier Character 7
5 Fallopian Tube, Right ♀ Oviduct Salpinx Uterine tube **6 Fallopian Tube, Left** ♀ *See 5 Fallopian Tube, Right* **7 Fallopian Tubes, Bilateral** ♀ **9 Uterus** ♀ Fundus uteri Myometrium Perimetrium Uterine cornu **C Cervix** ♀ **G Vagina** ♀	**Ø Open** **3 Percutaneous** **4 Percutaneous Endoscopic** **7 Via Natural or Artificial Opening** **8 Via Natural or Artificial Opening Endoscopic**	**D Intraluminal Device** **Z No Device**	**Z No Qualifier**
K Hymen ♀	**Ø Open** **3 Percutaneous** **4 Percutaneous Endoscopic** **7 Via Natural or Artificial Opening** **8 Via Natural or Artificial Opening Endoscopic** **X External**	**D Intraluminal Device** **Z No Device**	**Z No Qualifier**

Non-OR ØU7C[Ø,3,4,7,8][D,Z]Z
Non-OR ØU7G[7,8][D,Z]Z

♀ All body part, approach, device, and qualifier values

Ø Medical and Surgical
U Female Reproductive System
8 Division Definition: Cutting into a body part, without draining fluids and/or gases from the body part, in order to separate or transect a body part

Explanation: All or a portion of the body part is separated into two or more portions

Body Part Character 4	Approach Character 5	Device Character 6	Qualifier Character 7
Ø Ovary, Right ♀ **1 Ovary, Left** ♀ **2 Ovaries, Bilateral** ♀ **4 Uterine Supporting Structure** ♀ Broad ligament Infundibulopelvic ligament Ovarian ligament Round ligament of uterus	**Ø Open** **3 Percutaneous** **4 Percutaneous Endoscopic**	**Z No Device**	**Z No Qualifier**
K Hymen ♀	**7 Via Natural or Artificial Opening** **8 Via Natural or Artificial Opening Endoscopic** **X External**	**Z No Device**	**Z No Qualifier**

Non-OR ØU8K[7,8,X]ZZ

♀ All body part, approach, device, and qualifier values

Ø Medical and Surgical
U Female Reproductive System
9 Drainage Definition: Taking or letting out fluids and/or gases from a body part
Explanation: The qualifier DIAGNOSTIC is used to identify drainage procedures that are biopsies

Body Part Character 4	Approach Character 5	Device Character 6	Qualifier Character 7
Ø Ovary, Right ♀ 1 Ovary, Left ♀ 2 Ovaries, Bilateral ♀	Ø Open 3 Percutaneous 4 Percutaneous Endoscopic 8 Via Natural or Artificial Opening Endoscopic	Ø Drainage Device	Z No Qualifier
Ø Ovary, Right ♀ 1 Ovary, Left ♀ 2 Ovaries, Bilateral ♀	Ø Open 3 Percutaneous 4 Percutaneous Endoscopic 8 Via Natural or Artificial Opening Endoscopic	Z No Device	X Diagnostic Z No Qualifier
Ø Ovary, Right ♀ 1 Ovary, Left ♀ 2 Ovaries, Bilateral ♀	X External	Z No Device	Z No Qualifier
4 Uterine Supporting Structure ♀ Broad ligament Infundibulopelvic ligament Ovarian ligament Round ligament of uterus	Ø Open 3 Percutaneous 4 Percutaneous Endoscopic 8 Via Natural or Artificial Opening Endoscopic	Ø Drainage Device	Z No Qualifier
4 Uterine Supporting Structure ♀ Broad ligament Infundibulopelvic ligament Ovarian ligament Round ligament of uterus	Ø Open 3 Percutaneous 4 Percutaneous Endoscopic 8 Via Natural or Artificial Opening Endoscopic	Z No Device	X Diagnostic Z No Qualifier
5 Fallopian Tube, Right ♀ Oviduct Salpinx Uterine tube 6 Fallopian Tube, Left ♀ *See 5 Fallopian Tube, Right* 7 Fallopian Tubes, Bilateral ♀ 9 Uterus ♀ Fundus uteri Myometrium Perimetrium Uterine cornu C Cervix ♀ F Cul-de-sac ♀	Ø Open 3 Percutaneous 4 Percutaneous Endoscopic 7 Via Natural or Artificial Opening 8 Via Natural or Artificial Opening Endoscopic	Ø Drainage Device	Z No Qualifier
5 Fallopian Tube, Right ♀ Oviduct Salpinx Uterine tube 6 Fallopian Tube, Left ♀ *See 5 Fallopian Tube, Right* 7 Fallopian Tubes, Bilateral ♀ 9 Uterus ♀ Fundus uteri Myometrium Perimetrium Uterine cornu C Cervix ♀ F Cul-de-sac ♀	Ø Open 3 Percutaneous 4 Percutaneous Endoscopic 7 Via Natural or Artificial Opening 8 Via Natural or Artificial Opening Endoscopic	Z No Device	X Diagnostic Z No Qualifier

ØU9 Continued on next page

Non-OR ØU9[Ø,1,2][3,8]ØZ
Non-OR ØU9[Ø,1,2][3,8]ZZ
Non-OR ØU9[Ø,1,2]8ZX
Non-OR ØU94[3,8]ØZ
Non-OR ØU94[3,8]ZZ
Non-OR ØU948ZX
Non-OR ØU9[5,6,7,9,C]3ØZ
Non-OR ØU9F[3,4]ØZ
Non-OR ØU9[5,6,7][3,4,7,8]ZZ
Non-OR ØU9[9,C]3ZZ
Non-OR ØU9F[3,4]ZZ
♀ All body part, approach, device, and qualifier values

Ø **Medical and Surgical**
U **Female Reproductive System**
9 **Drainage** Definition: Taking or letting out fluids and/or gases from a body part

Explanation: The qualifier DIAGNOSTIC is used to identify drainage procedures that are biopsies

ØU9 Continued

Body Part Character 4	Approach Character 5	Device Character 6	Qualifier Character 7
G Vagina ♀ K Hymen ♀	Ø Open 3 Percutaneous 4 Percutaneous Endoscopic 7 Via Natural or Artificial Opening 8 Via Natural or Artificial Opening Endoscopic X External	Ø Drainage Device	Z No Qualifier
G Vagina ♀ K Hymen ♀	Ø Open 3 Percutaneous 4 Percutaneous Endoscopic 7 Via Natural or Artificial Opening 8 Via Natural or Artificial Opening Endoscopic X External	Z No Device	X Diagnostic Z No Qualifier
J Clitoris ♀ L Vestibular Gland ♀ Bartholin's (greater vestibular) gland Greater vestibular (Bartholin's) gland Paraurethral (Skene's) gland Skene's (paraurethral) gland M Vulva ♀ Labia majora Labia minora	Ø Open X External	Ø Drainage Device	Z No Qualifier
J Clitoris ♀ L Vestibular Gland ♀ Bartholin's (greater vestibular) gland Greater vestibular (Bartholin's) gland Paraurethral (Skene's) gland Skene's (paraurethral) gland M Vulva ♀ Labia majora Labia minora	Ø Open X External	Z No Device	X Diagnostic Z No Qualifier

Non-OR ØU9G3ØZ
Non-OR ØU9K[Ø,3,4,7,8,X]ØZ
Non-OR ØU9G3ZZ
Non-OR ØU9K[Ø,3,4,7,8,X]ZZ
Non-OR ØU9L[Ø,X]ØZ
Non-OR ØU9L[Ø,X]ZZ
♀ All body part, approach, device, and qualifier values

Female Reproductive System

ØU9–ØU9

Ø Medical and Surgical
U Female Reproductive System
B Excision Definition: Cutting out or off, without replacement, a portion of a body part
Explanation: The qualifier DIAGNOSTIC is used to identify excision procedures that are biopsies

Body Part Character 4	Approach Character 5	Device Character 6	Qualifier Character 7
Ø Ovary, Right ♀ **1 Ovary, Left** ♀ **2 Ovaries, Bilateral** ♀ **4 Uterine Supporting Structure** ♀ Broad ligament Infundibulopelvic ligament Ovarian ligament Round ligament of uterus **5 Fallopian Tube, Right** ♀ Oviduct Salpinx Uterine tube **6 Fallopian Tube, Left** ♀ *See 5 Fallopian Tube, Right* **7 Fallopian Tubes, Bilateral** ♀ **9 Uterus** ♀ Fundus uteri Myometrium Perimetrium Uterine cornu **C Cervix** ♀ **F Cul-de-sac** ♀	**Ø Open** **3 Percutaneous** **4 Percutaneous Endoscopic** **7 Via Natural or Artificial Opening** **8 Via Natural or Artificial Opening Endoscopic**	**Z No Device**	**X Diagnostic** **Z No Qualifier**
G Vagina ♀ **K Hymen** ♀	**Ø Open** **3 Percutaneous** **4 Percutaneous Endoscopic** **7 Via Natural or Artificial Opening** **8 Via Natural or Artificial Opening Endoscopic** **X External**	**Z No Device**	**X Diagnostic** **Z No Qualifier**
J Clitoris ♀ **L Vestibular Gland** ♀ Bartholin's (greater vestibular) gland Greater vestibular (Bartholin's) gland Paraurethral (Skene's) gland Skene's (paraurethral) gland **M Vulva** ♀ Labia majora Labia minora	**Ø Open** **X External**	**Z No Device**	**X Diagnostic** **Z No Qualifier**

♀ All body part, approach, device, and qualifier values

Ø Medical and Surgical
U Female Reproductive System
C Extirpation Definition: Taking or cutting out solid matter from a body part

Explanation: The solid matter may be an abnormal byproduct of a biological function or a foreign body; it may be imbedded in a body part or in the lumen of a tubular body part. The solid matter may or may not have been previously broken into pieces.

Body Part Character 4	Approach Character 5	Device Character 6	Qualifier Character 7
Ø Ovary, Right ♀ **1** Ovary, Left ♀ **2** Ovaries, Bilateral ♀ **4** Uterine Supporting Structure ♀ Broad ligament Infundibulopelvic ligament Ovarian ligament Round ligament of uterus	**Ø** Open **3** Percutaneous **4** Percutaneous Endoscopic **8** Via Natural or Artificial Opening Endoscopic	**Z** No Device	**Z** No Qualifier
5 Fallopian Tube, Right ♀ Oviduct Salpinx Uterine tube **6** Fallopian Tube, Left ♀ *See 5 Fallopian Tube, Right* **7** Fallopian Tubes, Bilateral ♀ **9** Uterus ♀ Fundus uteri Myometrium Perimetrium Uterine cornu **B** Endometrium ♀ **C** Cervix ♀ **F** Cul-de-sac ♀	**Ø** Open **3** Percutaneous **4** Percutaneous Endoscopic **7** Via Natural or Artificial Opening **8** Via Natural or Artificial Opening Endoscopic	**Z** No Device	**Z** No Qualifier
G Vagina ♀ **K** Hymen ♀	**Ø** Open **3** Percutaneous **4** Percutaneous Endoscopic **7** Via Natural or Artificial Opening **8** Via Natural or Artificial Opening Endoscopic **X** External	**Z** No Device	**Z** No Qualifier
J Clitoris ♀ **L** Vestibular Gland ♀ Bartholin's (greater vestibular) gland Greater vestibular (Bartholin's) gland Paraurethral (Skene's) gland Skene's (paraurethral) gland **M** Vulva ♀ Labia majora Labia minora	**Ø** Open **X** External	**Z** No Device	**Z** No Qualifier

Non-OR ØUC9[7,8]ZZ
Non-OR ØUCG[7,8,X]ZZ
Non-OR ØUCK[Ø,3,4,7,8,X]ZZ
Non-OR ØUCMXZZ
♀ All body part, approach, device, and qualifier values

Ø Medical and Surgical
U Female Reproductive System
D Extraction Definition: Pulling or stripping out or off all or a portion of a body part by the use of force

Explanation: The qualifier DIAGNOSTIC is used to identify extraction procedures that are biopsies

Body Part Character 4	Approach Character 5	Device Character 6	Qualifier Character 7
B Endometrium ♀	**7** Via Natural or Artificial Opening **8** Via Natural or Artificial Opening Endoscopic	**Z** No Device	**X** Diagnostic **Z** No Qualifier
N Ova ♀	**Ø** Open **3** Percutaneous **4** Percutaneous Endoscopic	**Z** No Device	**Z** No Qualifier

♀ All body part, approach, device, and qualifier values

Ø Medical and Surgical
U Female Reproductive System
F Fragmentation Definition: Breaking solid matter in a body part into pieces

Explanation: Physical force (e.g., manual, ultrasonic) applied directly or indirectly is used to break the solid matter into pieces. The solid matter may be an abnormal byproduct of a biological function or a foreign body. The pieces of solid matter are not taken out.

Body Part Character 4	Approach Character 5	Device Character 6	Qualifier Character 7
5 Fallopian Tube, Right NC♀ Oviduct Salpinx Uterine tube 6 Fallopian Tube, Left NC♀ *See 5 Fallopian Tube, Right* 7 Fallopian Tubes, Bilateral NC♀ 9 Uterus NC♀ Fundus uteri Myometrium Perimetrium Uterine cornu	Ø Open 3 Percutaneous 4 Percutaneous Endoscopic 7 Via Natural or Artificial Opening 8 Via Natural or Artificial Opening Endoscopic X External	Z No Device	Z No Qualifier

Non-OR ØUF[5,6,7,9]XZZ
NC ØUF[5,6,7,9]XZZ
♀ All body part, approach, device, and qualifier values

Ø Medical and Surgical
U Female Reproductive System
H Insertion Definition: Putting in a nonbiological appliance that monitors, assists, performs, or prevents a physiological function but does not physically take the place of a body part

Explanation: None

Body Part Character 4	Approach Character 5	Device Character 6	Qualifier Character 7
3 Ovary ♀	Ø Open 3 Percutaneous 4 Percutaneous Endoscopic	3 Infusion Device Y Other Device	Z No Qualifier
3 Ovary ♀	7 Via Natural or Artificial Opening 8 Via Natural or Artificial Opening Endoscopic	Y Other Device	Z No Qualifier
8 Fallopian Tube ♀ D Uterus and Cervix ♀ H Vagina and Cul-de-sac ♀	Ø Open 3 Percutaneous 4 Percutaneous Endoscopic 7 Via Natural or Artificial Opening 8 Via Natural or Artificial Opening Endoscopic	3 Infusion Device Y Other Device	Z No Qualifier
9 Uterus ♀ Fundus uteri Myometrium Perimetrium Uterine cornu	Ø Open 7 Via Natural or Artificial Opening 8 Via Natural or Artificial Opening Endoscopic	H Contraceptive Device	Z No Qualifier
C Cervix ♀	Ø Open 3 Percutaneous 4 Percutaneous Endoscopic	1 Radioactive Element	Z No Qualifier
C Cervix ♀	7 Via Natural or Artificial Opening 8 Via Natural or Artificial Opening Endoscopic	1 Radioactive Element H Contraceptive Device	Z No Qualifier
F Cul-de-sac ♀	7 Via Natural or Artificial Opening 8 Via Natural or Artificial Opening Endoscopic	G Intraluminal Device, Pessary	Z No Qualifier
G Vagina ♀	Ø Open 3 Percutaneous 4 Percutaneous Endoscopic X External	1 Radioactive Element	Z No Qualifier
G Vagina ♀	7 Via Natural or Artificial Opening 8 Via Natural or Artificial Opening Endoscopic	1 Radioactive Element G Intraluminal Device, Pessary	Z No Qualifier

Non-OR ØUH3[Ø,3,4][3,Y]Z
Non-OR ØUH3[7,8]YZ
Non-OR ØUH[8,D][Ø,3,4,7,8][3,Y]Z
Non-OR ØUHH[3,4]YZ
Non-OR ØUHH[7,8][3,Y]Z
Non-OR ØUH9[Ø,7,8]HZ
Non-OR ØUHC[7,8]HZ
Non-OR ØUHF[7,8]GZ
Non-OR ØUHG[7,8]GZ
♀ All body part, approach, device, and qualifier values

Ø Medical and Surgical
U Female Reproductive System
J Inspection Definition: Visually and/or manually exploring a body part

Explanation: Visual exploration may be performed with or without optical instrumentation. Manual exploration may be performed directly or through intervening body layers.

Body Part Character 4	Approach Character 5	Device Character 6	Qualifier Character 7
3 Ovary ♀	Ø Open 3 Percutaneous 4 Percutaneous Endoscopic 8 Via Natural or Artificial Opening Endoscopic X External	Z No Device	Z No Qualifier
8 Fallopian Tube ♀ D Uterus and Cervix ♀ H Vagina and Cul-de-sac ♀	Ø Open 3 Percutaneous 4 Percutaneous Endoscopic 7 Via Natural or Artificial Opening 8 Via Natural or Artificial Opening Endoscopic X External	Z No Device	Z No Qualifier
M Vulva ♀ Labia majora Labia minora	Ø Open X External	Z No Device	Z No Qualifier

Non-OR ØUJ3[3,8,X]ZZ
Non-OR ØUJ[8,D,H][3,7,8,X]ZZ
Non-OR ØUJMXZZ
♀ All body part, approach, device, and qualifier values

Ø Medical and Surgical
U Female Reproductive System
L Occlusion Definition: Completely closing an orifice or the lumen of a tubular body part

Explanation: The orifice can be a natural orifice or an artificially created orifice

Body Part Character 4	Approach Character 5	Device Character 6	Qualifier Character 7
5 Fallopian Tube, Right ♀ Oviduct Salpinx Uterine tube 6 Fallopian Tube, Left ♀ *See 5 Fallopian Tube, Right* 7 Fallopian Tubes, Bilateral NC ♀	Ø Open 3 Percutaneous 4 Percutaneous Endoscopic	C Extraluminal Device D Intraluminal Device Z No Device	Z No Qualifier
5 Fallopian Tube, Right ♀ Oviduct Salpinx Uterine tube 6 Fallopian Tube, Left ♀ *See 5 Fallopian Tube, Right* 7 Fallopian Tubes, Bilateral NC ♀	7 Via Natural or Artificial Opening 8 Via Natural or Artificial Opening Endoscopic	D Intraluminal Device Z No Device	Z No Qualifier
F Cul-de-sac ♀ G Vagina ♀	7 Via Natural or Artificial Opening 8 Via Natural or Artificial Opening Endoscopic	D Intraluminal Device Z No Device	Z No Qualifier

NC ØUL7[Ø,3,4][C,D,Z]Z with principal or secondary diagnosis of Z3Ø.2
NC ØUL7[7,8][D,Z]Z with principal or secondary diagnosis of Z3Ø.2
♀ All body part, approach, device, and qualifier values

Female Reproductive System

ØUJ–ØUL

Ø Medical and Surgical
U Female Reproductive System
M Reattachment Definition: Putting back in or on all or a portion of a separated body part to its normal location or other suitable location
Explanation: Vascular circulation and nervous pathways may or may not be reestablished

Body Part Character 4	Approach Character 5	Device Character 6	Qualifier Character 7
Ø Ovary, Right ♀ **1 Ovary, Left** ♀ **2 Ovaries, Bilateral** ♀ **4 Uterine Supporting Structure** ♀ Broad ligament Infundibulopelvic ligament Ovarian ligament Round ligament of uterus **5 Fallopian Tube, Right** ♀ Oviduct Salpinx Uterine tube **6 Fallopian Tube, Left** ♀ *See 5 Fallopian Tube, Right* **7 Fallopian Tubes, Bilateral** ♀ **9 Uterus** ♀ Fundus uteri Myometrium Perimetrium Uterine cornu **C Cervix** ♀ **F Cul-de-sac** ♀ **G Vagina** ♀	**Ø Open** **4 Percutaneous Endoscopic**	**Z No Device**	**Z No Qualifier**
J Clitoris ♀ **M Vulva** ♀ Labia majora Labia minora	**X External**	**Z No Device**	**Z No Qualifier**
K Hymen ♀	**Ø Open** **4 Percutaneous Endoscopic** **X External**	**Z No Device**	**Z No Qualifier**

♀ All body part, approach, device, and qualifier values

Ø Medical and Surgical
U Female Reproductive System
N Release Definition: Freeing a body part from an abnormal physical constraint by cutting or by the use of force
Explanation: Some of the restraining tissue may be taken out but none of the body part is taken out

Body Part Character 4	Approach Character 5	Device Character 6	Qualifier Character 7
Ø Ovary, Right ♀ **1** Ovary, Left ♀ **2** Ovaries, Bilateral ♀ **4** Uterine Supporting Structure ♀ Broad ligament Infundibulopelvic ligament Ovarian ligament Round ligament of uterus	**Ø** Open **3** Percutaneous **4** Percutaneous Endoscopic **8** Via Natural or Artificial Opening Endoscopic	**Z** No Device	**Z** No Qualifier
5 Fallopian Tube, Right ♀ Oviduct Salpinx Uterine tube **6** Fallopian Tube, Left ♀ *See 5 Fallopian Tube, Right* **7** Fallopian Tubes, Bilateral ♀ **9** Uterus ♀ Fundus uteri Myometrium Perimetrium Uterine cornu **C** Cervix ♀ **F** Cul-de-sac ♀	**Ø** Open **3** Percutaneous **4** Percutaneous Endoscopic **7** Via Natural or Artificial Opening **8** Via Natural or Artificial Opening Endoscopic	**Z** No Device	**Z** No Qualifier
G Vagina ♀ **K** Hymen ♀	**Ø** Open **3** Percutaneous **4** Percutaneous Endoscopic **7** Via Natural or Artificial Opening **8** Via Natural or Artificial Opening Endoscopic **X** External	**Z** No Device	**Z** No Qualifier
J Clitoris ♀ **L** Vestibular Gland ♀ Bartholin's (greater vestibular) gland Greater vestibular (Bartholin's) gland Paraurethral (Skene's) gland Skene's (paraurethral) gland **M** Vulva ♀ Labia majora Labia minora	**Ø** Open **X** External	**Z** No Device	**Z** No Qualifier

♀ All body part, approach, device, and qualifier values

Female Reproductive System

Ø Medical and Surgical
U Female Reproductive System
P Removal Definition: Taking out or off a device from a body part

Explanation: If a device is taken out and a similar device put in without cutting or puncturing the skin or mucous membrane, the procedure is coded to the root operation CHANGE. Otherwise, the procedure for taking out the device is coded to the root operation REMOVAL.

Body Part Character 4	Approach Character 5	Device Character 6	Qualifier Character 7
3 Ovary ♀	Ø Open 3 Percutaneous 4 Percutaneous Endoscopic	Ø Drainage Device 3 Infusion Device Y Other Device	Z No Qualifier
3 Ovary ♀	7 Via Natural or Artificial Opening 8 Via Natural or Artificial Opening Endoscopic	Y Other Device	Z No Qualifier
3 Ovary ♀	X External	Ø Drainage Device 3 Infusion Device	Z No Qualifier
8 Fallopian Tube ♀	Ø Open 3 Percutaneous 4 Percutaneous Endoscopic 7 Via Natural or Artificial Opening 8 Via Natural or Artificial Opening Endoscopic	Ø Drainage Device 3 Infusion Device 7 Autologous Tissue Substitute C Extraluminal Device D Intraluminal Device J Synthetic Substitute K Nonautologous Tissue Substitute Y Other Device	Z No Qualifier
8 Fallopian Tube ♀	X External	Ø Drainage Device 3 Infusion Device D Intraluminal Device	Z No Qualifier
D Uterus and Cervix ♀	Ø Open 3 Percutaneous 4 Percutaneous Endoscopic 7 Via Natural or Artificial Opening 8 Via Natural or Artificial Opening Endoscopic	Ø Drainage Device 1 Radioactive Element 3 Infusion Device 7 Autologous Tissue Substitute C Extraluminal Device D Intraluminal Device H Contraceptive Device J Synthetic Substitute K Nonautologous Tissue Substitute Y Other Device	Z No Qualifier
D Uterus and Cervix ♀	X External	Ø Drainage Device 3 Infusion Device D Intraluminal Device H Contraceptive Device	Z No Qualifier
H Vagina and Cul-de-sac ♀	Ø Open 3 Percutaneous 4 Percutaneous Endoscopic 7 Via Natural or Artificial Opening 8 Via Natural or Artificial Opening Endoscopic	Ø Drainage Device 1 Radioactive Element 3 Infusion Device 7 Autologous Tissue Substitute D Intraluminal Device J Synthetic Substitute K Nonautologous Tissue Substitute Y Other Device	Z No Qualifier
H Vagina and Cul-de-sac ♀	X External	Ø Drainage Device 1 Radioactive Element 3 Infusion Device D Intraluminal Device	Z No Qualifier
M Vulva ♀ Labia majora Labia minora	Ø Open	Ø Drainage Device 7 Autologous Tissue Substitute J Synthetic Substitute K Nonautologous Tissue Substitute	Z No Qualifier
M Vulva ♀ Labia majora Labia minora	X External	Ø Drainage Device	Z No Qualifier

Non-OR ØUP3[3,4]YZ
Non-OR ØUP3[7,8]YZ
Non-OR ØUP3X[Ø,3]Z
Non-OR ØUP8[3,4]YZ
Non-OR ØUP8[7,8][Ø,3,D,Y]Z
Non-OR ØUP8X[Ø,3,D]Z
Non-OR ØUPD[3,4][C,Y]Z
Non-OR ØUPD[7,8][Ø,3,C,D,H,Y]Z
Non-OR ØUPDX[Ø,3,D,H]Z
Non-OR ØUPH[3,4]YZ
Non-OR ØUPH[7,8][Ø,3,D,Y]Z
Non-OR ØUPHX[Ø,1,3,D]Z
Non-OR ØUPMXØZ
♀ All body part, approach, device, and qualifier values

ØUP–ØUP

Ø Medical and Surgical
U Female Reproductive System
Q Repair Definition: Restoring, to the extent possible, a body part to its normal anatomic structure and function
Explanation: Used only when the method to accomplish the repair is not one of the other root operations

Body Part Character 4	Approach Character 5	Device Character 6	Qualifier Character 7
Ø Ovary, Right ♀ **1** Ovary, Left ♀ **2** Ovaries, Bilateral ♀ **4** Uterine Supporting Structure ♀ Broad ligament Infundibulopelvic ligament Ovarian ligament Round ligament of uterus	**Ø** Open **3** Percutaneous **4** Percutaneous Endoscopic **8** Via Natural or Artificial Opening Endoscopic	**Z** No Device	**Z** No Qualifier
5 Fallopian Tube, Right ♀ Oviduct Salpinx Uterine tube **6** Fallopian Tube, Left ♀ *See 5 Fallopian Tube, Right* **7** Fallopian Tubes, Bilateral ♀ **9** Uterus ♀ Fundus uteri Myometrium Perimetrium Uterine cornu **C** Cervix ♀ **F** Cul-de-sac ♀	**Ø** Open **3** Percutaneous **4** Percutaneous Endoscopic **7** Via Natural or Artificial Opening **8** Via Natural or Artificial Opening Endoscopic	**Z** No Device	**Z** No Qualifier
G Vagina ♀ **K** Hymen ♀	**Ø** Open **3** Percutaneous **4** Percutaneous Endoscopic **7** Via Natural or Artificial Opening **8** Via Natural or Artificial Opening Endoscopic **X** External	**Z** No Device	**Z** No Qualifier
J Clitoris ♀ **L** Vestibular Gland ♀ Bartholin's (greater vestibular) gland Greater vestibular (Bartholin's) gland Paraurethral (Skene's) gland Skene's (paraurethral) gland **M** Vulva ♀ Labia majora Labia minora	**Ø** Open **X** External	**Z** No Device	**Z** No Qualifier

Non-OR ØUQG[7,X]ZZ
Non-OR ØUQKXZZ
Non-OR ØUQMXZZ
♀ All body part, approach, device, and qualifier values

Ø Medical and Surgical
U Female Reproductive System
S Reposition Definition: Moving to its normal location, or other suitable location, all or a portion of a body part
Explanation: The body part is moved to a new location from an abnormal location, or from a normal location where it is not functioning correctly. The body part may or may not be cut out or off to be moved to the new location.

Body Part Character 4	Approach Character 5	Device Character 6	Qualifier Character 7
Ø Ovary, Right ♀ **1** Ovary, Left ♀ **2** Ovaries, Bilateral ♀ **4** Uterine Supporting Structure ♀ Broad ligament Infundibulopelvic ligament Ovarian ligament Round ligament of uterus **5** Fallopian Tube, Right ♀ Oviduct Salpinx Uterine tube **6** Fallopian Tube, Left ♀ *See 5 Fallopian Tube, Right* **7** Fallopian Tubes, Bilateral ♀ **C** Cervix ♀ **F** Cul-de-sac ♀	**Ø** Open **4** Percutaneous Endoscopic **8** Via Natural or Artificial Opening Endoscopic	**Z** No Device	**Z** No Qualifier
9 Uterus ♀ Fundus uteri Myometrium Perimetrium Uterine cornu **G** Vagina ♀	**Ø** Open **4** Percutaneous Endoscopic **7** Via Natural or Artificial Opening **8** Via Natural or Artificial Opening Endoscopic **X** External	**Z** No Device	**Z** No Qualifier

Non-OR ØUS9XZZ
♀ All body part, approach, device, and qualifier values

Female Reproductive System

ØUQ–ØUS

Ø Medical and Surgical
U Female Reproductive System
T Resection Definition: Cutting out or off, without replacement, all of a body part
Explanation: None

Body Part Character 4	Approach Character 5	Device Character 6	Qualifier Character 7
Ø Ovary, Right ♀ **1** Ovary, Left ♀ **2** Ovaries, Bilateral ⊞♀ **5** Fallopian Tube, Right ♀ Oviduct Salpinx Uterine tube **6** Fallopian Tube, Left ♀ *See 5 Fallopian Tube, Right* **7** Fallopian Tubes, Bilateral ⊞♀	**Ø** Open **4** Percutaneous Endoscopic **7** Via Natural or Artificial Opening **8** Via Natural or Artificial Opening Endoscopic **F** Via Natural or Artificial Opening With Percutaneous Endoscopic Assistance	**Z** No Device	**Z** No Qualifier
4 Uterine Supporting Structure ⊞♀ Broad ligament Infundibulopelvic ligament Ovarian ligament Round ligament of uterus **C** Cervix ⊞♀ **F** Cul-de-sac ♀ **G** Vagina ⊞♀	**Ø** Open **4** Percutaneous Endoscopic **7** Via Natural or Artificial Opening **8** Via Natural or Artificial Opening Endoscopic	**Z** No Device	**Z** No Qualifier
9 Uterus ⊞♀ Fundus uteri Myometrium Perimetrium Uterine cornu	**Ø** Open **4** Percutaneous Endoscopic **7** Via Natural or Artificial Opening **8** Via Natural or Artificial Opening Endoscopic **F** Via Natural or Artificial Opening With Percutaneous Endoscopic Assistance	**Z** No Device	**L** Supracervical **Z** No Qualifier
J Clitoris ♀ **L** Vestibular Gland ♀ Bartholin's (greater vestibular) gland Greater vestibular (Bartholin's) gland Paraurethral (Skene's) gland Skene's (paraurethral) gland **M** Vulva ⊞♀ Labia majora Labia minora	**Ø** Open **X** External	**Z** No Device	**Z** No Qualifier
K Hymen ♀	**Ø** Open **4** Percutaneous Endoscopic **7** Via Natural or Artificial Opening **8** Via Natural or Artificial Opening Endoscopic **X** External	**Z** No Device	**Z** No Device

♀ All body part, approach, device, and qualifier values

See Appendix L for Procedure Combinations
⊞ ØUT[2,7]ØZZ
⊞ ØUT[4,C][Ø,4,7,8]ZZ
⊞ ØUTGØZZ
⊞ ØUT9[Ø,4,7,8,F]ZZ
⊞ ØUTM[Ø,X]ZZ

Ø Medical and Surgical
U Female Reproductive System
U Supplement Definition: Putting in or on biological or synthetic material that physically reinforces and/or augments the function of a portion of a body part

Explanation: The biological material is non-living, or is living and from the same individual. The body part may have been previously replaced, and the SUPPLEMENT procedure is performed to physically reinforce and/or augment the function of the replaced body part.

Body Part Character 4	Approach Character 5	Device Character 6	Qualifier Character 7
4 Uterine Supporting Structure ♀ Broad ligament Infundibulopelvic ligament Ovarian ligament Round ligament of uterus	**Ø** Open **4** Percutaneous Endoscopic	**7** Autologous Tissue Substitute **J** Synthetic Substitute **K** Nonautologous Tissue Substitute	**Z** No Qualifier
5 Fallopian Tube, Right ♀ Oviduct Salpinx Uterine tube **6** Fallopian Tube, Left ♀ *See 5 Fallopian Tube, Right* **7** Fallopian Tubes, Bilateral ♀ **F** Cul-de-sac ♀	**Ø** Open **4** Percutaneous Endoscopic **7** Via Natural or Artificial Opening **8** Via Natural or Artificial Opening Endoscopic	**7** Autologous Tissue Substitute **J** Synthetic Substitute **K** Nonautologous Tissue Substitute	**Z** No Qualifier
G Vagina ♀ **K** Hymen ♀	**Ø** Open **4** Percutaneous Endoscopic **7** Via Natural or Artificial Opening **8** Via Natural or Artificial Opening Endoscopic **X** External	**7** Autologous Tissue Substitute **J** Synthetic Substitute **K** Nonautologous Tissue Substitute	**Z** No Qualifier
J Clitoris ♀ **M** Vulva ♀ Labia majora Labia minora	**Ø** Open **X** External	**7** Autologous Tissue Substitute **J** Synthetic Substitute **K** Nonautologous Tissue Substitute	**Z** No Qualifier

♀ All body part, approach, device, and qualifier values

Ø Medical and Surgical
U Female Reproductive System
V Restriction Definition: Partially closing an orifice or the lumen of a tubular body part

Explanation: The orifice can be a natural orifice or an artificially created orifice

Body Part Character 4	Approach Character 5	Device Character 6	Qualifier Character 7
C Cervix ♀	**Ø** Open **3** Percutaneous **4** Percutaneous Endoscopic	**C** Extraluminal Device **D** Intraluminal Device **Z** No Device	**Z** No Qualifier
C Cervix ♀	**7** Via Natural or Artificial Opening **8** Via Natural or Artificial Opening Endoscopic	**D** Intraluminal Device **Z** No Device	**Z** No Qualifier

♀ All body part, approach, device, and qualifier values

Ø Medical and Surgical
U Female Reproductive System
W Revision Definition: Correcting, to the extent possible, a portion of a malfunctioning device or the position of a displaced device

Explanation: Revision can include correcting a malfunctioning or displaced device by taking out or putting in components of the device such as a screw or pin

Body Part Character 4	Approach Character 5	Device Character 6	Qualifier Character 7
3 Ovary ♀	Ø Open 3 Percutaneous 4 Percutaneous Endoscopic	Ø Drainage Device 3 Infusion Device Y Other Device	Z No Qualifier
3 Ovary ♀	7 Via Natural or Artificial Opening 8 Via Natural or Artificial Opening Endoscopic	Y Other Device	Z No Qualifier
3 Ovary ♀	X External	Ø Drainage Device 3 Infusion Device	Z No Qualifier
8 Fallopian Tube ♀	Ø Open 3 Percutaneous 4 Percutaneous Endoscopic 7 Via Natural or Artificial Opening 8 Via Natural or Artificial Opening Endoscopic	Ø Drainage Device 3 Infusion Device 7 Autologous Tissue Substitute C Extraluminal Device D Intraluminal Device J Synthetic Substitute K Nonautologous Tissue Substitute Y Other Device	Z No Qualifier
8 Fallopian Tube ♀	X External	Ø Drainage Device 3 Infusion Device 7 Autologous Tissue Substitute C Extraluminal Device D Intraluminal Device J Synthetic Substitute K Nonautologous Tissue Substitute	Z No Qualifier
D Uterus and Cervix ♀	Ø Open 3 Percutaneous 4 Percutaneous Endoscopic 7 Via Natural or Artificial Opening 8 Via Natural or Artificial Opening Endoscopic	Ø Drainage Device 1 Radioactive Element 3 Infusion Device 7 Autologous Tissue Substitute C Extraluminal Device D Intraluminal Device H Contraceptive Device J Synthetic Substitute K Nonautologous Tissue Substitute Y Other Device	Z No Qualifier
D Uterus and Cervix ♀	X External	Ø Drainage Device 3 Infusion Device 7 Autologous Tissue Substitute C Extraluminal Device D Intraluminal Device H Contraceptive Device J Synthetic Substitute K Nonautologous Tissue Substitute	Z No Qualifier
H Vagina and Cul-de-sac ♀	Ø Open 3 Percutaneous 4 Percutaneous Endoscopic 7 Via Natural or Artificial Opening 8 Via Natural or Artificial Opening Endoscopic	Ø Drainage Device 1 Radioactive Element 3 Infusion Device 7 Autologous Tissue Substitute D Intraluminal Device J Synthetic Substitute K Nonautologous Tissue Substitute Y Other Device	Z No Qualifier
H Vagina and Cul-de-sac ♀	X External	Ø Drainage Device 3 Infusion Device 7 Autologous Tissue Substitute D Intraluminal Device J Synthetic Substitute K Nonautologous Tissue Substitute	Z No Qualifier
M Vulva ♀ Labia majora Labia minora	Ø Open X External	Ø Drainage Device 7 Autologous Tissue Substitute J Synthetic Substitute K Nonautologous Tissue Substitute	Z No Qualifier

Non-OR ØUW3[3,4]YZ
Non-OR ØUW3[7,8]YZ
Non-OR ØUW3X[Ø,3]Z
Non-OR ØUW8[3,4,7,8]YZ
Non-OR ØUW8X[Ø,3,7,C,D,J,K]Z
Non-OR ØUWD[3,4,7,8]YZ
Non-OR ØUWDX[Ø,3,7,C,D,H,J,K]Z
Non-OR ØUWH[3,4,7,8]YZ
Non-OR ØUWHX[Ø,3,7,D,J,K]Z
Non-OR ØUWMX[Ø,7,J,K]Z
♀ All body part, approach, device, and qualifier values

Ø Medical and Surgical
U Female Reproductive System
Y Transplantation Definition: Putting in or on all or a portion of a living body part taken from another individual or animal to physically take the place and/or function of all or a portion of a similar body part

Explanation: The native body part may or may not be taken out, and the transplanted body part may take over all or a portion of its function

Body Part Character 4	Approach Character 5	Device Character 6	Qualifier Character 7
Ø Ovary, Right ♀ 1 Ovary, Left ♀ 9 Uterus ♀	Ø Open	Z No Device	Ø Allogeneic 1 Syngeneic 2 Zooplastic

♀ All body part, approach, device, and qualifier values

Male Reproductive System ØV1–ØVX

Character Meanings

This Character Meaning table is provided as a guide to assist the user in the identification of character members that may be found in this section of code tables. It **SHOULD NOT** be used to build a PCS code.

Operation–Character 3	Body Part–Character 4	Approach–Character 5	Device–Character 6	Qualifier–Character 7
1 Bypass	Ø Prostate	Ø Open	Ø Drainage Device	D Urethra
2 Change	1 Seminal Vesicle, Right	3 Percutaneous	1 Radioactive Element	J Epididymis, Right
5 Destruction	2 Seminal Vesicle, Left	4 Percutaneous Endoscopic	3 Infusion Device	K Epididymis, Left
7 Dilation	3 Seminal Vesicles, Bilateral	7 Via Natural or Artificial Opening	7 Autologous Tissue Substitute	N Vas Deferens, Right
9 Drainage	4 Prostate and Seminal Vesicles	8 Via Natural or Artificial Opening Endoscopic	C Extraluminal Device	P Vas Deferens, Left
B Excision	5 Scrotum	X External	D Intraluminal Device	S Penis
C Extirpation	6 Tunica Vaginalis, Right		J Synthetic Substitute	X Diagnostic
H Insertion	7 Tunica Vaginalis, Left		K Nonautologous Tissue Substitute	Z No Qualifier
J Inspection	8 Scrotum and Tunica Vaginalis		Y Other Device	
L Occlusion	9 Testis, Right		Z No Device	
M Reattachment	B Testis, Left			
N Release	C Testes, Bilateral			
P Removal	D Testis			
Q Repair	F Spermatic Cord, Right			
R Replacement	G Spermatic Cord, Left			
S Reposition	H Spermatic Cords, Bilateral			
T Resection	J Epididymis, Right			
U Supplement	K Epididymis, Left			
W Revision	L Epididymis, Bilateral			
X Transfer	M Epididymis and Spermatic Cord			
	N Vas Deferens, Right			
	P Vas Deferens, Left			
	Q Vas Deferens, Bilateral			
	R Vas Deferens			
	S Penis			
	T Prepuce			

AHA Coding Clinic for table ØVB
2016, 1Q, 23 Transurethral resection of ejaculatory ducts
2014, 4Q, 33 Radical prostatectomy

AHA Coding Clinic for table ØVP
2016, 2Q, 28 Removal of multi-component inflatable penile prosthesis with placement of new malleable device

AHA Coding Clinic for table ØVT
2014, 4Q, 33 Radical prostatectomy

AHA Coding Clinic for table ØVU
2016, 2Q, 28 Removal of multi-component inflatable penile prosthesis with placement of new malleable device
2015, 3Q, 25 Placement of inflatable penile prosthesis

Male Reproductive System

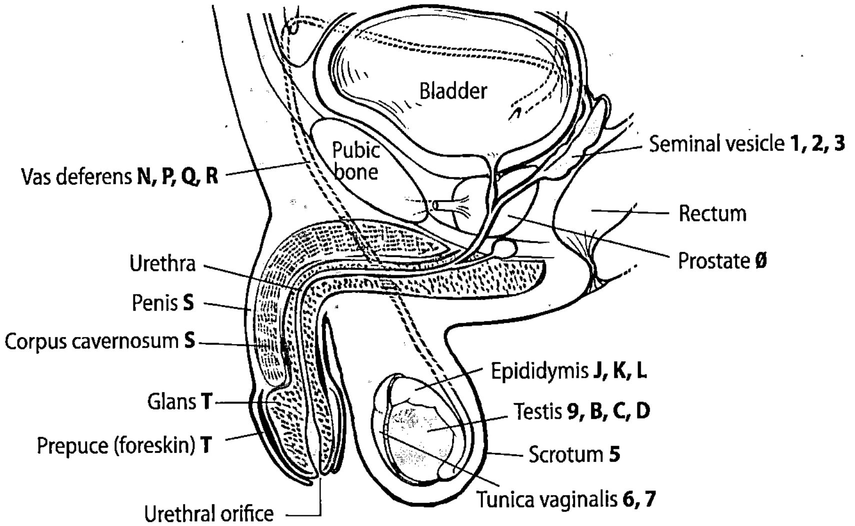

Penis

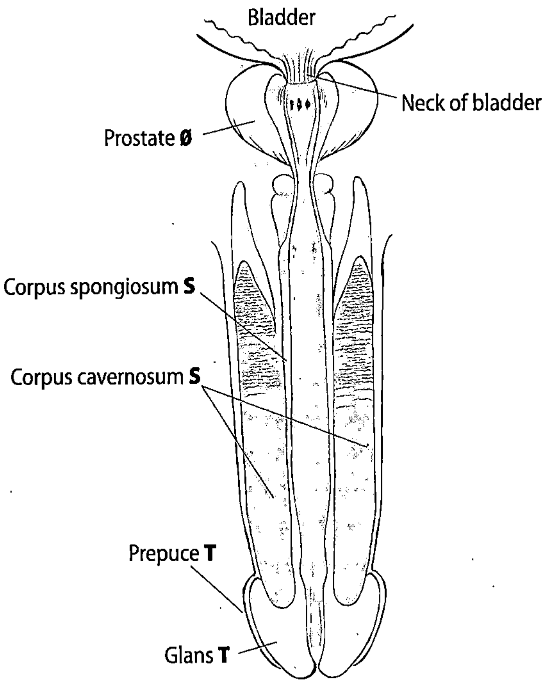

Ø Medical and Surgical
V Male Reproductive System
1 Bypass Definition: Altering the route of passage of the contents of a tubular body part
Explanation: Rerouting contents of a body part to a downstream area of the normal route, to a similar route and body part, or to an abnormal route and dissimilar body part. Includes one or more anastomoses, with or without the use of a device.

Body Part Character 4	Approach Character 5	Device Character 6	Qualifier Character 7
N Vas Deferens, Right ♂ Ductus deferens Ejaculatory duct **P** Vas Deferens, Left ♂ *See N Vas Deferens, Right* **Q** Vas Deferens, Bilateral ♂ *See N Vas Deferens, Right*	**Ø** Open **4** Percutaneous Endoscopic	**7** Autologous Tissue Substitute **J** Synthetic Substitute **K** Nonautologous Tissue Substitute **Z** No Device	**J** Epididymis, Right **K** Epididymis, Left **N** Vas Deferens, Right **P** Vas Deferens, Left

♂ All body part, approach, device, and qualifier values

Ø Medical and Surgical
V Male Reproductive System
2 Change Definition: Taking out or off a device from a body part and putting back an identical or similar device in or on the same body part without cutting or puncturing the skin or a mucous membrane
Explanation: All CHANGE procedures are coded using the approach EXTERNAL

Body Part Character 4	Approach Character 5	Device Character 6	Qualifier Character 7
4 Prostate and Seminal Vesicles ♂ **8** Scrotum and Tunica Vaginalis ♂ **D** Testis ♂ **M** Epididymis and Spermatic Cord ♂ **R** Vas Deferens ♂ Ductus deferens Ejaculatory duct **S** Penis ♂ Corpus cavernosum Corpus spongiosum	**X** External	**Ø** Drainage Device **Y** Other Device	**Z** No Qualifier

Non-OR All body part, approach, device, and qualifier values
♂ All body part, approach, device, and qualifier values

Ø Medical and Surgical
V Male Reproductive System
5 Destruction Definition: Physical eradication of all or a portion of a body part by the direct use of energy, force, or a destructive agent
Explanation: None of the body part is physically taken out

Body Part Character 4	Approach Character 5	Device Character 6	Qualifier Character 7
Ø Prostate ♂	**Ø** Open **3** Percutaneous **4** Percutaneous Endoscopic **7** Via Natural or Artificial Opening **8** Via Natural or Artificial Opening Endoscopic	**Z** No Device	**Z** No Qualifier
1 Seminal Vesicle, Right ♂ **2** Seminal Vesicle, Left ♂ **3** Seminal Vesicles, Bilateral ♂ **6** Tunica Vaginalis, Right ♂ **7** Tunica Vaginalis, Left ♂ **9** Testis, Right ♂ **B** Testis, Left ♂ **C** Testes, Bilateral ♂	**Ø** Open **3** Percutaneous **4** Percutaneous Endoscopic	**Z** No Device	**Z** No Qualifier
5 Scrotum ♂ **S** Penis ♂ Corpus cavernosum Corpus spongiosum **T** Prepuce ♂ Foreskin Glans penis	**Ø** Open **3** Percutaneous **4** Percutaneous Endoscopic **X** External	**Z** No Device	**Z** No Qualifier
F Spermatic Cord, Right ♂ **G** Spermatic Cord, Left ♂ **H** Spermatic Cords, Bilateral ♂ **J** Epididymis, Right ♂ **K** Epididymis, Left ♂ **L** Epididymis, Bilateral ♂ **N** Vas Deferens, Right NC ♂ Ductus deferens Ejaculatory duct **P** Vas Deferens, Left NC ♂ *See N Vas Deferens, Right* **Q** Vas Deferens, Bilateral NC ♂ *See N Vas Deferens, Right*	**Ø** Open **3** Percutaneous **4** Percutaneous Endoscopic **8** Via Natural or Artificial Opening Endoscopic	**Z** No Device	**Z** No Qualifier

Non-OR ØV55[Ø,3,4,X]ZZ
Non-OR ØV5[N,P,Q][Ø,3,4,8]ZZ
NC ØV5[N,P,Q][Ø,3,4]ZZ with principal or secondary diagnosis of Z3Ø.2
♂ All body part, approach, device, and qualifier values

Ø Medical and Surgical
V Male Reproductive System
7 Dilation Definition: Expanding an orifice or the lumen of a tubular body part

Explanation: The orifice can be a natural orifice or an artificially created orifice. Accomplished by stretching a tubular body part using intraluminal pressure or by cutting part of the orifice or wall of the tubular body part.

Body Part Character 4	Approach Character 5	Device Character 6	Qualifier Character 7
N Vas Deferens, Right ♂ Ductus deferens Ejaculatory duct P Vas Deferens, Left ♂ *See N Vas Deferens, Right* Q Vas Deferens, Bilateral ♂ *See N Vas Deferens, Right*	Ø Open 3 Percutaneous 4 Percutaneous Endoscopic	D Intraluminal Device Z No Device	Z No Qualifier

♂ All body part, approach, device, and qualifier values

Ø Medical and Surgical
V Male Reproductive System
9 Drainage Definition: Taking or letting out fluids and/or gases from a body part

Explanation: The qualifier DIAGNOSTIC is used to identify drainage procedures that are biopsies

Body Part Character 4	Approach Character 5	Device Character 6	Qualifier Character 7
Ø Prostate ♂	Ø Open 3 Percutaneous 4 Percutaneous Endoscopic 7 Via Natural or Artificial Opening 8 Via Natural or Artificial Opening Endoscopic	Ø Drainage Device	Z No Qualifier
Ø Prostate ♂	Ø Open 3 Percutaneous 4 Percutaneous Endoscopic 7 Via Natural or Artificial Opening 8 Via Natural or Artificial Opening Endoscopic	Z No Device	X Diagnostic Z No Qualifier
1 Seminal Vesicle, Right ♂ 2 Seminal Vesicle, Left ♂ 3 Seminal Vesicles, Bilateral ♂ 6 Tunica Vaginalis, Right ♂ 7 Tunica Vaginalis, Left ♂ 9 Testis, Right ♂ B Testis, Left ♂ C Testes, Bilateral ♂ F Spermatic Cord, Right ♂ G Spermatic Cord, Left ♂ H Spermatic Cords, Bilateral ♂ J Epididymis, Right ♂ K Epididymis, Left ♂ L Epididymis, Bilateral ♂ N Vas Deferens, Right ♂ Ductus deferens Ejaculatory duct P Vas Deferens, Left ♂ *See N Vas Deferens, Right* Q Vas Deferens, Bilateral ♂ *See N Vas Deferens, Right*	Ø Open 3 Percutaneous 4 Percutaneous Endoscopic	Ø Drainage Device	Z No Qualifier

ØV9 Continued on next page

Non-OR ØV9Ø[3,4]ØZ
Non-OR ØV9Ø[3,4]Z[X,Z]
Non-OR ØV9Ø[7,8]ZX
Non-OR ØV9[1,2,3,9,B,C][3,4]ØZ
Non-OR ØV9[6,7,F,G,H,N,P,Q][Ø,3,4]ØZ
Non-OR ØV9[J,K,L]3ØZ
♂ All body part, approach, device, and qualifier values

Ø Medical and Surgical
V Male Reproductive System
9 Drainage Definition: Taking or letting out fluids and/or gases from a body part
Explanation: The qualifier DIAGNOSTIC is used to identify drainage procedures that are biopsies

ØV9 Continued

Body Part Character 4	Approach Character 5	Device Character 6	Qualifier Character 7
1 Seminal Vesicle, Right ♂ 2 Seminal Vesicle, Left ♂ 3 Seminal Vesicles, Bilateral ♂ 6 Tunica Vaginalis, Right ♂ 7 Tunica Vaginalis, Left ♂ 9 Testis, Right ♂ B Testis, Left ♂ C Testes, Bilateral ♂ F Spermatic Cord, Right ♂ G Spermatic Cord, Left ♂ H Spermatic Cords, Bilateral ♂ J Epididymis, Right ♂ K Epididymis, Left ♂ L Epididymis, Bilateral ♂ N Vas Deferens, Right ♂ Ductus deferens Ejaculatory duct P Vas Deferens, Left ♂ *See N Vas Deferens, Right* Q Vas Deferens, Bilateral ♂ *See N Vas Deferens, Right*	Ø Open 3 Percutaneous 4 Percutaneous Endoscopic	Z No Device	X Diagnostic Z No Qualifier
5 Scrotum ♂ S Penis ♂ Corpus cavernosum Corpus spongiosum T Prepuce ♂ Foreskin Glans penis	Ø Open 3 Percutaneous 4 Percutaneous Endoscopic X External	Ø Drainage Device	Z No Qualifier
5 Scrotum ♂ S Penis ♂ Corpus cavernosum Corpus spongiosum T Prepuce ♂ Foreskin Glans penis	Ø Open 3 Percutaneous 4 Percutaneous Endoscopic X External	Z No Device	X Diagnostic Z No Qualifier

Non-OR ØV9[1,2,3,9,B,C][3,4]Z[X,Z]
Non-OR ØV9[6,7,F,G,H,J,K,L,N,P,Q][Ø,3,4]ZX
Non-OR ØV9[6,7,F,G,H,N,P,Q][Ø,3,4]ZZ
Non-OR ØV9[J,K,L]3ZZ
Non-OR ØV95[Ø,3,4,X]ØZ
Non-OR ØV9[S,T]3ØZ
Non-OR ØV95[Ø,3,4,X]Z[X,Z]
Non-OR ØV9[S,T]3ZZ
♂ All body part, approach, device, and qualifier values

Male Reproductive System

Ø Medical and Surgical
V Male Reproductive System
B Excision Definition: Cutting out or off, without replacement, a portion of a body part
Explanation: The qualifier DIAGNOSTIC is used to identify excision procedures that are biopsies

Body Part Character 4	Approach Character 5	Device Character 6	Qualifier Character 7
Ø Prostate ♂	**Ø** Open **3** Percutaneous **4** Percutaneous Endoscopic **7** Via Natural or Artificial Opening **8** Via Natural or Artificial Opening Endoscopic	**Z** No Device	**X** Diagnostic **Z** No Qualifier
1 Seminal Vesicle, Right ♂ **2** Seminal Vesicle, Left ♂ **3** Seminal Vesicles, Bilateral ♂ **6** Tunica Vaginalis, Right ♂ **7** Tunica Vaginalis, Left ♂ **9** Testis, Right ♂ **B** Testis, Left ♂ **C** Testes, Bilateral ♂	**Ø** Open **3** Percutaneous **4** Percutaneous Endoscopic	**Z** No Device	**X** Diagnostic **Z** No Qualifier
5 Scrotum ♂ **S** Penis ♂ Corpus cavernosum Corpus spongiosum **T** Prepuce ♂ Foreskin Glans penis	**Ø** Open **3** Percutaneous **4** Percutaneous Endoscopic **X** External	**Z** No Device	**X** Diagnostic **Z** No Qualifier
F Spermatic Cord, Right ♂ **G** Spermatic Cord, Left ♂ **H** Spermatic Cords, Bilateral ♂ **J** Epididymis, Right ♂ **K** Epididymis, Left ♂ **L** Epididymis, Bilateral ♂ **N** Vas Deferens, Right NC ♂ Ductus deferens Ejaculatory duct **P** Vas Deferens, Left NC ♂ *See N Vas Deferens, Right* **Q** Vas Deferens, Bilateral NC ♂ *See N Vas Deferens, Right*	**Ø** Open **3** Percutaneous **4** Percutaneous Endoscopic **8** Via Natural or Artificial Opening Endoscopic	**Z** No Device	**X** Diagnostic **Z** No Qualifier

Non-OR ØVBØ[3,4,7,8]ZX
Non-OR ØVB[1,2,3,9,B,C][3,4]ZX
Non-OR ØVB[6,7][Ø,3,4]ZX
Non-OR ØVB5[Ø,3,4,X]Z[X,Z]
Non-OR ØVB[F,G,H,J,K,L][Ø,3,4,8]ZX
Non-OR ØVB[N,P,Q][Ø,3,4,8]Z[X,Z]
NC ØVB[N,P,Q][Ø,3,4]ZZ with principal or secondary diagnosis of Z3Ø.2
♂ All body part, approach, device, and qualifier values

Ø Medical and Surgical
V Male Reproductive System
C Extirpation Definition: Taking or cutting out solid matter from a body part

Explanation: The solid matter may be an abnormal byproduct of a biological function or a foreign body; it may be imbedded in a body part or in the lumen of a tubular body part. The solid matter may or may not have been previously broken into pieces.

Body Part Character 4	Approach Character 5	Device Character 6	Qualifier Character 7
Ø Prostate ♂	Ø Open 3 Percutaneous 4 Percutaneous Endoscopic 7 Via Natural or Artificial Opening 8 Via Natural or Artificial Opening Endoscopic	Z No Device	Z No Qualifier
1 Seminal Vesicle, Right ♂ 2 Seminal Vesicle, Left ♂ 3 Seminal Vesicles, Bilateral ♂ 6 Tunica Vaginalis, Right ♂ 7 Tunica Vaginalis, Left ♂ 9 Testis, Right ♂ B Testis, Left ♂ C Testes, Bilateral ♂ F Spermatic Cord, Right ♂ G Spermatic Cord, Left ♂ H Spermatic Cords, Bilateral ♂ J Epididymis, Right ♂ K Epididymis, Left ♂ L Epididymis, Bilateral ♂ N Vas Deferens, Right ♂ Ductus deferens Ejaculatory duct P Vas Deferens, Left ♂ *See N Vas Deferens, Right* Q Vas Deferens, Bilateral ♂ *See N Vas Deferens, Right*	Ø Open 3 Percutaneous 4 Percutaneous Endoscopic	Z No Device	Z No Qualifier
5 Scrotum ♂ S Penis ♂ Corpus cavernosum Corpus spongiosum T Prepuce ♂ Foreskin Glans penis	Ø Open 3 Percutaneous 4 Percutaneous Endoscopic X External	Z No Device	Z No Qualifier

Non-OR ØVC[6,7,N,P,Q][Ø,3,4]ZZ
Non-OR ØVC5[Ø,3,4,X]ZZ
Non-OR ØVCSXZZ
♂ All body part, approach, device, and qualifier values

Ø Medical and Surgical
V Male Reproductive System
H Insertion Definition: Putting in a nonbiological appliance that monitors, assists, performs, or prevents a physiological function but does not physically take the place of a body part

Explanation: None

Body Part Character 4	Approach Character 5	Device Character 6	Qualifier Character 7
Ø Prostate ♂	**Ø** Open **3** Percutaneous **4** Percutaneous Endoscopic **7** Via Natural or Artificial Opening **8** Via Natural or Artificial Opening Endoscopic	**1** Radioactive Element	**Z** No Qualifier
4 Prostate and Seminal Vesicles ♂ **8** Scrotum and Tunica Vaginalis ♂ **D** Testis ♂ **M** Epididymis and Spermatic Cord ♂ **R** Vas Deferens ♂ Ductus deferens Ejaculatory duct	**Ø** Open **3** Percutaneous **4** Percutaneous Endoscopic **7** Via Natural or Artificial Opening **8** Via Natural or Artificial Opening Endoscopic	**3** Infusion Device **Y** Other Device	**Z** No Qualifier
S Penis ♂ Corpus cavernosum Corpus spongiosum	**Ø** Open **3** Percutaneous **4** Percutaneous Endoscopic	**3** Infusion Device **Y** Other Device	**Z** No Qualifier
S Penis ♂ Corpus cavernosum Corpus spongiosum	**7** Via Natural or Artificial Opening **8** Via Natural or Artificial Opening Endoscopic	**Y** Other Device	**Z** No Qualifier
S Penis ♂ Corpus cavernosum Corpus spongiosum	**X** External	**3** Infusion Device	**Z** No Qualifier

Non-OR ØVH[4,8,D,M,R][Ø,3,4,7,8][3,Y]Z
Non-OR ØVHS[Ø,3,4][3,Y]Z
Non-OR ØVHS[7,8]YZ
Non-OR ØVHSX3Z
♂ All body part, approach, device, and qualifier values

Ø Medical and Surgical
V Male Reproductive System
J Inspection Definition: Visually and/or manually exploring a body part

Explanation: Visual exploration may be performed with or without optical instrumentation. Manual exploration may be performed directly or through intervening body layers.

Body Part Character 4	Approach Character 5	Device Character 6	Qualifier Character 7
4 Prostate and Seminal Vesicles ♂ **8** Scrotum and Tunica Vaginalis ♂ **D** Testis ♂ **M** Epididymis and Spermatic Cord ♂ **R** Vas Deferens ♂ Ductus deferens Ejaculatory duct **S** Penis ♂ Corpus cavernosum Corpus spongiosum	**Ø** Open **3** Percutaneous **4** Percutaneous Endoscopic **X** External	**Z** No Device	**Z** No Qualifier

Non-OR ØVJ[4,D,M,R][3,X]ZZ
Non-OR ØVJ[8,S][Ø,3,4,X]ZZ
♂ All body part, approach, device, and qualifier values

Ø Medical and Surgical
V Male Reproductive System
L Occlusion Definition: Completely closing an orifice or the lumen of a tubular body part

Explanation: The orifice can be a natural orifice or an artificially created orifice

Body Part Character 4	Approach Character 5	Device Character 6	Qualifier Character 7
F Spermatic Cord, Right NC ♂ **G** Spermatic Cord, Left NC ♂ **H** Spermatic Cords, Bilateral NC ♂ **N** Vas Deferens, Right NC ♂ Ductus deferens Ejaculatory duct **P** Vas Deferens, Left NC ♂ *See N Vas Deferens, Right* **Q** Vas Deferens, Bilateral NC ♂ *See N Vas Deferens, Right*	**Ø** Open **3** Percutaneous **4** Percutaneous Endoscopic **8** Via Natural or Artificial Opening Endoscopic	**C** Extraluminal Device **D** Intraluminal Device **Z** No Device	**Z** No Qualifier

Non-OR ØVL[F,G,H][Ø,3,4,8][C,D,Z]Z
Non-OR ØVL[N,P,Q][Ø,3,4,8][C,Z]Z
NC ØVL[F,G,H][Ø,3,4][C,D,Z]Z with principal or secondary diagnosis of Z3Ø.2
NC ØVL[N,P,Q][Ø,3,4][C,Z]Z with principal or secondary diagnosis of Z3Ø.2
♂ All body part, approach, device, and qualifier values

Ø Medical and Surgical
V Male Reproductive System
M Reattachment Definition: Putting back in or on all or a portion of a separated body part to its normal location or other suitable location
Explanation: Vascular circulation and nervous pathways may or may not be reestablished

Body Part Character 4	Approach Character 5	Device Character 6	Qualifier Character 7
5 Scrotum ♂ **S** Penis ♂ Corpus cavernosum Corpus spongiosum	**X** External	**Z** No Device	**Z** No Qualifier
6 Tunica Vaginalis, Right ♂ **7** Tunica Vaginalis, Left ♂ **9** Testis, Right ♂ **B** Testis, Left ♂ **C** Testes, Bilateral ♂ **F** Spermatic Cord, Right ♂ **G** Spermatic Cord, Left ♂ **H** Spermatic Cords, Bilateral ♂	**Ø** Open **4** Percutaneous Endoscopic	**Z** No Device	**Z** No Qualifier

♂ All body part, approach, device, and qualifier values

Ø Medical and Surgical
V Male Reproductive System
N Release Definition: Freeing a body part from an abnormal physical constraint by cutting or by the use of force
Explanation: Some of the restraining tissue may be taken out but none of the body part is taken out

Body Part Character 4	Approach Character 5	Device Character 6	Qualifier Character 7
Ø Prostate ♂	**Ø** Open **3** Percutaneous **4** Percutaneous Endoscopic **7** Via Natural or Artificial Opening **8** Via Natural or Artificial Opening Endoscopic	**Z** No Device	**Z** No Qualifier
1 Seminal Vesicle, Right ♂ **2** Seminal Vesicle, Left ♂ **3** Seminal Vesicles, Bilateral ♂ **6** Tunica Vaginalis, Right ♂ **7** Tunica Vaginalis, Left ♂ **9** Testis, Right ♂ **B** Testis, Left ♂ **C** Testes, Bilateral ♂	**Ø** Open **3** Percutaneous **4** Percutaneous Endoscopic	**Z** No Device	**Z** No Qualifier
5 Scrotum ♂ **S** Penis ♂ Corpus cavernosum Corpus spongiosum **T** Prepuce ♂ Foreskin Glans penis	**Ø** Open **3** Percutaneous **4** Percutaneous Endoscopic **X** External	**Z** No Device	**Z** No Qualifier
F Spermatic Cord, Right ♂ **G** Spermatic Cord, Left ♂ **H** Spermatic Cords, Bilateral ♂ **J** Epididymis, Right ♂ **K** Epididymis, Left ♂ **L** Epididymis, Bilateral ♂ **N** Vas Deferens, Right ♂ Ductus deferens Ejaculatory duct **P** Vas Deferens, Left ♂ *See N Vas Deferens, Right* **Q** Vas Deferens, Bilateral ♂ *See N Vas Deferens, Right*	**Ø** Open **3** Percutaneous **4** Percutaneous Endoscopic **8** Via Natural or Artificial Opening Endoscopic	**Z** No Device	**Z** No Qualifier

Non-OR ØVN[9,B,C][Ø,3,4]ZZ
Non-OR ØVNT[Ø,3,4,X]ZZ

♂ All body part, approach, device, and qualifier values

Ø Medical and Surgical
V Male Reproductive System
P Removal Definition: Taking out or off a device from a body part

Explanation: If a device is taken out and a similar device put in without cutting or puncturing the skin or mucous membrane, the procedure is coded to the root operation CHANGE. Otherwise, the procedure for taking out the device is coded to the root operation REMOVAL.

Body Part Character 4	Approach Character 5	Device Character 6	Qualifier Character 7
4 Prostate and Seminal Vesicles ♂	Ø Open 3 Percutaneous 4 Percutaneous Endoscopic 7 Via Natural or Artificial Opening 8 Via Natural or Artificial Opening Endoscopic	Ø Drainage Device 1 Radioactive Element 3 Infusion Device 7 Autologous Tissue Substitute J Synthetic Substitute K Nonautologous Tissue Substitute Y Other Device	Z No Qualifier
4 Prostate and Seminal Vesicles ♂	X External	Ø Drainage Device 1 Radioactive Element 3 Infusion Device	Z No Qualifier
8 Scrotum and Tunica Vaginalis ♂ D Testis ♂ S Penis ♂ Corpus cavernosum Corpus spongiosum	Ø Open 3 Percutaneous 4 Percutaneous Endoscopic 7 Via Natural or Artificial Opening 8 Via Natural or Artificial Opening Endoscopic	Ø Drainage Device 3 Infusion Device 7 Autologous Tissue Substitute J Synthetic Substitute K Nonautologous Tissue Substitute Y Other Device	Z No Qualifier
8 Scrotum and Tunica Vaginalis ♂ D Testis ♂ S Penis ♂ Corpus cavernosum Corpus spongiosum	X External	Ø Drainage Device 3 Infusion Device	Z No Qualifier
M Epididymis and Spermatic Cord ♂	Ø Open 3 Percutaneous 4 Percutaneous Endoscopic 7 Via Natural or Artificial Opening 8 Via Natural or Artificial Opening Endoscopic	Ø Drainage Device 3 Infusion Device 7 Autologous Tissue Substitute C Extraluminal Device J Synthetic Substitute K Nonautologous Tissue Substitute Y Other Device	Z No Qualifier
M Epididymis and Spermatic Cord ♂	X External	Ø Drainage Device 3 Infusion Device	Z No Qualifier
R Vas Deferens ♂ Ductus deferens Ejaculatory duct	Ø Open 3 Percutaneous 4 Percutaneous Endoscopic 7 Via Natural or Artificial Opening 8 Via Natural or Artificial Opening Endoscopic	Ø Drainage Device 3 Infusion Device 7 Autologous Tissue Substitute C Extraluminal Device D Intraluminal Device J Synthetic Substitute K Nonautologous Tissue Substitute Y Other Device	Z No Qualifier
R Vas Deferens ♂ Ductus deferens Ejaculatory duct	X External	Ø Drainage Device 3 Infusion Device D Intraluminal Device	Z No Qualifier

Non-OR ØVP4[3,4]YZ
Non-OR ØVP4[7,8][Ø,3,Y]Z
Non-OR ØVP4X[Ø,1,3]Z
Non-OR ØVP8[Ø,3,4,7,8][Ø,3,7,J,K,Y]Z
Non-OR ØVP[D,S][3,4]YZ
Non-OR ØVP[D,S][7,8][Ø,3,Y]Z
Non-OR ØVP[8,D,S]X[Ø,3]Z
Non-OR ØVPM[3,4]YZ
Non-OR ØVPM[7,8][Ø,3,Y]Z
Non-OR ØVPMX[Ø,3]Z
Non-OR ØVPR[Ø,3,4][Ø,3,7,C,J,K,Y]Z
Non-OR ØVPR[7,8][Ø,3,7,C,D,J,K,Y]Z
Non-OR ØVPRX[Ø,3,D]Z
♂ All body part, approach, device, and qualifier values

Ø Medical and Surgical
V Male Reproductive System
Q Repair Definition: Restoring, to the extent possible, a body part to its normal anatomic structure and function
Explanation: Used only when the method to accomplish the repair is not one of the other root operations

Body Part Character 4	Approach Character 5	Device Character 6	Qualifier Character 7
Ø Prostate ♂	Ø Open 3 Percutaneous 4 Percutaneous Endoscopic 7 Via Natural or Artificial Opening 8 Via Natural or Artificial Opening Endoscopic	Z No Device	Z No Qualifier
1 Seminal Vesicle, Right ♂ 2 Seminal Vesicle, Left ♂ 3 Seminal Vesicles, Bilateral ♂ 6 Tunica Vaginalis, Right ♂ 7 Tunica Vaginalis, Left ♂ 9 Testis, Right ♂ B Testis, Left ♂ C Testes, Bilateral ♂	Ø Open 3 Percutaneous 4 Percutaneous Endoscopic	Z No Device	Z No Qualifier
5 Scrotum ♂ S Penis ♂ Corpus cavernosum Corpus spongiosum T Prepuce ♂ Foreskin Glans penis	Ø Open 3 Percutaneous 4 Percutaneous Endoscopic X External	Z No Device	Z No Qualifier
F Spermatic Cord, Right ♂ G Spermatic Cord, Left ♂ H Spermatic Cords, Bilateral ♂ J Epididymis, Right ♂ K Epididymis, Left ♂ L Epididymis, Bilateral ♂ N Vas Deferens, Right ♂ Ductus deferens Ejaculatory duct P Vas Deferens, Left ♂ *See N Vas Deferens, Right* Q Vas Deferens, Bilateral ♂ *See N Vas Deferens, Right*	Ø Open 3 Percutaneous 4 Percutaneous Endoscopic 8 Via Natural or Artificial Opening Endoscopic	Z No Device	Z No Qualifier

Non-OR ØVQ[6,7][Ø,3,4]ZZ
Non-OR ØVQ5[Ø,3,4,X]ZZ

♂ All body part, approach, device, and qualifier values

Ø Medical and Surgical
V Male Reproductive System
R Replacement Definition: Putting in or on biological or synthetic material that physically takes the place and/or function of all or a portion of a body part
Explanation: The body part may have been taken out or replaced, or may be taken out, physically eradicated, or rendered nonfunctional during the REPLACEMENT procedure. A REMOVAL procedure is coded for taking out the device used in a previous replacement procedure.

Body Part Character 4	Approach Character 5	Device Character 6	Qualifier Character 7
9 Testis, Right ♂ B Testis, Left ♂ C Testes, Bilateral ♂	Ø Open	J Synthetic Substitute	Z No Qualifier

♂ All body part, approach, device, and qualifier values

Ø Medical and Surgical
V Male Reproductive System
S Reposition Definition: Moving to its normal location, or other suitable location, all or a portion of a body part
Explanation: The body part is moved to a new location from an abnormal location, or from a normal location where it is not functioning correctly. The body part may or may not be cut out or off to be moved to the new location.

Body Part Character 4	Approach Character 5	Device Character 6	Qualifier Character 7
9 Testis, Right ♂ B Testis, Left ♂ C Testes, Bilateral ♂ F Spermatic Cord, Right ♂ G Spermatic Cord, Left ♂ H Spermatic Cords, Bilateral ♂	Ø Open 3 Percutaneous 4 Percutaneous Endoscopic 8 Via Natural or Artificial Opening Endoscopic	Z No Device	Z No Qualifier

♂ All body part, approach, device, and qualifier values

Ø Medical and Surgical
V Male Reproductive System
T Resection Definition: Cutting out or off, without replacement, all of a body part

Explanation: None

Body Part Character 4	Approach Character 5	Device Character 6	Qualifier Character 7
Ø Prostate ⊞♂	**Ø** Open **4** Percutaneous Endoscopic **7** Via Natural or Artificial Opening **8** Via Natural or Artificial Opening Endoscopic	**Z** No Device	**Z** No Qualifier
1 Seminal Vesicle, Right ♂ **2** Seminal Vesicle, Left ♂ **3** Seminal Vesicles, Bilateral ⊞♂ **6** Tunica Vaginalis, Right ♂ **7** Tunica Vaginalis, Left ♂ **9** Testis, Right ♂ **B** Testis, Left ♂ **C** Testes, Bilateral ♂ **F** Spermatic Cord, Right ♂ **G** Spermatic Cord, Left ♂ **H** Spermatic Cords, Bilateral ♂ **J** Epididymis, Right ♂ **K** Epididymis, Left ♂ **L** Epididymis, Bilateral ♂ **N** Vas Deferens, Right NC♂ Ductus deferens Ejaculatory duct **P** Vas Deferens, Left NC♂ *See N Vas Deferens, Right* **Q** Vas Deferens, Bilateral NC♂ *See N Vas Deferens, Right*	**Ø** Open **4** Percutaneous Endoscopic	**Z** No Device	**Z** No Qualifier
5 Scrotum ♂ **S** Penis ♂ Corpus cavernosum Corpus spongiosum **T** Prepuce ♂ Foreskin Glans penis	**Ø** Open **4** Percutaneous Endoscopic **X** External	**Z** No Device	**Z** No Qualifier

Non-OR ØVT[N,P,Q][Ø,4]ZZ
Non-OR ØVT[5,T][Ø,4,X]ZZ
NC ØVT[N,P,Q][Ø,4]ZZ with principal or secondary diagnosis of Z3Ø.2
♂ All body part, approach, device, and qualifier values

See Appendix L for Procedure Combinations
⊞ ØVTØ[Ø,4,7,8]ZZ
⊞ ØVT3[Ø,4]ZZ

Ø Medical and Surgical
V Male Reproductive System
U Supplement Definition: Putting in or on biological or synthetic material that physically reinforces and/or augments the function of a portion of a body part

Explanation: The biological material is non-living, or is living and from the same individual. The body part may have been previously replaced, and the SUPPLEMENT procedure is performed to physically reinforce and/or augment the function of the replaced body part.

Body Part Character 4	Approach Character 5	Device Character 6	Qualifier Character 7
1 Seminal Vesicle, Right ♂ **2** Seminal Vesicle, Left ♂ **3** Seminal Vesicles, Bilateral ♂ **6** Tunica Vaginalis, Right ♂ **7** Tunica Vaginalis, Left ♂ **F** Spermatic Cord, Right ♂ **G** Spermatic Cord, Left ♂ **H** Spermatic Cords, Bilateral ♂ **J** Epididymis, Right ♂ **K** Epididymis, Left ♂ **L** Epididymis, Bilateral ♂ **N** Vas Deferens, Right ♂ Ductus deferens Ejaculatory duct **P** Vas Deferens, Left ♂ *See N Vas Deferens, Right* **Q** Vas Deferens, Bilateral ♂ *See N Vas Deferens, Right*	**Ø** Open **4** Percutaneous Endoscopic **8** Via Natural or Artificial Opening Endoscopic	**7** Autologous Tissue Substitute **J** Synthetic Substitute **K** Nonautologous Tissue Substitute	**Z** No Qualifier
5 Scrotum ♂ **S** Penis ♂ Corpus cavernosum Corpus spongiosum **T** Prepuce ♂ Foreskin Glans penis	**Ø** Open **4** Percutaneous Endoscopic **X** External	**7** Autologous Tissue Substitute **J** Synthetic Substitute **K** Nonautologous Tissue Substitute	**Z** No Qualifier
9 Testis, Right ♂ **B** Testis, Left ♂ **C** Testes, Bilateral ♂	**Ø** Open	**7** Autologous Tissue Substitute **J** Synthetic Substitute **K** Nonautologous Tissue Substitute	**Z** No Qualifier

Non-OR ØVUSX[7,J,K]Z

♂ All body part, approach, device, and qualifier values

Ø Medical and Surgical
V Male Reproductive System
W Revision Definition: Correcting, to the extent possible, a portion of a malfunctioning device or the position of a displaced device

Explanation: Revision can include correcting a malfunctioning or displaced device by taking out or putting in components of the device such as a screw or pin

Body Part Character 4	Approach Character 5	Device Character 6	Qualifier Character 7
4 Prostate and Seminal Vesicles ♂ 8 Scrotum and Tunica Vaginalis ♂ D Testis ♂ S Penis ♂ Corpus cavernosum Corpus spongiosum	Ø Open 3 Percutaneous 4 Percutaneous Endoscopic 7 Via Natural or Artificial Opening 8 Via Natural or Artificial Opening Endoscopic	Ø Drainage Device 3 Infusion Device 7 Autologous Tissue Substitute J Synthetic Substitute K Nonautologous Tissue Substitute Y Other Device	Z No Qualifier
4 Prostate and Seminal Vesicles ♂ 8 Scrotum and Tunica Vaginalis ♂ D Testis ♂ S Penis ♂ Corpus cavernosum Corpus spongiosum	X External	Ø Drainage Device 3 Infusion Device 7 Autologous Tissue Substitute J Synthetic Substitute K Nonautologous Tissue Substitute	Z No Qualifier
M Epididymis and Spermatic Cord ♂	Ø Open 3 Percutaneous 4 Percutaneous Endoscopic 7 Via Natural or Artificial Opening 8 Via Natural or Artificial Opening Endoscopic	Ø Drainage Device 3 Infusion Device 7 Autologous Tissue Substitute C Extraluminal Device J Synthetic Substitute K Nonautologous Tissue Substitute Y Other Device	Z No Qualifier
M Epididymis and Spermatic Cord ♂	X External	Ø Drainage Device 3 Infusion Device 7 Autologous Tissue Substitute C Extraluminal Device J Synthetic Substitute K Nonautologous Tissue Substitute	Z No Qualifier
R Vas Deferens ♂ Ductus deferens Ejaculatory duct	Ø Open 3 Percutaneous 4 Percutaneous Endoscopic 7 Via Natural or Artificial Opening 8 Via Natural or Artificial Opening Endoscopic	Ø Drainage Device 3 Infusion Device 7 Autologous Tissue Substitute C Extraluminal Device D Intraluminal Device J Synthetic Substitute K Nonautologous Tissue Substitute Y Other Device	Z No Qualifier
R Vas Deferens ♂ Ductus deferens Ejaculatory duct	X External	Ø Drainage Device 3 Infusion Device 7 Autologous Tissue Substitute C Extraluminal Device D Intraluminal Device J Synthetic Substitute K Nonautologous Tissue Substitute	Z No Qualifier

Non-OR ØVW[4,D,S][3,4,7,8]YZ
Non-OR ØVW8[Ø,3,4,7,8][Ø,3,7,J,K,Y]Z
Non-OR ØVW[4,8,D,S]X[Ø,3,7,J,K]Z
Non-OR ØVWM[3,4,7,8]YZ
Non-OR ØVWMX[Ø,3,7,C,J,K]Z
Non-OR ØVWR[Ø,3,4,7,8][Ø,3,7,C,D,J,K,Y]Z
Non-OR ØVWRX[Ø,3,7,C,D,J,K]Z
♂ All body part, approach, device, and qualifier values

Ø Medical and Surgical
V Male Reproductive System
X Transfer Definition: Moving, without taking out, all or a portion of a body part to another location to take over the function of all or a portion of a body part

Explanation: The body part transferred remains connected to its vascular and nervous supply

Body Part Character 4	Approach Character 5	Device Character 6	Qualifier Character 7
T Prepuce ♂ Foreskin Glans penis	Ø Open X External	Z No Device	D Urethra S Penis

♂ All body part, approach, device, and qualifier values

Anatomical Regions, General ØWØ–ØWY

Character Meanings

This Character Meaning table is provided as a guide to assist the user in the identification of character members that may be found in this section of code tables. It **SHOULD NOT** be used to build a PCS code.

Operation–Character 3	Body Region–Character 4	Approach–Character 5	Device–Character 6	Qualifier–Character 7
Ø Alteration	Ø Head	Ø Open	Ø Drainage Device	Ø Vagina OR Allogeneic
1 Bypass	1 Cranial Cavity	3 Percutaneous	1 Radioactive Element	1 Penis OR Syngeneic
2 Change	2 Face	4 Percutaneous Endoscopic	3 Infusion Device	2 Stoma
3 Control	3 Oral Cavity and Throat	7 Via Natural or Artificial Opening	7 Autologous Tissue Substitute	4 Cutaneous
4 Creation	4 Upper Jaw	8 Via Natural or Artificial Opening Endoscopic	J Synthetic Substitute	9 Pleural Cavity, Right
8 Division	5 Lower Jaw	X External	K Nonautologous Tissue Substitute	B Pleural Cavity, Left
9 Drainage	6 Neck		Y Other Device	G Peritoneal Cavity
B Excision	8 Chest Wall		Z No Device	J Pelvic Cavity
C Extirpation	9 Pleural Cavity, Right			W Upper Vein
F Fragmentation	B Pleural Cavity, Left			X Diagnostic
H Insertion	C Mediastinum			Y Lower Vein
J Inspection	D Pericardial Cavity			Z No Qualifier
M Reattachment	F Abdominal Wall			
P Removal	G Peritoneal Cavity			
Q Repair	H Retroperitoneum			
U Supplement	J Pelvic Cavity			
W Revision	K Upper Back			
Y Transplantation	L Lower Back			
	M Perineum, Male			
	N Perineum, Female			
	P Gastrointestinal Tract			
	Q Respiratory Tract			
	R Genitourinary Tract			

AHA Coding Clinic for table ØWØ
2015, 1Q, 31 Bilateral browpexy

AHA Coding Clinic for table ØW1
2015, 2Q, 36 Insertion of infusion device into peritoneal cavity
2013, 4Q, 126-127 Creation of percutaneous cutaneoperitoneal fistula

AHA Coding Clinic for table ØW3
2018, 1Q, 19 Argon plasma coagulation of duodenal arteriovenous malformation
2018, 1Q, 19 Control of epistaxis via silver nitrate cauterization
2017, 4Q, 57-58 Added approach values - Transorifice esophageal vein banding
2017, 4Q, 105 Control of gastrointestinal bleeding
2017, 4Q, 106 Control of bleeding of external naris using suture
2017, 4Q, 106 Nasal packing for epistaxis
2016, 4Q, 99-100 Root operation Control
2014, 4Q, 44 Bakri balloon for control of postpartum hemorrhage
2013, 3Q, 23 Control of intraoperative bleeding

AHA Coding Clinic for table ØW4
2016, 4Q, 101 Root operation Creation

AHA Coding Clinic for table ØW9
2017, 3Q, 12 Therapeutic and diagnostic paracentesis
2017, 2Q, 16 Incision and drainage of floor of mouth

AHA Coding Clinic for table ØWB
2017, 2Q, 16 Excision of floor of mouth
2016, 1Q, 21 Excision of urachal mass
2013, 4Q, 119 Excision of inclusion cyst of perineum

AHA Coding Clinic for table ØWC
2017, 2Q, 16 Excision of floor of mouth

AHA Coding Clinic for table ØWH
2018, 1Q, 25 Intrauterine brachytherapy & placement of tandems & ovoids
2017, 4Q, 104 Intrauterine brachytherapy & placement of tandems & ovoids
2016, 2Q, 14 Insertion of peritoneal totally implantable venous access device
2015, 2Q, 36 Insertion of infusion device into peritoneal cavity

AHA Coding Clinic for table ØWJ
2016, 4Q, 58 Longitudinal vaginal septum
2013, 2Q, 36 Insertion of ventriculoperitoneal shunt with laparoscopic assistance

AHA Coding Clinic for table ØWQ
2017, 4Q, 106 Control of bleeding of external naris using suture
2017, 3Q, 8 Removal of silo and closure of gastroschisis
2016, 3Q, 3-7 Stoma creation & takedown procedures
2014, 4Q, 38 Abdominoplasty and abdominal wall plication for hernia repair
2014, 3Q, 28 Ileostomy takedown and parastomal hernia repair

AHA Coding Clinic for table ØWU
2017, 3Q, 8 First stage of gastroschisis repair with silo placement
2016, 3Q, 40 Omentoplasty
2015, 2Q, 29 Placement of Ioban™ antimicrobial drape over surgical wound
2014, 4Q, 39 Abdominal component release with placement of mesh for hernia repair
2012, 4Q, 101 Rib resection with reconstruction of anterior chest wall

AHA Coding Clinic for table ØWW
2015, 2Q, 9 Revision of ventriculoperitoneal (VP) shunt

AHA Coding Clinic for table ØWY
2016, 4Q, 112-113 Transplantation

Ø Medical and Surgical
W Anatomical Regions, General
Ø Alteration Definition: Modifying the anatomic structure of a body part without affecting the function of the body part
Explanation: Principal purpose is to improve appearance

Body Part Character 4	Approach Character 5	Device Character 6	Qualifier Character 7
Ø Head 2 Face 4 Upper Jaw 5 Lower Jaw 6 Neck 8 Chest Wall F Abdominal Wall K Upper Back L Lower Back M Perineum, Male ♂ N Perineum, Female ♀	Ø Open 3 Percutaneous 4 Percutaneous Endoscopic	7 Autologous Tissue Substitute J Synthetic Substitute K Nonautologous Tissue Substitute Z No Device	Z No Qualifier

♂ ØWØM[Ø,3,4][7,J,K,Z]Z
♀ ØWØN[Ø,3,4][7,J,K,Z]Z

Ø Medical and Surgical
W Anatomical Regions, General
1 Bypass Definition: Altering the route of passage of the contents of a tubular body part
Explanation: Rerouting contents of a body part to a downstream area of the normal route, to a similar route and body part, or to an abnormal route and dissimilar body part. Includes one or more anastomoses, with or without the use of a device.

Body Part Character 4	Approach Character 5	Device Character 6	Qualifier Character 7
1 Cranial Cavity	Ø Open	J Synthetic Substitute	9 Pleural Cavity, Right B Pleural Cavity, Left G Peritoneal Cavity J Pelvic Cavity
9 Pleural Cavity, Right B Pleural Cavity, Left G Peritoneal Cavity J Pelvic Cavity Retropubic space	Ø Open 3 Percutaneous 4 Percutaneous Endoscopic	J Synthetic Substitute	4 Cutaneous 9 Pleural Cavity, Right B Pleural Cavity, Left G Peritoneal Cavity J Pelvic Cavity W Upper Vein Y Lower Vein

Non-OR ØW1[9,B][Ø,4]J[4,G,Y]
Non-OR ØW1G[Ø,4]J[9,B,G,J]
Non-OR ØW1J[Ø,4]J[4,Y]
Non-OR ØW1[9,B,J]3J4

Ø Medical and Surgical
W Anatomical Regions, General
2 Change Definition: Taking out or off a device from a body part and putting back an identical or similar device in or on the same body part without cutting or puncturing the skin or a mucous membrane
Explanation: All CHANGE procedures are coded using the approach EXTERNAL

Body Part Character 4	Approach Character 5	Device Character 6	Qualifier Character 7
Ø Head 1 Cranial Cavity 2 Face 4 Upper Jaw 5 Lower Jaw 6 Neck 8 Chest Wall 9 Pleural Cavity, Right B Pleural Cavity, Left C Mediastinum Mediastinal cavity Mediastinal space D Pericardial Cavity F Abdominal Wall G Peritoneal Cavity H Retroperitoneum Retroperitoneal cavity Retroperitoneal space J Pelvic Cavity Retropubic space K Upper Back L Lower Back M Perineum, Male ♂ N Perineum, Female ♀	X External	Ø Drainage Device Y Other Device	Z No Qualifier

Non-OR All body part, approach, device, and qualifier values
♂ ØW2MX[Ø,Y]Z
♀ ØW2NX[Ø,Y]Z

Ø Medical and Surgical
W Anatomical Regions, General
3 Control Definition: Stopping, or attempting to stop, postprocedural or other acute bleeding
Explanation: The site of the bleeding is coded as an anatomical region and not to a specific body part

Body Part Character 4	Approach Character 5	Device Character 6	Qualifier Character 7
Ø Head 1 Cranial Cavity 2 Face 4 Upper Jaw 5 Lower Jaw 6 Neck 8 Chest Wall 9 Pleural Cavity, Right B Pleural Cavity, Left C Mediastinum Mediastinal cavity Mediastinal space D Pericardial Cavity F Abdominal Wall G Peritoneal Cavity H Retroperitoneum Retroperitoneal cavity Retroperitoneal space J Pelvic Cavity Retropubic space K Upper Back L Lower Back M Perineum, Male ♂ N Perineum, Female ♀	Ø Open 3 Percutaneous 4 Percutaneous Endoscopic	Z No Device	Z No Qualifier
3 Oral Cavity and Throat	Ø Open 3 Percutaneous 4 Percutaneous Endoscopic 7 Via Natural or Artificial Opening 8 Via Natural or Artificial Opening Endoscopic X External	Z No Device	Z No Qualifier
P Gastrointestinal Tract Q Respiratory Tract R Genitourinary Tract	Ø Open 3 Percutaneous 4 Percutaneous Endoscopic 7 Via Natural or Artificial Opening 8 Via Natural or Artificial Opening Endoscopic	Z No Device	Z No Qualifier

Non-OR ØW3GØZZ
Non-OR ØW3P8ZZ
♂ ØW3M[Ø,3,4]ZZ
♀ ØW3N[Ø,3,4]ZZ

Ø Medical and Surgical
W Anatomical Regions, General
4 Creation Definition: Putting in or on biological or synthetic material to form a new body part that to the extent possible replicates the anatomic structure or function of an absent body part
Explanation: Used for gender reassignment surgery and corrective procedures in individuals with congenital anomalies

Body Part Character 4	Approach Character 5	Device Character 6	Qualifier Character 7
M Perineum, Male ♂	Ø Open	7 Autologous Tissue Substitute J Synthetic Substitute K Nonautologous Tissue Substitute	Ø Vagina
N Perineum, Female ♀	Ø Open	7 Autologous Tissue Substitute J Synthetic Substitute K Nonautologous Tissue Substitute	1 Penis

♂ ØW4MØ[7,J,K]Ø
♀ ØW4NØ[7,J,K]1

Ø Medical and Surgical
W Anatomical Regions, General
8 Division Definition: Cutting into a body part, without draining fluids and/or gases from the body part, in order to separate or transect a body part
Explanation: All or a portion of the body part is separated into two or more portions

Body Part Character 4	Approach Character 5	Device Character 6	Qualifier Character 7
N Perineum, Female ♀	X External	Z No Device	Z No Qualifier

Non-OR ØW8NXZZ
♀ ØW8NXZZ

Ø Medical and Surgical
W Anatomical Regions, General
9 Drainage Definition: Taking or letting out fluids and/or gases from a body part
Explanation: The qualifier DIAGNOSTIC is used to identify drainage procedures that are biopsies

Body Part Character 4	Approach Character 5	Device Character 6	Qualifier Character 7
Ø Head 1 Cranial Cavity 2 Face 3 Oral Cavity and Throat 4 Upper Jaw 5 Lower Jaw 6 Neck 8 Chest Wall 9 Pleural Cavity, Right B Pleural Cavity, Left C Mediastinum Mediastinal cavity Mediastinal space D Pericardial Cavity F Abdominal Wall G Peritoneal Cavity H Retroperitoneum Retroperitoneal cavity Retroperitoneal space J Pelvic Cavity Retropubic space K Upper Back L Lower Back M Perineum, Male ♂ N Perineum, Female ♀	Ø Open 3 Percutaneous 4 Percutaneous Endoscopic	Ø Drainage Device	Z No Qualifier
Ø Head 1 Cranial Cavity 2 Face 3 Oral Cavity and Throat 4 Upper Jaw 5 Lower Jaw 6 Neck 8 Chest Wall 9 Pleural Cavity, Right B Pleural Cavity, Left C Mediastinum Mediastinal cavity Mediastinal space D Pericardial Cavity F Abdominal Wall G Peritoneal Cavity H Retroperitoneum Retroperitoneal cavity Retroperitoneal space J Pelvic Cavity Retropubic space K Upper Back L Lower Back M Perineum, Male ♂ N Perineum, Female ♀	Ø Open 3 Percutaneous 4 Percutaneous Endoscopic	Z No Device	X Diagnostic Z No Qualifier

Non-OR ØW9[Ø,8,9,B,K,L,M]ØØZ
Non-OR ØW9[Ø,1,2,3,4,5,6,8,9,B,C,D,F,G,H,J,K,L,M,N]3ØZ
Non-OR ØW9[Ø,1,8,D,F,G,K,L,M]4ØZ
Non-OR ØW9[Ø,2,3,4,5,6,8,9,B,K,L,M,N]ØZX
Non-OR ØW9[Ø,1,2,3,4,5,6,8,9,B,C,D,G,K,L,M,N]3ZX
Non-OR ØW9[Ø,1,2,3,4,5,6,8,9,B,C,D,K,L,M,N]4ZX
Non-OR ØW9[Ø,8,9,B,K,L,M]ØZZ
Non-OR ØW9[Ø,1,2,3,4,5,6,8,9,B,C,D,F,G,H,J,K,L,M,N]3ZZ
Non-OR ØW9[Ø,1,8,D,F,G,K,L,M]4ZZ

♂ ØW9M[Ø,3,4]ØZ
♂ ØW9M[Ø,3,4]Z[X,Z]
♀ ØW9N[Ø,3,4]ØZ
♀ ØW9N[Ø,3]Z[X,Z]
♀ ØW9N4ZZ

Ø Medical and Surgical
W Anatomical Regions, General
B Excision Definition: Cutting out or off, without replacement, a portion of a body part

Explanation: The qualifier DIAGNOSTIC is used to identify excision procedures that are biopsies

Body Part Character 4	Approach Character 5	Device Character 6	Qualifier Character 7
Ø Head 2 Face 3 Oral Cavity and Throat 4 Upper Jaw 5 Lower Jaw 8 Chest Wall K Upper Back L Lower Back M Perineum, Male ♂ N Perineum, Female ♀	Ø Open 3 Percutaneous 4 Percutaneous Endoscopic X External	Z No Device	X Diagnostic Z No Qualifier
6 Neck F Abdominal Wall	Ø Open 3 Percutaneous 4 Percutaneous Endoscopic	Z No Device	X Diagnostic Z No Qualifier
6 Neck F Abdominal Wall	X External	Z No Device	2 Stoma X Diagnostic Z No Qualifier
C Mediastinum Mediastinal cavity Mediastinal space H Retroperitoneum Retroperitoneal cavity Retroperitoneal space	Ø Open 3 Percutaneous 4 Percutaneous Endoscopic	Z No Device	X Diagnostic Z No Qualifier

Non-OR ØWB[Ø,2,4,5,8,K,L,M][Ø,3,4,X]ZX
Non-OR ØWB6[Ø,3,4]ZX
Non-OR ØWB6XZX
Non-OR ØWB[C,H][3,4]ZX

♂ ØWBM[Ø,3,4,X]Z[X,Z]
♀ ØWBN[Ø,3,4,X]Z[X,Z]

Ø Medical and Surgical
W Anatomical Regions, General
C Extirpation Definition: Taking or cutting out solid matter from a body part

Explanation: The solid matter may be an abnormal byproduct of a biological function or a foreign body; it may be imbedded in a body part or in the lumen of a tubular body part. The solid matter may or may not have been previously broken into pieces.

Body Part Character 4	Approach Character 5	Device Character 6	Qualifier Character 7
1 Cranial Cavity 3 Oral Cavity and Throat 9 Pleural Cavity, Right B Pleural Cavity, Left C Mediastinum Mediastinal cavity Mediastinal space D Pericardial Cavity G Peritoneal Cavity H Retroperitoneum Retroperitoneal cavity Retroperitoneal space J Pelvic Cavity Retropubic space	Ø Open 3 Percutaneous 4 Percutaneous Endoscopic X External	Z No Device	Z No Qualifier
P Gastrointestinal Tract Q Respiratory Tract R Genitourinary Tract	Ø Open 3 Percutaneous 4 Percutaneous Endoscopic 7 Via Natural or Artificial Opening 8 Via Natural or Artificial Opening Endoscopic X External	Z No Device	Z No Qualifier

Non-OR ØWC[1,3]XZZ
Non-OR ØWC[9,B][Ø,3,4,X]ZZ
Non-OR ØWC[C,D,G,H,J]XZZ
Non-OR ØWC[P,R][7,8,X]ZZ
Non-OR ØWCQ[Ø,3,4,X]ZZ

Ø Medical and Surgical
W Anatomical Regions, General
F Fragmentation Definition: Breaking solid matter in a body part into pieces

Explanation: Physical force (e.g., manual, ultrasonic) applied directly or indirectly is used to break the solid matter into pieces. The solid matter may be an abnormal byproduct of a biological function or a foreign body. The pieces of solid matter are not taken out.

Body Part Character 4	Approach Character 5	Device Character 6	Qualifier Character 7
1 Cranial Cavity NC 3 Oral Cavity and Throat NC 9 Pleural Cavity, Right NC B Pleural Cavity, Left NC C Mediastinum NC Mediastinal cavity Mediastinal space D Pericardial Cavity G Peritoneal Cavity NC J Pelvic Cavity NC Retropubic space	Ø Open 3 Percutaneous 4 Percutaneous Endoscopic X External	Z No Device	Z No Qualifier
P Gastrointestinal Tract NC Q Respiratory Tract NC R Genitourinary Tract	Ø Open 3 Percutaneous 4 Percutaneous Endoscopic 7 Via Natural or Artificial Opening 8 Via Natural or Artificial Opening Endoscopic X External	Z No Device	Z No Qualifier

DRG Non-OR ØWFRXZZ
Non-OR ØWF[1,3,9,B,C,G]XZZ
Non-OR ØWFJ[Ø,3,4,X]ZZ
Non-OR ØWFP[Ø,3,4,7,8,X]ZZ
Non-OR ØWFQXZZ
Non-OR ØWFR[Ø,3,4,7,8]ZZ
NC ØWF[1,3,9,B,C,G,J]XZZ
NC ØWF[P,Q]XZZ

Ø Medical and Surgical
W Anatomical Regions, General
H Insertion Definition: Putting in a nonbiological appliance that monitors, assists, performs, or prevents a physiological function but does not physically take the place of a body part

Explanation: None

Body Part Character 4	Approach Character 5	Device Character 6	Qualifier Character 7
Ø Head 1 Cranial Cavity 2 Face 3 Oral Cavity and Throat 4 Upper Jaw 5 Lower Jaw 6 Neck 8 Chest Wall 9 Pleural Cavity, Right B Pleural Cavity, Left C Mediastinum Mediastinal cavity Mediastinal space D Pericardial Cavity F Abdominal Wall G Peritoneal Cavity H Retroperitoneum Retroperitoneal cavity Retroperitoneal space J Pelvic Cavity Retropubic space K Upper Back L Lower Back M Perineum, Male N Perineum, Female ♀	Ø Open 3 Percutaneous 4 Percutaneous Endoscopic	1 Radioactive Element 3 Infusion Device Y Other Device	Z No Qualifier
P Gastrointestinal Tract Q Respiratory Tract R Genitourinary Tract	Ø Open 3 Percutaneous 4 Percutaneous Endoscopic 7 Via Natural or Artificial Opening 8 Via Natural or Artificial Opening Endoscopic	1 Radioactive Element 3 Infusion Device Y Other Device	Z No Qualifier

DRG Non-OR ØWH[Ø,2,4,5,6,K,L,M][Ø,3,4][3,Y]Z
Non-OR ØWH1[Ø,3,4]3Z
Non-OR ØWH[8,9,B][Ø,3,4][3,Y]Z
Non-OR ØWHPØYZ
Non-OR ØWHP[3,4,7,8][3,Y]Z
Non-OR ØWHQ[Ø,7,8][3,Y]Z
Non-OR ØWHR[Ø,3,4,7,8][3,Y]Z
♀ ØWHN[Ø,3,4][3,Y]Z

Ø Medical and Surgical
W Anatomical Regions, General
J Inspection Definition: Visually and/or manually exploring a body part
Explanation: Visual exploration may be performed with or without optical instrumentation. Manual exploration may be performed directly or through intervening body layers.

Body Part Character 4	Approach Character 5	Device Character 6	Qualifier Character 7
Ø Head 2 Face 3 Oral Cavity and Throat 4 Upper Jaw 5 Lower Jaw 6 Neck 8 Chest Wall F Abdominal Wall K Upper Back L Lower Back M Perineum, Male ♂ N Perineum, Female ♀	Ø Open 3 Percutaneous 4 Percutaneous Endoscopic X External	Z No Device	Z No Qualifier
1 Cranial Cavity 9 Pleural Cavity, Right B Pleural Cavity, Left C Mediastinum Mediastinal cavity Mediastinal space D Pericardial Cavity G Peritoneal Cavity H Retroperitoneum Retroperitoneal cavity Retroperitoneal space J Pelvic Cavity Retropubic space	Ø Open 3 Percutaneous 4 Percutaneous Endoscopic	Z No Device	Z No Qualifier
P Gastrointestinal Tract Q Respiratory Tract R Genitourinary Tract	Ø Open 3 Percutaneous 4 Percutaneous Endoscopic 7 Via Natural or Artificial Opening 8 Via Natural or Artificial Opening Endoscopic	Z No Device	Z No Qualifier

DRG Non-OR ØWJ[Ø,2,4,5,K,L]ØZZ
DRG Non-OR ØWJM[Ø,4]ZZ
Non-OR ØWJ3ØZZ
Non-OR ØWJ[Ø,2,3,4,5,6,8,F,K,L,M,N][3,X]ZZ
Non-OR ØWJ[Ø,2,3,4,5,K,L]4ZZ
Non-OR ØWJDØZZ
Non-OR ØWJ[1,9,B,C,D,G,H,J]3ZZ
Non-OR ØWJ[P,Q,R][3,7,8]ZZ
♂ ØWJM[Ø,3,4,X]ZZ
♀ ØWJN[Ø,3,4,X]ZZ

Ø Medical and Surgical
W Anatomical Regions, General
M Reattachment Definition: Putting back in or on all or a portion of a separated body part to its normal location or other suitable location
Explanation: Vascular circulation and nervous pathways may or may not be reestablished

Body Part Character 4	Approach Character 5	Device Character 6	Qualifier Character 7
2 Face 4 Upper Jaw 5 Lower Jaw 6 Neck 8 Chest Wall F Abdominal Wall K Upper Back L Lower Back M Perineum, Male ♂ N Perineum, Female ♀	Ø Open	Z No Device	Z No Qualifier

♂ ØWMMØZZ
♀ ØWMNØZZ

Ø Medical and Surgical
W Anatomical Regions, General
P Removal Definition: Taking out or off a device from a body part

Explanation: If a device is taken out and a similar device put in without cutting or puncturing the skin or mucous membrane, the procedure is coded to the root operation CHANGE. Otherwise, the procedure for taking out the device is coded to the root operation REMOVAL.

Body Part Character 4	Approach Character 5	Device Character 6	Qualifier Character 7
Ø Head 2 Face 4 Upper Jaw 5 Lower Jaw 6 Neck 8 Chest Wall C Mediastinum Mediastinal cavity Mediastinal space F Abdominal Wall K Upper Back L Lower Back M Perineum, Male ♂ N Perineum, Female ♀	Ø Open 3 Percutaneous 4 Percutaneous Endoscopic X External	Ø Drainage Device 1 Radioactive Element 3 Infusion Device 7 Autologous Tissue Substitute J Synthetic Substitute K Nonautologous Tissue Substitute Y Other Device	Z No Qualifier
1 Cranial Cavity 9 Pleural Cavity, Right B Pleural Cavity, Left G Peritoneal Cavity J Pelvic Cavity Retropubic space	Ø Open 3 Percutaneous 4 Percutaneous Endoscopic	Ø Drainage Device 1 Radioactive Element 3 Infusion Device J Synthetic Substitute Y Other Device	Z No Qualifier
1 Cranial Cavity 9 Pleural Cavity, Right B Pleural Cavity, Left G Peritoneal Cavity J Pelvic Cavity Retropubic space	X External	Ø Drainage Device 1 Radioactive Element 3 Infusion Device	Z No Qualifier
D Pericardial Cavity H Retroperitoneum Retroperitoneal cavity Retroperitoneal space	Ø Open 3 Percutaneous 4 Percutaneous Endoscopic	Ø Drainage Device 1 Radioactive Element 3 Infusion Device Y Other Device	Z No Qualifier
D Pericardial Cavity H Retroperitoneum Retroperitoneal cavity Retroperitoneal space	X External	Ø Drainage Device 1 Radioactive Element 3 Infusion Device	Z No Qualifier
P Gastrointestinal Tract Q Respiratory Tract R Genitourinary Tract	Ø Open 3 Percutaneous 4 Percutaneous Endoscopic 7 Via Natural or Artificial Opening 8 Via Natural or Artificial Opening Endoscopic X External	1 Radioactive Element 3 Infusion Device Y Other Device	Z No Qualifier

Non-OR ØWP[Ø,2,4,5,6,8][Ø,3,4,X][Ø,1,3,7,J,K,Y]Z
Non-OR ØWP[C,F]X[Ø,1,3,7,J,K,Y]Z
Non-OR ØWP[K,L][Ø,3,4,X][Ø,1,3,7,J,K,Y]Z
Non-OR ØWPM[Ø,3,4][Ø,1,3,J,Y]Z
Non-OR ØWPMX[Ø,1,3,Y]Z
Non-OR ØWPNX[Ø,1,3,7,J,K,Y]Z
Non-OR ØWP1[Ø,3,4]3Z
Non-OR ØWP[9,B,J][Ø,3,4][Ø,1,3,J,Y]Z
Non-OR ØWP[1,9,B,G,J]X[Ø,1,3]Z
Non-OR ØWP[D,H]X[Ø,1,3]Z
Non-OR ØWPP[3,4,7,8,X][1,3,Y]Z
Non-OR ØWPQ73Z
Non-OR ØWPQ8[3,Y]Z
Non-OR ØWPQ[Ø,X][1,3,Y]Z
Non-OR ØWPR[Ø,3,4,7,8,X][1,3,Y]Z

♂ ØWPM[Ø,3,4,X][Ø,1,3,7,J,K,Y]Z
♀ ØWPN[Ø,3,4,X][Ø,1,3,7,J,K,Y]Z

Ø Medical and Surgical
W Anatomical Regions, General
Q Repair Definition: Restoring, to the extent possible, a body part to its normal anatomic structure and function
Explanation: Used only when the method to accomplish the repair is not one of the other root operations

Body Part Character 4	Approach Character 5	Device Character 6	Qualifier Character 7
Ø Head **2** Face **3** Oral Cavity and Throat **4** Upper Jaw **5** Lower Jaw **8** Chest Wall **K** Upper Back **L** Lower Back **M** Perineum, Male ♂ **N** Perineum, Female ♀	**Ø** Open **3** Percutaneous **4** Percutaneous Endoscopic **X** External	**Z** No Device	**Z** No Qualifier
6 Neck **F** Abdominal Wall	**Ø** Open **3** Percutaneous **4** Percutaneous Endoscopic	**Z** No Device	**Z** No Qualifier
6 Neck **F** Abdominal Wall ⊞	**X** External	**Z** No Device	**2** Stoma **Z** No Qualifier
C Mediastinum Mediastinal cavity Mediastinal space	**Ø** Open **3** Percutaneous **4** Percutaneous Endoscopic	**Z** No Device	**Z** No Qualifier

Non-OR ØWQNXZZ
♂ ØWQM[Ø,3,4,X]ZZ
♀ ØWQN[Ø,3,4,X]ZZ

See Appendix L for Procedure Combinations
⊞ ØWQFXZ[2,Z]

Ø Medical and Surgical
W Anatomical Regions, General
U Supplement Definition: Putting in or on biological or synthetic material that physically reinforces and/or augments the function of a portion of a body part
Explanation: The biological material is non-living, or is living and from the same individual. The body part may have been previously replaced, and the SUPPLEMENT procedure is performed to physically reinforce and/or augment the function of the replaced body part.

Body Part Character 4	Approach Character 5	Device Character 6	Qualifier Character 7
Ø Head **2** Face **4** Upper Jaw **5** Lower Jaw **6** Neck **8** Chest Wall **C** Mediastinum Mediastinal cavity Mediastinal space **F** Abdominal Wall **K** Upper Back **L** Lower Back **M** Perineum, Male ♂ **N** Perineum, Female ♀	**Ø** Open **4** Percutaneous Endoscopic	**7** Autologous Tissue Substitute **J** Synthetic Substitute **K** Nonautologous Tissue Substitute	**Z** No Qualifier

♂ ØWUM[Ø,4][7,J,K]Z
♀ ØWUN[Ø,4][7,J,K]Z

Ø Medical and Surgical
W Anatomical Regions, General
W Revision Definition: Correcting, to the extent possible, a portion of a malfunctioning device or the position of a displaced device

Explanation: Revision can include correcting a malfunctioning or displaced device by taking out or putting in components of the device such as a screw or pin

Body Part Character 4	Approach Character 5	Device Character 6	Qualifier Character 7
Ø Head 2 Face 4 Upper Jaw 5 Lower Jaw 6 Neck 8 Chest Wall C Mediastinum Mediastinal cavity Mediastinal space F Abdominal Wall K Upper Back L Lower Back M Perineum, Male ♂ N Perineum, Female ♀	Ø Open 3 Percutaneous 4 Percutaneous Endoscopic X External	Ø Drainage Device 1 Radioactive Element 3 Infusion Device 7 Autologous Tissue Substitute J Synthetic Substitute K Nonautologous Tissue Substitute Y Other Device	Z No Qualifier
1 Cranial Cavity 9 Pleural Cavity, Right B Pleural Cavity, Left G Peritoneal Cavity J Pelvic Cavity Retropubic space	Ø Open 3 Percutaneous 4 Percutaneous Endoscopic X External	Ø Drainage Device 1 Radioactive Element 3 Infusion Device J Synthetic Substitute Y Other Device	Z No Qualifier
D Pericardial Cavity H Retroperitoneum Retroperitoneal cavity Retroperitoneal space	Ø Open 3 Percutaneous 4 Percutaneous Endoscopic X External	Ø Drainage Device 1 Radioactive Element 3 Infusion Device Y Other Device	Z No Qualifier
P Gastrointestinal Tract Q Respiratory Tract R Genitourinary Tract	Ø Open 3 Percutaneous 4 Percutaneous Endoscopic 7 Via Natural or Artificial Opening 8 Via Natural or Artificial Opening Endoscopic X External	1 Radioactive Element 3 Infusion Device Y Other Device	Z No Qualifier

DRG Non-OR ØWW[Ø,2,4,5,6,K,L][Ø,3,4][Ø,1,3,7,J,K,Y]Z
DRG Non-OR ØWWM[Ø,3,4][Ø,1,3,J,Y]Z
Non-OR ØWW[Ø,2,4,5,6,C,F,K,L,M,N]X[Ø,1,3,7,J,K,Y]Z
Non-OR ØWW8[Ø,3,4,X][Ø,1,3,7,J,K,Y]Z
Non-OR ØWW[1,G,J]X[Ø,1,3,J,Y]Z
Non-OR ØWW[9,B][Ø,3,4,X][Ø,1,3,J,Y]Z
Non-OR ØWW[D,H]X[Ø,1,3,Y]Z
Non-OR ØWWP[3,4,7,8,X][1,3,Y]Z
Non-OR ØWWQ[Ø,X][1,3,Y]Z
Non-OR ØWWR[Ø,3,4,7,8,X][1,3,Y]Z
♂ ØWWM[Ø,3,4,X][Ø,1,3,7,K,Y]Z
♀ ØWWN[Ø,3,4,X][Ø,1,3,7,K,Y]Z

Ø Medical and Surgical
W Anatomical Regions, General
Y Transplantation Definition: Putting in or on all or a portion of a living body part taken from another individual or animal to physically take the place and/or function of all or a portion of a similar body part

Explanation: The native body part may or may not be taken out, and the transplanted body part may take over all or a portion of its function

Body Part Character 4	Approach Character 5	Device Character 6	Qualifier Character 7
2 Face	Ø Open	Z No Device	Ø Allogeneic 1 Syngeneic

Anatomical Regions, Upper Extremities ØXØ–ØXY

Character Meanings

This Character Meaning table is provided as a guide to assist the user in the identification of character members that may be found in this section of code tables. It **SHOULD NOT** be used to build a PCS code.

Operation–Character 3	Body Part–Character 4	Approach–Character 5	Device–Character 6	Qualifier–Character 7
Ø Alteration	Ø Forequarter, Right	Ø Open	Ø Drainage Device	Ø Complete OR Allogeneic
2 Change	1 Forequarter, Left	3 Percutaneous	1 Radioactive Element	1 High OR Syngeneic
3 Control	2 Shoulder Region, Right	4 Percutaneous Endoscopic	3 Infusion Device	2 Mid
6 Detachment	3 Shoulder Region, Left	X External	7 Autologous Tissue Substitute	3 Low
9 Drainage	4 Axilla, Right		J Synthetic Substitute	4 Complete 1st Ray
B Excision	5 Axilla, Left		K Nonautologous Tissue Substitute	5 Complete 2nd Ray
H Insertion	6 Upper Extremity, Right		Y Other Device	6 Complete 3rd Ray
J Inspection	7 Upper Extremity, Left		Z No Device	7 Complete 4th Ray
M Reattachment	8 Upper Arm, Right			8 Complete 5th Ray
P Removal	9 Upper Arm, Left			9 Partial 1st Ray
Q Repair	B Elbow Region, Right			B Partial 2nd Ray
R Replacement	C Elbow Region, Left			C Partial 3rd Ray
U Supplement	D Lower Arm, Right			D Partial 4th Ray
W Revision	F Lower Arm, Left			F Partial 5th Ray
X Transfer	G Wrist Region, Right			L Thumb, Right
Y Transplantation	H Wrist Region, Left			M Thumb, Left
	J Hand, Right			N Toe, Right
	K Hand, Left			P Toe, Left
	L Thumb, Right			X Diagnostic
	M Thumb, Left			Z No Qualifier
	N Index Finger, Right			
	P Index Finger, Left			
	Q Middle Finger, Right			
	R Middle Finger, Left			
	S Ring Finger, Right			
	T Ring Finger, Left			
	V Little Finger, Right			
	W Little Finger, Left			

AHA Coding Clinic for table ØX3
2016, 4Q, 99 Root operation Control
2015, 1Q, 35 Evacuation of hematoma for control of postprocedural bleeding
2013, 3Q, 23 Control of intraoperative bleeding

AHA Coding Clinic for table ØX6
2017, 2Q, 3-4 Qualifiers for the root operation detachment
2017, 2Q, 18 Removal of polydactyl digits
2017, 1Q, 52 Further distal phalangeal amputation
2016, 3Q, 33 Traumatic amputation of fingers with further revision amputation

AHA Coding Clinic for table ØXH
2017, 2Q, 20 Exchange of intramedullary antibiotic impregnated spacer

AHA Coding Clinic for table ØXP
2017, 2Q, 20 Exchange of intramedullary antibiotic impregnated spacer

AHA Coding Clinic for table ØXY
2016, 4Q, 112-113 Transplantation

Detachment Qualifier Descriptions

Qualifier Definition	Upper Arm	Lower Arm
1 **High:** Amputation at the proximal portion of the shaft of the:	Humerus	Radius/Ulna
2 **Mid:** Amputation at the middle portion of the shaft of the:	Humerus	Radius/Ulna
3 **Low:** Amputation at the distal portion of the shaft of the:	Humerus	Radius/Ulna

Qualifier Definition	Hand
Ø Complete 1st through 5th Rays Ray: digit of hand or foot with corresponding metacarpus or metatarsus	Through carpo-metacarpal joint, **Wrist**
4 Complete 1st Ray	Through carpo-metacarpal joint, **Thumb**
5 Complete 2nd Ray	Through carpo-metacarpal joint, **Index Finger**
6 Complete 3rd Ray	Through carpo-metacarpal joint, **Middle Finger**
7 Complete 4th Ray	Through carpo-metacarpal joint, **Ring Finger**
8 Complete 5th Ray	Through carpo-metacarpal joint, **Little Finger**
9 Partial 1st Ray	Anywhere along shaft or head of metacarpal bone, **Thumb**
B Partial 2nd Ray	Anywhere along shaft or head of metacarpal bone, **Index Finger**
C Partial 3rd Ray	Anywhere along shaft or head of metacarpal bone, **Middle Finger**
D Partial 4th Ray	Anywhere along shaft or head of metacarpal bone, **Ring Finger**
F Partial 5th Ray	Anywhere along shaft or head of metacarpal bone, **Little Finger**

Qualifier Definition	Thumb/Finger
Ø Complete	At the metacarpophalangeal joint
1 High	Anywhere along the proximal phalanx
2 Mid	Through the proximal interphalangeal joint or anywhere along the middle phalanx
3 Low	Through the distal interphalangeal joint or anywhere along the distal phalanx

Ø Medical and Surgical
X Anatomical Regions, Upper Extremities
Ø Alteration Definition: Modifying the anatomic structure of a body part without affecting the function of the body part
Explanation: Principal purpose is to improve appearance

Body Part Character 4	Approach Character 5	Device Character 6	Qualifier Character 7
2 Shoulder Region, Right 3 Shoulder Region, Left 4 Axilla, Right 5 Axilla, Left 6 Upper Extremity, Right 7 Upper Extremity, Left 8 Upper Arm, Right 9 Upper Arm, Left B Elbow Region, Right C Elbow Region, Left D Lower Arm, Right F Lower Arm, Left G Wrist Region, Right H Wrist Region, Left	Ø Open 3 Percutaneous 4 Percutaneous Endoscopic	7 Autologous Tissue Substitute J Synthetic Substitute K Nonautologous Tissue Substitute Z No Device	Z No Qualifier

Ø Medical and Surgical
X Anatomical Regions, Upper Extremities
2 Change Definition: Taking out or off a device from a body part and putting back an identical or similar device in or on the same body part without cutting or puncturing the skin or a mucous membrane
Explanation: All CHANGE procedures are coded using the approach EXTERNAL

Body Part Character 4	Approach Character 5	Device Character 6	Qualifier Character 7
6 Upper Extremity, Right 7 Upper Extremity, Left	X External	Ø Drainage Device Y Other Device	Z No Qualifier

Non-OR All body part, approach, device, and qualifier values

Ø Medical and Surgical
X Anatomical Regions, Upper Extremities
3 Control Definition: Stopping, or attempting to stop, postprocedural or other acute bleeding
Explanation: The site of the bleeding is coded as an anatomical region and not to a specific body part

Body Part Character 4	Approach Character 5	Device Character 6	Qualifier Character 7
2 Shoulder Region, Right 3 Shoulder Region, Left 4 Axilla, Right 5 Axilla, Left 6 Upper Extremity, Right 7 Upper Extremity, Left 8 Upper Arm, Right 9 Upper Arm, Left B Elbow Region, Right C Elbow Region, Left D Lower Arm, Right F Lower Arm, Left G Wrist Region, Right H Wrist Region, Left J Hand, Right K Hand, Left	Ø Open 3 Percutaneous 4 Percutaneous Endoscopic	Z No Device	Z No Qualifier

Ø Medical and Surgical
X Anatomical Regions, Upper Extremities
6 Detachment Definition: Cutting off all or a portion of the upper or lower extremities

Explanation: The body part value is the site of the detachment, with a qualifier if applicable to further specify the level where the extremity was detached

Body Part Character 4	Approach Character 5	Device Character 6	Qualifier Character 7
Ø Forequarter, Right 1 Forequarter, Left 2 Shoulder Region, Right 3 Shoulder Region, Left B Elbow Region, Right C Elbow Region, Left	Ø Open	Z No Device	Z No Qualifier
8 Upper Arm, Right 9 Upper Arm, Left D Lower Arm, Right F Lower Arm, Left	Ø Open	Z No Device	1 High 2 Mid 3 Low
J Hand, Right K Hand, Left	Ø Open	Z No Device	Ø Complete 4 Complete 1st Ray 5 Complete 2nd Ray 6 Complete 3rd Ray 7 Complete 4th Ray 8 Complete 5th Ray 9 Partial 1st Ray B Partial 2nd Ray C Partial 3rd Ray D Partial 4th Ray F Partial 5th Ray
L Thumb, Right M Thumb, Left N Index Finger, Right P Index Finger, Left Q Middle Finger, Right R Middle Finger, Left S Ring Finger, Right T Ring Finger, Left V Little Finger, Right W Little Finger, Left	Ø Open	Z No Device	Ø Complete 1 High 2 Mid 3 Low

Ø Medical and Surgical
X Anatomical Regions, Upper Extremities
9 Drainage Definition: Taking or letting out fluids and/or gases from a body part
Explanation: The qualifier DIAGNOSTIC is used to identify drainage procedures that are biopsies

Body Part Character 4	Approach Character 5	Device Character 6	Qualifier Character 7
2 Shoulder Region, Right 3 Shoulder Region, Left 4 Axilla, Right 5 Axilla, Left 6 Upper Extremity, Right 7 Upper Extremity, Left 8 Upper Arm, Right 9 Upper Arm, Left B Elbow Region, Right C Elbow Region, Left D Lower Arm, Right F Lower Arm, Left G Wrist Region, Right H Wrist Region, Left J Hand, Right K Hand, Left	Ø Open 3 Percutaneous 4 Percutaneous Endoscopic	Ø Drainage Device	Z No Qualifier
2 Shoulder Region, Right 3 Shoulder Region, Left 4 Axilla, Right 5 Axilla, Left 6 Upper Extremity, Right 7 Upper Extremity, Left 8 Upper Arm, Right 9 Upper Arm, Left B Elbow Region, Right C Elbow Region, Left D Lower Arm, Right F Lower Arm, Left G Wrist Region, Right H Wrist Region, Left J Hand, Right K Hand, Left	Ø Open 3 Percutaneous 4 Percutaneous Endoscopic	Z No Device	X Diagnostic Z No Qualifier

Non-OR All body part, approach, device, and qualifier values

Ø Medical and Surgical
X Anatomical Regions, Upper Extremities
B Excision Definition: Cutting out or off, without replacement, a portion of a body part
Explanation: The qualifier DIAGNOSTIC is used to identify excision procedures that are biopsies

Body Part Character 4	Approach Character 5	Device Character 6	Qualifier Character 7
2 Shoulder Region, Right 3 Shoulder Region, Left 4 Axilla, Right 5 Axilla, Left 6 Upper Extremity, Right 7 Upper Extremity, Left 8 Upper Arm, Right 9 Upper Arm, Left B Elbow Region, Right C Elbow Region, Left D Lower Arm, Right F Lower Arm, Left G Wrist Region, Right H Wrist Region, Left J Hand, Right K Hand, Left	Ø Open 3 Percutaneous 4 Percutaneous Endoscopic	Z No Device	X Diagnostic Z No Qualifier

Non-OR ØXB[2,3,4,5,6,7,8,9,B,C,D,F,G,H,J,K][Ø,3,4]ZX

Ø Medical and Surgical
X Anatomical Regions, Upper Extremities
H Insertion Definition: Putting in a nonbiological appliance that monitors, assists, performs, or prevents a physiological function but does not physically take the place of a body part

Explanation: None

Body Part Character 4	Approach Character 5	Device Character 6	Qualifier Character 7
2 Shoulder Region, Right 3 Shoulder Region, Left 4 Axilla, Right 5 Axilla, Left 6 Upper Extremity, Right 7 Upper Extremity, Left 8 Upper Arm, Right 9 Upper Arm, Left B Elbow Region, Right C Elbow Region, Left D Lower Arm, Right F Lower Arm, Left G Wrist Region, Right H Wrist Region, Left J Hand, Right K Hand, Left	Ø Open 3 Percutaneous 4 Percutaneous Endoscopic	1 Radioactive Element 3 Infusion Device Y Other Device	Z No Qualifier

DRG Non-OR ØXH[2,3,4,5,6,7,8,9,B,C,D,F,G,H,J,K][Ø,3,4][3,Y]Z

Ø Medical and Surgical
X Anatomical Regions, Upper Extremities
J Inspection Definition: Visually and/or manually exploring a body part

Explanation: Visual exploration may be performed with or without optical instrumentation. Manual exploration may be performed directly or through intervening body layers.

Body Part Character 4	Approach Character 5	Device Character 6	Qualifier Character 7
2 Shoulder Region, Right 3 Shoulder Region, Left 4 Axilla, Right 5 Axilla, Left 6 Upper Extremity, Right 7 Upper Extremity, Left 8 Upper Arm, Right 9 Upper Arm, Left B Elbow Region, Right C Elbow Region, Left D Lower Arm, Right F Lower Arm, Left G Wrist Region, Right H Wrist Region, Left J Hand, Right K Hand, Left	Ø Open 3 Percutaneous 4 Percutaneous Endoscopic X External	Z No Device	Z No Qualifier

DRG Non-OR ØXJ[2,3,4,5,6,7,8,9,B,C,D,F,G,H,J,K]ØZZ
Non-OR ØXJ[2,3,4,5,6,7,8,9,B,C,D,F,G,H][3,4,X]ZZ
Non-OR ØXJ[J,K][3,X]ZZ

Ø Medical and Surgical
X Anatomical Regions, Upper Extremities
M Reattachment Definition: Putting back in or on all or a portion of a separated body part to its normal location or other suitable location
Explanation: Vascular circulation and nervous pathways may or may not be reestablished

Body Part Character 4	Approach Character 5	Device Character 6	Qualifier Character 7
Ø Forequarter, Right 1 Forequarter, Left 2 Shoulder Region, Right 3 Shoulder Region, Left 4 Axilla, Right 5 Axilla, Left 6 Upper Extremity, Right 7 Upper Extremity, Left 8 Upper Arm, Right 9 Upper Arm, Left B Elbow Region, Right C Elbow Region, Left D Lower Arm, Right F Lower Arm, Left G Wrist Region, Right H Wrist Region, Left J Hand, Right K Hand, Left L Thumb, Right M Thumb, Left N Index Finger, Right P Index Finger, Left Q Middle Finger, Right R Middle Finger, Left S Ring Finger, Right T Ring Finger, Left V Little Finger, Right W Little Finger, Left	Ø Open	Z No Device	Z No Qualifier

Ø Medical and Surgical
X Anatomical Regions, Upper Extremities
P Removal Definition: Taking out or off a device from a body part
Explanation: If a device is taken out and a similar device put in without cutting or puncturing the skin or mucous membrane, the procedure is coded to the root operation CHANGE. Otherwise, the procedure for taking out the device is coded to the root operation REMOVAL.

Body Part Character 4	Approach Character 5	Device Character 6	Qualifier Character 7
6 Upper Extremity, Right 7 Upper Extremity, Left	Ø Open 3 Percutaneous 4 Percutaneous Endoscopic X External	Ø Drainage Device 1 Radioactive Element 3 Infusion Device 7 Autologous Tissue Substitute J Synthetic Substitute K Nonautologous Tissue Substitute Y Other Device	Z No Qualifier

Non-OR All body part, approach, device, and qualifier values

Ø Medical and Surgical
X Anatomical Regions, Upper Extremities
Q Repair Definition: Restoring, to the extent possible, a body part to its normal anatomic structure and function
Explanation: Used only when the method to accomplish the repair is not one of the other root operations

Body Part Character 4	Approach Character 5	Device Character 6	Qualifier Character 7
2 Shoulder Region, Right 3 Shoulder Region, Left 4 Axilla, Right 5 Axilla, Left 6 Upper Extremity, Right 7 Upper Extremity, Left 8 Upper Arm, Right 9 Upper Arm, Left B Elbow Region, Right C Elbow Region, Left D Lower Arm, Right F Lower Arm, Left G Wrist Region, Right H Wrist Region, Left J Hand, Right K Hand, Left L Thumb, Right M Thumb, Left N Index Finger, Right P Index Finger, Left Q Middle Finger, Right R Middle Finger, Left S Ring Finger, Right T Ring Finger, Left V Little Finger, Right W Little Finger, Left	Ø Open 3 Percutaneous 4 Percutaneous Endoscopic X External	Z No Device	Z No Qualifier

Ø Medical and Surgical
X Anatomical Regions, Upper Extremities
R Replacement Definition: Putting in or on biological or synthetic material that physically takes the place and/or function of all or a portion of a body part
Explanation: The body part may have been taken out or replaced, or may be taken out, physically eradicated, or rendered nonfunctional during the REPLACEMENT procedure. A REMOVAL procedure is coded for taking out the device used in a previous replacement procedure.

Body Part Character 4	Approach Character 5	Device Character 6	Qualifier Character 7
L Thumb, Right M Thumb, Left	Ø Open 4 Percutaneous Endoscopic	7 Autologous Tissue Substitute	N Toe, Right P Toe, Left

Ø Medical and Surgical
X Anatomical Regions, Upper Extremities
U Supplement Definition: Putting in or on biological or synthetic material that physically reinforces and/or augments the function of a portion of a body part

Explanation: The biological material is non-living, or is living and from the same individual. The body part may have been previously replaced, and the SUPPLEMENT procedure is performed to physically reinforce and/or augment the function of the replaced body part.

Body Part Character 4	Approach Character 5	Device Character 6	Qualifier Character 7
2 Shoulder Region, Right 3 Shoulder Region, Left 4 Axilla, Right 5 Axilla, Left 6 Upper Extremity, Right 7 Upper Extremity, Left 8 Upper Arm, Right 9 Upper Arm, Left B Elbow Region, Right C Elbow Region, Left D Lower Arm, Right F Lower Arm, Left G Wrist Region, Right H Wrist Region, Left J Hand, Right K Hand, Left L Thumb, Right M Thumb, Left N Index Finger, Right P Index Finger, Left Q Middle Finger, Right R Middle Finger, Left S Ring Finger, Right T Ring Finger, Left V Little Finger, Right W Little Finger, Left	Ø Open 4 Percutaneous Endoscopic	7 Autologous Tissue Substitute J Synthetic Substitute K Nonautologous Tissue Substitute	Z No Qualifier

Ø Medical and Surgical
X Anatomical Regions, Upper Extremities
W Revision Definition: Correcting, to the extent possible, a portion of a malfunctioning device or the position of a displaced device

Explanation: Revision can include correcting a malfunctioning or displaced device by taking out or putting in components of the device such as a screw or pin

Body Part Character 4	Approach Character 5	Device Character 6	Qualifier Character 7
6 Upper Extremity, Right 7 Upper Extremity, Left	Ø Open 3 Percutaneous 4 Percutaneous Endoscopic X External	Ø Drainage Device 3 Infusion Device 7 Autologous Tissue Substitute J Synthetic Substitute K Nonautologous Tissue Substitute Y Other Device	Z No Qualifier

DRG Non-OR ØXW[6,7][Ø,3,4][Ø,3,7,J,K,Y]Z
Non-OR ØXW[6,7]X[Ø,3,7,J,K,Y]Z

Ø Medical and Surgical
X Anatomical Regions, Upper Extremities
X Transfer Definition: Moving, without taking out, all or a portion of a body part to another location to take over the function of all or a portion of a body part

Explanation: The body part transferred remains connected to its vascular and nervous supply

Body Part Character 4	Approach Character 5	Device Character 6	Qualifier Character 7
N Index Finger, Right	Ø Open	Z No Device	L Thumb, Right
P Index Finger, Left	Ø Open	Z No Device	M Thumb, Left

Ø Medical and Surgical
X Anatomical Regions, Upper Extremities
Y Transplantation Definition: Putting in or on all or a portion of a living body part taken from another individual or animal to physically take the place and/or function of all or a portion of a similar body part

Explanation: The native body part may or may not be taken out, and the transplanted body part may take over all or a portion of its function

Body Part Character 4	Approach Character 5	Device Character 6	Qualifier Character 7
J Hand, Right K Hand, Left	Ø Open	Z No Device	Ø Allogeneic 1 Syngeneic

Anatomical Regions, Lower Extremities ØYØ–ØYW

Character Meanings

This Character Meaning table is provided as a guide to assist the user in the identification of character members that may be found in this section of code tables. It **SHOULD NOT** be used to build a PCS code.

Operation–Character 3		Body Part–Character 4		Approach–Character 5		Device–Character 6		Qualifier–Character 7	
Ø	Alteration	Ø	Buttock, Right	Ø	Open	Ø	Drainage Device	Ø	Complete
2	Change	1	Buttock, Left	3	Percutaneous	1	Radioactive Element	1	High
3	Control	2	Hindquarter, Right	4	Percutaneous Endoscopic	3	Infusion Device	2	Mid
6	Detachment	3	Hindquarter, Left	X	External	7	Autologous Tissue Substitute	3	Low
9	Drainage	4	Hindquarter, Bilateral			J	Synthetic Substitute	4	Complete 1st Ray
B	Excision	5	Inguinal Region, Right			K	Nonautologous Tissue Substitute	5	Complete 2nd Ray
H	Insertion	6	Inguinal Region, Left			Y	Other Device	6	Complete 3rd Ray
J	Inspection	7	Femoral Region, Right			Z	No Device	7	Complete 4th Ray
M	Reattachment	8	Femoral Region, Left					8	Complete 5th Ray
P	Removal	9	Lower Extremity, Right					9	Partial 1st Ray
Q	Repair	A	Inguinal Region, Bilateral					B	Partial 2nd Ray
U	Supplement	B	Lower Extremity, Left					C	Partial 3rd Ray
W	Revision	C	Upper Leg, Right					D	Partial 4th Ray
		D	Upper Leg, Left					F	Partial 5th Ray
		E	Femoral Region, Bilateral					X	Diagnostic
		F	Knee Region, Right					Z	No Qualifier
		G	Knee Region, Left						
		H	Lower Leg, Right						
		J	Lower Leg, Left						
		K	Ankle Region, Right						
		L	Ankle Region, Left						
		M	Foot, Right						
		N	Foot, Left						
		P	1st Toe, Right						
		Q	1st Toe, Left						
		R	2nd Toe, Right						
		S	2nd Toe, Left						
		T	3rd Toe, Right						
		U	3rd Toe, Left						
		V	4th Toe, Right						
		W	4th Toe, Left						
		X	5th Toe, Right						
		Y	5th Toe, Left						

AHA Coding Clinic for table ØY3

2016, 4Q, 99 Root operation Control
2013, 3Q, 23 Control of intraoperative bleeding

AHA Coding Clinic for table ØY6

2017, 2Q, 3-4 Qualifiers for the root operation detachment
2017, 1Q, 22 Chopart amputation of foot
2015, 2Q, 28 Partial amputation of hallux at interphalangeal Joint
2015, 1Q, 28 Mid-foot amputation

AHA Coding Clinic for table ØY9

2015, 1Q, 22 Incision and drainage of abscess of femoropopliteal bypass site
2015, 1Q, 22 Incision and drainage of groin abscess

Detachment Qualifier Descriptions

Qualifier Definition	Upper Leg	Lower Leg
1 **High:** Amputation at the proximal portion of the shaft of the:	Femur	Tibia/Fibula
2 **Mid:** Amputation at the middle portion of the shaft of the:	Femur	Tibia/Fibula
3 **Low:** Amputation at the distal portion of the shaft of the:	Femur	Tibia/Fibula

Qualifier Definition	Foot
Ø Complete 1st through 5th Rays Ray: digit of hand or foot with corresponding metacarpus or metatarsus	Through tarso-metatarsal Joint, **Ankle**
4 Complete 1st Ray	Through tarso-metatarsal joint, **Great Toe**
5 Complete 2nd Ray	Through tarso-metatarsal joint, **2nd Toe**
6 Complete 3rd Ray	Through tarso-metatarsal joint, **3rd Toe**
7 Complete 4th Ray	Through tarso-metatarsal joint, **4th Toe**
8 Complete 5th Ray	Through tarso-metatarsal joint, **Little Toe**
9 Partial 1st Ray	Anywhere along shaft or head of metatarsal bone, **Great Toe**
B Partial 2nd Ray	Anywhere along shaft or head of metatarsal bone, **2nd Toe**
C Partial 3rd Ray	Anywhere along shaft or head of metatarsal bone, **3rd Toe**
D Partial 4th Ray	Anywhere along shaft or head of metatarsal bone, **4th Toe**
F Partial 5th Ray	Anywhere along shaft or head of metatarsal bone, **Little Toe**

Qualifier Definition	Toe
Ø Complete	At the metatarsal-phalangeal joint
1 High	Anywhere along the proximal phalanx
2 Mid	Through the proximal interphalangeal joint or anywhere along the middle phalanx
3 Low	Through the distal interphalangeal joint or anywhere along the distal phalanx

Ø Medical and Surgical
Y Anatomical Regions, Lower Extremities
Ø Alteration Definition: Modifying the anatomic structure of a body part without affecting the function of the body part
Explanation: Principal purpose is to improve appearance

Body Part Character 4	Approach Character 5	Device Character 6	Qualifier Character 7
Ø Buttock, Right 1 Buttock, Left 9 Lower Extremity, Right B Lower Extremity, Left C Upper Leg, Right D Upper Leg, Left F Knee Region, Right G Knee Region, Left H Lower Leg, Right J Lower Leg, Left K Ankle Region, Right L Ankle Region, Left	Ø Open 3 Percutaneous 4 Percutaneous Endoscopic	7 Autologous Tissue Substitute J Synthetic Substitute K Nonautologous Tissue Substitute Z No Device	Z No Qualifier

Ø Medical and Surgical
Y Anatomical Regions, Lower Extremities
2 Change Definition: Taking out or off a device from a body part and putting back an identical or similar device in or on the same body part without cutting or puncturing the skin or a mucous membrane
Explanation: All CHANGE procedures are coded using the approach EXTERNAL

Body Part Character 4	Approach Character 5	Device Character 6	Qualifier Character 7
9 Lower Extremity, Right B Lower Extremity, Left	X External	Ø Drainage Device Y Other Device	Z No Qualifier

Non-OR All body part, approach, device, and qualifier values

Ø Medical and Surgical
Y Anatomical Regions, Lower Extremities
3 Control Definition: Stopping, or attempting to stop, postprocedural or other acute bleeding
Explanation: The site of the bleeding is coded as an anatomical region and not to a specific body part

Body Part Character 4	Approach Character 5	Device Character 6	Qualifier Character 7
Ø Buttock, Right 1 Buttock, Left 5 Inguinal Region, Right Inguinal canal Inguinal triangle 6 Inguinal Region, Left *See 5 Inguinal Region, Right* 7 Femoral Region, Right 8 Femoral Region, Left 9 Lower Extremity, Right B Lower Extremity, Left C Upper Leg, Right D Upper Leg, Left F Knee Region, Right G Knee Region, Left H Lower Leg, Right J Lower Leg, Left K Ankle Region, Right L Ankle Region, Left M Foot, Right N Foot, Left	Ø Open 3 Percutaneous 4 Percutaneous Endoscopic	Z No Device	Z No Qualifier

Ø Medical and Surgical
Y Anatomical Regions, Lower Extremities
6 Detachment Definition: Cutting off all or a portion of the upper or lower extremities

Explanation: The body part value is the site of the detachment, with a qualifier if applicable to further specify the level where the extremity was detached

Body Part Character 4	Approach Character 5	Device Character 6	Qualifier Character 7
2 Hindquarter, Right 3 Hindquarter, Left 4 Hindquarter, Bilateral 7 Femoral Region, Right 8 Femoral Region, Left F Knee Region, Right G Knee Region, Left	Ø Open	Z No Device	Z No Qualifier
C Upper Leg, Right D Upper Leg, Left H Lower Leg, Right J Lower Leg, Left	Ø Open	Z No Device	1 High 2 Mid 3 Low
M Foot, Right N Foot, Left	Ø Open	Z No Device	Ø Complete 4 Complete 1st Ray 5 Complete 2nd Ray 6 Complete 3rd Ray 7 Complete 4th Ray 8 Complete 5th Ray 9 Partial 1st Ray B Partial 2nd Ray C Partial 3rd Ray D Partial 4th Ray F Partial 5th Ray
P 1st Toe, Right Hallux Q 1st Toe, Left *See 1st Toe, Right* R 2nd Toe, Right S 2nd Toe, Left T 3rd Toe, Right U 3rd Toe, Left V 4th Toe, Right W 4th Toe, Left X 5th Toe, Right Y 5th Toe, Left	Ø Open	Z No Device	Ø Complete 1 High 2 Mid 3 Low

Ø Medical and Surgical
Y Anatomical Regions, Lower Extremities
9 Drainage Definition: Taking or letting out fluids and/or gases from a body part
Explanation: The qualifier DIAGNOSTIC is used to identify drainage procedures that are biopsies

Body Part Character 4	Approach Character 5	Device Character 6	Qualifier Character 7
Ø Buttock, Right **1** Buttock, Left **5** Inguinal Region, Right Inguinal canal Inguinal triangle **6** Inguinal Region, Left *See 5 Inguinal Region, Right* **7** Femoral Region, Right **8** Femoral Region, Left **9** Lower Extremity, Right **B** Lower Extremity, Left **C** Upper Leg, Right **D** Upper Leg, Left **F** Knee Region, Right **G** Knee Region, Left **H** Lower Leg, Right **J** Lower Leg, Left **K** Ankle Region, Right **L** Ankle Region, Left **M** Foot, Right **N** Foot, Left	**Ø** Open **3** Percutaneous **4** Percutaneous Endoscopic	**Ø** Drainage Device	**Z** No Qualifier
Ø Buttock, Right **1** Buttock, Left **5** Inguinal Region, Right Inguinal canal Inguinal triangle **6** Inguinal Region, Left *See 5 Inguinal Region, Right* **7** Femoral Region, Right **8** Femoral Region, Left **9** Lower Extremity, Right **B** Lower Extremity, Left **C** Upper Leg, Right **D** Upper Leg, Left **F** Knee Region, Right **G** Knee Region, Left **H** Lower Leg, Right **J** Lower Leg, Left **K** Ankle Region, Right **L** Ankle Region, Left **M** Foot, Right **N** Foot, Left	**Ø** Open **3** Percutaneous **4** Percutaneous Endoscopic	**Z** No Device	**X** Diagnostic **Z** No Qualifier

Non-OR ØY9[Ø,1,7,8,9,B,C,D,F,G,H,J,K,L,M,N][Ø,3,4]ØZ
Non-OR ØY9[5,6]3ØZ
Non-OR ØY9[Ø,1,7,8,9,B,C,D,F,G,H,J,K,L,M,N][Ø,3,4]Z[X,Z]
Non-OR ØY9[5,6]3ZZ

Ø Medical and Surgical
Y Anatomical Regions, Lower Extremities
B Excision Definition: Cutting out or off, without replacement, a portion of a body part
Explanation: The qualifier DIAGNOSTIC is used to identify excision procedures that are biopsies

Body Part Character 4	Approach Character 5	Device Character 6	Qualifier Character 7
Ø Buttock, Right 1 Buttock, Left 5 Inguinal Region, Right Inguinal canal Inguinal triangle 6 Inguinal Region, Left *See 5 Inguinal Region, Right* 7 Femoral Region, Right 8 Femoral Region, Left 9 Lower Extremity, Right B Lower Extremity, Left C Upper Leg, Right D Upper Leg, Left F Knee Region, Right G Knee Region, Left H Lower Leg, Right J Lower Leg, Left K Ankle Region, Right L Ankle Region, Left M Foot, Right N Foot, Left	Ø Open 3 Percutaneous 4 Percutaneous Endoscopic	Z No Device	X Diagnostic Z No Qualifier

Non-OR ØYB[Ø,1,9,B,C,D,F,G,H,J,K,L,M,N][Ø,3,4]ZX

Ø Medical and Surgical
Y Anatomical Regions, Lower Extremities
H Insertion Definition: Putting in a nonbiological appliance that monitors, assists, performs, or prevents a physiological function but does not physically take the place of a body part
Explanation: None

Body Part Character 4	Approach Character 5	Device Character 6	Qualifier Character 7
Ø Buttock, Right 1 Buttock, Left 5 Inguinal Region, Right Inguinal canal Inguinal triangle 6 Inguinal Region, Left *See 5 Inguinal Region, Right* 7 Femoral Region, Right 8 Femoral Region, Left 9 Lower Extremity, Right B Lower Extremity, Left C Upper Leg, Right D Upper Leg, Left F Knee Region, Right G Knee Region, Left H Lower Leg, Right J Lower Leg, Left K Ankle Region, Right L Ankle Region, Left M Foot, Right N Foot, Left	Ø Open 3 Percutaneous 4 Percutaneous Endoscopic	1 Radioactive Element 3 Infusion Device Y Other Device	Z No Qualifier

DRG Non-OR ØYH[Ø,1,5,6,7,8,9,B,C,D,F,G,H,J,K,L,M,N][Ø,3,4][3,Y]Z

Ø Medical and Surgical
Y Anatomical Regions, Lower Extremities
J Inspection Definition: Visually and/or manually exploring a body part

Explanation: Visual exploration may be performed with or without optical instrumentation. Manual exploration may be performed directly or through intervening body layers.

Body Part Character 4	Approach Character 5	Device Character 6	Qualifier Character 7
Ø Buttock, Right **1** Buttock, Left **5** Inguinal Region, Right Inguinal canal Inguinal triangle **6** Inguinal Region, Left *See 5 Inguinal Region, Right* **7** Femoral Region, Right **8** Femoral Region, Left **9** Lower Extremity, Right **A** Inguinal Region, Bilateral *See 5 Inguinal Region, Right* **B** Lower Extremity, Left **C** Upper Leg, Right **D** Upper Leg, Left **E** Femoral Region, Bilateral **F** Knee Region, Right **G** Knee Region, Left **H** Lower Leg, Right **J** Lower Leg, Left **K** Ankle Region, Right **L** Ankle Region, Left **M** Foot, Right **N** Foot, Left	**Ø** Open **3** Percutaneous **4** Percutaneous Endoscopic **X** External	**Z** No Device	**Z** No Qualifier

DRG Non-OR ØYJ[Ø,1,8,9,B,C,D,E,F,G,H,J,K,L,M,N]ØZZ
Non-OR ØYJ[Ø,1,9,B,C,D,F,G,H,J,K,L,M,N][3,4,X]ZZ
Non-OR ØYJ[5,6,7,8,A,E][3,X]ZZ

Ø Medical and Surgical
Y Anatomical Regions, Lower Extremities
M Reattachment Definition: Putting back in or on all or a portion of a separated body part to its normal location or other suitable location
Explanation: Vascular circulation and nervous pathways may or may not be reestablished

Body Part Character 4	Approach Character 5	Device Character 6	Qualifier Character 7
Ø Buttock, Right 1 Buttock, Left 2 Hindquarter, Right 3 Hindquarter, Left 4 Hindquarter, Bilateral 5 Inguinal Region, Right Inguinal canal Inguinal triangle 6 Inguinal Region, Left *See 5 Inguinal Region, Right* 7 Femoral Region, Right 8 Femoral Region, Left 9 Lower Extremity, Right B Lower Extremity, Left C Upper Leg, Right D Upper Leg, Left F Knee Region, Right G Knee Region, Left H Lower Leg, Right J Lower Leg, Left K Ankle Region, Right L Ankle Region, Left M Foot, Right N Foot, Left P 1st Toe, Right Hallux Q 1st Toe, Left *See 1st Toe, Right* R 2nd Toe, Right S 2nd Toe, Left T 3rd Toe, Right U 3rd Toe, Left V 4th Toe, Right W 4th Toe, Left X 5th Toe, Right Y 5th Toe, Left	Ø Open	Z No Device	Z No Qualifier

Ø Medical and Surgical
Y Anatomical Regions, Lower Extremities
P Removal Definition: Taking out or off a device from a body part
Explanation: If a device is taken out and a similar device put in without cutting or puncturing the skin or mucous membrane, the procedure is coded to the root operation CHANGE. Otherwise, the procedure for taking out the device is coded to the root operation REMOVAL.

Body Part Character 4	Approach Character 5	Device Character 6	Qualifier Character 7
9 Lower Extremity, Right B Lower Extremity, Left	Ø Open 3 Percutaneous 4 Percutaneous Endoscopic X External	Ø Drainage Device 1 Radioactive Element 3 Infusion Device 7 Autologous Tissue Substitute J Synthetic Substitute K Nonautologous Tissue Substitute Y Other Device	Z No Qualifier

Non-OR All body part, approach, device, and qualifier values

Ø Medical and Surgical
Y Anatomical Regions, Lower Extremities
Q Repair Definition: Restoring, to the extent possible, a body part to its normal anatomic structure and function
Explanation: Used only when the method to accomplish the repair is not one of the other root operations

Body Part Character 4	Approach Character 5	Device Character 6	Qualifier Character 7
Ø Buttock, Right **1** Buttock, Left **5** Inguinal Region, Right Inguinal canal Inguinal triangle **6** Inguinal Region, Left *See 5 Inguinal Region, Right* **7** Femoral Region, Right **8** Femoral Region, Left **9** Lower Extremity, Right **A** Inguinal Region, Bilateral *See 5 Inguinal Region, Right* **B** Lower Extremity, Left **C** Upper Leg, Right **D** Upper Leg, Left **E** Femoral Region, Bilateral **F** Knee Region, Right **G** Knee Region, Left **H** Lower Leg, Right **J** Lower Leg, Left **K** Ankle Region, Right **L** Ankle Region, Left **M** Foot, Right **N** Foot, Left **P** 1st Toe, Right Hallux **Q** 1st Toe, Left *See 1st Toe, Right* **R** 2nd Toe, Right **S** 2nd Toe, Left **T** 3rd Toe, Right **U** 3rd Toe, Left **V** 4th Toe, Right **W** 4th Toe, Left **X** 5th Toe, Right **Y** 5th Toe, Left	**Ø** Open **3** Percutaneous **4** Percutaneous Endoscopic **X** External	**Z** No Device	**Z** No Qualifier

Non-OR ØYQ[5,6,7,8,A,E]XZZ

Ø Medical and Surgical
Y Anatomical Regions, Lower Extremities
U Supplement Definition: Putting in or on biological or synthetic material that physically reinforces and/or augments the function of a portion of a body part

Explanation: The biological material is non-living, or is living and from the same individual. The body part may have been previously replaced, and the SUPPLEMENT procedure is performed to physically reinforce and/or augment the function of the replaced body part.

Body Part Character 4	Approach Character 5	Device Character 6	Qualifier Character 7
Ø Buttock, Right 1 Buttock, Left 5 Inguinal Region, Right Inguinal canal Inguinal triangle 6 Inguinal Region, Left *See 5 Inguinal Region, Right* 7 Femoral Region, Right 8 Femoral Region, Left 9 Lower Extremity, Right A Inguinal Region, Bilateral *See 5 Inguinal Region, Right* B Lower Extremity, Left C Upper Leg, Right D Upper Leg, Left E Femoral Region, Bilateral F Knee Region, Right G Knee Region, Left H Lower Leg, Right J Lower Leg, Left K Ankle Region, Right L Ankle Region, Left M Foot, Right N Foot, Left P 1st Toe, Right Hallux Q 1st Toe, Left *See 1st Toe, Right* R 2nd Toe, Right S 2nd Toe, Left T 3rd Toe, Right U 3rd Toe, Left V 4th Toe, Right W 4th Toe, Left X 5th Toe, Right Y 5th Toe, Left	Ø Open 4 Percutaneous Endoscopic	7 Autologous Tissue Substitute J Synthetic Substitute K Nonautologous Tissue Substitute	Z No Qualifier

Ø Medical and Surgical
Y Anatomical Regions, Lower Extremities
W Revision Definition: Correcting, to the extent possible, a portion of a malfunctioning device or the position of a displaced device

Explanation: Revision can include correcting a malfunctioning or displaced device by taking out or putting in components of the device such as a screw or pin

Body Part Character 4	Approach Character 5	Device Character 6	Qualifier Character 7
9 Lower Extremity, Right B Lower Extremity, Left	Ø Open 3 Percutaneous 4 Percutaneous Endoscopic X External	Ø Drainage Device 3 Infusion Device 7 Autologous Tissue Substitute J Synthetic Substitute K Nonautologous Tissue Substitute Y Other Device	Z No Qualifier

DRG Non-OR ØYW[9,B][Ø,3,4][Ø,3,7,J,K,Y]Z
Non-OR ØYW[9,B]X[Ø,3,7,J,K,Y]Z

Obstetrics 1Ø2–1ØY

Character Meanings

This Character Meaning table is provided as a guide to assist the user in the identification of character members that may be found in this section of code tables. It **SHOULD NOT** be used to build a PCS code.

Ø: Pregnancy

Operation–Character 3	Body Part–Character 4	Approach–Character 5	Device–Character 6	Qualifier–Character 7
2 Change	Ø Products of Conception	Ø Open	3 Monitoring Electrode	Ø High
9 Drainage	1 Products of Conception, Retained	3 Percutaneous	Y Other Device	1 Low
A Abortion	2 Products of Conception, Ectopic	4 Percutaneous Endoscopic	Z No Device	2 Extraperitoneal
D Extraction		7 Via Natural or Artificial Opening		3 Low Forceps
E Delivery		8 Via Natural or Artificial Opening Endoscopic		4 Mid Forceps
H Insertion		X External		5 High Forceps
J Inspection				6 Vacuum
P Removal				7 Internal Version
Q Repair				8 Other
S Reposition				9 Fetal Blood OR Manual
T Resection				A Fetal Cerebrospinal Fluid
Y Transplantation				B Fetal Fluid, Other
				C Amniotic Fluid, Therapeutic
				D Fluid, Other
				E Nervous System
				F Cardiovascular System
				G Lymphatics & Hemic
				H Eye
				J Ear, Nose & Sinus
				K Respiratory System
				L Mouth & Throat
				M Gastrointestinal System
				N Hepatobiliary & Pancreas
				P Endocrine System
				Q Skin
				R Musculoskeletal System
				S Urinary System
				T Female Reproductive System
				U Amniotic Fluid, Diagnostic
				V Male Reproductive System
				W Laminaria
				X Abortifacient
				Y Other Body System
				Z No Qualifier

AHA Coding Clinic for table 1Ø9

2014, 3Q, 12 Fetoscopic laser photocoagulation and laser microseptostomy for twin-twin transfusion syndrome
2014, 2Q, 9 Pitocin administration to augment labor

AHA Coding Clinic for table 1ØD

2018, 2Q, 17 High transverse cesarean section
2016, 1Q, 9 Vaginal delivery assisted by vacuum and low forceps extraction
2014, 4Q, 43 Cesarean delivery assisted by vacuum extraction
2014, 4Q, 43 Vacuum dilation and curettage for blighted ovum

AHA Coding Clinic for table 1ØE

2017, 3Q, 5 Delivery of placenta
2016, 2Q, 34 Assisted vaginal delivery
2014, 4Q, 17 RH (D) alloimmunization (sensitization)
2014, 2Q, 9 Pitocin administration to augment labor

AHA Coding Clinic for table 1ØH

2013, 2Q, 36 Intrauterine pressure monitor

AHA Coding Clinic for table 1ØQ

2014, 3Q, 12 Fetoscopic laser photocoagulation and laser microseptostomy for twin-twin transfusion syndrome

AHA Coding Clinic for table 1ØT

2015, 3Q, 31 Laparoscopic partial salpingectomy for ectopic pregnancy

1 Obstetrics
Ø Pregnancy
2 Change Definition: Taking out or off a device from a body part and putting back an identical or similar device in or on the same body part without cutting or puncturing the skin or a mucous membrane

Explanation: None

Body Part Character 4	Approach Character 5	Device Character 6	Qualifier Character 7
Ø Products of Conception ♀	7 Via Natural or Artificial Opening	3 Monitoring Electrode Y Other Device	Z No Qualifier

Non-OR All body part, approach, device, and qualifier values
♀ All body part, approach, device, and qualifier values

1 Obstetrics
Ø Pregnancy
9 Drainage Definition: Taking or letting out fluids and/or gases from a body part

Explanation: None

Body Part Character 4	Approach Character 5	Device Character 6	Qualifier Character 7
Ø Products of Conception ♀	Ø Open 3 Percutaneous 4 Percutaneous Endoscopic 7 Via Natural or Artificial Opening 8 Via Natural or Artificial Opening Endoscopic	Z No Device	9 Fetal Blood A Fetal Cerebrospinal Fluid B Fetal Fluid, Other C Amniotic Fluid, Therapeutic D Fluid, Other U Amniotic Fluid, Diagnostic

Non-OR All body part, approach, device, and qualifier values
♀ All body part, approach, device, and qualifier values

1 Obstetrics
Ø Pregnancy
A Abortion Definition: Artificially terminating a pregnancy

Explanation: None

Body Part Character 4	Approach Character 5	Device Character 6	Qualifier Character 7
Ø Products of Conception ♀	Ø Open 3 Percutaneous 4 Percutaneous Endoscopic 8 Via Natural or Artificial Opening Endoscopic	Z No Device	Z No Qualifier
Ø Products of Conception ♀	7 Via Natural or Artificial Opening	Z No Device	6 Vacuum W Laminaria X Abortifacient Z No Qualifier

DRG Non-OR 1ØAØ7Z6
Non-OR 1ØAØ7Z[W,X]
♀ All body part, approach, device, and qualifier values

1 Obstetrics
Ø Pregnancy
D Extraction Definition: Pulling or stripping out or off all or a portion of a body part by the use of force

Explanation: None

Body Part Character 4	Approach Character 5	Device Character 6	Qualifier Character 7
Ø Products of Conception ♀	Ø Open	Z No Device	Ø High 1 Low 2 Extraperitoneal
Ø Products of Conception ♀	7 Via Natural or Artificial Opening	Z No Device	3 Low Forceps 4 Mid Forceps 5 High Forceps 6 Vacuum 7 Internal Version 8 Other
1 Products of Conception, Retained ♀	7 Via Natural or Artificial Opening 8 Via Natural or Artificial Opening Endoscopic	Z No Device	9 Manual Z No Qualifier
2 Products of Conception, Ectopic ♀	7 Via Natural or Artificial Opening 8 Via Natural or Artificial Opening Endoscopic	Z No Device	Z No Qualifier

DRG Non-OR 1ØDØ7Z[3,4,5,6,7,8]
♀ All body part, approach, device, and qualifier values

1 Obstetrics
Ø Pregnancy
E Delivery Definition: Assisting the passage of the products of conception from the genital canal
Explanation: None

Body Part Character 4	Approach Character 5	Device Character 6	Qualifier Character 7
Ø Products of Conception ♀	X External	Z No Device	Z No Qualifier

DRG Non-OR 1ØEØXZZ
♀ All body part, approach, device, and qualifier values

1 Obstetrics
Ø Pregnancy
H Insertion Definition: Putting in a nonbiological appliance that monitors, assists, performs, or prevents a physiological function but does not physically take the place of a body part
Explanation: None

Body Part Character 4	Approach Character 5	Device Character 6	Qualifier Character 7
Ø Products of Conception ♀	Ø Open 7 Via Natural or Artificial Opening	3 Monitoring Electrode Y Other Device	Z No Qualifier

Non-OR 1ØHØ7[3,Y]Z
♀ All body part, approach, device, and qualifier values

1 Obstetrics
Ø Pregnancy
J Inspection Definition: Visually and/or manually exploring a body part
Explanation: Visual exploration may be performed with or without optical instrumentation. Manual exploration may be performed directly or through intervening body layers.

Body Part Character 4	Approach Character 5	Device Character 6	Qualifier Character 7
Ø Products of Conception ♀ 1 Products of Conception, Retained ♀ 2 Products of Conception, Ectopic ♀	Ø Open 3 Percutaneous 4 Percutaneous Endoscopic 7 Via Natural or Artificial Opening 8 Via Natural or Artificial Opening Endoscopic X External	Z No Device	Z No Qualifier

Non-OR All body part, approach, device, and qualifier values
♀ All body part, approach, device, and qualifier values

1 Obstetrics
Ø Pregnancy
P Removal Definition: Taking out or off a device from a body part, region or orifice
Explanation: If a device is taken out and a similar device put in without cutting or puncturing the skin or mucous membrane, the procedure is coded to the root operation CHANGE. Otherwise, the procedure for taking out a device is coded to the root operation REMOVAL.

Body Part Character 4	Approach Character 5	Device Character 6	Qualifier Character 7
Ø Products of Conception ♀	Ø Open 7 Via Natural or Artificial Opening	3 Monitoring Electrode Y Other Device	Z No Qualifier

♀ All body part, approach, device, and qualifier values

1 Obstetrics
Ø Pregnancy
Q Repair Definition: Restoring, to the extent possible, a body part to its normal anatomic structure and function
Explanation: Used only when the method to accomplish the repair is not one of the other root operations

Body Part Character 4	Approach Character 5	Device Character 6	Qualifier Character 7
Ø Products of Conception ♀	Ø Open 3 Percutaneous 4 Percutaneous Endoscopic 7 Via Natural or Artificial Opening 8 Via Natural or Artificial Opening Endoscopic	Y Other Device Z No Device	E Nervous System F Cardiovascular System G Lymphatics and Hemic H Eye J Ear, Nose and Sinus K Respiratory System L Mouth and Throat M Gastrointestinal System N Hepatobiliary and Pancreas P Endocrine System Q Skin R Musculoskeletal System S Urinary System T Female Reproductive System V Male Reproductive System Y Other Body System

♀ All body part, approach, device, and qualifier values

1 Obstetrics
0 Pregnancy
S Reposition Definition: Moving to its normal location, or other suitable location, all or a portion of a body part

Explanation: The body part is moved to a new location from an abnormal location, or from a normal location where it is not functioning correctly. The body part may or may not be cut out or off to be moved to the new location.

Body Part Character 4	Approach Character 5	Device Character 6	Qualifier Character 7
0 Products of Conception ♀	7 Via Natural or Artificial Opening X External	Z No Device	Z No Qualifier
2 Products of Conception, Ectopic ♀	0 Open 3 Percutaneous 4 Percutaneous Endoscopic 7 Via Natural or Artificial Opening 8 Via Natural or Artificial Opening Endoscopic	Z No Device	Z No Qualifier

DRG Non-OR 10S07ZZ
Non-OR 10S0XZZ

♀ All body part, approach, device, and qualifier values

1 Obstetrics
0 Pregnancy
T Resection Definition: Cutting out or off, without replacement, all of a body part

Explanation: None

Body Part Character 4	Approach Character 5	Device Character 6	Qualifier Character 7
2 Products of Conception, Ectopic ♀	0 Open 3 Percutaneous 4 Percutaneous Endoscopic 7 Via Natural or Artificial Opening 8 Via Natural or Artificial Opening Endoscopic	Z No Device	Z No Qualifier

♀ All body part, approach, device, and qualifier values

1 Obstetrics
0 Pregnancy
Y Transplantation Definition: Putting in or on all or a portion of a living body part taken from another individual or animal to physically take the place and/or function of all or a portion of a similar body part

Explanation: The native body part may or may not be taken out, and the transplanted body part may take over all or a portion of its function

Body Part Character 4	Approach Character 5	Device Character 6	Qualifier Character 7
0 Products of Conception ♀	3 Percutaneous 4 Percutaneous Endoscopic 7 Via Natural or Artificial Opening	Z No Device	E Nervous System F Cardiovascular System G Lymphatics and Hemic H Eye J Ear, Nose and Sinus K Respiratory System L Mouth and Throat M Gastrointestinal System N Hepatobiliary and Pancreas P Endocrine System Q Skin R Musculoskeletal System S Urinary System T Female Reproductive System V Male Reproductive System Y Other Body System

♀ All body part, approach, device, and qualifier values

Placement 2WØ–2Y5

Character Meanings

This Character Meaning table is provided as a guide to assist the user in the identification of character members that may be found in this section of code tables. It **SHOULD NOT** be used to build a PCS code.

W: Anatomical Regions

Operation–Character 3	Body Region–Character 4	Approach–Character 5	Device–Character 6	Qualifier–Character 7
Ø Change	Ø Head	X External	Ø Traction Apparatus	Z No Qualifier
1 Compression	1 Face		1 Splint	
2 Dressing	2 Neck		2 Cast	
3 Immobilization	3 Abdominal Wall		3 Brace	
4 Packing	4 Chest Wall		4 Bandage	
5 Removal	5 Back		5 Packing Material	
6 Traction	6 Inguinal Region, Right		6 Pressure Dressing	
	7 Inguinal Region, Left		7 Intermittent Pressure Device	
	8 Upper Extremity, Right		9 Wire	
	9 Upper Extremity, Left		Y Other Device	
	A Upper Arm, Right		Z No Device	
	B Upper Arm, Left			
	C Lower Arm, Right			
	D Lower Arm, Left			
	E Hand, Right			
	F Hand, Left			
	G Thumb, Right			
	H Thumb, Left			
	J Finger, Right			
	K Finger, Left			
	L Lower Extremity, Right			
	M Lower Extremity, Left			
	N Upper Leg, Right			
	P Upper Leg, Left			
	Q Lower Leg, Right			
	R Lower Leg, Left			
	S Foot, Right			
	T Foot, Left			
	U Toe, Right			
	V Toe, Left			

Y: Anatomical Orifices

Operation–Character 3	Body Orifice–Character 4	Approach–Character 5	Device–Character 6	Qualifier–Character 7
Ø Change	Ø Mouth and Pharynx	X External	5 Packing Material	Z No Qualifier
4 Packing	1 Nasal			
5 Removal	2 Ear			
	3 Anorectal			
	4 Female Genital Tract			
	5 Urethra			

AHA Coding Clinic for table 2W6
2015, 2Q, 35 Application of tongs to reduce and stabilize cervical fracture
2013, 2Q, 39 Application of cervical tongs for reduction of cervical fracture

AHA Coding Clinic for table 2Y4
2017, 4Q, 106 Nasal packing for epistaxis

2 Placement
W Anatomical Regions
Ø Change Definition: Taking out or off a device from a body part and putting back an identical or similar device in or on the same body part without cutting or puncturing the skin or a mucous membrane

Body Region Character 4	Approach Character 5	Device Character 6	Qualifier Character 7
Ø Head 2 Neck 3 Abdominal Wall 4 Chest Wall 5 Back 6 Inguinal Region, Right 7 Inguinal Region, Left 8 Upper Extremity, Right 9 Upper Extremity, Left A Upper Arm, Right B Upper Arm, Left C Lower Arm, Right D Lower Arm, Left E Hand, Right F Hand, Left G Thumb, Right H Thumb, Left J Finger, Right K Finger, Left L Lower Extremity, Right M Lower Extremity, Left N Upper Leg, Right P Upper Leg, Left Q Lower Leg, Right R Lower Leg, Left S Foot, Right T Foot, Left U Toe, Right V Toe, Left	X External	Ø Traction Apparatus 1 Splint 2 Cast 3 Brace 4 Bandage 5 Packing Material 6 Pressure Dressing 7 Intermittent Pressure Device Y Other Device	Z No Qualifier
1 Face	X External	Ø Traction Apparatus 1 Splint 2 Cast 3 Brace 4 Bandage 5 Packing Material 6 Pressure Dressing 7 Intermittent Pressure Device 9 Wire Y Other Device	Z No Qualifier

2 Placement
W Anatomical Regions
1 Compression Definition: Putting pressure on a body region

Body Region Character 4	Approach Character 5	Device Character 6	Qualifier Character 7
Ø Head 1 Face 2 Neck 3 Abdominal Wall 4 Chest Wall 5 Back 6 Inguinal Region, Right 7 Inguinal Region, Left 8 Upper Extremity, Right 9 Upper Extremity, Left A Upper Arm, Right B Upper Arm, Left C Lower Arm, Right D Lower Arm, Left E Hand, Right F Hand, Left G Thumb, Right H Thumb, Left J Finger, Right K Finger, Left L Lower Extremity, Right M Lower Extremity, Left N Upper Leg, Right P Upper Leg, Left Q Lower Leg, Right R Lower Leg, Left S Foot, Right T Foot, Left U Toe, Right V Toe, Left	X External	6 Pressure Dressing 7 Intermittent Pressure Device	Z No Qualifier

2 Placement
W Anatomical Regions
2 Dressing Definition: Putting material on a body region for protection

Body Region Character 4	Approach Character 5	Device Character 6	Qualifier Character 7
Ø Head 1 Face 2 Neck 3 Abdominal Wall 4 Chest Wall 5 Back 6 Inguinal Region, Right 7 Inguinal Region, Left 8 Upper Extremity, Right 9 Upper Extremity, Left A Upper Arm, Right B Upper Arm, Left C Lower Arm, Right D Lower Arm, Left E Hand, Right F Hand, Left G Thumb, Right H Thumb, Left J Finger, Right K Finger, Left L Lower Extremity, Right M Lower Extremity, Left N Upper Leg, Right P Upper Leg, Left Q Lower Leg, Right R Lower Leg, Left S Foot, Right T Foot, Left U Toe, Right V Toe, Left	X External	4 Bandage	Z No Qualifier

2 Placement
W Anatomical Regions
3 Immobilization Definition: Limiting or preventing motion of a body region

Body Region Character 4	Approach Character 5	Device Character 6	Qualifier Character 7
Ø Head 2 Neck 3 Abdominal Wall 4 Chest Wall 5 Back 6 Inguinal Region, Right 7 Inguinal Region, Left 8 Upper Extremity, Right 9 Upper Extremity, Left A Upper Arm, Right B Upper Arm, Left C Lower Arm, Right D Lower Arm, Left E Hand, Right F Hand, Left G Thumb, Right H Thumb, Left J Finger, Right K Finger, Left L Lower Extremity, Right M Lower Extremity, Left N Upper Leg, Right P Upper Leg, Left Q Lower Leg, Right R Lower Leg, Left S Foot, Right T Foot, Left U Toe, Right V Toe, Left	X External	1 Splint 2 Cast 3 Brace Y Other Device	Z No Qualifier
1 Face	X External	1 Splint 2 Cast 3 Brace 9 Wire Y Other Device	Z No Qualifier

2 Placement
W Anatomical Regions
4 Packing Definition: Putting material in a body region or orifice

Body Region Character 4	Approach Character 5	Device Character 6	Qualifier Character 7
Ø Head 1 Face 2 Neck 3 Abdominal Wall 4 Chest Wall 5 Back 6 Inguinal Region, Right 7 Inguinal Region, Left 8 Upper Extremity, Right 9 Upper Extremity, Left A Upper Arm, Right B Upper Arm, Left C Lower Arm, Right D Lower Arm, Left E Hand, Right F Hand, Left G Thumb, Right H Thumb, Left J Finger, Right K Finger, Left L Lower Extremity, Right M Lower Extremity, Left N Upper Leg, Right P Upper Leg, Left Q Lower Leg, Right R Lower Leg, Left S Foot, Right T Foot, Left U Toe, Right V Toe, Left	X External	5 Packing Material	Z No Qualifier

2 Placement
W Anatomical Regions
5 Removal Definition: Taking out or off a device from a body part

Body Region Character 4	Approach Character 5	Device Character 6	Qualifier Character 7
Ø Head 2 Neck 3 Abdominal Wall 4 Chest Wall 5 Back 6 Inguinal Region, Right 7 Inguinal Region, Left 8 Upper Extremity, Right 9 Upper Extremity, Left A Upper Arm, Right B Upper Arm, Left C Lower Arm, Right D Lower Arm, Left E Hand, Right F Hand, Left G Thumb, Right H Thumb, Left J Finger, Right K Finger, Left L Lower Extremity, Right M Lower Extremity, Left N Upper Leg, Right P Upper Leg, Left Q Lower Leg, Right R Lower Leg, Left S Foot, Right T Foot, Left U Toe, Right V Toe, Left	X External	Ø Traction Apparatus 1 Splint 2 Cast 3 Brace 4 Bandage 5 Packing Material 6 Pressure Dressing 7 Intermittent Pressure Device Y Other Device	Z No Qualifier
1 Face	X External	Ø Traction Apparatus 1 Splint 2 Cast 3 Brace 4 Bandage 5 Packing Material 6 Pressure Dressing 7 Intermittent Pressure Device 9 Wire Y Other Device	Z No Qualifier

2 Placement
W Anatomical Regions
6 Traction Definition: Exerting a pulling force on a body region in a distal direction

Body Region Character 4	Approach Character 5	Device Character 6	Qualifier Character 7
Ø Head 1 Face 2 Neck 3 Abdominal Wall 4 Chest Wall 5 Back 6 Inguinal Region, Right 7 Inguinal Region, Left 8 Upper Extremity, Right 9 Upper Extremity, Left A Upper Arm, Right B Upper Arm, Left C Lower Arm, Right D Lower Arm, Left E Hand, Right F Hand, Left G Thumb, Right H Thumb, Left J Finger, Right K Finger, Left L Lower Extremity, Right M Lower Extremity, Left N Upper Leg, Right P Upper Leg, Left Q Lower Leg, Right R Lower Leg, Left S Foot, Right T Foot, Left U Toe, Right V Toe, Left	X External	Ø Traction Apparatus Z No Device	Z No Qualifier

2 Placement
Y Anatomical Orifices
Ø Change Definition: Taking out or off a device from a body part and putting back an identical or similar device in or on the same body part without cutting or puncturing the skin or a mucous membrane

Body Region Character 4	Approach Character 5	Device Character 6	Qualifier Character 7
Ø Mouth and Pharynx 1 Nasal 2 Ear 3 Anorectal 4 Female Genital Tract ♀ 5 Urethra	X External	5 Packing Material	Z No Qualifier

♀ 2YØ4X5Z

2 Placement
Y Anatomical Orifices
4 Packing Definition: Putting material in a body region or orifice

Body Region Character 4	Approach Character 5	Device Character 6	Qualifier Character 7
Ø Mouth and Pharynx 1 Nasal 2 Ear 3 Anorectal 4 Female Genital Tract ♀ 5 Urethra	X External	5 Packing Material	Z No Qualifier

♀ 2Y44X5Z

2 Placement
Y Anatomical Orifices
5 Removal Definition: Taking out or off a device from a body part

Body Region Character 4	Approach Character 5	Device Character 6	Qualifier Character 7
Ø Mouth and Pharynx 1 Nasal 2 Ear 3 Anorectal 4 Female Genital Tract ♀ 5 Urethra	X External	5 Packing Material	Z No Qualifier

♀ 2Y54X5Z

Administration 3Ø2–3E1

Character Meanings

This Character Meaning table is provided as a guide to assist the user in the identification of character members that may be found in this section of code tables. It **SHOULD NOT** be used to build a PCS code.

Ø: Circulatory

Operation–Character 3	Body System/Region – Character 4	Approach–Character 5	Substance–Character 6	Qualifier–Character 7
2 Transfusion	3 Peripheral Vein	Ø Open	A Stem Cells, Embryonic	Ø Autologous
	4 Central Vein	3 Percutaneous	B 4-Factor Prothrombin Complex Concentrate	1 Nonautologous
	5 Peripheral Artery	7 Via Natural or Artificial Opening	G Bone Marrow	2 Allogeneic, Related
	6 Central Artery		H Whole Blood	3 Allogeneic, Unrelated
	7 Products of Conception, Circulatory		J Serum Albumin	4 Allogeneic, Unspecified
	8 Vein		K Frozen Plasma	Z No Qualifier
			L Fresh Plasma	
			M Plasma Cryoprecipitate	
			N Red Blood Cells	
			P Frozen Red Cells	
			Q White Cells	
			R Platelets	
			S Globulin	
			T Fibrinogen	
			V Antihemophilic Factors	
			W Factor IX	
			X Stem Cells, Cord Blood	
			Y Stem Cells, Hematopoietic	

C: Indwelling Device

Operation–Character 3	Body System/Region – Character 4	Approach–Character 5	Substance–Character 6	Qualifier–Character 7
1 Irrigation	Z None	X External	8 Irrigating Substance	Z No Qualifier

Continued on next page

E: Physiological Systems and Anatomical Regions

Administration Character Meanings Continued

Operation–Character 3	Body System/Region–Character 4	Approach–Character 5	Substance–Character 6	Qualifier–Character 7
Ø Introduction	Ø Skin and Mucous Membranes	Ø Open	Ø Antineoplastic	Ø Autologous OR Influenza Vaccine
1 Irrigation	1 Subcutaneous Tissue	3 Percutaneous	1 Thrombolytic	1 Nonautologous
	2 Muscle	4 Percutaneous Endoscopic	2 Anti-infective	2 High-dose Interleukin-2
	3 Peripheral Vein	7 Via Natural or Artificial Opening	3 Anti-inflammatory	3 Low-dose Interleukin-2
	4 Central Vein	8 Via Natural or Artificial Opening Endoscopic	4 Serum, Toxoid and Vaccine	4 Liquid Brachytherapy Radioisotope
	5 Peripheral Artery	X External	5 Adhesion Barrier	5 Other Antineoplastic
	6 Central Artery		6 Nutritional Substance	6 Recombinant Human-activated Protein C
	7 Coronary Artery		7 Electrolytic and Water Balance Substance	7 Other Thrombolytic
	8 Heart		8 Irrigating Substance	8 Oxazolidinones
	9 Nose		9 Dialysate	9 Other Anti-infective
	A Bone Marrow		A Stem Cells, Embryonic	A Anti-infective Envelope
	B Ear		B Anesthetic Agent	B Recombinant Bone Morphogenetic Protein
	C Eye		E Stem Cells, Somatic	C Other Substance
	D Mouth and Pharynx		F Intracirculatory Anesthetic	D Nitric Oxide
	E Products of Conception		G Other Therapeutic Substance	F Other Gas
	F Respiratory Tract		H Radioactive Substance	G Insulin
	G Upper GI		K Other Diagnostic Substance	H Human B-type Natriuretic Peptide
	H Lower GI		L Sperm	J Other Hormone
	J Biliary and Pancreatic Tract		M Pigment	K Immunostimulator
	K Genitourinary Tract		N Analgesics, Hypnotics, Sedatives	L Immunosuppressive
	L Pleural Cavity		P Platelet Inhibitor	M Monoclonal Antibody
	M Peritoneal Cavity		Q Fertilized Ovum	N Blood Brain Barrier Disruption
	N Male Reproductive		R Antiarrhythmic	P Clofarabine
	P Female Reproductive		S Gas	Q Glucarpidase
	Q Cranial Cavity and Brain		T Destructive Agent	X Diagnostic
	R Spinal Canal		U Pancreatic Islet Cells	Z No Qualifier
	S Epidural Space		V Hormone	
	T Peripheral Nerves and Plexi		W Immunotherapeutic	
	U Joints		X Vasopressor	
	V Bones			
	W Lymphatics			
	X Cranial Nerves			
	Y Pericardial Cavity			

AHA Coding Clinic for table 3Ø2
2016, 4Q, 113 Bone marrow and stem cell transfusion (Transplantation)

AHA Coding Clinic for table 3EØ
2018, 1Q, 8 Placement of bone morphogenetic protein & spinal fusion surgery
2017, 2Q, 14 Infusion of tPA into pleural cavity
2017, 1Q, 37 Injection of glue into enteric fistula tract
2016, 4Q, 113-114 Substances applied to cranial cavity and brain
2016, 3Q, 29 Closure of bilateral alveolar clefts
2016, 1Q, 20 Metatarsophalangeal joint resection arthroplasty
2015, 3Q, 24 Esophagogastroduodenoscopy with epinephrine injection for control of bleeding
2015, 3Q, 29 Placement of adhesion barrier
2015, 2Q, 29 Insertion of nasogastric tube for drainage and feeding
2015, 2Q, 31 Thoracoscopic talc pleurodesis
2015, 1Q, 31 Intrathecal chemotherapy
2015, 1Q, 38 Chemoembolization of the hepatic artery
2014, 4Q, 16 Administration of RH (D) immunoglobulin
2014, 4Q, 17 RH (D) alloimmunization (sensitization)
2014, 4Q, 19 Ultrasound accelerated thrombolysis
2014, 4Q, 34 Resection of brain malignancy with implantation of chemotherapeutic wafer
2014, 4Q, 38 Placement of saline and seprafilm solution into abdominal cavity
2014, 3Q, 26 Coil embolization of gastroduodenal artery with chemoembolization of hepatic artery
2014, 2Q, 8 Medical induction of labor with Cervidil tampon insertion
2014, 2Q, 10 Prophylactic Neulasta injection for infection prevention
2013, 4Q, 124 Administration of tPA for stroke treatment prior to transfer
2013, 1Q, 27 Injection of sclerosing agent into an esophageal varix

AHA Coding Clinic for table 3E1
2017, 3Q, 14 Bronchoscopy with suctioning and washings for removal of mucus plug

3 Administration
Ø Circulatory
2 Transfusion Definition: Putting in blood or blood products

Body System/Region Character 4	Approach Character 5	Substance Character 6	Qualifier Character 7
3 Peripheral Vein NC 4 Central Vein NC	Ø Open 3 Percutaneous	A Stem Cells, Embryonic	Z No Qualifier
3 Peripheral Vein NC 4 Central Vein NC	Ø Open 3 Percutaneous	G Bone Marrow X Stem Cells, Cord Blood Y Stem Cells, Hematopoietic	Ø Autologous 2 Allogeneic, Related 3 Allogeneic, Unrelated 4 Allogeneic, Unspecified
3 Peripheral Vein 4 Central Vein	Ø Open 3 Percutaneous	H Whole Blood J Serum Albumin K Frozen Plasma L Fresh Plasma M Plasma Cryoprecipitate N Red Blood Cells P Frozen Red Cells Q White Cells R Platelets S Globulin T Fibrinogen V Antihemophilic Factors W Factor IX	Ø Autologous 1 Nonautologous
5 Peripheral Artery NC 6 Central Artery NC	Ø Open 3 Percutaneous	G Bone Marrow H Whole Blood J Serum Albumin K Frozen Plasma L Fresh Plasma M Plasma Cryoprecipitate N Red Blood Cells P Frozen Red Cells Q White Cells R Platelets S Globulin T Fibrinogen V Antihemophilic Factors W Factor IX X Stem Cells, Cord Blood Y Stem Cells, Hematopoietic	Ø Autologous 1 Nonautologous
7 Products of Conception, Circulatory ♀	3 Percutaneous 7 Via Natural or Artificial Opening	H Whole Blood J Serum Albumin K Frozen Plasma L Fresh Plasma M Plasma Cryoprecipitate N Red Blood Cells P Frozen Red Cells Q White Cells R Platelets S Globulin T Fibrinogen V Antihemophilic Factors W Factor IX	1 Nonautologous
8 Vein	Ø Open 3 Percutaneous	B 4-Factor Prothrombin Complex Concentrate	1 Nonautologous

Valid OR 3Ø2[3,4]ØAZ
Valid OR 3Ø2[3,4]Ø[G,X,Y][Ø,2,3,4]
Valid OR 3Ø2[3,4]3[G,X,Y][2,3,4]
Valid OR 3Ø2[5,6]Ø[G,X,Y][Ø,1]
DRG-Non-OR 3Ø2[3,4]3AZ
DRG-Non-OR 3Ø2[3,4]3[G,X,Y]Ø
DRG-Non-OR 3Ø2[5,6]3[G,X,Y][Ø,1]
NC 3Ø2[3,4][Ø,3]AZ Only when reported with PDx or SDx of C91.ØØ, C92.ØØ, C92.1Ø, C92.11, C92.4Ø, C92.5Ø, C92.6Ø, C92.AØ, C93.ØØ, C94.ØØ, C95.ØØ
NC 3Ø2[3,4][Ø,3][G,Y]Ø Only when reported with PDx or SDx of C91.ØØ, C92.ØØ, C92.1Ø, C92.11, C92.4Ø, C92.5Ø, C92.6Ø, C92.AØ, C93.ØØ, C94.ØØ, C95.ØØ
NC 3Ø2[3,4][Ø,3][G,Y][2,3,4]
NC 3Ø2[5,6][Ø,3][G,Y]Ø Only when reported with PDx or SDx of C91.ØØ, C92.ØØ, C92.1Ø, C92.11, C92.4Ø, C92.5Ø, C92.6Ø, C92.AØ, C93.ØØ, C94.ØØ, C95.ØØ
NC 3Ø2[5,6][Ø,3][G,Y]1 Only when reported with PDx or SDx of C9Ø.ØØ or C9Ø.Ø1
♀ 3Ø27[3,7][H,J,K,L,M,N,P,Q,R,S,T,V,W]1

3 Administration
C Indwelling Device
1 Irrigation Definition: Putting in or on a cleansing substance

Body System/Region Character 4	Approach Character 5	Substance Character 6	Qualifier Character 7
Z None	X External	8 Irrigating Substance	Z No Qualifier

Administration

3 **Administration**
E **Physiological Systems and Anatomical Regions**
Ø **Introduction** Definition: Putting in or on a therapeutic, diagnostic, nutritional, physiological, or prophylactic substance except blood or blood products

Body System/Region Character 4	Approach Character 5	Substance Character 6	Qualifier Character 7
Ø Skin and Mucous Membranes	X External	Ø Antineoplastic	5 Other Antineoplastic M Monoclonal Antibody
Ø Skin and Mucous Membranes	X External	2 Anti-infective	8 Oxazolidinones 9 Other Anti-infective
Ø Skin and Mucous Membranes	X External	3 Anti-inflammatory 4 Serum, Toxoid and Vaccine B Anesthetic Agent K Other Diagnostic Substance M Pigment N Analgesics, Hypnotics, Sedatives T Destructive Agent	Z No Qualifier
Ø Skin and Mucous Membranes	X External	G Other Therapeutic Substance	C Other Substance
1 Subcutaneous Tissue	Ø Open	2 Anti-infective	A Anti-Infective Envelope
1 Subcutaneous Tissue	3 Percutaneous	Ø Antineoplastic	5 Other Antineoplastic M Monoclonal Antibody
1 Subcutaneous Tissue	3 Percutaneous	2 Anti-infective	8 Oxazolidinones 9 Other Anti-infective A Anti-Infective Envelope
1 Subcutaneous Tissue	3 Percutaneous	3 Anti-inflammatory 6 Nutritional Substance 7 Electrolytic and Water Balance Substance B Anesthetic Agent H Radioactive Substance K Other Diagnostic Substance N Analgesics, Hypnotics, Sedatives T Destructive Agent	Z No Qualifier
1 Subcutaneous Tissue	3 Percutaneous	4 Serum, Toxoid and Vaccine	Ø Influenza Vaccine Z No Qualifier
1 Subcutaneous Tissue	3 Percutaneous	G Other Therapeutic Substance	C Other Substance
1 Subcutaneous Tissue	3 Percutaneous	V Hormone	G Insulin J Other Hormone
2 Muscle	3 Percutaneous	Ø Antineoplastic	5 Other Antineoplastic M Monoclonal Antibody
2 Muscle	3 Percutaneous	2 Anti-infective	8 Oxazolidinones 9 Other Anti-infective
2 Muscle	3 Percutaneous	3 Anti-inflammatory 6 Nutritional Substance 7 Electrolytic and Water Balance Substance B Anesthetic Agent H Radioactive Substance K Other Diagnostic Substance N Analgesics, Hypnotics, Sedatives T Destructive Agent	Z No Qualifier
2 Muscle	3 Percutaneous	4 Serum, Toxoid and Vaccine	Ø Influenza Vaccine Z No Qualifier
2 Muscle	3 Percutaneous	G Other Therapeutic Substance	C Other Substance
3 Peripheral Vein	Ø Open	Ø Antineoplastic	2 High-dose Interleukin-2 3 Low-dose Interleukin-2 5 Other Antineoplastic M Monoclonal Antibody P Clofarabine
3 Peripheral Vein	Ø Open	1 Thrombolytic	6 Recombinant Human-activated Protein C 7 Other Thrombolytic
3 Peripheral Vein	Ø Open	2 Anti-infective	8 Oxazolidinones 9 Other Anti-infective

3EØ Continued on next page

DRG Non-OR 3EØ3ØØ2
DRG Non-OR 3EØ3Ø17

3 **Administration**
E **Physiological Systems and Anatomical Regions**
Ø **Introduction** Definition: Putting in or on a therapeutic, diagnostic, nutritional, physiological, or prophylactic substance except blood or blood products

3EØ Continued

Body System/Region Character 4	Approach Character 5	Substance Character 6	Qualifier Character 7
3 Peripheral Vein	Ø Open	3 Anti-inflammatory 4 Serum, Toxoid and Vaccine 6 Nutritional Substance 7 Electrolytic and Water Balance Substance F Intracirculatory Anesthetic H Radioactive Substance K Other Diagnostic Substance N Analgesics, Hypnotics, Sedatives P Platelet Inhibitor R Antiarrhythmic T Destructive Agent X Vasopressor	Z No Qualifier
3 Peripheral Vein	Ø Open	G Other Therapeutic Substance	C Other Substance N Blood Brain Barrier Disruption
3 Peripheral Vein	Ø Open	U Pancreatic Islet Cells	Ø Autologous 1 Nonautologous
3 Peripheral Vein	Ø Open	V Hormone	G Insulin H Human B-type Natriuretic Peptide J Other Hormone
3 Peripheral Vein	Ø Open	W Immunotherapeutic	K Immunostimulator L Immunosuppressive
3 Peripheral Vein	3 Percutaneous	Ø Antineoplastic	2 High-dose Interleukin-2 3 Low-dose Interleukin-2 5 Other Antineoplastic M Monoclonal Antibody P Clofarabine
3 Peripheral Vein	3 Percutaneous	1 Thrombolytic	6 Recombinant Human-activated Protein C 7 Other Thrombolytic
3 Peripheral Vein	3 Percutaneous	2 Anti-infective	8 Oxazolidinones 9 Other Anti-infective
3 Peripheral Vein	3 Percutaneous	3 Anti-inflammatory 4 Serum, Toxoid and Vaccine 6 Nutritional Substance 7 Electrolytic and Water Balance Substance F Intracirculatory Anesthetic H Radioactive Substance K Other Diagnostic Substance N Analgesics, Hypnotics, Sedatives P Platelet Inhibitor R Antiarrhythmic T Destructive Agent X Vasopressor	Z No Qualifier
3 Peripheral Vein	3 Percutaneous	G Other Therapeutic Substance	C Other Substance N Blood Brain Barrier Disruption Q Glucarpidase
3 Peripheral Vein	3 Percutaneous	U Pancreatic Islet Cells	Ø Autologous 1 Nonautologous
3 Peripheral Vein	3 Percutaneous	V Hormone	G Insulin H Human B-type Natriuretic Peptide J Other Hormone
3 Peripheral Vein	3 Percutaneous	W Immunotherapeutic	K Immunostimulator L Immunosuppressive
4 Central Vein	Ø Open	Ø Antineoplastic	2 High-dose Interleukin-2 3 Low-dose Interleukin-2 5 Other Antineoplastic M Monoclonal Antibody P Clofarabine

3EØ Continued on next page

Valid OR	3EØ3ØTZ	DRG Non-OR	3EØ3317
DRG Non-OR	3EØ3ØU[Ø,1]	DRG Non-OR	3EØ33U[Ø,1]
DRG Non-OR	3EØ33Ø2	DRG Non-OR	3EØ4ØØ2

3EØ Continued

3 **Administration**
E **Physiological Systems and Anatomical Regions**
Ø **Introduction** Definition: Putting in or on a therapeutic, diagnostic, nutritional, physiological, or prophylactic substance except blood or blood products

Body System/Region Character 4	Approach Character 5	Substance Character 6	Qualifier Character 7
4 Central Vein	Ø Open	1 Thrombolytic	6 Recombinant Human-activated Protein C 7 Other Thrombolytic
4 Central Vein	Ø Open	2 Anti-infective	8 Oxazolidinones 9 Other Anti-infective
4 Central Vein	Ø Open	3 Anti-inflammatory 4 Serum, Toxoid and Vaccine 6 Nutritional Substance 7 Electrolytic and Water Balance Substance F Intracirculatory Anesthetic H Radioactive Substance K Other Diagnostic Substance N Analgesics, Hypnotics, Sedatives P Platelet Inhibitor R Antiarrhythmic T Destructive Agent X Vasopressor	Z No Qualifier
4 Central Vein	Ø Open	G Other Therapeutic Substance	C Other Substance N Blood Brain Barrier Disruption
4 Central Vein	Ø Open	V Hormone	G Insulin H Human B-type Natriuretic Peptide J Other Hormone
4 Central Vein	Ø Open	W Immunotherapeutic	K Immunostimulator L Immunosuppressive
4 Central Vein	3 Percutaneous	Ø Antineoplastic	2 High-dose Interleukin-2 3 Low-dose Interleukin-2 5 Other Antineoplastic M Monoclonal Antibody P Clofarabine
4 Central Vein	3 Percutaneous	1 Thrombolytic	6 Recombinant Human-activated Protein C 7 Other Thrombolytic
4 Central Vein	3 Percutaneous	2 Anti-infective	8 Oxazolidinones 9 Other Anti-infective
4 Central Vein	3 Percutaneous	3 Anti-inflammatory 4 Serum, Toxoid and Vaccine 6 Nutritional Substance 7 Electrolytic and Water Balance Substance F Intracirculatory Anesthetic H Radioactive Substance K Other Diagnostic Substance N Analgesics, Hypnotics, Sedatives P Platelet Inhibitor R Antiarrhythmic T Destructive Agent X Vasopressor	Z No Qualifier
4 Central Vein	3 Percutaneous	G Other Therapeutic Substance	C Other Substance N Blood Brain Barrier Disruption Q Glucarpidase
4 Central Vein	3 Percutaneous	V Hormone	G Insulin H Human B-type Natriuretic Peptide J Other Hormone
4 Central Vein	3 Percutaneous	W Immunotherapeutic	K Immunostimulator L Immunosuppressive
5 Peripheral Artery 6 Central Artery	Ø Open 3 Percutaneous	Ø Antineoplastic	2 High-dose Interleukin-2 3 Low-dose Interleukin-2 5 Other Antineoplastic M Monoclonal Antibody P Clofarabine

3EØ Continued on next page

Valid OR 3EØ4ØTZ
DRG Non-OR 3EØ4Ø17
DRG Non-OR 3EØ43Ø2
DRG Non-OR 3EØ4317
DRG Non-OR 3EØ[5,6][Ø,3]Ø2

3 Administration
E Physiological Systems and Anatomical Regions
Ø Introduction Definition: Putting in or on a therapeutic, diagnostic, nutritional, physiological, or prophylactic substance except blood or blood products

3EØ Continued

Body System/Region Character 4	Approach Character 5	Substance Character 6	Qualifier Character 7
5 Peripheral Artery 6 Central Artery	Ø Open 3 Percutaneous	1 Thrombolytic	6 Recombinant Human-activated Protein C 7 Other Thrombolytic
5 Peripheral Artery 6 Central Artery	Ø Open 3 Percutaneous	2 Anti-infective	8 Oxazolidinones 9 Other Anti-infective
5 Peripheral Artery 6 Central Artery	Ø Open 3 Percutaneous	3 Anti-inflammatory 4 Serum, Toxoid and Vaccine 6 Nutritional Substance 7 Electrolytic and Water Balance Substance F Intracirculatory Anesthetic H Radioactive Substance K Other Diagnostic Substance N Analgesics, Hypnotics, Sedatives P Platelet Inhibitor R Antiarrhythmic T Destructive Agent X Vasopressor	Z No Qualifier
5 Peripheral Artery 6 Central Artery	Ø Open 3 Percutaneous	G Other Therapeutic Substance	C Other Substance N Blood Brain Barrier Disruption
5 Peripheral Artery 6 Central Artery	Ø Open 3 Percutaneous	V Hormone	G Insulin H Human B-type Natriuretic Peptide J Other Hormone
5 Peripheral Artery 6 Central Artery	Ø Open 3 Percutaneous	W Immunotherapeutic	K Immunostimulator L Immunosuppressive
7 Coronary Artery 8 Heart	Ø Open 3 Percutaneous	1 Thrombolytic	6 Recombinant Human-activated Protein C 7 Other Thrombolytic
7 Coronary Artery 8 Heart	Ø Open 3 Percutaneous	G Other Therapeutic Substance	C Other Substance
7 Coronary Artery 8 Heart	Ø Open 3 Percutaneous	K Other Diagnostic Substance P Platelet Inhibitor	Z No Qualifier
7 Coronary Artery 8 Heart	4 Percutaneous Endoscopic	G Other Therapeutic Substance	C Other Substance
9 Nose	3 Percutaneous 7 Via Natural or Artificial Opening X External	Ø Antineoplastic	5 Other Antineoplastic M Monoclonal Antibody
9 Nose	3 Percutaneous 7 Via Natural or Artificial Opening X External	2 Anti-infective	8 Oxazolidinones 9 Other Anti-infective
9 Nose	3 Percutaneous 7 Via Natural or Artificial Opening X External	3 Anti-inflammatory 4 Serum, Toxoid and Vaccine B Anesthetic Agent H Radioactive Substance K Other Diagnostic Substance N Analgesics, Hypnotics, Sedatives T Destructive Agent	Z No Qualifier
9 Nose	3 Percutaneous 7 Via Natural or Artificial Opening X External	G Other Therapeutic Substance	C Other Substance
A Bone Marrow	3 Percutaneous	Ø Antineoplastic	5 Other Antineoplastic M Monoclonal Antibody
A Bone Marrow	3 Percutaneous	G Other Therapeutic Substance	C Other Substance
B Ear	3 Percutaneous 7 Via Natural or Artificial Opening X External	Ø Antineoplastic	4 Liquid Brachytherapy Radioisotope 5 Other Antineoplastic M Monoclonal Antibody
B Ear	3 Percutaneous 7 Via Natural or Artificial Opening X External	2 Anti-infective	8 Oxazolidinones 9 Other Anti-infective

3EØ Continued on next page

DRG Non-OR 3EØ[5,6][Ø,3]17
DRG Non-OR 3EØ8[Ø,3]17

3EØ Continued

3 Administration
E Physiological Systems and Anatomical Regions
Ø Introduction Definition: Putting in or on a therapeutic, diagnostic, nutritional, physiological, or prophylactic substance except blood or blood products

Body System/Region Character 4	Approach Character 5	Substance Character 6	Qualifier Character 7
B Ear	3 Percutaneous 7 Via Natural or Artificial Opening X External	3 Anti-inflammatory B Anesthetic Agent H Radioactive Substance K Other Diagnostic Substance N Analgesics, Hypnotics, Sedatives T Destructive Agent	Z No Qualifier
B Ear	3 Percutaneous 7 Via Natural or Artificial Opening X External	G Other Therapeutic Substance	C Other Substance
C Eye	3 Percutaneous 7 Via Natural or Artificial Opening X External	Ø Antineoplastic	4 Liquid Brachytherapy Radioisotope 5 Other Antineoplastic M Monoclonal Antibody
C Eye	3 Percutaneous 7 Via Natural or Artificial Opening X External	2 Anti-infective	8 Oxazolidinones 9 Other Anti-infective
C Eye	3 Percutaneous 7 Via Natural or Artificial Opening X External	3 Anti-inflammatory B Anesthetic Agent H Radioactive Substance K Other Diagnostic Substance M Pigment N Analgesics, Hypnotics, Sedatives T Destructive Agent	Z No Qualifier
C Eye	3 Percutaneous 7 Via Natural or Artificial Opening X External	G Other Therapeutic Substance	C Other Substance
C Eye	3 Percutaneous 7 Via Natural or Artificial Opening X External	S Gas	F Other Gas
D Mouth and Pharynx	3 Percutaneous 7 Via Natural or Artificial Opening X External	Ø Antineoplastic	4 Liquid Brachytherapy Radioisotope 5 Other Antineoplastic M Monoclonal Antibody
D Mouth and Pharynx	3 Percutaneous 7 Via Natural or Artificial Opening X External	2 Anti-infective	8 Oxazolidinones 9 Other Anti-infective
D Mouth and Pharynx	3 Percutaneous 7 Via Natural or Artificial Opening X External	3 Anti-inflammatory 4 Serum, Toxoid and Vaccine 6 Nutritional Substance 7 Electrolytic and Water Balance Substance B Anesthetic Agent H Radioactive Substance K Other Diagnostic Substance N Analgesics, Hypnotics, Sedatives R Antiarrhythmic T Destructive Agent	Z No Qualifier
D Mouth and Pharynx	3 Percutaneous 7 Via Natural or Artificial Opening X External	G Other Therapeutic Substance	C Other Substance
E Products of Conception ♀ G Upper GI H Lower GI K Genitourinary Tract N Male Reproductive ♂	3 Percutaneous 7 Via Natural or Artificial Opening 8 Via Natural or Artificial Opening Endoscopic	Ø Antineoplastic	4 Liquid Brachytherapy Radioisotope 5 Other Antineoplastic M Monoclonal Antibody
E Products of Conception ♀ G Upper GI H Lower GI K Genitourinary Tract N Male Reproductive ♂	3 Percutaneous 7 Via Natural or Artificial Opening 8 Via Natural or Artificial Opening Endoscopic	2 Anti-infective	8 Oxazolidinones 9 Other Anti-infective

3EØ Continued on next page

♂ All approach, substance, and qualifier values for body system/region (character 4) with this icon
♀ All approach, substance, and qualifier values for body system/region (character 4) with this icon

3 Administration
E Physiological Systems and Anatomical Regions
Ø Introduction Definition: Putting in or on a therapeutic, diagnostic, nutritional, physiological, or prophylactic substance except blood or blood products

3EØ Continued

Body System/Region Character 4	Approach Character 5	Substance Character 6	Qualifier Character 7
E Products of Conception ♀ G Upper GI H Lower GI K Genitourinary Tract N Male Reproductive ♂	3 Percutaneous 7 Via Natural or Artificial Opening 8 Via Natural or Artificial Opening Endoscopic	3 Anti-inflammatory 6 Nutritional Substance 7 Electrolytic and Water Balance Substance B Anesthetic Agent H Radioactive Substance K Other Diagnostic Substance N Analgesics, Hypnotics, Sedatives T Destructive Agent	Z No Qualifier
E Products of Conception ♀ G Upper GI H Lower GI K Genitourinary Tract N Male Reproductive ♂	3 Percutaneous 7 Via Natural or Artificial Opening 8 Via Natural or Artificial Opening Endoscopic	G Other Therapeutic Substance	C Other Substance
E Products of Conception ♀ G Upper GI H Lower GI K Genitourinary Tract N Male Reproductive ♂	3 Percutaneous 7 Via Natural or Artificial Opening 8 Via Natural or Artificial Opening Endoscopic	S Gas	F Other Gas
E Products of Conception ♀ G Upper GI H Lower GI K Genitourinary Tract N Male Reproductive ♂	4 Percutaneous Endoscopic	G Other Therapeutic Substance	C Other Substance
F Respiratory Tract	3 Percutaneous 7 Via Natural or Artificial Opening 8 Via Natural or Artificial Opening Endoscopic	Ø Antineoplastic	4 Liquid Brachytherapy Radioisotope 5 Other Antineoplastic M Monoclonal Antibody
F Respiratory Tract	3 Percutaneous 7 Via Natural or Artificial Opening 8 Via Natural or Artificial Opening Endoscopic	2 Anti-infective	8 Oxazolidinones 9 Other Anti-infective
F Respiratory Tract	3 Percutaneous 7 Via Natural or Artificial Opening 8 Via Natural or Artificial Opening Endoscopic	3 Anti-inflammatory 6 Nutritional Substance 7 Electrolytic and Water Balance Substance B Anesthetic Agent H Radioactive Substance K Other Diagnostic Substance N Analgesics, Hypnotics, Sedatives T Destructive Agent	Z No Qualifier
F Respiratory Tract	3 Percutaneous 7 Via Natural or Artificial Opening 8 Via Natural or Artificial Opening Endoscopic	G Other Therapeutic Substance	C Other Substance
F Respiratory Tract	3 Percutaneous 7 Via Natural or Artificial Opening 8 Via Natural or Artificial Opening Endoscopic	S Gas	D Nitric Oxide F Other Gas
F Respiratory Tract	4 Percutaneous Endoscopic	G Other Therapeutic Substance	C Other Substance
J Biliary and Pancreatic Tract	3 Percutaneous 7 Via Natural or Artificial Opening 8 Via Natural or Artificial Opening Endoscopic	Ø Antineoplastic	4 Liquid Brachytherapy Radioisotope 5 Other Antineoplastic M Monoclonal Antibody

3EØ Continued on next page

♂ All approach, substance, and qualifier values for body system/region (character 4) with this icon
♀ All approach, substance, and qualifier values for body system/region (character 4) with this icon

3EØ Continued

3 Administration
E Physiological Systems and Anatomical Regions
Ø Introduction Definition: Putting in or on a therapeutic, diagnostic, nutritional, physiological, or prophylactic substance except blood or blood products

Body System/Region Character 4	Approach Character 5	Substance Character 6	Qualifier Character 7
J Biliary and Pancreatic Tract	3 Percutaneous 7 Via Natural or Artificial Opening 8 Via Natural or Artificial Opening Endoscopic	2 Anti-infective	8 Oxazolidinones 9 Other Anti-infective
J Biliary and Pancreatic Tract	3 Percutaneous 7 Via Natural or Artificial Opening 8 Via Natural or Artificial Opening Endoscopic	3 Anti-inflammatory 6 Nutritional Substance 7 Electrolytic and Water Balance Substance B Anesthetic Agent H Radioactive Substance K Other Diagnostic Substance N Analgesics, Hypnotics, Sedatives T Destructive Agent	Z No Qualifier
J Biliary and Pancreatic Tract	3 Percutaneous 7 Via Natural or Artificial Opening 8 Via Natural or Artificial Opening Endoscopic	G Other Therapeutic Substance	C Other Substance
J Biliary and Pancreatic Tract	3 Percutaneous 7 Via Natural or Artificial Opening 8 Via Natural or Artificial Opening Endoscopic	S Gas	F Other Gas
J Biliary and Pancreatic Tract	3 Percutaneous 7 Via Natural or Artificial Opening 8 Via Natural or Artificial Opening Endoscopic	U Pancreatic Islet Cells	Ø Autologous 1 Nonautologous
J Biliary and Pancreatic Tract	4 Percutaneous Endoscopic	G Other Therapeutic Substance	C Other Substance
L Pleural Cavity M Peritoneal Cavity	Ø Open	5 Adhesion Barrier	Z No Qualifier
L Pleural Cavity M Peritoneal Cavity	3 Percutaneous	Ø Antineoplastic	4 Liquid Brachytherapy Radioisotope 5 Other Antineoplastic M Monoclonal Antibody
L Pleural Cavity M Peritoneal Cavity	3 Percutaneous	2 Anti-infective	8 Oxazolidinones 9 Other Anti-infective
L Pleural Cavity M Peritoneal Cavity	3 Percutaneous	3 Anti-inflammatory 5 Adhesion Barrier 6 Nutritional Substance 7 Electrolytic and Water Balance Substance B Anesthetic Agent H Radioactive Substance K Other Diagnostic Substance N Analgesics, Hypnotics, Sedatives T Destructive Agent	Z No Qualifier
L Pleural Cavity M Peritoneal Cavity	3 Percutaneous	G Other Therapeutic Substance	C Other Substance
L Pleural Cavity M Peritoneal Cavity	3 Percutaneous	S Gas	F Other Gas
L Pleural Cavity M Peritoneal Cavity	4 Percutaneous Endoscopic	5 Adhesion Barrier	Z No Qualifier
L Pleural Cavity M Peritoneal Cavity	4 Percutaneous Endoscopic	G Other Therapeutic Substance	C Other Substance
L Pleural Cavity M Peritoneal Cavity	7 Via Natural or Artificial Opening	Ø Antineoplastic	4 Liquid Brachytherapy Radioisotope 5 Other Antineoplastic M Monoclonal Antibody
L Pleural Cavity M Peritoneal Cavity	7 Via Natural or Artificial Opening	S Gas	F Other Gas
P Female Reproductive ♀	Ø Open	5 Adhesion Barrier	Z No Qualifier
P Female Reproductive ♀	3 Percutaneous	Ø Antineoplastic	4 Liquid Brachytherapy Radioisotope 5 Other Antineoplastic M Monoclonal Antibody
P Female Reproductive ♀	3 Percutaneous	2 Anti-infective	8 Oxazolidinones 9 Other Anti-infective

3EØ Continued on next page

DRG Non-OR 3EØJ[3,7,8]U[Ø,1]
♀ All approach, substance, and qualifier values for body system/region (character 4) with this icon

3 **Administration**
E **Physiological Systems and Anatomical Regions**
Ø **Introduction** Definition: Putting in or on a therapeutic, diagnostic, nutritional, physiological, or prophylactic substance except blood or blood products

3EØ Continued

Body System/Region Character 4	Approach Character 5	Substance Character 6	Qualifier Character 7
P Female Reproductive ♀	3 Percutaneous	3 Anti-inflammatory 5 Adhesion Barrier 6 Nutritional Substance 7 Electrolytic and Water Balance Substance B Anesthetic Agent H Radioactive Substance K Other Diagnostic Substance L Sperm N Analgesics, Hypnotics, Sedatives T Destructive Agent V Hormone	Z No Qualifier
P Female Reproductive ♀	3 Percutaneous	G Other Therapeutic Substance	C Other Substance
P Female Reproductive ♀	3 Percutaneous	Q Fertilized Ovum	Ø Autologous 1 Nonautologous
P Female Reproductive ♀	3 Percutaneous	S Gas	F Other Gas
P Female Reproductive ♀	4 Percutaneous Endoscopic	5 Adhesion Barrier	Z No Qualifier
P Female Reproductive ♀	4 Percutaneous Endoscopic	G Other Therapeutic Substance	C Other Substance
P Female Reproductive ♀	7 Via Natural or Artificial Opening	Ø Antineoplastic	4 Liquid Brachytherapy Radioisotope 5 Other Antineoplastic M Monoclonal Antibody
P Female Reproductive ♀	7 Via Natural or Artificial Opening	2 Anti-infective	8 Oxazolidinones 9 Other Anti-infective
P Female Reproductive ♀	7 Via Natural or Artificial Opening	3 Anti-inflammatory 6 Nutritional Substance 7 Electrolytic and Water Balance Substance B Anesthetic Agent H Radioactive Substance K Other Diagnostic Substance L Sperm N Analgesics, Hypnotics, Sedatives T Destructive Agent V Hormone	Z No Qualifier
P Female Reproductive ♀	7 Via Natural or Artificial Opening	G Other Therapeutic Substance	C Other Substance
P Female Reproductive ♀	7 Via Natural or Artificial Opening	Q Fertilized Ovum	Ø Autologous 1 Nonautologous
P Female Reproductive ♀	7 Via Natural or Artificial Opening	S Gas	F Other Gas
P Female Reproductive ♀	8 Via Natural or Artificial Opening Endoscopic	Ø Antineoplastic	4 Liquid Brachytherapy Radioisotope 5 Other Antineoplastic M Monoclonal Antibody
P Female Reproductive ♀	8 Via Natural or Artificial Opening Endoscopic	2 Anti-infective	8 Oxazolidinones 9 Other Anit-infection
P Female Reproductive ♀	8 Via Natural or Artificial Opening Endoscopic	3 Anti-inflammatory 6 Nutritional Substance 7 Electrolytic and Water Balance Substance B Anesthetic Agent H Radioactive Substance K Other Diagnostic Substance N Analgesics, Hypnotics, Sedative T Destructive Agent	Z No Qualifier
P Female Reproductive ♀	8 Via Natural or Artificial Opening Endoscopic	G Other Therapeutic Substance	C Other Substance
P Female Reproductive ♀	8 Via Natural or Artificial Opening Endoscopic	S Gas	F Other Gas
Q Cranial Cavity and Brain	Ø Open 3 Percutaneous	Ø Antineoplastic	4 Liquid Brachytherapy Radioisotope 5 Other Antineoplastic M Monoclonal Antibody
Q Cranial Cavity and Brain	Ø Open 3 Percutaneous	2 Anti-infective	8 Oxazolidinones 9 Other Anti-infective

3EØ Continued on next page

Valid OR 3EØP3Q[Ø,1]
Valid OR 3EØP7Q[Ø,1]
DRG Non-OR 3EØQ[Ø,3]Ø5
♀ All approach, substance, and qualifier values for body system/region (character 4) with this icon

3EØ Continued

3 **Administration**
E **Physiological Systems and Anatomical Regions**
Ø **Introduction** Definition: Putting in or on a therapeutic, diagnostic, nutritional, physiological, or prophylactic substance except blood or blood products

Body System/Region Character 4	Approach Character 5	Substance Character 6	Qualifier Character 7
Q Cranial Cavity and Brain	Ø Open 3 Percutaneous	3 Anti-inflammatory 6 Nutritional Substance 7 Electrolytic and Water Balance Substance A Stem Cells, Embryonic B Anesthetic Agent H Radioactive Substance K Other Diagnostic Substance N Analgesics, Hypnotics, Sedatives T Destructive Agent	Z No Qualifier
Q Cranial Cavity and Brain	Ø Open 3 Percutaneous	E Stem Cells, Somatic	Ø Autologous 1 Nonautologous
Q Cranial Cavity and Brain	Ø Open 3 Percutaneous	G Other Therapeutic Substance	C Other Substance
Q Cranial Cavity and Brain	Ø Open 3 Percutaneous	S Gas	F Other Gas
Q Cranial Cavity and Brain	7 Via Natural or Artificial Opening	Ø Antineoplastic	4 Liquid Brachytherapy Radioisotope 5 Other Antineoplastic M Monoclonal Antibody
Q Cranial Cavity and Brain	7 Via Natural or Artificial Opening	S Gas	F Other Gas
R Spinal Canal	Ø Open	A Stem Cells, Embryonic	Z No Qualifier
R Spinal Canal	Ø Open	E Stem Cells, Somatic	Ø Autologous 1 Nonautologous
R Spinal Canal	3 Percutaneous	Ø Antineoplastic	2 High-dose Interleukin-2 3 Low-dose Interleukin-2 4 Liquid Brachytherapy Radioisotope 5 Other Antineoplastic M Monoclonal Antibody
R Spinal Canal	3 Percutaneous	2 Anti-infective	8 Oxazolidinones 9 Other Anti-infective
R Spinal Canal	3 Percutaneous	3 Anti-inflammatory 6 Nutritional Substance 7 Electrolytic and Water Balance Substance A Stem Cells, Embryonic B Anesthetic Agent H Radioactive Substance K Other Diagnostic Substance N Analgesics, Hypnotics, Sedatives T Destructive Agent	Z No Qualifier
R Spinal Canal	3 Percutaneous	E Stem Cells, Somatic	Ø Autologous 1 Nonautologous
R Spinal Canal	3 Percutaneous	G Other Therapeutic Substance	C Other Substance
R Spinal Canal	3 Percutaneous	S Gas	F Other Gas
R Spinal Canal	7 Via Natural or Artificial Opening	S Gas	F Other Gas
S Epidural Space	3 Percutaneous	Ø Antineoplastic	2 High-dose Interleukin-2 3 Low-dose Interleukin-2 4 Liquid Brachytherapy Radioisotope 5 Other Antineoplastic M Monoclonal Antibody
S Epidural Space	3 Percutaneous	2 Anti-infective	8 Oxazolidinones 9 Other Anti-infective
S Epidural Space	3 Percutaneous	3 Anti-inflammatory 6 Nutritional Substance 7 Electrolytic and Water Balance Substance B Anesthetic Agent H Radioactive Substance K Other Diagnostic Substance N Analgesics, Hypnotics, Sedatives T Destructive Agent	Z No Qualifier

3EØ Continued on next page

DRG Non-OR 3EØQ7Ø5
DRG Non-OR 3EØR3Ø2
DRG Non-OR 3EØS3Ø2

3 Administration
E Physiological Systems and Anatomical Regions
Ø Introduction Definition: Putting in or on a therapeutic, diagnostic, nutritional, physiological, or prophylactic substance except blood or blood products

3EØ Continued

Body System/Region Character 4	Approach Character 5	Substance Character 6	Qualifier Character 7
S Epidural Space	3 Percutaneous	G Other Therapeutic Substance	C Other Substance
S Epidural Space	3 Percutaneous	S Gas	F Other Gas
S Epidural Space	7 Via Natural or Artificial Opening	S Gas	F Other Gas
T Peripheral Nerves and Plexi X Cranial Nerves	3 Percutaneous	3 Anti-inflammatory B Anesthetic Agent T Destructive Agent	Z No Qualifier
T Peripheral Nerves and Plexi X Cranial Nerves	3 Percutaneous	G Other Therapeutic Substance	C Other Substance
U Joints	Ø Open	2 Anti-infective	8 Oxazolidinones 9 Other Anti-infective
U Joints	Ø Open	G Other Therapeutic Substance	B Recombinant Bone Morphogenetic Protein
U Joints	3 Percutaneous	Ø Antineoplastic	4 Liquid Brachytherapy Radioisotope 5 Other Antineoplastic M Monoclonal Antibody
U Joints	3 Percutaneous	2 Anti-infective	8 Oxazolidinones 9 Other Anti-infective
U Joints	3 Percutaneous	3 Anti-inflammatory 6 Nutritional Substance 7 Electrolytic and Water Balance Substance B Anesthetic Agent H Radioactive Substance K Other Diagnostic Substance N Analgesics, Hypnotics, Sedatives T Destructive Agent	Z No Qualifier
U Joints	3 Percutaneous	G Other Therapeutic Substance	B Recombinant Bone Morphogenetic Protein C Other Substance
U Joints	3 Percutaneous	S Gas	F Other Gas
U Joints	4 Percutaneous Endoscopic	G Other Therapeutic Substance	C Other Substance
V Bones	Ø Open	G Other Therapeutic Substance	B Recombinant Bone Morphogenetic Protein
V Bones	3 Percutaneous	Ø Antineoplastic	5 Other Antineoplastic M Monoclonal Antibody
V Bones	3 Percutaneous	2 Anti-infective	8 Oxazolidinones 9 Other Anti-infective
V Bones	3 Percutaneous	3 Anti-inflammatory 6 Nutritional Substance 7 Electrolytic and Water Balance Substance B Anesthetic Agent H Radioactive Substance K Other Diagnostic Substance N Analgesics, Hypnotics, Sedatives T Destructive Agent	Z No Qualifier
V Bones	3 Percutaneous	G Other Therapeutic Substance	B Recombinant Bone Morphogenetic Protein C Other Substance
W Lymphatics	3 Percutaneous	Ø Antineoplastic	5 Other Antineoplastic M Monoclonal Antibody
W Lymphatics	3 Percutaneous	2 Anti-infective	8 Oxazolidinones 9 Other Anti-infective
W Lymphatics	3 Percutaneous	3 Anti-inflammatory 6 Nutritional Substance 7 Electrolytic and Water Balance Substance B Anesthetic Agent H Radioactive Substance K Other Diagnostic Substance N Analgesics, Hypnotics, Sedatives T Destructive Agent	Z No Qualifier

3EØ Continued on next page

3EØ Continued

3 Administration
E Physiological Systems and Anatomical Regions
Ø Introduction Definition: Putting in or on a therapeutic, diagnostic, nutritional, physiological, or prophylactic substance except blood or blood products

Body System/Region Character 4	Approach Character 5	Substance Character 6	Qualifier Character 7
W Lymphatics	**3** Percutaneous	**G** Other Therapeutic Substance	**C** Other Substance
Y Pericardial Cavity	**3** Percutaneous	**Ø** Antineoplastic	**4** Liquid Brachytherapy Radioisotope **5** Other Antineoplastic **M** Monoclonal Antibody
Y Pericardial Cavity	**3** Percutaneous	**2** Anti-infective	**8** Oxazolidinones **9** Other Anti-infective
Y Pericardial Cavity	**3** Percutaneous	**3** Anti-inflammatory **6** Nutritional Substance **7** Electrolytic and Water Balance Substance **B** Anesthetic Agent **H** Radioactive Substance **K** Other Diagnostic Substance **N** Analgesics, Hypnotics, Sedatives **T** Destructive Agent	**Z** No Qualifier
Y Pericardial Cavity	**3** Percutaneous	**G** Other Therapeutic Substance	**C** Other Substance
Y Pericardial Cavity	**3** Percutaneous	**S** Gas	**F** Other Gas
Y Pericardial Cavity	**4** Percutaneous Endoscopic	**G** Other Therapeutic Substance	**C** Other Substance
Y Pericardial Cavity	**7** Via Natural or Artificial Opening	**Ø** Antineoplastic	**4** Liquid Brachytherapy Radioisotope **5** Other Antineoplastic **M** Monoclonal Antibody
Y Pericardial Cavity	**7** Via Natural or Artificial Opening	**S** Gas	**F** Other Gas

3 Administration
E Physiological Systems and Anatomical Regions
1 Irrigation Definition: Putting in or on a cleansing substance

Body System/Region Character 4	Approach Character 5	Substance Character 6	Qualifier Character 7
Ø Skin and Mucous Membranes **C** Eye	**3** Percutaneous **X** External	**8** Irrigating Substance	**X** Diagnostic **Z** No Qualifier
9 Nose **B** Ear **F** Respiratory Tract **G** Upper GI **H** Lower GI **J** Biliary and Pancreatic Tract **K** Genitourinary Tract **N** Male Reproductive ♂ **P** Female Reproductive ♀	**3** Percutaneous **7** Via Natural or Artificial Opening **8** Via Natural or Artificial Opening Endoscopic	**8** Irrigating Substance	**X** Diagnostic **Z** No Qualifier
L Pleural Cavity **Q** Cranial Cavity and Brain **R** Spinal Canal **S** Epidural Space **U** Joints **Y** Pericardial Cavity	**3** Percutaneous	**8** Irrigating Substance	**X** Diagnostic **Z** No Qualifier
M Peritoneal Cavity	**3** Percutaneous	**8** Irrigating Substance	**X** Diagnostic **Z** No Qualifier
M Peritoneal Cavity	**3** Percutaneous	**9** Dialysate	**Z** No Qualifier

♂ 3E1N[3,7,8]8[X,Z]
♀ 3E1P[3,7,8]8[X,Z]

Measurement and Monitoring 4AØ–4BØ

Character Meanings

This Character Meaning table is provided as a guide to assist the user in the identification of character members that may be found in this section of code tables. It **SHOULD NOT** be used to build a PCS code.

A: Physiological Systems

Operation–Character 3	Body System–Character 4	Approach–Character 5	Function/Device–Character 6	Qualifier–Character 7
Ø Measurement	Ø Central Nervous	Ø Open	Ø Acuity	Ø Central
1 Monitoring	1 Peripheral Nervous	3 Percutaneous	1 Capacity	1 Peripheral
	2 Cardiac	4 Percutaneous Endoscopic	2 Conductivity	2 Portal
	3 Arterial	7 Via Natural or Artificial Opening	3 Contractility	3 Pulmonary
	4 Venous	8 Via Natural or Artificial Opening Endoscopic	4 Electrical Activity	4 Stress
	5 Circulatory	X External	5 Flow	5 Ambulatory
	6 Lymphatic		6 Metabolism	6 Right Heart
	7 Visual		7 Mobility	7 Left Heart
	8 Olfactory		8 Motility	8 Bilateral
	9 Respiratory		9 Output	9 Sensory
	B Gastrointestinal		B Pressure	A Guidance
	C Biliary		C Rate	B Motor
	D Urinary		D Resistance	C Coronary
	F Musculoskeletal		F Rhythm	D Intracranial
	G Skin and Breast		G Secretion	F Other Thoracic
	H Products of Conception, Cardiac		H Sound	G Intraoperative
	J Products of Conception, Nervous		J Pulse	H Indocyanine Green Dye
	Z None		K Temperature	Z No Qualifier
			L Volume	
			M Total Activity	
			N Sampling and Pressure	
			P Action Currents	
			Q Sleep	
			R Saturation	
			S Vascular Perfusion	

B: Physiological Devices

Operation–Character 3	Body System–Character 4	Approach–Character 5	Function/Device–Character 6	Qualifier–Character 7
Ø Measurement	Ø Central Nervous	X External	S Pacemaker	Z No Qualifier
	1 Peripheral Nervous		T Defibrillator	
	2 Cardiac		V Stimulator	
	9 Respiratory			
	F Musculoskeletal			

AHA Coding Clinic for table 4AØ
2018, 1Q, 12 Percutaneous balloon valvuloplasty & cardiac catheterization with ventriculogram
2016, 3Q, 37 Fractional flow reserve
2015, 3Q, 29 Approach value for esophageal electrophysiology study

AHA Coding Clinic for table 4A1
2016, 4Q, 114 Fluorescence vascular angiography
2016, 2Q, 29 Decompressive craniectomy with cryopreservation and storage of bone flap
2016, 2Q, 33 Monitoring of arterial pressure & pulse
2015, 3Q, 35 Swan Ganz catheterization
2015, 2Q, 14 Intraoperative EMG monitoring via endotracheal tube
2015, 1Q, 26 Intraoperative monitoring using Sentio MMG®
2014, 4Q, 28 Removal and replacement of displaced growing rods

4 Measurement and Monitoring
A Physiological Systems
Ø Measurement Definition: Determining the level of a physiological or physical function at a point in time

Body System Character 4	Approach Character 5	Function/Device Character 6	Qualifier Character 7
Ø Central Nervous	Ø Open	2 Conductivity 4 Electrical Activity B Pressure	Z No Qualifier
Ø Central Nervous	3 Percutaneous 7 Via Natural or Artificial Opening 8 Via Natural or Artificial Opening Endoscopic	4 Electrical Activity	Z No Qualifier
Ø Central Nervous	3 Percutaneous 7 Via Natural or Artificial Opening 8 Via Natural or Artificial Opening Endoscopic	B Pressure K Temperature R Saturation	D Intracranial
Ø Central Nervous	X External	2 Conductivity 4 Electrical Activity	Z No Qualifier
1 Peripheral Nervous	Ø Open 3 Percutaneous 7 Via Natural or Artificial Opening 8 Via Natural or Artificial Opening Endoscopic X External	2 Conductivity	9 Sensory B Motor
1 Peripheral Nervous	Ø Open 3 Percutaneous 7 Via Natural or Artificial Opening 8 Via Natural or Artificial Opening Endoscopic X External	4 Electrical Activity	Z No Qualifier
2 Cardiac	Ø Open 3 Percutaneous 7 Via Natural or Artificial Opening 8 Via Natural or Artificial Opening Endoscopic	4 Electrical Activity 9 Output C Rate F Rhythm H Sound P Action Currents	Z No Qualifier
2 Cardiac	Ø Open 3 Percutaneous 7 Via Natural or Artificial Opening 8 Via Natural or Artificial Opening Endoscopic	N Sampling and Pressure	6 Right Heart 7 Left Heart 8 Bilateral
2 Cardiac	X External	4 Electrical Activity	A Guidance Z No Qualifier
2 Cardiac	X External	9 Output C Rate F Rhythm H Sound P Action Currents	Z No Qualifier
2 Cardiac	X External	M Total Activity	4 Stress
3 Arterial	Ø Open 3 Percutaneous	5 Flow J Pulse	1 Peripheral 3 Pulmonary C Coronary
3 Arterial	Ø Open 3 Percutaneous	B Pressure	1 Peripheral 3 Pulmonary C Coronary F Other Thoracic
3 Arterial	Ø Open 3 Percutaneous	H Sound R Saturation	1 Peripheral
3 Arterial	X External	5 Flow B Pressure H Sound J Pulse R Saturation	1 Peripheral

4AØ Continued on next page

DRG Non-OR 4AØ2[3,7,8]FZ
DRG Non-OR 4AØ2[Ø,3,7,8]N[6,7,8]

4 Measurement and Monitoring
A Physiological Systems
Ø Measurement Definition: Determining the level of a physiological or physical function at a point in time

4AØ Continued

Body System Character 4	Approach Character 5	Function/Device Character 6	Qualifier Character 7
4 Venous	**Ø** Open **3** Percutaneous	**5** Flow **B** Pressure **J** Pulse	**Ø** Central **1** Peripheral **2** Portal **3** Pulmonary
4 Venous	**Ø** Open **3** Percutaneous	**R** Saturation	**1** Peripheral
4 Venous	**X** External	**5** Flow **B** Pressure **J** Pulse **R** Saturation	**1** Peripheral
5 Circulatory	**X** External	**L** Volume	**Z** No Qualifier
6 Lymphatic	**Ø** Open **3** Percutaneous **7** Via Natural or Artificial Opening **8** Via Natural or Artificial Opening Endoscopic	**5** Flow **B** Pressure	**Z** No Qualifier
7 Visual	**X** External	**Ø** Acuity **7** Mobility **B** Pressure	**Z** No Qualifier
8 Olfactory	**X** External	**Ø** Acuity	**Z** No Qualifier
9 Respiratory	**7** Via Natural or Artificial Opening **8** Via Natural or Artificial Opening Endoscopic **X** External	**1** Capacity **5** Flow **C** Rate **D** Resistance **L** Volume **M** Total Activity	**Z** No Qualifier
B Gastrointestinal	**7** Via Natural or Artificial Opening **8** Via Natural or Artificial Opening Endoscopic	**8** Motility **B** Pressure **G** Secretion	**Z** No Qualifier
C Biliary	**3** Percutaneous **4** Percutaneous Endoscopic **7** Via Natural or Artificial Opening **8** Via Natural or Artificial Opening Endoscopic	**5** Flow **B** Pressure	**Z** No Qualifier
D Urinary	**7** Via Natural or Artificial Opening **8** Via Natural or Artificial Opening Endoscopic	**3** Contractility **5** Flow **B** Pressure **D** Resistance **L** Volume	**Z** No Qualifier
F Musculoskeletal	**3** Percutaneous **X** External	**3** Contractility	**Z** No Qualifier
H Products of Conception, Cardiac ♀	**7** Via Natural or Artificial Opening **8** Via Natural or Artificial Opening Endoscopic **X** External	**4** Electrical Activity **C** Rate **F** Rhythm **H** Sound	**Z** No Qualifier
J Products of Conception, Nervous ♀	**7** Via Natural or Artificial Opening **8** Via Natural or Artificial Opening Endoscopic **X** External	**2** Conductivity **4** Electrical Activity **B** Pressure	**Z** No Qualifier
Z None	**7** Via Natural or Artificial Opening	**6** Metabolism **K** Temperature	**Z** No Qualifier
Z None	**X** External	**6** Metabolism **K** Temperature **Q** Sleep	**Z** No Qualifier

Valid OR	4AØ6Ø[5,B]Z	♀	4AØH[7,8,X][4,C,F,H]Z
Valid OR	4AØC4[5,B]Z	♀	4AØJ[7,8,X][2,4,B]Z

Measurement and Monitoring

4AØ–4AØ

Measurement and Monitoring

4 Measurement and Monitoring
A Physiological Systems
1 Monitoring Definition: Determining the level of a physiological or physical function repetitively over a period of time

Body System Character 4	Approach Character 5	Function/Device Character 6	Qualifier Character 7
Ø Central Nervous	Ø Open	2 Conductivity B Pressure	Z No Qualifier
Ø Central Nervous	Ø Open	4 Electrical Activity	G Intraoperative Z No Qualifier
Ø Central Nervous	3 Percutaneous 7 Via Natural or Artificial Opening 8 Via Natural or Artificial Opening Endoscopic	4 Electrical Activity	G Intraoperative Z No Qualifier
Ø Central Nervous	3 Percutaneous 7 Via Natural or Artificial Opening 8 Via Natural or Artificial Opening Endoscopic	B Pressure K Temperature R Saturation	D Intracranial
Ø Central Nervous	X External	2 Conductivity	Z No Qualifier
Ø Central Nervous	X External	4 Electrical Activity	G Intraoperative Z No Qualifier
1 Peripheral Nervous	Ø Open 3 Percutaneous 7 Via Natural or Artificial Opening 8 Via Natural or Artificial Opening Endoscopic X External	2 Conductivity	9 Sensory B Motor
1 Peripheral Nervous	Ø Open 3 Percutaneous 7 Via Natural or Artificial Opening 8 Via Natural or Artificial Opening Endoscopic X External	4 Electrical Activity	G Intraoperative Z No Qualifier
2 Cardiac	Ø Open 3 Percutaneous 7 Via Natural or Artificial Opening 8 Via Natural or Artificial Opening Endoscopic	4 Electrical Activity 9 Output C Rate F Rhythm H Sound	Z No Qualifier
2 Cardiac	X External	4 Electrical Activity	5 Ambulatory Z No Qualifier
2 Cardiac	X External	9 Output C Rate F Rhythm H Sound	Z No Qualifier
2 Cardiac	X External	M Total Activity	4 Stress
2 Cardiac	X External	S Vascular Perfusion	H Indocyanine Green Dye
3 Arterial	Ø Open 3 Percutaneous	5 Flow B Pressure J Pulse	1 Peripheral 3 Pulmonary C Coronary
3 Arterial	Ø Open 3 Percutaneous	H Sound R Saturation	1 Peripheral
3 Arterial	X External	5 Flow B Pressure H Sound J Pulse R Saturation	1 Peripheral
4 Venous	Ø Open 3 Percutaneous	5 Flow B Pressure J Pulse	Ø Central 1 Peripheral 2 Portal 3 Pulmonary
4 Venous	Ø Open 3 Percutaneous	R Saturation	Ø Central 2 Portal 3 Pulmonary
4 Venous	X External	5 Flow B Pressure J Pulse	1 Peripheral
6 Lymphatic	Ø Open 3 Percutaneous 7 Via Natural or Artificial Opening 8 Via Natural or Artificial Opening Endoscopic	5 Flow B Pressure	Z No Qualifier

4A1 Continued on next page

Valid OR 4A16Ø[5,B]Z

4A1 Continued

4 Measurement and Monitoring
A Physiological Systems
1 Monitoring Definition: Determining the level of a physiological or physical function repetitively over a period of time

Body System Character 4	Approach Character 5	Function/Device Character 6	Qualifier Character 7
9 Respiratory	**7** Via Natural or Artificial Opening **X** External	**1** Capacity **5** Flow **C** Rate **D** Resistance **L** Volume	**Z** No Qualifier
B Gastrointestinal	**7** Via Natural or Artificial Opening **8** Via Natural or Artificial Opening Endoscopic	**8** Motility **B** Pressure **G** Secretion	**Z** No Qualifier
B Gastrointestinal	**X** External	**S** Vascular Perfusion	**H** Indocyanine Green Dye
D Urinary	**7** Via Natural or Artificial Opening **8** Via Natural or Artificial Opening Endoscopic	**3** Contractility **5** Flow **B** Pressure **D** Resistance **L** Volume	**Z** No Qualifier
G Skin and Breast	**X** External	**S** Vascular Perfusion	**H** Indocyanine Green Dye
H Products of Conception, Cardiac ♀	**7** Via Natural or Artificial Opening **8** Via Natural or Artificial Opening Endoscopic **X** External	**4** Electrical Activity **C** Rate **F** Rhythm **H** Sound	**Z** No Qualifier
J Products of Conception, Nervous ♀	**7** Via Natural or Artificial Opening **8** Via Natural or Artificial Opening Endoscopic **X** External	**2** Conductivity **4** Electrical Activity **B** Pressure	**Z** No Qualifier
Z None	**7** Via Natural or Artificial Opening	**K** Temperature	**Z** No Qualifier
Z None	**X** External	**K** Temperature **Q** Sleep	**Z** No Qualifier

♀ 4A1H[7,8,X][4,C,F,H]Z
♀ 4A1J[7,8,X][2,4,B]Z

4 Measurement and Monitoring
B Physiological Devices
Ø Measurement Definition: Determining the level of a physiological or physical function at a point in time

Body System Character 4	Approach Character 5	Function/Device Character 6	Qualifier Character 7
Ø Central Nervous **1** Peripheral Nervous **F** Musculoskeletal	**X** External	**V** Stimulator	**Z** No Qualifier
2 Cardiac	**X** External	**S** Pacemaker **T** Defibrillator	**Z** No Qualifier
9 Respiratory	**X** External	**S** Pacemaker	**Z** No Qualifier

Extracorporeal or Systemic Assistance and Performance 5AØ–5A2

Character Meanings

This Character Meaning table is provided as a guide to assist the user in the identification of character members that may be found in this section of code tables. It **SHOULD NOT** be used to build a PCS code.

A: Physiological Systems

Operation–Character 3		Body System–Character 4		Duration–Character 5		Function–Character 6		Qualifier–Character 7	
Ø	Assistance	2	Cardiac	Ø	Single	Ø	Filtration	Ø	Balloon Pump
1	Performance	5	Circulatory	1	Intermittent	1	Output	1	Hyperbaric
2	Restoration	9	Respiratory	2	Continuous	2	Oxygenation	2	Manual
		C	Biliary	3	Less than 24 Consecutive Hours	3	Pacing	4	Nonmechanical
		D	Urinary	4	24-96 Consecutive Hours	4	Rhythm	5	Pulsatile Compression
				5	Greater than 96 Consecutive Hours	5	Ventilation	6	Other Pump
				6	Multiple			7	Continuous Positive Airway Pressure
				7	Intermittent, Less than 6 Hours per Day			8	Intermittent Positive Airway Pressure
				8	Prolonged Intermittent, 6-18 hours per Day			9	Continuous Negative Airway Pressure
				9	Continuous, Greater than 18 hours per Day			B	Intermittent Negative Airway Pressure
								C	Supersaturated
								D	Impeller Pump
								F	Membrane, Central
								G	Membrane, Peripheral Veno-arterial
								H	Membrane, Peripheral Veno-venous
								Z	No Qualifier

AHA Coding Clinic for table 5AØ

2018, 2Q, 3-5 Intra-aortic balloon pump
2017, 4Q, 43-44 Insertion of external heart assist devices
2017, 3Q, 18 Intra-aortic balloon pump removal
2017, 1Q, 10-11 External heart assist device
2017, 1Q, 29 Newborn resuscitation using positive pressure ventilation
2017, 1Q, 29 Newborn noninvasive ventilation
2016, 4Q, 137-139 Heart assist device systems
2014, 4Q, 9 Mechanical ventilation
2014, 3Q, 19 Ablation of ventricular tachycardia with Impella® support
2013, 3Q, 18 Heart transplant surgery

AHA Coding Clinic for table 5A1

2018, 1Q, 13 Mechanical ventilation using patient's equipment
2017, 4Q, 71-73 Hemodialysis and renal replacement therapy
2017, 3Q, 7 Senning procedure (arterial switch)
2017, 1Q, 19 Norwood Sano procedure
2016, 1Q, 27 Aortocoronary bypass graft utilizing Y-graft
2016, 1Q, 28 Extracorporeal liver assist device
2016, 1Q, 29 Duration of hemodialysis
2015, 4Q, 22-24 Congenital heart corrective procedures
2014, 4Q, 3-10 Mechanical ventilation
2014, 4Q, 11-15 Sequencing of mechanical ventilation with other procedures
2014, 3Q, 16 Repair of Tetralogy of Fallot
2014, 3Q, 20 MAZE procedure performed with coronary artery bypass graft
2014, 1Q, 10 Repair of thoracic aortic aneurysm & coronary artery bypass graft
2013, 3Q, 18 Heart transplant surgery

5 Extracorporeal or Systemic Assistance and Performance
A Physiological Systems
Ø Assistance Definition: Taking over a portion of a physiological function by extracorporeal means

Body System Character 4	Duration Character 5	Function Character 6	Qualifier Character 7
2 Cardiac	1 Intermittent 2 Continuous	1 Output	Ø Balloon Pump 5 Pulsatile Compression 6 Other Pump D Impeller Pump
5 Circulatory	1 Intermittent 2 Continuous	2 Oxygenation	1 Hyperbaric C Supersaturated
9 Respiratory	2 Continuous	Ø Filtration	Z No Qualifier
9 Respiratory	3 Less than 24 Consecutive Hours 4 24-96 Consecutive Hours 5 Greater than 96 Consecutive Hours	5 Ventilation	7 Continuous Positive Airway Pressure 8 Intermittent Positive Airway Pressure 9 Continuous Negative Airway Pressure B Intermittent Negative Airway Pressure Z No Qualifier

Valid OR 5AØ2[1,2]1[Ø,6,D]

5 Extracorporeal or Systemic Assistance and Performance
A Physiological Systems
1 Performance Definition: Completely taking over a physiological function by extracorporeal means

Body System Character 4	Duration Character 5	Function Character 6	Qualifier Character 7
2 Cardiac	Ø Single	1 Output	2 Manual
2 Cardiac	1 Intermittent	3 Pacing	Z No Qualifier
2 Cardiac	2 Continuous	1 Output 3 Pacing	Z No Qualifier
5 Circulatory	2 Continuous	2 Oxygenation	F Membrane, Central G Membrane, Peripheral Veno-arterial H Membrane, Peripheral Veno-venous
9 Respiratory	Ø Single	5 Ventilation	4 Nonmechanical
9 Respiratory	3 Less than 24 Consecutive Hours 4 24-96 Consecutive Hours 5 Greater than 96 Consecutive Hours	5 Ventilation	Z No Qualifier
C Biliary	Ø Single 6 Multiple	Ø Filtration	Z No Qualifier
D Urinary	7 Intermittent, Less than 6 Hours per day 8 Prolonged Intermittent, 6-18 Hours per day 9 Continuous, Greater than 18 Hours per day	Ø Filtration	Z No Qualifier

Valid OR 5A1522[F,G,H]
DRG Non-OR 5A19[3,4,5]5Z
Note: For code 5A1955Z, length of stay must be > 4 consecutive days.

5 Extracorporeal or Systemic Assistance and Performance
A Physiological Systems
2 Restoration Definition: Returning, or attempting to return, a physiological function to its original state by extracorporeal means.

Body System Character 4	Duration Character 5	Function Character 6	Qualifier Character 7
2 Cardiac	Ø Single	4 Rhythm	Z No Qualifier

Extracorporeal or Systemic Therapies 6AØ–6AB

Character Meanings

This Character Meaning table is provided as a guide to assist the user in the identification of character members that may be found in this section of code tables. It **SHOULD NOT** be used to build a PCS code.

A: Physiological Systems

Operation–Character 3		Body System–Character 4		Duration–Character 5		Qualifier–Character 6		Qualifier–Character 7	
Ø	Atmospheric Control	Ø	Skin	Ø	Single	B	Donor Organ	Ø	Erythrocytes
1	Decompression	1	Urinary	1	Multiple	Z	No Qualifier	1	Leukocytes
2	Electromagnetic Therapy	2	Central Nervous					2	Platelets
3	Hyperthermia	3	Musculoskeletal					3	Plasma
4	Hypothermia	5	Circulatory					4	Head and Neck Vessels
5	Pheresis	B	Respiratory System					5	Heart
6	Phototherapy	F	Hepatobiliary System and Pancreas					6	Peripheral Vessels
7	Ultrasound Therapy	T	Urinary System					7	Other Vessels
8	Ultraviolet Light Therapy	Z	None					T	Stem Cells, Cord Blood
9	Shock Wave Therapy							V	Stem Cells, Hematopoietic
B	Perfusion							Z	No Qualifier

AHA Coding Clinic for table 6A7
2014, 4Q, 19 Ultrasound accelerated thrombolysis

AHA Coding Clinic for table 6AB
2016, 4Q, 115 Donor organ perfusion

6 Extracorporeal or Systemic Therapies
A Physiological Systems
Ø Atmospheric Control Definition: Extracorporeal control of atmospheric pressure and composition

Body System Character 4	Duration Character 5	Qualifier Character 6	Qualifier Character 7
Z None	Ø Single 1 Multiple	Z No Qualifier	Z No Qualifier

6 Extracorporeal or Systemic Therapies
A Physiological Systems
1 Decompression Definition: Extracorporeal elimination of undissolved gas from body fluids

Body System Character 4	Duration Character 5	Qualifier Character 6	Qualifier Character 7
5 Circulatory	Ø Single 1 Multiple	Z No Qualifier	Z No Qualifier

6 Extracorporeal or Systemic Therapies
A Physiological Systems
2 Electromagnetic Therapy Definition: Extracorporeal treatment by electromagnetic rays

Body System Character 4	Duration Character 5	Qualifier Character 6	Qualifier Character 7
1 Urinary 2 Central Nervous	Ø Single 1 Multiple	Z No Qualifier	Z No Qualifier

6 Extracorporeal or Systemic Therapies
A Physiological Systems
3 Hyperthermia Definition: Extracorporeal raising of body temperature

Body System Character 4	Duration Character 5	Qualifier Character 6	Qualifier Character 7
Z None	Ø Single 1 Multiple	Z No Qualifier	Z No Qualifier

6 Extracorporeal or Systemic Therapies
A Physiological Systems
4 Hypothermia Definition: Extracorporeal lowering of body temperature

Body System Character 4	Duration Character 5	Qualifier Character 6	Qualifier Character 7
Z None	Ø Single 1 Multiple	Z No Qualifier	Z No Qualifier

6 Extracorporeal or Systemic Therapies
A Physiological Systems
5 Pheresis Definition: Extracorporeal separation of blood products

Body System Character 4	Duration Character 5	Qualifier Character 6	Qualifier Character 7
5 Circulatory	Ø Single 1 Multiple	Z No Qualifier	Ø Erythrocytes 1 Leukocytes 2 Platelets 3 Plasma T Stem Cells, Cord Blood V Stem Cells, Hematopoietic

6 Extracorporeal or Systemic Therapies
A Physiological Systems
6 Phototherapy Definition: Extracorporeal treatment by light rays

Body System Character 4	Duration Character 5	Qualifier Character 6	Qualifier Character 7
Ø Skin 5 Circulatory	Ø Single 1 Multiple	Z No Qualifier	Z No Qualifier

6 Extracorporeal or Systemic Therapies
A Physiological Systems
7 Ultrasound Therapy Definition: Extracorporeal treatment by ultrasound

Body System Character 4	Duration Character 5	Qualifier Character 6	Qualifier Character 7
5 Circulatory	Ø Single 1 Multiple	Z No Qualifier	4 Head and Neck Vessels 5 Heart 6 Peripheral Vessels 7 Other Vessels Z No Qualifier

6 Extracorporeal or Systemic Therapies
A Physiological Systems
8 Ultraviolet Light Therapy Definition: Extracorporeal treatment by ultraviolet light

Body System Character 4	Duration Character 5	Qualifier Character 6	Qualifier Character 7
Ø Skin	Ø Single 1 Multiple	Z No Qualifier	Z No Qualifier

6 Extracorporeal or Systemic Therapies
A Physiological Systems
9 Shock Wave Therapy Definition: Extracorporeal treatment by shock waves

Body System Character 4	Duration Character 5	Qualifier Character 6	Qualifier Character 7
3 Musculoskeletal	Ø Single 1 Multiple	Z No Qualifier	Z No Qualifier

6 Extracorporeal or Systemic Therapies
A Physiological Systems
B Perfusion Definition: Extracorporeal treatment by diffusion of therapeutic fluid

Body System Character 4	Duration Character 5	Qualifier Character 6	Qualifier Character 7
5 Circulatory B Respiratory System F Hepatobiliary System and Pancreas T Urinary System	Ø Single	B Donor Organ	Z No Qualifier

Osteopathic 7WØ

Character Meanings

This Character Meaning table is provided as a guide to assist the user in the identification of character members that may be found in this section of code tables. It **SHOULD NOT** be used to build a PCS code.

W: Anatomical Regions

Operation–Character 3	Body Region–Character 4	Approach–Character 5	Method–Character 6	Qualifier–Character 7
Ø Treatment	Ø Head	X External	Ø Articulatory-Raising	Z None
	1 Cervical		1 Fascial Release	
	2 Thoracic		2 General Mobilization	
	3 Lumbar		3 High Velocity-Low Amplitude	
	4 Sacrum		4 Indirect	
	5 Pelvis		5 Low Velocity-High Amplitude	
	6 Lower Extremities		6 Lymphatic Pump	
	7 Upper Extremities		7 Muscle Energy-Isometric	
	8 Rib Cage		8 Muscle Energy-Isotonic	
	9 Abdomen		9 Other Method	

7 Osteopathic
W Anatomical Regions
Ø Treatment Definition: Manual treatment to eliminate or alleviate somatic dysfunction and related disorders

Body Region Character 4	Approach Character 5	Method Character 6	Qualifier Character 7
Ø Head **1** Cervical **2** Thoracic **3** Lumbar **4** Sacrum **5** Pelvis **6** Lower Extremities **7** Upper Extremities **8** Rib Cage **9** Abdomen	**X** External	**Ø** Articulatory-Raising **1** Fascial Release **2** General Mobilization **3** High Velocity-Low Amplitude **4** Indirect **5** Low Velocity-High Amplitude **6** Lymphatic Pump **7** Muscle Energy-Isometric **8** Muscle Energy-Isotonic **9** Other Method	**Z** None

Other Procedures 8CØ–8EØ

Character Meanings

This Character Meaning table is provided as a guide to assist the user in the identification of character members that may be found in this section of code tables. It **SHOULD NOT** be used to build a PCS code.

C: Indwelling Devices

Operation–Character 3	Body Region–Character 4	Approach–Character 5	Method–Character 6	Qualifier–Character 7
Ø Other procedures	1 Nervous System	X External	6 Collection	J Cerebrospinal Fluid
	2 Circulatory System			K Blood
				L Other Fluid

E: Physiological Systems and Anatomical Regions

Operation–Character 3	Body Region–Character 4	Approach–Character 5	Method–Character 6	Qualifier–Character 7
Ø Other Procedures	1 Nervous System	Ø Open	Ø Acupuncture	Ø Anesthesia
	2 Circulatory System	3 Percutaneous	1 Therapeutic Massage	1 In Vitro Fertilization
	9 Head and Neck Region	4 Percutaneous Endoscopic	6 Collection	2 Breast Milk
	H Integumentary System and Breast	7 Via Natural or Artificial Opening	B Computer Assisted Procedure	3 Sperm
	K Musculoskeletal System	8 Via Natural or Artificial Opening Endoscopic	C Robotic Assisted Procedure	4 Yoga Therapy
	U Female Reproductive System	X External	D Near Infrared Spectroscopy	5 Meditation
	V Male Reproductive System		Y Other Method	6 Isolation
	W Trunk Region			7 Examination
	X Upper Extremity			8 Suture Removal
	Y Lower Extremity			9 Piercing
	Z None			C Prostate
				D Rectum
				F With Fluoroscopy
				G With Computerized Tomography
				H With Magnetic Resonance Imaging
				Z No Qualifier

AHA Coding Clinic for table 8EØ

2015, 1Q, 33 Robotic-assisted laparoscopic hysterectomy converted to open procedure
2014, 4Q, 33 Radical prostatectomy

8 Other Procedures
C Indwelling Device
Ø Other Procedures Definition: Methodologies which attempt to remediate or cure a disorder or disease

Body Region Character 4	Approach Character 5	Method Character 6	Qualifier Character 7
1 Nervous System	X External	6 Collection	J Cerebrospinal Fluid L Other Fluid
2 Circulatory System	X External	6 Collection	K Blood L Other Fluid

8 Other Procedures
E Physiological Systems and Anatomical Regions
Ø Other Procedures Definition: Methodologies which attempt to remediate or cure a disorder or disease

Body Region Character 4	Approach Character 5	Method Character 6	Qualifier Character 7
1 Nervous System U Female Reproductive System ♀	X External	Y Other Method	7 Examination
2 Circulatory System	3 Percutaneous	D Near Infrared Spectroscopy	Z No Qualifier
9 Head and Neck Region W Trunk Region	Ø Open 3 Percutaneous 4 Percutaneous Endoscopic 7 Via Natural or Artificial Opening 8 Via Natural or Artificial Opening Endoscopic	C Robotic Assisted Procedure	Z No Qualifier
9 Head and Neck Region W Trunk Region	X External	B Computer Assisted Procedure	F With Fluoroscopy G With Computerized Tomography H With Magnetic Resonance Imaging Z No Qualifier
9 Head and Neck Region W Trunk Region	X External	C Robotic Assisted Procedure	Z No Qualifier
9 Head and Neck Region W Trunk Region	X External	Y Other Method	8 Suture Removal
H Integumentary System and Breast	3 Percutaneous	Ø Acupuncture	Ø Anesthesia Z No Qualifier
H Integumentary System and Breast ♀	X External	6 Collection	2 Breast Milk
H Integumentary System and Breast	X External	Y Other Method	9 Piercing
K Musculoskeletal System	X External	1 Therapeutic Massage	Z No Qualifier
K Musculoskeletal System	X External	Y Other Method	7 Examination
V Male Reproductive System ♂	X External	1 Therapeutic Massage	C Prostate D Rectum
V Male Reproductive System ♂	X External	6 Collection	3 Sperm
X Upper Extremity Y Lower Extremity	Ø Open 3 Percutaneous 4 Percutaneous Endoscopic	C Robotic Assisted Procedure	Z No Qualifier
X Upper Extremity Y Lower Extremity	X External	B Computer Assisted Procedure	F With Fluoroscopy G With Computerized Tomography H With Magnetic Resonance Imaging Z No Qualifier
X Upper Extremity Y Lower Extremity	X External	C Robotic Assisted Procedure	Z No Qualifier
X Upper Extremity Y Lower Extremity	X External	Y Other Method	8 Suture Removal
Z None	X External	Y Other Method	1 In Vitro Fertilization 4 Yoga Therapy 5 Meditation 6 Isolation

♂ 8EØVX1C
♂ 8EØVX63
♀ 8EØUXY7
♀ 8EØHX62

Chiropractic 9WB

Character Meanings

This Character Meaning table is provided as a guide to assist the user in the identification of character members that may be found in this section of code tables. It **SHOULD NOT** be used to build a PCS code.

W: Anatomical Regions

Operation–Character 3	Body Region–Character 4	Approach–Character 5	Method–Character 6	Qualifier–Character 7
B Manipulation	Ø Head	X External	B Non-Manual	Z None
	1 Cervical		C Indirect Visceral	
	2 Thoracic		D Extra-Articular	
	3 Lumbar		F Direct Visceral	
	4 Sacrum		G Long Lever Specific Contact	
	5 Pelvis		H Short Lever Specific Contact	
	6 Lower Extremities		J Long and Short Lever Specific Contact	
	7 Upper Extremities		K Mechanically Assisted	
	8 Rib Cage		L Other Method	
	9 Abdomen			

9 Chiropractic
W Anatomical Regions
B Manipulation Definition: Manual procedure that involves a directed thrust to move a joint past the physiological range of motion, without exceeding the anatomical limit

Body Region Character 4	Approach Character 5	Method Character 6	Qualifier Character 7
Ø Head **1** Cervical **2** Thoracic **3** Lumbar **4** Sacrum **5** Pelvis **6** Lower Extremities **7** Upper Extremities **8** Rib Cage **9** Abdomen	**X** External	**B** Non-Manual **C** Indirect Visceral **D** Extra-Articular **F** Direct Visceral **G** Long Lever Specific Contact **H** Short Lever Specific Contact **J** Long and Short Lever Specific Contact **K** Mechanically Assisted **L** Other Method	**Z** None

Imaging BØØ–BY4

Character Meanings

This Character Meaning table is provided as a guide to assist the user in the identification of character members that may be found in this section of code tables. It **SHOULD NOT** be used to build a PCS code.

Body System–Character 2	Type–Character 3	Body Part–Character 4	Contrast–Character 5	Qualifier–Character 6	Qualifier–Character 7
Ø Central Nervous System	Ø Plain Radiography	See next page	Ø High Osmolar	Ø Unenhanced and Enhanced	Ø Intraoperative
2 Heart	1 Fluoroscopy		1 Low Osmolar	1 Laser	1 Densitometry
3 Upper Arteries	2 Computerized Tomography (CT Scan)		Y Other Contrast	2 Intravascular Optical Coherence	3 Intravascular
4 Lower Arteries	3 Magnetic Resonance Imaging (MRI)		Z None	Z None	4 Transesophageal
5 Veins	4 Ultrasonography				A Guidance
7 Lymphatic System					Z None
8 Eye					
9 Ear, Nose, Mouth and Throat					
B Respiratory System					
D Gastrointestinal System					
F Hepatobiliary System and Pancreas					
G Endocrine System					
H Skin, Subcutaneous Tissue and Breast					
L Connective Tissue					
N Skull and Facial Bones					
P Non-Axial Upper Bones					
Q Non-Axial Lower Bones					
R Axial Skeleton, Except Skull and Facial Bones					
T Urinary System					
U Female Reproductive System					
V Male Reproductive System					
W Anatomical Regions					
Y Fetus and Obstetrical					

Continued on next page

Body Part—Character 4 Meanings

Continued from previous page

Body System–Character 2	Body Part– Character 4	
Ø Central Nervous System	Ø Brain	9 Sella Turcica/Pituitary Gland
	7 Cisterna	B Spinal Cord
	8 Cerebral Ventricle(s)	C Acoustic Nerves
2 Heart	Ø Coronary Artery, Single	7 Internal Mammary Bypass Graft, Right
	1 Coronary Arteries, Multiple	8 Internal Mammary Bypass Graft, Left
	2 Coronary Artery Bypass Graft, Single	B Heart with Aorta
	3 Coronary Artery Bypass Grafts, Multiple	C Pericardium
	4 Heart, Right	D Pediatric Heart
	5 Heart, Left	F Bypass Graft, Other
	6 Heart, Right and Left	
3 Upper Arteries	Ø Thoracic Aorta	G Vertebral Arteries, Bilateral
	1 Brachiocephalic-Subclavian Artery, Right	H Upper Extremity Arteries, Right
	2 Subclavian Artery, Left	J Upper Extremity Arteries, Left
	3 Common Carotid Artery, Right	K Upper Extremity Arteries, Bilateral
	4 Common Carotid Artery, Left	L Intercostal and Bronchial Arteries
	5 Common Carotid Arteries, Bilateral	M Spinal Arteries
	6 Internal Carotid Artery, Right	N Upper Arteries, Other
	7 Internal Carotid Artery, Left	P Thoraco-Abdominal Aorta
	8 Internal Carotid Arteries, Bilateral	Q Cervico-Cerebral Arch
	9 External Carotid Artery, Right	R Intracranial Arteries
	B External Carotid Artery, Left	S Pulmonary Artery, Right
	C External Carotid Arteries, Bilateral	T Pulmonary Artery, Left
	D Vertebral Artery, Right	U Pulmonary Trunk
	F Vertebral Artery, Left	V Ophthalmic Arteries
4 Lower Arteries	Ø Abdominal Aorta	C Pelvic Arteries
	1 Celiac Artery	D Aorta and Bilateral Lower Extremity Arteries
	2 Hepatic Artery	F Lower Extremity Arteries, Right
	3 Splenic Arteries	G Lower Extremity Arteries, Left
	4 Superior Mesenteric Artery	H Lower Extremity Arteries, Bilateral
	5 Inferior Mesenteric Artery	J Lower Arteries, Other
	6 Renal Artery, Right	K Celiac and Mesenteric Arteries
	7 Renal Artery, Left	L Femoral Artery
	8 Renal Arteries, Bilateral	M Renal Artery Transplant
	9 Lumbar Arteries	N Penile Arteries
	B Intra-Abdominal Arteries, Other	
5 Veins	Ø Epidural Veins	G Pelvic (Iliac) Veins, Left
	1 Cerebral and Cerebellar Veins	H Pelvic (Iliac) Veins, Bilateral
	2 Intracranial Sinuses	J Renal Vein, Right
	3 Jugular Veins, Right	K Renal Vein, Left
	4 Jugular Veins, Left	L Renal Veins, Bilateral
	5 Jugular Veins, Bilateral	M Upper Extremity Veins, Right
	6 Subclavian Vein, Right	N Upper Extremity Veins, Left
	7 Subclavian Vein, Left	P Upper Extremity Veins, Bilateral
	8 Superior Vena Cava	Q Pulmonary Vein, Right
	9 Inferior Vena Cava	R Pulmonary Vein, Left
	B Lower Extremity Veins, Right	S Pulmonary Veins, Bilateral
	C Lower Extremity Veins, Left	T Portal and Splanchnic Veins
	D Lower Extremity Veins, Bilateral	V Veins, Other
	F Pelvic (Iliac) Veins, Right	W Dialysis Shunt/Fistula
7 Lymphatic System	Ø Abdominal/Retroperitoneal Lymphatics, Unilateral	7 Upper Extremity Lymphatics, Bilateral
	1 Abdominal/Retroperitoneal Lymphatics, Bilateral	8 Lower Extremity Lymphatics, Right
	4 Lymphatics, Head and Neck	9 Lower Extremity Lymphatics, Left
	5 Upper Extremity Lymphatics, Right	B Lower Extremity Lymphatics, Bilateral
	6 Upper Extremity Lymphatics, Left	C Lymphatics, Pelvic
8 Eye	Ø Lacrimal Duct, Right	4 Optic Foramina, Left
	1 Lacrimal Duct, Left	5 Eye, Right
	2 Lacrimal Ducts, Bilateral	6 Eye, Left
	3 Optic Foramina, Right	7 Eyes, Bilateral
9 Ear, Nose, Mouth and Throat	Ø Ear	B Salivary Gland, Right
	2 Paranasal Sinuses	C Salivary Gland, Left
	4 Parotid Gland, Right	D Salivary Glands, Bilateral
	5 Parotid Gland, Left	F Nasopharynx/Oropharynx
	6 Parotid Glands, Bilateral	G Pharynx and Epiglottis
	7 Submandibular Gland, Right	H Mastoids
	8 Submandibular Gland, Left	J Larynx
	9 Submandibular Glands, Bilateral	
B Respiratory System	2 Lung, Right	9 Tracheobronchial Trees, Bilateral
	3 Lung, Left	B Pleura
	4 Lungs, Bilateral	C Mediastinum
	6 Diaphragm	D Upper Airways
	7 Tracheobronchial Tree, Right	F Trachea/Airways
	8 Tracheobronchial Tree, Left	G Lung Apices

Continued on next page

Continued from previous page

Body System–Character 2	Body Part–Character 4	
D Gastrointestinal System	1 Esophagus 2 Stomach 3 Small Bowel 4 Colon 5 Upper GI 6 Upper GI and Small Bowel	7 Gastrointestinal Tract 8 Appendix 9 Duodenum B Mouth/Oropharynx C Rectum
F Hepatobiliary System and Pancreas	Ø Bile Ducts 1 Biliary and Pancreatic Ducts 2 Gallbladder 3 Gallbladder and Bile Ducts 4 Gallbladder, Bile Ducts and Pancreatic Ducts	5 Liver 6 Liver and Spleen 7 Pancreas 8 Pancreatic Ducts C Hepatobiliary System, All
G Endocrine System	Ø Adrenal Gland, Right 1 Adrenal Gland, Left 2 Adrenal Glands, Bilateral	3 Parathyroid Glands 4 Thyroid Gland
H Skin, Subcutaneous Tissue and Breast	Ø Breast, Right 1 Breast, Left 2 Breasts, Bilateral 3 Single Mammary Duct, Right 4 Single Mammary Duct, Left 5 Multiple Mammary Ducts, Right 6 Multiple Mammary Ducts, Left 7 Extremity, Upper 8 Extremity, Lower	9 Abdominal Wall B Chest Wall C Head and Neck D Subcutaneous Tissue, Head/Neck F Subcutaneous Tissue, Upper Extremity G Subcutaneous Tissue, Thorax H Subcutaneous Tissue, Abdomen and Pelvis J Subcutaneous Tissue, Lower Extremity
L Connective Tissue	Ø Connective Tissue, Upper Extremity 1 Connective Tissue, Lower Extremity	2 Tendons, Upper Extremity 3 Tendons, Lower Extremity
N Skull and Facial Bones	Ø Skull 1 Orbit, Right 2 Orbit, Left 3 Orbits, Bilateral 4 Nasal Bones 5 Facial Bones 6 Mandible 7 Temporomandibular Joint, Right 8 Temporomandibular Joint, Left	9 Temporomandibular Joints, Bilateral B Zygomatic Arch, Right C Zygomatic Arch, Left D Zygomatic Arches, Bilateral F Temporal Bones G Tooth, Single H Teeth, Multiple J Teeth, All
P Non-Axial Upper Bones	Ø Sternoclavicular Joint, Right 1 Sternoclavicular Joint, Left 2 Sternoclavicular Joints, Bilateral 3 Acromioclavicular Joints, Bilateral 4 Clavicle, Right 5 Clavicle, Left 6 Scapula, Right 7 Scapula, Left 8 Shoulder, Right 9 Shoulder, Left A Humerus, Right B Humerus, Left C Hand/Finger Joint, Right D Hand/Finger Joint, Left E Upper Arm, Right F Upper Arm, Left G Elbow, Right	H Elbow, Left J Forearm, Right K Forearm, Left L Wrist, Right M Wrist, Left N Hand, Right P Hand, Left Q Hands and Wrists, Bilateral R Finger(s), Right S Finger(s), Left T Upper Extremity, Right U Upper Extremity, Left V Upper Extremities, Bilateral W Thorax X Ribs, Right Y Ribs, Left
Q Non-Axial Lower Bones	Ø Hip, Right 1 Hip, Left 2 Hips, Bilateral 3 Femur, Right 4 Femur, Left 7 Knee, Right 8 Knee, Left 9 Knees, Bilateral B Tibia/Fibula, Right C Tibia/Fibula, Left D Lower Leg, Right F Lower Leg, Left G Ankle, Right	H Ankle, Left J Calcaneus, Right K Calcaneus, Left L Foot, Right M Foot, Left P Toe(s), Right Q Toe(s), Left R Lower Extremity, Right S Lower Extremity, Left V Patella, Right W Patella, Left X Foot/Toe Joint, Right Y Foot/Toe Joint, Left
R Axial Skeleton, Except Skull and Facial Bones	Ø Cervical Spine 1 Cervical Disc(s) 2 Thoracic Disc(s) 3 Lumbar Disc(s) 4 Cervical Facet Joint(s) 5 Thoracic Facet Joint(s) 6 Lumbar Facet Joint(s) 7 Thoracic Spine	8 Thoracolumbar Joint 9 Lumbar Spine B Lumbosacral Joint C Pelvis D Sacroiliac Joints F Sacrum and Coccyx G Whole Spine H Sternum

Continued on next page

Continued from previous page

Body System–Character 2	Body Part– Character 4	
T Urinary System	Ø Bladder 1 Kidney, Right 2 Kidney, Left 3 Kidneys, Bilateral 4 Kidneys, Ureters and Bladder 5 Urethra 6 Ureter, Right 7 Ureter, Left	8 Ureters, Bilateral 9 Kidney Transplant B Bladder and Urethra C Ileal Diversion Loop D Kidney, Ureter and Bladder, Right F Kidney, Ureter and Bladder, Left G Ileal Loop, Ureters and Kidneys J Kidneys and Bladder
U Female Reproductive System	Ø Fallopian Tube, Right 1 Fallopian Tube, Left 2 Fallopian Tubes, Bilateral 3 Ovary, Right 4 Ovary, Left 5 Ovaries, Bilateral	6 Uterus 8 Uterus and Fallopian Tubes 9 Vagina B Pregnant Uterus C Uterus and Ovaries
V Male Reproductive System	Ø Corpora Cavernosa 1 Epididymis, Right 2 Epididymis, Left 3 Prostate 4 Scrotum 5 Testicle, Right	6 Testicle, Left 7 Testicles, Bilateral 8 Vasa Vasorum 9 Prostate and Seminal Vesicles B Penis
W Anatomical Regions	Ø Abdomen 1 Abdomen and Pelvis 3 Chest 4 Chest and Abdomen 5 Chest, Abdomen and Pelvis 8 Head 9 Head and Neck B Long Bones, All C Lower Extremity	F Neck G Pelvic Region H Retroperitoneum J Upper Extremity K Whole Body L Whole Skeleton M Whole Body, Infant P Brachial Plexus
Y Fetus and Obstetrical	Ø Fetal Head 1 Fetal Heart 2 Fetal Thorax 3 Fetal Abdomen 4 Fetal Spine 5 Fetal Extremities 6 Whole Fetus 7 Fetal Umbilical Cord	8 Placenta 9 First Trimester, Single Fetus B First Trimester, Multiple Gestation C Second Trimester, Single Fetus D Second Trimester, Multiple Gestation F Third Trimester, Single Fetus G Third Trimester, Multiple Gestation

AHA Coding Clinic for table B21
2018, 1Q, 12 Percutaneous balloon valvuloplasty & cardiac catheterization with ventriculogram
2016, 3Q, 36 Type of contrast medium for angiography (high osmolar, low osmolar, and other)

AHA Coding Clinic for table B41
2015, 3Q, 9 Aborted endovascular stenting of superficial femoral artery

AHA Coding Clinic for table B51
2015, 4Q, 30 Vascular access devices

AHA Coding Clinic for table BF4
2014, 3Q, 15 Drainage of pancreatic pseudocyst

B Imaging
Ø Central Nervous System
Ø Plain Radiography Definition: Planar display of an image developed from the capture of external ionizing radiation on photographic or photoconductive plate

Body Part Character 4	Contrast Character 5	Qualifier Character 6	Qualifier Character 7
B Spinal Cord	Ø High Osmolar 1 Low Osmolar Y Other Contrast Z None	Z None	Z None

B Imaging
Ø Central Nervous System
1 Fluoroscopy Definition: Single plane or bi-plane real time display of an image developed from the capture of external ionizing radioation on a fluorescent screen. The image may also be stored by either digital or analog means.

Body Part Character 4	Contrast Character 5	Qualifier Character 6	Qualifier Character 7
B Spinal Cord	Ø High Osmolar 1 Low Osmolar Y Other Contrast Z None	Z None	Z None

B Imaging
Ø Central Nervous System
2 Computerized Tomography (CT Scan) Definition: Computer reformatted digital display of multiplanar images developed from the capture of multiple exposures of external ionizing radiation

Body Part Character 4	Contrast Character 5	Qualifier Character 6	Qualifier Character 7
Ø Brain 7 Cisterna 8 Cerebral Ventricle(s) 9 Sella Turcica/Pituitary Gland B Spinal Cord	Ø High Osmolar 1 Low Osmolar Y Other Contrast	Ø Unenhanced and Enhanced Z None	Z None
Ø Brain 7 Cisterna 8 Cerebral Ventricle(s) 9 Sella Turcica/Pituitary Gland B Spinal Cord	Z None	Z None	Z None

B Imaging
Ø Central Nervous System
3 Magnetic Resonance Imaging (MRI) Definition: Computer reformatted digital display of multiplanar images developed from the capture of radio-frequency signals emitted by nuclei in a body site excited within a magnetic field

Body Part Character 4	Contrast Character 5	Qualifier Character 6	Qualifier Character 7
Ø Brain 9 Sella Turcica/Pituitary Gland B Spinal Cord C Acoustic Nerves	Y Other Contrast	Ø Unenhanced and Enhanced Z None	Z None
Ø Brain 9 Sella Turcica/Pituitary Gland B Spinal Cord C Acoustic Nerves	Z None	Z None	Z None

B Imaging
Ø Central Nervous System
4 Ultrasonography Definition: Real time display of images of anatomy or flow information developed from the capture of relected and attenuated high frequency sound waves

Body Part Character 4	Contrast Character 5	Qualifier Character 6	Qualifier Character 7
Ø Brain B Spinal Cord	Z None	Z None	Z None

B Imaging
2 Heart
Ø Plain Radiography Definition: Planar display of an image developed from the capture of external ionizing radiation on photographic or photoconductive plate

Body Part Character 4	Contrast Character 5	Qualifier Character 6	Qualifier Character 7
Ø Coronary Artery, Single 1 Coronary Arteries, Multiple 2 Coronary Artery Bypass Graft, Single 3 Coronary Artery Bypass Grafts, Multiple 4 Heart, Right 5 Heart, Left 6 Heart, Right and Left 7 Internal Mammary Bypass Graft, Right 8 Internal Mammary Bypass Graft, Left F Bypass Graft, Other	Ø High Osmolar 1 Low Osmolar Y Other Contrast	Z None	Z None

DRG Non-OR All body part, contrast, and qualifier values

B Imaging
2 Heart
1 Fluoroscopy Definition: Single plane or bi-plane real time display of an image developed from the capture of external ionizing radioation on a fluorescent screen. The image may also be stored by either digital or analog means.

Body Part Character 4	Contrast Character 5	Qualifier Character 6	Qualifier Character 7
Ø Coronary Artery, Single 1 Coronary Arteries, Multiple 2 Coronary Artery Bypass Graft, Single 3 Coronary Artery Bypass Grafts, Multiple	Ø High Osmolar 1 Low Osmolar Y Other Contrast	1 Laser	Ø Intraoperative
Ø Coronary Artery, Single 1 Coronary Arteries, Multiple 2 Coronary Artery Bypass Graft, Single 3 Coronary Artery Bypass Grafts, Multiple	Ø High Osmolar 1 Low Osmolar Y Other Contrast	Z None	Z None
4 Heart, Right 5 Heart, Left 6 Heart, Right and Left 7 Internal Mammary Bypass Graft, Right 8 Internal Mammary Bypass Graft, Left F Bypass Graft, Other	Ø High Osmolar 1 Low Osmolar Y Other Contrast	Z None	Z None

DRG Non-OR All body part, contrast, and qualifier values

B Imaging
2 Heart
2 Computerized Tomography (CT Scan) Definition: Computer reformatted digital display of multiplanar images developed from the capture of multiple exposures of external ionizing radiation

Body Part Character 4	Contrast Character 5	Qualifier Character 6	Qualifier Character 7
1 Coronary Arteries, Multiple 3 Coronary Artery Bypass Grafts, Multiple 6 Heart, Right and Left	Ø High Osmolar 1 Low Osmolar Y Other Contrast	Ø Unenhanced and Enhanced Z None	Z None
1 Coronary Arteries, Multiple 3 Coronary Artery Bypass Grafts, Multiple 6 Heart, Right and Left	Z None	2 Intravascular Optical Coherence Z None	Z None

B Imaging
2 Heart
3 Magnetic Resonance Imaging (MRI) Definition: Computer reformatted digital display of multiplanar images developed from the capture of radio-frequency signals emitted by nuclei in a body site excited within a magnetic field

Body Part Character 4	Contrast Character 5	Qualifier Character 6	Qualifier Character 7
1 Coronary Arteries, Multiple 3 Coronary Artery Bypass Grafts, Multiple 6 Heart, Right and Left	Y Other Contrast	Ø Unenhanced and Enhanced Z None	Z None
1 Coronary Arteries, Multiple 3 Coronary Artery Bypass Grafts, Multiple 6 Heart, Right and Left	Z None	Z None	Z None

B Imaging
2 Heart
4 Ultrasonography Definition: Real time display of images of anatomy or flow information developed from the capture of relected and attenuated high frequency sound waves

Body Part Character 4	Contrast Character 5	Qualifier Character 6	Qualifier Character 7
Ø Coronary Artery, Single 1 Coronary Arteries, Multiple 4 Heart, Right 5 Heart, Left 6 Heart, Right and Left B Heart with Aorta C Pericardium D Pediatric Heart	Y Other Contrast	Z None	Z None
Ø Coronary Artery, Single 1 Coronary Arteries, Multiple 4 Heart, Right 5 Heart, Left 6 Heart, Right and Left B Heart with Aorta C Pericardium D Pediatric Heart	Z None	Z None	3 Intravascular 4 Transesophageal Z None

B Imaging
3 Upper Arteries
Ø Plain Radiography Definition: Planar display of an image developed from the capture of external ionizing radiation on photographic or photoconductive plate

Body Part Character 4	Contrast Character 5	Qualifier Character 6	Qualifier Character 7
Ø Thoracic Aorta 1 Brachiocephalic-Subclavian Artery, Right 2 Subclavian Artery, Left 3 Common Carotid Artery, Right 4 Common Carotid Artery, Left 5 Common Carotid Arteries, Bilateral 6 Internal Carotid Artery, Right 7 Internal Carotid Artery, Left 8 Internal Carotid Arteries, Bilateral 9 External Carotid Artery, Right B External Carotid Artery, Left C External Carotid Arteries, Bilateral D Vertebral Artery, Right F Vertebral Artery, Left G Vertebral Arteries, Bilateral H Upper Extremity Arteries, Right J Upper Extremity Arteries, Left K Upper Extremity Arteries, Bilateral L Intercostal and Bronchial Arteries M Spinal Arteries N Upper Arteries, Other P Thoraco-Abdominal Aorta Q Cervico-Cerebral Arch R Intracranial Arteries S Pulmonary Artery, Right T Pulmonary Artery, Left	Ø High Osmolar 1 Low Osmolar Y Other Contrast Z None	Z None	Z None

Imaging

B Imaging
3 Upper Arteries
1 Fluoroscopy Definition: Single plane or bi-plane real time display of an image developed from the capture of external ionizing radiation on a fluorescent screen. The image may also be stored by either digital or analog means.

Body Part Character 4	Contrast Character 5	Qualifier Character 6	Qualifier Character 7
Ø Thoracic Aorta 1 Brachiocephalic-Subclavian Artery, Right 2 Subclavian Artery, Left 3 Common Carotid Artery, Right 4 Common Carotid Artery, Left 5 Common Carotid Arteries, Bilateral 6 Internal Carotid Artery, Right 7 Internal Carotid Artery, Left 8 Internal Carotid Arteries, Bilateral 9 External Carotid Artery, Right B External Carotid Artery, Left C External Carotid Arteries, Bilateral D Vertebral Artery, Right F Vertebral Artery, Left G Vertebral Arteries, Bilateral H Upper Extremity Arteries, Right J Upper Extremity Arteries, Left K Upper Extremity Arteries, Bilateral L Intercostal and Bronchial Arteries M Spinal Arteries N Upper Arteries, Other P Thoraco-Abdominal Aorta Q Cervico-Cerebral Arch R Intracranial Arteries S Pulmonary Artery, Right T Pulmonary Artery, Left U Pulmonary Trunk	Ø High Osmolar 1 Low Osmolar Y Other Contrast	1 Laser	Ø Intraoperative
Ø Thoracic Aorta 1 Brachiocephalic-Subclavian Artery, Right 2 Subclavian Artery, Left 3 Common Carotid Artery, Right 4 Common Carotid Artery, Left 5 Common Carotid Arteries, Bilateral 6 Internal Carotid Artery, Right 7 Internal Carotid Artery, Left 8 Internal Carotid Arteries, Bilateral 9 External Carotid Artery, Right B External Carotid Artery, Left C External Carotid Arteries, Bilateral D Vertebral Artery, Right F Vertebral Artery, Left G Vertebral Arteries, Bilateral H Upper Extremity Arteries, Right J Upper Extremity Arteries, Left K Upper Extremity Arteries, Bilateral L Intercostal and Bronchial Arteries M Spinal Arteries N Upper Arteries, Other P Thoraco-Abdominal Aorta Q Cervico-Cerebral Arch R Intracranial Arteries S Pulmonary Artery, Right T Pulmonary Artery, Left U Pulmonary Trunk	Ø High Osmolar 1 Low Osmolar Y Other Contrast	Z None	Z None

B31 Continued on next page

B Imaging
3 Upper Arteries
1 Fluoroscopy Definition: Single plane or bi-plane real time display of an image developed from the capture of external ionizing radiation on a fluorescent screen. The image may also be stored by either digital or analog means.

B31 Continued

Body Part Character 4	Contrast Character 5	Qualifier Character 6	Qualifier Character 7
Ø Thoracic Aorta 1 Brachiocephalic-Subclavian Artery, Right 2 Subclavian Artery, Left 3 Common Carotid Artery, Right 4 Common Carotid Artery, Left 5 Common Carotid Arteries, Bilateral 6 Internal Carotid Artery, Right 7 Internal Carotid Artery, Left 8 Internal Carotid Arteries, Bilateral 9 External Carotid Artery, Right B External Carotid Artery, Left C External Carotid Arteries, Bilateral D Vertebral Artery, Right F Vertebral Artery, Left G Vertebral Arteries, Bilateral H Upper Extremity Arteries, Right J Upper Extremity Arteries, Left K Upper Extremity Arteries, Bilateral L Intercostal and Bronchial Arteries M Spinal Arteries N Upper Arteries, Other P Thoraco-Abdominal Aorta Q Cervico-Cerebral Arch R Intracranial Arteries S Pulmonary Artery, Right T Pulmonary Artery, Left U Pulmonary Trunk	Z None	Z None	Z None

B Imaging
3 Upper Arteries
2 Computerized Tomography (CT Scan) Definition: Computer reformatted digital display of multiplanar images developed from the capture of multiple exposures of external ionizing radiation

Body Part Character 4	Contrast Character 5	Qualifier Character 6	Qualifier Character 7
Ø Thoracic Aorta 5 Common Carotid Arteries, Bilateral 8 Internal Carotid Arteries, Bilateral G Vertebral Arteries, Bilateral R Intracranial Arteries S Pulmonary Artery, Right T Pulmonary Artery, Left	Ø High Osmolar 1 Low Osmolar Y Other Contrast	Z None	Z None
Ø Thoracic Aorta 5 Common Carotid Arteries, Bilateral 8 Internal Carotid Arteries, Bilateral G Vertebral Arteries, Bilateral R Intracranial Arteries S Pulmonary Artery, Right T Pulmonary Artery, Left	Z None	2 Intravascular Optical Coherence Z None	Z None

B Imaging
3 Upper Arteries
3 Magnetic Resonance Imaging (MRI) Definition: Computer reformatted digital display of multiplanar images developed from the capture of radio-frequency signals emitted by nuclei in a body site excited within a magnetic field

Body Part Character 4	Contrast Character 5	Qualifier Character 6	Qualifier Character 7
Ø Thoracic Aorta 5 Common Carotid Arteries, Bilateral 8 Internal Carotid Arteries, Bilateral G Vertebral Arteries, Bilateral H Upper Extremity Arteries, Right J Upper Extremity Arteries, Left K Upper Extremity Arteries, Bilateral M Spinal Arteries Q Cervico-Cerebral Arch R Intracranial Arteries	Y Other Contrast	Ø Unenhanced and Enhanced Z None	Z None
Ø Thoracic Aorta 5 Common Carotid Arteries, Bilateral 8 Internal Carotid Arteries, Bilateral G Vertebral Arteries, Bilateral H Upper Extremity Arteries, Right J Upper Extremity Arteries, Left K Upper Extremity Arteries, Bilateral M Spinal Arteries Q Cervico-Cerebral Arch R Intracranial Arteries	Z None	Z None	Z None

B Imaging
3 Upper Arteries
4 Ultrasonography Definition: Real time display of images of anatomy or flow information developed from the capture of relected and attenuated high frequency sound waves

Body Part Character 4	Contrast Character 5	Qualifier Character 6	Qualifier Character 7
Ø Thoracic Aorta 1 Brachiocephalic-Subclavian Artery, Right 2 Subclavian Artery, Left 3 Common Carotid Artery, Right 4 Common Carotid Artery, Left 5 Common Carotid Arteries, Bilateral 6 Internal Carotid Artery, Right 7 Internal Carotid Artery, Left 8 Internal Carotid Arteries, Bilateral H Upper Extremity Arteries, Right J Upper Extremity Arteries, Left K Upper Extremity Arteries, Bilateral R Intracranial Arteries S Pulmonary Artery, Right T Pulmonary Artery, Left V Ophthalmic Arteries	Z None	Z None	3 Intravascular Z None

B Imaging
4 Lower Arteries
Ø Plain Radiography Definition: Planar display of an image developed from the capture of external ionizing radiation on photographic or photoconductive plate

Body Part Character 4	Contrast Character 5	Qualifier Character 6	Qualifier Character 7
Ø Abdominal Aorta 2 Hepatic Artery 3 Splenic Arteries 4 Superior Mesenteric Artery 5 Inferior Mesenteric Artery 6 Renal Artery, Right 7 Renal Artery, Left 8 Renal Arteries, Bilateral 9 Lumbar Arteries B Intra-Abdominal Arteries, Other C Pelvic Arteries D Aorta and Bilateral Lower Extremity Arteries F Lower Extremity Arteries, Right G Lower Extremity Arteries, Left J Lower Arteries, Other M Renal Artery Transplant	Ø High Osmolar 1 Low Osmolar Y Other Contrast	Z None	Z None

B Imaging
4 Lower Arteries
1 Fluoroscopy Definition: Single plane or bi-plane real time display of an image developed from the capture of external ionizing radiation on a fluorescent screen. The image may also be stored by either digital or analog means.

Body Part Character 4	Contrast Character 5	Qualifier Character 6	Qualifier Character 7
Ø Abdominal Aorta 2 Hepatic Artery 3 Splenic Arteries 4 Superior Mesenteric Artery 5 Inferior Mesenteric Artery 6 Renal Artery, Right 7 Renal Artery, Left 8 Renal Arteries, Bilateral 9 Lumbar Arteries B Intra-Abdominal Arteries, Other C Pelvic Arteries D Aorta and Bilateral Lower Extremity Arteries F Lower Extremity Arteries, Right G Lower Extremity Arteries, Left J Lower Arteries, Other	Ø High Osmolar 1 Low Osmolar Y Other Contrast	1 Laser	Ø Intraoperative
Ø Abdominal Aorta 2 Hepatic Artery 3 Splenic Arteries 4 Superior Mesenteric Artery 5 Inferior Mesenteric Artery 6 Renal Artery, Right 7 Renal Artery, Left 8 Renal Arteries, Bilateral 9 Lumbar Arteries B Intra-Abdominal Arteries, Other C Pelvic Arteries D Aorta and Bilateral Lower Extremity Arteries F Lower Extremity Arteries, Right G Lower Extremity Arteries, Left J Lower Arteries, Other	Ø High Osmolar 1 Low Osmolar Y Other Contrast	Z None	Z None
Ø Abdominal Aorta 2 Hepatic Artery 3 Splenic Arteries 4 Superior Mesenteric Artery 5 Inferior Mesenteric Artery 6 Renal Artery, Right 7 Renal Artery, Left 8 Renal Arteries, Bilateral 9 Lumbar Arteries B Intra-Abdominal Arteries, Other C Pelvic Arteries D Aorta and Bilateral Lower Extremity Arteries F Lower Extremity Arteries, Right G Lower Extremity Arteries, Left J Lower Arteries, Other	Z None	Z None	Z None

B Imaging
4 Lower Arteries
2 Computerized Tomography (CT Scan) Definition: Computer reformatted digital display of multiplanar images developed from the capture of multiple exposures of external ionizing radiation

Body Part Character 4	Contrast Character 5	Qualifier Character 6	Qualifier Character 7
Ø Abdominal Aorta 1 Celiac Artery 4 Superior Mesenteric Artery 8 Renal Arteries, Bilateral C Pelvic Arteries F Lower Extremity Arteries, Right G Lower Extremity Arteries, Left H Lower Extremity Arteries, Bilateral M Renal Artery Transplant	Ø High Osmolar 1 Low Osmolar Y Other Contrast	Z None	Z None
Ø Abdominal Aorta 1 Celiac Artery 4 Superior Mesenteric Artery 8 Renal Arteries, Bilateral C Pelvic Arteries F Lower Extremity Arteries, Right G Lower Extremity Arteries, Left H Lower Extremity Arteries, Bilateral M Renal Artery Transplant	Z None	2 Intravascular Optical Coherence Z None	Z None

B Imaging
4 Lower Arteries
3 Magnetic Resonance Imaging (MRI) Definition: Computer reformatted digital display of multiplanar images developed from the capture of radio-frequency signals emitted by nuclei in a body site excited within a magnetic field

Body Part Character 4	Contrast Character 5	Qualifier Character 6	Qualifier Character 7
Ø Abdominal Aorta 1 Celiac Artery 4 Superior Mesenteric Artery 8 Renal Arteries, Bilateral C Pelvic Arteries F Lower Extremity Arteries, Right G Lower Extremity Arteries, Left H Lower Extremity Arteries, Bilateral	Y Other Contrast	Ø Unenhanced and Enhanced Z None	Z None
Ø Abdominal Aorta 1 Celiac Artery 4 Superior Mesenteric Artery 8 Renal Arteries, Bilateral C Pelvic Arteries F Lower Extremity Arteries, Right G Lower Extremity Arteries, Left H Lower Extremity Arteries, Bilateral	Z None	Z None	Z None

B Imaging
4 Lower Arteries
4 Ultrasonography Definition: Real time display of images of anatomy or flow information developed from the capture of relected and attenuated high frequency sound waves

Body Part Character 4	Contrast Character 5	Qualifier Character 6	Qualifier Character 7
Ø Abdominal Aorta 4 Superior Mesenteric Artery 5 Inferior Mesenteric Artery 6 Renal Artery, Right 7 Renal Artery, Left 8 Renal Arteries, Bilateral B Intra-Abdominal Arteries, Other F Lower Extremity Arteries, Right G Lower Extremity Arteries, Left H Lower Extremity Arteries, Bilateral K Celiac and Mesenteric Arteries L Femoral Artery N Penile Arteries	Z None	Z None	3 Intravascular Z None

B Imaging
5 Veins
Ø Plain Radiography Definition: Planar display of an image developed from the capture of external ionizing radiation on photographic or photoconductive plate

Body Part Character 4	Contrast Character 5	Qualifier Character 6	Qualifier Character 7
Ø Epidural Veins 1 Cerebral and Cerebellar Veins 2 Intracranial Sinuses 3 Jugular Veins, Right 4 Jugular Veins, Left 5 Jugular Veins, Bilateral 6 Subclavian Vein, Right 7 Subclavian Vein, Left 8 Superior Vena Cava 9 Inferior Vena Cava B Lower Extremity Veins, Right C Lower Extremity Veins, Left D Lower Extremity Veins, Bilateral F Pelvic (Iliac) Veins, Right G Pelvic (Iliac) Veins, Left H Pelvic (Iliac) Veins, Bilateral J Renal Vein, Right K Renal Vein, Left L Renal Veins, Bilateral M Upper Extremity Veins, Right N Upper Extremity Veins, Left P Upper Extremity Veins, Bilateral Q Pulmonary Vein, Right R Pulmonary Vein, Left S Pulmonary Veins, Bilateral T Portal and Splanchnic Veins V Veins, Other W Dialysis Shunt/Fistula	Ø High Osmolar 1 Low Osmolar Y Other Contrast	Z None	Z None

B Imaging
5 Veins
1 Fluoroscopy Definition: Single plane or bi-plane real time display of an image developed from the capture of external ionizing radioation on a fluorescent screen. The image may also be stored by either digital or analog means.

Body Part Character 4	Contrast Character 5	Qualifier Character 6	Qualifier Character 7
Ø Epidural Veins 1 Cerebral and Cerebellar Veins 2 Intracranial Sinuses 3 Jugular Veins, Right 4 Jugular Veins, Left 5 Jugular Veins, Bilateral 6 Subclavian Vein, Right 7 Subclavian Vein, Left 8 Superior Vena Cava 9 Inferior Vena Cava B Lower Extremity Veins, Right C Lower Extremity Veins, Left D Lower Extremity Veins, Bilateral F Pelvic (Iliac) Veins, Right G Pelvic (Iliac) Veins, Left H Pelvic (Iliac) Veins, Bilateral J Renal Vein, Right K Renal Vein, Left L Renal Veins, Bilateral M Upper Extremity Veins, Right N Upper Extremity Veins, Left P Upper Extremity Veins, Bilateral Q Pulmonary Vein, Right R Pulmonary Vein, Left S Pulmonary Veins, Bilateral T Portal and Splanchnic Veins V Veins, Other W Dialysis Shunt/Fistula	Ø High Osmolar 1 Low Osmolar Y Other Contrast Z None	Z None	A Guidance Z None

B Imaging
5 Veins
2 Computerized Tomography (CT Scan) Definition: Computer reformatted digital display of multiplanar images developed from the capture of multiple exposures of external ionizing radiation

Body Part Character 4	Contrast Character 5	Qualifier Character 6	Qualifier Character 7
2 Intracranial Sinuses 8 Superior Vena Cava 9 Inferior Vena Cava F Pelvic (Iliac) Veins, Right G Pelvic (Iliac) Veins, Left H Pelvic (Iliac) Veins, Bilateral J Renal Vein, Right K Renal Vein, Left L Renal Veins, Bilateral Q Pulmonary Vein, Right R Pulmonary Vein, Left S Pulmonary Veins, Bilateral T Portal and Splanchnic Veins	Ø High Osmolar 1 Low Osmolar Y Other Contrast	Ø Unenhanced and Enhanced Z None	Z None
2 Intracranial Sinuses 8 Superior Vena Cava 9 Inferior Vena Cava F Pelvic (Iliac) Veins, Right G Pelvic (Iliac) Veins, Left H Pelvic (Iliac) Veins, Bilateral J Renal Vein, Right K Renal Vein, Left L Renal Veins, Bilateral Q Pulmonary Vein, Right R Pulmonary Vein, Left S Pulmonary Veins, Bilateral T Portal and Splanchnic Veins	Z None	2 Intravascular Optical Coherence Z None	Z None

B Imaging
5 Veins
3 Magnetic Resonance Imaging (MRI) Definition: Computer reformatted digital display of multiplanar images developed from the capture of radio-frequency signals emitted by nuclei in a body site excited within a magnetic field

Body Part Character 4	Contrast Character 5	Qualifier Character 6	Qualifier Character 7
1 Cerebral and Cerebellar Veins 2 Intracranial Sinuses 5 Jugular Veins, Bilateral 8 Superior Vena Cava 9 Inferior Vena Cava B Lower Extremity Veins, Right C Lower Extremity Veins, Left D Lower Extremity Veins, Bilateral H Pelvic (Iliac) Veins, Bilateral L Renal Veins, Bilateral M Upper Extremity Veins, Right N Upper Extremity Veins, Left P Upper Extremity Veins, Bilateral S Pulmonary Veins, Bilateral T Portal and Splanchnic Veins V Veins, Other	Y Other Contrast	Ø Unenhanced and Enhanced Z None	Z None
1 Cerebral and Cerebellar Veins 2 Intracranial Sinuses 5 Jugular Veins, Bilateral 8 Superior Vena Cava 9 Inferior Vena Cava B Lower Extremity Veins, Right C Lower Extremity Veins, Left D Lower Extremity Veins, Bilateral H Pelvic (Iliac) Veins, Bilateral L Renal Veins, Bilateral M Upper Extremity Veins, Right N Upper Extremity Veins, Left P Upper Extremity Veins, Bilateral S Pulmonary Veins, Bilateral T Portal and Splanchnic Veins V Veins, Other	Z None	Z None	Z None

B Imaging
5 Veins
4 Ultrasonography Definition: Real time display of images of anatomy or flow information developed from the capture of relected and attenuated high frequency sound waves

Body Part Character 4	Contrast Character 5	Qualifier Character 6	Qualifier Character 7
3 Jugular Veins, Right 4 Jugular Veins, Left 6 Subclavian Vein, Right 7 Subclavian Vein, Left 8 Superior Vena Cava 9 Inferior Vena Cava B Lower Extremity Veins, Right C Lower Extremity Veins, Left D Lower Extremity Veins, Bilateral J Renal Vein, Right K Renal Vein, Left L Renal Veins, Bilateral M Upper Extremity Veins, Right N Upper Extremity Veins, Left P Upper Extremity Veins, Bilateral T Portal and Splanchnic Veins	Z None	Z None	3 Intravascular A Guidance Z None

B Imaging
7 Lymphatic System
Ø Plain Radiography Definition: Planar display of an image developed from the capture of external ionizing radiation on photographic or photoconductive plate

Body Part Character 4	Contrast Character 5	Qualifier Character 6	Qualifier Character 7
Ø Abdominal/Retroperitoneal Lymphatics, Unilateral 1 Abdominal/Retroperitoneal Lymphatics, Bilateral 4 Lymphatics, Head and Neck 5 Upper Extremity Lymphatics, Right 6 Upper Extremity Lymphatics, Left 7 Upper Extremity Lymphatics, Bilateral 8 Lower Extremity Lymphatics, Right 9 Lower Extremity Lymphatics, Left B Lower Extremity Lymphatics, Bilateral C Lymphatics, Pelvic	Ø High Osmolar 1 Low Osmolar Y Other Contrast	Z None	Z None

B Imaging
8 Eye
Ø Plain Radiography Definition: Planar display of an image developed from the capture of external ionizing radiation on photographic or photoconductive plate

Body Part Character 4	Contrast Character 5	Qualifier Character 6	Qualifier Character 7
Ø Lacrimal Duct, Right 1 Lacrimal Duct, Left 2 Lacrimal Ducts, Bilateral	Ø High Osmolar 1 Low Osmolar Y Other Contrast	Z None	Z None
3 Optic Foramina, Right 4 Optic Foramina, Left 5 Eye, Right 6 Eye, Left 7 Eyes, Bilateral	Z None	Z None	Z None

B Imaging
8 Eye
2 Computerized Tomography (CT Scan) Definition: Computer reformatted digital display of multiplanar images developed from the capture of multiple exposures of external ionizing radiation

Body Part Character 4	Contrast Character 5	Qualifier Character 6	Qualifier Character 7
5 Eye, Right 6 Eye, Left 7 Eyes, Bilateral	Ø High Osmolar 1 Low Osmolar Y Other Contrast	Ø Unenhanced and Enhanced Z None	Z None
5 Eye, Right 6 Eye, Left 7 Eyes, Bilateral	Z None	Z None	Z None

B Imaging
8 Eye
3 Magnetic Resonance Imaging (MRI) Definition: Computer reformatted digital display of multiplanar images developed from the capture of radio-frequency signals emitted by nuclei in a body site excited within a magnetic field

Body Part Character 4	Contrast Character 5	Qualifier Character 6	Qualifier Character 7
5 Eye, Right 6 Eye, Left 7 Eyes, Bilateral	Y Other Contrast	Ø Unenhanced and Enhanced Z None	Z None
5 Eye, Right 6 Eye, Left 7 Eyes, Bilateral	Z None	Z None	Z None

B Imaging
8 Eye
4 Ultrasonography Definition: Real time display of images of anatomy or flow information developed from the capture of relected and attenuated high frequency sound waves

Body Part Character 4	Contrast Character 5	Qualifier Character 6	Qualifier Character 7
5 Eye, Right 6 Eye, Left 7 Eyes, Bilateral	Z None	Z None	Z None

B Imaging
9 Ear, Nose, Mouth and Throat
Ø Plain Radiography Definition: Planar display of an image developed from the capture of external ionizing radiation on photographic or photoconductive plate

Body Part Character 4	Contrast Character 5	Qualifier Character 6	Qualifier Character 7
2 Paranasal Sinuses F Nasopharynx/Oropharynx H Mastoids	Z None	Z None	Z None
4 Parotid Gland, Right 5 Parotid Gland, Left 6 Parotid Glands, Bilateral 7 Submandibular Gland, Right 8 Submandibular Gland, Left 9 Submandibular Glands, Bilateral B Salivary Gland, Right C Salivary Gland, Left D Salivary Glands, Bilateral	Ø High Osmolar 1 Low Osmolar Y Other Contrast	Z None	Z None

B Imaging
9 Ear, Nose, Mouth and Throat
1 Fluoroscopy Definition: Single plane or bi-plane real time display of an image developed from the capture of external ionizing radioation on a fluorescent screen. The image may also be stored by either digital or analog means.

Body Part Character 4	Contrast Character 5	Qualifier Character 6	Qualifier Character 7
G Pharynx and Epiglottis J Larynx	Y Other Contrast Z None	Z None	Z None

B Imaging
9 Ear, Nose, Mouth and Throat
2 Computerized Tomography (CT Scan) Definition: Computer reformatted digital display of multiplanar images developed from the capture of multiple exposures of external ionizing radiation

Body Part Character 4	Contrast Character 5	Qualifier Character 6	Qualifier Character 7
Ø Ear 2 Paranasal Sinuses 6 Parotid Glands, Bilateral 9 Submandibular Glands, Bilateral D Salivary Glands, Bilateral F Nasopharynx/Oropharynx J Larynx	Ø High Osmolar 1 Low Osmolar Y Other Contrast	Ø Unenhanced and Enhanced Z None	Z None
Ø Ear 2 Paranasal Sinuses 6 Parotid Glands, Bilateral 9 Submandibular Glands, Bilateral D Salivary Glands, Bilateral F Nasopharynx/Oropharynx J Larynx	Z None	Z None	Z None

B Imaging
9 Ear, Nose, Mouth and Throat
3 Magnetic Resonance Imaging (MRI) Definition: Computer reformatted digital display of multiplanar images developed from the capture of radio-frequency signals emitted by nuclei in a body site excited within a magnetic field

Body Part Character 4	Contrast Character 5	Qualifier Character 6	Qualifier Character 7
Ø Ear 2 Paranasal Sinuses 6 Parotid Glands, Bilateral 9 Submandibular Glands, Bilateral D Salivary Glands, Bilateral F Nasopharynx/Oropharynx J Larynx	Y Other Contrast	Ø Unenhanced and Enhanced Z None	Z None
Ø Ear 2 Paranasal Sinuses 6 Parotid Glands, Bilateral 9 Submandibular Glands, Bilateral D Salivary Glands, Bilateral F Nasopharynx/Oropharynx J Larynx	Z None	Z None	Z None

B Imaging
B Respiratory System
Ø Plain Radiography Definition: Planar display of an image developed from the capture of external ionizing radiation on photographic or photoconductive plate

Body Part Character 4	Contrast Character 5	Qualifier Character 6	Qualifier Character 7
7 Tracheobronchial Tree, Right 8 Tracheobronchial Tree, Left 9 Tracheobronchial Trees, Bilateral	Y Other Contrast	Z None	Z None
D Upper Airways	Z None	Z None	Z None

B Imaging
B Respiratory System
1 Fluoroscopy Definition: Single plane or bi-plane real time display of an image developed from the capture of external ionizing radioation on a fluorescent screen. The image may also be stored by either digital or analog means.

Body Part Character 4	Contrast Character 5	Qualifier Character 6	Qualifier Character 7
2 Lung, Right 3 Lung, Left 4 Lungs, Bilateral 6 Diaphragm C Mediastinum D Upper Airways	Z None	Z None	Z None
7 Tracheobronchial Tree, Right 8 Tracheobronchial Tree, Left 9 Tracheobronchial Trees, Bilateral	Y Other Contrast	Z None	Z None

B Imaging
B Respiratory System
2 Computerized Tomography (CT Scan) Definition: Computer reformatted digital display of multiplanar images developed from the capture of multiple exposures of external ionizing radiation

Body Part Character 4	Contrast Character 5	Qualifier Character 6	Qualifier Character 7
4 Lungs, Bilateral 7 Tracheobronchial Tree, Right 8 Tracheobronchial Tree, Left 9 Tracheobronchial Trees, Bilateral F Trachea/Airways	Ø High Osmolar 1 Low Osmolar Y Other Contrast	Ø Unenhanced and Enhanced Z None	Z None
4 Lungs, Bilateral 7 Tracheobronchial Tree, Right 8 Tracheobronchial Tree, Left 9 Tracheobronchial Trees, Bilateral F Trachea/Airways	Z None	Z None	Z None

B Imaging
B Respiratory System
3 Magnetic Resonance Imaging (MRI) Definition: Computer reformatted digital display of multiplanar images developed from the capture of radio-frequency signals emitted by nuclei in a body site excited within a magnetic field

Body Part Character 4	Contrast Character 5	Qualifier Character 6	Qualifier Character 7
G Lung Apices	Y Other Contrast	Ø Unenhanced and Enhanced Z None	Z None
G Lung Apices	Z None	Z None	Z None

B Imaging
B Respiratory System
4 Ultrasonography Definition: Real time display of images of anatomy or flow information developed from the capture of relected and attenuated high frequency sound waves

Body Part Character 4	Contrast Character 5	Qualifier Character 6	Qualifier Character 7
B Pleura C Mediastinum	Z None	Z None	Z None

B Imaging
D Gastrointestinal System
1 Fluoroscopy Definition: Single plane or bi-plane real time display of an image developed from the capture of external ionizing radioation on a fluorescent screen. The image may also be stored by either digital or analog means.

Body Part Character 4	Contrast Character 5	Qualifier Character 6	Qualifier Character 7
1 Esophagus 2 Stomach 3 Small Bowel 4 Colon 5 Upper GI 6 Upper GI and Small Bowel 9 Duodenum B Mouth/Oropharynx	Y Other Contrast Z None	Z None	Z None

B Imaging
D Gastrointestinal System
2 Computerized Tomography (CT Scan) Definition: Computer reformatted digital display of multiplanar images developed from the capture of multiple exposures of external ionizing radiation

Body Part Character 4	Contrast Character 5	Qualifier Character 6	Qualifier Character 7
4 Colon	Ø High Osmolar 1 Low Osmolar Y Other Contrast	Ø Unenhanced and Enhanced Z None	Z None
4 Colon	Z None	Z None	Z None

B Imaging
D Gastrointestinal System
4 Ultrasonography Definition: Real time display of images of anatomy or flow information developed from the capture of relected and attenuated high frequency sound waves

Body Part Character 4	Contrast Character 5	Qualifier Character 6	Qualifier Character 7
1 Esophagus 2 Stomach 7 Gastrointestinal Tract 8 Appendix 9 Duodenum C Rectum	Z None	Z None	Z None

B Imaging
F Hepatobiliary System and Pancreas
Ø Plain Radiography Definition: Planar display of an image developed from the capture of external ionizing radiation on photographic or photoconductive plate

Body Part Character 4	Contrast Character 5	Qualifier Character 6	Qualifier Character 7
Ø Bile Ducts 3 Gallbladder and Bile Ducts C Hepatobiliary System, All	Ø High Osmolar 1 Low Osmolar Y Other Contrast	Z None	Z None

B Imaging
F Hepatobiliary System and Pancreas
1 Fluoroscopy Definition: Single plane or bi-plane real time display of an image developed from the capture of external ionizing radioation on a fluorescent screen. The image may also be stored by either digital or analog means.

Body Part Character 4	Contrast Character 5	Qualifier Character 6	Qualifier Character 7
Ø Bile Ducts 1 Biliary and Pancreatic Ducts 2 Gallbladder 3 Gallbladder and Bile Ducts 4 Gallbladder, Bile Ducts and Pancreatic Ducts 8 Pancreatic Ducts	Ø High Osmolar 1 Low Osmolar Y Other Contrast	Z None	Z None

B Imaging
F Hepatobiliary System and Pancreas
2 Computerized Tomography (CT Scan) Definition: Computer reformatted digital display of multiplanar images developed from the capture of multiple exposures of external ionizing radiation

Body Part Character 4	Contrast Character 5	Qualifier Character 6	Qualifier Character 7
5 Liver 6 Liver and Spleen 7 Pancreas C Hepatobiliary System, All	Ø High Osmolar 1 Low Osmolar Y Other Contrast	Ø Unenhanced and Enhanced Z None	Z None
5 Liver 6 Liver and Spleen 7 Pancreas C Hepatobiliary System, All	Z None	Z None	Z None

B Imaging
F Hepatobiliary System and Pancreas
3 Magnetic Resonance Imaging (MRI) Definition: Computer reformatted digital display of multiplanar images developed from the capture of radio-frequency signals emitted by nuclei in a body site excited within a magnetic field

Body Part Character 4	Contrast Character 5	Qualifier Character 6	Qualifier Character 7
5 Liver 6 Liver and Spleen 7 Pancreas	Y Other Contrast	Ø Unenhanced and Enhanced Z None	Z None
5 Liver 6 Liver and Spleen 7 Pancreas	Z None	Z None	Z None

B Imaging
F Hepatobiliary System and Pancreas
4 Ultrasonography Definition: Real time display of images of anatomy or flow information developed from the capture of relected and attenuated high frequency sound waves

Body Part Character 4	Contrast Character 5	Qualifier Character 6	Qualifier Character 7
Ø Bile Ducts 2 Gallbladder 3 Gallbladder and Bile Ducts 5 Liver 6 Liver and Spleen 7 Pancreas C Hepatobiliary System, All	Z None	Z None	Z None

B Imaging
G Endocrine System
2 Computerized Tomography (CT Scan) Definition: Computer reformatted digital display of multiplanar images developed from the capture of multiple exposures of external ionizing radiation

Body Part Character 4	Contrast Character 5	Qualifier Character 6	Qualifier Character 7
2 Adrenal Glands, Bilateral 3 Parathyroid Glands 4 Thyroid Gland	Ø High Osmolar 1 Low Osmolar Y Other Contrast	Ø Unenhanced and Enhanced Z None	Z None
2 Adrenal Glands, Bilateral 3 Parathyroid Glands 4 Thyroid Gland	Z None	Z None	Z None

B Imaging
G Endocrine System
3 Magnetic Resonance Imaging (MRI) Definition: Computer reformatted digital display of multiplanar images developed from the capture of radio-frequency signals emitted by nuclei in a body site excited within a magnetic field

Body Part Character 4	Contrast Character 5	Qualifier Character 6	Qualifier Character 7
2 Adrenal Glands, Bilateral 3 Parathyroid Glands 4 Thyroid Gland	Y Other Contrast	Ø Unenhanced and Enhanced Z None	Z None
2 Adrenal Glands, Bilateral 3 Parathyroid Glands 4 Thyroid Gland	Z None	Z None	Z None

B Imaging
G Endocrine System
4 Ultrasonography Definition: Real time display of images of anatomy or flow information developed from the capture of relected and attenuated high frequency sound waves

Body Part Character 4	Contrast Character 5	Qualifier Character 6	Qualifier Character 7
Ø Adrenal Gland, Right 1 Adrenal Gland, Left 2 Adrenal Glands, Bilateral 3 Parathyroid Glands 4 Thyroid Gland	Z None	Z None	Z None

B Imaging
H Skin, Subcutaneous Tissue and Breast
Ø Plain Radiography Definition: Planar display of an image developed from the capture of external ionizing radiation on photographic or photoconductive plate

Body Part Character 4	Contrast Character 5	Qualifier Character 6	Qualifier Character 7
Ø Breast, Right 1 Breast, Left 2 Breasts, Bilateral	Z None	Z None	Z None
3 Single Mammary Duct, Right 4 Single Mammary Duct, Left 5 Multiple Mammary Ducts, Right 6 Multiple Mammary Ducts, Left	Ø High Osmolar 1 Low Osmolar Y Other Contrast Z None	Z None	Z None

B Imaging
H Skin, Subcutaneous Tissue and Breast
3 Magnetic Resonance Imaging (MRI) Definition: Computer reformatted digital display of multiplanar images developed from the capture of radio-frequency signals emitted by nuclei in a body site excited within a magnetic field

Body Part Character 4	Contrast Character 5	Qualifier Character 6	Qualifier Character 7
Ø Breast, Right 1 Breast, Left 2 Breasts, Bilateral D Subcutaneous Tissue, Head/Neck F Subcutaneous Tissue, Upper Extremity G Subcutaneous Tissue, Thorax H Subcutaneous Tissue, Abdomen and Pelvis J Subcutaneous Tissue, Lower Extremity	Y Other Contrast	Ø Unenhanced and Enhanced Z None	Z None
Ø Breast, Right 1 Breast, Left 2 Breasts, Bilateral D Subcutaneous Tissue, Head/Neck F Subcutaneous Tissue, Upper Extremity G Subcutaneous Tissue, Thorax H Subcutaneous Tissue, Abdomen and Pelvis J Subcutaneous Tissue, Lower Extremity	Z None	Z None	Z None

B Imaging
H Skin, Subcutaneous Tissue and Breast
4 Ultrasonography Definition: Real time display of images of anatomy or flow information developed from the capture of relected and attenuated high frequency sound waves

Body Part Character 4	Contrast Character 5	Qualifier Character 6	Qualifier Character 7
Ø Breast, Right 1 Breast, Left 2 Breasts, Bilateral 7 Extremity, Upper 8 Extremity, Lower 9 Abdominal Wall B Chest Wall C Head and Neck	Z None	Z None	Z None

B Imaging
L Connective Tissue
3 Magnetic Resonance Imaging (MRI) Definition: Computer reformatted digital display of multiplanar images developed from the capture of radio-frequency signals emitted by nuclei in a body site excited within a magnetic field

Body Part Character 4	Contrast Character 5	Qualifier Character 6	Qualifier Character 7
Ø Connective Tissue, Upper Extremity 1 Connective Tissue, Lower Extremity 2 Tendons, Upper Extremity 3 Tendons, Lower Extremity	Y Other Contrast	Ø Unenhanced and Enhanced Z None	Z None
Ø Connective Tissue, Upper Extremity 1 Connective Tissue, Lower Extremity 2 Tendons, Upper Extremity 3 Tendons, Lower Extremity	Z None	Z None	Z None

B Imaging
L Connective Tissue
4 Ultrasonography Definition: Real time display of images of anatomy or flow information developed from the capture of relected and attenuated high frequency sound waves

Body Part Character 4	Contrast Character 5	Qualifier Character 6	Qualifier Character 7
Ø Connective Tissue, Upper Extremity 1 Connective Tissue, Lower Extremity 2 Tendons, Upper Extremity 3 Tendons, Lower Extremity	Z None	Z None	Z None

B Imaging
N Skull and Facial Bones
Ø Plain Radiography Definition: Planar display of an image developed from the capture of external ionizing radiation on photographic or photoconductive plate

Body Part Character 4	Contrast Character 5	Qualifier Character 6	Qualifier Character 7
Ø Skull 1 Orbit, Right 2 Orbit, Left 3 Orbits, Bilateral 4 Nasal Bones 5 Facial Bones 6 Mandible B Zygomatic Arch, Right C Zygomatic Arch, Left D Zygomatic Arches, Bilateral G Tooth, Single H Teeth, Multiple J Teeth, All	Z None	Z None	Z None
7 Temporomandibular Joint, Right 8 Temporomandibular Joint, Left 9 Temporomandibular Joints, Bilateral	Ø High Osmolar 1 Low Osmolar Y Other Contrast Z None	Z None	Z None

B Imaging
N Skull and Facial Bones
1 Fluoroscopy Definition: Single plane or bi-plane real time display of an image developed from the capture of external ionizing radioation on a fluorescent screen. The image may also be stored by either digital or analog means.

Body Part Character 4	Contrast Character 5	Qualifier Character 6	Qualifier Character 7
7 Temporomandibular Joint, Right 8 Temporomandibular Joint, Left 9 Temporomandibular Joints, Bilateral	Ø High Osmolar 1 Low Osmolar Y Other Contrast Z None	Z None	Z None

B Imaging
N Skull and Facial Bones
2 Computerized Tomography (CT Scan) Definition: Computer reformatted digital display of multiplanar images developed from the capture of multiple exposures of external ionizing radiation

Body Part Character 4	Contrast Character 5	Qualifier Character 6	Qualifier Character 7
Ø Skull 3 Orbits, Bilateral 5 Facial Bones 6 Mandible 9 Temporomandibular Joints, Bilateral F Temporal Bones	Ø High Osmolar 1 Low Osmolar Y Other Contrast Z None	Z None	Z None

B Imaging
N Skull and Facial Bones
3 Magnetic Resonance Imaging (MRI) Definition: Computer reformatted digital display of multiplanar images developed from the capture of radio-frequency signals emitted by nuclei in a body site excited within a magnetic field

Body Part Character 4	Contrast Character 5	Qualifier Character 6	Qualifier Character 7
9 Temporomandibular Joints, Bilateral	Y Other Contrast Z None	Z None	Z None

B Imaging
P Non-Axial Upper Bones
Ø Plain Radiography Definition: Planar display of an image developed from the capture of external ionizing radiation on photographic or photoconductive plate

Body Part Character 4	Contrast Character 5	Qualifier Character 6	Qualifier Character 7
Ø Sternoclavicular Joint, Right 1 Sternoclavicular Joint, Left 2 Sternoclavicular Joints, Bilateral 3 Acromioclavicular Joints, Bilateral 4 Clavicle, Right 5 Clavicle, Left 6 Scapula, Right 7 Scapula, Left A Humerus, Right B Humerus, Left E Upper Arm, Right F Upper Arm, Left J Forearm, Right K Forearm, Left N Hand, Right P Hand, Left R Finger(s), Right S Finger(s), Left X Ribs, Right Y Ribs, Left	Z None	Z None	Z None
8 Shoulder, Right 9 Shoulder, Left C Hand/Finger Joint, Right D Hand/Finger Joint, Left G Elbow, Right H Elbow, Left L Wrist, Right M Wrist, Left	Ø High Osmolar 1 Low Osmolar Y Other Contrast Z None	Z None	Z None

B Imaging
P Non-Axial Upper Bones
1 Fluoroscopy Definition: Single plane or bi-plane real time display of an image developed from the capture of external ionizing radioation on a fluorescent screen. The image may also be stored by either digital or analog means.

Body Part Character 4	Contrast Character 5	Qualifier Character 6	Qualifier Character 7
Ø Sternoclavicular Joint, Right 1 Sternoclavicular Joint, Left 2 Sternoclavicular Joints, Bilateral 3 Acromioclavicular Joints, Bilateral 4 Clavicle, Right 5 Clavicle, Left 6 Scapula, Right 7 Scapula, Left A Humerus, Right B Humerus, Left E Upper Arm, Right F Upper Arm, Left J Forearm, Right K Forearm, Left N Hand, Right P Hand, Left R Finger(s), Right S Finger(s), Left X Ribs, Right Y Ribs, Left	Z None	Z None	Z None
8 Shoulder, Right 9 Shoulder, Left L Wrist, Right M Wrist, Left	Ø High Osmolar 1 Low Osmolar Y Other Contrast Z None	Z None	Z None
C Hand/Finger Joint, Right D Hand/Finger Joint, Left G Elbow, Right H Elbow, Left	Ø High Osmolar 1 Low Osmolar Y Other Contrast	Z None	Z None

B Imaging
P Non-Axial Upper Bones
2 Computerized Tomography (CT Scan) Definition: Computer reformatted digital display of multiplanar images developed from the capture of multiple exposures of external ionizing radiation

Body Part Character 4	Contrast Character 5	Qualifier Character 6	Qualifier Character 7
Ø Sternoclavicular Joint, Right 1 Sternoclavicular Joint, Left W Thorax	Ø High Osmolar 1 Low Osmolar Y Other Contrast	Z None	Z None
2 Sternoclavicular Joints, Bilateral 3 Acromioclavicular Joints, Bilateral 4 Clavicle, Right 5 Clavicle, Left 6 Scapula, Right 7 Scapula, Left 8 Shoulder, Right 9 Shoulder, Left A Humerus, Right B Humerus, Left E Upper Arm, Right F Upper Arm, Left G Elbow, Right H Elbow, Left J Forearm, Right K Forearm, Left L Wrist, Right M Wrist, Left N Hand, Right P Hand, Left Q Hands and Wrists, Bilateral R Finger(s), Right S Finger(s), Left T Upper Extremity, Right U Upper Extremity, Left V Upper Extremities, Bilateral X Ribs, Right Y Ribs, Left	Ø High Osmolar 1 Low Osmolar Y Other Contrast Z None	Z None	Z None
C Hand/Finger Joint, Right D Hand/Finger Joint, Left	Z None	Z None	Z None

B Imaging
P Non-Axial Upper Bones
3 Magnetic Resonance Imaging (MRI) Definition: Computer reformatted digital display of multiplanar images developed from the capture of radio-frequency signals emitted by nuclei in a body site excited within a magnetic field

Body Part Character 4	Contrast Character 5	Qualifier Character 6	Qualifier Character 7
8 Shoulder, Right 9 Shoulder, Left C Hand/Finger Joint, Right D Hand/Finger Joint, Left E Upper Arm, Right F Upper Arm, Left G Elbow, Right H Elbow, Left J Forearm, Right K Forearm, Left L Wrist, Right M Wrist, Left	Y Other Contrast	Ø Unenhanced and Enhanced Z None	Z None
8 Shoulder, Right 9 Shoulder, Left C Hand/Finger Joint, Right D Hand/Finger Joint, Left E Upper Arm, Right F Upper Arm, Left G Elbow, Right H Elbow, Left J Forearm, Right K Forearm, Left L Wrist, Right M Wrist, Left	Z None	Z None	Z None

B Imaging
P Non-Axial Upper Bones
4 Ultrasonography Definition: Real time display of images of anatomy or flow information developed from the capture of relected and attenuated high frequency sound waves

Body Part Character 4	Contrast Character 5	Qualifier Character 6	Qualifier Character 7
8 Shoulder, Right 9 Shoulder, Left G Elbow, Right H Elbow, Left L Wrist, Right M Wrist, Left N Hand, Right P Hand, Left	Z None	Z None	1 Densitometry Z None

B Imaging
Q Non-Axial Lower Bones
Ø Plain Radiography Definition: Planar display of an image developed from the capture of external ionizing radiation on photographic or photoconductive plate

Body Part Character 4	Contrast Character 5	Qualifier Character 6	Qualifier Character 7
Ø Hip, Right 1 Hip, Left	Ø High Osmolar 1 Low Osmolar Y Other Contrast	Z None	Z None
Ø Hip, Right 1 Hip, Left	Z None	Z None	1 Densitometry Z None
3 Femur, Right 4 Femur, Left	Z None	Z None	1 Densitometry Z None
7 Knee, Right 8 Knee, Left G Ankle, Right H Ankle, Left	Ø High Osmolar 1 Low Osmolar Y Other Contrast Z None	Z None	Z None
D Lower Leg, Right F Lower Leg, Left J Calcaneus, Right K Calcaneus, Left L Foot, Right M Foot, Left P Toe(s), Right Q Toe(s), Left V Patella, Right W Patella, Left	Z None	Z None	Z None
X Foot/Toe Joint, Right Y Foot/Toe Joint, Left	Ø High Osmolar 1 Low Osmolar Y Other Contrast	Z None	Z None

B Imaging
Q Non-Axial Lower Bones
1 Fluoroscopy Definition: Single plane or bi-plane real time display of an image developed from the capture of external ionizing radioation on a fluorescent screen. The image may also be stored by either digital or analog means.

Body Part Character 4	Contrast Character 5	Qualifier Character 6	Qualifier Character 7
Ø Hip, Right 1 Hip, Left 7 Knee, Right 8 Knee, Left G Ankle, Right H Ankle, Left X Foot/Toe Joint, Right Y Foot/Toe Joint, Left	Ø High Osmolar 1 Low Osmolar Y Other Contrast Z None	Z None	Z None
3 Femur, Right 4 Femur, Left D Lower Leg, Right F Lower Leg, Left J Calcaneus, Right K Calcaneus, Left L Foot, Right M Foot, Left P Toe(s), Right Q Toe(s), Left V Patella, Right W Patella, Left	Z None	Z None	Z None

B Imaging
Q Non-Axial Lower Bones
2 Computerized Tomography (CT Scan) Definition: Computer reformatted digital display of multiplanar images developed from the capture of multiple exposures of external ionizing radiation

Body Part Character 4	Contrast Character 5	Qualifier Character 6	Qualifier Character 7
Ø Hip, Right 1 Hip, Left 3 Femur, Right 4 Femur, Left 7 Knee, Right 8 Knee, Left D Lower Leg, Right F Lower Leg, Left G Ankle, Right H Ankle, Left J Calcaneus, Right K Calcaneus, Left L Foot, Right M Foot, Left P Toe(s), Right Q Toe(s), Left R Lower Extremity, Right S Lower Extremity, Left V Patella, Right W Patella, Left X Foot/Toe Joint, Right Y Foot/Toe Joint, Left	Ø High Osmolar 1 Low Osmolar Y Other Contrast Z None	Z None	Z None
B Tibia/Fibula, Right C Tibia/Fibula, Left	Ø High Osmolar 1 Low Osmolar Y Other Contrast	Z None	Z None

B Imaging
Q Non-Axial Lower Bones
3 Magnetic Resonance Imaging (MRI) Definition: Computer reformatted digital display of multiplanar images developed from the capture of radio-frequency signals emitted by nuclei in a body site excited within a magnetic field

Body Part Character 4	Contrast Character 5	Qualifier Character 6	Qualifier Character 7
Ø Hip, Right 1 Hip, Left 3 Femur, Right 4 Femur, Left 7 Knee, Right 8 Knee, Left D Lower Leg, Right F Lower Leg, Left G Ankle, Right H Ankle, Left J Calcaneus, Right K Calcaneus, Left L Foot, Right M Foot, Left P Toe(s), Right Q Toe(s), Left V Patella, Right W Patella, Left	Y Other Contrast	Ø Unenhanced and Enhanced Z None	Z None
Ø Hip, Right 1 Hip, Left 3 Femur, Right 4 Femur, Left 7 Knee, Right 8 Knee, Left D Lower Leg, Right F Lower Leg, Left G Ankle, Right H Ankle, Left J Calcaneus, Right K Calcaneus, Left L Foot, Right M Foot, Left P Toe(s), Right Q Toe(s), Left V Patella, Right W Patella, Left	Z None	Z None	Z None

B Imaging
Q Non-Axial Lower Bones
4 Ultrasonography Definition: Real time display of images of anatomy or flow information developed from the capture of relected and attenuated high frequency sound waves

Body Part Character 4	Contrast Character 5	Qualifier Character 6	Qualifier Character 7
Ø Hip, Right 1 Hip, Left 2 Hips, Bilateral 7 Knee, Right 8 Knee, Left 9 Knees, Bilateral	Z None	Z None	Z None

B Imaging
R Axial Skeleton, Except Skull and Facial Bones
Ø Plain Radiography Definition: Planar display of an image developed from the capture of external ionizing radiation on photographic or photoconductive plate

Body Part Character 4	Contrast Character 5	Qualifier Character 6	Qualifier Character 7
Ø Cervical Spine **7** Thoracic Spine **9** Lumbar Spine **G** Whole Spine	**Z** None	**Z** None	**1** Densitometry **Z** None
1 Cervical Disc(s) **2** Thoracic Disc(s) **3** Lumbar Disc(s) **4** Cervical Facet Joint(s) **5** Thoracic Facet Joint(s) **6** Lumbar Facet Joint(s) **D** Sacroiliac Joints	**Ø** High Osmolar **1** Low Osmolar **Y** Other Contrast **Z** None	**Z** None	**Z** None
8 Thoracolumbar Joint **B** Lumbosacral Joint **C** Pelvis **F** Sacrum and Coccyx **H** Sternum	**Z** None	**Z** None	**Z** None

B Imaging
R Axial Skeleton, Except Skull and Facial Bones
1 Fluoroscopy Definition: Single plane or bi-plane real time display of an image developed from the capture of external ionizing radioation on a fluorescent screen. The image may also be stored by either digital or analog means.

Body Part Character 4	Contrast Character 5	Qualifier Character 6	Qualifier Character 7
Ø Cervical Spine **1** Cervical Disc(s) **2** Thoracic Disc(s) **3** Lumbar Disc(s) **4** Cervical Facet Joint(s) **5** Thoracic Facet Joint(s) **6** Lumbar Facet Joint(s) **7** Thoracic Spine **8** Thoracolumbar Joint **9** Lumbar Spine **B** Lumbosacral Joint **C** Pelvis **D** Sacroiliac Joints **F** Sacrum and Coccyx **G** Whole Spine **H** Sternum	**Ø** High Osmolar **1** Low Osmolar **Y** Other Contrast **Z** None	**Z** None	**Z** None

B Imaging
R Axial Skeleton, Except Skull and Facial Bones
2 Computerized Tomography (CT Scan) Definition: Computer reformatted digital display of multiplanar images developed from the capture of multiple exposures of external ionizing radiation

Body Part Character 4	Contrast Character 5	Qualifier Character 6	Qualifier Character 7
Ø Cervical Spine **7** Thoracic Spine **9** Lumbar Spine **C** Pelvis **D** Sacroiliac Joints **F** Sacrum and Coccyx	**Ø** High Osmolar **1** Low Osmolar **Y** Other Contrast **Z** None	**Z** None	**Z** None

B Imaging
R Axial Skeleton, Except Skull and Facial Bones
3 Magnetic Resonance Imaging (MRI) Definition: Computer reformatted digital display of multiplanar images developed from the capture of radio-frequency signals emitted by nuclei in a body site excited within a magnetic field

Body Part Character 4	Contrast Character 5	Qualifier Character 6	Qualifier Character 7
Ø Cervical Spine 1 Cervical Disc(s) 2 Thoracic Disc(s) 3 Lumbar Disc(s) 7 Thoracic Spine 9 Lumbar Spine C Pelvis F Sacrum and Coccyx	Y Other Contrast	Ø Unenhanced and Enhanced Z None	Z None
Ø Cervical Spine 1 Cervical Disc(s) 2 Thoracic Disc(s) 3 Lumbar Disc(s) 7 Thoracic Spine 9 Lumbar Spine C Pelvis F Sacrum and Coccyx	Z None	Z None	Z None

B Imaging
R Axial Skeleton, Except Skull and Facial Bones
4 Ultrasonography Definition: Real time display of images of anatomy or flow information developed from the capture of relected and attenuated high frequency sound waves

Body Part Character 4	Contrast Character 5	Qualifier Character 6	Qualifier Character 7
Ø Cervical Spine 7 Thoracic Spine 9 Lumbar Spine F Sacrum and Coccyx	Z None	Z None	Z None

B Imaging
T Urinary System
Ø Plain Radiography Definition: Planar display of an image developed from the capture of external ionizing radiation on photographic or photoconductive plate

Body Part Character 4	Contrast Character 5	Qualifier Character 6	Qualifier Character 7
Ø Bladder 1 Kidney, Right 2 Kidney, Left 3 Kidneys, Bilateral 4 Kidneys, Ureters and Bladder 5 Urethra 6 Ureter, Right 7 Ureter, Left 8 Ureters, Bilateral B Bladder and Urethra C Ileal Diversion Loop	Ø High Osmolar 1 Low Osmolar Y Other Contrast Z None	Z None	Z None

B Imaging
T Urinary System
1 Fluoroscopy Definition: Single plane or bi-plane real time display of an image developed from the capture of external ionizing radioation on a fluorescent screen. The image may also be stored by either digital or analog means.

Body Part Character 4	Contrast Character 5	Qualifier Character 6	Qualifier Character 7
Ø Bladder 1 Kidney, Right 2 Kidney, Left 3 Kidneys, Bilateral 4 Kidneys, Ureters and Bladder 5 Urethra 6 Ureter, Right 7 Ureter, Left B Bladder and Urethra C Ileal Diversion Loop D Kidney, Ureter and Bladder, Right F Kidney, Ureter and Bladder, Left G Ileal Loop, Ureters and Kidneys	Ø High Osmolar 1 Low Osmolar Y Other Contrast Z None	Z None	Z None

B Imaging
T Urinary System
2 Computerized Tomography (CT Scan) Definition: Computer reformatted digital display of multiplanar images developed from the capture of multiple exposures of external ionizing radiation

Body Part Character 4	Contrast Character 5	Qualifier Character 6	Qualifier Character 7
Ø Bladder 1 Kidney, Right 2 Kidney, Left 3 Kidneys, Bilateral 9 Kidney Transplant	Ø High Osmolar 1 Low Osmolar Y Other Contrast	Ø Unenhanced and Enhanced Z None	Z None
Ø Bladder 1 Kidney, Right 2 Kidney, Left 3 Kidneys, Bilateral 9 Kidney Transplant	Z None	Z None	Z None

B Imaging
T Urinary System
3 Magnetic Resonance Imaging (MRI) Definition: Computer reformatted digital display of multiplanar images developed from the capture of radio-frequency signals emitted by nuclei in a body site excited within a magnetic field

Body Part Character 4	Contrast Character 5	Qualifier Character 6	Qualifier Character 7
Ø Bladder 1 Kidney, Right 2 Kidney, Left 3 Kidneys, Bilateral 9 Kidney Transplant	Y Other Contrast	Ø Unenhanced and Enhanced Z None	Z None
Ø Bladder 1 Kidney, Right 2 Kidney, Left 3 Kidneys, Bilateral 9 Kidney Transplant	Z None	Z None	Z None

B Imaging
T Urinary System
4 Ultrasonography Definition: Real time display of images of anatomy or flow information developed from the capture of relected and attenuated high frequency sound waves

Body Part Character 4	Contrast Character 5	Qualifier Character 6	Qualifier Character 7
Ø Bladder 1 Kidney, Right 2 Kidney, Left 3 Kidneys, Bilateral 5 Urethra 6 Ureter, Right 7 Ureter, Left 8 Ureters, Bilateral 9 Kidney Transplant J Kidneys and Bladder	Z None	Z None	Z None

B Imaging
U Female Reproductive System
Ø Plain Radiography Definition: Planar display of an image developed from the capture of external ionizing radiation on photographic or photoconductive plate

Body Part Character 4	Contrast Character 5	Qualifier Character 6	Qualifier Character 7
Ø Fallopian Tube, Right ♀ 1 Fallopian Tube, Left ♀ 2 Fallopian Tubes, Bilateral ♀ 6 Uterus ♀ 8 Uterus and Fallopian Tubes ♀ 9 Vagina ♀	Ø High Osmolar 1 Low Osmolar Y Other Contrast	Z None	Z None

♀ All body part, contrast, and qualifier values

B Imaging
U Female Reproductive System
1 Fluoroscopy Definition: Single plane or bi-plane real time display of an image developed from the capture of external ionizing radioation on a fluorescent screen. The image may also be stored by either digital or analog means.

Body Part Character 4	Contrast Character 5	Qualifier Character 6	Qualifier Character 7
Ø Fallopian Tube, Right ♀ 1 Fallopian Tube, Left ♀ 2 Fallopian Tubes, Bilateral ♀ 6 Uterus ♀ 8 Uterus and Fallopian Tubes ♀ 9 Vagina ♀	Ø High Osmolar 1 Low Osmolar Y Other Contrast Z None	Z None	Z None

♀ All body part, contrast, and qualifier values

B Imaging
U Female Reproductive System
3 Magnetic Resonance Imaging (MRI) Definition: Computer reformatted digital display of multiplanar images developed from the capture of radio-frequency signals emitted by nuclei in a body site excited within a magnetic field

Body Part Character 4	Contrast Character 5	Qualifier Character 6	Qualifier Character 7
3 Ovary, Right ♀ 4 Ovary, Left ♀ 5 Ovaries, Bilateral ♀ 6 Uterus ♀ 9 Vagina ♀ B Pregnant Uterus ♀ C Uterus and Ovaries ♀	Y Other Contrast	Ø Unenhanced and Enhanced Z None	Z None
3 Ovary, Right ♀ 4 Ovary, Left ♀ 5 Ovaries, Bilateral ♀ 6 Uterus ♀ 9 Vagina ♀ B Pregnant Uterus ♀ C Uterus and Ovaries ♀	Z None	Z None	Z None

♀ All body part, contrast, and qualifier values

B Imaging
U Female Reproductive System
4 Ultrasonography Definition: Real time display of images of anatomy or flow information developed from the capture of relected and attenuated high frequency sound waves

Body Part Character 4	Contrast Character 5	Qualifier Character 6	Qualifier Character 7
Ø Fallopian Tube, Right ♀ 1 Fallopian Tube, Left ♀ 2 Fallopian Tubes, Bilateral ♀ 3 Ovary, Right ♀ 4 Ovary, Left ♀ 5 Ovaries, Bilateral ♀ 6 Uterus ♀ C Uterus and Ovaries ♀	Y Other Contrast Z None	Z None	Z None

♀ All body part, contrast, and qualifier values

B Imaging
V Male Reproductive System
Ø Plain Radiography Definition: Planar display of an image developed from the capture of external ionizing radiation on photographic or photoconductive plate

Body Part Character 4	Contrast Character 5	Qualifier Character 6	Qualifier Character 7
Ø Corpora Cavernosa ♂ 1 Epididymis, Right ♂ 2 Epididymis, Left ♂ 3 Prostate ♂ 5 Testicle, Right ♂ 6 Testicle, Left ♂ 8 Vasa Vasorum ♂	Ø High Osmolar 1 Low Osmolar Y Other Contrast	Z None	Z None

♂ All body part, contrast, and qualifier values

B Imaging
V Male Reproductive System
1 Fluoroscopy Definition: Single plane or bi-plane real time display of an image developed from the capture of external ionizing radioation on a fluorescent screen. The image may also be stored by either digital or analog means.

Body Part Character 4	Contrast Character 5	Qualifier Character 6	Qualifier Character 7
Ø Corpora Cavernosa ♂ 8 Vasa Vasorum ♂	Ø High Osmolar 1 Low Osmolar Y Other Contrast Z None	Z None	Z None

♂ All body part, contrast, and qualifier values

B Imaging
V Male Reproductive System
2 Computerized Tomography (CT Scan) Definition: Computer reformatted digital display of multiplanar images developed from the capture of multiple exposures of external ionizing radiation

Body Part Character 4	Contrast Character 5	Qualifier Character 6	Qualifier Character 7
3 Prostate ♂	Ø High Osmolar 1 Low Osmolar Y Other Contrast	Ø Unenhanced and Enhanced Z None	Z None
3 Prostate ♂	Z None	Z None	Z None

♂ BV23[Ø,Y][Ø,Z]Z
♂ BV231ØZ
♂ BV23ZZZ

B Imaging
V Male Reproductive System
3 Magnetic Resonance Imaging (MRI) Definition: Computer reformatted digital display of multiplanar images developed from the capture of radio-frequency signals emitted by nuclei in a body site excited within a magnetic field

Body Part Character 4	Contrast Character 5	Qualifier Character 6	Qualifier Character 7
Ø Corpora Cavernosa ♂ 3 Prostate ♂ 4 Scrotum ♂ 5 Testicle, Right ♂ 6 Testicle, Left ♂ 7 Testicles, Bilateral ♂	Y Other Contrast	Ø Unenhanced and Enhanced Z None	Z None
Ø Corpora Cavernosa ♂ 3 Prostate ♂ 4 Scrotum ♂ 5 Testicle, Right ♂ 6 Testicle, Left ♂ 7 Testicles, Bilateral ♂	Z None	Z None	Z None

♂ All body part, contrast, and qualifier values

B Imaging
V Male Reproductive System
4 Ultrasonography Definition: Real time display of images of anatomy or flow information developed from the capture of relected and attenuated high frequency sound waves

Body Part Character 4	Contrast Character 5	Qualifier Character 6	Qualifier Character 7
4 Scrotum ♂ 9 Prostate and Seminal Vesicles ♂ B Penis ♂	Z None	Z None	Z None

♂ All body part, contrast, and qualifier values

B Imaging
W Anatomical Regions
Ø Plain Radiography Definition: Planar display of an image developed from the capture of external ionizing radiation on photographic or photoconductive plate

Body Part Character 4	Contrast Character 5	Qualifier Character 6	Qualifier Character 7
Ø Abdomen 1 Abdomen and Pelvis 3 Chest B Long Bones, All C Lower Extremity J Upper Extremity K Whole Body L Whole Skeleton M Whole Body, Infant	Z None	Z None	Z None

Imaging (side tab)

B Imaging
W Anatomical Regions
1 Fluoroscopy Definition: Single plane or bi-plane real time display of an image developed from the capture of external ionizing radioation on a fluorescent screen. The image may also be stored by either digital or analog means.

Body Part Character 4	Contrast Character 5	Qualifier Character 6	Qualifier Character 7
1 Abdomen and Pelvis 9 Head and Neck C Lower Extremity J Upper Extremity	Ø High Osmolar 1 Low Osmolar Y Other Contrast Z None	Z None	Z None

B Imaging
W Anatomical Regions
2 Computerized Tomography (CT Scan) Definition: Computer reformatted digital display of multiplanar images developed from the capture of multiple exposures of external ionizing radiation

Body Part Character 4	Contrast Character 5	Qualifier Character 6	Qualifier Character 7
Ø Abdomen 1 Abdomen and Pelvis 4 Chest and Abdomen 5 Chest, Abdomen and Pelvis 8 Head 9 Head and Neck F Neck G Pelvic Region	Ø High Osmolar 1 Low Osmolar Y Other Contrast	Ø Unenhanced and Enhanced Z None	Z None
Ø Abdomen 1 Abdomen and Pelvis 4 Chest and Abdomen 5 Chest, Abdomen and Pelvis 8 Head 9 Head and Neck F Neck G Pelvic Region	Z None	Z None	Z None

B Imaging
W Anatomical Regions
3 Magnetic Resonance Imaging (MRI) Definition: Computer reformatted digital display of multiplanar images developed from the capture of radio-frequency signals emitted by nuclei in a body site excited within a magnetic field

Body Part Character 4	Contrast Character 5	Qualifier Character 6	Qualifier Character 7
Ø Abdomen 8 Head F Neck G Pelvic Region H Retroperitoneum P Brachial Plexus	Y Other Contrast	Ø Unenhanced and Enhanced Z None	Z None
Ø Abdomen 8 Head F Neck G Pelvic Region H Retroperitoneum P Brachial Plexus	Z None	Z None	Z None
3 Chest	Y Other Contrast	Ø Unenhanced and Enhanced Z None	Z None

B Imaging
W Anatomical Regions
4 Ultrasonography Definition: Real time display of images of anatomy or flow information developed from the capture of relected and attenuated high frequency sound waves

Body Part Character 4	Contrast Character 5	Qualifier Character 6	Qualifier Character 7
Ø Abdomen 1 Abdomen and Pelvis F Neck G Pelvic Region	Z None	Z None	Z None

BW1–BW4 (side tab)

B Imaging
Y Fetus and Obstetrical
3 Magnetic Resonance Imaging (MRI) Definition: Computer reformatted digital display of multiplanar images developed from the capture of radio-frequency signals emitted by nuclei in a body site excited within a magnetic field

Body Part Character 4	Contrast Character 5	Qualifier Character 6	Qualifier Character 7
Ø Fetal Head ♀ **1** Fetal Heart ♀ **2** Fetal Thorax ♀ **3** Fetal Abdomen ♀ **4** Fetal Spine ♀ **5** Fetal Extremities ♀ **6** Whole Fetus ♀	**Y** Other Contrast	**Ø** Unenhanced and Enhanced **Z** None	**Z** None
Ø Fetal Head ♀ **1** Fetal Heart ♀ **2** Fetal Thorax ♀ **3** Fetal Abdomen ♀ **4** Fetal Spine ♀ **5** Fetal Extremities ♀ **6** Whole Fetus ♀	**Z** None	**Z** None	**Z** None

♀ BY3[Ø,1,2,3,5,6]Y[Ø,Z]Z
♀ BY34YZZ
♀ BY3[Ø,1,2,3,4,5,6]ZZZ

B Imaging
Y Fetus and Obstetrical
4 Ultrasonography Definition: Real time display of images of anatomy or flow information developed from the capture of relected and attenuated high frequency sound waves

Body Part Character 4	Contrast Character 5	Qualifier Character 6	Qualifier Character 7
7 Fetal Umbilical Cord ♀ **8** Placenta ♀ **9** First Trimester, Single Fetus ♀ **B** First Trimester, Multiple Gestation ♀ **C** Second Trimester, Single Fetus ♀ **D** Second Trimester, Multiple Gestation ♀ **F** Third Trimester, Single Fetus ♀ **G** Third Trimester, Multiple Gestation ♀	**Z** None	**Z** None	**Z** None

♀ All body part, contrast, and qualifier values

Nuclear Medicine CØ1–CW7

Character Meanings

This Character Meaning table is provided as a guide to assist the user in the identification of character members that may be found in this section of code tables. It **SHOULD NOT** be used to build a PCS code.

Body System–Character 2	Type–Character 3	Body Part–Character 4	Radionuclide–Character 5	Qualifier–Character 6	Qualifier–Character 7
Ø Central Nervous System	1 Planar Nuclear Medicine Imaging	See below	1 Technetium 99m (Tc-99m)	Z None	Z None
2 Heart	2 Tomographic (Tomo) Nuclear Medicine Imaging		7 Cobalt 58 (Co-58)		
5 Veins	3 Positron Emission Tomographic (PET) Imaging		8 Samarium 153 (Sm-153)		
7 Lymphatic and Hematologic System	4 Nonimaging Nuclear Medicine Uptake		9 Krypton (Kr-81m)		
8 Eye	5 Nonimaging Nuclear Medicine Probe		B Carbon 11 (C-11)		
9 Ear, Nose, Mouth and Throat	6 Nonimaging Nuclear Medicine Assay		C Cobalt 57 (Co-57)		
B Respiratory System	7 Systemic Nuclear Medicine Therapy		D Indium 111 (In-111)		
D Gastrointestinal System			F Iodine 123 (I-123)		
F Hepatobiliary System and Pancreas			G Iodine 131 (I-131)		
G Endocrine System			H Iodine 125 (I-125)		
H Skin, Subcutaneous Tissue and Breast			K Fluorine 18 (F-18)		
P Musculoskeletal System			L Gallium 67 (Ga-67)		
T Urinary System			M Oxygen 15 (O-15)		
V Male Reproductive System			N Phosphorus 32 (P-32)		
W Anatomical Regions			P Strontium 89 (Sr-89)		
			Q Rubidium 82 (Rb-82)		
			R Nitrogen 13 (N-13)		
			S Thallium 2Ø1 (Tl-2Ø1)		
			T Xenon 127 (Xe-127)		
			V Xenon 133 (Xe-133)		
			W Chromium (Cr-51)		
			Y Other Radionuclide		
			Z None		

Body Part—Character 4 Meanings

Body System–Character 2	Body Part–Character 4
Ø Central Nervous System	Ø Brain 5 Cerebrospinal Fluid Y Central Nervous System
2 Heart	6 Heart, Right and Left G Myocardium Y Heart
5 Veins	B Lower Extremity Veins, Right C Lower Extremity Veins, Left D Lower Extremity Veins, Bilateral N Upper Extremity Veins, Right P Upper Extremity Veins, Left Q Upper Extremity Veins, Bilateral R Central Veins Y Veins

Continued on next page

Continued from previous page

Body System– Character 2	Body Part– Character 4
7 Lymphatic and Hematologic System	Ø Bone Marrow 2 Spleen 3 Blood 5 Lymphatics, Head and Neck D Lymphatics, Pelvic J Lymphatics, Head K Lymphatics, Neck L Lymphatics, Upper Chest M Lymphatics, Trunk N Lymphatics, Upper Extremity P Lymphatics, Lower Extremity Y Lymphatic and Hematologic System
8 Eye	9 Lacrimal Ducts, Bilateral Y Eye
9 Ear, Nose, Mouth and Throat	B Salivary Glands, Bilateral Y Ear, Nose, Mouth and Throat
B Respiratory System	2 Lungs and Bronchi Y Respiratory System
D Gastrointestinal System	5 Upper Gastrointestinal Tract 7 Gastrointestinal Tract Y Digestive System
F Hepatobiliary System and Pancreas	4 Gallbladder 5 Liver 6 Liver and Spleen C Hepatobiliary System, All Y Hepatobiliary System and Pancreas
G Endocrine System	1 Parathyroid Glands 2 Thyroid Gland 4 Adrenal Glands, Bilateral Y Endocrine System
H Skin, Subcutaneous Tissue and Breast	Ø Breast, Right 1 Breast, Left 2 Breasts, Bilateral Y Skin, Subcutaneous Tissue and Breast
P Musculoskeletal System	1 Skull 2 Cervical Spine 3 Skull and Cervical Spine 4 Thorax 5 Spine 6 Pelvis 7 Spine and Pelvis 8 Upper Extremity, Right 9 Upper Extremity, Left B Upper Extremities, Bilateral C Lower Extremity, Right D Lower Extremity, Left F Lower Extremities, Bilateral G Thoracic Spine H Lumbar Spine J Thoracolumbar Spine N Upper Extremities P Lower Extremities Y Musculoskeletal System, Other Z Musculoskeletal System, All
T Urinary System	3 Kidneys, Ureters and Bladder H Bladder and Ureters Y Urinary System
V Male Reproductive System	9 Testicles, Bilateral Y Male Reproductive System
W Anatomical Regions	Ø Abdomen 1 Abdomen and Pelvis 3 Chest 4 Chest and Abdomen 6 Chest and Neck B Head and Neck D Lower Extremity G Thyroid J Pelvic Region M Upper Extremity N Whole Body Y Anatomical Regions, Multiple Z Anatomical Region, Other

C Nuclear Medicine
Ø Central Nervous System
1 Planar Nuclear Medicine Imaging Definition: Introduction of radioactive materials into the body for single plane display of images developed from the capture of radioactive emissions

Body Part Character 4	Radionuclide Character 5	Qualifier Character 6	Qualifier Character 7
Ø Brain	1 Technetium 99m (Tc-99m) Y Other Radionuclide	Z None	Z None
5 Cerebrospinal Fluid	D Indium 111 (In-111) Y Other Radionuclide	Z None	Z None
Y Central Nervous System	Y Other Radionuclide	Z None	Z None

C Nuclear Medicine
Ø Central Nervous System
2 Tomographic (Tomo) Nuclear Medicine Imaging Definition: Introduction of radioactive materials into the body for three dimensional display of images developed from the capture of radioactive emissions

Body Part Character 4	Radionuclide Character 5	Qualifier Character 6	Qualifier Character 7
Ø Brain	1 Technetium 99m (Tc-99m) F Iodine 123 (I-123) S Thallium 201 (Tl-201) Y Other Radionuclide	Z None	Z None
5 Cerebrospinal Fluid	D Indium 111 (In-111) Y Other Radionuclide	Z None	Z None
Y Central Nervous System	Y Other Radionuclide	Z None	Z None

C Nuclear Medicine
Ø Central Nervous System
3 Positron Emission Tomographic (PET) Imaging Definition: Introduction of radioactive materials into the body for three dimensional display of images developed from the simultaneous capture, 180 degrees apart, of radioactive emissions

Body Part Character 4	Radionuclide Character 5	Qualifier Character 6	Qualifier Character 7
Ø Brain	B Carbon 11 (C-11) K Fluorine 18 (F-18) M Oxygen 15 (O-15) Y Other Radionuclide	Z None	Z None
Y Central Nervous System	Y Other Radionuclide	Z None	Z None

C Nuclear Medicine
Ø Central Nervous System
5 Nonimaging Nuclear Medicine Probe Definition: Introduction of radioactive materials into the body for the study of distribution and fate of certain substances by the detection of radioactive emissions; or, alternatively, measurement of absorption of radioactive emissions from an external source

Body Part Character 4	Radionuclide Character 5	Qualifier Character 6	Qualifier Character 7
Ø Brain	V Xenon 133 (Xe-133) Y Other Radionuclide	Z None	Z None
Y Central Nervous System	Y Other Radionuclide	Z None	Z None

C Nuclear Medicine
2 Heart
1 Planar Nuclear Medicine Imaging Definition: Introduction of radioactive materials into the body for single plane display of images developed from the capture of radioactive emissions

Body Part Character 4	Radionuclide Character 5	Qualifier Character 6	Qualifier Character 7
6 Heart, Right and Left	1 Technetium 99m (Tc-99m) Y Other Radionuclide	Z None	Z None
G Myocardium	1 Technetium 99m (Tc-99m) D Indium 111 (In-111) S Thallium 201 (Tl-201) Y Other Radionuclide Z None	Z None	Z None
Y Heart	Y Other Radionuclide	Z None	Z None

C Nuclear Medicine
2 Heart
2 Tomographic (Tomo) Nuclear Medicine Imaging Definition: Introduction of radioactive materials into the body for three dimensional display of images developed from the capture of radioactive emissions

Body Part Character 4	Radionuclide Character 5	Qualifier Character 6	Qualifier Character 7
6 Heart, Right and Left	1 Technetium 99m (Tc-99m) Y Other Radionuclide	Z None	Z None
G Myocardium	1 Technetium 99m (Tc-99m) D Indium 111 (In-111) K Fluorine 18 (F-18) S Thallium 201 (Tl-201) Y Other Radionuclide Z None	Z None	Z None
Y Heart	Y Other Radionuclide	Z None	Z None

C Nuclear Medicine
2 Heart
3 Positron Emission Tomographic (PET) Imaging Definition: Introduction of radioactive materials into the body for three dimensional display of images developed from the simultaneous capture, 180 degrees apart, of radioactive emissions

Body Part Character 4	Radionuclide Character 5	Qualifier Character 6	Qualifier Character 7
G Myocardium	K Fluorine 18 (F-18) M Oxygen 15 (O-15) Q Rubidium 82 (Rb-82) R Nitrogen 13 (N-13) Y Other Radionuclide	Z None	Z None
Y Heart	Y Other Radionuclide	Z None	Z None

C Nuclear Medicine
2 Heart
5 Nonimaging Nuclear Medicine Probe Definition: Introduction of radioactive materials into the body for the study of distribution and fate of certain substances by the detection of radioactive emissions; or, alternatively, measurement of absorption of radioactive emissions from an external source

Body Part Character 4	Radionuclide Character 5	Qualifier Character 6	Qualifier Character 7
6 Heart, Right and Left	1 Technetium 99m (Tc-99m) Y Other Radionuclide	Z None	Z None
Y Heart	Y Other Radionuclide	Z None	Z None

C Nuclear Medicine
5 Veins
1 Planar Nuclear Medicine Imaging Definition: Introduction of radioactive materials into the body for single plane display of images developed from the capture of radioactive emissions

Body Part Character 4	Radionuclide Character 5	Qualifier Character 6	Qualifier Character 7
B Lower Extremity Veins, Right C Lower Extremity Veins, Left D Lower Extremity Veins, Bilateral N Upper Extremity Veins, Right P Upper Extremity Veins, Left Q Upper Extremity Veins, Bilateral R Central Veins	1 Technetium 99m (Tc-99m) Y Other Radionuclide	Z None	Z None
Y Veins	Y Other Radionuclide	Z None	Z None

C Nuclear Medicine
7 Lymphatic and Hematologic System
1 Planar Nuclear Medicine Imaging Definition: Introduction of radioactive materials into the body for single plane display of images developed from the capture of radioactive emissions

Body Part Character 4	Radionuclide Character 5	Qualifier Character 6	Qualifier Character 7
Ø Bone Marrow	1 Technetium 99m (Tc-99m) D Indium 111 (In-111) Y Other Radionuclide	Z None	Z None
2 Spleen 5 Lymphatics, Head and Neck D Lymphatics, Pelvic J Lymphatics, Head K Lymphatics, Neck L Lymphatics, Upper Chest M Lymphatics, Trunk N Lymphatics, Upper Extremity P Lymphatics, Lower Extremity	1 Technetium 99m (Tc-99m) Y Other Radionuclide	Z None	Z None
3 Blood	D Indium 111 (In-111) Y Other Radionuclide	Z None	Z None
Y Lymphatic and Hematologic System	Y Other Radionuclide	Z None	Z None

C Nuclear Medicine
7 Lymphatic and Hematologic System
2 Tomographic (Tomo) Nuclear Medicine Imaging Definition: Introduction of radioactive materials into the body for three dimensional display of images developed from the capture of radioactive emissions

Body Part Character 4	Radionuclide Character 5	Qualifier Character 6	Qualifier Character 7
2 Spleen	1 Technetium 99m (Tc-99m) Y Other Radionuclide	Z None	Z None
Y Lymphatic and Hematologic System	Y Other Radionuclide	Z None	Z None

C Nuclear Medicine
7 Lymphatic and Hematologic System
5 Nonimaging Nuclear Medicine Probe Definition: Introduction of radioactive materials into the body for the study of distribution and fate of certain substances by the detection of radioactive emissions; or, alternatively, measurement of absorption of radioactive emissions from an external source

Body Part Character 4	Radionuclide Character 5	Qualifier Character 6	Qualifier Character 7
5 Lymphatics, Head and Neck D Lymphatics, Pelvic J Lymphatics, Head K Lymphatics, Neck L Lymphatics, Upper Chest M Lymphatics, Trunk N Lymphatics, Upper Extremity P Lymphatics, Lower Extremity	1 Technetium 99m (Tc-99m) Y Other Radionuclide	Z None	Z None
Y Lymphatic and Hematologic System	Y Other Radionuclide	Z None	Z None

C Nuclear Medicine
7 Lymphatic and Hematologic System
6 Nonimaging Nuclear Medicine Assay Definition: Introduction of radioactive materials into the body for the study of body fluids and blood elements, by the detection of radioactive emissions

Body Part Character 4	Radionuclide Character 5	Qualifier Character 6	Qualifier Character 7
3 Blood	1 Technetium 99m (Tc-99m) 7 Cobalt 58 (Co-58) C Cobalt 57 (Co-57) D Indium 111 (In-111) H Iodine 125 (I-125) W Chromium (Cr-51) Y Other Radionuclide	Z None	Z None
Y Lymphatic and Hematologic System	Y Other Radionuclide	Z None	Z None

C Nuclear Medicine
8 Eye
1 Planar Nuclear Medicine Imaging Definition: Introduction of radioactive materials into the body for single plane display of images developed from the capture of radioactive emissions

Body Part Character 4	Radionuclide Character 5	Qualifier Character 6	Qualifier Character 7
9 Lacrimal Ducts, Bilateral	**1** Technetium 99m (Tc-99m) **Y** Other Radionuclide	**Z** None	**Z** None
Y Eye	**Y** Other Radionuclide	**Z** None	**Z** None

C Nuclear Medicine
9 Ear, Nose, Mouth and Throat
1 Planar Nuclear Medicine Imaging Definition: Introduction of radioactive materials into the body for single plane display of images developed from the capture of radioactive emissions

Body Part Character 4	Radionuclide Character 5	Qualifier Character 6	Qualifier Character 7
B Salivary Glands, Bilateral	**1** Technetium 99m (Tc-99m) **Y** Other Radionuclide	**Z** None	**Z** None
Y Ear, Nose, Mouth and Throat	**Y** Other Radionuclide	**Z** None	**Z** None

C Nuclear Medicine
B Respiratory System
1 Planar Nuclear Medicine Imaging Definition: Introduction of radioactive materials into the body for single plane display of images developed from the capture of radioactive emissions

Body Part Character 4	Radionuclide Character 5	Qualifier Character 6	Qualifier Character 7
2 Lungs and Bronchi	**1** Technetium 99m (Tc-99m) **9** Krypton (Kr-81m) **T** Xenon 127 (Xe-127) **V** Xenon 133 (Xe-133) **Y** Other Radionuclide	**Z** None	**Z** None
Y Respiratory System	**Y** Other Radionuclide	**Z** None	**Z** None

C Nuclear Medicine
B Respiratory System
2 Tomographic (Tomo) Nuclear Medicine Imaging Definition: Introduction of radioactive materials into the body for three dimensional display of images developed from the capture of radioactive emissions

Body Part Character 4	Radionuclide Character 5	Qualifier Character 6	Qualifier Character 7
2 Lungs and Bronchi	**1** Technetium 99m (Tc-99m) **9** Krypton (Kr-81m) **Y** Other Radionuclide	**Z** None	**Z** None
Y Respiratory System	**Y** Other Radionuclide	**Z** None	**Z** None

C Nuclear Medicine
B Respiratory System
3 Positron Emission Tomographic (PET) Imaging Definition: Introduction of radioactive materials into the body for three dimensional display of images developed from the simultaneous capture, 180 degrees apart, of radioactive emissions

Body Part Character 4	Radionuclide Character 5	Qualifier Character 6	Qualifier Character 7
2 Lungs and Bronchi	**K** Fluorine 18 (F-18) **Y** Other Radionuclide	**Z** None	**Z** None
Y Respiratory System	**Y** Other Radionuclide	**Z** None	**Z** None

C Nuclear Medicine
D Gastrointestinal System
1 Planar Nuclear Medicine Imaging Definition: Introduction of radioactive materials into the body for single plane display of images developed from the capture of radioactive emissions

Body Part Character 4	Radionuclide Character 5	Qualifier Character 6	Qualifier Character 7
5 Upper Gastrointestinal Tract **7** Gastrointestinal Tract	**1** Technetium 99m (Tc-99m) **D** Indium 111 (In-111) **Y** Other Radionuclide	**Z** None	**Z** None
Y Digestive System	**Y** Other Radionuclide	**Z** None	**Z** None

C Nuclear Medicine
D Gastrointestinal System
2 Tomographic (Tomo) Nuclear Medicine Imaging Definition: Introduction of radioactive materials into the body for three dimensional display of images developed from the capture of radioactive emissions

Body Part Character 4	Radionuclide Character 5	Qualifier Character 6	Qualifier Character 7
7 Gastrointestinal Tract	1 Technetium 99m (Tc-99m) D Indium 111 (In-111) Y Other Radionuclide	Z None	Z None
Y Digestive System	Y Other Radionuclide	Z None	Z None

C Nuclear Medicine
F Hepatobiliary System and Pancreas
1 Planar Nuclear Medicine Imaging Definition: Introduction of radioactive materials into the body for single plane display of images developed from the capture of radioactive emissions

Body Part Character 4	Radionuclide Character 5	Qualifier Character 6	Qualifier Character 7
4 Gallbladder 5 Liver 6 Liver and Spleen C Hepatobiliary System, All	1 Technetium 99m (Tc-99m) Y Other Radionuclide	Z None	Z None
Y Hepatobiliary System and Pancreas	Y Other Radionuclide	Z None	Z None

C Nuclear Medicine
F Hepatobiliary System and Pancreas
2 Tomographic (Tomo) Nuclear Medicine Imaging Definition: Introduction of radioactive materials into the body for three dimensional display of images developed from the capture of radioactive emissions

Body Part Character 4	Radionuclide Character 5	Qualifier Character 6	Qualifier Character 7
4 Gallbladder 5 Liver 6 Liver and Spleen	1 Technetium 99m (Tc-99m) Y Other Radionuclide	Z None	Z None
Y Hepatobiliary System and Pancreas	Y Other Radionuclide	Z None	Z None

C Nuclear Medicine
G Endocrine System
1 Planar Nuclear Medicine Imaging Definition: Introduction of radioactive materials into the body for single plane display of images developed from the capture of radioactive emissions

Body Part Character 4	Radionuclide Character 5	Qualifier Character 6	Qualifier Character 7
1 Parathyroid Glands	1 Technetium 99m (Tc-99m) S Thallium 201 (Tl-201) Y Other Radionuclide	Z None	Z None
2 Thyroid Gland	1 Technetium 99m (Tc-99m) F Iodine 123 (I-123) G Iodine 131 (I-131) Y Other Radionuclide	Z None	Z None
4 Adrenal Glands, Bilateral	G Iodine 131 (I-131) Y Other Radionuclide	Z None	Z None
Y Endocrine System	Y Other Radionuclide	Z None	Z None

C Nuclear Medicine
G Endocrine System
2 Tomographic (Tomo) Nuclear Medicine Imaging Definition: Introduction of radioactive materials into the body for three dimensional display of images developed from the capture of radioactive emissions

Body Part Character 4	Radionuclide Character 5	Qualifier Character 6	Qualifier Character 7
1 Parathyroid Glands	1 Technetium 99m (Tc-99m) S Thallium 201 (Tl-201) Y Other Radionuclide	Z None	Z None
Y Endocrine System	Y Other Radionuclide	Z None	Z None

C Nuclear Medicine
G Endocrine System
4 Nonimaging Nuclear Medicine Uptake Definition: Introduction of radioactive materials into the body for measurements of organ function, from the detection of radioactive emmissions

Body Part Character 4	Radionuclide Character 5	Qualifier Character 6	Qualifier Character 7
2 Thyroid Gland	1 Technetium 99m (Tc-99m) F Iodine 123 (I-123) G Iodine 131 (I-131) Y Other Radionuclide	Z None	Z None
Y Endocrine System	Y Other Radionuclide	Z None	Z None

C Nuclear Medicine
H Skin, Subcutaneous Tissue and Breast
1 Planar Nuclear Medicine Imaging Definition: Introduction of radioactive materials into the body for single plane display of images developed from the capture of radioactive emissions

Body Part Character 4	Radionuclide Character 5	Qualifier Character 6	Qualifier Character 7
0 Breast, Right 1 Breast, Left 2 Breasts, Bilateral	1 Technetium 99m (Tc-99m) S Thallium 201 (Tl-201) Y Other Radionuclide	Z None	Z None
Y Skin, Subcutaneous Tissue and Breast	Y Other Radionuclide	Z None	Z None

C Nuclear Medicine
H Skin, Subcutaneous Tissue and Breast
2 Tomographic (Tomo) Nuclear Medicine Imaging Definition: Introduction of radioactive materials into the body for three dimensional display of images developed from the capture of radioactive emissions

Body Part Character 4	Radionuclide Character 5	Qualifier Character 6	Qualifier Character 7
0 Breast, Right 1 Breast, Left 2 Breasts, Bilateral	1 Technetium 99m (Tc-99m) S Thallium 201 (Tl-201) Y Other Radionuclide	Z None	Z None
Y Skin, Subcutaneous Tissue and Breast	Y Other Radionuclide	Z None	Z None

C Nuclear Medicine
P Musculoskeletal System
1 Planar Nuclear Medicine Imaging Definition: Introduction of radioactive materials into the body for single plane display of images developed from the capture of radioactive emissions

Body Part Character 4	Radionuclide Character 5	Qualifier Character 6	Qualifier Character 7
1 Skull 4 Thorax 5 Spine 6 Pelvis 7 Spine and Pelvis 8 Upper Extremity, Right 9 Upper Extremity, Left B Upper Extremities, Bilateral C Lower Extremity, Right D Lower Extremity, Left F Lower Extremities, Bilateral Z Musculoskeletal System, All	1 Technetium 99m (Tc-99m) Y Other Radionuclide	Z None	Z None
Y Musculoskeletal System, Other	Y Other Radionuclide	Z None	Z None

C Nuclear Medicine
P Musculoskeletal System
2 Tomographic (Tomo) Nuclear Medicine Imaging Definition: Introduction of radioactive materials into the body for three dimensional display of images developed from the capture of radioactive emissions

Body Part Character 4	Radionuclide Character 5	Qualifier Character 6	Qualifier Character 7
1 Skull 2 Cervical Spine 3 Skull and Cervical Spine 4 Thorax 6 Pelvis 7 Spine and Pelvis 8 Upper Extremity, Right 9 Upper Extremity, Left B Upper Extremities, Bilateral C Lower Extremity, Right D Lower Extremity, Left F Lower Extremities, Bilateral G Thoracic Spine H Lumbar Spine J Thoracolumbar Spine	1 Technetium 99m (Tc-99m) Y Other Radionuclide	Z None	Z None
Y Musculoskeletal System, Other	Y Other Radionuclide	Z None	Z None

C Nuclear Medicine
P Musculoskeletal System
5 Nonimaging Nuclear Medicine Probe Definition: Introduction of radioactive materials into the body for the study of distribution and fate of certain substances by the detection of radioactive emissions; or, alternatively, measurement of absorption of radioactive emissions from an external source

Body Part Character 4	Radionuclide Character 5	Qualifier Character 6	Qualifier Character 7
5 Spine N Upper Extremities P Lower Extremities	Z None	Z None	Z None
Y Musculoskeletal System, Other	Y Other Radionuclide	Z None	Z None

C Nuclear Medicine
T Urinary System
1 Planar Nuclear Medicine Imaging Definition: Introduction of radioactive materials into the body for single plane display of images developed from the capture of radioactive emissions

Body Part Character 4	Radionuclide Character 5	Qualifier Character 6	Qualifier Character 7
3 Kidneys, Ureters and Bladder	1 Technetium 99m (Tc-99m) F Iodine 123 (I-123) G Iodine 131 (I-131) Y Other Radionuclide	Z None	Z None
H Bladder and Ureters	1 Technetium 99m (Tc-99m) Y Other Radionuclide	Z None	Z None
Y Urinary System	Y Other Radionuclide	Z None	Z None

C Nuclear Medicine
T Urinary System
2 Tomographic (Tomo) Nuclear Medicine Imaging Definition: Introduction of radioactive materials into the body for three dimensional display of images developed from the capture of radioactive emissions

Body Part Character 4	Radionuclide Character 5	Qualifier Character 6	Qualifier Character 7
3 Kidneys, Ureters and Bladder	1 Technetium 99m (Tc-99m) Y Other Radionuclide	Z None	Z None
Y Urinary System	Y Other Radionuclide	Z None	Z None

C Nuclear Medicine
T Urinary System
6 Nonimaging Nuclear Medicine Assay Definition: Introduction of radioactive materials into the body for the study of body fluids and blood elements, by the detection of radioactive emissions

Body Part Character 4	Radionuclide Character 5	Qualifier Character 6	Qualifier Character 7
3 Kidneys, Ureters and Bladder	1 Technetium 99m (Tc-99m) F Iodine 123 (I-123) G Iodine 131 (I-131) H Iodine 125 (I-125) Y Other Radionuclide	Z None	Z None
Y Urinary System	Y Other Radionuclide	Z None	Z None

C Nuclear Medicine
V Male Reproductive System
1 Planar Nuclear Medicine Imaging Definition: Introduction of radioactive materials into the body for single plane display of images developed from the capture of radioactive emissions

Body Part Character 4	Radionuclide Character 5	Qualifier Character 6	Qualifier Character 7
9 Testicles, Bilateral ♂	1 Technetium 99m (Tc-99m) Y Other Radionuclide	Z None	Z None
Y Male Reproductive System ♂	Y Other Radionuclide	Z None	Z None

♂ All body part, radionuclide, and qualifier values

C Nuclear Medicine
W Anatomical Regions
1 Planar Nuclear Medicine Imaging Definition: Introduction of radioactive materials into the body for single plane display of images developed from the capture of radioactive emissions

Body Part Character 4	Radionuclide Character 5	Qualifier Character 6	Qualifier Character 7
Ø Abdomen 1 Abdomen and Pelvis 4 Chest and Abdomen 6 Chest and Neck B Head and Neck D Lower Extremity J Pelvic Region M Upper Extremity N Whole Body	1 Technetium 99m (Tc-99m) D Indium 111 (In-111) F Iodine 123 (I-123) G Iodine 131 (I-131) L Gallium 67 (Ga-67) S Thallium 201 (Tl-201) Y Other Radionuclide	Z None	Z None
3 Chest	1 Technetium 99m (Tc-99m) D Indium 111 (In-111) F Iodine 123 (I-123) G Iodine 131 (I-131) K Fluorine 18 (F-18) L Gallium 67 (Ga-67) S Thallium 201 (Tl-201) Y Other Radionuclide	Z None	Z None
Y Anatomical Regions, Multiple	Y Other Radionuclide	Z None	Z None
Z Anatomical Region, Other	Z None	Z None	Z None

C Nuclear Medicine
W Anatomical Regions
2 Tomographic (Tomo) Nuclear Medicine Imaging Definition: Introduction of radioactive materials into the body for three dimensional display of images developed from the capture of radioactive emissions

Body Part Character 4	Radionuclide Character 5	Qualifier Character 6	Qualifier Character 7
Ø Abdomen 1 Abdomen and Pelvis 3 Chest 4 Chest and Abdomen 6 Chest and Neck B Head and Neck D Lower Extremity J Pelvic Region M Upper Extremity	1 Technetium 99m (Tc-99m) D Indium 111 (In-111) F Iodine 123 (I-123) G Iodine 131 (I-131) K Fluorine 18 (F-18) L Gallium 67 (Ga-67) S Thallium 201 (Tl-201) Y Other Radionuclide	Z None	Z None
Y Anatomical Regions, Multiple	Y Other Radionuclide	Z None	Z None

C Nuclear Medicine
W Anatomical Regions
3 Positron Emission Tomographic (PET) Imaging Definition: Introduction of radioactive materials into the body for three dimensional display of images developed from the simultaneous capture, 180 degrees apart, of radioactive emissions

Body Part Character 4	Radionuclide Character 5	Qualifier Character 6	Qualifier Character 7
N Whole Body	Y Other Radionuclide	Z None	Z None

C Nuclear Medicine
W Anatomical Regions
5 Nonimaging Nuclear Medicine Probe Definition: Introduction of radioactive materials into the body for the study of distribution and fate of certain substances by the detection of radioactive emissions; or, alternatively, measurement of absorption of radioactive emissions from an external source

Body Part Character 4	Radionuclide Character 5	Qualifier Character 6	Qualifier Character 7
Ø Abdomen **1** Abdomen and Pelvis **3** Chest **4** Chest and Abdomen **6** Chest and Neck **B** Head and Neck **D** Lower Extremity **J** Pelvic Region **M** Upper Extremity	**1** Technetium 99m (Tc-99m) **D** Indium 111 (In-111) **Y** Other Radionuclide	**Z** None	**Z** None

C Nuclear Medicine
W Anatomical Regions
7 Systemic Nuclear Medicine Therapy Definition: Introduction of unsealed radioactive materials into the body for treatment

Body Part Character 4	Radionuclide Character 5	Qualifier Character 6	Qualifier Character 7
Ø Abdomen **3** Chest	**N** Phosphorus 32 (P-32) **Y** Other Radionuclide	**Z** None	**Z** None
G Thyroid	**G** Iodine 131 (I-131) **Y** Other Radionuclide	**Z** None	**Z** None
N Whole Body	**8** Samarium 153 (Sm-153) **G** Iodine 131 (I-131) **N** Phosphorus 32 (P-32) **P** Strontium 89 (Sr-89) **Y** Other Radionuclide	**Z** None	**Z** None
Y Anatomical Regions, Multiple	**Y** Other Radionuclide	**Z** None	**Z** None

Radiation Therapy DØØ–DWY

Character Meanings

This Character Meaning table is provided as a guide to assist the user in the identification of character members that may be found in this section of code tables. It **SHOULD NOT** be used to build a PCS code.

Body System–Character 2	Modality–Character 3	Treatment Site–Character 4	Modality Qualifier–Character 5	Isotope–Character 6	Qualifier–Character 7
Ø Central and Peripheral Nervous System	Ø Beam Radiation	See next page	Ø Photons <1 MeV	7 Cesium 137 (Cs-137)	Ø Intraoperative
7 Lymphatic and Hematologic System	1 Brachytherapy		1 Photons 1 - 1Ø MeV	8 Iridium 192 (Ir-192)	Z None
8 Eye	2 Stereotactic Radiosurgery		2 Photons >1Ø MeV	9 Iodine 125 (I-125)	
9 Ear, Nose, Mouth and Throat	Y Other Radiation		3 Electrons	B Palladium 1Ø3 (Pd-1Ø3)	
B Respiratory System			4 Heavy Particles (Protons, Ions)	C Californium 252 (Cf-252)	
D Gastrointestinal System			5 Neutrons	D Iodine 131 (I-131)	
F Hepatobiliary System and Pancreas			6 Neutron Capture	F Phosphorus 32 (P-32)	
G Endocrine System			7 Contact Radiation	G Strontium 89 (Sr-89)	
H Skin			8 Hyperthermia	H Strontium 9Ø (Sr-9Ø)	
M Breast			9 High Dose Rate (HDR)	Y Other Isotope	
P Musculoskeletal System			B Low Dose Rate (LDR)	Z None	
T Urinary System			C Intraoperative Radiation Therapy (IORT)		
U Female Reproductive System			D Stereotactic Other Photon Radiosurgery		
V Male Reproductive System			F Plaque Radiation		
W Anatomical Regions			G Isotope Administration		
			H Stereotactic Particulate Radiosurgery		
			J Stereotactic Gamma Beam Radiosurgery		
			K Laser Interstitial Thermal Therapy		

Treatment Site—Character 4 Meanings

Body System– Character 2	Treatment Site– Character 4	
Ø Central and Peripheral Nervous System	Ø Brain 1 Brain Stem 6 Spinal Cord 7 Peripheral Nerve	
7 Lymphatic and Hematologic System	Ø Bone Marrow 1 Thymus 2 Spleen 3 Lymphatics, Neck 4 Lymphatics, Axillary	5 Lymphatics, Thorax 6 Lymphatics, Abdomen 7 Lymphatics, Pelvis 8 Lymphatics, Inguinal
8 Eye	Ø Eye	
9 Ear, Nose, Mouth and Throat	Ø Ear 1 Nose 3 Hypopharynx 4 Mouth 5 Tongue 6 Salivary Glands 7 Sinuses	8 Hard Palate 9 Soft Palate B Larynx C Pharynx D Nasopharynx F Oropharynx
B Respiratory System	Ø Trachea 1 Bronchus 2 Lung 5 Pleura	6 Mediastinum 7 Chest Wall 8 Diaphragm
D Gastrointestinal System	Ø Esophagus 1 Stomach 2 Duodenum 3 Jejunum	4 Ileum 5 Colon 7 Rectum 8 Anus
F Hepatobiliary System and Pancreas	Ø Liver 1 Gallbladder	2 Bile Ducts 3 Pancreas
G Endocrine System	Ø Pituitary Gland 1 Pineal Body 2 Adrenal Glands	4 Parathyroid Glands 5 Thyroid
H Skin	2 Skin, Face 3 Skin, Neck 4 Skin, Arm 5 Skin, Hand 6 Skin, Chest	7 Skin, Back 8 Skin, Abdomen 9 Skin, Buttock B Skin, Leg C Skin, Foot
M Breast	Ø Breast, Left 1 Breast, Right	
P Musculoskeletal System	Ø Skull 2 Maxilla 3 Mandible 4 Sternum 5 Rib(s) 6 Humerus	7 Radius/Ulna 8 Pelvic Bones 9 Femur B Tibia/Fibula C Other Bone
T Urinary System	Ø Kidney 1 Ureter	2 Bladder 3 Urethra
U Female Reproductive System	Ø Ovary 1 Cervix 2 Uterus	
V Male Reproductive System	Ø Prostate 1 Testis	
W Anatomical Regions	1 Head and Neck 2 Chest 3 Abdomen	4 Hemibody 5 Whole Body 6 Pelvic Region

AHA Coding Clinic for table DU1
2017, 4Q, 104 Intrauterine brachytherapy & placement of tandems & ovoids

D Radiation Therapy
Ø Central and Peripheral Nervous System
Ø Beam Radiation

Treatment Site Character 4	Modality Qualifier Character 5	Isotope Character 6	Qualifier Character 7
Ø Brain 1 Brain Stem 6 Spinal Cord 7 Peripheral Nerve	Ø Photons <1 MeV 1 Photons 1- 10 MeV 2 Photons >10 MeV 4 Heavy Particles (Protons, Ions) 5 Neutrons 6 Neutron Capture	Z None	Z None
Ø Brain 1 Brain Stem 6 Spinal Cord 7 Peripheral Nerve	3 Electrons	Z None	Ø Intraoperative Z None

D Radiation Therapy
Ø Central and Peripheral Nervous System
1 Brachytherapy

Treatment Site Character 4	Modality Qualifier Character 5	Isotope Character 6	Qualifier Character 7
Ø Brain 1 Brain Stem 6 Spinal Cord 7 Peripheral Nerve	9 High Dose Rate (HDR) B Low Dose Rate (LDR)	7 Cesium 137 (Cs-137) 8 Iridium 192 (Ir-192) 9 Iodine 125 (I-125) B Palladium 103 (Pd-103) C Californium 252 (Cf-252) Y Other Isotope	Z None

D Radiation Therapy
Ø Central and Peripheral Nervous System
2 Stereotactic Radiosurgery

Treatment Site Character 4	Modality Qualifier Character 5	Isotope Character 6	Qualifier Character 7
Ø Brain 1 Brain Stem 6 Spinal Cord 7 Peripheral Nerve	D Stereotactic Other Photon Radiosurgery H Stereotactic Particulate Radiosurgery J Stereotactic Gamma Beam Radiosurgery	Z None	Z None

DRG Non-OR All treatment site, modality, isotope, and qualifier values

D Radiation Therapy
Ø Central and Peripheral Nervous System
Y Other Radiation

Treatment Site Character 4	Modality Qualifier Character 5	Isotope Character 6	Qualifier Character 7
Ø Brain 1 Brain Stem 6 Spinal Cord 7 Peripheral Nerve	7 Contact Radiation 8 Hyperthermia F Plaque Radiation K Laser Interstitial Thermal Therapy	Z None	Z None

Valid OR DØY[Ø,1,6,7]KZZ

D Radiation Therapy
7 Lymphatic and Hematologic System
Ø Beam Radiation

Treatment Site Character 4	Modality Qualifier Character 5	Isotope Character 6	Qualifier Character 7
Ø Bone Marrow 1 Thymus 2 Spleen 3 Lymphatics, Neck 4 Lymphatics, Axillary 5 Lymphatics, Thorax 6 Lymphatics, Abdomen 7 Lymphatics, Pelvis 8 Lymphatics, Inguinal	Ø Photons <1 MeV 1 Photons 1-10 MeV 2 Photons >10 MeV 4 Heavy Particles (Protons, Ions) 5 Neutrons 6 Neutron Capture	Z None	Z None
Ø Bone Marrow 1 Thymus 2 Spleen 3 Lymphatics, Neck 4 Lymphatics, Axillary 5 Lymphatics, Thorax 6 Lymphatics, Abdomen 7 Lymphatics, Pelvis 8 Lymphatics, Inguinal	3 Electrons	Z None	Ø Intraoperative Z None

D Radiation Therapy
7 Lymphatic and Hematologic System
1 Brachytherapy

Treatment Site Character 4	Modality Qualifier Character 5	Isotope Character 6	Qualifier Character 7
Ø Bone Marrow 1 Thymus 2 Spleen 3 Lymphatics, Neck 4 Lymphatics, Axillary 5 Lymphatics, Thorax 6 Lymphatics, Abdomen 7 Lymphatics, Pelvis 8 Lymphatics, Inguinal	9 High Dose Rate (HDR) B Low Dose Rate (LDR)	7 Cesium 137 (Cs-137) 8 Iridium 192 (Ir-192) 9 Iodine 125 (I-125) B Palladium 103 (Pd-103) C Californium 252 (Cf-252) Y Other Isotope	Z None

D Radiation Therapy
7 Lymphatic and Hematologic System
2 Stereotactic Radiosurgery

Treatment Site Character 4	Modality Qualifier Character 5	Isotope Character 6	Qualifier Character 7
Ø Bone Marrow 1 Thymus 2 Spleen 3 Lymphatics, Neck 4 Lymphatics, Axillary 5 Lymphatics, Thorax 6 Lymphatics, Abdomen 7 Lymphatics, Pelvis 8 Lymphatics, Inguinal	D Stereotactic Other Photon Radiosurgery H Stereotactic Particulate Radiosurgery J Stereotactic Gamma Beam Radiosurgery	Z None	Z None

DRG Non-OR All treatment site, modality, isotope, and qualifier values

D Radiation Therapy
7 Lymphatic and Hematologic System
Y Other Radiation

Treatment Site Character 4	Modality Qualifier Character 5	Isotope Character 6	Qualifier Character 7
Ø Bone Marrow 1 Thymus 2 Spleen 3 Lymphatics, Neck 4 Lymphatics, Axillary 5 Lymphatics, Thorax 6 Lymphatics, Abdomen 7 Lymphatics, Pelvis 8 Lymphatics, Inguinal	8 Hyperthermia F Plaque Radiation	Z None	Z None

D Radiation Therapy
8 Eye
Ø Beam Radiation

Treatment Site Character 4	Modality Qualifier Character 5	Isotope Character 6	Qualifier Character 7
Ø Eye	Ø Photons <1 MeV 1 Photons 1-10 MeV 2 Photons >10 MeV 4 Heavy Particles (Protons, Ions) 5 Neutrons 6 Neutron Capture	Z None	Z None
Ø Eye	3 Electrons	Z None	Ø Intraoperative Z None

D Radiation Therapy
8 Eye
1 Brachytherapy

Treatment Site Character 4	Modality Qualifier Character 5	Isotope Character 6	Qualifier Character 7
Ø Eye	9 High Dose Rate (HDR) B Low Dose Rate (LDR)	7 Cesium 137 (Cs-137) 8 Iridium 192 (Ir-192) 9 Iodine 125 (I-125) B Palladium 103 (Pd-103) C Californium 252 (Cf-252) Y Other Isotope	Z None

D Radiation Therapy
8 Eye
2 Stereotactic Radiosurgery

Treatment Site Character 4	Modality Qualifier Character 5	Isotope Character 6	Qualifier Character 7
Ø Eye	D Stereotactic Other Photon Radiosurgery H Stereotactic Particulate Radiosurgery J Stereotactic Gamma Beam Radiosurgery	Z None	Z None

DRG Non-OR All treatment site, modality, isotope, and qualifier values

D Radiation Therapy
8 Eye
Y Other Radiation

Treatment Site Character 4	Modality Qualifier Character 5	Isotope Character 6	Qualifier Character 7
Ø Eye	7 Contact Radiation 8 Hyperthermia F Plaque Radiation	Z None	Z None

D Radiation Therapy
9 Ear, Nose, Mouth and Throat
0 Beam Radiation

Treatment Site Character 4	Modality Qualifier Character 5	Isotope Character 6	Qualifier Character 7
0 Ear 1 Nose 3 Hypopharynx 4 Mouth 5 Tongue 6 Salivary Glands 7 Sinuses 8 Hard Palate 9 Soft Palate B Larynx D Nasopharynx F Oropharynx	0 Photons <1 MeV 1 Photons 1-10 MeV 2 Photons >10 MeV 4 Heavy Particles (Protons, Ions) 5 Neutrons 6 Neutron Capture	Z None	Z None
0 Ear 1 Nose 3 Hypopharynx 4 Mouth 5 Tongue 6 Salivary Glands 7 Sinuses 8 Hard Palate 9 Soft Palate B Larynx D Nasopharynx F Oropharynx	3 Electrons	Z None	0 Intraoperative Z None

D Radiation Therapy
9 Ear, Nose, Mouth and Throat
1 Brachytherapy

Treatment Site Character 4	Modality Qualifier Character 5	Isotope Character 6	Qualifier Character 7
0 Ear 1 Nose 3 Hypopharynx 4 Mouth 5 Tongue 6 Salivary Glands 7 Sinuses 8 Hard Palate 9 Soft Palate B Larynx D Nasopharynx F Oropharynx	9 High Dose Rate (HDR) B Low Dose Rate (LDR)	7 Cesium 137 (Cs-137) 8 Iridium 192 (Ir-192) 9 Iodine 125 (I-125) B Palladium 103 (Pd-103) C Californium 252 (Cf-252) Y Other Isotope	Z None

D Radiation Therapy
9 Ear, Nose, Mouth and Throat
2 Stereotactic Radiosurgery

Treatment Site Character 4	Modality Qualifier Character 5	Isotope Character 6	Qualifier Character 7
0 Ear 1 Nose 4 Mouth 5 Tongue 6 Salivary Glands 7 Sinuses 8 Hard Palate 9 Soft Palate B Larynx C Pharynx D Nasopharynx	D Stereotactic Other Photon Radiosurgery H Stereotactic Particulate Radiosurgery J Stereotactic Gamma Beam Radiosurgery	Z None	Z None

DRG Non-OR All treatment site, modality, isotope, and qualifier values

D Radiation Therapy
9 Ear, Nose, Mouth and Throat
Y Other Radiation

Treatment Site Character 4	Modality Qualifier Character 5	Isotope Character 6	Qualifier Character 7
Ø Ear 1 Nose 5 Tongue 6 Salivary Glands 7 Sinuses 8 Hard Palate 9 Soft Palate	7 Contact Radiation 8 Hyperthermia F Plaque Radiation	Z None	Z None
3 Hypopharynx F Oropharynx	7 Contact Radiation 8 Hyperthermia	Z None	Z None
4 Mouth B Larynx D Nasopharynx	7 Contact Radiation 8 Hyperthermia C Intraoperative Radiation Therapy (IORT) F Plaque Radiation	Z None	Z None
C Pharynx	C Intraoperative Radiation Therapy (IORT) F Plaque Radiation	Z None	Z None

D Radiation Therapy
B Respiratory System
Ø Beam Radiation

Treatment Site Character 4	Modality Qualifier Character 5	Isotope Character 6	Qualifier Character 7
Ø Trachea 1 Bronchus 2 Lung 5 Pleura 6 Mediastinum 7 Chest Wall 8 Diaphragm	Ø Photons <1 MeV 1 Photons 1-10 MeV 2 Photons >10 MeV 4 Heavy Particles (Protons, Ions) 5 Neutrons 6 Neutron Capture	Z None	Z None
Ø Trachea 1 Bronchus 2 Lung 5 Pleura 6 Mediastinum 7 Chest Wall 8 Diaphragm	3 Electrons	Z None	Ø Intraoperative Z None

D Radiation Therapy
B Respiratory System
1 Brachytherapy

Treatment Site Character 4	Modality Qualifier Character 5	Isotope Character 6	Qualifier Character 7
Ø Trachea 1 Bronchus 2 Lung 5 Pleura 6 Mediastinum 7 Chest Wall 8 Diaphragm	9 High Dose Rate (HDR) B Low Dose Rate (LDR)	7 Cesium 137 (Cs-137) 8 Iridium 192 (Ir-192) 9 Iodine 125 (I-125) B Palladium 103 (Pd-103) C Californium 252 (Cf-252) Y Other Isotope	Z None

D Radiation Therapy
B Respiratory System
2 Stereotactic Radiosurgery

Treatment Site Character 4	Modality Qualifier Character 5	Isotope Character 6	Qualifier Character 7
Ø Trachea 1 Bronchus 2 Lung 5 Pleura 6 Mediastinum 7 Chest Wall 8 Diaphragm	D Stereotactic Other Photon Radiosurgery H Stereotactic Particulate Radiosurgery J Stereotactic Gamma Beam Radiosurgery	Z None	Z None

DRG Non-OR All treatment site, modality, isotope, and qualifier values

D Radiation Therapy
B Respiratory System
Y Other Radiation

Treatment Site Character 4	Modality Qualifier Character 5	Isotope Character 6	Qualifier Character 7
Ø Trachea 1 Bronchus 2 Lung 5 Pleura 6 Mediastinum 7 Chest Wall 8 Diaphragm	7 Contact Radiation 8 Hyperthermia F Plaque Radiation K Laser Interstitial Thermal Therapy	Z None	Z None

Valid OR DBY[Ø,1,2,5,6,7,8]KZZ

D Radiation Therapy
D Gastrointestinal System
Ø Beam Radiation

Treatment Site Character 4	Modality Qualifier Character 5	Isotope Character 6	Qualifier Character 7
Ø Esophagus 1 Stomach 2 Duodenum 3 Jejunum 4 Ileum 5 Colon 7 Rectum	Ø Photons <1 MeV 1 Photons 1-10 MeV 2 Photons >10 MeV 4 Heavy Particles (Protons, Ions) 5 Neutrons 6 Neutron Capture	Z None	Z None
Ø Esophagus 1 Stomach 2 Duodenum 3 Jejunum 4 Ileum 5 Colon 7 Rectum	3 Electrons	Z None	Ø Intraoperative Z None

D Radiation Therapy
D Gastrointestinal System
1 Brachytherapy

Treatment Site Character 4	Modality Qualifier Character 5	Isotope Character 6	Qualifier Character 7
Ø Esophagus 1 Stomach 2 Duodenum 3 Jejunum 4 Ileum 5 Colon 7 Rectum	9 High Dose Rate (HDR) B Low Dose Rate (LDR)	7 Cesium 137 (Cs-137) 8 Iridium 192 (Ir-192) 9 Iodine 125 (I-125) B Palladium 103 (Pd-103) C Californium 252 (Cf-252) Y Other Isotope	Z None

D Radiation Therapy
D Gastrointestinal System
2 Stereotactic Radiosurgery

Treatment Site Character 4	Modality Qualifier Character 5	Isotope Character 6	Qualifier Character 7
Ø Esophagus 1 Stomach 2 Duodenum 3 Jejunum 4 Ileum 5 Colon 7 Rectum	D Stereotactic Other Photon Radiosurgery H Stereotactic Particulate Radiosurgery J Stereotactic Gamma Beam Radiosurgery	Z None	Z None

DRG Non-OR All treatment site, modality, isotope, and qualifier values

D Radiation therapy
D Gastrointestinal System
Y Other Radiation

Treatment Site Character 4	Modality Qualifier Character 5	Isotope Character 6	Qualifier Character 7
Ø Esophagus	7 Contact Radiation 8 Hyperthermia F Plaque Radiation K Laser Interstitial Thermal Therapy	Z None	Z None
1 Stomach 2 Duodenum 3 Jejunum 4 Ileum 5 Colon 7 Rectum	7 Contact Radiation 8 Hyperthermia C Intraoperative Radiation Therapy (IORT) F Plaque Radiation K Laser Interstitial Thermal Therapy	Z None	Z None
8 Anus	C Intraoperative Radiation Therapy (IORT) F Plaque Radiation K Laser Interstitial Thermal Therapy	Z None	Z None

Valid OR DDYØKZZ
Valid OR DDY[1,2,3,4,5,7]KZZ
Valid OR DDY8KZZ

D Radiation Therapy
F Hepatobiliary System and Pancreas
Ø Beam Radiation

Treatment Site Character 4	Modality Qualifier Character 5	Isotope Character 6	Qualifier Character 7
Ø Liver 1 Gallbladder 2 Bile Ducts 3 Pancreas	Ø Photons <1 MeV 1 Photons 1-10 MeV 2 Photons >10 MeV 4 Heavy Particles (Protons, Ions) 5 Neutrons 6 Neutron Capture	Z None	Z None
Ø Liver 1 Gallbladder 2 Bile Ducts 3 Pancreas	3 Electrons	Z None	Ø Intraoperative Z None

D Radiation Therapy
F Hepatobiliary System and Pancreas
1 Brachytherapy

Treatment Site Character 4	Modality Qualifier Character 5	Isotope Character 6	Qualifier Character 7
Ø Liver 1 Gallbladder 2 Bile Ducts 3 Pancreas	9 High Dose Rate (HDR) B Low Dose Rate (LDR)	7 Cesium 137 (Cs-137) 8 Iridium 192 (Ir-192) 9 Iodine 125 (I-125) B Palladium 103 (Pd-103) C Californium 252 (Cf-252) Y Other Isotope	Z None

D Radiation Therapy
F Hepatobiliary System and Pancreas
2 Stereotactic Radiosurgery

Treatment Site Character 4	Modality Qualifier Character 5	Isotope Character 6	Qualifier Character 7
Ø Liver 1 Gallbladder 2 Bile Ducts 3 Pancreas	D Stereotactic Other Photon Radiosurgery H Stereotactic Particulate Radiosurgery J Stereotactic Gamma Beam Radiosurgery	Z None	Z None

DRG Non-OR All treatment site, modality, isotope, and qualifier values

D Radiation Therapy
F Hepatobiliary System and Pancreas
Y Other Radiation

Treatment Site Character 4	Modality Qualifier Character 5	Isotope Character 6	Qualifier Character 7
Ø Liver 1 Gallbladder 2 Bile Ducts 3 Pancreas	7 Contact Radiation 8 Hyperthermia C Intraoperative Radiation Therapy (IORT) F Plaque Radiation K Laser Interstitial Thermal Therapy	Z None	Z None

Valid OR DFY[Ø,1,2,3]KZZ

D Radiation Therapy
G Endocrine System
Ø Beam Radiation

Treatment Site Character 4	Modality Qualifier Character 5	Isotope Character 6	Qualifier Character 7
Ø Pituitary Gland 1 Pineal Body 2 Adrenal Glands 4 Parathyroid Glands 5 Thyroid	Ø Photons <1 MeV 1 Photons 1-10 MeV 2 Photons >10 MeV 5 Neutrons 6 Neutron Capture	Z None	Z None
Ø Pituitary Gland 1 Pineal Body 2 Adrenal Glands 4 Parathyroid Glands 5 Thyroid	3 Electrons	Z None	Ø Intraoperative Z None

D Radiation Therapy
G Endocrine System
1 Brachytherapy

Treatment Site Character 4	Modality Qualifier Character 5	Isotope Character 6	Qualifier Character 7
Ø Pituitary Gland 1 Pineal Body 2 Adrenal Glands 4 Parathyroid Glands 5 Thyroid	9 High Dose Rate (HDR) B Low Dose Rate (LDR)	7 Cesium 137 (Cs-137) 8 Iridium 192 (Ir-192) 9 Iodine 125 (I-125) B Palladium 103 (Pd-103) C Californium 252 (Cf-252) Y Other Isotope	Z None

D Radiation Therapy
G Endocrine System
2 Stereotactic Radiosurgery

Treatment Site Character 4	Modality Qualifier Character 5	Isotope Character 6	Qualifier Character 7
Ø Pituitary Gland 1 Pineal Body 2 Adrenal Glands 4 Parathyroid Glands 5 Thyroid	D Stereotactic Other Photon Radiosurgery H Stereotactic Particulate Radiosurgery J Stereotactic Gamma Beam Radiosurgery	Z None	Z None

DRG Non-OR All treatment site, modality, isotope, and qualifier values

D Radiation therapy
G Endocrine System
Y Other Radiation

Treatment Site Character 4	Modality Qualifier Character 5	Isotope Character 6	Qualifier Character 7
Ø Pituitary Gland 1 Pineal Body 2 Adrenal Glands 4 Parathyroid Glands 5 Thyroid	7 Contact Radiation 8 Hyperthermia F Plaque Radiation K Laser Interstitial Thermal Therapy	Z None	Z None

Valid OR DGY[Ø,1,2,4,5]KZZ

D Radiation Therapy
H Skin
Ø Beam Radiation

Treatment Site Character 4	Modality Qualifier Character 5	Isotope Character 6	Qualifier Character 7
2 Skin, Face 3 Skin, Neck 4 Skin, Arm 6 Skin, Chest 7 Skin, Back 8 Skin, Abdomen 9 Skin, Buttock B Skin, Leg	Ø Photons <1 MeV 1 Photons 1-10 MeV 2 Photons >10 MeV 4 Heavy Particles (Protons, Ions) 5 Neutrons 6 Neutron Capture	Z None	Z None
2 Skin, Face 3 Skin, Neck 4 Skin, Arm 6 Skin, Chest 7 Skin, Back 8 Skin, Abdomen 9 Skin, Buttock B Skin, Leg	3 Electrons	Z None	Ø Intraoperative Z None

D Radiation Therapy
H Skin
Y Other Radiation

Treatment Site Character 4	Modality Qualifier Character 5	Isotope Character 6	Qualifier Character 7
2 Skin, Face 3 Skin, Neck 4 Skin, Arm 6 Skin, Chest 7 Skin, Back 8 Skin, Abdomen 9 Skin, Buttock B Skin, Leg	7 Contact Radiation 8 Hyperthermia F Plaque Radiation	Z None	Z None
5 Skin, Hand C Skin, Foot	F Plaque Radiation	Z None	Z None

D Radiation Therapy
M Breast
Ø Beam Radiation

Treatment Site Character 4	Modality Qualifier Character 5	Isotope Character 6	Qualifier Character 7
Ø Breast, Left 1 Breast, Right	Ø Photons <1 MeV 1 Photons 1-10 MeV 2 Photons >10 MeV 4 Heavy Particles (Protons, Ions) 5 Neutrons 6 Neutron Capture	Z None	Z None
Ø Breast, Left 1 Breast, Right	3 Electrons	Z None	Ø Intraoperative Z None

D Radiation Therapy
M Breast
1 Brachytherapy

Treatment Site Character 4	Modality Qualifier Character 5	Isotope Character 6	Qualifier Character 7
Ø Breast, Left 1 Breast, Right	9 High Dose Rate (HDR) B Low Dose Rate (LDR)	7 Cesium 137 (Cs-137) 8 Iridium 192 (Ir-192) 9 Iodine 125 (I-125) B Palladium 103 (Pd-103) C Californium 252 (Cf-252) Y Other Isotope	Z None

D Radiation Therapy
M Breast
2 Stereotactic Radiosurgery

Treatment Site Character 4	Modality Qualifier Character 5	Isotope Character 6	Qualifier Character 7
Ø Breast, Left 1 Breast, Right	D Stereotactic Other Photon Radiosurgery H Stereotactic Particulate Radiosurgery J Stereotactic Gamma Beam Radiosurgery	Z None	Z None

DRG Non-OR All treatment site, modality, isotope, and qualifier values

D Radiation Therapy
M Breast
Y Other Radiation

Treatment Site Character 4	Modality Qualifier Character 5	Isotope Character 6	Qualifier Character 7
Ø Breast, Left 1 Breast, Right	7 Contact Radiation 8 Hyperthermia F Plaque Radiation K Laser Interstitial Thermal Therapy	Z None	Z None

Valid OR DMY[Ø,1]KZZ

D Radiation Therapy
P Musculoskeletal System
Ø Beam Radiation

Treatment Site Character 4	Modality Qualifier Character 5	Isotope Character 6	Qualifier Character 7
Ø Skull 2 Maxilla 3 Mandible 4 Sternum 5 Rib(s) 6 Humerus 7 Radius/Ulna 8 Pelvic Bones 9 Femur B Tibia/Fibula C Other Bone	Ø Photons <1 MeV 1 Photons 1-10 MeV 2 Photons >10 MeV 4 Heavy Particles (Protons, Ions) 5 Neutrons 6 Neutron Capture	Z None	Z None
Ø Skull 2 Maxilla 3 Mandible 4 Sternum 5 Rib(s) 6 Humerus 7 Radius/Ulna 8 Pelvic Bones 9 Femur B Tibia/Fibula C Other Bone	3 Electrons	Z None	Ø Intraoperative Z None

D Radiation Therapy
P Musculoskeletal System
Y Other Radiation

Treatment Site Character 4	Modality Qualifier Character 5	Isotope Character 6	Qualifier Character 7
Ø Skull 2 Maxilla 3 Mandible 4 Sternum 5 Rib(s) 6 Humerus 7 Radius/Ulna 8 Pelvic Bones 9 Femur B Tibia/Fibula C Other Bone	7 Contact Radiation 8 Hyperthermia F Plaque Radiation	Z None	Z None

D Radiation Therapy
T Urinary System
Ø Beam Radiation

Treatment Site Character 4	Modality Qualifier Character 5	Isotope Character 6	Qualifier Character 7
Ø Kidney 1 Ureter 2 Bladder 3 Urethra	Ø Photons <1 MeV 1 Photons 1-10 MeV 2 Photons >10 MeV 4 Heavy Particles (Protons, Ions) 5 Neutrons 6 Neutron Capture	Z None	Z None
Ø Kidney 1 Ureter 2 Bladder 3 Urethra	3 Electrons	Z None	Ø Intraoperative Z None

D Radiation Therapy
T Urinary System
1 Brachytherapy

Treatment Site Character 4	Modality Qualifier Character 5	Isotope Character 6	Qualifier Character 7
Ø Kidney 1 Ureter 2 Bladder 3 Urethra	9 High Dose Rate (HDR) B Low Dose Rate (LDR)	7 Cesium 137 (Cs-137) 8 Iridium 192 (Ir-192) 9 Iodine 125 (I-125) B Palladium 103 (Pd-103) C Californium 252 (Cf-252) Y Other Isotope	Z None

D Radiation Therapy
T Urinary System
2 Stereotactic Radiosurgery

Treatment Site Character 4	Modality Qualifier Character 5	Isotope Character 6	Qualifier Character 7
Ø Kidney 1 Ureter 2 Bladder 3 Urethra	D Stereotactic Other Photon Radiosurgery H Stereotactic Particulate Radiosurgery J Stereotactic Gamma Beam Radiosurgery	Z None	Z None

DRG Non-OR All treatment site, modality, isotope, and qualifier values

D Radiation Therapy
T Urinary System
Y Other Radiation

Treatment Site Character 4	Modality Qualifier Character 5	Isotope Character 6	Qualifier Character 7
Ø Kidney 1 Ureter 2 Bladder 3 Urethra	7 Contact Radiation 8 Hyperthermia C Intraoperative Radiation Therapy (IORT) F Plaque Radiation	Z None	Z None

D Radiation Therapy
U Female Reproductive System
Ø Beam Radiation

Treatment Site Character 4	Modality Qualifier Character 5	Isotope Character 6	Qualifier Character 7
Ø Ovary ♀ 1 Cervix ♀ 2 Uterus ♀	Ø Photons <1 MeV 1 Photons 1-10 MeV 2 Photons >10 MeV 4 Heavy Particles (Protons, Ions) 5 Neutrons 6 Neutron Capture	Z None	Z None
Ø Ovary ♀ 1 Cervix ♀ 2 Uterus ♀	3 Electrons	Z None	Ø Intraoperative Z None

♀ All treatment site, modality, isotope, and qualifier values

D Radiation Therapy
U Female Reproductive System
1 Brachytherapy

Treatment Site Character 4	Modality Qualifier Character 5	Isotope Character 6	Qualifier Character 7
Ø Ovary ♀ 1 Cervix ♀ 2 Uterus ♀	9 High Dose Rate (HDR) B Low Dose Rate (LDR)	7 Cesium 137 (Cs-137) 8 Iridium 192 (Ir-192) 9 Iodine 125 (I-125) B Palladium 103 (Pd-103) C Californium 252 (Cf-252) Y Other Isotope	Z None

♀ All treatment site, modality, isotope, and qualifier values

D Radiation Therapy
U Female Reproductive System
2 Stereotactic Radiosurgery

Treatment Site Character 4	Modality Qualifier Character 5	Isotope Character 6	Qualifier Character 7
Ø Ovary ♀ 1 Cervix ♀ 2 Uterus ♀	D Stereotactic Other Photon Radiosurgery H Stereotactic Particulate Radiosurgery J Stereotactic Gamma Beam Radiosurgery	Z None	Z None

DRG Non-OR All treatment site, modality, isotope, and qualifier values
♀ All treatment site, modality, isotope, and qualifier values

D Radiation Therapy
U Female Reproductive System
Y Other Radiation

Treatment Site Character 4	Modality Qualifier Character 5	Isotope Character 6	Qualifier Character 7
Ø Ovary ♀ 1 Cervix ♀ 2 Uterus ♀	7 Contact Radiation 8 Hyperthermia C Intraoperative Radiation Therapy (IORT) F Plaque Radiation	Z None	Z None

♀ All treatment site, modality, isotope, and qualifier values

D Radiation Therapy
V Male Reproductive System
Ø Beam Radiation

Treatment Site Character 4	Modality Qualifier Character 5	Isotope Character 6	Qualifier Character 7
Ø Prostate ♂ 1 Testis ♂	Ø Photons <1 MeV 1 Photons 1-10 MeV 2 Photons >10 MeV 4 Heavy Particles (Protons, Ions) 5 Neutrons 6 Neutron Capture	Z None	Z None
Ø Prostate ♂ 1 Testis ♂	3 Electrons	Z None	Ø Intraoperative Z None

♂ All treatment site, modality, isotope, and qualifier values

D Radiation Therapy
V Male Reproductive System
1 Brachytherapy

Treatment Site Character 4	Modality Qualifier Character 5	Isotope Character 6	Qualifier Character 7
Ø Prostate ♂ 1 Testis ♂	9 High Dose Rate (HDR) B Low Dose Rate (LDR)	7 Cesium 137 (Cs-137) 8 Iridium 192 (Ir-192) 9 Iodine 125 (I-125) B Palladium 103 (Pd-103) C Californium 252 (Cf-252) Y Other Isotope	Z None

♂ All treatment site, modality, isotope, and qualifier values

D Radiation Therapy
V Male Reproductive System
2 Stereotactic Radiosurgery

Treatment Site Character 4	Modality Qualifier Character 5	Isotope Character 6	Qualifier Character 7
Ø Prostate ♂ 1 Testis ♂	D Stereotactic Other Photon Radiosurgery H Stereotactic Particulate Radiosurgery J Stereotactic Gamma Beam Radiosurgery	Z None	Z None

DRG Non-OR All treatment site, modality, isotope, and qualifier values
♂ All treatment site, modality, isotope, and qualifier values

D Radiation Therapy
V Male Reproductive System
Y Other Radiation

Treatment Site Character 4	Modality Qualifier Character 5	Isotope Character 6	Qualifier Character 7
Ø Prostate ♂	7 Contact Radiation 8 Hyperthermia C Intraoperative Radiation Therapy (IORT) F Plaque Radiation K Laser Interstitial Thermal Therapy	Z None	Z None
1 Testis ♂	7 Contact Radiation 8 Hyperthermia F Plaque Radiation	Z None	Z None

Valid OR DVYØKZZ
♂ All treatment site, modality, isotope, and qualifier values

D Radiation Therapy
W Anatomical Regions
Ø Beam Radiation

Treatment Site Character 4	Modality Qualifier Character 5	Isotope Character 6	Qualifier Character 7
1 Head and Neck 2 Chest 3 Abdomen 4 Hemibody 5 Whole Body 6 Pelvic Region	Ø Photons <1 MeV 1 Photons 1 - 10 MeV 2 Photons >10 MeV 4 Heavy Particles (Protons, Ions) 5 Neutrons 6 Neutron Capture	Z None	Z None
1 Head and Neck 2 Chest 3 Abdomen 4 Hemibody 5 Whole Body 6 Pelvic Region	3 Electrons	Z None	Ø Intraoperative Z None

D Radiation Therapy
W Anatomical Regions
1 Brachytherapy

Treatment Site Character 4	Modality Qualifier Character 5	Isotope Character 6	Qualifier Character 7
1 Head and Neck 2 Chest 3 Abdomen 6 Pelvic Region	9 High Dose Rate (HDR) B Low Dose Rate (LDR)	7 Cesium 137 (Cs-137) 8 Iridium 192 (Ir-192) 9 Iodine 125 (I-125) B Palladium 103 (Pd-103) C Californium 252 (Cf-252) Y Other Isotope	Z None

D Radiation Therapy
W Anatomical Regions
2 Stereotactic Radiosurgery

Treatment Site Character 4	Modality Qualifier Character 5	Isotope Character 6	Qualifier Character 7
1 Head and Neck 2 Chest 3 Abdomen 6 Pelvic Region	D Stereotactic Other Photon Radiosurgery H Stereotactic Particulate Radiosurgery J Stereotactic Gamma Beam Radiosurgery	Z None	Z None

DRG Non-OR All treatment site, modality, isotope, and qualifier values

D Radiation Therapy
W Anatomical Regions
Y Other Radiation

Treatment Site Character 4	Modality Qualifier Character 5	Isotope Character 6	Qualifier Character 7
1 Head and Neck 2 Chest 3 Abdomen 4 Hemibody 6 Pelvic Region	7 Contact Radiation 8 Hyperthermia F Plaque Radiation	Z None	Z None
5 Whole Body	7 Contact Radiation 8 Hyperthermia F Plaque Radiation	Z None	Z None
5 Whole Body	G Isotope Administration	D Iodine 131 (I-131) F Phosphorus 32 (P-32) G Strontium 89 (Sr-89) H Strontium 90 (Sr-90) Y Other Isotope	Z None

Physical Rehabilitation and Diagnostic Audiology FØØ–F15

Character Meanings

This Character Meaning table is provided as a guide to assist the user in the identification of character members that may be found in this section of code tables. It **SHOULD NOT** be used to build a PCS code.

Ø: Rehabilitation

Type–Character 3	Body System/Region–Character 4	Type Qualifier–Character 5	Equipment–Character 6	Qualifier–Character 7
Ø Speech Assessment	Ø Neurological System - Head and Neck	See next page	1 Audiometer	Z None
1 Motor and/or Nerve Function Assessment	1 Neurological System - Upper Back / Upper Extremity		2 Sound Field / Booth	
2 Activities of Daily Living Assessment	2 Neurological System - Lower Back / Lower Extremity		4 Electroacoustic Immitance/ Acoustic Reflex	
6 Speech Treatment	3 Neurological System - Whole Body		5 Hearing Aid Selection / Fitting / Test	
7 Motor Treatment	4 Circulatory System - Head and Neck		7 Electrophysiologic	
8 Activities of Daily Living Treatment	5 Circulatory System - Upper Back / Upper Extremity		8 Vestibular / Balance	
9 Hearing Treatment	6 Circulatory System - Lower Back / Lower Extremity		9 Cochlear Implant	
B Cochlear Implant Treatment	7 Circulatory System - Whole Body		B Physical Agents	
C Vestibular Treatment	8 Respiratory System - Head and Neck		C Mechanical	
D Device Fitting	9 Respiratory System - Upper Back / Upper Extremity		D Electrotherapeutic	
F Caregiver Training	B Respiratory System - Lower Back / Lower Extremity		E Orthosis	
	C Respiratory System - Whole Body		F Assistive, Adaptive, Supportive or Protective	
	D Integumentary System - Head and Neck		G Aerobic Endurance and Conditioning	
	F Integumentary System - Upper Back / Upper Extremity		H Mechanical or Electromechanical	
	G Integumentary System - Lower Back / Lower Extremity		J Somatosensory	
	H Integumentary System - Whole Body		K Audiovisual	
	J Musculoskeletal System - Head and Neck		L Assistive Listening	
	K Musculoskeletal System - Upper Back / Upper Extremity		M Augmentative / Alternative Communication	
	L Musculoskeletal System - Lower Back / Lower Extremity		N Biosensory Feedback	
	M Musculoskeletal System - Whole Body		P Computer	
	N Genitourinary System		Q Speech Analysis	
	Z None		S Voice Analysis	
			T Aerodynamic Function	
			U Prosthesis	
			V Speech Prosthesis	
			W Swallowing	
			X Cerumen Management	
			Y Other Equipment	
			Z None	

Continued on next page

Ø: Rehabilitation
Type Qualifier—Character 5 Meanings

Continued from previous page

Type–Character 3	Type Qualifier–Character 5
Ø Speech Assessment	Ø Filtered Speech 1 Speech Threshold 2 Speech/Word Recognition 3 Staggered Spondaic Word 4 Sensorineural Acuity Level 5 Synthetic Sentence Identification 6 Speech and/or Language Screening 7 Nonspoken Language 8 Receptive/Expressive Language 9 Articulation/Phonology B Motor Speech C Aphasia D Fluency F Voice G Communicative/Cognitive Integration Skills H Bedside Swallowing and Oral Function J Instrumental Swallowing and Oral Function K Orofacial Myofunctional L Augmentative/Alternative Communication System M Voice Prosthetic N Non-invasive Instrumental Status P Oral Peripheral Mechanism Q Performance Intensity Phonetically Balanced Speech Discrimination R Brief Tone Stimuli S Distorted Speech T Dichotic Stimuli V Temporal Ordering of Stimuli W Masking Patterns X Other Specified Central Auditory Processing
1 Motor and/or Nerve Function Assessment	Ø Muscle Performance 1 Integumentary Integrity 2 Visual Motor Integration 3 Coordination/Dexterity 4 Motor Function 5 Range of Motion and Joint Integrity 6 Sensory Awareness/Processing/Integrity 7 Facial Nerve Function 9 Somatosensory Evoked Potentials B Bed Mobility C Transfer D Gait and/or Balance F Wheelchair Mobility G Reflex Integrity
2 Activities of Daily Living Assessment	Ø Bathing/Showering 1 Dressing 2 Feeding/Eating 3 Grooming/Personal Hygiene 4 Home Management 5 Perceptual Processing 6 Psychosocial Skills 7 Aerobic Capacity and Endurance 8 Anthropometric Characteristics 9 Cranial Nerve Integrity B Environmental, Home and Work Barriers C Ergonomics and Body Mechanics D Neuromotor Development F Pain G Ventilation, Respiration and Circulation H Vocational Activities and Functional Community or Work Reintegration Skills
6 Speech Treatment	Ø Nonspoken Language 1 Speech-Language Pathology and Related Disorders Counseling 2 Speech-Language Pathology and Related Disorders Prevention 3 Aphasia 4 Articulation/Phonology 5 Aural Rehabilitation 6 Communicative/Cognitive Integration Skills 7 Fluency 8 Motor Speech 9 Orofacial Myofunctional B Receptive/Expressive Language C Voice D Swallowing Dysfunction
7 Motor Treatment	Ø Range of Motion and Joint Mobility 1 Muscle Performance 2 Coordination/Dexterity 3 Motor Function 4 Wheelchair Mobility 5 Bed Mobility 6 Therapeutic Exercise 7 Manual Therapy Techniques 8 Transfer Training 9 Gait Training/Functional Ambulation
8 Activities of Daily Living Treatment	Ø Bathing/Showering Techniques 1 Dressing Techniques 2 Grooming/Personal Hygiene 3 Feeding/Eating 4 Home Management 5 Wound Management 6 Psychosocial Skills 7 Vocational Activities and Functional Community or Work Reintegration Skills
9 Hearing Treatment	Ø Hearing and Related Disorders Counseling 1 Hearing and Related Disorders Prevention 2 Auditory Processing 3 Cerumen Management
B Cochlear Implant Treatment	Ø Cochlear Implant Rehabilitation
C Vestibular Treatment	Ø Vestibular 1 Perceptual Processing 2 Visual Motor Integration 3 Postural Control
D Device Fitting	Ø Tinnitus Masker 1 Monaural Hearing Aid 2 Binaural Hearing Aid 3 Augmentative/Alternative Communication System 4 Voice Prosthetic 5 Assistive Listening Device 6 Dynamic Orthosis 7 Static Orthosis 8 Prosthesis 9 Assistive, Adaptive, Supportive or Protective Devices
F Caregiver Training	Ø Bathing/Showering Technique 1 Dressing 2 Feeding and Eating 3 Grooming/Personal Hygiene 4 Bed Mobility 5 Transfer 6 Wheelchair Mobility 7 Therapeutic Exercise 8 Airway Clearance Techniques 9 Wound Management B Vocational Activities and Functional Community or Work Reintegration Skills C Gait Training/Functional Ambulation D Application, Proper Use and Care of Assistive, Adaptive, Supportive or Protective Devices F Application, Proper Use and Care of Orthoses G Application, Proper Use and Care of Prosthesis H Home Management J Communication Skills

1: Diagnostic Audiology

Type–Character 3	Body System/Region–Character 4	Type Qualifier–Character 5	Equipment–Character 6	Qualifer–Character 7
3 Hearing Assessment	Z None	See below	Ø Occupational Hearing	Z None
4 Hearing Aid Assessment			1 Audiometer	
5 Vestibular Assessment			2 Sound Field / Booth	
			3 Tympanometer	
			4 Electroacoustic Immitance / Acoustic Reflex	
			5 Hearing Aid Selection / Fitting / Test	
			6 Otoacoustic Emission (OAE)	
			7 Electrophysiologic	
			8 Vestibular / Balance	
			9 Cochlear Implant	
			K Audiovisual	
			L Assistive Listening	
			P Computer	
			Y Other Equipment	
			Z None	

1: Diagnostic Audiology
Type Qualifier—Character 5 Meanings

Type–Character 3	Type Qualifier–Character 5
3 Hearing Assessment	Ø Hearing Screening 1 Pure Tone Audiometry, Air 2 Pure Tone Audiometry, Air and Bone 3 Bekesy Audiometry 4 Conditioned Play Audiometry 5 Select Picture Audiometry 6 Visual Reinforcement Audiometry 7 Alternate Binaural or Monaural Loudness Balance 8 Tone Decay 9 Short Increment Sensitivity Index B Stenger C Pure Tone Stenger D Tympanometry F Eustachian Tube Function G Acoustic Reflex Patterns H Acoustic Reflex Threshold J Acoustic Reflex Decay K Electrocochleography L Auditory Evoked Potentials M Evoked Otoacoustic Emissions, Screening N Evoked Otoacoustic Emissions, Diagnostic P Aural Rehabilitation Status Q Auditory Processing
4 Hearing Aid Assessment	Ø Cochlear Implant 1 Ear Canal Probe Microphone 2 Monaural Hearing Aid 3 Binaural Hearing Aid 4 Assistive Listening System/Device Selection 5 Sensory Aids 6 Binaural Electroacoustic Hearing Aid Check 7 Ear Protector Attentuation 8 Monaural Electroacoustic Hearing Aid Check
5 Vestibular Assessment	Ø Bithermal, Bionaural Caloric Irrigation 1 Bithermal, Monaural Caloric Irrigation 2 Unithermal Binaural Screen 3 Oscillating Tracking 4 Sinusoidal Vertical Axis Rotational 5 Dix-Hallpike Dynamic 6 Computerized Dynamic Posturography 7 Tinnitus Masker

Physical Rehabilitation and Diagnostic Audiology Physical Rehabilitation and Diagnostic Audiology

F Physical Rehabilitation and Diagnostic Audiology
Ø Rehabilitation
Ø Speech Assessment Definition: Measurement of speech and related functions

Body System/Region Character 4	Type Qualifier Character 5	Equipment Character 6	Qualifier Character 7
3 Neurological System - Whole Body	G Communicative/Cognitive Integration Skills	K Audiovisual M Augmentative / Alternative Communication P Computer Y Other Equipment Z None	Z None
Z None	Ø Filtered Speech 3 Staggered Spondaic Word Q Performance Intensity Phonetically Balanced Speech Discrimination R Brief Tone Stimuli S Distorted Speech T Dichotic Stimuli V Temporal Ordering of Stimuli W Masking Patterns	1 Audiometer 2 Sound Field / Booth K Audiovisual Z None	Z None
Z None	1 Speech Threshold 2 Speech/Word Recognition	1 Audiometer 2 Sound Field / Booth 9 Cochlear Implant K Audiovisual Z None	Z None
Z None	4 Sensorineural Acuity Level	1 Audiometer 2 Sound Field / Booth Z None	Z None
Z None	5 Synthetic Sentence Identification	1 Audiometer 2 Sound Field / Booth 9 Cochlear Implant K Audiovisual	Z None
Z None	6 Speech and/or Language Screening 7 Nonspoken Language 8 Receptive/Expressive Language C Aphasia G Communicative/Cognitive Integration Skills L Augmentative/Alternative Communication System	K Audiovisual M Augmentative / Alternative Communication P Computer Y Other Equipment Z None	Z None
Z None	9 Articulation/Phonology	K Audiovisual P Computer Q Speech Analysis Y Other Equipment Z None	Z None
Z None	B Motor Speech	K Audiovisual N Biosensory Feedback P Computer Q Speech Analysis T Aerodynamic Function Y Other Equipment Z None	Z None
Z None	D Fluency	K Audiovisual N Biosensory Feedback P Computer Q Speech Analysis S Voice Analysis T Aerodynamic Function Y Other Equipment Z None	Z None
Z None	F Voice	K Audiovisual N Biosensory Feedback P Computer S Voice Analysis T Aerodynamic Function Y Other Equipment Z None	Z None

FØØ Continued on next page

DRG Non-OR All body system/region, type qualifier, equipment, and qualifier values

F Physical Rehabilitation and Diagnostic Audiology
Ø Rehabilitation
Ø Speech Assessment Definition: Measurement of speech and related functions

FØØ Continued

Body System/Region Character 4	Type Qualifier Character 5	Equipment Character 6	Qualifier Character 7
Z None	H Bedside Swallowing and Oral Function P Oral Peripheral Mechanism	Y Other Equipment Z None	Z None
Z None	J Instrumental Swallowing and Oral Function	T Aerodynamic Function W Swallowing Y Other Equipment	Z None
Z None	K Orofacial Myofunctional	K Audiovisual P Computer Y Other Equipment Z None	Z None
Z None	M Voice Prosthetic	K Audiovisual P Computer S Voice Analysis V Speech Prosthesis Y Other Equipment Z None	Z None
Z None	N Non-invasive Instrumental Status	N Biosensory Feedback P Computer Q Speech Analysis S Voice Analysis T Aerodynamic Function Y Other Equipment	Z None
Z None	X Other Specified Central Auditory Processing	Z None	Z None

DRG Non-OR All body system/region, type qualifier, equipment, and qualifier values

F Physical Rehabilitation and Diagnostic Audiology
Ø Rehabilitation
1 Motor and/or Nerve Function Assessment Definition: Measurement of motor, nerve, and related functions

Body System/Region Character 4	Type Qualifier Character 5	Equipment Character 6	Qualifier Character 7
Ø Neurological System - Head and Neck 1 Neurological System - Upper Back/ Upper Extremity 2 Neurological System - Lower Back/ Lower Extremity 3 Neurological System - Whole Body	Ø Muscle Performance	E Orthosis F Assistive, Adaptive, Supportive or Protective U Prosthesis Y Other Equipment Z None	Z None
Ø Neurological System - Head and Neck 1 Neurological System - Upper Back/ Upper Extremity 2 Neurological System - Lower Back/ Lower Extremity 3 Neurological System - Whole Body	1 Integumentary Integrity 3 Coordination/Dexterity 4 Motor Function G Reflex Integrity	Z None	Z None
Ø Neurological System - Head and Neck 1 Neurological System - Upper Back/ Upper Extremity 2 Neurological System - Lower Back/ Lower Extremity 3 Neurological System - Whole Body	5 Range of Motion and Joint Integrity 6 Sensory Awareness/Processing/ Integrity	Y Other Equipment Z None	Z None
D Integumentary System - Head and Neck F Integumentary System - Upper Back/ Upper Extremity G Integumentary System - Lower Back/ Lower Extremity H Integumentary System - Whole Body J Musculoskeletal System - Head and Neck K Musculoskeletal System - Upper Back/ Upper Extremity L Musculoskeletal System - Lower Back/ Lower Extremity M Musculoskeletal System - Whole Body	Ø Muscle Performance	E Orthosis F Assistive, Adaptive, Supportive or Protective U Prosthesis Y Other Equipment Z None	Z None

FØ1 Continued on next page

DRG Non-OR All body system/region, type qualifier, equipment, and qualifier values

FØ1 Continued

F Physical Rehabilitation and Diagnostic Audiology
Ø Rehabilitation
1 Motor and/or Nerve Function Assessment Definition: Measurement of motor, nerve, and related functions

Body System/Region Character 4	Type Qualifier Character 5	Equipment Character 6	Qualifier Character 7
D Integumentary System - Head and Neck F Integumentary System - Upper Back/ Upper Extremity G Integumentary System - Lower Back/ Lower Extremity H Integumentary System - Whole Body J Musculoskeletal System - Head and Neck K Musculoskeletal System - Upper Back/ Upper Extremity L Musculoskeletal System - Lower Back/ Lower Extremity M Musculoskeletal System - Whole Body	1 Integumentary Integrity	Z None	Z None
D Integumentary System - Head and Neck F Integumentary System - Upper Back/ Upper Extremity G Integumentary System - Lower Back/ Lower Extremity H Integumentary System - Whole Body J Musculoskeletal System - Head and Neck K Musculoskeletal System - Upper Back/ Upper Extremity L Musculoskeletal System - Lower Back/ Lower Extremity M Musculoskeletal System - Whole Body	5 Range of Motion and Joint Integrity 6 Sensory Awareness/Processing/ Integrity	Y Other Equipment Z None	Z None
N Genitourinary System	Ø Muscle Performance	E Orthosis F Assistive, Adaptive, Supportive or Protective U Prosthesis Y Other Equipment Z None	Z None
Z None	2 Visual Motor Integration	K Audiovisual M Augmentative / Alternative Communication N Biosensory Feedback P Computer Q Speech Analysis S Voice Analysis Y Other Equipment Z None	Z None
Z None	7 Facial Nerve Function	7 Electrophysiologic	Z None
Z None	9 Somatosensory Evoked Potentials	J Somatosensory	Z None
Z None	B Bed Mobility C Transfer F Wheelchair Mobility	E Orthosis F Assistive, Adaptive, Supportive or Protective U Prosthesis Z None	Z None
Z None	D Gait and/or Balance	E Orthosis F Assistive, Adaptive, Supportive or Protective U Prosthesis Y Other Equipment Z None	Z None

DRG Non-OR All body system/region, type qualifier, equipment, and qualifier values

F Physical Rehabilitation and Diagnostic Audiology
Ø Rehabilitation
2 Activities of Daily Living Assessment Definition: Measurement of functional level for activities of daily living

Body System/Region Character 4	Type Qualifier Character 5	Equipment Character 6	Qualifier Character 7
Ø Neurological System - Head and Neck	9 Cranial Nerve Integrity D Neuromotor Development	Y Other Equipment Z None	Z None
1 Neurological System - Upper Back/ Upper Extremity 2 Neurological System - Lower Back/ Lower Extremity 3 Neurological System - Whole Body	D Neuromotor Development	Y Other Equipment Z None	Z None
4 Circulatory System - Head and Neck 5 Circulatory System - Upper Back/ Upper Extremity 6 Circulatory System - Lower Back/ Lower Extremity 8 Respiratory System - Head and Neck 9 Respiratory System - Upper Back/ Upper Extremity B Respiratory System - Lower Back/ Lower Extremity	G Ventilation, Respiration and Circulation	C Mechanical G Aerobic Endurance and Conditioning Y Other Equipment Z None	Z None
7 Circulatory System - Whole Body C Respiratory System - Whole Body	7 Aerobic Capacity and Endurance	E Orthosis G Aerobic Endurance and Conditioning U Prosthesis Y Other Equipment Z None	Z None
7 Circulatory System - Whole Body C Respiratory System - Whole Body	G Ventilation, Respiration and Circulation	C Mechanical G Aerobic Endurance and Conditioning Y Other Equipment Z None	Z None
Z None	Ø Bathing/Showering 1 Dressing 3 Grooming/Personal Hygiene 4 Home Management	E Orthosis F Assistive, Adaptive, Supportive or Protective U Prosthesis Z None	Z None
Z None	2 Feeding/Eating 8 Anthropometric Characteristics F Pain	Y Other Equipment Z None	Z None
Z None	5 Perceptual Processing	K Audiovisual M Augmentative / Alternative Communication N Biosensory Feedback P Computer Q Speech Analysis S Voice Analysis Y Other Equipment Z None	Z None
Z None	6 Psychosocial Skills	Z None	Z None
Z None	B Environmental, Home and Work Barriers C Ergonomics and Body Mechanics	E Orthosis F Assistive, Adaptive, Supportive or Protective U Prosthesis Y Other Equipment Z None	Z None
Z None	H Vocational Activities and Functional Community or Work Reintegration Skills	E Orthosis F Assistive, Adaptive, Supportive or Protective G Aerobic Endurance and Conditioning U Prosthesis Y Other Equipment Z None	Z None

DRG Non-OR All body system/region, type qualifier, equipment, and qualifier values

F Physical Rehabilitation and Diagnostic Audiology
Ø Rehabilitation
6 Speech Treatment Definition: Application of techniques to improve, augment, or compensate for speech and related functional impairment

Body System/Region Character 4	Type Qualifier Character 5	Equipment Character 6	Qualifier Character 7
3 Neurological System - Whole Body	6 Communicative/Cognitive Integration Skills	K Audiovisual M Augmentative / Alternative Communication P Computer Y Other Equipment Z None	Z None
Z None	Ø Nonspoken Language 3 Aphasia 6 Communicative/Cognitive Integration Skills	K Audiovisual M Augmentative / Alternative Communication P Computer Y Other Equipment Z None	Z None
Z None	1 Speech-Language Pathology and Related Disorders Counseling 2 Speech-Language Pathology and Related Disorders Prevention	K Audiovisual Z None	Z None
Z None	4 Articulation/Phonology	K Audiovisual P Computer Q Speech Analysis T Aerodynamic Function Y Other Equipment Z None	Z None
Z None	5 Aural Rehabilitation	K Audiovisual L Assistive Listening M Augmentative / Alternative Communication N Biosensory Feedback P Computer Q Speech Analysis S Voice Analysis Y Other Equipment Z None	Z None
Z None	7 Fluency	4 Electroacoustic Immitance / Acoustic Reflex K Audiovisual N Biosensory Feedback Q Speech Analysis S Voice Analysis T Aerodynamic Function Y Other Equipment Z None	Z None
Z None	8 Motor Speech	K Audiovisual N Biosensory Feedback P Computer Q Speech Analysis S Voice Analysis T Aerodynamic Function Y Other Equipment Z None	Z None
Z None	9 Orofacial Myofunctional	K Audiovisual P Computer Y Other Equipment Z None	Z None
Z None	B Receptive/Expressive Language	K Audiovisual L Assistive Listening M Augmentative / Alternative Communication P Computer Y Other Equipment Z None	Z None

FØ6 Continued on next page

DRG Non-OR All body system/region, type qualifier, equipment, and qualifier values

F Physical Rehabilitation and Diagnostic Audiology
0 Rehabilitation
6 Speech Treatment Definition: Application of techniques to improve, augment, or compensate for speech and related functional impairment

F06 Continued

Body System/Region Character 4	Type Qualifier Character 5	Equipment Character 6	Qualifier Character 7
Z None	C Voice	K Audiovisual N Biosensory Feedback P Computer S Voice Analysis T Aerodynamic Function V Speech Prosthesis Y Other Equipment Z None	Z None
Z None	D Swallowing Dysfunction	M Augmentative / Alternative Communication T Aerodynamic Function V Speech Prosthesis Y Other Equipment Z None	Z None

DRG Non-OR All body system/region, type qualifier, equipment, and qualifier values

F Physical Rehabilitation and Diagnostic Audiology
Ø Rehabilitation
7 Motor Treatment Definition: Exercise or activities to increase or facilitate motor function

Body System/Region Character 4	Type Qualifier Character 5	Equipment Character 6	Qualifier Character 7
Ø Neurological System - Head and Neck 1 Neurological System - Upper Back/Upper Extremity 2 Neurological System - Lower Back/Lower Extremity 3 Neurological System - Whole Body D Integumentary System - Head and Neck F Integumentary System - Upper Back/Upper Extremity G Integumentary System - Lower Back/Lower Extremity H Integumentary System - Whole Body J Musculoskeletal System - Head and Neck K Musculoskeletal System - Upper Back/Upper Extremity L Musculoskeletal System - Lower Back/Lower Extremity M Musculoskeletal System - Whole Body	Ø Range of Motion and Joint Mobility 1 Muscle Performance 2 Coordination/Dexterity 3 Motor Function	E Orthosis F Assistive, Adaptive, Supportive or Protective U Prosthesis Y Other Equipment Z None	Z None
Ø Neurological System - Head and Neck 1 Neurological System - Upper Back/Upper Extremity 2 Neurological System - Lower Back/Lower Extremity 3 Neurological System - Whole Body D Integumentary System - Head and Neck F Integumentary System - Upper Back/Upper Extremity G Integumentary System - Lower Back/Lower Extremity H Integumentary System - Whole Body J Musculoskeletal System - Head and Neck K Musculoskeletal System - Upper Back/Upper Extremity L Musculoskeletal System - Lower Back/Lower Extremity M Musculoskeletal System - Whole Body	6 Therapeutic Exercise	B Physical Agents C Mechanical D Electrotherapeutic E Orthosis F Assistive, Adaptive, Supportive or Protective G Aerobic Endurance and Conditioning H Mechanical or Electromechanical U Prosthesis Y Other Equipment Z None	Z None
Ø Neurological System - Head and Neck 1 Neurological System - Upper Back/Upper Extremity 2 Neurological System - Lower Back/Lower Extremity 3 Neurological System - Whole Body D Integumentary System - Head and Neck F Integumentary System - Upper Back/Upper Extremity G Integumentary System - Lower Back/Lower Extremity H Integumentary System - Whole Body J Musculoskeletal System - Head and Neck K Musculoskeletal System - Upper Back/Upper Extremity L Musculoskeletal System - Lower Back/Lower Extremity M Musculoskeletal System - Whole Body	7 Manual Therapy Techniques	Z None	Z None

FØ7 Continued on next page

DRG Non-OR All body system/region, type qualifier, equipment, and qualifier values

F **Physical Rehabilitation and Diagnostic Audiology**
0 **Rehabilitation**
7 **Motor Treatment** Definition: Exercise or activities to increase or facilitate motor function

F07 Continued

Body System/Region Character 4	Type Qualifier Character 5	Equipment Character 6	Qualifier Character 7
4 Circulatory System - Head and Neck 5 Circulatory System - Upper Back / Upper Extremity 6 Circulatory System - Lower Back / Lower Extremity 7 Circulatory System - Whole Body 8 Respiratory System - Head and Neck 9 Respiratory System - Upper Back / Upper Extremity B Respiratory System - Lower Back / Lower Extremity C Respiratory System - Whole Body	6 Therapeutic Exercise	B Physical Agents C Mechanical D Electrotherapeutic E Orthosis F Assistive, Adaptive, Supportive or Protective G Aerobic Endurance and Conditioning H Mechanical or Electromechanical U Prosthesis Y Other Equipment Z None	Z None
N Genitourinary System	1 Muscle Performance	E Orthosis F Assistive, Adaptive, Supportive or Protective U Prosthesis Y Other Equipment Z None	Z None
N Genitourinary System	6 Therapeutic Exercise	B Physical Agents C Mechanical D Electrotherapeutic E Orthosis F Assistive, Adaptive, Supportive or Protective G Aerobic Endurance and Conditioning H Mechanical or Electromechanical U Prosthesis Y Other Equipment Z None	Z None
Z None	4 Wheelchair Mobility	D Electrotherapeutic E Orthosis F Assistive, Adaptive, Supportive or Protective U Prosthesis Y Other Equipment Z None	Z None
Z None	5 Bed Mobility	C Mechanical E Orthosis F Assistive, Adaptive, Supportive or Protective U Prosthesis Y Other Equipment Z None	Z None
Z None	8 Transfer Training	C Mechanical D Electrotherapeutic E Orthosis F Assistive, Adaptive, Supportive or Protective U Prosthesis Y Other Equipment Z None	Z None
Z None	9 Gait Training/Functional Ambulation	C Mechanical D Electrotherapeutic E Orthosis F Assistive, Adaptive, Supportive or Protective G Aerobic Endurance and Conditioning U Prosthesis Y Other Equipment Z None	Z None

DRG Non-OR All body system/region, type qualifier, equipment, and qualifier values

F Physical Rehabilitation and Diagnostic Audiology
Ø Rehabilitation
8 Activities of Daily Living Treatment Definition: Exercise or activities to facilitate functional competence for activities of daily living

Body System/Region Character 4	Type Qualifier Character 5	Equipment Character 6	Qualifier Character 7
D Integumentary System - Head and Neck F Integumentary System - Upper Back/Upper Extremity G Integumentary System - Lower Back/Lower Extremity H Integumentary System - Whole Body J Musculoskeletal System - Head and Neck K Musculoskeletal System - Upper Back/Upper Extremity L Musculoskeletal System - Lower Back/Lower Extremity M Musculoskeletal System - Whole Body	5 Wound Management	B Physical Agents C Mechanical D Electrotherapeutic E Orthosis F Assistive, Adaptive, Supportive or Protective U Prosthesis Y Other Equipment Z None	Z None
Z None	Ø Bathing/Showering Techniques 1 Dressing Techniques 2 Grooming/Personal Hygiene	E Orthosis F Assistive, Adaptive, Supportive or Protective U Prosthesis Y Other Equipment Z None	Z None
Z None	3 Feeding/Eating	C Mechanical D Electrotherapeutic E Orthosis F Assistive, Adaptive, Supportive or Protective U Prosthesis Y Other Equipment Z None	Z None
Z None	4 Home Management	D Electrotherapeutic E Orthosis F Assistive, Adaptive, Supportive or Protective U Prosthesis Y Other Equipment Z None	Z None
Z None	6 Psychosocial Skills	Z None	Z None
Z None	7 Vocational Activities and Functional Community or Work Reintegration Skills	B Physical Agents C Mechanical D Electrotherapeutic E Orthosis F Assistive, Adaptive, Supportive or Protective G Aerobic Endurance and Conditioning U Prosthesis Y Other Equipment Z None	Z None

DRG Non-OR All body system/region, type qualifier, equipment, and qualifier values

F Physical Rehabilitation and Diagnostic Audiology
Ø Rehabilitation
9 Hearing Treatment Definition: Application of techniques to improve, augment, or compensate for hearing and related functional impairment

Body System/Region Character 4	Type Qualifier Character 5	Equipment Character 6	Qualifier Character 7
Z None	Ø Hearing and Related Disorders Counseling 1 Hearing and Related Disorders Prevention	K Audiovisual Z None	Z None
Z None	2 Auditory Processing	K Audiovisual L Assistive Listening P Computer Y Other Equipment Z None	Z None
Z None	3 Cerumen Management	X Cerumen Management Z None	Z None

DRG Non-OR All body system/region, type qualifier, equipment, and qualifier values

F Physical Rehabilitation and Diagnostic Audiology
Ø Rehabilitation
B Cochlear Implant Treatment Definition: Application of techniques to improve the communication abilities of individuals with cochlear implant

Body System/Region Character 4	Type Qualifier Character 5	Equipment Character 6	Qualifier Character 7
Z None	Ø Cochlear Implant Rehabilitation	1 Audiometer 2 Sound Field / Booth 9 Cochlear Implant K Audiovisual P Computer Y Other Equipment	Z None

DRG Non-OR All body system/region, type qualifier, equipment, and qualifier values

F Physical Rehabilitation and Diagnostic Audiology
Ø Rehabilitation
C Vestibular Treatment Definition: Application of techniques to improve, augment, or compensate for vestibular and related functional impairment

Body System/Region Character 4	Type Qualifier Character 5	Equipment Character 6	Qualifier Character 7
3 Neurological System - Whole Body H Integumentary System - Whole Body M Musculoskeletal System - Whole Body	3 Postural Control	E Orthosis F Assistive, Adaptive, Supportive or Protective U Prosthesis Y Other Equipment Z None	Z None
Z None	Ø Vestibular	8 Vestibular / Balance Z None	Z None
Z None	1 Perceptual Processing 2 Visual Motor Integration	K Audiovisual L Assistive Listening N Biosensory Feedback P Computer Q Speech Analysis S Voice Analysis T Aerodynamic Function Y Other Equipment Z None	Z None

DRG Non-OR All body system/region, type qualifier, equipment, and qualifier values

F Physical Rehabilitation and Diagnostic Audiology
Ø Rehabilitation
D Device Fitting Definition: Fitting of a device designed to facilitate or support achievement of a higher level of function

Body System/Region Character 4	Type Qualifier Character 5	Equipment Character 6	Qualifier Character 7
Z None	Ø Tinnitus Masker	5 Hearing Aid Selection / Fitting / Test Z None	Z None
Z None	1 Monaural Hearing Aid 2 Binaural Hearing Aid 5 Assistive Listening Device	1 Audiometer 2 Sound Field / Booth 5 Hearing Aid Selection / Fitting / Test K Audiovisual L Assistive Listening Z None	Z None
Z None	3 Augmentative/Alternative Communication System	M Augmentative / Alternative Communication	Z None
Z None	4 Voice Prosthetic	S Voice Analysis V Speech Prosthesis	Z None
Z None	6 Dynamic Orthosis 7 Static Orthosis 8 Prosthesis 9 Assistive, Adaptive,Supportive or Protective Devices	E Orthosis F Assistive, Adaptive, Supportive or Protective U Prosthesis Z None	Z None

DRG Non-OR FØDZØ[5,Z]Z
DRG Non-OR FØDZ[1, 2,5][1,2,5, K,L,Z]Z
DRG Non-OR FØDZ3MZ
DRG Non-OR FØDZ4[S,V]Z
DRG Non-OR FØDZ[6,7][E,F,U,Z]Z
DRG Non-OR FØDZ8[E,F,U]Z

F Physical Rehabilitation and Diagnostic Audiology
Ø Rehabilitation
F Caregiver Training Definition: Training in activities to support patient's optimal level of function

Body System/Region Character 4	Type Qualifier Character 5	Equipment Character 6	Qualifier Character 7
Z None	Ø Bathing/Showering Technique 1 Dressing 2 Feeding and Eating 3 Grooming/Personal Hygiene 4 Bed Mobility 5 Transfer 6 Wheelchair Mobility 7 Therapeutic Exercise 8 Airway Clearance Techniques 9 Wound Management B Vocational Activities and Functional Community or Work Reintegration Skills C Gait Training/Functional Ambulation D Application, Proper Use and Care of Devices F Application, Proper Use and Care of Orthoses G Application, Proper Use and Care of Prosthesis H Home Management	E Orthosis F Assistive, Adaptive, Supportive or Protective U Prosthesis Z None	Z None
Z None	J Communication Skills	K Audiovisual L Assistive Listening M Augmentative / Alternative Communication P Computer Z None	Z None

DRG Non-OR All body system/region, type qualifier, equipment, and qualifier values

F Physical Rehabilitation and Diagnostic Audiology
1 Diagnostic Audiology
3 Hearing Assessment Definition: Measurement of hearing and related functions

Body System/Region Character 4	Type Qualifier Character 5	Equipment Character 6	Qualifier Character 7
Z None	Ø Hearing Screening	Ø Occupational Hearing 1 Audiometer 2 Sound Field / Booth 3 Tympanometer 8 Vestibular / Balance 9 Cochlear Implant Z None	Z None
Z None	1 Pure Tone Audiometry, Air 2 Pure Tone Audiometry, Air and Bone	Ø Occupational Hearing 1 Audiometer 2 Sound Field / Booth Z None	Z None
Z None	3 Bekesy Audiometry 6 Visual Reinforcement Audiometry 9 Short Increment Sensitivity Index B Stenger C Pure Tone Stenger	1 Audiometer 2 Sound Field / Booth Z None	Z None
Z None	4 Conditioned Play Audiometry 5 Select Picture Audiometry	1 Audiometer 2 Sound Field / Booth K Audiovisual Z None	Z None
Z None	7 Alternate Binaural or Monaural Loudness Balance	1 Audiometer K Audiovisual Z None	Z None
Z None	8 Tone Decay D Tympanometry F Eustachian Tube Function G Acoustic Reflex Patterns H Acoustic Reflex Threshold J Acoustic Reflex Decay	3 Tympanometer 4 Electroacoustic Immitance / Acoustic Reflex Z None	Z None
Z None	K Electrocochleography L Auditory Evoked Potentials	7 Electrophysiologic Z None	Z None
Z None	M Evoked Otoacoustic Emissions, Screening N Evoked Otoacoustic Emissions, Diagnostic	6 Otoacoustic Emission (OAE) Z None	Z None
Z None	P Aural Rehabilitation Status	1 Audiometer 2 Sound Field / Booth 4 Electroacoustic Immitance / Acoustic Reflex 9 Cochlear Implant K Audiovisual L Assistive Listening P Computer Z None	Z None
Z None	Q Auditory Processing	K Audiovisual P Computer Y Other Equipment Z None	Z None

F Physical Rehabilitation and Diagnostic Audiology
1 Diagnostic Audiology
4 Hearing Aid Assessment Definition: Measurement of the appropriateness and/or effectiveness of a hearing device

Body System/Region Character 4	Type Qualifier Character 5	Equipment Character 6	Qualifier Character 7
Z None	Ø Cochlear Implant	1 Audiometer 2 Sound Field / Booth 3 Tympanometer 4 Electroacoustic Immitance / Acoustic Reflex 5 Hearing Aid Selection / Fitting / Test 7 Electrophysiologic 9 Cochlear Implant K Audiovisual L Assistive Listening P Computer Y Other Equipment Z None	Z None
Z None	1 Ear Canal Probe Microphone 6 Binaural Electroacoustic Hearing Aid Check 8 Monaural Electroacoustic Hearing Aid Check	5 Hearing Aid Selection / Fitting / Test Z None	Z None
Z None	2 Monaural Hearing Aid 3 Binaural Hearing Aid	1 Audiometer 2 Sound Field / Booth 3 Tympanometer 4 Electroacoustic Immitance / Acoustic Reflex 5 Hearing Aid Selection / Fitting / Test K Audiovisual L Assistive Listening P Computer Z None	Z None
Z None	4 Assistive Listening System/Device Selection	1 Audiometer 2 Sound Field / Booth 3 Tympanometer 4 Electroacoustic Immitance / Acoustic Reflex K Audiovisual L Assistive Listening Z None	Z None
Z None	5 Sensory Aids	1 Audiometer 2 Sound Field / Booth 3 Tympanometer 4 Electroacoustic Immitance / Acoustic Reflex 5 Hearing Aid Selection / Fitting / Test K Audiovisual L Assistive Listening Z None	Z None
Z None	7 Ear Protector Attentuation	Ø Occupational Hearing Z None	Z None

F Physical Rehabilitation and Diagnostic Audiology
1 Diagnostic Audiology
5 Vestibular Assessment Definition: Measurement of the vestibular system and related functions

Body System/Region Character 4	Type Qualifier Character 5	Equipment Character 6	Qualifier Character 7
Z None	Ø Bithermal, Binaural Caloric Irrigation 1 Bithermal, Monaural Caloric Irrigation 2 Unithermal Binaural Screen 3 Oscillating Tracking 4 Sinusoidal Vertical Axis Rotational 5 Dix-Hallpike Dynamic 6 Computerized Dynamic Posturography	8 Vestibular / Balance Z None	Z None
Z None	7 Tinnitus Masker	5 Hearing Aid Selection / Fitting / Test Z None	Z None

Mental Health GZ1–GZJ

Character Meanings

This Character Meaning table is provided as a guide to assist the user in the identification of character members that may be found in this section of code tables. It **SHOULD NOT** be used to build a PCS code.

Z: None

Type–Character 3	Qualifier–Character 4	Qualifier–Character 5	Qualifier–Character 6	Qualifier–Character 7
1 Psychological Tests	Ø Developmental 1 Personality and Behavioral 2 Intellectual and Psychoeducational 3 Neuropsychological 4 Neurobehavioral and Cognitive Status	Z None	Z None	Z None
2 Crisis Intervention	Z None			
3 Medication Management	Z None			
5 Individual Psychotherapy	Ø Interactive 1 Behavioral 2 Cognitive 3 Interpersonal 4 Psychoanalysis 5 Psychodynamic 6 Supportive 8 Cognitive-Behavioral 9 Psychophysiological			
6 Counseling	Ø Educational 1 Vocational 3 Other Counseling			
7 Family Psychotherapy	2 Other Family Psychotherapy			
B Electroconvulsive Therapy	Ø Unilateral-Single Seizure 1 Unilateral-Multiple Seizure 2 Bilateral-Single Seizure 3 Bilateral-Multiple Seizure 4 Other Electroconvulsive Therapy			
C Biofeedback	9 Other Biofeedback			
F Hypnosis	Z None			
G Narcosynthesis	Z None			
H Group Psychotherapy	Z None			
J Light Therapy	Z None			

G Mental Health
Z None
1 Psychological Tests Definition: The administration and interpretation of standardized psychological tests and measurement instruments for the assessment of psychological function

Qualifier Character 4	Qualifier Character 5	Qualifier Character 6	Qualifier Character 7
Ø Developmental 1 Personality and Behavioral 2 Intellectual and Psychoeducational 3 Neuropsychological 4 Neurobehavioral and Cognitive Status	Z None	Z None	Z None

G Mental Health
Z None
2 Crisis Intervention Definition: Treatment of a traumatized, acutely disturbed or distressed individual for the purpose of short-term stabilization

Qualifier Character 4	Qualifier Character 5	Qualifier Character 6	Qualifier Character 7
Z None	Z None	Z None	Z None

G Mental Health
Z None
3 Medication Management Definition: Monitoring and adjusting the use of medications for the treatment of a mental health disorder

Qualifier Character 4	Qualifier Character 5	Qualifier Character 6	Qualifier Character 7
Z None	Z None	Z None	Z None

G Mental Health
Z None
5 Individual Psychotherapy Definition: Treatment of an individual with a mental health disorder by behavioral, cognitive, psychoanalytic, psychodynamic or psychophysiological means to improve functioning or well-being

Qualifier Character 4	Qualifier Character 5	Qualifier Character 6	Qualifier Character 7
Ø Interactive 1 Behavioral 2 Cognitive 3 Interpersonal 4 Psychoanalysis 5 Psychodynamic 6 Supportive 8 Cognitive-Behavioral 9 Psychophysiological	Z None	Z None	Z None

G Mental Health
Z None
6 Counseling Definition: The application of psychological methods to treat an individual with normal developmental issues and psychological problems in order to increase function, improve well-being, alleviate distress, maladjustment or resolve crises

Qualifier Character 4	Qualifier Character 5	Qualifier Character 6	Qualifier Character 7
Ø Educational 1 Vocational 3 Other Counseling	Z None	Z None	Z None

G Mental Health
Z None
7 Family Psychotherapy Definition: Treatment that includes one or more family members of an individual with a mental health disorder by behavioral, cognitive, psychoanalytic, psychodynamic or psychophysiological means to improve functioning or well-being

Explanation: Remediation of emotional or behavioral problems presented by one or more family members in cases where psychotherapy with more than one family member is indicated

Qualifier Character 4	Qualifier Character 5	Qualifier Character 6	Qualifier Character 7
2 Other Family Psychotherapy	Z None	Z None	Z None

G Mental Health
Z None
B Electroconvulsive Therapy Definition: The application of controlled electrical voltages to treat a mental health disorder

Qualifier Character 4	Qualifier Character 5	Qualifier Character 6	Qualifier Character 7
Ø Unilateral-Single Seizure 1 Unilateral-Multiple Seizure 2 Bilateral-Single Seizure 3 Bilateral-Multiple Seizure 4 Other Electroconvulsive Therapy	Z None	Z None	Z None

G Mental Health
Z None
C Biofeedback Definition: Provision of information from the monitoring and regulating of physiological processes in conjunction with cognitive-behavioral techniques to improve patient functioning or well-being

Qualifier Character 4	Qualifier Character 5	Qualifier Character 6	Qualifier Character 7
9 Other Biofeedback	Z None	Z None	Z None

G Mental Health
Z None
F Hypnosis Definition: Induction of a state of heightened suggestibility by auditory, visual and tactile techniques to elicit an emotional or behavioral response

Qualifier Character 4	Qualifier Character 5	Qualifier Character 6	Qualifier Character 7
Z None	Z None	Z None	Z None

G Mental Health
Z None
G Narcosynthesis Definition: Administration of intravenous barbiturates in order to release suppressed or repressed thoughts

Qualifier Character 4	Qualifier Character 5	Qualifier Character 6	Qualifier Character 7
Z None	Z None	Z None	Z None

G Mental Health
Z None
H Group Psychotherapy Definition: Treatment of two or more individuals with a mental health disorder by behavioral, cognitive, psychoanalytic, psychodynamic or psychophysiological means to improve functioning or well-being

Qualifier Character 4	Qualifier Character 5	Qualifier Character 6	Qualifier Character 7
Z None	Z None	Z None	Z None

G Mental Health
Z None
J Light Therapy Definition: Application of specialized light treatments to improve functioning or well-being

Qualifier Character 4	Qualifier Character 5	Qualifier Character 6	Qualifier Character 7
Z None	Z None	Z None	Z None

Substance Abuse Treatment HZ2–HZ9

Character Meanings

This Character Meaning table is provided as a guide to assist the user in the identification of character members that may be found in this section of code tables. It **SHOULD NOT** be used to build a PCS code.

Z: None

Type–Character 3	Qualifier–Character 4	Qualifier–Character 5	Qualifier–Character 6	Qualifier–Character 7
2 Detoxification Services	Z None	Z None	Z None	Z None
3 Individual Counseling	Ø Cognitive			
	1 Behavioral			
	2 Cognitive-Behavioral			
	3 12-Step			
	4 Interpersonal			
	5 Vocational			
	6 Psychoeducation			
	7 Motivational Enhancement			
	8 Confrontational			
	9 Continuing Care			
	B Spiritual			
	C Pre/Post-Test Infectious Disease			
4 Group Counseling	Ø Cognitive			
	1 Behavioral			
	2 Cognitive-Behavioral			
	3 12-Step			
	4 Interpersonal			
	5 Vocational			
	6 Psychoeducation			
	7 Motivational Enhancement			
	8 Confrontational			
	9 Continuing Care			
	B Spiritual			
	C Pre/Post-Test Infectious Disease			
5 Individual Psychotherapy	Ø Cognitive			
	1 Behavioral			
	2 Cognitive-Behavioral			
	3 12-Step			
	4 Interpersonal			
	5 Interactive			
	6 Psychoeducation			
	7 Motivational Enhancement			
	8 Confrontational			
	9 Supportive			
	B Psychoanalysis			
	C Psychodynamic			
	D Psychophysiological			
6 Family Counseling	3 Other Family Counseling			
8 Medication Management	Ø Nicotine Replacement			
	1 Methadone Maintenance			
	2 Levo-alpha-acetyl-methadol (LAAM)			
	3 Antabuse			
	4 Naltrexone			
	5 Naloxone			
	6 Clonidine			
	7 Bupropion			
	8 Psychiatric Medication			
	9 Other Replacement Medication			
9 Pharmacotherapy	Ø Nicotine Replacement			
	1 Methadone Maintenance			
	2 Levo-alpha-acetyl-methadol (LAAM)			
	3 Antabuse			
	4 Naltrexone			
	5 Naloxone			
	6 Clonidine			
	7 Bupropion			
	8 Psychiatric Medication			
	9 Other Replacement Medication			

H Substance Abuse Treatment
Z None
2 Detoxification Services Definition: Detoxification from alcohol and/or drugs
Explanation: Not a treatment modality, but helps the patient stabilize physically and psychologically until the body becomes free of drugs and the effects of alcohol

Qualifier Character 4	Qualifier Character 5	Qualifier Character 6	Qualifier Character 7
Z None	Z None	Z None	Z None

H Substance Abuse Treatment
Z None
3 Individual Counseling Definition: The application of psychological methods to treat an individual with addictive behavior
Explanation: Comprised of several different techniques, which apply various strategies to address drug addiction

Qualifier Character 4	Qualifier Character 5	Qualifier Character 6	Qualifier Character 7
Ø Cognitive 1 Behavioral 2 Cognitive-Behavioral 3 12-Step 4 Interpersonal 5 Vocational 6 Psychoeducation 7 Motivational Enhancement 8 Confrontational 9 Continuing Care B Spiritual C Pre/Post-Test Infectious Disease	Z None	Z None	Z None

DRG Non-OR HZ3[Ø,1,2,3,4,5,6,7,8,9,B]ZZZ

H Substance Abuse Treatment
Z None
4 Group Counseling Definition: The application of psychological methods to treat two or more individuals with addictive behavior
Explanation: Provides structured group counseling sessions and healing power through the connection with others

Qualifier Character 4	Qualifier Character 5	Qualifier Character 6	Qualifier Character 7
Ø Cognitive 1 Behavioral 2 Cognitive-Behavioral 3 12-Step 4 Interpersonal 5 Vocational 6 Psychoeducation 7 Motivational Enhancement 8 Confrontational 9 Continuing Care B Spiritual C Pre/Post-Test Infectious Disease	Z None	Z None	Z None

DRG Non-OR HZ4[Ø,1,2,3,4,5,6,7,8,9,B]ZZZ

H Substance Abuse Treatment
Z None
5 Individual Psychotherapy Definition: Treatment of an individual with addictive behavior by behavioral, cognitive, psychoanalytic, psychodynamic or psychophysiological means

Qualifier Character 4	Qualifier Character 5	Qualifier Character 6	Qualifier Character 7
Ø Cognitive 1 Behavioral 2 Cognitive-Behavioral 3 12-Step 4 Interpersonal 5 Interactive 6 Psychoeducation 7 Motivational Enhancement 8 Confrontational 9 Supportive B Psychoanalysis C Psychodynamic D Psychophysiological	Z None	Z None	Z None

DRG Non-OR For all qualifier values

H Substance Abuse Treatment
Z None
6 Family Counseling Definition: The application of psychological methods that includes one or more family members to treat an individual with addictive behavior

Explanation: Provides support and education for family members of addicted individuals. Family member participation is seen as a critical area of substance abuse treatment

Qualifier Character 4	Qualifier Character 5	Qualifier Character 6	Qualifier Character 7
3 Other Family Counseling	Z None	Z None	Z None

H Substance Abuse Treatment
Z None
8 Medication Management Definition: Monitoring or adjusting the use of replacement medications for the treatment of addiction

Qualifier Character 4	Qualifier Character 5	Qualifier Character 6	Qualifier Character 7
0 Nicotine Replacement 1 Methadone Maintenance 2 Levo-alpha-acetyl-methadol (LAAM) 3 Antabuse 4 Naltrexone 5 Naloxone 6 Clonidine 7 Bupropion 8 Psychiatric Medication 9 Other Replacement Medication	Z None	Z None	Z None

H Substance Abuse Treatment
Z None
9 Pharmacotherapy Definition: The use of replacement medications for the treatment of addiction

Qualifier Character 4	Qualifier Character 5	Qualifier Character 6	Qualifier Character 7
0 Nicotine Replacement 1 Methadone Maintenance 2 Levo-alpha-acetyl-methadol (LAAM) 3 Antabuse 4 Naltrexone 5 Naloxone 6 Clonidine 7 Bupropion 8 Psychiatric Medication 9 Other Replacement Medication	Z None	Z None	Z None

New Technology X2A–XYØ

AHA Coding Clinic for all tables in the New Technology Section
2015, 4Q, 8-11

AHA Coding Clinic for table X2A
2016, 4Q, 115-116 Cerebral embolic filtration

AHA Coding Clinic for table X2C
2016, 4Q, 82-83 Coronary artery, number of arteries
2015, 4Q, 8-14 New Section X codes—New Technology procedures

AHA Coding Clinic for table X2R
2016, 4Q, 116 Aortic valve rapid deployment
2015, 4Q, 8-12 New Section X codes—New Technology procedures

AHA Coding Clinic for table XHR
2016, 4Q, 116 Application of wound matrix

AHA Coding Clinic for table XKØ
2017, 4Q, 74 Intramuscular autologous bone marrow cell therapy

AHA Coding Clinic for table XNS
2017, 4Q, 74-75 Magnetic growth rods
2016, 4Q, 117 Placement of magnetic growth rods

AHA Coding Clinic for table XRG
2017, 4Q, 76 Radiolucent porous interbody fusion device

AHA Coding Clinic for table XWØ
2015, 4Q, 8-15 New Section X codes—New Technology procedures

AHA Coding Clinic for table XYØ
2017, 4Q, 78 Intraoperative treatment of vascular grafts

X New Technology
2 Cardiovascular System
A Assistance Definition: Taking over a portion of a physiological function by extracorporeal means
Explanation: None

Body Part Character 4	Approach Character 5	Device/Substance/Technology Character 6	Qualifier Character 7
5 Innominate Artery and Left Common Carotid Artery	3 Percutaneous	1 Cerebral Embolic Filtration, Dual Filter	2 New Technology Group 2

X New Technology
2 Cardiovascular System
C Extirpation Definition: Taking or cutting out solid matter from a body part
Explanation: The solid matter may be an abnormal byproduct of a biological function or a foreign body; it may be imbedded in a body part or in the lumen of a tubular body part. The solid matter may or may not have been previously broken into pieces.

Body Part Character 4	Approach Character 5	Device/Substance/Technology Character 6	Qualifier Character 7
Ø Coronary Artery, One Artery 1 Coronary Artery, Two Arteries 2 Coronary Artery, Three Arteries 3 Coronary Artery, Four or More Arteries	3 Percutaneous	6 Orbital Atherectomy Technology	1 New Technology Group 1

Valid OR All body part, approach, device/substance/technology, and qualifier values

X New Technology
2 Cardiovascular System
R Replacement Definition: Putting in or on biological or synthetic material that physically takes the place and/or function of all or a portion of a body part
Explanation: The body part may have been taken out or replaced, or may be taken out, physically eradicated, or rendered nonfunctional during the REPLACEMENT procedure. A REMOVAL procedure is coded for taking out the device used in a previous replacement procedure

Body Part Character 4	Approach Character 5	Device/Substance/Technology Character 6	Qualifier Character 7
F Aortic Valve	Ø Open 3 Percutaneous 4 Percutaneous Endoscopic	3 Zooplastic Tissue, Rapid Deployment Technique	2 New Technology Group 2

Valid OR All body part, approach, device/substance/technology, and qualifier values

X New Technology
H Skin, Subcutaneous Tissue, Fascia and Breast
R Replacement Definition: Putting in or on biological or synthetic material that physically takes the place and/or function of all or a portion of a body part
Explanation: The body part may have been taken out or replaced, or may be taken out, physically eradicated, or rendered nonfunctional during the REPLACEMENT procedure. A REMOVAL procedure is coded for taking out the device used in a previous replacement procedure

Body Part Character 4	Approach Character 5	Device/Substance/Technology Character 6	Qualifier Character 7
P Skin	X External	L Skin Substitute, Porcine Liver Derived	2 New Technology Group 2

Valid OR All body part, approach, device/substance/technology, and qualifier values

X New Technology
K Muscles, Tendons, Bursae and Ligaments
Ø Introduction Definition: Putting in or on a therapeutic, diagnostic, nutritional, physiological, or prophylactic substance except blood or blood products
Explanation: None

Body Part Character 4	Approach Character 5	Device/Substance/Technology Character 6	Qualifier Character 7
2 Muscle	3 Percutaneous	Ø Concentrated Bone Marrow Aspirate	3 New Technology Group 3

X New Technology
N Bones
S Reposition Definition: Moving to its normal location, or other suitable location, all or a portion of a body part
Explanation: The body part is moved to a new location from an abnormal location, or from a normal location where it is not functioning correctly. The body part may or may not be cut out or off to be moved to the new location.

Body Part Character 4	Approach Character 5	Device/Substance/Technology Character 6	Qualifier Character 7
Ø Lumbar Vertebra 3 Cervical Vertebra 4 Thoracic Vertebra	Ø Open 3 Percutaneous	3 Magnetically Controlled Growth Rod(s)	2 New Technology Group 2

Valid OR All body part, approach, device/substance/technology, and qualifier values

X New Technology
R Joints
2 Monitoring Definition: Determining the level of a physiological or physical function repetitively over a period of time
Explanation: None

Body Part Character 4	Approach Character 5	Device/Substance/Technology Character 6	Qualifier Character 7
G Knee Joint, Right H Knee Joint, Left	Ø Open	2 Intraoperative Knee Replacement Sensor	1 New Technology Group 1

Valid OR All body part, approach, device/substance/technology, and qualifier values

X New Technology
R Joints
G Fusion Definition: Joining together portions of an articular body part rendering the articular body part immobile
Explanation: The body part is joined together by fixation device, bone graft, or other means

Body Part Character 4	Approach Character 5	Device/Substance/Technology Character 6	Qualifier Character 7
Ø Occipital-cervical Joint	Ø Open	9 Interbody Fusion Device, Nanotextured Surface	2 New Technology Group 2
Ø Occipital-cervical Joint	Ø Open	F Interbody Fusion Device, Radiolucent Porous	3 New Technology Group 3
1 Cervical Vertebral Joint	Ø Open	9 Interbody Fusion Device, Nanotextured Surface	2 New Technology Group 2
1 Cervical Vertebral Joint	Ø Open	F Interbody Fusion Device, Radiolucent Porous	3 New Technology Group 3
2 Cervical Vertebral Joints, 2 or more	Ø Open	9 Interbody Fusion Device, Nanotextured Surface	2 New Technology Group 2
2 Cervical Vertebral Joints, 2 or more	Ø Open	F Interbody Fusion Device, Radiolucent Porous	3 New Technology Group 3
4 Cervicothoracic Vertebral Joint	Ø Open	9 Interbody Fusion Device, Nanotextured Surface	2 New Technology Group 2
4 Cervicothoracic Vertebral Joint	Ø Open	F Interbody Fusion Device, Radiolucent Porous	3 New Technology Group 3
6 Thoracic Vertebral Joint	Ø Open	9 Interbody Fusion Device, Nanotextured Surface	2 New Technology Group 2
6 Thoracic Vertebral Joint	Ø Open	F Interbody Fusion Device, Radiolucent Porous	3 New Technology Group 3
7 Thoracic Vertebral Joints, 2 to 7 ⊞	Ø Open	9 Interbody Fusion Device, Nanotextured Surface	2 New Technology Group 2
7 Thoracic Vertebral Joints, 2 to 7 ⊞	Ø Open	F Interbody Fusion Device, Radiolucent Porous	3 New Technology Group 3
8 Thoracic Vertebral Joints, 8 or more	Ø Open	9 Interbody Fusion Device, Nanotextured Surface	2 New Technology Group 2
8 Thoracic Vertebral Joints, 8 or more	Ø Open	F Interbody Fusion Device, Radiolucent Porous	3 New Technology Group 3
A Thoracolumbar Vertebral Joint	Ø Open	9 Interbody Fusion Device, Nanotextured Surface	2 New Technology Group 2
A Thoracolumbar Vertebral Joint	Ø Open	F Interbody Fusion Device, Radiolucent Porous	3 New Technology Group 3
B Lumbar Vertebral Joint	Ø Open	9 Interbody Fusion Device, Nanotextured Surface	2 New Technology Group 2
B Lumbar Vertebral Joint	Ø Open	F Interbody Fusion Device, Radiolucent Porous	3 New Technology Group 3
C Lumbar Vertebral Joints, 2 or more ⊞	Ø Open	9 Interbody Fusion Device, Nanotextured Surface	2 New Technology Group 2
C Lumbar Vertebral Joints, 2 or more ⊞	Ø Open	F Interbody Fusion Device, Radiolucent Porous	3 New Technology Group 3
D Lumbosacral Joint	Ø Open	9 Interbody Fusion Device, Nanotextured Surface	2 New Technology Group 2
D Lumbosacral Joint	Ø Open	F Interbody Fusion Device, Radiolucent Porous	3 New Technology Group 3

Valid OR All body part, approach, device/substance/technology, and qualifier values

HAC XRG[Ø,1,2,4,6,7,8,A,B,C,D]Ø92 when reported with SDx K68.11 or T81.4XXA or T84.6Ø-T84.619, T84.63-T84.7 with 7th character A

HAC XRG[Ø,1,2,4,6,7,8,A,B,C,D]ØF3 when reported with SDx K68.11 or T81.4XXA or T84.6Ø-T84.619, T84.63-T84.7 with 7th character A

See Appendix L for Procedure Combinations
⊞ XRG7Ø92
⊞ XRG7ØF3
⊞ XRGCØ92
⊞ XRGCØF3

X New Technology
V Male Reproductive System
5 Destruction Definition: Physical eradication of all or a portion of a body part by the direct use of energy, force, or a destructive agent
Explanation: None of the body part is physically taken out

Body Part Character 4	Approach Character 5	Device/Substance/Technology Character 6	Qualifier Character 7
Ø Prostate	8 Via Natural or Artificial Opening Endoscopic	A Robotic Waterjet Ablation	4 New Technology Group 4

X New Technology
W Anatomical Regions
Ø Introduction Definition: Putting in or on a therapeutic, diagnostic, nutritional, physiological, or prophylactic substance except blood or blood products
Explanation: None

Body Part Character 4	Approach Character 5	Device/Substance/Technology Character 6	Qualifier Character 7
3 Peripheral Vein	3 Percutaneous	2 Ceftazidime-Avibactam Anti-infective 3 Idarucizumab, Dabigatran Reversal Agent 4 Isavuconazole Anti- infective 5 Blinatumomab Antineoplastic Immunotherapy	1 New Technology Group 1
3 Peripheral Vein	3 Percutaneous	7 Andexanet Alfa, Factor Xa Inhibitor Reversal Agent 9 Defibrotide Sodium Anticoagulant	2 New Technology Group 2
3 Peripheral Vein	3 Percutaneous	A Bezlotoxumab Monoclonal Antibody B Cytarabine and Daunorubicin Liposome Antineoplastic C Engineered Autologous Chimeric Antigen Receptor T-cell Immunotherapy F Other New Technology Therapeutic Substance	3 New Technology Group 3
3 Peripheral Vein	3 Percutaneous	G Plazomicin Anti-infective H Synthetic Human Angiotensin II	4 New Technology Group 4
4 Central Vein	3 Percutaneous	2 Ceftazidime-Avibactam Anti-infective 3 Idarucizumab, Dabigatran Reversal Agent 4 Isavuconazole Anti- infective 5 Blinatumomab Antineoplastic Immunotherapy	1 New Technology Group 1
4 Central Vein	3 Percutaneous	7 Andexanet Alfa, Factor Xa Inhibitor Reversal Agent 9 Defibrotide Sodium Anticoagulant	2 New Technology Group 2
4 Central Vein	3 Percutaneous	A Bezlotoxumab Monoclonal Antibody B Cytarabine and Daunorubicin Liposome Antineoplastic C Engineered Autologous Chimeric Antigen Receptor T-cell Immunotherapy F Other New Technology Therapeutic Substance	3 New Technology Group 3
4 Central Vein	3 Percutaneous	G Plazomicin Anti-infective H Synthetic Human Angiotensin II	4 New Technology Group 4
D Mouth and Pharynx	X External	8 Uridine Triacetate	2 New Technology Group 2

X New Technology
Y Extracorporeal
Ø Introduction Definition: Putting in or on a therapeutic, diagnostic, nutritional, physiological, or prophylactic substance except blood or blood products
Explanation: None

Body Part Character 4	Approach Character 5	Device/Substance/Technology Character 6	Qualifier Character 7
V Vein Graft	X External	8 Endothelial Damage Inhibitor	3 New Technology Group 3

Appendixes

Appendix A: Components of the Medical and Surgical Approach Definitions

ICD-10-PCS Value	Definition	Access Location	Method	Type of Instrumentation	Example
Open (Ø)	Cutting through the skin or mucous membrane and any other body layers necessary to expose the site of the procedure	Skin or mucous membrane, any other body layers	Cutting	None	Abdominal hysterectomy
Percutaneous (3)	Entry, by puncture or minor incision, of instrumentation through the skin or mucous membrane and any other body layers necessary to reach the site of the procedure	Skin or mucous membrane, any other body layers	Puncture or minor incision	Without visualization	Needle biopsy of liver, Liposuction
Percutaneous endoscopic (4)	Entry, by puncture or minor incision, of instrumentation through the skin or mucous membrane and any other body layers necessary to reach and visualize the site of the procedure	Skin or mucous membrane, any other body layers	Puncture or minor incision	With visualization	Arthroscopy, Laparoscopic cholecystectomy
Via natural or artificial opening (7)	Entry of instrumentation through a natural or artificial external opening to reach the site of the procedure	Natural or artificial external opening	Direct entry	Without visualization	Endotracheal tube insertion, Foley catheter placement
Via natural or artificial opening endoscopic (8)	Entry of instrumentation through a natural or artificial external opening to reach and visualize the site of the procedure	Natural or artificial external opening	Direct entry	With visualization	Sigmoidoscopy, EGD, ERCP
Via natural or artificial opening with percutaneous endoscopic assistance (F)	Entry of instrumentation through a natural or artificial external opening and entry, by puncture or minor incision, of instrumentation through the skin or mucous membrane and any other body layers necessary to aid in the performance of the procedure	Skin or mucous membrane, any other body layers	Direct entry with puncture or minor incision for instrumentation only	With visualization	Laparoscopic-assisted vaginal hysterectomy
External (X)	Procedures performed directly on the skin or mucous membrane and procedures performed indirectly by the application of external force through the skin or mucous membrane	Skin or mucous membrane	Direct or indirect application	None	Closed fracture reduction, Resection of tonsils

Open (Ø)

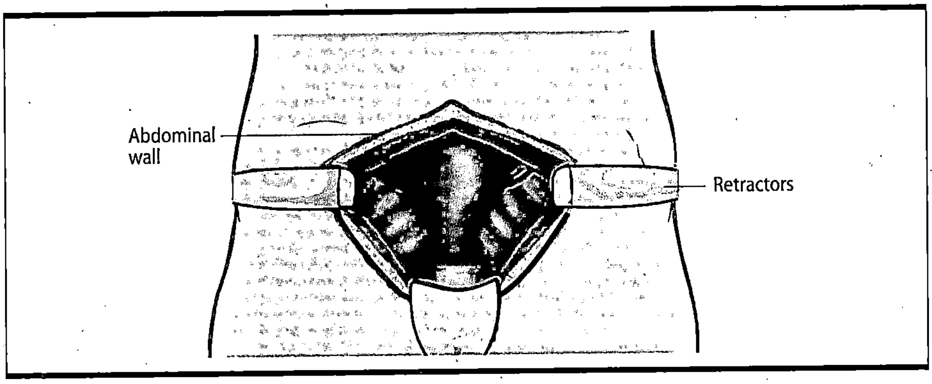

Percutaneous (3)

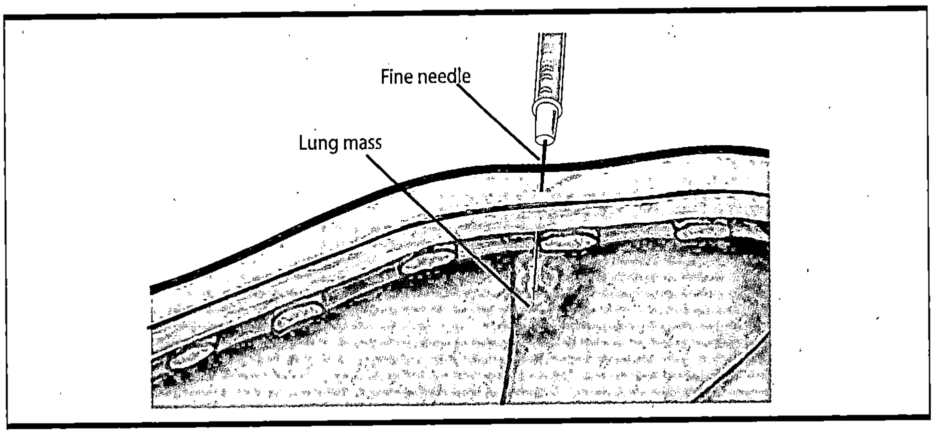

Percutaneous Endoscopic (4)

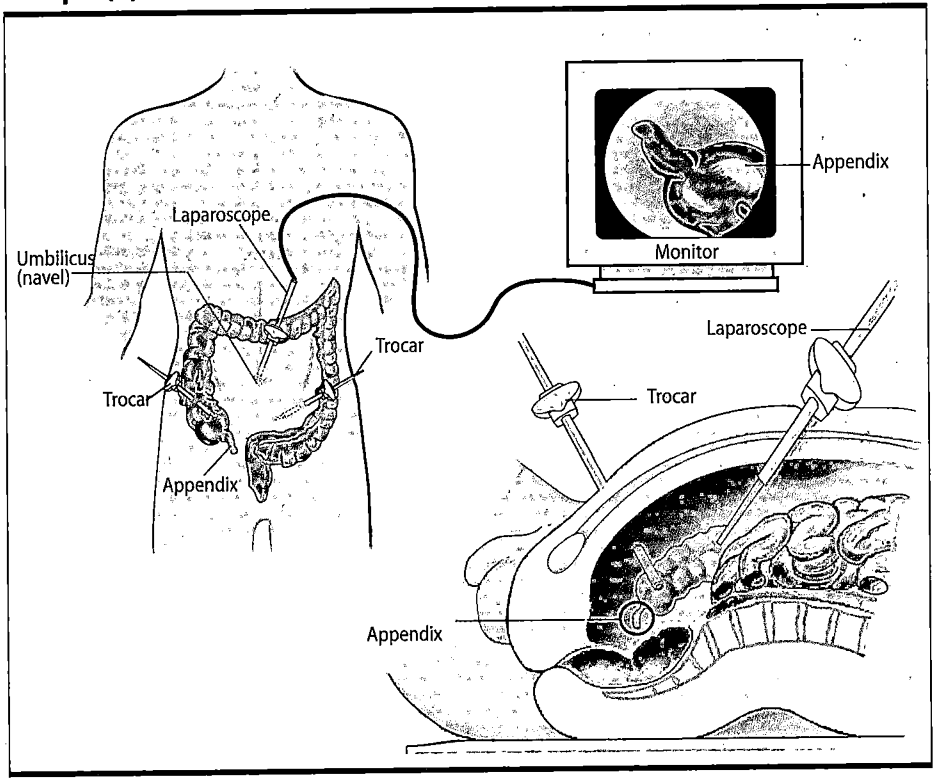

Via Natural or Artificial Opening (7)

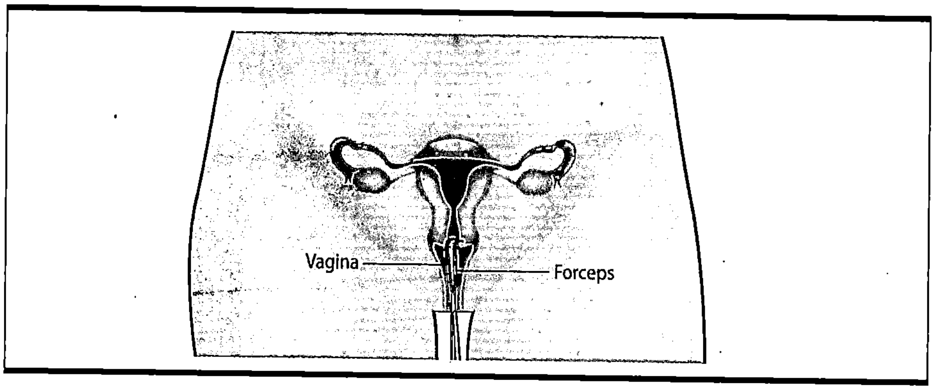

Via Natural or Artificial Opening, Endoscopic (8)

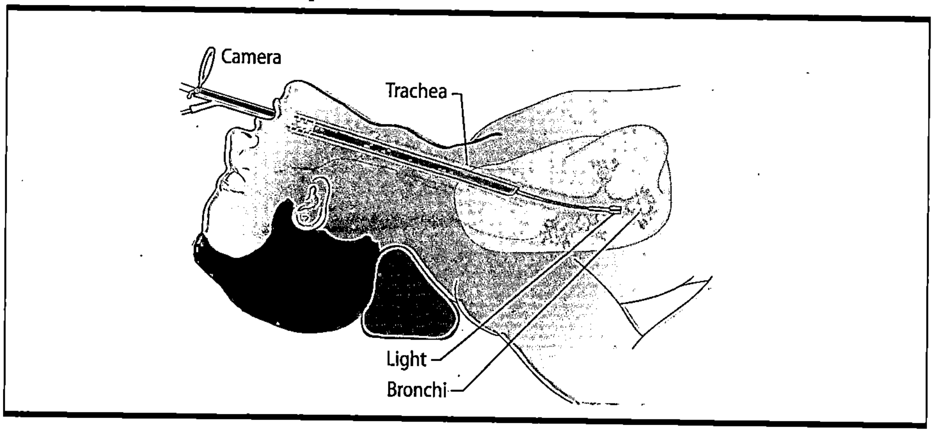

Via Natural or Artificial Opening with Percutaneous Endoscopic Assistance (F)

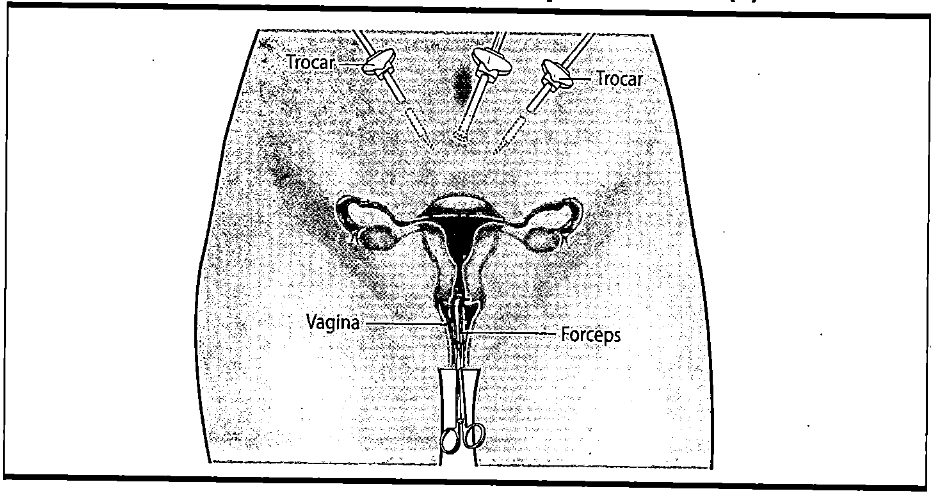

External (X)

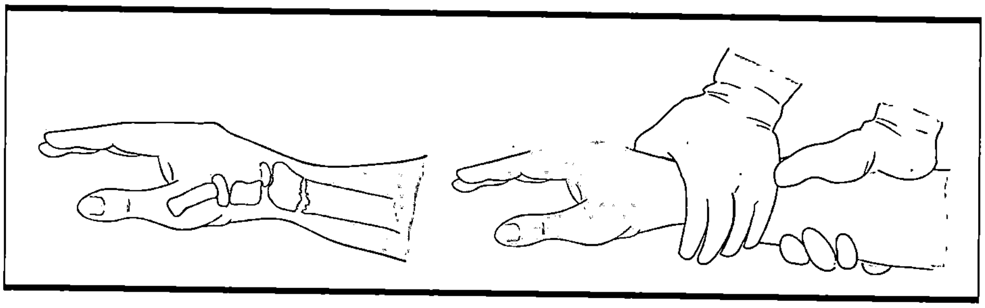

Appendix B: Root Operation Definitions

Ø Medical and Surgical

ICD-10-PCS Value		Definition	
Ø	Alteration	Definition:	Modifying the anatomic structure of a body part without affecting the function of the body part
		Explanation:	Principal purpose is to improve appearance
		Examples:	Face lift, breast augmentation
1	Bypass	Definition:	Altering the route of passage of the contents of a tubular body part
		Explanation:	Rerouting contents of a body part to a downstream area of the normal route, to a similar route and body part, or to an abnormal route and dissimilar body part. Includes one or more anastomoses, with or without the use of a device.
		Examples:	Coronary artery bypass, colostomy formation
2	Change	Definition:	Taking out or off a device from a body part and putting back an identical or similar device in or on the same body part without cutting or puncturing the skin or a mucous membrane
		Explanation:	All CHANGE procedures are coded using the approach EXTERNAL
		Example:	Urinary catheter change, gastrostomy tube change
3	Control	Definition:	Stopping, or attempting to stop, postprocedural or other acute bleeding
		Explanation:	The site of the bleeding is coded as an anatomical region and not to a specific body part
		Examples:	Control of post-prostatectomy hemorrhage, control of intracranial subdural hemorrhage, control of bleeding duodenal ulcer, control of retroperitoneal hemorrhage
4	Creation	Definition:	Putting in or on biological or synthetic material to form a new body part that to the extent possible replicates the anatomic structure or function of an absent body part
		Explanation:	Used for gender reassignment surgery and corrective procedures in individuals with congenital anomalies
		Examples:	Creation of vagina in a male, creation of right and left atrioventricular valve from common atrioventricular valve
5	Destruction	Definition:	Physical eradication of all or a portion of a body part by the direct use of energy, force, or a destructive agent
		Explanation:	None of the body part is physically taken out
		Examples:	Fulguration of rectal polyp, cautery of skin lesion
6	Detachment	Definition:	Cutting off all or a portion of the upper or lower extremities
		Explanation:	The body part value is the site of the detachment, with a qualifier if applicable to further specify the level where the extremity was detached
		Examples:	Below knee amputation, disarticulation of shoulder
7	Dilation	Definition:	Expanding an orifice or the lumen of a tubular body part
		Explanation:	The orifice can be a natural orifice or an artificially created orifice. Accomplished by stretching a tubular body part using intraluminal pressure or by cutting part of the orifice or wall of the tubular body part.
		Examples:	Percutaneous transluminal angioplasty, internal urethrotomy
8	Division	Definition:	Cutting into a body part, without draining fluids and/or gases from the body part, in order to separate or transect a body part
		Explanation:	All or a portion of the body part is separated into two or more portions
		Examples:	Spinal cordotomy, osteotomy
9	Drainage	Definition:	Taking or letting out fluids and/or gases from a body part
		Explanation:	The qualifier DIAGNOSTIC is used to identify drainage procedures that are biopsies
		Examples:	Thoracentesis, incision and drainage
B	Excision	Definition:	Cutting out or off, without replacement, a portion of a body part
		Explanation:	The qualifier DIAGNOSTIC is used to identify excision procedures that are biopsies
		Examples:	Partial nephrectomy, liver biopsy
C	Extirpation	Definition:	Taking or cutting out solid matter from a body part
		Explanation:	The solid matter may be an abnormal byproduct of a biological function or a foreign body; it may be imbedded in a body part or in the lumen of a tubular body part. The solid matter may or may not have been previously broken into pieces.
		Examples:	Thrombectomy, choledocholithotomy

Continued on next page

Ø Medical and Surgical

Continued from previous page

ICD-10-PCS Value		Definition	
D	Extraction	Definition:	Pulling or stripping out or off all or a portion of a body part by the use of force
		Explanation:	The qualifier DIAGNOSTIC is used to identify extractions that are biopsies
		Examples:	Dilation and curettage, vein stripping
F	Fragmentation	Definition:	Breaking solid matter in a body part into pieces
		Explanation:	Physical force (e.g., manual, ultrasonic) applied directly or indirectly is used to break the solid matter into pieces. The solid matter may be an abnormal byproduct of a biological function or a foreign body. The pieces of solid matter are not taken out.
		Examples:	Extracorporeal shockwave lithotripsy, transurethral lithotripsy
G	Fusion	Definition:	Joining together portions of an articular body part rendering the articular body part immobile
		Explanation:	The body part is joined together by fixation device, bone graft, or other means
		Examples:	Spinal fusion, ankle arthrodesis
H	Insertion	Definition:	Putting in a nonbiological appliance that monitors, assists, performs, or prevents a physiological function but does not physically take the place of a body part
		Explanation:	None
		Examples:	Insertion of radioactive implant, insertion of central venous catheter
J	Inspection	Definition:	Visually and/or manually exploring a body part
		Explanation:	Visual exploration may be performed with or without optical instrumentation. Manual exploration may be performed directly or through intervening body layers.
		Examples:	Diagnostic arthroscopy, exploratory laparotomy
K	Map	Definition:	Locating the route of passage of electrical impulses and/or locating functional areas in a body part
		Explanation:	Applicable only to the cardiac conduction mechanism and the central nervous system
		Examples:	Cardiac mapping, cortical mapping
L	Occlusion	Definition:	Completely closing an orifice or lumen of a tubular body part
		Explanation:	The orifice can be a natural orifice or an artificially created orifice
		Examples:	Fallopian tube ligation, ligation of inferior vena cava
M	Reattachment	Definition:	Putting back in or on all or a portion of a separated body part to its normal location or other suitable location
		Explanation:	Vascular circulation and nervous pathways may or may not be reestablished
		Examples:	Reattachment of hand, reattachment of avulsed kidney
N	Release	Definition:	Freeing a body part from an abnormal physical constraint by cutting or by use of force
		Explanation:	Some of the restraining tissue may be taken out but none of the body part is taken out
		Examples:	Adhesiolysis, carpal tunnel release
P	Removal	Definition:	Taking out or off a device from a body part
		Explanation:	If a device is taken out and a similar device put in without cutting or puncturing the skin or mucous membrane, the procedure is coded to the root operation CHANGE. Otherwise, the procedure for taking out a device is coded to the root operation REMOVAL.
		Examples:	Drainage tube removal, cardiac pacemaker removal
Q	Repair	Definition:	Restoring, to the extent possible, a body part to its normal anatomic structure and function
		Explanation:	Used only when the method to accomplish the repair is not one of the other root operations
		Examples:	Colostomy takedown, suture of laceration
R	Replacement	Definition:	Putting in or on biological or synthetic material that physically takes the place and/or function of all or a portion of a body part
		Explanation:	The body part may have been taken out or replaced, or may be taken out, physically eradicated, or rendered nonfunctional during the REPLACEMENT procedure. A REMOVAL procedure is coded for taking out the device used in a previous replacement procedure.
		Examples:	Total hip replacement, bone graft, free skin graft
S	Reposition	Definition:	Moving to its normal location, or other suitable location, all or a portion of a body part
		Explanation:	The body part is moved to a new location from an abnormal location, or from a normal location where it is not functioning correctly. The body part may or may not be cut out or off to be moved to the new location.
		Examples:	Reposition of undescended testicle, fracture reduction

Continued on next page

Appendix B: Root Operation Definitions

Ø Medical and Surgical			*Continued from previous page*
ICD-10-PCS Value		**Definition**	
T	Resection	Definition:	Cutting out or off, without replacement, all of a body part
		Explanation:	None
		Examples:	Total nephrectomy, total lobectomy of lung
V	Restriction	Definition:	Partially closing an orifice or the lumen of a tubular body part
		Explanation:	The orifice can be a natural orifice or an artificially created orifice
		Examples:	Esophagogastric fundoplication, cervical cerclage
W	Revision	Definition:	Correcting, to the extent possible, a portion of a malfunctioning device or the position of a displaced device
		Explanation:	Revision can include correcting a malfunctioning or displaced device by taking out or putting in components of the device such as a screw or pin
		Examples:	Adjustment of position of pacemaker lead, recementing of hip prosthesis
U	Supplement	Definition:	Putting in or on biological or synthetic material that physically reinforces and/or augments the function of a portion of a body part
		Explanation:	The biological material is non-living, or is living and from the same individual. The body part may have been previously replaced, and the SUPPLEMENT procedure is performed to physically reinforce and/or augment the function of the replaced body part.
		Examples:	Herniorrhaphy using mesh, free nerve graft, mitral valve ring annuloplasty, put a new acetabular liner in a previous hip replacement
X	Transfer	Definition:	Moving, without taking out, all or a portion of a body part to another location to take over the function of all or a portion of a body part
		Explanation:	The body part transferred remains connected to its vascular and nervous supply
		Examples:	Tendon transfer, skin pedicle flap transfer
Y	Transplantation	Definition:	Putting in or on all or a portion of a living body part taken from another individual or animal to physically take the place and/or function of all or a portion of a similar body part
		Explanation:	The native body part may or may not be taken out, and the transplanted body part may take over all or a portion of its function
		Examples:	Kidney transplant, heart transplant

Root Operation Definitions for Other Sections

1 Obstetrics			
ICD-10-PCS Value		**Definition**	
2	Change	Definition:	Taking out or off a device from a body part and putting back an identical or similar device in or on the same body part without cutting or puncturing the skin or a mucous membrane
		Explanation:	None
		Examples:	Replacement of fetal scalp electrode
9	Drainage	Definition:	Taking or letting out fluids and/or gases from a body part
		Explanation:	None
		Examples:	Biopsy of amniotic fluid
A	Abortion	Definition:	Artificially terminating a pregnancy
		Explanation:	None
		Examples:	Transvaginal abortion using vacuum aspiration technique
D	Extraction	Definition:	Pulling or stripping out or off all or a portion of a body part by the use of force
		Explanation:	None
		Examples:	Low-transverse C-section
E	Delivery	Definition:	Assisting the passage of the products of conception from the genital canal
		Explanation:	None
		Examples:	Manually-assisted delivery
H	Insertion	Definition:	Putting in a nonbiological appliance that monitors, assists, performs, or prevents a physiological function but does not physically take the place of a body part
		Explanation:	None
		Examples:	Placement of fetal scalp electrode

Continued on next page

1 Obstetrics

Continued from previous page

ICD-10-PCS Value		Definition	
J	Inspection	Definition:	Visually and/or manually exploring a body part
		Explanation:	Visual exploration may be performed with or without optical instrumentation. Manual exploration may be performed directly or through intervening body layers.
		Examples:	Bimanual pregnancy exam
P	Removal	Definition:	Taking out or off a device from a body part, region or orifice
		Explanation:	If a device is taken out and a similar device put in without cutting or puncturing the skin or mucous membrane, the procedure is coded to the root operation CHANGE. Otherwise, the procedure for taking out a device is coded to the root operation REMOVAL.
		Examples:	Removal of fetal monitoring electrode
Q	Repair	Definition:	Restoring, to the extent possible, a body part to its normal anatomic structure and function
		Explanation:	Used only when the method to accomplish the repair is not one of the other root operations
		Examples:	In utero repair of congenital diaphragmatic hernia
S	Reposition	Definition:	Moving to its normal location, or other suitable location, all or a portion of a body part
		Explanation:	The body part is moved to a new location from an abnormal location, or from a normal location where it is not functioning correctly. The body part may or may not be cut out or off to be moved to the new location..
		Examples:	External version of fetus
T	Resection	Definition:	Cutting out or off, without replacement, all of a body part
		Explanation:	None
		Examples:	Total excision of tubal pregnancy
Y	Transplantation	Definition:	Putting in or on all or a portion of a living body part taken from another individual or animal to physically take the place and/or function of all or a portion of a similar body part
		Explanation:	The native body part may or may not be taken out, and the transplanted body part may take over all or a portion of its function
		Examples:	In utero fetal kidney transplant

2 Placement

ICD-10-PCS Value		Definition	
Ø	Change	Definition:	Taking out or off a device from a body part and putting back an identical or similar device in or on the same body part without cutting or puncturing the skin or a mucous membrane
		Examples:	Change of vaginal packing
1	Compression	Definition:	Putting pressure on a body region
		Examples:	Placement of pressure dressing on abdominal wall
2	Dressing	Definition:	Putting material on a body region for protection
		Examples:	Application of sterile dressing to head wound
3	Immobilization	Definition:	Limiting or preventing motion of a body region
		Examples:	Placement of splint on left finger
4	Packing	Definition:	Putting material in a body region or orifice
		Examples:	Placement of nasal packing
5	Removal	Definition:	Taking out or off a device from a body part
		Examples:	Removal of stereotactic head frame
6	Traction	Definition:	Exerting a pulling force on a body region in a distal direction
		Examples:	Lumbar traction using motorized split-traction table

3 Administration

ICD-10-PCS Value		Definition	
Ø	Introduction	Definition:	Putting in or on a therapeutic, diagnostic, nutritional, physiological, or prophylactic substance except blood or blood products
		Examples:	Nerve block injection to median nerve
1	Irrigation	Definition:	Putting in or on a cleansing substance
		Examples:	Flushing of eye
2	Transfusion	Definition:	Putting in blood or blood products
		Examples:	Transfusion of cell saver red cells into central venous line

4 Measurement and Monitoring

ICD-10-PCS Value		Definition	
Ø	Measurement	Definition:	Determining the level of a physiological or physical function at a point in time
		Examples:	External electrocardiogram(EKG), single reading
1	Monitoring	Definition:	Determining the level of a physiological or physical function repetitively over a period of time
		Examples:	Urinary pressure monitoring

5 Extracorporeal or Systemic Assistance and Performance

ICD-10-PCS Value		Definition	
Ø	Assistance	Definition:	Taking over a portion of a physiological function by extracorporeal means
		Examples:	Hyperbaric oxygenation of wound
1	Performance	Definition:	Completely taking over a physiological function by extracorporeal means
		Examples:	Cardiopulmonary bypass in conjunction with CABG
2	Restoration	Definition:	Returning, or attempting to return, a physiological function to its original state by extracorporeal means
		Examples:	Attempted cardiac defibrillation, unsuccessful

6 Extracorporeal or Systemic Therapies

ICD-10-PCS Value		Definition	
Ø	Atmospheric Control	Definition:	Extracorporeal control of atmospheric pressure and composition
		Examples:	Antigen-free air conditioning, series treatment
1	Decompression	Definition:	Extracorporeal elimination of undissolved gas from body fluids
		Examples:	Hyperbaric decompression treatment, single
2	Electromagnetic Therapy	Definition:	Extracorporeal treatment by electromagnetic rays
		Examples:	TMS (transcranial magnetic stimulation), series treatment
3	Hyperthermia	Definition:	Extracorporeal raising of body temperature
		Examples:	None
4	Hypothermia	Definition:	Extracorporeal lowering of body temperature
		Examples:	Whole body hypothermia treatment for temperature imbalances, series
5	Pheresis	Definition:	Extracorporeal separation of blood products
		Examples:	Therapeutic leukopheresis, single treatment
6	Phototherapy	Definition:	Extracorporeal treatment by light rays
		Examples:	Phototherapy of circulatory system, series treatment
7	Ultrasound Therapy	Definition:	Extracorporeal treatment by ultrasound
		Examples:	Therapeutic ultrasound of peripheral vessels, single treatment
8	Ultraviolet Light Therapy	Definition:	Extracorporeal treatment by ultraviolet light
		Examples:	Ultraviolet light phototherapy, series treatment
9	Shock Wave Therapy	Definition:	Extracorporeal treatment by shock waves
		Examples:	Shockwave therapy of plantar fascia, single treatment
B	Perfusion	Definition:	Extracorporeal treatment by diffusion of therapeutic fluid
		Examples:	Perfusion of donor liver while preparing transplant patient

7 Osteopathic

ICD-10-PCS Value		Definition	
Ø	Treatment	Definition:	Manual treatment to eliminate or alleviate somatic dysfunction and related disorders
		Examples:	Fascial release of abdomen, osteopathic treatment

8 Other Procedures

ICD-10-PCS Value		Definition	
Ø	Other Procedures	Definition:	Methodologies which attempt to remediate or cure a disorder or disease
		Examples:	Acupuncture, yoga therapy

9 Chiropractic

ICD-10-PCS Value		Definition	
B	Manipulation	Definition:	Manual procedure that involves a directed thrust to move a joint past the physiological range of motion, without exceeding the anatomical limit
		Examples:	Chiropractic treatment of cervical spine, short lever specific contact

Note: Sections B-H (Imaging through Substance Abuse Treatment) do not include root operations. The character 3 position represents type of procedure, therefore those definitions are not included in this appendix. See appendix I for definitions of the type (character 3) or type qualifiers (character 5) that provide details of the procedures performed.

Appendix C: Comparison of Medical and Surgical Root Operations

Note: the character associated with each operation appears in parentheses after its title.

Procedures That Take Out Some or All of a Body Part

Root Operation	Objective of Procedure	Site of Procedure	Example
Destruction (5)	Eradicating without taking out or replacement	Some/all of a body part	Fulguration of endometrium
Detachment (6)	Cutting out/off without replacement	Extremity only, any level	Amputation above elbow
Excision (B)	Cutting out/off without replacement	Some of a body part	Breast lumpectomy
Extraction (D)	Pulling out or off without replacement	Some/all of a body part	Suction D&C
Resection (T)	Cutting out/off without replacement	All of a body part	Total mastectomy

Procedures That Put in/Put Back or Move Some/All of a Body Part

Root Operation	Objective of Procedure	Site of Procedure	Example
Reattachment (M)	Putting back a detached body part	Some/all of a body part	Reattach finger
Reposition (S)	Moving a body part to normal or other suitable location	Some/all of a body part	Move undescended testicle
Transfer (X)	Moving a body part to function for a similar body part	Some/all of a body part	Skin pedicle transfer flap
Transplantation (Y)	Putting in a living body part from a person/animal	Some/all of a body part	Kidney transplant

Procedures That Take Out or Eliminate Solid Matter, Fluids, or Gases From a Body Part

Root Operation	Objective of Procedure	Site of Procedure	Example
Drainage (9)	Taking or letting out	Fluids and/or gases from a body part	Incision and drainage
Extirpation (C)	Taking or cutting out	Solid matter in a body part	Thrombectomy
Fragmentation (F)	Breaking into pieces	Solid matter within a body part	Lithotripsy

Procedures That Involve Only Examination of Body Parts and Regions

Root Operation	Objective of Procedure	Site of Procedure	Example
Inspection (J)	Visual/manual exploration	Some/all of a body part	Diagnostic cystoscopy Exploratory laparoscopy
Map (K)	Locating electrical impulse route/functional areas	Brain/cardiac conduction mechanism	Cardiac mapping

Procedures That Alter the Diameter/Route of a Tubular Body Part

Root Operation	Objective of Procedure	Site of Procedure	Example
Bypass (1)	Altering route of passage of contents	Tubular body part	Coronary artery bypass graft (CABG)
Dilation (7)	Expanding natural or artificially created orifice/lumen	Tubular body part	Percutaneous transluminal coronary angioplasty (PTCA)
Occlusion (L)	Completely closing natural or artificially created orifice/lumen	Tubular body part	Fallopian tube ligation
Restriction (V)	Partially closing natural or artificially created orifice/lumen	Tubular body part	Gastroesophageal fundoplication

Procedures That Always Involve Devices

Root Operation	Objective of Procedure	Site of Procedure	Example
Change (2) DVC	Exchanging device w/out cutting/puncturing	In/on a body part	Gastrostomy tube change
Insertion (H) DVC	Putting in nonbiological device	In/on a body part	Central line insertion
Removal (P) DVC	Taking out device	In/on a body part	Central line removal
Replacement (R) DVC	Putting in device that replaces a body part	Some/all of a body part	Total hip replacement
Revision (W) DVC	Correcting a malfunctioning/displaced device	In/on a body part	Revision of pacemaker
Supplement (U) DVC	Putting in device that reinforces or augments a body part	In/on a body part	Abdominal wall herniorrhaphy using mesh

DVC = Device involved in root operation

Procedures Involving Cutting or Separation Only

Root Operation	Objective of Procedure	Site of Procedure	Example
Division (8)	Cutting into/separating	A body part	Neurotomy
Release (N)	Freeing a body part from constraint	Around a body part	Adhesiolysis

Procedures That Define Other Repairs

Root Operation	Objective of Procedure	Site of Procedure	Example
Control (3)	Stopping/attempting to stop postprocedural or other acute bleeding	Anatomical region	Post-prostatectomy bleeding control, control subdural hemorrhage, bleeding ulcer, retroperitoneal hemorrhage
Repair (Q)	Restoring body part to its normal structure/function	Some/all of a body part	Suture laceration

Procedures That Define Other Objectives

Root Operation	Objective of Procedure	Site of Procedure	Example
Alteration (Ø)	Modifying body part for cosmetic purposes without affecting function	Some/all of a body part	Face lift
Creation (4)	Using biological or synthetic material to form a new body part that replicates the anatomic structure or function of a missing body part	Perineum, valve	Sex change/artificial vagina/penis, atrioventricular valve creation
Fusion (G)	Unification or immobilization	Joint or articular body part	Spinal fusion

Appendix D: Body Part Key

Term	ICD-10-PCS Value
Abdominal aortic plexus	Abdominal Sympathetic Nerve
Abdominal esophagus	Esophagus, Lower
Abductor hallucis muscle	Foot Muscle, Right
	Foot Muscle, Left
Accessory cephalic vein	Cephalic Vein, Right
	Cephalic Vein, Left
Accessory obturator nerve	Lumbar Plexus
Accessory phrenic nerve	Phrenic nerve
Accessory spleen	Spleen
Acetabulofemoral joint	Hip Joint, Right
	Hip Joint, Left
Achilles tendon	Lower Leg Tendon, Right
	Lower Leg Tendon, Left
Acromioclavicular ligament	Shoulder Bursa and Ligament, Right
	Shoulder Bursa and Ligament, Left
Acromion (process)	Scapula, Right
	Scapula, Left
Adductor brevis muscle	Upper Leg Muscle, Right
	Upper Leg Muscle, Left
Adductor hallucis muscle	Foot Muscle, Right
	Foot Muscle, Left
Adductor longus muscle	Upper Leg Muscle, Right
	Upper Leg Muscle, Left
Adductor magnus muscle	Upper Leg Muscle, Right
	Upper Leg Muscle, Left
Adenohypophysis	Pituitary Gland
Alar ligament of axis	Head and Neck Bursa and Ligament
Alveolar process of mandible	Mandible, Right
	Mandible, Left
Alveolar process of maxilla	Maxilla
Anal orifice	Anus
Anatomical snuffbox	Lower Arm and Wrist Muscle, Right
	Lower Arm and Wrist Muscle, Left
Angular artery	Face Artery
Angular vein	Face Vein, Right
	Face Vein, Left
Annular ligament	Elbow Bursa and Ligament, Right
	Elbow Bursa and Ligament, Left
Anorectal junction	Rectum
Ansa cervicalis	Cervical Plexus
Antebrachial fascia	Subcutaneous Tissue and Fascia, Right Lower Arm
	Subcutaneous Tissue and Fascia, Left Lower Arm
Anterior (pectoral) lymph node	Lymphatic, Right Axillary
	Lymphatic, Left Axillary
Anterior cerebral artery	Intracranial Artery
Anterior cerebral vein	Intracranial Vein
Anterior choroidal artery	Intracranial Artery
Anterior circumflex humeral artery	Axillary Artery, Right
	Axillary Artery, Left
Anterior communicating artery	Intracranial Artery

Term	ICD-10-PCS Value
Anterior cruciate ligament (ACL)	Knee Bursa and Ligament, Right
	Knee Bursa and Ligament, Left
Anterior crural nerve	Femoral Nerve
Anterior facial vein	Face Vein, Right
	Face Vein, Left
Anterior intercostal artery	Internal Mammary Artery, Right
	Internal Mammary Artery, Left
Anterior interosseous nerve	Median Nerve
Anterior lateral malleolar artery	Anterior Tibial Artery, Right
	Anterior Tibial Artery, Left
Anterior lingual gland	Minor Salivary Gland
Anterior medial malleolar artery	Anterior Tibial Artery, Right
	Anterior Tibial Artery, Left
Anterior spinal artery	Vertebral Artery, Right
	Vertebral Artery, Left
Anterior tibial recurrent artery	Anterior Tibial Artery, Right
	Anterior Tibial Artery, Left
Anterior ulnar recurrent artery	Ulnar Artery, Right
	Ulnar Artery, Left
Anterior vagal trunk	Vagus Nerve
Anterior vertebral muscle	Neck Muscle, Right
	Neck Muscle, Left
Antihelix	External Ear, Right
	External Ear, Left
	External Ear, Bilateral
Antitragus	External Ear, Right
	External Ear, Left
	External Ear, Bilateral
Antrum of Highmore	Maxillary Sinus, Right
	Maxillary Sinus, Left
Aortic annulus	Aortic Valve
Aortic arch	Thoracic Aorta, Ascending/Arch
Aortic intercostal artery	Upper Artery
Apical (subclavicular) lymph node	Lymphatic, Right Axillary
	Lymphatic, Left Axillary
Apneustic center	Pons
Aqueduct of Sylvius	Cerebral Ventricle
Aqueous humour	Anterior Chamber, Right
	Anterior Chamber, Left
Arachnoid mater, intracranial	Cerebral Meninges
Arachnoid mater, spinal	Spinal Meninges
Arcuate artery	Foot Artery, Right
	Foot Artery, Left
Areola	Nipple, Right
	Nipple, Left
Arterial canal (duct)	Pulmonary Artery, Left
Aryepiglottic fold	Larynx
Arytenoid cartilage	Larynx
Arytenoid muscle	Neck Muscle, Right
	Neck Muscle, Left
Ascending aorta	Thoracic Aorta, Ascending/Arch

Term	ICD-10-PCS Value
Ascending palatine artery	Face Artery
Ascending pharyngeal artery	External Carotid Artery, Right
	External Carotid Artery, Left
Atlantoaxial joint	Cervical Vertebral Joint
Atrioventricular node	Conduction Mechanism
Atrium dextrum cordis	Atrium, Right
Atrium pulmonale	Atrium, Left
Auditory tube	Eustachian Tube, Right
	Eustachian Tube, Left
Auerbach's (myenteric)plexus	Abdominal Sympathetic Nerve
Auricle	External Ear, Right
	External Ear, Left
	External Ear, Bilateral
Auricularis muscle	Head Muscle
Axillary fascia	Subcutaneous Tissue and Fascia, Right Upper Arm
	Subcutaneous Tissue and Fascia, Left Upper Arm
Axillary nerve	Brachial Plexus
Bartholin's (greater vestibular) gland	Vestibular Gland
Basal (internal) cerebral vein	Intracranial Vein
Basal nuclei	Basal Ganglia
Base of tongue	Pharynx
Basilar artery	Intracranial Artery
Basis pontis	Pons
Biceps brachii muscle	Upper Arm Muscle, Right
	Upper Arm Muscle, Left
Biceps femoris muscle	Upper Leg Muscle, Right
	Upper Leg Muscle, Left
Bicipital aponeurosis	Subcutaneous Tissue and Fascia, Right Lower Arm
	Subcutaneous Tissue and Fascia, Left Lower Arm
Bicuspid valve	Mitral Valve
Body of femur	Femoral Shaft, Right
	Femoral Shaft, Left
Body of fibula	Fibula, Right
	Fibula, Left
Bony labyrinth	Inner Ear, Right
	Inner Ear, Left
Bony orbit	Orbit, Right
	Orbit, Left
Bony vestibule	Inner Ear, Right
	Inner Ear, Left
Botallo's duct	Pulmonary Artery, Left
Brachial (lateral) lymph node	Lymphatic, Right Axillary
	Lymphatic, Left Axillary
Brachialis muscle	Upper Arm Muscle, Right
	Upper Arm Muscle, Left
Brachiocephalic artery	Innominate Artery
Brachiocephalic trunk	Innominate Artery
Brachiocephalic vein	Innominate Vein, Right
	Innominate Vein, Left

Term	ICD-10-PCS Value
Brachioradialis muscle	Lower Arm and Wrist Muscle, Right
	Lower Arm and Wrist Muscle, Left
Broad ligament	Uterine Supporting Structure
Bronchial artery	Upper Artery
Bronchus intermedius	Main Bronchus, Right
Buccal gland	Buccal Mucosa
Buccinator lymph node	Lymphatic, Head
Buccinator muscle	Facial Muscle
Bulbospongiosus muscle	Perineum Muscle
Bulbourethral (Cowper's) gland	Urethra
Bundle of His	Conduction Mechanism
Bundle of Kent	Conduction Mechanism
Calcaneocuboid joint	Tarsal Joint, Right
	Tarsal Joint, Left
Calcaneocuboid ligament	Foot Bursa and Ligament, Right
	Foot Bursa and Ligament, Left
Calcaneofibular ligament	Ankle Bursa and Ligament, Right
	Ankle Bursa and Ligament, Left
Calcaneus	Tarsal, Right
	Tarsal, Left
Capitate bone	Carpal, Right
	Carpal, Left
Cardia	Esophagogastric Junction
Cardiac plexus	Thoracic Sympathetic Nerve
Cardioesophageal junction	Esophagogastric Junction
Caroticotympanic artery	Internal Carotid Artery, Right
	Internal Carotid Artery, Left
Carotid glomus	Carotid Body, Right
	Carotid Body, Left
	Carotid Bodies, Bilateral
Carotid sinus	Internal Carotid Artery, Right
	Internal Carotid Artery, Left
Carotid sinus nerve	Glossopharyngeal Nerve
Carpometacarpal ligament	Hand Bursa and Ligament, Right
	Hand Bursa and Ligament, Left
Cauda equina	Lumbar Spinal Cord
Cavernous plexus	Head and Neck Sympathetic Nerve
Celiac ganglion	Abdominal Sympathetic Nerve
Celiac (solar) plexus	Abdominal Sympathetic Nerve
Celiac lymph node	Lymphatic, Aortic
Celiac trunk	Celiac Artery
Central axillary lymph node	Lymphatic, Right Axillary
	Lymphatic, Left Axillary
Cerebral aqueduct (Sylvius)	Cerebral Ventricle
Cerebrum	Brain
Cervical esophagus	Esophagus, Upper
Cervical facet joint	Cervical Vertebral Joint
	Cervical Vertebral Joints, 2 or more
Cervical ganglion	Head and Neck Sympathetic Nerve
Cervical interspinous ligament	Head and Neck Bursa and Ligament
Cervical intertransverse ligament	Head and Neck Bursa and Ligament

Term	ICD-10-PCS Value
Cervical ligamentum flavum	Head and Neck Bursa and Ligament
Cervical lymph node	Lymphatic, Right Neck
	Lymphatic, Left Neck
Cervicothoracic facet joint	Cervicothoracic Vertebral Joint
Choana	Nasopharynx
Chondroglossus muscle	Tongue, Palate, Pharynx Muscle
Chorda tympani	Facial Nerve
Choroid plexus	Cerebral Ventricle
Ciliary body	Eye, Right
	Eye, Left
Ciliary ganglion	Head and Neck Sympathetic Nerve
Circle of Willis	Intracranial Artery
Circumflex iliac artery	Femoral Artery, Right
	Femoral Artery, Left
Claustrum	Basal Ganglia
Coccygeal body	Coccygeal Glomus
Coccygeus muscle	Trunk Muscle, Right
	Trunk Muscle, Left
Cochlea	Inner Ear, Right
	Inner Ear, Left
Cochlear nerve	Acoustic Nerve
Columella	Nasal Mucosa and Soft Tissue
Common digital vein	Foot Vein, Right
	Foot Vein, Left
Common facial vein	Face Vein, Right
	Face Vein, Left
Common fibular nerve	Peroneal Nerve
Common hepatic artery	Hepatic Artery
Common iliac (subaortic) lymph node	Lymphatic, Pelvis
Common interosseous artery	Ulnar Artery, Right
	Ulnar Artery, Left
Common peroneal nerve	Peroneal Nerve
Condyloid process	Mandible, Right
	Mandible, Left
Conus arteriosus	Ventricle, Right
Conus medullaris	Lumbar Spinal Cord
Coracoacromial ligament	Shoulder Bursa and Ligament, Right
	Shoulder Bursa and Ligament, Left
Coracobrachialis muscle	Upper Arm Muscle, Right
	Upper Arm Muscle, Left
Coracoclavicular ligament	Shoulder Bursa and Ligament, Right
	Shoulder Bursa and Ligament, Left
Coracohumeral ligament	Shoulder Bursa and Ligament, Right
	Shoulder Bursa and Ligament, Left
Coracoid process	Scapula, Right
	Scapula, Left
Corniculate cartilage	Larynx
Corpus callosum	Brain
Corpus cavernosum	Penis
Corpus spongiosum	Penis
Corpus striatum	Basal Ganglia
Corrugator supercilii muscle	Facial Muscle

Term	ICD-10-PCS Value
Costocervical trunk	Subclavian Artery, Right
	Subclavian Artery, Left
Costoclavicular ligament	Shoulder Bursa and Ligament, Right
	Shoulder Bursa and Ligament, Left
Costotransverse joint	Thoracic Vertebral Joint
Costotransverse ligament	Rib(s) Bursa and Ligament
Costovertebral joint	Thoracic Vertebral Joint
Costoxiphoid ligament	Sternum Bursa and Ligament
Cowper's (bulbourethral) gland	Urethra
Cremaster muscle	Perineum Muscle
Cribriform plate	Ethmoid Bone, Right
	Ethmoid Bone, Left
Cricoid cartilage	Trachea
Cricothyroid artery	Thyroid Artery, Right
	Thyroid Artery, Left
Cricothyroid muscle	Neck Muscle, Right
	Neck Muscle, Left
Crural fascia	Subcutaneous Tissue and Fascia, Right Upper Leg
	Subcutaneous Tissue and Fascia, Left Upper Leg
Cubital lymph node	Lymphatic, Right Upper Extremity
	Lymphatic, Left Upper Extremity
Cubital nerve	Ulnar Nerve
Cuboid bone	Tarsal, Right
	Tarsal, Left
Cuboideonavicular joint	Tarsal Joint, Right
	Tarsal Joint, Left
Culmen	Cerebellum
Cuneiform cartilage	Larynx
Cuneonavicular joint	Tarsal Joint, Right
	Tarsal Joint, Left
Cuneonavicular ligament	Foot Bursa and Ligament, Right
	Foot Bursa and Ligament, Left
Cutaneous (transverse) cervical nerve	Cervical Plexus
Deep cervical fascia	Subcutaneous Tissue and Fascia, Right Neck
	Subcutaneous Tissue and Fascia, Left Neck
Deep cervical vein	Vertebral Vein, Right
	Vertebral Vein, Left
Deep circumflex iliac artery	External Iliac Artery, Right
	External Iliac Artery, Left
Deep facial vein	Face Vein, Right
	Face Vein, Left
Deep femoral artery	Femoral Artery, Right
	Femoral Artery, Left
Deep femoral (profunda femoris) vein	Femoral Vein, Right
	Femoral Vein, Left
Deep palmar arch	Hand Artery, Right
	Hand Artery, Left
Deep transverse perineal muscle	Perineum Muscle
Deferential artery	Internal Iliac Artery, Right
	Internal Iliac Artery, Left

Term	ICD-10-PCS Value
Deltoid fascia	Subcutaneous Tissue and Fascia, Right Upper Arm
	Subcutaneous Tissue and Fascia, Left Upper Arm
Deltoid ligament	Ankle Bursa and Ligament, Right
	Ankle Bursa and Ligament, Left
Deltoid muscle	Shoulder Muscle, Right
	Shoulder Muscle, Left
Deltopectoral (infraclavicular) lymph node	Lymphatic, Right Upper Extremity
	Lymphatic, Left Upper Extremity
Dens	Cervical Vertebra
Denticulate (dentate) ligament	Spinal Meninges
Depressor anguli oris muscle	Facial Muscle
Depressor labii inferioris muscle	Facial Muscle
Depressor septi nasi muscle	Facial Muscle
Depressor supercilii muscle	Facial Muscle
Dermis	Skin
Descending genicular artery	Femoral Artery, Right
	Femoral Artery, Left
Diaphragma sellae	Dura Mater
Distal humerus	Humeral Shaft, Right
	Humeral Shaft, Left
Distal humerus, involving joint	Elbow Joint, Right
	Elbow Joint, Left
Distal radioulnar joint	Wrist Joint, Right
	Wrist Joint, Left
Dorsal digital nerve	Radial Nerve
Dorsal metacarpal vein	Hand Vein, Right
	Hand Vein, Left
Dorsal metatarsal artery	Foot Artery, Right
	Foot Artery, Left
Dorsal metatarsal vein	Foot Vein, Right
	Foot Vein, Left
Dorsal scapular artery	Subclavian Artery, Right
	Subclavian Artery, Left
Dorsal scapular nerve	Brachial Plexus
Dorsal venous arch	Foot Vein, Right
	Foot Vein, Left
Dorsalis pedis artery	Anterior Tibial Artery, Right
	Anterior Tibial Artery, Left
Duct of Santorini	Pancreatic Duct, Accessory
Duct of Wirsung	Pancreatic Duct
Ductus deferens	Vas Deferens, Right
	Vas Deferens, Left
	Vas Deferens, Bilateral
	Vas Deferens
Duodenal ampulla	Ampulla of Vater
Duodenojejunal flexure	Jejunum
Dura mater, intracranial	Dura Mater
Dura mater, spinal	Spinal Meninges
Dural venous sinus	Intracranial Vein

Term	ICD-10-PCS Value
Earlobe	External Ear, Right
	External Ear, Left
	External Ear, Bilateral
Eighth cranial nerve	Acoustic Nerve
Ejaculatory duct	Vas Deferens, Right
	Vas Deferens, Left
	Vas Deferens, Bilateral
	Vas Deferens
Eleventh cranial nerve	Accessory Nerve
Encephalon	Brain
Ependyma	Cerebral Ventricle
Epidermis	Skin
Epidural space, spinal	Spinal Canal
Epiploic foramen	Peritoneum
Epithalamus	Thalamus
Epitroclear lymph node	Lymphatic, Right Upper Extremity
	Lymphatic, Left Upper Extremity
Erector spinae muscle	Trunk Muscle, Right
	Trunk Muscle, Left
Esophageal artery	Upper Artery
Esophageal plexus	Thoracic Sympathetic Nerve
Ethmoidal air cell	Ethmoid Sinus, Right
	Ethmoid Sinus, Left
Extensor carpi radialis muscle	Lower Arm and Wrist Muscle, Right
Extensor carpi ulnaris muscle	Lower Arm and Wrist Muscle, Left
Extensor digitorum brevis muscle	Foot Muscle, Right
	Foot Muscle, Left
Extensor digitorum longus muscle	Lower Leg Muscle, Right
	Lower Leg Muscle, Left
Extensor hallucis brevis muscle	Foot Muscle, Right
	Foot Muscle, Left
Extensor hallucis longus muscle	Lower Leg Muscle, Right
	Lower Leg Muscle, Left
External anal sphincter	Anal Sphincter
External auditory meatus	External Auditory Canal, Right
	External Auditory Canal, Left
External maxillary artery	Face Artery
External naris	Nasal Mucosa and Soft Tissue
External oblique aponeurosis	Subcutaneous Tissue and Fascia, Trunk
External oblique muscle	Abdomen Muscle, Right
	Abdomen Muscle, Left
External popliteal nerve	Peroneal Nerve
External pudendal artery	Femoral Artery, Right
	Femoral Artery, Left
External pudenal vein	Saphenous Vein, Right
	Saphenous Vein, Left
External urethral sphincter	Urethra
Extradural space, intracranial	Epidural Space, Intracranial
Extradural space, spinal	Spinal Canal
Facial artery	Face Artery
False vocal cord	Larynx
Falx cerebri	Dura Mater

Term	ICD-10-PCS Value
Fascia lata	Subcutaneous Tissue and Fascia, Right Upper Leg
	Subcutaneous Tissue and Fascia, Left Upper Leg
Femoral head	Upper Femur, Right
	Upper Femur, Left
Femoral lymph node	Lymphatic, Right Lower Extremity
	Lymphatic, Left Lower Extremity
Femoropatellar joint	Knee Joint, Right
	Knee Joint, Left
	Knee Joint, Femoral Surface, Right
	Knee Joint, Femoral Surface, Left
Femorotibial joint	Knee Joint, Right
	Knee Joint, Left
	Knee Joint, Tibial Surface, Right
	Knee Joint, Tibial Surface, Left
Fibular artery	Peroneal Artery, Right
	Peroneal Artery, Left
Fibularis brevis muscle	Lower Leg Muscle, Right
	Lower Leg Muscle, Left
Fibularis longus muscle	Lower Leg Muscle, Right
	Lower Leg Muscle, Left
Fifth cranial nerve	Trigeminal Nerve
Filum terminale	Spinal Meninges
First cranial nerve	Olfactory Nerve
First intercostal nerve	Brachial Plexus
Flexor carpi radialis muscle	Lower Arm and Wrist Muscle, Right
	Lower Arm and Wrist Muscle, Left
Flexor carpi ulnaris muscle	Lower Arm and Wrist Muscle, Right
	Lower Arm and Wrist Muscle, Left
Flexor digitorum brevis muscle	Foot Muscle, Right
	Foot Muscle, Left
Flexor digitorum longus muscle	Lower Leg Muscle, Right
	Lower Leg Muscle, Left
Flexor hallucis brevis muscle	Foot Muscle, Right
	Foot Muscle, Left
Flexor hallucis longus muscle	Lower Leg Muscle, Right
	Lower Leg Muscle, Left
Flexor pollicis longus muscle	Lower Arm and Wrist Muscle, Right
	Lower Arm and Wrist Muscle, Left
Foramen magnum	Occipital Bone
Foramen of Monro (intraventricular)	Cerebral Ventricle
Foreskin	Prepuce
Fossa of Rosenmuller	Nasopharynx
Fourth cranial nerve	Trochlear Nerve
Fourth ventricle	Cerebral Ventricle
Fovea	Retina, Right
	Retina, Left
Frenulum labii inferioris	Lower Lip
Frenulum labii superioris	Upper Lip
Frenulum linguae	Tongue
Frontal lobe	Cerebral Hemisphere
Frontal vein	Face Vein, Right
	Face Vein, Left

Term	ICD-10-PCS Value
Fundus uteri	Uterus
Galea aponeurotica	Subcutaneous Tissue and Fascia, Scalp
Ganglion impar (ganglion of Walther)	Sacral Sympathetic Nerve
Gasserian ganglion	Trigeminal Nerve
Gastric lymph node	Lymphatic, Aortic
Gastric plexus	Abdominal Sympathetic Nerve
Gastrocnemius muscle	Lower Leg Muscle, Right
	Lower Leg Muscle, Left
Gastrocolic ligament	Omentum
Gastrocolic omentum	Omentum
Gastroduodenal artery	Hepatic Artery
Gastroesophageal (GE) junction	Esophagogastric Junction
Gastrohepatic omentum	Omentum
Gastrophrenic ligament	Omentum
Gastrosplenic ligament	Omentum
Gemellus muscle	Hip Muscle, Right
	Hip Muscle, Left
Geniculate ganglion	Facial Nerve
Geniculate nucleus	Thalamus
Genioglossus muscle	Tongue, Palate, Pharynx Muscle
Genitofemoral nerve	Lumbar Plexus
Glans penis	Prepuce
Glenohumeral joint	Shoulder Joint, Right
	Shoulder Joint, Left
Glenohumeral ligament	Shoulder Bursa and Ligament, Right
	Shoulder Bursa and Ligament, Left
Glenoid fossa (of scapula)	Glenoid Cavity, Right
	Glenoid Cavity, Left
Glenoid ligament (labrum)	Shoulder Joint, Right
	Shoulder Joint, Left
Globus pallidus	Basal Ganglia
Glossoepiglottic fold	Epiglottis
Glottis	Larynx
Gluteal lymph node	Lymphatic, Pelvis
Gluteal vein	Hypogastric Vein, Right
	Hypogastric Vein, Left
Gluteus maximus muscle	Hip Muscle, Right
	Hip Muscle, Left
Gluteus medius muscle	Hip Muscle, Right
	Hip Muscle, Left
Gluteus minimus muscle	Hip Muscle, Right
	Hip Muscle, Left
Gracilis muscle	Upper Leg Muscle, Right
	Upper Leg Muscle, Left
Great auricular nerve	Cervical Plexus
Great cerebral vein	Intracranial Vein
Great(er) saphenous vein	Saphenous Vein, Right
	Saphenous Vein, Left
Greater alar cartilage	Nasal Mucosa and Soft Tissue
Greater occipital nerve	Cervical Nerve
Greater omentum	Omentum
Greater splanchnic nerve	Thoracic Sympathetic Nerve

Term	ICD-10-PCS Value
Greater superficial petrosal nerve	Facial Nerve
Greater trochanter	Upper Femur, Right
	Upper Femur, Left
Greater tuberosity	Humeral Head, Right
	Humeral Head, Left
Greater vestibular (Bartholin's) gland	Vestibular Gland
Greater wing	Sphenoid Bone
Hallux	1st Toe, Right
	1st Toe, Left
Hamate bone	Carpal, Right
	Carpal, Left
Head of fibula	Fibula, Right
	Fibula, Left
Helix	External Ear, Right
	External Ear, Left
	External Ear, Bilateral
Hepatic artery proper	Hepatic Artery
Hepatic flexure	Transverse Colon
Hepatic lymph node	Lymphatic, Aortic
Hepatic plexus	Abdominal Sympathetic Nerve
Hepatic portal vein	Portal Vein
Hepatogastric ligament	Omentum
Hepatopancreatic ampulla	Ampulla of Vater
Humeroradial joint	Elbow Joint, Right
	Elbow Joint, Left
Humeroulnar joint	Elbow Joint, Right
	Elbow Joint, Left
Humerus, distal	Humeral Shaft, Right
	Humeral Shaft, Left
Hyoglossus muscle	Tongue, Palate, Pharynx Muscle
Hyoid artery	Thyroid Artery, Right
	Thyroid Artery, Left
Hypogastric artery	Internal Iliac Artery, Right
	Internal Iliac Artery, Left
Hypopharynx	Pharynx
Hypophysis	Pituitary Gland
Hypothenar muscle	Hand Muscle, Right
	Hand Muscle, Left
Ileal artery	Superior Mesenteric Artery
Ileocolic artery	Superior Mesenteric Artery
Ileocolic vein	Colic Vein
Iliac crest	Pelvic Bone, Right
	Pelvic Bone, Left
Iliac fascia	Subcutaneous Tissue and Fascia, Right Upper Leg
	Subcutaneous Tissue and Fascia, Left Upper Leg
Iliac lymph node	Lymphatic, Pelvis
Iliacus muscle	Hip Muscle, Right
	Hip Muscle, Left
Iliofemoral ligament	Hip Bursa and Ligament, Right
	Hip Bursa and Ligament, Left
Iliohypogastric nerve	Lumbar Plexus
Ilioinguinal nerve	Lumbar Plexus

Term	ICD-10-PCS Value
Iliolumbar artery	Internal Iliac Artery, Right
	Internal Iliac Artery, Left
Iliolumbar ligament	Lower Spine Bursa and Ligament
Iliotibial tract (band)	Subcutaneous Tissue and Fascia, Right Upper Leg
	Subcutaneous Tissue and Fascia, Left Upper Leg
Ilium	Pelvic Bone, Right
	Pelvic Bone, Left
Incus	Auditory Ossicle, Right
	Auditory Ossicle, Left
Inferior cardiac nerve	Thoracic Sympathetic Nerve
Inferior cerebellar vein	Intracranial Vein
Inferior cerebral vein	Intracranial Vein
Inferior epigastric artery	External Iliac Artery, Right
	External Iliac Artery, Left
Inferior epigastric lymph node	Lymphatic, Pelvis
Inferior genicular artery	Popliteal Artery, Right
	Popliteal Artery, Left
Inferior gluteal artery	Internal Iliac Artery, Right
	Internal Iliac Artery, Left
Inferior gluteal nerve	Sacral Plexus
Inferior hypogastric plexus	Abdominal Sympathetic Nerve
Inferior labial artery	Face Artery
Inferior longitudinal muscle	Tongue, Palate, Pharynx Muscle
Inferior mesenteric ganglion	Abdominal Sympathetic Nerve
Inferior mesenteric lymph node	Lymphatic, Mesenteric
Inferior mesenteric plexus	Abdominal Sympathetic Nerve
Inferior oblique muscle	Extraocular Muscle, Right
	Extraocular Muscle, Left
Inferior pancreaticoduodenal artery	Superior Mesenteric Artery
Inferior phrenic artery	Abdominal Aorta
Inferior rectus muscle	Extraocular Muscle, Right
	Extraocular Muscle, Left
Inferior suprarenal artery	Renal Artery, Right
	Renal Artery, Left
Inferior tarsal plate	Lower Eyelid, Right
	Lower Eyelid, Left
Inferior thyroid vein	Innominate Vein, Right
	Innominate Vein, Left
Inferior tibiofibular joint	Ankle Joint, Right
	Ankle Joint, Left
Inferior turbinate	Nasal Turbinate
Inferior ulnar collateral artery	Brachial Artery, Right
	Brachial Artery, Left
Inferior vesical artery	Internal Iliac Artery, Right
	Internal Iliac Artery, Left
Infraauricular lymph node	Lymphatic, Head
Infraclavicular (deltopectoral) lymph node	Lymphatic, Right Upper Extremity
	Lymphatic, Left Upper Extremity

Term	ICD-10-PCS Value
Infrahyoid muscle	Neck Muscle, Right
	Neck Muscle, Left
Infraparotid lymph node	Lymphatic, Head
Infraspinatus fascia	Subcutaneous Tissue and Fascia, Right Upper Arm
	Subcutaneous Tissue and Fascia, Left Upper Arm
Infraspinatus muscle	Shoulder Muscle, Right
	Shoulder Muscle, Left
Infundibulopelvic ligament	Uterine Supporting Structure
Inguinal canal	Inguinal Region, Right
	Inguinal Region, Left
	Inguinal Region, Bilateral
Inguinal triangle	Inguinal Region, Right
	Inguinal Region, Left
	Inguinal Region, Bilateral
Interatrial septum	Atrial Septum
Intercarpal joint	Carpal Joint, Right
	Carpal Joint, Left
Intercarpal ligament	Hand Bursa and Ligament, Right
	Hand Bursa and Ligament, Left
Interclavicular ligament	Shoulder Bursa and Ligament, Right
	Shoulder Bursa and Ligament, Left
Intercostal lymph node	Lymphatic, Thorax
Intercostal muscle	Thorax Muscle, Right
	Thorax Muscle, Left
Intercostal nerve	Thoracic Nerve
Intercostobrachial nerve	Thoracic Nerve
Intercuneiform joint	Tarsal Joint, Right
	Tarsal Joint, Left
Intercuneiform ligament	Foot Bursa and Ligament, Right
	Foot Bursa and Ligament, Left
Intermediate bronchus	Main Bronchus, Right
Intermediate cuneiform bone	Tarsal, Right
	Tarsal, Left
Internal anal sphincter	Anal Sphincter
Internal (basal) cerebral vein	Intracranial Vein
Internal carotid artery, intracranial portion	Intracranial Artery
Internal carotid plexus	Head and Neck Sympathetic Nerve
Internal iliac vein	Hypogastric Vein, Right
	Hypogastric Vein, Left
Internal maxillary artery	External Carotid Artery, Right
	External Carotid Artery, Left
Internal naris	Nasal Mucosa and Soft Tissue
Internal oblique muscle	Abdomen Muscle, Right
	Abdomen Muscle, Left
Internal pudendal artery	Internal Iliac Artery, Right
	Internal Iliac Artery, Left
Internal pudendal vein	Hypogastric Vein, Right
	Hypogastric Vein, Left

Term	ICD-10-PCS Value
Internal thoracic artery	Internal Mammary Artery, Right
	Internal Mammary Artery, Left
	Subclavian Artery, Right
	Subclavian Artery, Left
Internal urethral sphincter	Urethra
Interphalangeal (IP) joint	Finger Phalangeal Joint, Right
	Finger Phalangeal Joint, Left
	Toe Phalangeal Joint, Right
	Toe Phalangeal Joint, Left
Interphalangeal ligament	Foot Bursa and Ligament, Right
	Foot Bursa and Ligament, Left
	Hand Bursa and Ligament, Right
	Hand Bursa and Ligament, Left
Interspinalis muscle	Trunk Muscle, Right
	Trunk Muscle, Left
Interspinous ligament, cervical	Head and Neck Bursa and Ligament
Interspinous ligament, lumbar	Lower Spine Bursa and Ligament
Interspinous ligament, thoracic	Upper Spine Bursa and Ligament
Intertransversarius muscle	Trunk Muscle, Right
	Trunk Muscle, Left
Intertransverse ligament, cervical	Head and Neck Bursa and Ligament
Intertransverse ligament, lumbar	Lower Spine Bursa and Ligament
Intertransverse ligament, thoracic	Upper Spine Bursa and Ligament
Interventricular foramen (Monro)	Cerebral Ventricle
Interventricular septum	Ventricular Septum
Intestinal lymphatic trunk	Cisterna Chyli
Ischiatic nerve	Sciatic Nerve
Ischiocavernosus muscle	Perineum Muscle
Ischiofemoral ligament	Hip Bursa and Ligament, Right
	Hip Bursa and Ligament, Left
Ischium	Pelvic Bone, Right
	Pelvic Bone, Left
Jejunal artery	Superior Mesenteric Artery
Jugular body	Glomus Jugulare
Jugular lymph node	Lymphatic, Right Neck
	Lymphatic, Left Neck
Labia majora	Vulva
Labia minora	Vulva
Labial gland	Upper Lip
	Lower Lip
Lacrimal canaliculus	Lacrimal Duct, Right
	Lacrimal Duct, Left
Lacrimal punctum	Lacrimal Duct, Right
	Lacrimal Duct, Left
Lacrimal sac	Lacrimal Duct, Right
	Lacrimal Duct, Left
Laryngopharynx	Pharynx
Lateral (brachial) lymph node	Lymphatic, Right Axillary
	Lymphatic, Left Axillary

Term	ICD-10-PCS Value
Lateral canthus	Upper Eyelid, Right
	Upper Eyelid, Left
Lateral collateral ligament (LCL)	Knee Bursa and Ligament, Right
	Knee Bursa and Ligament, Left
Lateral condyle of femur	Lower Femur, Right
	Lower Femur, Left
Lateral condyle of tibia	Tibia, Right
	Tibia, Left
Lateral cuneiform bone	Tarsal, Right
	Tarsal, Left
Lateral epicondyle of femur	Lower Femur, Right
	Lower Femur, Left
Lateral epicondyle of humerus	Humeral Shaft, Right
	Humeral Shaft, Left
Lateral femoral cutaneous nerve	Lumbar Plexus
Lateral malleolus	Fibula, Right
	Fibula, Left
Lateral meniscus	Knee Joint, Right
	Knee Joint, Left
Lateral nasal cartilage	Nasal Mucosa and Soft Tissue
Lateral plantar artery	Foot Artery, Right
	Foot Artery, Left
Lateral plantar nerve	Tibial Nerve
Lateral rectus muscle	Extraocular Muscle, Right
	Extraocular Muscle, Left
Lateral sacral artery	Internal Iliac Artery, Right
	Internal Iliac Artery, Left
Lateral sacral vein	Hypogastric Vein, Right
	Hypogastric Vein, Left
Lateral sural cutaneous nerve	Peroneal Nerve
Lateral tarsal artery	Foot Artery, Right
	Foot Artery, Left
Lateral temporo-mandibular ligament	Head and Neck Bursa and Ligament
Lateral thoracic artery	Axillary Artery, Right
	Axillary Artery, Left
Latissimus dorsi muscle	Trunk Muscle, Right
	Trunk Muscle, Left
Least splanchnic nerve	Thoracic Sympathetic Nerve
Left ascending lumbar vein	Hemiazygos Vein
Left atrioventricular valve	Mitral Valve
Left auricular appendix	Atrium, Left
Left colic vein	Colic Vein
Left coronary sulcus	Heart, Left
Left gastric artery	Gastric Artery
Left gastroepiploic artery	Splenic Artery
Left gastroepiploic vein	Splenic Vein
Left inferior phrenic vein	Renal Vein, Left
Left inferior pulmonary vein	Pulmonary Vein, Left
Left jugular trunk	Thoracic Duct
Left lateral ventricle	Cerebral Ventricle
Left ovarian vein	Renal Vein, Left
Left second lumbar vein	Renal Vein, Left

Term	ICD-10-PCS Value
Left subclavian trunk	Thoracic Duct
Left subcostal vein	Hemiazygos Vein
Left superior pulmonary vein	Pulmonary Vein, Left
Left suprarenal vein	Renal Vein, Left
Left testicular vein	Renal Vein, Left
Leptomeninges, intracranial	Cerebral Meninges
Leptomeninges, spinal	Spinal Meninges
Lesser alar cartilage	Nasal Mucosa and Soft Tissue
Lesser occipital nerve	Cervical Plexus
Lesser omentum	Omentum
Lesser saphenous vein	Saphenous Vein, Right
	Saphenous Vein, Left
Lesser splanchnic nerve	Thoracic Sympathetic Nerve
Lesser trochanter	Upper Femur, Right
	Upper Femur, Left
Lesser tuberosity	Humeral Head, Right
	Humeral Head, Left
Lesser wing	Sphenoid Bone
Levator anguli oris muscle	Facial Muscle
Levator ani muscle	Perineum Muscle
Levator labii superioris alaeque nasi muscle	Facial Muscle
Levator labii superioris muscle	Facial Muscle
Levator palpebrae superioris muscle	Upper Eyelid, Right
	Upper Eyelid, Left
Levator scapulae muscle	Neck Muscle, Right
	Neck Muscle, Left
Levator veli palatini muscle	Tongue, Palate, Pharynx Muscle
Levatores costarum muscle	Thorax Muscle, Right
	Thorax Muscle, Left
Ligament of head of fibula	Knee Bursa and Ligament, Right
	Knee Bursa and Ligament, Left
Ligament of the lateral malleolus	Ankle Bursa and Ligament, Right
	Ankle Bursa and Ligament, Left
Ligamentum flavum, cervical	Head and Neck Bursa and Ligament
Ligamentum flavum, lumbar	Lower Spine Bursa and Ligament
Ligamentum flavum, thoracic	Upper Spine Bursa and Ligament
Lingual artery	External Carotid Artery, Right
	External Carotid Artery, Left
Lingual tonsil	Pharynx
Locus ceruleus	Pons
Long thoracic nerve	Brachial Plexus
Lumbar artery	Abdominal Aorta
Lumbar facet joint	Lumbar Vertebral Joint
Lumbar ganglion	Lumbar Sympathetic Nerve
Lumbar lymph node	Lymphatic, Aortic
Lumbar lymphatic trunk	Cisterna Chyli
Lumbar splanchnic nerve	Lumbar Sympathetic Nerve
Lumbosacral facet joint	Lumbosacral Joint
Lumbosacral trunk	Lumbar Nerve

Term	ICD-10-PCS Value
Lunate bone	Carpal, Right
	Carpal, Left
Lunotriquetral ligament	Hand Bursa and Ligament, Right
	Hand Bursa and Ligament, Left
Macula	Retina, Right
	Retina, Left
Malleus	Auditory Ossicle, Right
	Auditory Ossicle, Left
Mammary duct	Breast, Right
	Breast, Left
	Breast, Bilateral
Mammary gland	Breast, Right
	Breast, Left
	Breast, Bilateral
Mammillary body	Hypothalamus
Mandibular nerve	Trigeminal Nerve
Mandibular notch	Mandible, Right
	Mandible, Left
Manubrium	Sternum
Masseter muscle	Head Muscle
Masseteric fascia	Subcutaneous Tissue and Fascia, Face
Mastoid (postauricular) lymph node	Lymphatic, Right Neck
	Lymphatic, Left Neck
Mastoid air cells	Mastoid Sinus, Right
	Mastoid Sinus, Left
Mastoid process	Temporal Bone, Right
	Temporal Bone, Left
Maxillary artery	External Carotid Artery, Right
	External Carotid Artery, Left
Maxillary nerve	Trigeminal Nerve
Medial canthus	Lower Eyelid, Right
	Lower Eyelid, Left
Medial collateral ligament (MCL)	Knee Bursa and Ligament, Right
	Knee Bursa and Ligament, Left
Medial condyle of femur	Lower Femur, Right
	Lower Femur, Left
Medial condyle of tibia	Tibia, Right
	Tibia, Left
Medial cuneiform bone	Tarsal, Right
	Tarsal, Left
Medial epicondyle of femur	Lower Femur, Right
	Lower Femur, Left
Medial epicondyle of humerus	Humeral Shaft, Right
	Humeral Shaft, Left
Medial malleolus	Tibia, Right
	Tibia, Left
Medial meniscus	Knee Joint, Right
	Knee Joint, Left
Medial plantar artery	Foot Artery, Right
	Foot Artery, Left
Medial plantar nerve	Tibial Nerve
Medial popliteal nerve	Tibial Nerve
Medial rectus muscle	Extraocular Muscle, Right
	Extraocular Muscle, Left

Term	ICD-10-PCS Value
Medial sural cutaneous nerve	Tibial Nerve
Median antebrachial vein	Basilic Vein, Right
	Basilic Vein, Left
Median cubital vein	Basilic Vein, Right
	Basilic Vein, Left
Median sacral artery	Abdominal Aorta
Mediastinal cavity	Mediastinum
Mediastinal lymph node	Lymphatic, Thorax
Mediastinal space	Mediastinum
Meissner's (submucous) plexus	Abdominal Sympathetic Nerve
Membranous urethra	Urethra
Mental foramen	Mandible, Right
	Mandible, Left
Mentalis muscle	Facial Muscle
Mesoappendix	Mesentery
Mesocolon	Mesentery
Metacarpal ligament	Hand Bursa and Ligament, Right
	Hand Bursa and Ligament, Left
Metacarpophalangeal ligament	Hand Bursa and Ligament, Right
	Hand Bursa and Ligament, Left
Metatarsal ligament	Foot Bursa and Ligament, Right
	Foot Bursa and Ligament, Left
Metatarsophalangeal ligament	Foot Bursa and Ligament, Right
	Foot Bursa and Ligament, Left
Metatarsophalangeal (MTP) joint	Metatarsal-Phalangeal Joint, Right
	Metatarsal-Phalangeal Joint, Left
Metathalamus	Thalamus
Midcarpal joint	Carpal Joint, Right
	Carpal Joint, Left
Middle cardiac nerve	Thoracic Sympathetic Nerve
Middle cerebral artery	Intracranial Artery
Middle cerebral vein	Intracranial Vein
Middle colic vein	Colic Vein
Middle genicular artery	Popliteal Artery, Right
	Popliteal Artery, Left
Middle hemorrhoidal vein	Hypogastric Vein, Right
	Hypogastric Vein, Left
Middle rectal artery	Internal Iliac Artery, Right
	Internal Iliac Artery, Left
Middle suprarenal artery	Abdominal Aorta
Middle temporal artery	Temporal Artery, Right
	Temporal Artery, Left
Middle turbinate	Nasal Turbinate
Mitral annulus	Mitral Valve
Molar gland	Buccal Mucosa
Musculocutaneous nerve	Brachial Plexus
Musculophrenic artery	Internal Mammary Artery, Right
	Internal Mammary Artery, Left
Musculospiral nerve	Radial Nerve
Myelencephalon	Medulla Oblongata
Myenteric (Auerbach's) plexus	Abdominal Sympathetic Nerve
Myometrium	Uterus

Term	ICD-10-PCS Value
Nail bed	Finger Nail
	Toe Nail
Nail plate	Finger Nail
	Toe Nail
Nasal cavity	Nasal Mucosa and Soft Tissue
Nasal concha	Nasal Turbinate
Nasalis muscle	Facial Muscle
Nasolacrimal duct	Lacrimal Duct, Right
	Lacrimal Duct, Left
Navicular bone	Tarsal, Right
	Tarsal, Left
Neck of femur	Upper Femur, Right
	Upper Femur, Left
Neck of humerus (anatomical) (surgical)	Humeral Head, Right
	Humeral Head, Left
Nerve to the stapedius	Facial Nerve
Neurohypophysis	Pituitary Gland
Ninth cranial nerve	Glossopharyngeal Nerve
Nostril	Nasal Mucosa and Soft Tissue
Obturator artery	Internal Iliac Artery, Right
	Internal Iliac Artery, Left
Obturator lymph node	Lymphatic, Pelvis
Obturator muscle	Hip Muscle, Right
	Hip Muscle, Left
Obturator nerve	Lumbar Plexus
Obturator vein	Hypogastric Vein, Right
	Hypogastric Vein, Left
Obtuse margin	Heart, Left
Occipital artery	External Carotid Artery, Right
	External Carotid Artery, Left
Occipital lobe	Cerebral Hemisphere
Occipital lymph node	Lymphatic, Right Neck
	Lymphatic, Left Neck
Occipitofrontalis muscle	Facial Muscle
Odontoid process	Cervical Vertebra
Olecranon bursa	Elbow Bursa and Ligament, Right
	Elbow Bursa and Ligament, Left
Olecranon process	Ulna, Right
	Ulna, Left
Olfactory bulb	Olfactory Nerve
Ophthalmic artery	Intracranial Artery
Ophthalmic nerve	Trigeminal Nerve
Ophthalmic vein	Intracranial Vein
Optic chiasma	Optic Nerve
Optic disc	Retina, Right
	Retina, Left
Optic foramen	Sphenoid Bone
Orbicularis oculi muscle	Upper Eyelid, Right
	Upper Eyelid, Left
Orbicularis oris muscle	Facial Muscle
Orbital fascia	Subcutaneous Tissue and Fascia, Face
Orbital portion of ethmoid bone	Orbit, Right
	Orbit, Left

Term	ICD-10-PCS Value
Orbital portion of frontal bone	Orbit, Right
	Orbit, Left
Orbital portion of lacrimal bone	Orbit, Right
	Orbit, Left
Orbital portion of maxilla	Orbit, Right
	Orbit, Left
Orbital portion of palatine bone	Orbit, Right
	Orbit, Left
Orbital portion of sphenoid bone	Orbit, Right
	Orbit, Left
Orbital portion of zygomatic bone	Orbit, Right
	Orbit, Left
Oropharynx	Pharynx
Otic ganglion	Head and Neck Sympathetic Nerve
Oval window	Middle Ear, Right
	Middle Ear, Left
Ovarian artery	Abdominal Aorta
Ovarian ligament	Uterine Supporting Structure
Oviduct	Fallopian Tube, Right
	Fallopian Tube, Left
Palatine gland	Buccal Mucosa
Palatine tonsil	Tonsils
Palatine uvula	Uvula
Palatoglossal muscle	Tongue, Palate, Pharynx Muscle
Palatopharyngeal muscle	Tongue, Palate, Pharynx Muscle
Palmar (volar) digital vein	Hand Vein, Right
	Hand Vein, Left
Palmar (volar) metacarpal vein	Hand Vein, Right
	Hand Vein, Left
Palmar cutaneous nerve	Median Nerve
	Radial Nerve
Palmar fascia (aponeurosis)	Subcutaneous Tissue and Fascia, Right Hand
	Subcutaneous Tissue and Fascia, Left Hand
Palmar interosseous muscle	Hand Muscle, Right
	Hand Muscle, Left
Palmar ulnocarpal ligament	Wrist Bursa and Ligament, Right
	Wrist Bursa and Ligament, Left
Palmaris longus muscle	Lower Arm and Wrist Muscle, Right
	Lower Arm and Wrist Muscle, Left
Pancreatic artery	Splenic Artery
Pancreatic plexus	Abdominal Sympathetic Nerve
Pancreatic vein	Splenic Vein
Pancreaticosplenic lymph node	Lymphatic, Aortic
Paraaortic lymph node	Lymphatic, Aortic
Pararectal lymph node	Lymphatic, Mesenteric
Parasternal lymph node	Lymphatic, Thorax
Paratracheal lymph node	Lymphatic, Thorax
Paraurethral (Skene's) gland	Vestibular Gland
Parietal lobe	Cerebral Hemisphere
Parotid lymph node	Lymphatic, Head
Parotid plexus	Facial Nerve

Term	ICD-10-PCS Value
Pars flaccida	Tympanic Membrane, Right
	Tympanic Membrane, Left
Patellar ligament	Knee Bursa and Ligament, Right
	Knee Bursa and Ligament, Left
Patellar tendon	Knee Tendon, Right
	Knee Tendon, Left
Patellofemoral joint	Knee Joint, Right
	Knee Joint, Left
	Knee Joint, Femoral Surface, Right
	Knee Joint, Femoral Surface, Left
Pectineus muscle	Upper Leg Muscle, Right
	Upper Leg Muscle, Left
Pectoral (anterior) lymph node	Lymphatic, Right Axillary
	Lymphatic, Left Axillary
Pectoral fascia	Subcutaneous Tissue and Fascia, Chest
Pectoralis major muscle	Thorax Muscle, Right
	Thorax Muscle, Left
Pectoralis minor muscle	Thorax Muscle, Right
	Thorax Muscle, Left
Pelvic splanchnic nerve	Abdominal Sympathetic Nerve
	Sacral Sympathetic Nerve
Penile urethra	Urethra
Pericardiophrenic artery	Internal Mammary Artery, Right
	Internal Mammary Artery, Left
Perimetrium	Uterus
Peroneus brevis muscle	Lower Leg Muscle, Right
	Lower Leg Muscle, Left
Peroneus longus muscle	Lower Leg Muscle, Right
	Lower Leg Muscle, Left
Petrous part of temporal bone	Temporal Bone, Right
	Temporal Bone, Left
Pharyngeal constrictor muscle	Tongue, Palate, Pharynx Muscle
Pharyngeal plexus	Vagus Nerve
Pharyngeal recess	Nasopharynx
Pharyngeal tonsil	Adenoids
Pharyngotympanic tube	Eustachian Tube, Right
	Eustachian Tube, Left
Pia mater, intracranial	Cerebral Meninges
Pia mater, spinal	Spinal Meninges
Pinna	External Ear, Right
	External Ear, Left
	External Ear, Bilateral
Piriform recess (sinus)	Pharynx
Piriformis muscle	Hip Muscle, Right
	Hip Muscle, Left
Pisiform bone	Carpal, Right
	Carpal, Left
Pisohamate ligament	Hand Bursa and Ligament, Right
	Hand Bursa and Ligament, Left
Pisometacarpal ligament	Hand Bursa and Ligament, Right
	Hand Bursa and Ligament, Left
Plantar digital vein	Foot Vein, Right
	Foot Vein, Left

Term	ICD-10-PCS Value
Plantar fascia (aponeurosis)	Subcutaneous Tissue and Fascia, Right Foot
	Subcutaneous Tissue and Fascia, Left Foot
Plantar metatarsal vein	Foot Vein, Right
	Foot Vein, Left
Plantar venous arch	Foot Vein, Right
	Foot Vein, Left
Platysma muscle	Neck Muscle, Right
	Neck Muscle, Left
Plica semilunaris	Conjunctiva, Right
	Conjunctiva, Left
Pneumogastric nerve	Vagus Nerve
Pneumotaxic center	Pons
Pontine tegmentum	Pons
Popliteal ligament	Knee Bursa and Ligament, Right
	Knee Bursa and Ligament, Left
Popliteallymph node	Lymphatic, Left Lower Extremity
	Lymphatic, Right Lower Extremity
Popliteal vein	Femoral Vein, Right
	Femoral Vein, Left
Popliteus muscle	Lower Leg Muscle, Right
	Lower Leg Muscle, Left
Postauricular (mastoid) lymph node	Lymphatic, Right Neck
	Lymphatic, Left Neck
Postcava	Inferior Vena Cava
Posterior (subscapular) lymph node	Lymphatic, Right Axillary
	Lymphatic, Left Axillary
Posterior auricular artery	External Carotid Artery, Right
	External Carotid Artery, Left
Posterior auricular nerve	Facial Nerve
Posterior auricular vein	External Jugular Vein, Right
	External Jugular Vein, Left
Posterior cerebral artery	Intracranial Artery
Posterior chamber	Eye, Right
	Eye, Left
Posterior circumflex humeral artery	Axillary Artery, Right
	Axillary Artery, Left
Posterior communicating artery	Intracranial Artery
Posterior cruciate ligament (PCL)	Knee Bursa and Ligament, Right
	Knee Bursa and Ligament, Left
Posterior facial (retromandibular) vein	Face Vein, Right
	Face Vein, Left
Posterior femoral cutaneous nerve	Sacral Plexus
Posterior inferior cerebellar artery (PICA)	Intracranial Artery
Posterior interosseous nerve	Radial Nerve
Posterior labial nerve	Pudendal Nerve
Posterior scrotal nerve	Pudendal Nerve
Posterior spinal artery	Vertebral Artery, Right
	Vertebral Artery, Left
Posterior tibial recurrent artery	Anterior Tibial Artery, Right
	Anterior Tibial Artery, Left
Posterior ulnar recurrent artery	Ulnar Artery, Right
	Ulnar Artery, Left

Term	ICD-10-PCS Value
Posterior vagal trunk	Vagus Nerve
Preauricular lymph node	Lymphatic, Head
Precava	Superior Vena Cava
Prepatellar bursa	Knee Bursa and Ligament, Right
	Knee Bursa and Ligament, Left
Pretracheal fascia	Subcutaneous Tissue and Fascia, Right Neck
	Subcutaneous Tissue and Fascia, Left Neck
Prevertebral fascia	Subcutaneous Tissue and Fascia, Right Neck
	Subcutaneous Tissue and Fascia, Left Neck
Princeps pollicis artery	Hand Artery, Right
	Hand Artery, Left
Procerus muscle	Facial Muscle
Profunda brachii	Brachial Artery, Right
	Brachial Artery, Left
Profunda femoris (deep femoral) vein	Femoral Vein, Right
	Femoral Vein, Left
Pronator quadratus muscle	Lower Arm and Wrist Muscle, Right
	Lower Arm and Wrist Muscle, Left
Pronator teres muscle	Lower Arm and Wrist Muscle, Right
	Lower Arm and Wrist Muscle, Left
Prostatic urethra	Urethra
Proximal radioulnar joint	Elbow Joint, Right
	Elbow Joint, Left
Psoas muscle	Hip Muscle, Right
	Hip Muscle, Left
Pterygoid muscle	Head Muscle
Pterygoid process	Sphenoid Bone
Pterygopalatine (sphenopalatine) ganglion	Head and Neck Sympathetic Nerve
Pubis	Pelvic Bone, Right
	Pelvic Bone, Left
Pubofemoral ligament	Hip Bursa and Ligament, Right
	Hip Bursa and Ligament, Left
Pudendal nerve	Sacral Plexus
Pulmoaortic canal	Pulmonary Artery, Left
Pulmonary annulus	Pulmonary Valve
Pulmonary plexus	Thoracic Sympathetic Nerve
	Vagus Nerve
Pulmonic valve	Pulmonary Valve
Pulvinar	Thalamus
Pyloric antrum	Stomach, Pylorus
Pyloric canal	Stomach, Pylorus
Pyloric sphincter	Stomach, Pylorus
Pyramidalis muscle	Abdomen Muscle, Right
	Abdomen Muscle, Left
Quadrangular cartilage	Nasal Septum
Quadrate lobe	Liver
Quadratus femoris muscle	Hip Muscle, Right
	Hip Muscle, Left
Quadratus lumborum muscle	Trunk Muscle, Right
	Trunk Muscle, Left
Quadratus plantae muscle	Foot Muscle, Right
	Foot Muscle, Left

Term	ICD-10-PCS Value
Quadriceps (femoris)	Upper Leg Muscle, Right
	Upper Leg Muscle, Left
Radial collateral carpal ligament	Wrist Bursa and Ligament, Right
	Wrist Bursa and Ligament, Left
Radial collateral ligament	Elbow Bursa and Ligament, Right
	Elbow Bursa and Ligament, Left
Radial notch	Ulna, Right
	Ulna, Left
Radial recurrent artery	Radial Artery, Right
	Radial Artery, Left
Radial vein	Brachial Vein, Right
	Brachial Vein, Left
Radialis indicis	Hand Artery, Right
	Hand Artery, Left
Radiocarpal joint	Wrist Joint, Right
	Wrist Joint, Left
Radiocarpal ligament	Wrist Bursa and Ligament, Right
	Wrist Bursa and Ligament, Left
Radioulnar ligament	Wrist Bursa and Ligament, Right
	Wrist Bursa and Ligament, Left
Rectosigmoid junction	Sigmoid Colon
Rectus abdominis muscle	Abdomen Muscle, Right
	Abdomen Muscle, Left
Rectus femoris muscle	Upper Leg Muscle, Right
	Upper Leg Muscle, Left
Recurrent laryngeal nerve	Vagus Nerve
Renal calyx	Kidney, Right
	Kidney, Left
	Kidneys, Bilateral
	Kidney
Renal capsule	Kidney, Right
	Kidney, Left
	Kidneys, Bilateral
	Kidney
Renal cortex	Kidney, Right
	Kidney, Left
	Kidneys, Bilateral
	Kidney
Renal plexus	Abdominal Sympathetic Nerve
Renal segment	Kidney, Right
	Kidney, Left
	Kidneys, Bilateral
	Kidney
Renal segmental artery	Renal Artery, Right
	Renal Artery, Left
Retroperitoneal cavity	Retroperitoneum
Retroperitoneal lymph node	Lymphatic, Aortic
Retroperitoneal space	Retroperitoneum
Retropharyngeal lymph node	Lymphatic, Right Neck
	Lymphatic, Left Neck
Retropubic space	Pelvic Cavity
Rhinopharynx	Nasopharynx
Rhomboid major muscle	Trunk Muscle, Right
	Trunk Muscle, Left

Term	ICD-10-PCS Value
Rhomboid minor muscle	Trunk Muscle, Right
	Trunk Muscle, Left
Right ascending lumbar vein	Azygos Vein
Right atrioventricular valve	Tricuspid Valve
Right auricular appendix	Atrium, Right
Right colic vein	Colic Vein
Right coronary sulcus	Heart, Right
Right gastric artery	Gastric Artery
Right gastroepiploic vein	Superior Mesenteric Vein
Right inferior phrenic vein	Inferior Vena Cava
Right inferior pulmonary vein	Pulmonary Vein, Right
Right jugular trunk	Lymphatic, Right Neck
Right lateral ventricle	Cerebral Ventricle
Right lymphatic duct	Lymphatic, Right Neck
Right ovarian vein	Inferior Vena Cava
Right second lumbar vein	Inferior Vena Cava
Right subclavian trunk	Lymphatic, Right Neck
Right subcostal vein	Azygos Vein
Right superior pulmonary vein	Pulmonary Vein, Right
Right suprarenal vein	Inferior Vena Cava
Right testicular vein	Inferior Vena Cava
Rima glottidis	Larynx
Risorius muscle	Facial Muscle
Round ligament of uterus	Uterine Supporting Structure
Round window	Inner Ear, Right
	Inner Ear, Left
Sacral ganglion	Sacral Sympathetic Nerve
Sacral lymph node	Lymphatic, Pelvis
Sacral splanchnic nerve	Sacral Sympathetic Nerve
Sacrococcygeal ligament	Lower Spine Bursa and Ligament
Sacrococcygeal symphysis	Sacrococcygeal Joint
Sacroiliac ligament	Lower Spine Bursa and Ligament
Sacrospinous ligament	Lower Spine Bursa and Ligament
Sacrotuberous ligament	Lower Spine Bursa and Ligament
Salpingopharyngeus muscle	Tongue, Palate, Pharynx Muscle
Salpinx	Fallopian Tube, Right
	Fallopian Tube, Left
Saphenous nerve	Femoral Nerve
Sartorius muscle	Upper Leg Muscle, Right
	Upper Leg Muscle, Left
Scalene muscle	Neck Muscle, Right
	Neck Muscle, Left
Scaphoid bone	Carpal, Right
	Carpal, Left
Scapholunate ligament	Hand Bursa and Ligament, Right
	Hand Bursa and Ligament, Left
Scaphotrapezium ligament	Hand Bursa and Ligament, Right
	Hand Bursa and Ligament, Left
Scarpa's (vestibular) ganglion	Acoustic Nerve
Sebaceous gland	Skin

Term	ICD-10-PCS Value
Second cranial nerve	Optic Nerve
Sella turcica	Sphenoid Bone
Semicircular canal	Inner Ear, Right
	Inner Ear, Left
Semimembranosus muscle	Upper Leg Muscle, Right
	Upper Leg Muscle, Left
Semitendinosus muscle	Upper Leg Muscle, Right
	Upper Leg Muscle, Left
Septal cartilage	Nasal Septum
Serratus anterior muscle	Thorax Muscle, Right
	Thorax Muscle, Left
Serratus posterior muscle	Trunk Muscle, Right
	Trunk Muscle, Left
Seventh cranial nerve	Facial Nerve
Short gastric artery	Splenic Artery
Sigmoid artery	Inferior Mesenteric Artery
Sigmoid flexure	Sigmoid Colon
Sigmoid vein	Inferior Mesenteric Vein
Sinoatrial node	Conduction Mechanism
Sinus venosus	Atrium, Right
Sixth cranial nerve	Abducens Nerve
Skene's (paraurethral) gland	Vestibular Gland
Small saphenous vein	Saphenous Vein, Right
	Saphenous Vein, Left
Solar (celiac) plexus	Abdominal Sympathetic Nerve
Soleus muscle	Lower Leg Muscle, Right
	Lower Leg Muscle, Left
Sphenomandibular ligament	Head and Neck Bursa and Ligament
Sphenopalatine (pterygopalatine) ganglion	Head and Neck Sympathetic Nerve
Spinal nerve, cervical	Cervical Nerve
Spinal nerve, lumbar	Lumbar Nerve
Spinal nerve, sacral	Sacral Nerve
Spinal nerve, thoracic	Thoracic Nerve
Spinous process	Cervical Vertebra
	Lumbar Vertebra
	Thoracic Vertebra
Spiral ganglion	Acoustic Nerve
Splenic flexure	Transverse Colon
Splenic plexus	Abdominal Sympathetic Nerve
Splenius capitis muscle	Head Muscle
Splenius cervicis muscle	Neck Muscle, Right
	Neck Muscle, Left
Stapes	Auditory Ossicle, Right
	Auditory Ossicle, Left
Stellate ganglion	Head and Neck Sympathetic Nerve
Stensen's duct	Parotid Duct, Right
	Parotid Duct, Left
Sternoclavicular ligament	Shoulder Bursa and Ligament, Right
	Shoulder Bursa and Ligament, Left
Sternocleidomastoid artery	Thyroid Artery, Right
	Thyroid Artery, Left

Term	ICD-10-PCS Value
Sternocleidomastoid muscle	Neck Muscle, Right
	Neck Muscle, Left
Sternocostal ligament	Sternum Bursa and Ligament
Styloglossus muscle	Tongue, Palate, Pharynx Muscle
Stylomandibular ligament	Head and Neck Bursa and Ligament
Stylopharyngeus muscle	Tongue, Palate, Pharynx Muscle
Subacromial bursa	Shoulder Bursa and Ligament, Right
	Shoulder Bursa and Ligament, Left
Subaortic (common iliac) lymph node	Lymphatic, Pelvis
Subarachnoid space, spinal	Spinal Canal
Subclavicular (apical) lymph node	Lymphatic, Right Axillary
	Lymphatic, Left Axillary
Subclavius muscle	Thorax Muscle, Right
	Thorax Muscle, Left
Subclavius nerve	Brachial Plexus
Subcostal artery	Upper Artery
Subcostal muscle	Thorax Muscle, Right
	Thorax Muscle, Left
Subcostal nerve	Thoracic Nerve
Subdural space, spinal	Spinal Canal
Submandibular ganglion	Facial Nerve
	Head and Neck Sympathetic Nerve
Submandibular gland	Submaxillary Gland, Right
	Submaxillary Gland, Left
Submandibular lymph node	Lymphatic, Head
Submaxillary ganglion	Head and Neck Sympathetic Nerve
Submaxillary lymph node	Lymphatic, Head
Submental artery	Face Artery
Submental lymph node	Lymphatic, Head
Submucous (Meissner's) plexus	Abdominal Sympathetic Nerve
Suboccipital nerve	Cervical Nerve
Suboccipital venous plexus	Vertebral Vein, Right
	Vertebral Vein, Left
Subparotid lymph node	Lymphatic, Head
Subscapular aponeurosis	Subcutaneous Tissue and Fascia, Right Upper Arm
	Subcutaneous Tissue and Fascia, Left Upper Arm
Subscapular artery	Axillary Artery, Right
	Axillary Artery, Left
Subscapular (posterior) lymph node	Lymphatic, Right Axillary
	Lymphatic, Left Axillary
Subscapularis muscle	Shoulder Muscle, Right
	Shoulder Muscle, Left
Substantia nigra	Basal Ganglia
Subtalar (talocalcaneal) joint	Tarsal Joint, Right
	Tarsal Joint, Left
Subtalar ligament	Foot Bursa and Ligament, Right
	Foot Bursa and Ligament, Left
Subthalamic nucleus	Basal Ganglia
Superficial circumflex iliac vein	Saphenous Vein, Right
	Saphenous Vein, Left

Term	ICD-10-PCS Value
Superficial epigastric artery	Femoral Artery, Right
	Femoral Artery, Left
Superficial epigastric vein	Saphenous Vein, Right
	Saphenous Vein, Left
Superficial palmar arch	Hand Artery, Right
	Hand Artery, Left
Superficial palmar venous arch	Hand Vein, Right
	Hand Vein, Left
Superficial temporal artery	Temporal Artery, Right
	Temporal Artery, Left
Superficial transverse perineal muscle	Perineum Muscle
Superior cardiac nerve	Thoracic Sympathetic Nerve
Superior cerebellar vein	Intracranial Vein
Superior cerebral vein	Intracranial Vein
Superior clunic (cluneal) nerve	Lumbar Nerve
Superior epigastric artery	Internal Mammary Artery, Right
	Internal Mammary Artery, Left
Superior genicular artery	Popliteal Artery, Right
	Popliteal Artery, Left
Superior gluteal artery	Internal Iliac Artery, Right
	Internal Iliac Artery, Left
Superior gluteal nerve	Lumbar Plexus
Superior hypogastric plexus	Abdominal Sympathetic Nerve
Superior labial artery	Face Artery
Superior laryngeal artery	Thyroid Artery, Right
	Thyroid Artery, Left
Superior laryngeal nerve	Vagus Nerve
Superior longitudinal muscle	Tongue, Palate, Pharynx Muscle
Superior mesenteric ganglion	Abdominal Sympathetic Nerve
Superior mesenteric lymph node	Lymphatic, Mesenteric
Superior mesenteric plexus	Abdominal Sympathetic Nerve
Superior oblique muscle	Extraocular Muscle, Right
	Extraocular Muscle, Left
Superior olivary nucleus	Pons
Superior rectal artery	Inferior Mesenteric Artery
Superior rectal vein	Inferior Mesenteric Vein
Superior rectus muscle	Extraocular Muscle, Right
	Extraocular Muscle, Left
Superior tarsal plate	Upper Eyelid, Right
	Upper Eyelid, Left
Superior thoracic artery	Axillary Artery, Right
	Axillary Artery, Left
Superior thyroid artery	External Carotid Artery, Right
	External Carotid Artery, Left
	Thyroid Artery, Right
	Thyroid Artery, Left
Superior turbinate	Nasal Turbinate
Superior ulnar collateral artery	Brachial Artery, Right
	Brachial Artery, Left
Supraclavicular nerve	Cervical Plexus

Term	ICD-10-PCS Value
Supraclavicular (Virchow's) lymph node	Lymphatic, Right Neck
	Lymphatic, Left Neck
Suprahyoid lymph node	Lymphatic, Head
Suprahyoid muscle	Neck Muscle, Right
	Neck Muscle, Left
Suprainguinal lymph node	Lymphatic, Pelvis
Supraorbital vein	Face Vein, Right
	Face Vein, Left
Suprarenal gland	Adrenal Gland, Right
	Adrenal Gland, Left
	Adrenal Glands, Bilateral
	Adrenal Gland
Suprarenal plexus	Abdominal Sympathetic Nerve
Suprascapular nerve	Brachial Plexus
Supraspinatus fascia	Subcutaneous Tissue and Fascia, Right Upper Arm
	Subcutaneous Tissue and Fascia, Left Upper Arm
Supraspinatus muscle	Shoulder Muscle, Right
	Shoulder Muscle, Left
Supraspinous ligament	Upper Spine Bursa and Ligament
	Lower Spine Bursa and Ligament
Suprasternal notch	Sternum
Supratrochlear lymph node	Lymphatic, Right Upper Extremity
	Lymphatic, Left Upper Extremity
Sural artery	Popliteal Artery, Right
	Popliteal Artery, Left
Sweat gland	Skin
Talocalcaneal ligament	Foot Bursa and Ligament, Right
	Foot Bursa and Ligament, Left
Talocalcaneal (subtalar) joint	Tarsal Joint, Right
	Tarsal Joint, Left
Talocalcaneonavicular joint	Tarsal Joint, Right
	Tarsal Joint, Left
Talocalcaneonavicular ligament	Foot Bursa and Ligament, Right
	Foot Bursa and Ligament, Left
Talocrural joint	Ankle Joint, Right
	Ankle Joint, Left
Talofibular ligament	Ankle Bursa and Ligament, Right
	Ankle Bursa and Ligament, Left
Talus bone	Tarsal, Right
	Tarsal, Left
Tarsometatarsal ligament	Foot Bursa and Ligament, Right
	Foot Bursa and Ligament, Left
Temporal lobe	Cerebral Hemisphere
Temporalis muscle	Head Muscle
Temporoparietalis muscle	Head Muscle
Tensor fasciae latae muscle	Hip Muscle, Right
	Hip Muscle, Left
Tensor veli palatini muscle	Tongue, Palate, Pharynx Muscle
Tenth cranial nerve	Vagus Nerve
Tentorium cerebelli	Dura Mater
Teres major muscle	Shoulder Muscle, Right
	Shoulder Muscle, Left
Teres minor muscle	Shoulder Muscle, Right
	Shoulder Muscle, Left
Testicular artery	Abdominal Aorta
Thenar muscle	Hand Muscle, Right
	Hand Muscle, Left
Third cranial nerve	Oculomotor Nerve
Third occipital nerve	Cervical Nerve
Third ventricle	Cerebral Ventricle
Thoracic aortic plexus	Thoracic Sympathetic Nerve
Thoracic esophagus	Esophagus, Middle
Thoracic facet joint	Thoracic Vertebral Joint
Thoracic ganglion	Thoracic Sympathetic Nerve
Thoracoacromial artery	Axillary Artery, Right
	Axillary Artery, Left
Thoracolumbar facet joint	Thoracolumbar Vertebral Joint
Thymus gland	Thymus
Thyroarytenoid muscle	Neck Muscle, Right
	Neck Muscle, Left
Thyrocervical trunk	Thyroid Artery, Right
	Thyroid Artery, Left
Thyroid cartilage	Larynx
Tibialis anterior muscle	Lower Leg Muscle, Right
	Lower Leg Muscle, Left
Tibialis posterior muscle	Lower Leg Muscle, Right
	Lower Leg Muscle, Left
Tibiofemoral joint	Knee Joint, Right
	Knee Joint, Left
	Knee Joint, Tibial Surface, Right
	Knee Joint, Tibial Surface, Left
Tongue, base of	Pharynx
Tracheobronchial lymph node	Lymphatic, Thorax
Tragus	External Ear, Right
	External Ear, Left
	External Ear, Bilateral
Transversalis fascia	Subcutaneous Tissue and Fascia, Trunk
Transverse acetabular ligament	Hip Bursa and Ligament, Right
	Hip Bursa and Ligament, Left
Transverse (cutaneous) cervical nerve	Cervical Plexus
Transverse facial artery	Temporal Artery, Right
	Temporal Artery, Left
Transverse foramen	Cervical Vertebra
Transverse humeral ligament	Shoulder Bursa and Ligament, Right
	Shoulder Bursa and Ligament, Left
Transverse ligament of atlas	Head and Neck Bursa and Ligament
Transverse process	Cervical Vertebra
	Thoracic Vertebra
	Lumbar Vertebra
Transverse scapular ligament	Shoulder Bursa and Ligament, Right
	Shoulder Bursa and Ligament, Left
Transverse thoracis muscle	Thorax Muscle, Right
	Thorax Muscle, Left

Term	ICD-10-PCS Value
Transversospinalis muscle	Trunk Muscle, Right
	Trunk Muscle, Left
Transversus abdominis muscle	Abdomen Muscle, Right
	Abdomen Muscle, Left
Trapezium bone	Carpal, Right
	Carpal, Left
Trapezius muscle	Trunk Muscle, Right
	Trunk Muscle, Left
Trapezoid bone	Carpal, Right
	Carpal, Left
Triceps brachii muscle	Upper Arm Muscle, Right
	Upper Arm Muscle, Left
Tricuspid annulus	Tricuspid Valve
Trifacial nerve	Trigeminal Nerve
Trigone of bladder	Bladder
Triquetral bone	Carpal, Right
	Carpal, Left
Trochantericbursa	Hip Bursa and Ligament, Right
	Hip Bursa and Ligament, Left
Twelfth cranial nerve	Hypoglossal Nerve
Tympanic cavity	Middle Ear, Right
	Middle Ear, Left
Tympanic nerve	Glossopharyngeal Nerve
Tympanic part of temoporal bone	Temporal Bone, Right
	Temporal Bone, Left
Ulnar collateral carpal ligament	Wrist Bursa and Ligament, Right
	Wrist Bursa and Ligament, Left
Ulnar collateral ligament	Elbow Bursa and Ligament, Right
	Elbow Bursa and Ligament, Left
Ulnar notch	Radius, Right
	Radius, Left
Ulnar vein	Brachial Vein, Right
	Brachial Vein, Left
Umbilical artery	Internal Iliac Artery, Right
	Internal Iliac Artery, Left
	Lower Artery
Ureteral orifice	Ureter, Right
	Ureter, Left
	Ureters, Bilateral
	Ureter
Ureteropelvic junction (UPJ)	Kidney Pelvis, Right
	Kidney Pelvis, Left
Ureterovesical orifice	Ureter, Right
	Ureter, Left
	Ureters, Bilateral
	Ureter
Uterine artery	Internal Iliac Artery, Right
	Internal Iliac Artery, Left
Uterine cornu	Uterus
Uterine tube	Fallopian Tube, Right
	Fallopian Tube, Left
Uterine vein	Hypogastric Vein, Right
	Hypogastric Vein, Left
Vaginal artery	Internal Iliac Artery, Right
	Internal Iliac Artery, Left

Term	ICD-10-PCS Value
Vaginal vein	Hypogastric Vein, Right
	Hypogastric Vein, Left
Vastus intermedius muscle	Upper Leg Muscle, Right
	Upper Leg Muscle, Left
Vastus lateralis muscle	Upper Leg Muscle, Right
	Upper Leg Muscle, Left
Vastus medialis muscle	Upper Leg Muscle, Right
	Upper Leg Muscle, Left
Ventricular fold	Larynx
Vermiform appendix	Appendix
Vermilion border	Upper Lip
	Lower Lip
Vertebral arch	Cervical Vertebra
	Lumbar Vertebra
	Thoracic Vertebra
Vertebral body	Cervical Vertebra
	Lumbar Vertebra
	Thoracic Vertebra
Vertebral canal	Spinal Canal
Vertebral foramen	Cervical Vertebra
	Lumbar Vertebra
	Thoracic Vertebra
Vertebral lamina	Cervical Vertebra
	Lumbar Vertebra
	Thoracic Vertebra
Vertebral pedicle	Cervical Vertebra
	Lumbar Vertebra
	Thoracic Vertebra
Vesical vein	Hypogastric Vein, Right
	Hypogastric Vein, Left
Vestibular (Scarpa's) ganglion	Acoustic Nerve
Vestibular nerve	Acoustic Nerve
Vestibulocochlear nerve	Acoustic Nerve
Virchow's (supraclavicular) lymph node	Lymphatic, Right Neck
	Lymphatic, Left Neck
Vitreous body	Vitreous, Right
	Vitreous, Left
Vocal fold	Vocal Cord, Right
	Vocal Cord, Left
Volar (palmar) digital vein	Hand Vein, Right
	Hand Vein, Left
Volar (palmar) metacarpal vein	Hand Vein, Right
	Hand Vein, Left
Vomer bone	Nasal Septum
Vomer of nasal septum	Nasal Bone
Xiphoid process	Sternum
Zonule of Zinn	Lens, Right
	Lens, Left
Zygomatic process of frontal bone	Frontal Bone
Zygomatic process of temporal bone	Temporal Bone, Right
	Temporal Bone, Left
Zygomaticus muscle	Facial Muscle

Appendix E: Body Part Definitions

ICD-10-PCS Value	Definition
1st Toe, Left **1st Toe, Right**	**Includes:** Hallux
Abdomen Muscle, Left **Abdomen Muscle, Right**	**Includes:** External oblique muscle Internal oblique muscle Pyramidalis muscle Rectus abdominis muscle Transversus abdominis muscle
Abdominal Aorta	**Includes:** Inferior phrenic artery Lumbar artery Median sacral artery Middle suprarenal artery Ovarian artery Testicular artery
Abdominal Sympathetic Nerve	**Includes:** Abdominal aortic plexus Auerbach's (myenteric) plexus Celiac (solar) plexus Celiac ganglion Gastric plexus Hepatic plexus Inferior hypogastric plexus Inferior mesenteric ganglion Inferior mesenteric plexus Meissner's (submucous) plexus Myenteric (Auerbach's) plexus Pancreatic plexus Pelvic splanchnic nerve Renal plexus Solar (celiac) plexus Splenic plexus Submucous (Meissner's) plexus Superior hypogastric plexus Superior mesenteric ganglion Superior mesenteric plexus Suprarenal plexus
Abducens Nerve	**Includes:** Sixth cranial nerve
Accessory Nerve	**Includes:** Eleventh cranial nerve
Acoustic Nerve	**Includes:** Cochlear nerve Eighth cranial nerve Scarpa's (vestibular) ganglion Spiral ganglion Vestibular (Scarpa's) ganglion Vestibular nerve Vestibulocochlear nerve
Adenoids	**Includes:** Pharyngeal tonsil
Adrenal Gland **Adrenal Gland, Left** **Adrenal Gland, Right** **Adrenal Glands, Bilateral**	**Includes:** Suprarenal gland
Ampulla of Vater	**Includes:** Duodenal ampulla Hepatopancreatic ampulla
Anal Sphincter	**Includes:** External anal sphincter Internal anal sphincter

ICD-10-PCS Value	Definition
Ankle Bursa and Ligament, Left **Ankle Bursa and Ligament, Right**	**Includes:** Calcaneofibular ligament Deltoid ligament Ligament of the lateral malleolus Talofibular ligament
Ankle Joint, Left **Ankle Joint, Right**	**Includes:** Inferior tibiofibular joint Talocrural joint
Anterior Chamber, Left **Anterior Chamber, Right**	**Includes:** Aqueous humour
Anterior Tibial Artery, Left **Anterior Tibial Artery, Right**	**Includes:** Anterior lateral malleolar artery Anterior medial malleolar artery Anterior tibial recurrent artery Dorsalis pedis artery Posterior tibial recurrent artery
Anus	**Includes:** Anal orifice
Aortic Valve	**Includes:** Aortic annulus
Appendix	**Includes:** Vermiform appendix
Atrial Septum	**Includes:** Interatrial septum
Atrium, Left	**Includes:** Atrium pulmonale Left auricular appendix
Atrium, Right	**Includes:** Atrium dextrum cordis Right auricular appendix Sinus venosus
Auditory Ossicle, Left **Auditory Ossicle, Right**	**Includes:** Incus Malleus Stapes
Axillary Artery, Left **Axillary Artery, Right**	**Includes:** Anterior circumflex humeral artery Lateral thoracic artery Posterior circumflex humeral artery Subscapular artery Superior thoracic artery Thoracoacromial artery
Azygos Vein	**Includes:** Right ascending lumbar vein Right subcostal vein
Basal Ganglia	**Includes:** Basal nuclei Claustrum Corpus striatum Globus pallidus Substantia nigra Subthalamic nucleus
Basilic Vein, Left **Basilic Vein, Right**	**Includes:** Median antebrachial vein Median cubital vein
Bladder	**Includes:** Trigone of bladder
Brachial Artery, Left **Brachial Artery, Right**	**Includes:** Inferior ulnar collateral artery Profunda brachii Superior ulnar collateral artery

ICD-10-PCS Value	Definition
Brachial Plexus	**Includes:** Axillary nerve Dorsal scapular nerve First intercostal nerve Long thoracic nerve Musculocutaneous nerve Subclavius nerve Suprascapular nerve
Brachial Vein, Left **Brachial Vein, Right**	**Includes:** Radial vein Ulnar vein
Brain	**Includes:** Cerebrum Corpus callosum Encephalon
Breast, Bilateral **Breast, Left** **Breast, Right**	**Includes:** Mammary duct Mammary gland
Buccal Mucosa	**Includes:** Buccal gland Molar gland Palatine gland
Carotid Bodies, Bilateral **Carotid Body, Left** **Carotid Body, Right**	**Includes:** Carotid glomus
Carpal Joint, Left **Carpal Joint, Right**	**Includes:** Intercarpal joint Midcarpal joint
Carpal, Left **Carpal, Right**	**Includes:** Capitate bone Hamate bone Lunate bone Pisiform bone Scaphoid bone Trapezium bone Trapezoid bone Triquetral bone
Celiac Artery	**Includes:** Celiac trunk
Cephalic Vein, Left **Cephalic Vein, Right**	**Includes:** Accessory cephalic vein
Cerebellum	**Includes:** Culmen
Cerebral Hemisphere	**Includes:** Frontal lobe Occipital lobe Parietal lobe Temporal lobe
Cerebral Meninges	**Includes:** Arachnoid mater, intracranial Leptomeninges, intracranial Pia mater, intracranial
Cerebral Ventricle	**Includes:** Aqueduct of Sylvius Cerebral aqueduct (Sylvius) Choroid plexus Ependyma Foramen of Monro (intraventricular) Fourth ventricle Interventricular foramen (Monro) Left lateral ventricle Right lateral ventricle Third ventricle

ICD-10-PCS Value	Definition
Cervical Nerve	**Includes:** Greater occipital nerve Spinal nerve, cervical Suboccipital nerve Third occipital nerve
Cervical Plexus	**Includes:** Ansa cervicalis Cutaneous (transverse) cervical nerve Great auricular nerve Lesser occipital nerve Supraclavicular nerve Transverse (cutaneous) cervical nerve
Cervical Vertebra	**Includes:** Dens Odontoid process Spinous process Transverse foramen Transverse process Vertebral arch Vertebral body Vertebral foramen Vertebral lamina Vertebral pedicle
Cervical Vertebral Joint	**Includes:** Atlantoaxial joint Cervical facet joint
Cervical Vertebral Joints, 2 or more	**Includes:** Cervical facet joint
Cervicothoracic Vertebral Joint	**Includes:** Cervicothoracic facet joint
Cisterna Chyli	**Includes:** Intestinal lymphatic trunk Lumbar lymphatic trunk
Coccygeal Glomus	**Includes:** Coccygeal body
Colic Vein	**Includes:** Ileocolic vein Left colic vein Middle colic vein Right colic vein
Conduction Mechanism	**Includes:** Atrioventricular node Bundle of His Bundle of Kent Sinoatrial node
Conjunctiva, Left **Conjunctiva, Right**	**Includes:** Plica semilunaris
Dura Mater	**Includes:** Diaphragma sellae Dura mater, intracranial Falx cerebri Tentorium cerebelli
Elbow Bursa and Ligament, Left **Elbow Bursa and Ligament, Right**	**Includes:** Annular ligament Olecranon bursa Radial collateral ligament Ulnar collateral ligament
Elbow Joint, Left **Elbow Joint, Right**	**Includes:** Distal humerus, involving joint Humeroradial joint Humeroulnar joint Proximal radioulnar joint
Epidural Space, Intracranial	**Includes:** Extradural space, intracranial

ICD-10-PCS Value	Definition
Epiglottis	**Includes:** Glossoepiglottic fold
Esophagogastric Junction	**Includes:** Cardia Cardioesophageal junction Gastroesophageal (GE) junction
Esophagus, Lower	**Includes:** Abdominal esophagus
Esophagus, Middle	**Includes:** Thoracic esophagus
Esophagus, Upper	**Includes:** Cervical esophagus
Ethmoid Bone, Left **Ethmoid Bone, Right**	**Includes:** Cribriform plate
Ethmoid Sinus, Left **Ethmoid Sinus, Right**	**Includes:** Ethmoidal air cell
Eustachian Tube, Left **Eustachian Tube, Right**	**Includes:** Auditory tube Pharyngotympanic tube
External Auditory Canal, Left **External Auditory Canal, Right**	**Includes:** External auditory meatus
External Carotid Artery, Left **External Carotid Artery, Right**	**Includes:** Ascending pharyngeal artery Internal maxillary artery Lingual artery Maxillary artery Occipital artery Posterior auricular artery Superior thyroid artery
External Ear, Bilateral **External Ear, Left** **External Ear, Right**	**Includes:** Antihelix Antitragus Auricle Earlobe Helix Pinna Tragus
External Iliac Artery, Left **External Iliac Artery, Right**	**Includes:** Deep circumflex iliac artery Inferior epigastric artery
External Jugular Vein, Left **External Jugular Vein, Right**	**Includes:** Posterior auricular vein
Extraocular Muscle, Left **Extraocular Muscle, Right**	**Includes:** Inferior oblique muscle Inferior rectus muscle Lateral rectus muscle Medial rectus muscle Superior oblique muscle Superior rectus muscle
Eye, Left **Eye, Right**	**Includes:** Ciliary body Posterior chamber
Face Artery	**Includes:** Angular artery Ascending palatine artery External maxillary artery Facial artery Inferior labial artery Submental artery Superior labial artery

ICD-10-PCS Value	Definition
Face Vein, Left **Face Vein, Right**	**Includes:** Angular vein Anterior facial vein Common facial vein Deep facial vein Frontal vein Posterior facial (retromandibular) vein Supraorbital vein
Facial Muscle	**Includes:** Buccinator muscle Corrugator supercilii muscle Depressor anguli oris muscle Depressor labii inferioris muscle Depressor septi nasi muscle Depressor supercilii muscle Levator anguli oris muscle Levator labii superioris alaeque nasi muscle Levator labii superioris muscle Mentalis muscle Nasalis muscle Occipitofrontalis muscle Orbicularis oris muscle Procerus muscle Risorius muscle Zygomaticus muscle
Facial Nerve	**Includes:** Chorda tympani Geniculate ganglion Greater superficial petrosal nerve Nerve to the stapedius Parotid plexus Posterior auricular nerve Seventh cranial nerve Submandibular ganglion
Fallopian Tube, Left **Fallopian Tube, Right**	**Includes:** Oviduct Salpinx Uterine tube
Femoral Artery, Left **Femoral Artery, Right**	**Includes:** Circumflex iliac artery Deep femoral artery Descending genicular artery External pudendal artery Superficial epigastric artery
Femoral Nerve	**Includes:** Anterior crural nerve Saphenous nerve
Femoral Shaft, Left **Femoral Shaft, Right**	**Includes:** Body of femur
Femoral Vein, Left **Femoral Vein, Right**	**Includes:** Deep femoral (profunda femoris) vein Popliteal vein Profunda femoris (deep femoral) vein
Fibula, Left **Fibula, Right**	**Includes:** Body of fibula Head of fibula Lateral malleolus
Finger Nail	**Includes:** Nail bed Nail plate

ICD-10-PCS Value	Definition
Finger Phalangeal Joint, Left **Finger Phalangeal Joint, Right**	**Includes:** Interphalangeal (IP) joint
Foot Artery, Left **Foot Artery, Right**	**Includes:** Arcuate artery Dorsal metatarsal artery Lateral plantar artery Lateral tarsal artery Medial plantar artery
Foot Bursa and Ligament, Left **Foot Bursa and Ligament, Right**	**Includes:** Calcaneocuboid ligament Cuneonavicular ligament Intercuneiform ligament Interphalangeal ligament Metatarsal ligament Metatarsophalangeal ligament Subtalar ligament Talocalcaneal ligament Talocalcaneonavicular ligament Tarsometatarsal ligament
Foot Muscle, Left **Foot Muscle, Right**	**Includes:** Abductor hallucis muscle Adductor hallucis muscle Extensor digitorum brevis muscle Extensor hallucis brevis muscle Flexor digitorum brevis muscle Flexor hallucis brevis muscle Quadratus plantae muscle
Foot Vein, Left **Foot Vein, Right**	**Includes:** Common digital vein Dorsal metatarsal vein Dorsal venous arch Plantar digital vein Plantar metatarsal vein Plantar venous arch
Frontal Bone	**Includes:** Zygomatic process of frontal bone
Gastric Artery	**Includes:** Left gastric artery Right gastric artery
Glenoid Cavity, Left **Glenoid Cavity, Right**	**Includes:** Glenoid fossa (of scapula)
Glomus Jugulare	**Includes:** Jugular body
Glossopharyngeal Nerve	**Includes:** Carotid sinus nerve Ninth cranial nerve Tympanic nerve
Hand Artery, Left **Hand Artery, Right**	**Includes:** Deep palmar arch Princeps pollicis artery Radialis indicis Superficial palmar arch
Hand Bursa and Ligament, Left **Hand Bursa and Ligament, Right**	**Includes:** Carpometacarpal ligament Intercarpal ligament Interphalangeal ligament Lunotriquetral ligament Metacarpal ligament Metacarpophalangeal ligament Pisohamate ligament Pisometacarpal ligament Scapholunate ligament Scaphotrapezium ligament

ICD-10-PCS Value	Definition
Hand Muscle, Left **Hand Muscle, Right**	**Includes:** Hypothenar muscle Palmar interosseous muscle Thenar muscle
Hand Vein, Left **Hand Vein, Right**	**Includes:** Dorsal metacarpal vein Palmar (volar) digital vein Palmar (volar) metacarpal vein Superficial palmar venous arch Volar (palmar) digital vein Volar (palmar) metacarpal vein
Head and Neck Bursa and Ligament	**Includes:** Alar ligament of axis Cervical interspinous ligament Cervical intertransverse ligament Cervical ligamentum flavum Interspinous ligament, cervical Intertransverse ligament, cervical Lateral temporomandibular ligament Ligamentum flavum, cervical Sphenomandibular ligament Stylomandibular ligament Transverse ligament of atlas
Head and Neck Sympathetic Nerve	**Includes:** Cavernous plexus Cervical ganglion Ciliary ganglion Internal carotid plexus Otic ganglion Pterygopalatine (sphenopalatine) ganglion Sphenopalatine (pterygopalatine) ganglion Stellate ganglion Submandibular ganglion Submaxillary ganglion
Head Muscle	**Includes:** Auricularis muscle Masseter muscle Pterygoid muscle Splenius capitis muscle Temporalis muscle Temporoparietalis muscle
Heart, Left	**Includes:** Left coronary sulcus Obtuse margin
Heart, Right	**Includes:** Right coronary sulcus
Hemiazygos Vein	**Includes:** Left ascending lumbar vein Left subcostal vein
Hepatic Artery	**Includes:** Common hepatic artery Gastroduodenal artery Hepatic artery proper
Hip Bursa and Ligament, Left **Hip Bursa and Ligament, Right**	**Includes:** Iliofemoral ligament Ischiofemoral ligament Pubofemoral ligament Transverse acetabular ligament Trochanteric bursa
Hip Joint, Left **Hip Joint, Right**	**Includes:** Acetabulofemoral joint

ICD-10-PCS Value	Definition
Hip Muscle, Left **Hip Muscle, Right**	**Includes:** Gemellus muscle Gluteus maximus muscle Gluteus medius muscle Gluteus minimus muscle Iliacus muscle Obturator muscle Piriformis muscle Psoas muscle Quadratus femoris muscle Tensor fasciae latae muscle
Humeral Head, Left **Humeral Head, Right**	**Includes:** Greater tuberosity Lesser tuberosity Neck of humerus (anatomical)(surgical)
Humeral Shaft, Left **Humeral Shaft, Right**	**Includes:** Distal humerus Humerus, distal Lateral epicondyle of humerus Medial epicondyle of humerus
Hypogastric Vein, Left **Hypogastric Vein, Right**	**Includes:** Gluteal vein Internal iliac vein Internal pudendal vein Lateral sacral vein Middle hemorrhoidal vein Obturator vein Uterine vein Vaginal vein Vesical vein
Hypoglossal Nerve	**Includes:** Twelfth cranial nerve
Hypothalamus	**Includes:** Mammillary body
Inferior Mesenteric Artery	**Includes:** Sigmoid artery Superior rectal artery
Inferior Mesenteric Vein	**Includes:** Sigmoid vein Superior rectal vein
Inferior Vena Cava	**Includes:** Postcava Right inferior phrenic vein Right ovarian vein Right second lumbar vein Right suprarenal vein Right testicular vein
Inguinal Region, Bilateral **Inguinal Region, Left** **Inguinal Region, Right**	**Includes:** Inguinal canal Inguinal triangle
Inner Ear, Left **Inner Ear, Right**	**Includes:** Bony labyrinth Bony vestibule Cochlea Round window Semicircular canal
Innominate Artery	**Includes:** Brachiocephalic artery Brachiocephalic trunk
Innominate Vein, Left **Innominate Vein, Right**	**Includes:** Brachiocephalic vein Inferior thyroid vein
Internal Carotid Artery, Left **Internal Carotid Artery, Right**	**Includes:** Caroticotympanic artery Carotid sinus

ICD-10-PCS Value	Definition
Internal Iliac Artery, Left **Internal Iliac Artery, Right**	**Includes:** Deferential artery Hypogastric artery Iliolumbar artery Inferior gluteal artery Inferior vesical artery Internal pudendal artery Lateral sacral artery Middle rectal artery Obturator artery Superior gluteal artery Umbilical artery Uterine artery Vaginal artery
Internal Mammary Artery, Left **Internal Mammary Artery, Right**	**Includes:** Anterior intercostal artery Internal thoracic artery Musculophrenic artery Pericardiophrenic artery Superior epigastric artery
Intracranial Artery	**Includes:** Anterior cerebral artery Anterior choroidal artery Anterior communicating artery Basilar artery Circle of Willis Internal carotid artery, intracranial portion Middle cerebral artery Ophthalmic artery Posterior cerebral artery Posterior communicating artery Posterior inferior cerebellar artery (PICA)
Intracranial Vein	**Includes:** Anterior cerebral vein Basal (internal) cerebral vein Dural venous sinus Great cerebral vein Inferior cerebellar vein Inferior cerebral vein Internal (basal) cerebral vein Middle cerebral vein Ophthalmic vein Superior cerebellar vein Superior cerebral vein
Jejunum	**Includes:** Duodenojejunal flexure
Kidney	**Includes:** Renal calyx Renal capsule Renal cortex Renal segment
Kidney Pelvis, Left **Kidney Pelvis, Right**	**Includes:** Ureteropelvic junction (UPJ)
Kidney, Left **Kidney, Right** **Kidneys, Bilateral**	**Includes:** Renal calyx Renal capsule Renal cortex Renal segment

ICD-10-PCS Value	Definition
Knee Bursa and Ligament, Left Knee Bursa and Ligament, Right	**Includes:** Anterior cruciate ligament (ACL) Lateral collateral ligament (LCL) Ligament of head of fibula Medial collateral ligament (MCL) Patellar ligament Popliteal ligament Posterior cruciate ligament (PCL) Prepatellar bursa
Knee Joint, Femoral Surface, Left Knee Joint, Femoral Surface, Right	**Includes:** Femoropatellar joint Patellofemoral joint
Knee Joint, Left Knee Joint, Right	**Includes:** Femoropatellar joint Femorotibial joint Lateral meniscus Medial meniscus Patellofemoral joint Tibiofemoral joint
Knee Joint, Tibial Surface, Left Knee Joint, Tibial Surface, Right	**Includes:** Femorotibial joint Tibiofemoral joint
Knee Tendon, Left Knee Tendon, Right	**Includes:** Patellar tendon
Lacrimal Duct, Left Lacrimal Duct, Right	**Includes:** Lacrimal canaliculus Lacrimal punctum Lacrimal sac Nasolacrimal duct
Larynx	**Includes:** Aryepiglottic fold Arytenoid cartilage Corniculate cartilage Cuneiform cartilage False vocal cord Glottis Rima glottidis Thyroid cartilage Ventricular fold
Lens, Left Lens, Right	**Includes:** Zonule of Zinn
Liver	**Includes:** Quadrate lobe
Lower Arm and Wrist Muscle, Left Lower Arm and Wrist Muscle, Right	**Includes:** Anatomical snuffbox Brachioradialis muscle Extensor carpi radialis muscle Extensor carpi ulnaris muscle Flexor carpi radialis muscle Flexor carpi ulnaris muscle Flexor pollicis longus muscle Palmaris longus muscle Pronator quadratus muscle Pronator teres muscle
Lower Artery	**Includes:** Umbilical artery
Lower Eyelid, Left Lower Eyelid, Right	**Includes:** Inferior tarsal plate Medial canthus
Lower Femur, Left Lower Femur, Right	**Includes:** Lateral condyle of femur Lateral epicondyle of femur Medial condyle of femur Medial epicondyle of femur

ICD-10-PCS Value	Definition
Lower Leg Muscle, Left Lower Leg Muscle, Right	**Includes:** Extensor digitorum longus muscle Extensor hallucis longus muscle Fibularis brevis muscle Fibularis longus muscle Flexor digitorum longus muscle Flexor hallucis longus muscle Gastrocnemius muscle Peroneus brevis muscle Peroneus longus muscle Popliteus muscle Soleus muscle Tibialis anterior muscle Tibialis posterior muscle
Lower Leg Tendon, Left Lower Leg Tendon, Right	**Includes:** Achilles tendon
Lower Lip	**Includes:** Frenulum labii inferioris Labial gland Vermilion border
Lower Spine Bursa and Ligament	**Includes:** Iliolumbar ligament Interspinous ligament, lumbar Intertransverse ligament, lumbar Ligamentum flavum, lumbar Sacrococcygeal ligament Sacroiliac ligament Sacrospinous ligament Sacrotuberous ligament Supraspinous ligament
Lumbar Nerve	**Includes:** Lumbosacral trunk Spinal nerve, lumbar Superior clunic (cluneal) nerve
Lumbar Plexus	**Includes:** Accessory obturator nerve Genitofemoral nerve Iliohypogastric nerve Ilioinguinal nerve Lateral femoral cutaneous nerve Obturator nerve Superior gluteal nerve
Lumbar Spinal Cord	**Includes:** Cauda equina Conus medullaris
Lumbar Sympathetic Nerve	**Includes:** Lumbar ganglion Lumbar splanchnic nerve
Lumbar Vertebra	**Includes:** Spinous process Transverse process Vertebral arch Vertebral body Vertebral foramen Vertebral lamina Vertebral pedicle
Lumbar Vertebral Joint	**Includes:** Lumbar facet joint
Lumbosacral Joint	**Includes:** Lumbosacral facet joint

ICD-10-PCS Value	Definition
Lymphatic, Aortic	**Includes:** Celiac lymph node Gastric lymph node Hepatic lymph node Lumbar lymph node Pancreaticosplenic lymph node Paraaortic lymph node Retroperitoneal lymph node
Lymphatic, Head	**Includes:** Buccinator lymph node Infraauricular lymph node Infraparotid lymph node Parotid lymph node Preauricular lymph node Submandibular lymph node Submaxillary lymph node Submental lymph node Subparotid lymph node Suprahyoid lymph node
Lymphatic, Left Axillary	**Includes:** Anterior (pectoral) lymph node Apical (subclavicular) lymph node Brachial (lateral) lymph node Central axillary lymph node Lateral (brachial) lymph node Pectoral (anterior) lymph node Posterior (subscapular) lymph node Subclavicular (apical) lymph node Subscapular (posterior) lymph node
Lymphatic, Left Lower Extremity	**Includes:** Femoral lymph node Popliteal lymph node
Lymphatic, Left Neck	**Includes:** Cervical lymph node Jugular lymph node Mastoid (postauricular) lymph node Occipital lymph node Postauricular (mastoid) lymph node Retropharyngeal lymph node Supraclavicular (Virchow's) lymph node Virchow's (supraclavicular) lymph node
Lymphatic, Left Upper Extremity	**Includes:** Cubital lymph node Deltopectoral (infraclavicular) lymph node Epitrochlear lymph node Infraclavicular (deltopectoral) lymph node Supratrochlear lymph node
Lymphatic, Mesenteric	**Includes:** Inferior mesenteric lymph node Pararectal lymph node Superior mesenteric lymph node
Lymphatic, Pelvis	**Includes:** Common iliac (subaortic) lymph node Gluteal lymph node Iliac lymph node Inferior epigastric lymph node Obturator lymph node Sacral lymph node Subaortic (common iliac) lymph node Suprainguinal lymph node

ICD-10-PCS Value	Definition
Lymphatic, Right Axillary	**Includes:** Anterior (pectoral) lymph node Apical (subclavicular) lymph node Brachial (lateral) lymph node Central axillary lymph node Lateral (brachial) lymph node Pectoral (anterior) lymph node Posterior (subscapular) lymph node Subclavicular (apical) lymph node Subscapular (posterior) lymph node
Lymphatic, Right Lower Extremity	**Includes:** Femoral lymph node Popliteal lymph node
Lymphatic, Right Neck	**Includes:** Cervical lymph node Jugular lymph node Mastoid (postauricular) lymph node Occipital lymph node Postauricular (mastoid) lymph node Retropharyngeal lymph node Right jugular trunk Right lymphatic duct Right subclavian trunk Supraclavicular (Virchow's) lymph node Virchow's (supraclavicular) lymph node
Lymphatic, Right Upper Extremity	**Includes:** Cubital lymph node Deltopectoral (infraclavicular) lymph node Epitrochlear lymph node Infraclavicular (deltopectoral) lymph node Supratrochlear lymph node
Lymphatic, Thorax	**Includes:** Intercostal lymph node Mediastinal lymph node Parasternal lymph node Paratracheal lymph node Tracheobronchial lymph node
Main Bronchus, Right	**Includes:** Bronchus intermedius Intermediate bronchus
Mandible, Left **Mandible, Right**	**Includes:** Alveolar process of mandible Condyloid process Mandibular notch Mental foramen
Mastoid Sinus, Left **Mastoid Sinus, Right**	**Includes:** Mastoid air cells
Maxilla	**Includes:** Alveolar process of maxilla
Maxillary Sinus, Left **Maxillary Sinus, Right**	**Includes:** Antrum of Highmore
Median Nerve	**Includes:** Anterior interosseous nerve Palmar cutaneous nerve
Mediastinum	**Includes:** Mediastinal cavity Mediastinal space
Medulla Oblongata	**Includes:** Myelencephalon
Mesentery	**Includes:** Mesoappendix Mesocolon

ICD-10-PCS Value	Definition
Metatarsal-Phalangeal Joint, Left **Metatarsal-Phalangeal Joint, Right**	**Includes:** Metatarsophalangeal (MTP) joint
Middle Ear, Left **Middle Ear, Right**	**Includes:** Oval window Tympanic cavity
Minor Salivary Gland	**Includes:** Anterior lingual gland
Mitral Valve	**Includes:** Bicuspid valve Left atrioventricular valve Mitral annulus
Nasal Bone	**Includes:** Vomer of nasal septum
Nasal Mucosa and Soft Tissue	**Includes:** Columella External naris Greater alar cartilage Internal naris Lateral nasal cartilage Lesser alar cartilage Nasal cavity Nostril
Nasal Septum	**Includes:** Quadrangular cartilage Septal cartilage Vomer bone
Nasal Turbinate	**Includes:** Inferior turbinate Middle turbinate Nasal concha Superior turbinate
Nasopharynx	**Includes:** Choana Fossa of Rosenmuller Pharyngeal recess Rhinopharynx
Neck Muscle, Left **Neck Muscle, Right**	**Includes:** Anterior vertebral muscle Arytenoid muscle Cricothyroid muscle Infrahyoid muscle Levator scapulae muscle Platysma muscle Scalene muscle Splenius cervicis muscle Sternocleidomastoid muscle Suprahyoid muscle Thyroarytenoid muscle
Nipple, Left **Nipple, Right**	**Includes:** Areola
Occipital Bone	**Includes:** Foramen magnum
Oculomotor Nerve	**Includes:** Third cranial nerve
Olfactory Nerve	**Includes:** First cranial nerve Olfactory bulb

ICD-10-PCS Value	Definition
Omentum	**Includes:** Gastrocolic ligament Gastrocolic omentum Gastrohepatic omentum Gastrophrenic ligament Gastrosplenic ligament Greater Omentum Hepatogastric ligament Lesser Omentum
Optic Nerve	**Includes:** Optic chiasma Second cranial nerve
Orbit, Left **Orbit, Right**	**Includes:** Bony orbit Orbital portion of ethmoid bone Orbital portion of frontal bone Orbital portion of lacrimal bone Orbital portion of maxilla Orbital portion of palatine bone Orbital portion of sphenoid bone Orbital portion of zygomatic bone
Pancreatic Duct	**Includes:** Duct of Wirsung
Pancreatic Duct, Accessory	**Includes:** Duct of Santorini
Parotid Duct, Left **Parotid Duct, Right**	**Includes:** Stensen's duct
Pelvic Bone, Left **Pelvic Bone, Right**	**Includes:** Iliac crest Ilium Ischium Pubis
Pelvic Cavity	**Includes:** Retropubic space
Penis	**Includes:** Corpus cavernosum Corpus spongiosum
Perineum Muscle	**Includes:** Bulbospongiosus muscle Cremaster muscle Deep transverse perineal muscle Ischiocavernosus muscle Levator ani muscle Superficial transverse perineal muscle
Peritoneum	**Includes:** Epiploic foramen
Peroneal Artery, Left **Peroneal Artery, Right**	**Includes:** Fibular artery
Peroneal Nerve	**Includes:** Common fibular nerve Common peroneal nerve External popliteal nerve Lateral sural cutaneous nerve
Pharynx	**Includes:** Base of Tongue Hypopharynx Laryngopharynx Lingual tonsil Oropharynx Piriform recess (sinus) Tongue, base of
Phrenic Nerve	**Includes:** Accessory phrenic nerve

ICD-10-PCS Value	Definition
Pituitary Gland	**Includes:** Adenohypophysis Hypophysis Neurohypophysis
Pons	**Includes:** Apneustic center Basis pontis Locus ceruleus Pneumotaxic center Pontine tegmentum Superior olivary nucleus
Popliteal Artery, Left **Popliteal Artery, Right**	**Includes:** Inferior genicular artery Middle genicular artery Superior genicular artery Sural artery
Portal Vein	**Includes:** Hepatic portal vein
Prepuce	**Includes:** Foreskin Glans penis
Pudendal Nerve	**Includes:** Posterior labial nerve Posterior scrotal nerve
Pulmonary Artery, Left	**Includes:** Arterial canal (duct) Botallo's duct Pulmoaortic canal
Pulmonary Valve	**Includes:** Pulmonary annulus Pulmonic valve
Pulmonary Vein, Left	**Includes:** Left inferior pulmonary vein Left superior pulmonary vein
Pulmonary Vein, Right	**Includes:** Right inferior pulmonary vein Right superior pulmonary vein
Radial Artery, Left **Radial Artery, Right**	**Includes:** Radial recurrent artery
Radial Nerve	**Includes:** Dorsal digital nerve Musculospiral nerve Palmar cutaneous nerve Posterior interosseous nerve
Radius, Left **Radius, Right**	**Includes:** Ulnar notch
Rectum	**Includes:** Anorectal junction
Renal Artery, Left **Renal Artery, Right**	**Includes:** Inferior suprarenal artery Renal segmental artery
Renal Vein, Left	**Includes:** Left inferior phrenic vein Left ovarian vein Left second lumbar vein Left suprarenal vein Left testicular vein
Retina, Left **Retina, Right**	**Includes:** Fovea Macula Optic disc
Retroperitoneum	**Includes:** Retroperitoneal cavity Retroperitoneal space

ICD-10-PCS Value	Definition
Rib(s) Bursa and Ligament	**Includes:** Costotransverse ligament
Sacral Nerve	**Includes:** Spinal nerve, sacral
Sacral Plexus	**Includes:** Inferior gluteal nerve Posterior femoral cutaneous nerve Pudendal nerve
Sacral Sympathetic Nerve	**Includes:** Ganglion impar (ganglion of Walther) Pelvic splanchnic nerve Sacral ganglion Sacral splanchnic nerve
Sacrococcygeal Joint	**Includes:** Sacrococcygeal symphysis
Saphenous Vein, Left **Saphenous Vein, Right**	**Includes:** External pudendal vein Great(er) saphenous vein Lesser saphenous vein Small saphenous vein Superficial circumflex iliac vein Superficial epigastric vein
Scapula, Left **Scapula, Right**	**Includes:** Acromion (process) Coracoid process
Sciatic Nerve	**Includes:** Ischiatic nerve
Shoulder Bursa and Ligament, Left **Shoulder Bursa and Ligament, Right**	**Includes:** Acromioclavicular ligament Coracoacromial ligament Coracoclavicular ligament Coracohumeral ligament Costoclavicular ligament Glenohumeral ligament Interclavicular ligament Sternoclavicular ligament Subacromial bursa Transverse humeral ligament Transverse scapular ligament
Shoulder Joint, Left **Shoulder Joint, Right**	**Includes:** Glenohumeral joint Glenoid ligament (labrum)
Shoulder Muscle, Left **Shoulder Muscle, Right**	**Includes:** Deltoid muscle Infraspinatus muscle Subscapularis muscle Supraspinatus muscle Teres major muscle Teres minor muscle
Sigmoid Colon	**Includes:** Rectosigmoid junction Sigmoid flexure
Skin	**Includes:** Dermis Epidermis Sebaceous gland Sweat gland
Sphenoid Bone	**Includes:** Greater wing Lesser wing Optic foramen Pterygoid process Sella turcica

Appendix E: Body Part Definitions

ICD-10-PCS Value	Definition
Spinal Canal	**Includes:** Epidural space, spinal Extradural space, spinal Subarachnoid space, spinal Subdural space, spinal Vertebral canal
Spinal Meninges	**Includes:** Arachnoid mater, spinal Denticulate (dentate) ligament Dura mater, spinal Filum terminale Leptomeninges, spinal Pia mater, spinal
Spleen	**Includes:** Accessory spleen
Splenic Artery	**Includes:** Left gastroepiploic artery Pancreatic artery Short gastric artery
Splenic Vein	**Includes:** Left gastroepiploic vein Pancreatic vein
Sternum	**Includes:** Manubrium Suprasternal notch Xiphoid process
Sternum Bursa and Ligament	**Includes:** Costoxiphoid ligament Sternocostal ligament
Stomach, Pylorus	**Includes:** Pyloric antrum Pyloric canal Pyloric sphincter
Subclavian Artery, Left **Subclavian Artery, Right**	**Includes:** Costocervical trunk Dorsal scapular artery Internal thoracic artery
Subcutaneous Tissue and Fascia, Chest	**Includes:** Pectoral fascia
Subcutaneous Tissue and Fascia, Face	**Includes:** Masseteric fascia Orbital fascia
Subcutaneous Tissue and Fascia, Left Foot	**Includes:** Plantar fascia (aponeurosis)
Subcutaneous Tissue and Fascia, Left Hand	**Includes:** Palmar fascia (aponeurosis)
Subcutaneous Tissue and Fascia, Left Lower Arm	**Includes:** Antebrachial fascia Bicipital aponeurosis
Subcutaneous Tissue and Fascia, Left Neck	**Includes:** Deep cervical fascia Pretracheal fascia Prevertebral fascia
Subcutaneous Tissue and Fascia, Left Upper Arm	**Includes:** Axillary fascia Deltoid fascia Infraspinatus fascia Subscapular aponeurosis Supraspinatus fascia
Subcutaneous Tissue and Fascia, Left Upper Leg	**Includes:** Crural fascia Fascia lata Iliac fascia Iliotibial tract (band)
Subcutaneous Tissue and Fascia, Right Foot	**Includes:** Plantar fascia (aponeurosis)
Subcutaneous Tissue and Fascia, Right Hand	**Includes:** Palmar fascia (aponeurosis)
Subcutaneous Tissue and Fascia, Right Lower Arm	**Includes:** Antebrachial fascia Bicipital aponeurosis
Subcutaneous Tissue and Fascia, Right Neck	**Includes:** Deep cervical fascia Pretracheal fascia Prevertebral fascia
Subcutaneous Tissue and Fascia, Right Upper Arm	**Includes:** Axillary fascia Deltoid fascia Infraspinatus fascia Subscapular aponeurosis Supraspinatus fascia
Subcutaneous Tissue and Fascia, Right Upper Leg	**Includes:** Crural fascia Fascia lata Iliac fascia Iliotibial tract (band)
Subcutaneous Tissue and Fascia, Scalp	**Includes:** Galea aponeurotica
Subcutaneous Tissue and Fascia, Trunk	**Includes:** External oblique aponeurosis Transversalis fascia
Submaxillary Gland, Left **Submaxillary Gland, Right**	**Includes:** Submandibular gland
Superior Mesenteric Artery	**Includes:** Ileal artery Ileocolic artery Inferior pancreaticoduodenal artery Jejunal artery
Superior Mesenteric Vein	**Includes:** Right gastroepiploic vein
Superior Vena Cava	**Includes:** Precava
Tarsal Joint, Left **Tarsal Joint, Right**	**Includes:** Calcaneocuboid joint Cuboideonavicular joint Cuneonavicular joint Intercuneiform joint Subtalar (talocalcaneal) joint Talocalcaneal (subtalar) joint Talocalcaneonavicular joint
Tarsal, Left **Tarsal, Right**	**Includes:** Calcaneus Cuboid bone Intermediate cuneiform bone Lateral cuneiform bone Medial cuneiform bone Navicular bone Talus bone
Temporal Artery, Left **Temporal Artery, Right**	**Includes:** Middle temporal artery Superficial temporal artery Transverse facial artery
Temporal Bone, Left **Temporal Bone, Right**	**Includes:** Mastoid process Petrous part of temporal bone Tympanic part of temporal bone Zygomatic process of temporal bone

ICD-10-PCS Value	Definition
Thalamus	**Includes:** Epithalamus Geniculate nucleus Metathalamus Pulvinar
Thoracic Aorta, Ascending/Arch	**Includes:** Aortic arch Ascending aorta
Thoracic Duct	**Includes:** Left jugular trunk Left subclavian trunk
Thoracic Nerve	**Includes:** Intercostal nerve Intercostobrachial nerve Spinal nerve, thoracic Subcostal nerve
Thoracic Sympathetic Nerve	**Includes:** Cardiac plexus Esophageal plexus Greater splanchnic nerve Inferior cardiac nerve Least splanchnic nerve Lesser splanchnic nerve Middle cardiac nerve Pulmonary plexus Superior cardiac nerve Thoracic aortic plexus Thoracic ganglion
Thoracic Vertebra	**Includes:** Spinous process Transverse process Vertebral arch Vertebral body Vertebral foramen Vertebral lamina Vertebral pedicle
Thoracic Vertebral Joint	**Includes:** Costotransverse joint Costovertebral joint Thoracic facet joint
Thoracolumbar Vertebral Joint	**Includes:** Thoracolumbar facet joint
Thorax Muscle, Left **Thorax Muscle, Right**	**Includes:** Intercostal muscle Levatores costarum muscle Pectoralis major muscle Pectoralis minor muscle Serratus anterior muscle Subclavius muscle Subcostal muscle Transverse thoracis muscle
Thymus	**Includes:** Thymus gland
Thyroid Artery, Left **Thyroid Artery, Right**	**Includes:** Cricothyroid artery Hyoid artery Sternocleidomastoid artery Superior laryngeal artery Superior thyroid artery Thyrocervical trunk
Tibia, Left **Tibia, Right**	**Includes:** Lateral condyle of tibia Medial condyle of tibia Medial malleolus

ICD-10-PCS Value	Definition
Tibial Nerve	**Includes:** Lateral plantar nerve Medial plantar nerve Medial popliteal nerve Medial sural cutaneous nerve
Toe Nail	**Includes:** Nail bed Nail plate
Toe Phalangeal Joint, Left **Toe Phalangeal Joint, Right**	**Includes:** Interphalangeal (IP) joint
Tongue	**Includes:** Frenulum linguae
Tongue, Palate, Pharynx Muscle	**Includes:** Chondroglossus muscle Genioglossus muscle Hyoglossus muscle Inferior longitudinal muscle Levator veli palatini muscle Palatoglossal muscle Palatopharyngeal muscle Pharyngeal constrictor muscle Salpingopharyngeus muscle Styloglossus muscle Stylopharyngeus muscle Superior longitudinal muscle Tensor veli palatini muscle
Tonsils	**Includes:** Palatine tonsil
Trachea	**Includes:** Cricoid cartilage
Transverse Colon	**Includes:** Hepatic flexure Splenic flexure
Tricuspid Valve	**Includes:** Right atrioventricular valve Tricuspid annulus
Trigeminal Nerve	**Includes:** Fifth cranial nerve Gasserian ganglion Mandibular nerve Maxillary nerve Ophthalmic nerve Trifacial nerve
Trochlear Nerve	**Includes:** Fourth cranial nerve
Trunk Muscle, Left **Trunk Muscle, Right**	**Includes:** Coccygeus muscle Erector spinae muscle Interspinalis muscle Intertransversarius muscle Latissimus dorsi muscle Quadratus lumborum muscle Rhomboid major muscle Rhomboid minor muscle Serratus posterior muscle Transversospinalis muscle Trapezius muscle
Tympanic Membrane, Left **Tympanic Membrane, Right**	**Includes:** Pars flaccida
Ulna, Left **Ulna, Right**	**Includes:** Olecranon process Radial notch

ICD-10-PCS Value	Definition
Ulnar Artery, Left **Ulnar Artery, Right**	**Includes:** Anterior ulnar recurrent artery Common interosseous artery Posterior ulnar recurrent artery
Ulnar Nerve	**Includes:** Cubital nerve
Upper Arm Muscle, Left **Upper Arm Muscle, Right**	**Includes:** Biceps brachii muscle Brachialis muscle Coracobrachialis muscle Triceps brachii muscle
Upper Artery	**Includes:** Aortic intercostal artery Bronchial artery Esophageal artery Subcostal artery
Upper Eyelid, Left **Upper Eyelid, Right**	**Includes:** Lateral canthus Levator palpebrae superioris muscle Orbicularis oculi muscle Superior tarsal plate
Upper Femur, Left **Upper Femur, Right**	**Includes:** Femoral head Greater trochanter Lesser trochanter Neck of femur
Upper Leg Muscle, Left **Upper Leg Muscle, Right**	**Includes:** Adductor brevis muscle Adductor longus muscle Adductor magnus muscle Biceps femoris muscle Gracilis muscle Pectineus muscle Quadriceps (femoris) Rectus femoris muscle Sartorius muscle Semimembranosus muscle Semitendinosus muscle Vastus intermedius muscle Vastus lateralis muscle Vastus medialis muscle
Upper Lip	**Includes:** Frenulum labii superioris Labial gland Vermilion border
Upper Spine Bursa and Ligament	**Includes:** Interspinous ligament, thoracic Intertransverse ligament, thoracic Ligamentum flavum, thoracic Supraspinous ligament
Ureter **Ureter, Left** **Ureter, Right** **Ureters, Bilateral**	**Includes:** Ureteral orifice Ureterovesical orifice
Urethra	**Includes:** Bulbourethral (Cowper's) gland Cowper's (bulbourethral) gland External urethral sphincter Internal urethral sphincter Membranous urethra Penile urethra Prostatic urethra
Uterine Supporting Structure	**Includes:** Broad ligament Infundibulopelvic ligament Ovarian ligament Round ligament of uterus
Uterus	**Includes:** Fundus uteri Myometrium Perimetrium Uterine cornu
Uvula	**Includes:** Palatine uvula
Vagus Nerve	**Includes:** Anterior vagal trunk Pharyngeal plexus Pneumogastric nerve Posterior vagal trunk Pulmonary plexus Recurrent laryngeal nerve Superior laryngeal nerve Tenth cranial nerve
Vas Deferens **Vas Deferens, Bilateral** **Vas Deferens, Left** **Vas Deferens, Right**	**Includes:** Ductus deferens Ejaculatory duct
Ventricle, Right	**Includes:** Conus arteriosus
Ventricular Septum	**Includes:** Interventricular septum
Vertebral Artery, Left **Vertebral Artery, Right**	**Includes:** Anterior spinal artery Posterior spinal artery
Vertebral Vein, Left **Vertebral Vein, Right**	**Includes:** Deep cervical vein Suboccipital venous plexus
Vestibular Gland	**Includes:** Bartholin's (greater vestibular) gland Greater vestibular (Bartholin's) gland Paraurethral (Skene's) gland Skene's (paraurethral) gland
Vitreous, Left **Vitreous, Right**	**Includes:** Vitreous body
Vocal Cord, Left **Vocal Cord, Right**	**Includes:** Vocal fold
Vulva	**Includes:** Labia majora Labia minora
Wrist Bursa and Ligament, Left **Wrist Bursa and Ligament, Right**	**Includes:** Palmar ulnocarpal ligament Radial collateral carpal ligament Radiocarpal ligament Radioulnar ligament Ulnar collateral carpal ligament
Wrist Joint, Left **Wrist Joint, Right**	**Includes:** Distal radioulnar joint Radiocarpal joint

Appendix F: Device Key and Aggregation Table

Device Key

Term	ICD-10-PCS Value
3f (Aortic) Bioprosthesis valve	Zooplastic Tissue in Heart and Great Vessels
AbioCor® Total Replacement Heart	Synthetic Substitute
Absolute Pro Vascular (OTW) Self-Expanding Stent System	Intraluminal Device
Acculink (RX) Carotid Stent System	Intraluminal Device
Acellular Hydrated Dermis	Nonautologous Tissue Substitute
Acetabular cup	Liner in Lower Joints
Activa PC neurostimulator	Stimulator Generator, Multiple Array for Insertion in Subcutaneous Tissue and Fascia
Activa RC neurostimulator	Stimulator Generator, Multiple Array Rechargeable for Insertion in Subcutaneous Tissue and Fascia
Activa SC neurostimulator	Stimulator Generator, Single Array for Insertion in Subcutaneous Tissue and Fascia
ACUITY™ Steerable Lead	Cardiac Lead, Pacemaker for Insertion in Heart and Great Vessels Cardiac Lead, Defibrillator for Insertion in Heart and Great Vessels
Advisa (MRI)	Pacemaker, Dual Chamber for Insertion in Subcutaneous Tissue and Fascia
AFX® Endovascular AAA System	Intraluminal Device
AMPLATZER® Muscular VSD Occluder	Synthetic Substitute
AMS 800® Urinary Control System	Artificial Sphincter in Urinary System
AneuRx® AAA Advantage®	Intraluminal Device
Annuloplasty ring	Synthetic Substitute
Articulating Spacer (Antibiotic)	Articulating Spacer in Lower Joints
Artificial anal sphincter (AAS)	Artificial Sphincter in Gastrointestinal System
Artificial bowel sphincter (neosphincter)	Artificial Sphincter in Gastrointestinal System
Artificial urinary sphincter (AUS)	Artificial Sphincter in Urinary System
Ascenda Intrathecal Catheter	Infusion Device
Assurant (Cobalt) stent	Intraluminal Device
AtriClip LAA Exclusion System	Extraluminal Device
Attain Ability® Lead	Cardiac Lead, Pacemaker for Insertion in Heart and Great Vessels Cardiac Lead, Defibrillator for Insertion in Heart and Great Vessels
Attain StarFix® (OTW) Lead	Cardiac Lead, Pacemaker for Insertion in Heart and Great Vessels Cardiac Lead, Defibrillator for Insertion in Heart and Great Vessels
Autograft	Autologous Tissue Substitute
Autologous artery graft	Autologous Arterial Tissue in Heart and Great Vessels Autologous Arterial Tissue in Upper Arteries Autologous Arterial Tissue in Lower Arteries Autologous Arterial Tissue in Upper Veins Autologous Arterial Tissue in Lower Veins
Autologous vein graft	Autologous Venous Tissue in Heart and Great Vessels Autologous Venous Tissue in Upper Arteries Autologous Venous Tissue in Lower Arteries Autologous Venous Tissue in Upper Veins Autologous Venous Tissue in Lower Veins
Axial Lumbar Interbody Fusion System	Interbody Fusion Device in Lower Joints
AxiaLIF® System	Interbody Fusion Device in Lower Joints
BAK/C® Interbody Cervical Fusion System	Interbody Fusion Device in Upper Joints
Bard® Composix® (E/X)(LP) mesh	Synthetic Substitute
Bard® Composix® Kugel® patch	Synthetic Substitute
Bard® Dulex™ mesh	Synthetic Substitute
Bard® Ventralex™ hernia patch	Synthetic Substitute
Baroreflex Activation Therapy® (BAT®)	Stimulator Lead in Upper Arteries Stimulator Generator in Subcutaneous Tissue and Fascia
Berlin Heart Ventricular Assist Device	Implantable Heart Assist System in Heart and Great Vessels
Bioactive embolization coil(s)	Intraluminal Device, Bioactive in Upper Arteries
Biventricular external heart assist system	Short-term External Heart Assist System in Heart and Great Vessels
Blood glucose monitoring system	Monitoring Device
Bone anchored hearing device	Hearing Device, Bone Conduction for Insertion in Ear, Nose, Sinus Hearing Device, in Head and Facial Bones
Bone bank bone graft	Nonautologous Tissue Substitute
Bone screw (interlocking)(lag)(pedicle)(recessed)	Internal Fixation Device in Head and Facial Bones Internal Fixation Device in Upper Bones Internal Fixation Device in Lower Bones
Bovine pericardial valve	Zooplastic Tissue in Heart and Great Vessels
Bovine pericardium graft	Zooplastic Tissue in Heart and Great Vessels
Brachytherapy seeds	Radioactive Element
BRYAN® Cervical Disc System	Synthetic Substitute
BVS 5000 Ventricular Assist Device	Short-term External Heart Assist System in Heart and Great Vessels
Cardiac contractility modulation lead	Cardiac Lead in Heart and Great Vessels

Term	ICD-10-PCS Value
Cardiac event recorder	Monitoring Device
Cardiac resynchronization therapy (CRT) lead	Cardiac Lead, Pacemaker for Insertion in Heart and Great Vessels Cardiac Lead, Defibrillator for Insertion in Heart and Great Vessels
CardioMEMS® pressure sensor	Monitoring Device, Pressure Sensor for Insertion in Heart and Great Vessels
Carotid (artery) sinus (baroreceptor) lead	Stimulator Lead in Upper Arteries
Carotid WALLSTENT® Monorail® Endoprosthesis	Intraluminal Device
Centrimag® Blood Pump	Short-term External Heart Assist System in Heart and Great Vessels
Ceramic on ceramic bearing surface	Synthetic Substitute, Ceramic for Replacement in Lower Joints
Cesium-131 Collagen Implant	Radioactive Element, Cesium-131 Collagen Implant for Insertion in Central Nervous System and Cranial Nerves
Clamp and rod internal fixation system (CRIF)	Internal Fixation Device in Upper Bones Internal Fixation Device in Lower Bones
COALESCE® radiolucent interbody fusion device	Interbody Fusion Device, Radiolucent Porous in New Technology
CoAxia NeuroFlo catheter	Intraluminal Device
Cobalt/chromium head and polyethylene socket	Synthetic Substitute, Metal on Polyethylene for Replacement in Lower Joints
Cobalt/chromium head and socket	Synthetic Substitute, Metal for Replacement in Lower Joints
Cochlear implant (CI), multiple channel (electrode)	Hearing Device, Multiple Channel Cochlear Prosthesis for Insertion in Ear, Nose, Sinus
Cochlear implant (CI), single channel (electrode)	Hearing Device, Single Channel Cochlear Prosthesis for Insertion in Ear, Nose, Sinus
COGNIS® CRT-D	Cardiac Resynchronization Defibrillator Pulse Generator for Insertion in Subcutaneous Tissue and Fascia
COHERE® radiolucent interbody fusion device	Interbody Fusion Device, Radiolucent Porous in New Technology
Colonic Z-Stent®	Intraluminal Device
Complete (SE) stent	Intraluminal Device
Concerto II CRT-D	Cardiac Resynchronization Defibrillator Pulse Generator for Insertion in Subcutaneous Tissue and Fascia
CONSERVE® PLUS Total Resurfacing Hip System	Resurfacing Device in Lower Joints
Consulta CRT-D	Cardiac Resynchronization Defibrillator Pulse Generator for Insertion in Subcutaneous Tissue and Fascia
Consulta CRT-P	Cardiac Resynchronization Pacemaker Pulse Generator for Insertion in Subcutaneous Tissue and Fascia
CONTAK RENEWAL® 3 RF (HE) CRT-D	Cardiac Resynchronization Defibrillator Pulse Generator for Insertion in Subcutaneous Tissue and Fascia
Contegra Pulmonary Valved Conduit	Zooplastic Tissue in Heart and Great Vessels
Continuous Glucose Monitoring (CGM) device	Monitoring Device
Cook Biodesign® Fistula Plug(s)	Nonautologous Tissue Substitute

Term	ICD-10-PCS Value
Cook Biodesign® Hernia Graft(s)	Nonautologous Tissue Substitute
Cook Biodesign® Layered Graft(s)	Nonautologous Tissue Substitute
Cook Zenapro™ Layered Graft(s)	Nonautologous Tissue Substitute
Cook Zenith AAA Endovascular Graft	Intraluminal Device Intraluminal Device, Branched or Fenestrated, One or Two Arteries for Restriction in Lower Arteries Intraluminal Device, Branched or Fenestrated, Three or More Arteries for Restriction in Lower Arteries
CoreValve transcatheter aortic valve	Zooplastic Tissue in Heart and Great Vessels
Cormet Hip Resurfacing System	Resurfacing Device in Lower Joints
CoRoent® XL	Interbody Fusion Device in Lower Joints
Corox (OTW) Bipolar Lead	Cardiac Lead, Pacemaker for Insertion in Heart and Great Vessels Cardiac Lead, Defibrillator for Insertion in Heart and Great Vessels
Cortical strip neurostimulator lead	Neurostimulator Lead in Central Nervous System and Cranial Nerves
Cultured epidermal cell autograft	Autologous Tissue Substitute
CYPHER® Stent	Intraluminal Device, Drug-eluting in Heart and Great Vessels
Cystostomy tube	Drainage Device
DBS lead	Neurostimulator Lead in Central Nervous System and Cranial Nerves
DeBakey Left Ventricular Assist Device	Implantable Heart Assist System in Heart and Great Vessels
Deep brain neurostimulator lead	Neurostimulator Lead in Central Nervous System and Cranial Nerves
Delta frame external fixator	External Fixation Device, Hybrid for Insertion in Upper Bones External Fixation Device, Hybrid for Reposition in Upper Bones External Fixation Device, Hybrid for Insertion in Lower Bones External Fixation Device, Hybrid for Reposition in Lower Bones
Delta III Reverse shoulder prosthesis	Synthetic Substitute, Reverse Ball and Socket for Replacement in Upper Joints
Diaphragmatic pacemaker generator	Stimulator Generator in Subcutaneous Tissue and Fascia
Direct Lateral Interbody Fusion (DLIF) device	Interbody Fusion Device in Lower Joints
Driver stent (RX) (OTW)	Intraluminal Device
DuraHeart Left Ventricular Assist System	Implantable Heart Assist System in Heart and Great Vessels
Durata® Defibrillation Lead	Cardiac Lead, Defibrillator for Insertion in Heart and Great Vessels
Dynesys® Dynamic Stabilization System	Spinal Stabilization Device, Pedicle-Based for Insertion in Upper Joints Spinal Stabilization Device, Pedicle-Based for Insertion in Lower Joints
E-Luminexx™ (Biliary)(Vascular) Stent	Intraluminal Device
EDWARDS INTUITY Elite valve system	Zooplastic Tissue, Rapid Deployment Technique in New Technology

Term	ICD-10-PCS Value
Electrical bone growth stimulator (EBGS)	Bone Growth Stimulator in Head and Facial Bones Bone Growth Stimulator in Upper Bones Bone Growth Stimulator in Lower Bones
Electrical muscle stimulation (EMS) lead	Stimulator Lead in Muscles
Electronic muscle stimulator lead	Stimulator Lead in Muscles
Embolization coil(s)	Intraluminal Device
Endeavor® (III)(IV) (Sprint) Zotarolimus-eluting Coronary Stent System	Intraluminal Device, Drug-eluting in Heart and Great Vessels
Endologix AFX® Endovascular AAA System	Intraluminal Device
EndoSure® sensor	Monitoring Device, Pressure Sensor for Insertion in Heart and Great Vessels
ENDOTAK RELIANCE® (G) Defibrillation Lead	Cardiac Lead, Defibrillator for Insertion in Heart and Great Vessels
Endotracheal tube (cuffed)(double-lumen)	Intraluminal Device, Endotracheal Airway in Respiratory System
Endurant® Endovascular Stent Graft	Intraluminal Device
Endurant® II AAA stent graft system	Intraluminal Device
EnRhythm	Pacemaker, Dual Chamber for Insertion in Subcutaneous Tissue and Fascia
Enterra gastric neurostimulator	Stimulator Generator, Multiple Array for Insertion in Subcutaneous Tissue and Fascia
Epic™ Stented Tissue Valve (aortic)	Zooplastic Tissue in Heart and Great Vessels
Epicel® cultured epidermal autograft	Autologous Tissue Substitute
Esophageal obturator airway (EOA)	Intraluminal Device, Airway in Gastrointestinal System
Esteem® implantable hearing system	Hearing Device in Ear, Nose, Sinus
Evera (XT)(S)(DR/VR)	Defibrillator Generator for Insertion in Subcutaneous Tissue and Fascia
Everolimus-eluting coronary stent	Intraluminal Device, Drug-eluting in Heart and Great Vessels
Ex-PRESS™ mini glaucoma shunt	Synthetic Substitute
EXCLUDER® AAA Endoprosthesis	Intraluminal Device Intraluminal Device, Branched or Fenestrated, One or Two Arteries for Restriction in Lower Arteries Intraluminal Device, Branched or Fenestrated, Three or More Arteries for Restriction in Lower Arteries
EXCLUDER® IBE Endoprosthesis	Intraluminal Device, Branched or Fenestrated, One or Two Arteries for Restriction in Lower Arteries
Express® (LD) Premounted Stent System	Intraluminal Device
Express® Biliary SD Monorail® Premounted Stent System	Intraluminal Device
Express® SD Renal Monorail® Premounted Stent System	Intraluminal Device

Term	ICD-10-PCS Value
External fixator	External Fixation Device in Head and Facial Bones External Fixation Device in Upper Bones External Fixation Device in Lower Bones External Fixation Device in Upper Joints External Fixation Device in Lower Joints
EXtreme Lateral Interbody Fusion (XLIF) device	Interbody Fusion Device in Lower Joints
Facet replacement spinal stabilization device	Spinal Stabilization Device, Facet Replacement for Insertion in Upper Joints Spinal Stabilization Device, Facet Replacement for Insertion in Lower Joints
FLAIR® Endovascular Stent Graft	Intraluminal Device
Flexible Composite Mesh	Synthetic Substitute
Foley catheter	Drainage Device
Formula™ Balloon-Expandable Renal Stent System	Intraluminal Device
Freestyle (Stentless) Aortic Root Bioprosthesis	Zooplastic Tissue in Heart and Great Vessels
Fusion screw (compression)(lag)(locking)	Internal Fixation Device in Upper Joints Internal Fixation Device in Lower Joints
GammaTile™	Radioactive Element, Cesium-131 Collagen Implant for Insertion in Central Nervous System and Cranial Nerves
Gastric electrical stimulation (GES) lead	Stimulator Lead in Gastrointestinal System
Gastric pacemaker lead	Stimulator Lead in Gastrointestinal System
GORE EXCLUDER® AAA Endoprosthesis	Intraluminal Device Intraluminal Device, Branched or Fenestrated, One or Two Arteries for Restriction in Lower Arteries Intraluminal Device, Branched or Fenestrated, Three or More Arteries for Restriction in Lower Arteries
GORE EXCLUDER® IBE Endoprosthesis	Intraluminal Device, Branched or Fenestrated, One or Two Arteries for Restriction in Lower Arteries
GORE TAG® Thoracic Endoprosthesis	Intraluminal Device
GORE® DUALMESH®	Synthetic Substitute
Guedel airway	Intraluminal Device, Airway in Mouth and Throat
Hancock Bioprosthesis (aortic)(mitral) valve	Zooplastic Tissue in Heart and Great Vessels
Hancock Bioprosthetic Valved Conduit	Zooplastic Tissue in Heart and Great Vessels
HeartMate 3™ LVAS	Implantable Heart Assist System in Heart and Great Vessels
HeartMate II® Left Ventricular Assist Device (LVAD)	Implantable Heart Assist System in Heart and Great Vessels
HeartMate XVE® Left Ventricular Assist Device (LVAD)	Implantable Heart Assist System in Heart and Great Vessels
Herculink (RX) Elite Renal Stent System	Intraluminal Device

Term	ICD-10-PCS Value
Hip (joint) liner	Liner in Lower Joints
Holter valve ventricular shunt	Synthetic Substitute
Ilizarov external fixator	External Fixation Device, Ring for Insertion in Upper Bones External Fixation Device, Ring for Reposition in Upper Bones External Fixation Device, Ring for Insertion in Lower Bones External Fixation Device, Ring for Reposition in Lower Bones
Ilizarov-Vecklich device	External Fixation Device, Limb Lengthening for Insertion in Upper Bones External Fixation Device, Limb Lengthening for Insertion in Lower Bones
Impella® heart pump	Short-term External Heart Assist System in Heart and Great Vessels
Implantable cardioverter-defibrillator (ICD)	Defibrillator Generator for Insertion in Subcutaneous Tissue and Fascia
Implantable drug infusion pump (anti-spasmodic) (chemotherapy)(pain)	Infusion Device, Pump in Subcutaneous Tissue and Fascia
Implantable glucose monitoring device	Monitoring Device
Implantable hemodynamic monitor (IHM)	Monitoring Device, Hemodynamic for Insertion in Subcutaneous Tissue and Fascia
Implantable hemodynamic monitoring system (IHMS)	Monitoring Device, Hemodynamic for Insertion in Subcutaneous Tissue and Fascia
Implantable Miniature Telescope™ (IMT)	Synthetic Substitute, Intraocular Telescope for Replacement in Eye
Implanted (venous)(access) port	Vascular Access Device, Totally Implantable in Subcutaneous Tissue and Fascia
InDura, intrathecal catheter (1P) (spinal)	Infusion Device
Injection reservoir, port	Vascular Access Device, Totally Implantable in Subcutaneous Tissue and Fascia
Injection reservoir, pump	Infusion Device, Pump in Subcutaneous Tissue and Fascia
Interbody fusion (spine) cage	Interbody Fusion Device in Upper Joints Interbody Fusion Device in Lower Joints
Interspinous process spinal stabilization device	Spinal Stabilization Device, Interspinous Process for Insertion in Upper Joints Spinal Stabilization Device, Interspinous Process for Insertion in Lower Joints
InterStim® Therapy lead	Neurostimulator Lead in Peripheral Nervous System
InterStim® Therapy neurostimulator	Stimulator Generator, Single Array for Insertion in Subcutaneous Tissue and Fascia
Intramedullary (IM) rod (nail)	Internal Fixation Device, Intramedullary in Upper Bones Internal Fixation Device, Intramedullary in Lower Bones
Intramedullary skeletal kinetic distractor (ISKD)	Internal Fixation Device, Intramedullary in Upper Bones Internal Fixation Device, Intramedullary in Lower Bones
Intrauterine Device (IUD)	Contraceptive Device in Female Reproductive System
INTUITY Elite valve system, EDWARDS	Zooplastic Tissue, Rapid Deployment Technique in New Technology
Itrel (3)(4) neurostimulator	Stimulator Generator, Single Array for Insertion in Subcutaneous Tissue and Fascia
Joint fixation plate	Internal Fixation Device in Upper Joints Internal Fixation Device in Lower Joints
Joint liner (insert)	Liner in Lower Joints
Joint spacer (antibiotic)	Spacer in Upper Joints Spacer in Lower Joints
Kappa	Pacemaker, Dual Chamber for Insertion in Subcutaneous Tissue and Fascia
Kirschner wire (K-wire)	Internal Fixation Device in Head and Facial Bones Internal Fixation Device in Upper Bones Internal Fixation Device in Lower Bones Internal Fixation Device in Upper Joints Internal Fixation Device in Lower Joints
Knee (implant) insert	Liner in Lower Joints
Kuntscher nail	Internal Fixation Device, Intramedullary in Upper Bones Internal Fixation Device, Intramedullary in Lower Bones
LAP-BAND® adjustable gastric banding system	Extraluminal Device
LifeStent® (Flexstar)(XL) Vascular Stent System	Intraluminal Device
LIVIAN™ CRT-D	Cardiac Resynchronization Defibrillator Pulse Generator for Insertion in Subcutaneous Tissue and Fascia
Loop recorder, implantable	Monitoring Device
MAGEC® Spinal Bracing and Distraction System	Magnetically Controlled Growth Rod(s) in New Technology
Mark IV Breathing Pacemaker System	Stimulator Generator in Subcutaneous Tissue and Fascia
Maximo II DR (VR)	Defibrillator Generator for Insertion in Subcutaneous Tissue and Fascia
Maximo II DR CRT-D	Cardiac Resynchronization Defibrillator Pulse Generator for Insertion in Subcutaneous Tissue and Fascia
Medtronic Endurant® II AAA stent graft system	Intraluminal Device
Melody® transcatheter pulmonary valve	Zooplastic Tissue in Heart and Great Vessels
Metal on metal bearing surface	Synthetic Substitute, Metal for Replacement in Lower Joints
Micro-Driver stent (RX) (OTW)	Intraluminal Device
MicroMed HeartAssist	Implantable Heart Assist System in Heart and Great Vessels
Micrus CERECYTE microcoil	Intraluminal Device, Bioactive in Upper Arteries
MIRODERM™ Biologic Wound Matrix	Skin Substitute, Porcine Liver Derived in New Technology
MitraClip valve repair system	Synthetic Substitute

Term	ICD-10-PCS Value
Mitroflow® Aortic Pericardial Heart Valve	Zooplastic Tissue in Heart and Great Vessels
Mosaic Bioprosthesis (aortic) (mitral) valve	Zooplastic Tissue in Heart and Great Vessels
MULTI-LINK (VISION)(MINI-VISION)(ULTRA) Coronary Stent System	Intraluminal Device
nanoLOCK™ interbody fusion device	Interbody Fusion Device, Nanotextured Surface in New Technology
Nasopharyngeal airway (NPA)	Intraluminal Device, Airway in Ear, Nose, Sinus
Neuromuscular electrical stimulation (NEMS) lead	Stimulator Lead in Muscles
Neurostimulator generator, multiple channel	Stimulator Generator, Multiple Array for Insertion in Subcutaneous Tissue and Fascia
Neurostimulator generator, multiple channel rechargeable	Stimulator Generator, Multiple Array Rechargeable for Insertion in Subcutaneous Tissue and Fascia
Neurostimulator generator, single channel	Stimulator Generator, Single Array for Insertion in Subcutaneous Tissue and Fascia
Neurostimulator generator, single channel rechargeable	Stimulator Generator, Single Array Rechargeable for Insertion in Subcutaneous Tissue and Fascia
Neutralization plate	Internal Fixation Device in Head and Facial Bones Internal Fixation Device in Upper Bones Internal Fixation Device in Lower Bones
Nitinol framed polymer mesh	Synthetic Substitute
Non-tunneled central venous catheter	Infusion Device
Novacor Left Ventricular Assist Device	Implantable Heart Assist System in Heart and Great Vessels
Novation® Ceramic AHS® (Articulation Hip System)	Synthetic Substitute, Ceramic for Replacement in Lower Joints
Omnilink Elite Vascular Balloon Expandable Stent System	Intraluminal Device
Open Pivot Aortic Valve Graft (AVG)	Synthetic Substitute
Open Pivot (mechanical) Valve	Synthetic Substitute
Optimizer™ III implantable pulse generator	Contractility Modulation Device for Insertion in Subcutaneous Tissue and Fascia
Oropharyngeal airway (OPA)	Intraluminal Device, Airway in Mouth and Throat
Ovatio™ CRT-D	Cardiac Resynchronization Defibrillator Pulse Generator for Insertion in Subcutaneous Tissue and Fascia
OXINIUM	Synthetic Substitute, Oxidized Zirconium on Polyethylene for Replacement in Lower Joints
Paclitaxel-eluting coronary stent	Intraluminal Device, Drug-eluting in Heart and Great Vessels
Paclitaxel-eluting peripheral stent	Intraluminal Device, Drug-eluting in Upper Arteries Intraluminal Device, Drug-eluting in Lower Arteries
Partially absorbable mesh	Synthetic Substitute

Term	ICD-10-PCS Value
Pedicle-based dynamic stabilization device	Spinal Stabilization Device, Pedicle-Based for Insertion in Upper Joints Spinal Stabilization Device, Pedicle-Based for Insertion in Lower Joints
Perceval sutureless valve	Zooplastic Tissue, Rapid Deployment Technique in New Technology
Percutaneous endoscopic gastrojejunostomy (PEG/J) tube	Feeding Device in Gastrointestinal System
Percutaneous endoscopic gastrostomy (PEG) tube	Feeding Device in Gastrointestinal System
Percutaneous nephrostomy catheter	Drainage Device
Peripherally inserted central catheter (PICC)	Infusion Device
Pessary ring	Intraluminal Device, Pessary in Female Reproductive System
Phrenic nerve stimulator generator	Stimulator Generator in Subcutaneous Tissue and Fascia
Phrenic nerve stimulator lead	Diaphragmatic Pacemaker Lead in Respiratory System
PHYSIOMESH™ Flexible Composite Mesh	Synthetic Substitute
Pipeline™ Embolization device (PED)	Intraluminal Device
Polyethylene socket	Synthetic Substitute, Polyethylene for Replacement in Lower Joints
Polymethylmethacrylate (PMMA)	Synthetic Substitute
Polypropylene mesh	Synthetic Substitute
Porcine (bioprosthetic) valve	Zooplastic Tissue in Heart and Great Vessels
PRESTIGE® Cervical Disc	Synthetic Substitute
PrimeAdvanced neurostimulator (SureScan)(MRI Safe)	Stimulator Generator, Multiple Array for Insertion in Subcutaneous Tissue and Fascia
PROCEED™ Ventral Patch	Synthetic Substitute
Prodisc-C	Synthetic Substitute
Prodisc-L	Synthetic Substitute
PROLENE Polypropylene Hernia System (PHS)	Synthetic Substitute
Protecta XT CRT-D	Cardiac Resynchronization Defibrillator Pulse Generator for Insertion in Subcutaneous Tissue and Fascia
Protecta XT DR (XT VR)	Defibrillator Generator for Insertion in Subcutaneous Tissue and Fascia
Protégé® RX Carotid Stent System	Intraluminal Device
Pump reservoir	Infusion Device, Pump in Subcutaneous Tissue and Fascia
REALIZE® Adjustable Gastric Band	Extraluminal Device
Rebound HRD® (Hernia Repair Device)	Synthetic Substitute
RestoreAdvanced neurostimulator (SureScan)(MRI Safe)	Stimulator Generator, Multiple Array Rechargeable for Insertion in Subcutaneous Tissue and Fascia
RestoreSensor neurostimulator (SureScan)(MRI Safe)	Stimulator Generator, Multiple Array Rechargeable for Insertion in Subcutaneous Tissue and Fascia
RestoreUltra neurostimulator (SureScan)(MRI Safe)	Stimulator Generator, Multiple Array Rechargeable for Insertion in Subcutaneous Tissue and Fascia

Term	ICD-10-PCS Value
Reveal (DX)(XT)	Monitoring Device
Reverse® Shoulder Prosthesis	Synthetic Substitute, Reverse Ball and Socket for Replacement in Upper Joints
Revo MRI™ SureScan® pacemaker	Pacemaker, Dual Chamber for Insertion in Subcutaneous Tissue and Fascia
Rheos® System device	Stimulator Generator in Subcutaneous Tissue and Fascia
Rheos® System lead	Stimulator Lead in Upper Arteries
RNS System lead	Neurostimulator Lead in Central Nervous System and Cranial Nerves
RNS system neurostimulator generator	Neurostimulator Generator in Head and Facial Bones
Sacral nerve modulation (SNM) lead	Stimulator Lead in Urinary System
Sacral neuromodulation lead	Stimulator Lead in Urinary System
SAPIEN transcatheter aortic valve	Zooplastic Tissue in Heart and Great Vessels
Secura (DR) (VR)	Defibrillator Generator for Insertion in Subcutaneous Tissue and Fascia
Sheffield hybrid external fixator	External Fixation Device, Hybrid for Insertion in Upper Bones External Fixation Device, Hybrid for Reposition in Upper Bones External Fixation Device, Hybrid for Insertion in Lower Bones External Fixation Device, Hybrid for Reposition in Lower Bones
Sheffield ring external fixator	External Fixation Device, Ring for Insertion in Upper Bones External Fixation Device, Ring for Reposition in Upper Bones External Fixation Device, Ring for Insertion in Lower Bones External Fixation Device, Ring for Reposition in Lower Bones
Single lead pacemaker (atrium)(ventricle)	Pacemaker, Single Chamber for Insertion in Subcutaneous Tissue and Fascia
Single lead rate responsive pacemaker (atrium)(ventricle)	Pacemaker, Single Chamber Rate Responsive for Insertion in Subcutaneous Tissue and Fascia
Sirolimus-eluting coronary stent	Intraluminal Device, Drug-eluting in Heart and Great Vessels
SJM Biocor® Stented Valve System	Zooplastic Tissue in Heart and Great Vessels
Spacer, Articulating (Antibiotic)	Articulating Spacer in Lower Joints
Spacer, Static (Antibiotic)	Spacer in Lower Joints
Spinal cord neurostimulator lead	Neurostimulator Lead in Central Nervous System and Cranial Nerves
Spinal growth rods, magnetically controlled	Magnetically Controlled Growth Rod(s) in New Technology
Spiration IBV™ Valve System	Intraluminal Device, Endobronchial Valve in Respiratory System
Static Spacer (Antibiotic)	Spacer in Lower Joints
Stent, intraluminal (cardiovascular)(gastrointestinal)(hepatobiliary)(urinary)	Intraluminal Device
Stented tissue valve	Zooplastic Tissue in Heart and Great Vessels
Stratos LV	Cardiac Resynchronization Pacemaker Pulse Generator for Insertion in Subcutaneous Tissue and Fascia

Term	ICD-10-PCS Value
Subcutaneous injection reservoir, port	Vascular Access Device, Totally Implantable in Subcutaneous Tissue and Fascia
Subcutaneous injection reservoir, pump	Infusion Device, Pump in Subcutaneous Tissue and Fascia
Subdermal progesterone implant	Contraceptive Device in Subcutaneous Tissue and Fascia
Sutureless valve, Perceval	Zooplastic Tissue, Rapid Deployment Technique in New Technology
SynCardia Total Artificial Heart	Synthetic Substitute
Synchra CRT-P	Cardiac Resynchronization Pacemaker Pulse Generator for Insertion in Subcutaneous Tissue and Fascia
SyncroMed Pump	Infusion Device, Pump in Subcutaneous Tissue and Fascia
Talent® Converter	Intraluminal Device
Talent® Occluder	Intraluminal Device
Talent® Stent Graft (abdominal)(thoracic)	Intraluminal Device
TandemHeart® System	Short-term External Heart Assist System in Heart and Great Vessels
TAXUS® Liberté® Paclitaxel-eluting Coronary Stent System	Intraluminal Device, Drug-eluting in Heart and Great Vessels
Therapeutic occlusion coil(s)	Intraluminal Device
Thoracostomy tube	Drainage Device
Thoratec IVAD (Implantable Ventricular Assist Device)	Implantable Heart Assist System in Heart and Great Vessels
Thoratec Paracorporeal Ventricular Assist Device	Short-term External Heart Assist System in Heart and Great Vessels
Tibial insert	Liner in Lower Joints
Tissue bank graft	Nonautologous Tissue Substitute
Tissue expander (inflatable)(injectable)	Tissue Expander in Skin and Breast Tissue Expander in Subcutaneous Tissue and Fascia
Titanium Sternal Fixation System (TSFS)	Internal Fixation Device, Rigid Plate for Insertion in Upper Bones Internal Fixation Device, Rigid Plate for Reposition in Upper Bones
Total artificial (replacement) heart	Synthetic Substitute
Tracheostomy tube	Tracheostomy Device in Respiratory System
Trifecta™ Valve (aortic)	Zooplastic Tissue in Heart and Great Vessels
Tunneled central venous catheter	Vascular Access Device, Tunneled in Subcutaneous Tissue and Fascia
Tunneled spinal (intrathecal) catheter	Infusion Device
Two lead pacemaker	Pacemaker, Dual Chamber for Insertion in Subcutaneous Tissue and Fascia
Ultraflex™ Precision Colonic Stent System	Intraluminal Device
ULTRAPRO Hernia System (UHS)	Synthetic Substitute
ULTRAPRO Partially Absorbable Lightweight Mesh	Synthetic Substitute
ULTRAPRO Plug	Synthetic Substitute

Term	ICD-10-PCS Value
Ultrasonic osteogenic stimulator	Bone Growth Stimulator in Head and Facial Bones Bone Growth Stimulator in Upper Bones Bone Growth Stimulator in Lower Bones
Ultrasound bone healing system	Bone Growth Stimulator in Head and Facial Bones Bone Growth Stimulator in Upper Bones Bone Growth Stimulator in Lower Bones
Uniplanar external fixator	External Fixation Device, Monoplanar for Insertion in Upper Bones External Fixation Device, Monoplanar for Reposition in Upper Bones External Fixation Device, Monoplanar for Insertion in Lower Bones External Fixation Device, Monoplanar for Reposition in Lower Bones
Urinary incontinence stimulator lead	Stimulator Lead in Urinary System
Vaginal pessary	Intraluminal Device, Pessary in Female Reproductive System
Valiant Thoracic Stent Graft	Intraluminal Device
Vectra® Vascular Access Graft	Vascular Access Device, Tunneled in Subcutaneous Tissue and Fascia
Ventrio™ Hernia Patch	Synthetic Substitute
Versa	Pacemaker, Dual Chamber for Insertion in Subcutaneous Tissue and Fascia
Virtuoso (II) (DR) (VR)	Defibrillator Generator for Insertion in Subcutaneous Tissue and Fascia
Viva(XT)(S)	Cardiac Resynchronization Defibrillator Pulse Generator for Insertion in Subcutaneous Tissue and Fascia
WALLSTENT® Endoprosthesis	Intraluminal Device
X-STOP® Spacer	Spinal Stabilization Device, Interspinous Process for Insertion in Upper Joints Spinal Stabilization Device, Interspinous Process for Insertion in Lower Joints
Xact Carotid Stent System	Intraluminal Device
Xenograft	Zooplastic Tissue in Heart and Great Vessels
XIENCE Everolimus Eluting Coronary Stent System	Intraluminal Device, Drug-eluting in Heart and Great Vessels
XLIF® System	Interbody Fusion Device in Lower Joints
Zenith AAA Endovascular Graft	Intraluminal Device, Branched or Fenestrated, One or Two Arteries for Restriction in Lower Arteries Intraluminal Device, Branched or Fenestrated, Three or More Arteries for Restriction in Lower Arteries Intraluminal Device
Zenith Flex® AAA Endovascular Graft	Intraluminal Device
Zenith TX2® TAA Endovascular Graft	Intraluminal Device
Zenith® Renu™ AAA Ancillary Graft	Intraluminal Device
Zilver® PTX® (paclitaxel) Drug-Eluting Peripheral Stent	Intraluminal Device, Drug-eluting in Upper Arteries Intraluminal Device, Drug-eluting in Lower Arteries
Zimmer® NexGen® LPS Mobile Bearing Knee	Synthetic Substitute
Zimmer® NexGen® LPS-Flex Mobile Knee	Synthetic Substitute
Zotarolimus-eluting coronary stent	Intraluminal Device, Drug-eluting in Heart and Great Vessels

Device Aggregation Table

This table crosswalks specific device character value definitions for specific root operations in a specific body system to the more general device character value to be used when the root operation covers a wide range of body parts and the device character represents an entire family of devices.

Specific Device	for Operation	in Body System	General Device
Autologous Arterial Tissue (A)	All applicable	Heart and Great Vessels Lower Arteries Lower Veins Upper Arteries Upper Veins	7 Autologous Tissue Substitute
Autologous Venous Tissue (9)	All applicable	Heart and Great Vessels Lower Arteries Lower Veins Upper Arteries Upper Veins	7 Autologous Tissue Substitute
Cardiac Lead, Defibrillator (K)	Insertion	Heart and Great Vessels	M Cardiac Lead
Cardiac Lead, Pacemaker (J)	Insertion	Heart and Great Vessels	M Cardiac Lead
Cardiac Resynchronization Defibrillator Pulse Generator (9)	Insertion	Subcutaneous Tissue and Fascia	P Cardiac Rhythm Related Device
Cardiac Resynchronization Pacemaker Pulse Generator (7)	Insertion	Subcutaneous Tissue and Fascia	P Cardiac Rhythm Related Device
Contractility Modulation Device (A)	Insertion	Subcutaneous Tissue and Fascia	P Cardiac Rhythm Related Device
Defibrillator Generator (8)	Insertion	Subcutaneous Tissue and Fascia	P Cardiac Rhythm Related Device
Epiretinal Visual Prosthesis (5)	All applicable	Eye	J Synthetic Substitute
External Fixation Device, Hybrid (D)	Insertion	Lower Bones Upper Bones	5 External Fixation Device
External Fixation Device, Hybrid (D)	Reposition	Lower Bones Upper Bones	5 External Fixation Device
External Fixation Device, Limb Lengthening (8)	Insertion	Lower Bones Upper Bones	5 External Fixation Device
External Fixation Device, Monoplanar (B)	Insertion	Lower Bones Upper Bones	5 External Fixation Device
External Fixation Device, Monoplanar (B)	Reposition	Lower Bones Upper Bones	5 External Fixation Device
External Fixation Device, Ring (C)	Insertion	Lower Bones Upper Bones	5 External Fixation Device
External Fixation Device, Ring (C)	Reposition	Lower Bones Upper Bones	5 External Fixation Device
Hearing Device, Bone Conduction (4)	Insertion	Ear, Nose, Sinus	S Hearing Device
Hearing Device, Multiple Channel Cochlear Prosthesis (6)	Insertion	Ear, Nose, Sinus	S Hearing Device
Hearing Device, Single Channel Cochlear Prosthesis (5)	Insertion	Ear, Nose, Sinus	S Hearing Device
Internal Fixation Device, Intramedullary (6)	All applicable	Lower Bones Upper Bones	4 Internal Fixation Device
Internal Fixation Device, Rigid Plate (Ø)	Insertion	Upper Bones	4 Internal Fixation Device
Internal Fixation Device, Rigid Plate (Ø)	Reposition	Upper Bones	4 Internal Fixation Device
Intraluminal Device, Airway (B)	All applicable	Ear, Nose, Sinus Gastrointestinal System Mouth and Throat	D Intraluminal Device
Intraluminal Device, Bioactive (B)	All applicable	Upper Arteries	D Intraluminal Device
Intraluminal Device, Branched or Fenestrated, One or Two Arteries (E)	Restriction	Heart and Great Vessels Lower Arteries	D Intraluminal Device
Intraluminal Device, Branched or Fenestrated, Three or More Arteries (F)	Restriction	Heart and Great Vessels Lower Arteries	D Intraluminal Device
Intraluminal Device, Drug-eluting (4)	All applicable	Heart and Great Vessels Lower Arteries Upper Arteries	D Intraluminal Device
Intraluminal Device, Drug-eluting, Four or More (7)	All applicable	Heart and Great Vessels Lower Arteries Upper Arteries	D Intraluminal Device

Specific Device	for Operation	in Body System	General Device
Intraluminal Device, Drug-eluting, Three (6)	All applicable	Heart and Great Vessels Lower Arteries Upper Arteries	**D** Intraluminal Device
Intraluminal Device, Drug-eluting, Two (5)	All applicable	Heart and Great Vessels Lower Arteries Upper Arteries	**D** Intraluminal Device
Intraluminal Device, Endobronchial Valve (G)	All applicable	Respiratory System	**D** Intraluminal Device
Intraluminal Device, Endotracheal Airway (E)	All applicable	Respiratory System	**D** Intraluminal Device
Intraluminal Device, Four or More (G)	All applicable	Heart and Great Vessels Lower Arteries Upper Arteries	**D** Intraluminal Device
Intraluminal Device, Pessary (G)	All applicable	Female Reproductive System	**D** Intraluminal Device
Intraluminal Device, Radioactive (T)	All applicable	Heart and Great Vessels	**D** Intraluminal Device
Intraluminal Device, Three (F)	All applicable	Heart and Great Vessels Lower Arteries Upper Arteries	**D** Intraluminal Device
Intraluminal Device, Two (E)	All applicable	Heart and Great Vessels Lower Arteries Upper Arteries	**D** Intraluminal Device
Monitoring Device, Hemodynamic (Ø)	Insertion	Subcutaneous Tissue and Fascia	**2** Monitoring Device
Monitoring Device, Pressure Sensor (Ø)	Insertion	Heart and Great Vessels	**2** Monitoring Device
Pacemaker, Dual Chamber (6)	Insertion	Subcutaneous Tissue and Fascia	**P** Cardiac Rhythm Related Device
Pacemaker, Single Chamber (4)	Insertion	Subcutaneous Tissue and Fascia	**P** Cardiac Rhythm Related Device
Pacemaker, Single Chamber Rate Responsive (5)	Insertion	Subcutaneous Tissue and Fascia	**P** Cardiac Rhythm Related Device
Spinal Stabilization Device, Facet Replacement (D)	Insertion	Lower Joints Upper Joints	**4** Internal Fixation Device
Spinal Stabilization Device, Interspinous Process (B)	Insertion	Lower Joints Upper Joints	**4** Internal Fixation Device
Spinal Stabilization Device, Pedicle-Based (C)	Insertion	Lower Joints Upper Joints	**4** Internal Fixation Device
Stimulator Generator, Multiple Array (D)	Insertion	Subcutaneous Tissue and Fascia	**M** Stimulator Generator
Stimulator Generator, Multiple Array Rechargeable (E)	Insertion	Subcutaneous Tissue and Fascia	**M** Stimulator Generator
Stimulator Generator, Single Array (B)	Insertion	Subcutaneous Tissue and Fascia	**M** Stimulator Generator
Stimulator Generator, Single Array Rechargeable (C)	Insertion	Subcutaneous Tissue and Fascia	**M** Stimulator Generator
Synthetic Substitute, Ceramic (3)	Replacement	Lower Joints	**J** Synthetic Substitute
Synthetic Substitute, Ceramic on Polyethylene (4)	Replacement	Lower Joints	**J** Synthetic Substitute
Synthetic Substitute, Intraocular Telescope (Ø)	Replacement	Eye	**J** Synthetic Substitute
Synthetic Substitute, Metal (1)	Replacement	Lower Joints	**J** Synthetic Substitute
Synthetic Substitute, Metal on Polyethylene (2)	Replacement	Lower Joints	**J** Synthetic Substitute
Synthetic Substitute, Oxidized Zirconium on Polyethylene (6)	Replacement	Lower Joints	**J** Synthetic Substitute
Synthetic Substitute, Polyethylene (Ø)	Replacement	Lower Joints	**J** Synthetic Substitute
Synthetic Substitute, Reverse Ball and Socket (Ø)	Replacement	Upper Joints	**J** Synthetic Substitute

Appendix G: Device Definitions

ICD-10-PCS Value	Definition
Articulating Spacer in Lower Joints	**Includes:** Articulating Spacer (Antibiotic) Spacer, Articulating (Antibiotic)
Artificial Sphincter in Gastrointestinal System	**Includes:** Artificial anal sphincter (AAS) Artificial bowel sphincter (neosphincter)
Artificial Sphincter in Urinary System	**Includes:** AMS 800® Urinary Control System Artificial urinary sphincter (AUS)
Autologous Arterial Tissue in Heart and Great Vessels	**Includes:** Autologous artery graft
Autologous Arterial Tissue in Lower Arteries	**Includes:** Autologous artery graft
Autologous Arterial Tissue in Lower Veins	**Includes:** Autologous artery graft
Autologous Arterial Tissue in Upper Arteries	**Includes:** Autologous artery graft
Autologous Arterial Tissue in Upper Veins	**Includes:** Autologous artery graft
Autologous Tissue Substitute	**Includes:** Autograft Cultured epidermal cell autograft Epicel® cultured epidermal autograft
Autologous Venous Tissue in Heart and Great Vessels	**Includes:** Autologous vein graft
Autologous Venous Tissue in Lower Arteries	**Includes:** Autologous vein graft
Autologous Venous Tissue in Lower Veins	**Includes:** Autologous vein graft
Autologous Venous Tissue in Upper Arteries	**Includes:** Autologous vein graft
Autologous Venous Tissue in Upper Veins	**Includes:** Autologous vein graft
Bone Growth Stimulator in Head and Facial Bones	**Includes:** Electrical bone growth stimulator (EBGS) Ultrasonic osteogenic stimulator Ultrasound bone healing system
Bone Growth Stimulator in Lower Bones	**Includes:** Electrical bone growth stimulator (EBGS) Ultrasonic osteogenic stimulator Ultrasound bone healing system
Bone Growth Stimulator in Upper Bones	**Includes:** Electrical bone growth stimulator (EBGS) Ultrasonic osteogenic stimulator Ultrasound bone healing system
Cardiac Lead in Heart and Great Vessels	**Includes:** Cardiac contractility modulation lead

ICD-10-PCS Value	Definition
Cardiac Lead, Defibrillator for Insertion in Heart and Great Vessels	**Includes:** ACUITY™ Steerable Lead Attain Ability® lead Attain StarFix® (OTW) lead Cardiac resynchronization therapy (CRT) lead Corox (OTW) Bipolar Lead Durata® Defibrillation Lead ENDOTAK RELIANCE® (G) Defibrillation Lead
Cardiac Lead, Pacemaker for Insertion in Heart and Great Vessels	**Includes:** ACUITY™ Steerable Lead Attain Ability® lead Attain StarFix® (OTW) lead Cardiac resynchronization therapy (CRT) lead Corox (OTW) Bipolar Lead
Cardiac Resynchronization Defibrillator Pulse Generator for Insertion in Subcutaneous Tissue and Fascia	**Includes:** COGNIS® CRT-D Concerto II CRT-D Consulta CRT-D CONTAK RENEWA® 3 RF (HE) CRT-D LIVIAN™ CRT-D Maximo II DR CRT-D Ovatio™ CRT-D Protecta XT CRT-D Viva (XT)(S)
Cardiac Resynchronization Pacemaker Pulse Generator for Insertion in Subcutaneous Tissue and Fascia	**Includes:** Consulta CRT-P Stratos LV Synchra CRT-P
Contraceptive Device in Female Reproductive System	**Includes:** Intrauterine device (IUD)
Contraceptive Device in Subcutaneous Tissue and Fascia	**Includes:** Subdermal progesterone implant
Contractility Modulation Device for Insertion in Subcutaneous Tissue and Fascia	**Includes:** Optimizer™ III implantable pulse generator
Defibrillator Generator for Insertion in Subcutaneous Tissue and Fascia	**Includes:** Evera (XT)(S)(DR/VR) Implantable cardioverter-defibrillator (ICD) Maximo II DR (VR) Protecta XT DR (XT VR) Secura (DR) (VR) Virtuoso (II) (DR) (VR)
Diaphragmatic Pacemaker Lead in Respiratory System	**Includes:** Phrenic nerve stimulator lead
Drainage Device	**Includes:** Cystostomy tube Foley catheter Percutaneous nephrostomy catheter Thoracostomy tube
External Fixation Device in Head and Facial Bones	**Includes:** External fixator
External Fixation Device in Lower Bones	**Includes:** External fixator
External Fixation Device in Lower Joints	**Includes:** External fixator

ICD-10-PCS Value	Definition
External Fixation Device in Upper Bones	**Includes:** External fixator
External Fixation Device in Upper Joints	**Includes:** External fixator
External Fixation Device, Hybrid for Insertion in Lower Bones	**Includes:** Delta frame external fixator Sheffield hybrid external fixator
External Fixation Device, Hybrid for Insertion in Upper Bones	**Includes:** Delta frame external fixator Sheffield hybrid external fixator
External Fixation Device, Hybrid for Reposition in Lower Bones	**Includes:** Delta frame external fixator Sheffield hybrid external fixator
External Fixation Device, Hybrid for Reposition in Upper Bones	**Includes:** Delta frame external fixator Sheffield hybrid external fixator
External Fixation Device, Limb Lengthening for Insertion in Lower Bones	**Includes:** Ilizarov-Vecklich device
External Fixation Device, Limb Lengthening for Insertion in Upper Bones	**Includes:** Ilizarov-Vecklich device
External Fixation Device, Monoplanar for Insertion in Lower Bones	**Includes:** Uniplanar external fixator
External Fixation Device, Monoplanar for Insertion in Upper Bones	**Includes:** Uniplanar external fixator
External Fixation Device, Monoplanar for Reposition in Lower Bones	**Includes:** Uniplanar external fixator
External Fixation Device, Monoplanar for Reposition in Upper Bones	**Includes:** Uniplanar external fixator
External Fixation Device, Ring for Insertion in Lower Bones	**Includes:** Ilizarov external fixator Sheffield ring external fixator
External Fixation Device, Ring for Insertion in Upper Bones	**Includes:** Ilizarov external fixator Sheffield ring external fixator
External Fixation Device, Ring for Reposition in Lower Bones	**Includes:** Ilizarov external fixator Sheffield ring external fixator
External Fixation Device, Ring for Reposition in Upper Bones	**Includes:** Ilizarov external fixator Sheffield ring external fixator
Extraluminal Device	**Includes:** AtriClip LAA Exclusion System LAP-BAND® adjustable gastric banding system REALIZE® Adjustable Gastric Band
Feeding Device in Gastrointestinal System	**Includes:** Percutaneous endoscopic gastrojejunostomy (PEG/J) tube Percutaneous endoscopic gastrostomy (PEG) tube
Hearing Device in Ear, Nose, Sinus	**Includes:** Esteem® implantable hearing system
Hearing Device in Head and Facial Bones	**Includes:** Bone anchored hearing device

ICD-10-PCS Value	Definition
Hearing Device, Bone Conduction for Insertion in Ear, Nose, Sinus	**Includes:** Bone anchored hearing device
Hearing Device, Multiple Channel Cochlear Prosthesis for Insertion in Ear, Nose, Sinus	**Includes:** Cochlear implant (CI), multiple channel (electrode)
Hearing Device, Single Channel Cochlear Prosthesis for Insertion in Ear, Nose, Sinus	**Includes:** Cochlear implant (CI), single channel (electrode)
Implantable Heart Assist System in Heart and Great Vessels	**Includes:** Berlin Heart Ventricular Assist Device DeBakey Left Ventricular Assist Device DuraHeart Left Ventricular Assist System HeartMate 3™ LVAS HeartMate II® Left Ventricular Assist Device (LVAD) HeartMate XVE® Left Ventricular Assist Device (LVAD) MicroMed HeartAssist Novacor Left Ventricular Assist Device Thoratec IVAD (Implantable Ventricular Assist Device)
Infusion Device	**Includes:** Ascenda Intrathecal Catheter InDura, intrathecal catheter (1P) (spinal) Non-tunneled central venous catheter Peripherally inserted central catheter (PICC) Tunneled spinal (intrathecal) catheter
Infusion Device, Pump in Subcutaneous Tissue and Fascia	**Includes:** Implantable drug infusion pump (anti-spasmodic)(chemotherapy) (pain) Injection reservoir, pump Pump reservoir Subcutaneous injection reservoir, pump SynchroMed pump
Interbody Fusion Device in Lower Joints	**Includes:** Axial Lumbar Interbody Fusion System AxiaLIF® System CoRoent® XL Direct Lateral Interbody Fusion (DLIF) device EXtreme Lateral Interbody Fusion (XLIF) device Interbody fusion (spine) cage XLIF® System
Interbody Fusion Device in Upper Joints	**Includes:** BAK/C® Interbody Cervical Fusion System Interbody fusion (spine) cage
Interbody Fusion Device, Nanotextured Surface in New Technology	**Includes:** nanoLOCK™ interbody fusion device

ICD-10-PCS Value	Definition
Interbody Fusion Device, Radiolucent Porous in New Technology	**Includes:** COALESCE® radiolucent interbody fusion device COHERE® radiolucent interbody fusion device
Internal Fixation Device in Head and Facial Bones	**Includes:** Bone screw (interlocking)(lag)(pedicle)(recessed) Kirschner wire (K-wire) Neutralization plate
Internal Fixation Device in Lower Bones	**Includes:** Bone screw (interlocking)(lag)(pedicle)(recessed) Clamp and rod internal fixation system (CRIF) Kirschner wire (K-wire) Neutralization plate
Internal Fixation Device in Lower Joints	**Includes:** Fusion screw (compression)(lag)(locking) Joint fixation plate Kirschner wire (K-wire)
Internal Fixation Device in Upper Bones	**Includes:** Bone screw (interlocking)(lag)(pedicle)(recessed) Clamp and rod internal fixation system (CRIF) Kirschner wire (K-wire) Neutralization plate
Internal Fixation Device in Upper Joints	**Includes:** Fusion screw (compression)(lag)(locking) Joint fixation plate Kirschner wire (K-wire)
Internal Fixation Device, Intramedullary in Lower Bones	**Includes:** Intramedullary (IM) rod (nail) Intramedullary skeletal kinetic distractor (ISKD) Kuntscher nail
Internal Fixation Device, Intramedullary in Upper Bones	**Includes:** Intramedullary (IM) rod (nail) Intramedullary skeletal kinetic distractor (ISKD) Kuntscher nail
Internal Fixation Device, Rigid Plate for Insertion in Upper Bones	**Includes:** Titanium Sternal Fixation System (TSFS)
Internal Fixation Device, Rigid Plate for Reposition in Upper Bones	**Includes:** Titanium Sternal Fixation System (TSFS)

ICD-10-PCS Value	Definition
Intraluminal Device	**Includes:** Absolute Pro Vascular (OTW) Self-Expanding Stent System Acculink (RX) Carotid Stent System AFX® Endovascular AAA System AneuRx® AAA Advantage® Assurant (Cobalt) stent Carotid WALLSTENT® Monorail® Endoprosthesis CoAxia NeuroFlo catheter Colonic Z-Stent® Complete (SE) stent Cook Zenith AAA Endovascular Graft Driver stent (RX) (OTW) E-Luminexx™ (Biliary)(Vascular) Stent Embolization coil(s) Endologix AFX® Endovascular AAA System Endurant® Endovascular Stent Graft Endurant® II AAA stent graft system EXCLUDER® AAA Endoprosthesis Express® (LD) Premounted Stent System Express® Biliary SD Monorail® Premounted Stent System Express® SD Renal Monorail® Premounted Stent System FLAIR® Endovascular Stent Graft Formula™ Balloon-Expandable Renal Stent System GORE EXCLUDER® AAA Endoprosthesis GORE TAG® Thoracic Endoprosthesis Herculink (RX) Elite Renal Stent System LifeStent® (Flexstar)(XL) Vascular Stent System Medtronic Endurant® II AAA stent graft system Micro-Driver stent (RX) (OTW) MULTI-LINK (VISION)(MINI-VISION)(ULTRA) Coronary Stent System Omnilink Elite Vascular Balloon Expandable Stent System Pipeline™ Embolization device (PED) Protege® RX Carotid Stent System Stent, intraluminal (cardiovascular)(gastrointestinal)(hepatobiliary)(urinary) Talent® Converter Talent® Occluder Talent® Stent Graft (abdominal)(thoracic) Therapeutic occlusion coil(s) Ultraflex™ Precision Colonic Stent System Valiant Thoracic Stent Graft WALLSTENT® Endoprosthesis Xact Carotid Stent System Zenith AAA Endovascular Graft Zenith Flex® AAA Endovascular Graft Zenith TX2® TAA Endovascular Graft Zenith® Renu™ AAA Ancillary Graft
Intraluminal Device, Airway in Ear, Nose, Sinus	**Includes:** Nasopharyngeal airway (NPA)
Intraluminal Device, Airway in Gastrointestinal System	**Includes:** Esophageal obturator airway (EOA)

ICD-10-PCS Value	Definition
Intraluminal Device, Airway in Mouth and Throat	**Includes:** Guedel airway Oropharyngeal airway (OPA)
Intraluminal Device, Bioactive in Upper Arteries	**Includes:** Bioactive embolization coil(s) Micrus CERECYTE microcoil
Intraluminal Device, Branched or Fenestrated, One or Two Arteries for Restriction in Lower Arteries	**Includes:** Cook Zenith AAA Endovascular Graft EXCLUDER® AAA Endoprosthesis EXCLUDER® IBE Endoprosthesis GORE EXCLUDER® AAA Endoprosthesis GORE EXCLUDER®IBE Endoprosthesis Zenith AAA Endovascular Graft
Intraluminal Device, Branched or Fenestrated, Three or More Arteries for Restriction in Lower Arteries	**Includes:** Cook Zenith AAA Endovascular Graft EXCLUDER® AAA Endoprosthesis GORE EXCLUDER® AAA Endoprosthesis Zenith AAA Endovascular Graft
Intraluminal Device, Drug-eluting in Heart and Great Vessels	**Includes:** CYPHER® Stent Endeavor® (III)(IV) (Sprint) Zotarolimus-eluting Coronary Stent System Everolimus-eluting coronary stent Paclitaxel-eluting coronary stent Sirolimus-eluting coronary stent TAXUS® Liberte® Paclitaxel-eluting Coronary Stent System XIENCE Everolimus Eluting Coronary Stent System Zotarolimus-eluting coronary stent
Intraluminal Device, Drug-eluting in Lower Arteries	**Includes:** Paclitaxel-eluting peripheral stent Zilver® PTX® (paclitaxel) Drug-Eluting Peripheral Stent
Intraluminal Device, Drug-eluting in Upper Arteries	**Includes:** Paclitaxel-eluting peripheral stent Zilver® PTX® (paclitaxel) Drug-Eluting Peripheral Stent
Intraluminal Device, Endobronchial Valve in Respiratory System	**Includes:** Spiration IBV™ Valve System
Intraluminal Device, Endotracheal Airway in Respiratory System	**Includes:** Endotracheal tube (cuffed)(double-lumen)
Intraluminal Device, Pessary in Female Reproductive System	**Includes:** Pessary ring Vaginal pessary
Liner in Lower Joints	**Includes:** Acetabular cup Hip (joint) liner Joint liner (insert) Knee (implant) insert Tibial insert
Magnetically Controlled Growth Rod(s) in New Technology	**Includes:** MAGEC® Spinal Bracing and Distraction System Spinal growth rods, magnetically controlled

ICD-10-PCS Value	Definition
Monitoring Device	**Includes:** Blood glucose monitoring system Cardiac event recorder Continuous Glucose Monitoring (CGM) device Implantable glucose monitoring device Loop recorder, implantable Reveal (DX)(XT)
Monitoring Device, Hemodynamic for Insertion in Subcutaneous Tissue and Fascia	**Includes:** Implantable hemodynamic monitor (IHM) Implantable hemodynamic monitoring system (IHMS)
Monitoring Device, Pressure Sensor for Insertion in Heart and Great Vessels	**Includes:** CardioMEMS® pressure sensor EndoSure® sensor
Neurostimulator Generator in Head and Facial Bones	**Includes:** RNS system neurostimulator generator
Neurostimulator Lead in Central Nervous System and Cranial Nerves	**Includes:** Cortical strip neurostimulator lead DBS lead Deep brain neurostimulator lead RNS System lead Spinal cord neurostimulator lead
Neurostimulator Lead in Peripheral Nervous System	**Includes:** InterStim® Therapy lead
Nonautologous Tissue Substitute	**Includes:** Acellular Hydrated Dermis Bone bank bone graft Cook Biodesign® Fistula Plug(s) Cook Biodesign® Hernia Graft(s) Cook Biodesign® Layered Graft(s) Cook Zenapro™ Layered Graft(s) Tissue bank graft
Pacemaker, Dual Chamber for Insertion in Subcutaneous Tissue and Fascia	**Includes:** Advisa (MRI) EnRhythm Kappa Revo MRI™ SureScan® pacemaker Two lead pacemaker Versa
Pacemaker, Single Chamber for Insertion in Subcutaneous Tissue and Fascia	**Includes:** Single lead pacemaker (atrium)(ventricle)
Pacemaker, Single Chamber Rate Responsive for Insertion in Subcutaneous Tissue and Fascia	**Includes:** Single lead rate responsive pacemaker (atrium)(ventricle)
Radioactive Element	**Includes:** Brachytherapy seeds
Radioactive Element, Cesium-131 Collagen Implant for Insertion in Central Nervous System and Cranial Nerves	**Includes:** Cesium-131 Collagen Implant GammaTile™
Resurfacing Device in Lower Joints	**Includes:** CONSERVE® PLUS Total Resurfacing Hip System Cormet Hip Resurfacing System

ICD-10-PCS Value	Definition
Short-term External Heart Assist System in Heart and Great Vessels	**Includes:** Biventricular external heart assist system BVS 5000 Ventricular Assist Device Centrimag® Blood Pump Impella® heart pump TandemHeart® System Thoratec Paracorporeal Ventricular Assist Device
Skin Substitute, Porcine Liver Derived in New Technology	**Includes:** MIRODERM™ Biologic Wound Matrix
Spacer in Lower Joints	**Includes:** Joint spacer (antibiotic) Spacer, Static (Antibiotic) Static Spacer (Antibiotic)
Spacer in Upper Joints	**Includes:** Joint spacer (antibiotic)
Spinal Stabilization Device, Facet Replacement for Insertion in Lower Joints	**Includes:** Facet replacement spinal stabilization device
Spinal Stabilization Device, Facet Replacement for Insertion in Upper Joints	**Includes:** Facet replacement spinal stabilization device
Spinal Stabilization Device, Interspinous Process for Insertion in Lower Joints	**Includes:** Interspinous process spinal stabilization device X-STOP® Spacer
Spinal Stabilization Device, Interspinous Process for Insertion in Upper Joints	**Includes:** Interspinous process spinal stabilization device X-STOP® Spacer
Spinal Stabilization Device, Pedicle- Based for Insertion in Lower Joints	**Includes:** Dynesys® Dynamic Stabilization System Pedicle-based dynamic stabilization device
Spinal Stabilization Device, Pedicle-Based for Insertion in Upper Joints	**Includes:** Dynesys® Dynamic Stabilization System Pedicle-based dynamic stabilization device
Stimulator Generator in Subcutaneous Tissue and Fascia	**Includes:** Baroreflex Activation Therapy® (BAT®) Diaphragmatic pacemaker generator Mark IV Breathing Pacemaker System Phrenic nerve stimulator generator Rheos® System device
Stimulator Generator, Multiple Array for Insertion in Subcutaneous Tissue and Fascia	**Includes:** Activa PC neurostimulator Enterra gastric neurostimulator Neurostimulator generator, multiple channel PrimeAdvanced neurostimulator (SureScan)(MRI Safe)
Stimulator Generator, Multiple Array Rechargeable for Insertion in Subcutaneous Tissue and Fascia	**Includes:** Activa RC neurostimulator Neurostimulator generator, multiple channel rechargeable RestoreAdvanced neurostimulator (SureScan)(MRI Safe) RestoreSensor neurostimulator (SureScan)(MRI Safe) RestoreUltra neurostimulator (SureScan)(MRI Safe)
Stimulator Generator, Single Array for Insertion in Subcutaneous Tissue and Fascia	**Includes:** Activa SC neurostimulator InterStim® Therapy neurostimulator Itrel (3)(4) neurostimulator Neurostimulator generator, single channel
Stimulator Generator, Single Array Rechargeable for Insertion in Subcutaneous Tissue and Fascia	**Includes:** Neurostimulator generator, single channel rechargeable
Stimulator Lead in Gastrointestinal System	**Includes:** Gastric electrical stimulation (GES) lead Gastric pacemaker lead
Stimulator Lead in Muscles	**Includes:** Electrical muscle stimulation (EMS) lead Electronic muscle stimulator lead Neuromuscular electrical stimulation (NEMS) lead
Stimulator Lead in Upper Arteries	**Includes:** Baroreflex Activation Therapy® (BAT®) Carotid (artery) sinus (baroreceptor) lead Rheos® System lead
Stimulator Lead in Urinary System	**Includes:** Sacral nerve modulation (SNM) lead Sacral neuromodulation lead Urinary incontinence stimulator lead
Synthetic Substitute	**Includes:** AbioCor® Total Replacement Heart AMPLATZER® Muscular VSD Occluder Annuloplasty ring Bard® Composix® (E/X) (LP) mesh Bard® Composix® Kugel® patch Bard® Dulex™ mesh Bard® Ventralex™ hernia patch BRYAN® Cervical Disc System Ex-PRESS™ mini glaucoma shunt Flexible Composite Mesh GORE® DUALMESH® Holter valve ventricular shunt MitraClip valve repair system Nitinol framed polymer mesh Open Pivot (mechanical) valve Open Pivot Aortic Valve Graft (AVG) Partially absorbable mesh PHYSIOMESH™ Flexible Composite Mesh

Continued on next column

ICD-10-PCS Value	Definition
Synthetic Substitute (continued)	**Includes:** Polymethylmethacrylate (PMMA) Polypropylene mesh PRESTIGE® Cervical Disc PROCEED™ Ventral Patch Prodisc-C Prodisc-L PROLENE Polypropylene Hernia System (PHS) Rebound HRD® (Hernia Repair Device) SynCardia Total Artificial Heart Total artificial (replacement) heart ULTRAPRO Hernia System (UHS) ULTRAPRO Partially Absorbable Lightweight Mesh ULTRAPRO Plug Ventrio™ Hernia Patch Zimmer® NexGen® LPS Mobile Bearing Knee Zimmer® NexGen® LPS-Flex Mobile Knee
Synthetic Substitute, Ceramic for Replacement in Lower Joints	**Includes:** Ceramic on ceramic bearing surface Novation® Ceramic AHS® (Articulation Hip System)
Synthetic Substitute, Intraocular Telescope for Replacement in Eye	**Includes:** Implantable Miniature Telescope™ (IMT)
Synthetic Substitute, Metal for Replacement in Lower Joints	**Includes:** Cobalt/chromium head and socket Metal on metal bearing surface
Synthetic Substitute, Metal on Polyethylene for Replacement in Lower Joints	**Includes:** Cobalt/chromium head and polyethylene socket
Synthetic Substitute, Oxidized Zirconium on Polyethylene for Replacement in Lower Joints	**Includes:** OXINIUM
Synthetic Substitute, Polyethylene for Replacement in Lower Joints	**Includes:** Polyethylene socket
Synthetic Substitute, Reverse Ball and Socket for Replacement in Upper Joints	**Includes:** Delta III Reverse shoulder prosthesis Reverse® Shoulder Prosthesis
Tissue Expander in Skin and Breast	**Includes:** Tissue expander (inflatable) (injectable)

ICD-10-PCS Value	Definition
Tissue Expander in Subcutaneous Tissue and Fascia	**Includes:** Tissue expander (inflatable) (injectable)
Tracheostomy Device in Respiratory System	**Includes:** Tracheostomy tube
Vascular Access Device, Totally Implantable in Subcutaneous Tissue and Fascia	**Includes:** Implanted (venous)(access) port Injection reservoir, port Subcutaneous injection reservoir, port
Vascular Access Device, Tunneled in Subcutaneous Tissue and Fascia	**Includes:** Tunneled central venous catheter Vectra® Vascular Access Graft
Zooplastic Tissue in Heart and Great Vessels	**Includes:** 3f (Aortic) Bioprosthesis valve Bovine pericardial valve Bovine pericardium graft Contegra Pulmonary Valved Conduit CoreValve transcatheter aortic valve Epic™ Stented Tissue Valve (aortic) Freestyle (Stentless) Aortic Root Bioprosthesis Hancock Bioprosthesis (aortic) (mitral) valve Hancock Bioprosthetic Valved Conduit Melody® transcatheter pulmonary valve Mitroflow® Aortic Pericardial Heart Valve Mosaic Bioprosthesis (aortic) (mitral) valve Porcine (bioprosthetic) valve SAPIEN transcatheter aortic valve SJM Biocor® Stented Valve System Stented tissue valve Trifecta™ Valve (aortic) Xenograft
Zooplastic Tissue, Rapid Deployment Technique in New Technology	**Includes:** EDWARDS INTUITY Elite valve system INTUITY Elite valve system, EDWARDS Perceval sutureless valve Sutureless valve, Perceval

Appendix H: Substance Key/Substance Definitions

Substance Key

This table crosswalks a specific substance, listed by trade name or synonym, to the PCS value that would be used to represent that substance in either the Administration or New Technology section. The ICD-10-PCS value may be located in either the 6th-character Substance column or the 7th-character Qualifier column depending on the section/table to which it is classified. The most specific character is listed in the table.

Trade Name or Synonym	ICD-10-PCS Value	PCS Section
AIGISRx Antibacterial Envelope	Anti-Infective Envelope (A)	Administration (3)
Angiotensin II	Synthetic Human Angiotensin II	New technology (X)
Antimicrobial envelope	Anti-Infective Envelope (A)	Administration (3)
Axicabtagene Ciloeucel	Engineered Autologous Chimeric Antigen Receptor T-cell Immunotherapy (C)	New technology (X)
Bone morphogenetic protein 2 (BMP 2)	Recombinant Bone Morphogenetic Protein (B)	Administration (3)
CBMA (Concentrated Bone Marrow Aspirate)	Concentrated Bone Marrow Aspirate (Ø)	New technology (X)
Clolar	Clofarabine (P)	Administration (3)
Defitelio	Defibrotide Sodium Anticoagulant (9)	New technology (X)
DuraGraft® Endothelial Damage Inhibitor	Endothelial Damage Inhibitor (8)	New technology (X)
Factor Xa Inhibitor Reversal Agent, Andexanet Alfa	Andexanet Alfa, Factor Xa Inhibitor Reversal Agent (7)	New technology (X)
GIAPREZA™	Synthetic Human Angiotensin II	New technology (X)
Human angiotensin II, synthetic	Synthetic Human Angiotensin II	New technology (X)
Kcentra	4-Factor Prothrombin Complex Concentrate (B)	Administration (3)
KYMRIAH	Engineered Autologous Chimeric Antigen Receptor T-cell Immunotherapy	New technology (X)
Nesiritide	Human B-type Natriuretic Peptide (H)	Administration (3)
rhBMP-2	Recombinant Bone Morphogenetic Protein (B)	Administration (3)
Seprafilm	Adhesion Barrier (5)	Administration (3)
STELARA®	Other New Technology Therapeutic Substance (F)	New technology (X)
Tisagenlecleucel	Engineered Autologous Chimeric Antigen Receptor T-cell Immunotherapy	New technology (X)
Tissue Plasminogen Activator (tPA)(r- tPA)	Other Thrombolytic (7)	Administration (3)
Ustekinumab	Other New Technology Therapeutic Substance (F)	New technology (X)
Vistogard®	Uridine Triacetate (8)	New technology (X)
Voraxaze	Glucarpidase (Q)	Administration (3)
VYXEOS™	Cytarabine and Daunorubicin Liposome Antineoplastic (B)	New technology (X)
ZINPLAVA™	Bezlotoxumab Monoclonal Antibody (A)	New technology (X)
Zyvox	Oxazolidinones (8)	Administration (3)

Substance Definitions

This table crosswalks a PCS value, used in the Administration or New Technology section, to a specific substance. The specific substances are listed by trade name or synonym. The ICD-10-PCS value may be located in either the 6th-character Substance column or the 7th-character Qualifier column depending on the section/table to which it is classified.

ICD-10-PCS Value	Trade Name or Synonym	PCS Section
4-Factor Prothrombin Complex Concentrate (B)	**Includes:** Kcentra	Administration (3)
Adhesion Barrier (5)	**Includes:** Seprafilm	Administration (3)
Andexanet Alfa, Factor Xa Inhibitor Reversal Agent (7)	**Includes:** Factor Xa Inhibitor Reversal Agent, Andexanet Alfa	New technology (X)
Anti-Infective Envelope (A)	**Includes:** AIGISRx Antibacterial Envelope Antimicrobial envelope	Administration (3)
Bezlotoxumab Monoclonal Antibody (A)	**Includes:** ZINPLAVA™	New technology (X)
Clofarabine (P)	**Includes:** Clolar	Administration (3)
Concentrated Bone Marrow Aspirate (Ø)	**Includes:** CBMA (Concentrated Bone Marrow Aspirate)	New technology (X)
Cytarabine and Daunorubicin Liposome Antineoplastic (B)	**Includes:** VYXEOS™	New technology (X)
Defibrotide Sodium Anticoagulant (9)	**Includes:** Defitelio	New technology (X)
Endothelial Damage Inhibitor (8)	**Includes:** DuraGraft® Endothelial Damage Inhibitor	New technology (X)
Engineered Autologous Chimeric Antigen Receptor T-cell Immunotherapy (C)	**Includes:** Axicabtagene Ciloeucel KYMRIAH Tisagenlecleucel	New technology (X)
Glucarpidase (Q)	**Includes:** Voraxaze	Administration (3)
Human B-type Natriuretic Peptide (H)	**Includes:** Nesiritide	Administration (3)
Other New Technology Therapeutic Substance (F)	**Includes:** STELARA® Ustekinumab	New technology (X)
Other Thrombolytic (7)	**Includes:** Tissue Plasminogen Activator (tPA)(r-tPA)	Administration (3)
Oxazolidinones (8)	**Includes:** Zyvox	Administration (3)
Recombinant Bone Morphogenetic Protein (B)	**Includes:** Bone morphogenetic protein 2 (BMP 2) rhBMP-2	Administration (3)
Synthetic Human Angiotensin II	**Includes:** Angiotensin II GIAPREZA™ Human angiotensin II, synthetic	New technology (X)
Uridine Triacetate (8)	**Includes:** Vistogard®	New technology (X)

Appendix I: Sections B–H Character Definitions

Section B–Imaging

ICD-10-PCS Value (Character 3)	Definition
Computerized Tomography (CT Scan) (2)	Computer reformatted digital display of multiplanar images developed from the capture of multiple exposures of external ionizing radiation
Fluoroscopy (1)	Single plane or bi-plane real time display of an image developed from the capture of external ionizing radiation on a fluorescent screen. The image may also be stored by either digital or analog means.
Magnetic Resonance Imaging (MRI) (3)	Computer reformatted digital display of multiplanar images developed from the capture of radiofrequency signals emitted by nuclei in a body site excited within a magnetic field
Plain Radiography (Ø)	Planar display of an image developed from the capture of external ionizing radiation on photographic or photoconductive plate
Ultrasonography (4)	Real time display of images of anatomy or flow information developed from the capture of reflected and attenuated high frequency sound waves

Section C–Nuclear Medicine

ICD-10-PCS Value (Character 3)	Definition
Nonimaging Nuclear Medicine Assay (6)	Introduction of radioactive materials into the body for the study of body fluids and blood elements, by the detection of radioactive emissions
Nonimaging Nuclear Medicine Probe (5)	Introduction of radioactive materials into the body for the study of distribution and fate of certain substances by the detection of radioactive emissions; or, alternatively, measurement of absorption of radioactive emissions from an external source
Nonimaging Nuclear Medicine Uptake (4)	Introduction of radioactive materials into the body for measurements of organ function, from the detection of radioactive emissions
Planar Nuclear Medicine Imaging (1)	Introduction of radioactive materials into the body for single plane display of images developed from the capture of radioactive emissions
Positron Emission Tomographic (PET) Imaging (3)	Introduction of radioactive materials into the body for three dimensional display of images developed from the simultaneous capture, 18Ø degrees apart, of radioactive emissions
Systemic Nuclear Medicine Therapy (7)	Introduction of unsealed radioactive materials into the body for treatment
Tomographic (Tomo) Nuclear Medicine Imaging (2)	Introduction of radioactive materials into the body for three dimensional display of images developed from the capture of radioactive emissions

Section F–Physical Rehabilitation and Diagnostic Audiology

ICD-10-PCS Value (Character 3)	Definition
Activities of Daily Living Assessment (2)	Measurement of functional level for activities of daily living
Activities of Daily Living Treatment (8)	Exercise or activities to facilitate functional competence for activities of daily living
Caregiver Training (F)	Training in activities to support patient's optimal level of function
Cochlear Implant Treatment (B)	Application of techniques to improve the communication abilities of individuals with cochlear implant
Device Fitting (D)	Fitting of a device designed to facilitate or support achievement of a higher level of function
Hearing Aid Assessment (4)	Measurement of the appropriateness and/or effectiveness of a hearing device
Hearing Assessment (3)	Measurement of hearing and related functions
Hearing Treatment (9)	Application of techniques to improve, augment, or compensate for hearing and related functional impairment
Motor and/or Nerve Function Assessment (1)	Measurement of motor, nerve, and related functions
Motor Treatment (7)	Exercise or activities to increase or facilitate motor function

Continued on next page

Section F–Physical Rehabilitation and Diagnostic Audiology

Continued from previous page

ICD-10-PCS Value (Character 3)	Definition
Speech Assessment (Ø)	Measurement of speech and related functions
Speech Treatment (6)	Application of techniques to improve, augment, or compensate for speech and related functional impairment
Vestibular Assessment (5)	Measurement of the vestibular system and related functions
Vestibular Treatment (C)	Application of techniques to improve, augment, or compensate for vestibular and related functional impairment

Section F–Physical Rehabilitation and Diagnostic Audiology

ICD-10-PCS Value Qualifier (Character 5)	Definition
Acoustic Reflex Decay (J)	Measures reduction in size/strength of acoustic reflex over time Includes/Examples: Includes site of lesion test
Acoustic Reflex Patterns (G)	Defines site of lesion based upon presence/absence of acoustic reflexes with ipsilateral vs. contralateral stimulation
Acoustic Reflex Threshold (H)	Determines minimal intensity that acoustic reflex occurs with ipsilateral and/or contralateral stimulation
Aerobic Capacity and Endurance (7)	Measures autonomic responses to positional changes; perceived exertion, dyspnea or angina during activity; performance during exercise protocols; standard vital signs; and blood gas analysis or oxygen consumption
Alternate Binaural or Monaural Loudness Balance (7)	Determines auditory stimulus parameter that yields the same objective sensation Includes/Examples: Sound intensities that yield same loudness perception
Anthropometric Characteristics (B)	Measures edema, body fat composition, height, weight, length and girth
Aphasia (Assessment) (C)	Measures expressive and receptive speech and language function including reading and writing
Aphasia (Treatment) (3)	Applying techniques to improve, augment, or compensate for receptive/ expressive language impairments
Articulation/Phonology (Assessment) (9)	Measures speech production
Articulation/Phonology (Treatment) (4)	Applying techniques to correct, improve, or compensate for speech productive impairment
Assistive Listening Device (5)	Assists in use of effective and appropriate assistive listening device/system
Assistive Listening System/Device Selection (4)	Measures the effectiveness and appropriateness of assistive listening systems/devices
Assistive, Adaptive, Supportive or Protective Devices (9)	Explanation: Devices to facilitate or support achievement of a higher level of function in wheelchair mobility; bed mobility; transfer or ambulation ability; bath and showering ability; dressing; grooming; personal hygiene; play or leisure
Auditory Evoked Potentials (L)	Measures electric responses produced by the VIIIth cranial nerve and brainstem following auditory stimulation
Auditory Processing (Assessment) (Q)	Evaluates ability to receive and process auditory information and comprehension of spoken language
Auditory Processing (Treatment) (2)	Applying techniques to improve the receiving and processing of auditory information and comprehension of spoken language
Augmentative/Alternative Communication System (Assessment) (L)	Determines the appropriateness of aids, techniques, symbols, and/or strategies to augment or replace speech and enhance communication Includes/Examples: Includes the use of telephones, writing equipment, emergency equipment, and TDD
Augmentative/Alternative Communication System (Treatment) (3)	Includes/Examples: Includes augmentative communication devices and aids
Aural Rehabilitation (5)	Applying techniques to improve the communication abilities associated with hearing loss
Aural Rehabilitation Status (P)	Measures impact of a hearing loss including evaluation of receptive and expressive communication skills
Bathing/Showering (Ø)	Includes/Examples: Includes obtaining and using supplies; soaping, rinsing, and drying body parts; maintaining bathing position; and transferring to and from bathing positions

Continued on next page

Section F–Physical Rehabilitation and Diagnostic Audiology

Continued from previous page

ICD-10-PCS Value Qualifier (Character 5)	Definition
Bathing/Showering Techniques (Ø)	Activities to facilitate obtaining and using supplies, soaping, rinsing and drying body parts, maintaining bathing position, and transferring to and from bathing positions
Bed Mobility (Assessment) (B)	Transitional movement within bed
Bed Mobility (Treatment) (5)	Exercise or activities to facilitate transitional movements within bed
Bedside Swallowing and Oral Function (H)	Includes/Examples: Bedside swallowing includes assessment of sucking, masticating, coughing, and swallowing. Oral function includes assessment of musculature for controlled movements, structures, and functions to determine coordination and phonation.
Bekesy Audiometry (3)	Uses an instrument that provides a choice of discrete or continuously varying pure tones; choice of pulsed or continuous signal
Binaural Electroacoustic Hearing Aid Check (6)	Determines mechanical and electroacoustic function of bilateral hearing aids using hearing aid test box
Binaural Hearing Aid (Assessment) (3)	Measures the candidacy, effectiveness, and appropriateness of a hearing aid Explanation: Measures bilateral fit
Binaural Hearing Aid (Treatment) (2)	Explanation: Assists in achieving maximum understanding and performance
Bithermal, Binaural Caloric Irrigation (Ø)	Measures the rhythmic eye movements stimulated by changing the temperature of the vestibular system
Bithermal, Monaural Caloric Irrigation (1)	Measures the rhythmic eye movements stimulated by changing the temperature of the vestibular system in one ear
Brief Tone Stimuli (R)	Measures specific central auditory process
Cerumen Management (3)	Includes examination of external auditory canal and tympanic membrane and removal of cerumen from external ear canal
Cochlear Implant (Ø)	Measures candidacy for cochlear implant
Cochlear Implant Rehabilitation (Ø)	Applying techniques to improve the communication abilities of individuals with cochlear implant; includes programming the device, providing patients/families with information
Communicative/Cognitive Integration Skills (Assessment) (G)	Measures ability to use higher cortical functions Includes/Examples: Includes orientation, recognition, attention span, initiation and termination of activity, memory, sequencing, categorizing, concept formation, spatial operations, judgment, problem solving, generalization and pragmatic communication
Communicative/Cognitive Integration Skills (Treatment) (6)	Activities to facilitate the use of higher cortical functions Includes/Examples: Includes level of arousal, orientation, recognition, attention span, initiation and termination of activity, memory.sequencing, judgment and problem solving, learning and generalization, and pragmatic communication
Computerized Dynamic Posturography (6)	Measures the status of the peripheral and central vestibular system and the sensory/motor component of balance; evaluates the efficacy of vestibular rehabilitation
Conditioned Play Audiometry (4)	Behavioral measures using nonspeech and speech stimuli to obtain frequency-specific and ear-specific information on auditory status from the patient Explanation: Obtains speech reception threshold by having patient point to pictures of spondaic words
Coordination/Dexterity (Assessment) (3)	Measures large and small muscle groups for controlled goal-directed movements Explanation: Dexterity includes object manipulation
Coordination/Dexterity (Treatment) (2)	Exercise or activities to facilitate gross coordination and fine coordination
Cranial Nerve Integrity (9)	Measures cranial nerve sensory and motor functions, including tastes, smell and facial expression
Dichotic Stimuli (T)	Measures specific central auditory process
Distorted Speech (S)	Measures specific central auditory process
Dix-Hallpike Dynamic (5)	Measures nystagmus following Dix-Hallpike maneuver
Dressing (1)	Includes/Examples: Includes selecting clothing and accessories, obtaining clothing from storage, dressing, fastening and adjusting clothing and shoes, and applying and removing personal devices, prosthesis or orthosis

Continued on next page

Section F–Physical Rehabilitation and Diagnostic Audiology

Continued from previous page

ICD-10-PCS Value Qualifier (Character 5)	Definition
Dressing Techniques (1)	Activities to facilitate selecting clothing and accessories, dressing and undressing, adjusting clothing and shoes, applying and removing devices, prostheses or orthoses
Dynamic Orthosis (6)	Includes/Examples: Includes customized and prefabricated splints, inhibitory casts, spinal and other braces, and protective devices; allows motion through transfer of movement from other body parts or by use of outside forces
Ear Canal Probe Microphone (1)	Real ear measures
Ear Protector Attentuation (7)	Measures ear protector fit and effectiveness
Electrocochleography (K)	Measures the VIIIth cranial nerve action potential
Environmental, Home, Work Barriers (B)	Measures current and potential barriers to optimal function, including safety hazards, access problems and home or office design
Ergonomics and Body Mechanics (C)	Ergonomic measurement of job tasks, work hardening or work conditioning needs; functional capacity; and body mechanics
Eustachian Tube Function (F)	Measures eustachian tube function and patency of eustachian tube
Evoked Otoacoustic Emissions, Diagnostic (N)	Measures auditory evoked potentials in a diagnostic format
Evoked Otoacoustic Emissions, Screening (M)	Measures auditory evoked potentials in a screening format
Facial Nerve Function (7)	Measures electrical activity of the VIIth cranial nerve (facial nerve)
Feeding/Eating (Assessment) (2)	Includes/Examples: Includes setting up food, selecting and using utensils and tableware, bringing food or drink to mouth, cleaning face, hands, and clothing, and management of alternative methods of nourishment
Feeding/Eating (Treatment) (3)	Exercise or activities to facilitate setting up food, selecting and using utensils and tableware, bringing food or drink to mouth, cleaning face, hands, and clothing, and management of alternative methods of nourishment
Filtered Speech (Ø)	Uses high or low pass filtered speech stimuli to assess central auditory processing disorders, site of lesion testing
Fluency (Assessment) (D)	Measures speech fluency or stuttering
Fluency (Treatment) (7)	Applying techniques to improve and augment fluent speech
Gait and/or Balance (D)	Measures biomechanical, arthrokinematic and other spatial and temporal characteristics of gait and balance
Gait Training/Functional Ambulation (9)	Exercise or activities to facilitate ambulation on a variety of surfaces and in a variety of environments
Grooming/Personal Hygiene (Assessment) (3)	Includes/Examples: Includes ability to obtain and use supplies in a sequential fashion, general grooming, oral hygiene, toilet hygiene, personal care devices, including care for artificial airways
Grooming/Personal Hygiene (Treatment) (2)	Activities to facilitate obtaining and using supplies in a sequential fashion: general grooming, oral hygiene, toilet hygiene, cleaning body, and personal care devices, including artificial airways
Hearing and Related Disorders Counseling (Ø)	Provides patients/families/caregivers with information, support, referrals to facilitate recovery from a communication disorder Includes/Examples: Includes strategies for psychosocial adjustment to hearing loss for clients and families/caregivers
Hearing and Related Disorders Prevention (1)	Provides patients/families/caregivers with information and support to prevent communication disorders
Hearing Screening (Ø)	Pass/refer measures designed to identify need for further audiologic assessment
Home Management (Assessment) (4)	Obtaining and maintaining personal and household possessions and environment Includes/Examples: Includes clothing care, cleaning, meal preparation and cleanup, shopping, money management, household maintenance, safety procedures, and childcare/parenting
Home Management (Treatment) (4)	Activities to facilitate obtaining and maintaining personal household possessions and environment Includes/Examples: Includes clothing care, cleaning, meal preparation and clean-up, shopping, money management, household maintenance, safety procedures, childcare/parenting

Continued on next page

Section F–Physical Rehabilitation and Diagnostic Audiology

Continued from previous page

ICD-10-PCS Value Qualifier (Character 5)	Definition
Instrumental Swallowing and Oral Function (J)	Measures swallowing function using instrumental diagnostic procedures Explanation: Methods include videofluoroscopy, ultrasound, manometry, endoscopy
Integumentary Integrity (1)	Includes/Examples: Includes burns, skin conditions, ecchymosis, bleeding, blisters, scar tissue, wounds and other traumas, tissue mobility, turgor and texture
Manual Therapy Techniques (7)	Techniques in which the therapist uses his/her hands to administer skilled movements Includes/Examples: Includes connective tissue massage, joint mobilization and manipulation, manual lymph drainage, manual traction, soft tissue mobilization and manipulation
Masking Patterns (W)	Measures central auditory processing status
Monaural Electroacoustic Hearing Aid Check (8)	Determines mechanical and electroacoustic function of one hearing aid using hearing aid test box
Monaural Hearing Aid (Assessment) (2)	Measures the candidacy, effectiveness, and appropriateness of a hearing aid Explanation: Measures unilateral fit
Monaural Hearing Aid (Treatment) (1)	Explanation: Assists in achieving maximum understanding and performance
Motor Function (Assessment) (4)	Measures the body's functional and versatile movement patterns Includes/Examples: Includes motor assessment scales, analysis of head, trunk and limb movement, and assessment of motor learning
Motor Function (Treatment) (3)	Exercise or activities to facilitate crossing midline, laterality, bilateral integration, praxis, neuromuscular relaxation, inhibition, facilitation, motor function and motor learning
Motor Speech (Assessment) (B)	Measures neurological motor aspects of speech production
Motor Speech (Treatment) (8)	Applying techniques to improve and augment the impaired neurological motor aspects of speech production
Muscle Performance (Assessment) (Ø)	Measures muscle strength, power and endurance using manual testing, dynamometry or computer-assisted electromechanical muscle test; functional muscle strength, power and endurance; muscle pain, tone, or soreness; or pelvic-floor musculature Explanation: Muscle endurance refers to the ability to contract a muscle repeatedly over time
Muscle Performance (Treatment) (1)	Exercise or activities to increase the capacity of a muscle to do work in terms of strength, power, and/or endurance Explanation: Muscle strength is the force exerted to overcome resistance in one maximal effort. Muscle power is work produced per unit of time, or the product of strength and speed. Muscle endurance is the ability to contract a muscle repeatedly over time.
Neuromotor Development (D)	Measures motor development, righting and equilibrium reactions, and reflex and equilibrium reactions
Non-invasive Instrumental Status (N)	Instrumental measures of oral, nasal, vocal, and velopharyngeal functions as they pertain to speech production
Nonspoken Language (Assessment) (7)	Measures nonspoken language (print, sign, symbols) for communication
Nonspoken Language (Treatment) (Ø)	Applying techniques that improve, augment, or compensate spoken communication
Oral Peripheral Mechanism (P)	Structural measures of face, jaw, lips, tongue, teeth, hard and soft palate, pharynx as related to speech production
Orofacial Myofunctional (Assessment) (K)	Measures orofacial myofunctional patterns for speech and related functions
Orofacial Myofunctional (Treatment) (9)	Applying techniques to improve, alter, or augment impaired orofacial myofunctional patterns and related speech production errors
Oscillating Tracking (3)	Measures ability to visually track
Pain (F)	Measures muscle soreness, pain and soreness with joint movement, and pain perception Includes/Examples: Includes questionnaires, graphs, symptom magnification scales or visual analog scales
Perceptual Processing (Assessment) (5)	Measures stereognosis, kinesthesia, body schema, right-left discrimination, form constancy, position in space, visual closure, figure-ground, depth perception, spatial relations and topographical orientation

Continued on next page

Section F–Physical Rehabilitation and Diagnostic Audiology

Continued from previous page

ICD-10-PCS Value Qualifier (Character 5)	Definition
Perceptual Processing (Treatment) (1)	Exercise and activities to facilitate perceptual processing Explanation: Includes stereognosis, kinesthesia, body schema, right-left discrimination, form constancy, position in space, visual closure, figure-ground, depth perception, spatial relations, and topographical orientation Includes/Examples: Includes stereognosis, kinesthesia, body schema, right-left discrimination, form constancy, position in space, visual closure, figure-ground, depth perception, spatial relations, and topographical orientation
Performance Intensity Phonetically Balanced Speech Discrimination (Q)	Measures word recognition over varying intensity levels
Postural Control (3)	Exercise or activities to increase postural alignment and control
Prosthesis (8)	Explanation: Artificial substitutes for missing body parts that augment performance or function Includes/Examples: Limb prosthesis, ocular prosthesis
Psychosocial Skills (Assessment) (6)	The ability to interact in society and to process emotions Includes/Examples: Includes psychological (values, interests, self-concept); social (role performance, social conduct, interpersonal skills, self expression); self-management (coping skills, time management, self-control)
Psychosocial Skills (Treatment) (6)	The ability to interact in society and to process emotions Includes/Examples: Includes psychological (values, interests, self-concept); social (role performance, social conduct, interpersonal skills, self expression); self-management (coping skills, time management, self-control)
Pure Tone Audiometry, Air (1)	Air-conduction pure tone threshold measures with appropriate masking
Pure Tone Audiometry, Air and Bone (2)	Air-conduction and bone-conduction pure tone threshold measures with appropriate masking
Pure Tone Stenger (C)	Measures unilateral nonorganic hearing loss based on simultaneous presentation of pure tones of differing volume
Range of Motion and Joint Integrity (5)	Measures quantity, quality, grade, and classification of joint movement and/or mobility Explanation: Range of Motion is the space, distance or angle through which movement occurs at a joint or series of joints. Joint integrity is the conformance of joints to expected anatomic, biomechanical and kinematic norms.
Range of Motion and Joint Mobility (Ø)	Exercise or activities to increase muscle length and joint mobility
Receptive/Expressive Language (Assessment) (8)	Measures receptive and expressive language
Receptive/Expressive Language (Treatment) (B)	Applying techniques to improve and augment receptive/expressive language
Reflex Integrity (G)	Measures the presence, absence, or exaggeration of developmentally appropriate, pathologic or normal reflexes
Select Picture Audiometry (5)	Establishes hearing threshold levels for speech using pictures
Sensorineural Acuity Level (4)	Measures sensorineural acuity masking presented via bone conduction
Sensory Aids (5)	Determines the appropriateness of a sensory prosthetic device, other than a hearing aid or assistive listening system/device
Sensory Awareness/ Processing/ Integrity (6)	Includes/Examples: Includes light touch, pressure, temperature, pain, sharp/dull, proprioception, vestibular, visual, auditory, gustatory, and olfactory
Short Increment Sensitivity Index (9)	Measures the ear's ability to detect small intensity changes; site of lesion test requiring a behavioral response
Sinusoidal Vertical Axis Rotational (4)	Measures nystagmus following rotation
Somatosensory Evoked Potentials (9)	Measures neural activity from sites throughout the body
Speech/Language Screening (6)	Identifies need for further speech and/or language evaluation
Speech Threshold (1)	Measures minimal intensity needed to repeat spondaic words

Continued on next page

Section F–Physical Rehabilitation and Diagnostic Audiology

Continued from previous page

ICD-10-PCS Value Qualifier (Character 5)	Definition
Speech-Language Pathology and Related Disorders Counseling (1)	Provides patients/families with information, support, referrals to facilitate recovery from a communication disorder
Speech-Language Pathology and Related Disorders Prevention (2)	Applying techniques to avoid or minimize onset and/or development of a communication disorder
Speech/Word Recognition (2)	Measures ability to repeat/identify single syllable words; scores given as a percentage; includes word recognition/speech discrimination
Staggered Spondaic Word (3)	Measures central auditory processing site of lesion based upon dichotic presentation of spondaic words
Static Orthosis (7)	Includes/Examples: Includes customized and prefabricated splints, inhibitory casts, spinal and other braces, and protective devices; has no moving parts, maintains joint(s) in desired position
Stenger (B)	Measures unilateral nonorganic hearing loss based on simultaneous presentation of signals of differing volume
Swallowing Dysfunction (D)	Activities to improve swallowing function in coordination with respiratory function Includes/Examples: Includes function and coordination of sucking, mastication, coughing, swallowing
Synthetic Sentence Identification (5)	Measures central auditory dysfunction using identification of third order approximations of sentences and competing messages
Temporal Ordering of Stimuli (V)	Measures specific central auditory process
Therapeutic Exercise (6)	Exercise or activities to facilitate sensory awareness, sensory processing, sensory integration, balance training, conditioning, reconditioning Includes/Examples: Includes developmental activities, breathing exercises, aerobic endurance activities, aquatic exercises, stretching and ventilatory muscle training
Tinnitus Masker (Assessment) (7)	Determines candidacy for tinnitus masker
Tinnitus Masker (Treatment) (Ø)	Explanation: Used to verify physical fit, acoustic appropriateness, and benefit; assists in achieving maximum benefit
Tone Decay (8)	Measures decrease in hearing sensitivity to a tone; site of lesion test requiring a behavioral response
Transfer (C)	Transitional movement from one surface to another
Transfer Training (8)	Exercise or activities to facilitate movement from one surface to another
Tympanometry (D)	Measures the integrity of the middle ear; measures ease at which sound flows through the tympanic membrane while air pressure against the membrane is varied
Unithermal Binaural Screen (2)	Measures the rhythmic eye movements stimulated by changing the temperature of the vestibular system in both ears using warm water, screening format
Ventilation/Respiration/Circulation (G)	Measures ventilatory muscle strength, power and endurance, pulmonary function and ventilatory mechanics Includes/Examples: Includes ability to clear airway, activities that aggravate or relieve edema, pain, dyspnea or other symptoms, chest wall mobility, cardiopulmonary response to performance of ADL and IAD, cough and sputum, standard vital signs
Vestibular (Ø)	Applying techniques to compensate for balance disorders; includes habituation, exercise therapy, and balance retraining
Visual Motor Integration (Assessment) (2)	Coordinating the interaction of information from the eyes with body movement during activity
Visual Motor Integration (Treatment) (2)	Exercise or activities to facilitate coordinating the interaction of information from eyes with body movement during activity
Visual Reinforcement Audiometry (6)	Behavioral measures using nonspeech and speech stimuli to obtain frequency/ear-specific information on auditory status Includes/Examples: Includes a conditioned response of looking toward a visual reinforcer (e.g., lights, animated toy) every time auditory stimuli are heard
Vocational Activities and Functional Community or Work Reintegration Skills (Assessment) (H)	Measures environmental, home, work (job/school/play) barriers that keep patients from functioning optimally in their environment Includes/Examples: Includes assessment of vocational skills and interests, environment of work (job/school/play), injury potential and injury prevention or reduction, ergonomic stressors, transportation skills, and ability to access and use community resources

Continued on next page

Section F–Physical Rehabilitation and Diagnostic Audiology

Continued from previous page

ICD-10-PCS Value Qualifier (Character 5)	Definition
Vocational Activities and Functional Community or Work Reintegration Skills (Treatment) (7)	Activities to facilitate vocational exploration, body mechanics training, job acquisition, and environmental or work (job/school/play) task adaptation Includes/Examples: Includes injury prevention and reduction, ergonomic stressor reduction, job coaching and simulation, work hardening and conditioning, driving training, transportation skills, and use of community resources
Voice (Assessment) (F)	Measures vocal structure, function and production
Voice (Treatment) (C)	Applying techniques to improve voice and vocal function
Voice Prosthetic (Assessment) (M)	Determines the appropriateness of voice prosthetic/adaptive device to enhance or facilitate communication
Voice Prosthetic (Treatment) (4)	Includes/Examples: Includes electrolarynx, and other assistive, adaptive, supportive devices
Wheelchair Mobility (Assessment) (F)	Measures fit and functional abilities within wheelchair in a variety of environments
Wheelchair Mobility (Treatment) (4)	Management, maintenance and controlled operation of a wheelchair, scooter or other device, in and on a variety of surfaces and environments
Wound Management (5)	Includes/Examples: Includes non-selective and selective debridement (enzymes, autolysis, sharp debridement), dressings (wound coverings, hydrogel, vacuum-assisted closure), topical agents, etc.

Section G–Mental Health

ICD-10-PCS Value (Character 3)	Definition
Biofeedback (C)	Provision of information from the monitoring and regulating of physiological processes in conjunction with cognitive-behavioral techniques to improve patient functioning or well-being Includes/Examples: Includes EEG, blood pressure, skin temperature or peripheral blood flow, ECG, electrooculogram, EMG, respirometry or capnometry, GSR/EDR, perineometry to monitor/regulate bowel/bladder activity, electrogastrogram to monitor/regulate gastric motility
Counseling (6)	The application of psychological methods to treat an individual with normal developmental issues and psychological problems in order to increase function, improve well-being, alleviate distress, maladjustment or resolve crises
Crisis Intervention (2)	Treatment of a traumatized, acutely disturbed or distressed individual for the purpose of short-term stabilization Includes/Examples: Includes defusing, debriefing, counseling, psychotherapy and/or coordination of care with other providers or agencies
Electroconvulsive Therapy (B)	The application of controlled electrical voltages to treat a mental health disorder Includes/Examples: Includes appropriate sedation and other preparation of the individual
Family Psychotherapy (7)	Treatment that includes one or more family members of an individual with a mental health disorder by behavioral, cognitive, psychoanalytic, psychodynamic or psychophysiological means to improve functioning or well-being Explanation: Remediation of emotional or behavioral problems presented by one or more family members in cases where psychotherapy with more than one family member is indicated
Group Psychotherapy (H)	Treatment of two or more individuals with a mental health disorder by behavioral, cognitive, psychoanalytic, psychodynamic or psychophysiological means to improve functioning or well-being
Hypnosis (F)	Induction of a state of heightened suggestibility by auditory, visual and tactile techniques to elicit an emotional or behavioral response
Individual Psychotherapy (5)	Treatment of an individual with a mental health disorder by behavioral, cognitive, psychoanalytic, psychodynamic or psychophysiological means to improve functioning or well-being
Light Therapy (J)	Application of specialized light treatments to improve functioning or well-being
Medication Management (3)	Monitoring and adjusting the use of medications for the treatment of a mental health disorder
Narcosynthesis (G)	Administration of intravenous barbiturates in order to release suppressed or repressed thoughts
Psychological Tests (1)	The administration and interpretation of standardized psychological tests and measurement instruments for the assessment of psychological function

Continued on next page

Section G–Mental Health

ICD-10-PCS Value Qualifier (Character 4)	Definition
Behavioral (1)	Primarily to modify behavior Includes/Examples: Includes modeling and role playing, positive reinforcement of target behaviors, response cost, and training of self-management skills
Cognitive (2)	Primarily to correct cognitive distortions and errors
Cognitive-Behavioral (8)	Combining cognitive and behavioral treatment strategies to improve functioning Explanation: Maladaptive responses are examined to determine how cognitions relate to behavior patterns in response to an event. Uses learning principles and information-processing models.
Developmental (Ø)	Age-normed developmental status of cognitive, social and adaptive behavior skills
Intellectual and Psychoeducational (2)	Intellectual abilities, academic achievement and learning capabilities (including behaviors and emotional factors affecting learning)
Interactive (Ø)	Uses primarily physical aids and other forms of non-oral interaction with a patient who is physically, psychologically or developmentally unable to use ordinary language for communication Includes/Examples: Includes the use of toys in symbolic play
Interpersonal (3)	Helps an individual make changes in interpersonal behaviors to reduce psychological dysfunction Includes/Examples: Includes exploratory techniques, encouragement of affective expression, clarification of patient statements, analysis of communication patterns, use of therapy relationship and behavior change techniques
Neurobehavioral and Cognitive Status (4)	Includes neurobehavioral status exam, interview(s), and observation for the clinical assessment of thinking, reasoning and judgment, acquired knowledge, attention, memory, visual spatial abilities, language functions, and planning
Neuropsychological (3)	Thinking, reasoning and judgment, acquired knowledge, attention, memory, visual spatial abilities, language functions, planning
Personality and Behavioral (1)	Mood, emotion, behavior, social functioning, psychopathological conditions, personality traits and characteristics
Psychoanalysis (4)	Methods of obtaining a detailed account of past and present mental and emotional experiences to determine the source and eliminate or diminish the undesirable effects of unconscious conflicts Explanation: Accomplished by making the individual aware of their existence, origin, and inappropriate expression in emotions and behavior
Psychodynamic (5)	Exploration of past and present emotional experiences to understand motives and drives using insight-oriented techniques to reduce the undesirable effects of internal conflicts on emotions and behavior Explanation: Techniques include empathetic listening, clarifying self-defeating behavior patterns, and exploring adaptive alternatives
Psychophysiological (9)	Monitoring and alteration of physiological processes to help the individual associate physiological reactions combined with cognitive and behavioral strategies to gain improved control of these processes to help the individual cope more effectively
Supportive (6)	Formation of therapeutic relationship primarily for providing emotional support to prevent further deterioration in functioning during periods of particular stress Explanation: Often used in conjunction with other therapeutic approaches
Vocational (1)	Exploration of vocational interests, aptitudes and required adaptive behavior skills to develop and carry out a plan for achieving a successful vocational placement Includes/Examples: Includes enhancing work related adjustment and/or pursuing viable options in training education or preparation

Section H - Substance Abuse Treatment

ICD-10-PCS Value (Character 3)	Definition
Detoxification Services (2)	Detoxification from alcohol and/or drugs Explanation: Not a treatment modality, but helps the patient stabilize physically and psychologically until the body becomes free of drugs and the effects of alcohol
Family Counseling (6)	The application of psychological methods that includes one or more family members to treat an individual with addictive behavior Explanation: Provides support and education for family members of addicted individuals. Family member participation is seen as a critical area of substance abuse treatment.
Group Counseling (4)	The application of psychological methods to treat two or more individuals with addictive behavior Explanation: Provides structured group counseling sessions and healing power through the connection with others
Individual Counseling (3)	The application of psychological methods to treat an individual with addictive behavior Explanation: Comprised of several different techniques, which apply various strategies to address drug addiction
Individual Psychotherapy (5)	Treatment of an individual with addictive behavior by behavioral, cognitive, psychoanalytic, psychodynamic or psychophysiological means
Medication Management (8)	Monitoring and adjusting the use of replacement medications for the treatment of addiction
Pharmacotherapy (9)	The use of replacement medications for the treatment of addiction

Appendix J: Hospital Acquired Conditions

Hospital-acquired conditions (HACs) are conditions considered reasonably preventable through the application of evidence-based guidelines. Although it is the ICD-10-CM code that drives a HAC designation, in some cases a specific ICD-10-PCS code must also be present before that ICD-10-CM code can be considered a HAC. For example, the yellow color bar identifies ØJH63XZ as a HAC in the tabular section of this manual. In the annotation box below table ØJH it is noted that when the ICD-10-CM code J95.811 is reported as a secondary diagnosis, not present on admission, AND ØJH63XZ is also reported during that same admission, J95.811 would be considered a hospital-acquired condition. This resource provides all 14 HAC categories, as well as the specific ICD-10-CM codes and, when applicable, the specific ICD-10-PCS codes applicable to each category.

Note: The resource used to compile this list is the fiscal 2018 ICD-10 MS-DRG Definitions Manual Files v35. The most current version, v36, of ICD-10 MS-DRG Definitions Manual was not available at the time this book was printed. For the most current files related to IPPS please refer to the following: https://www.cms.gov/Medicare/Medicare-Fee-for-Service-Payment/AcuteInpatientPPS/IPPS-Regulations-and-Notices.html.

HAC 01: Foreign Object Retained After Surgery

Secondary diagnosis not POA:

T81.5ØØA
T81.5Ø1A
T81.5Ø2A
T81.5Ø3A
T81.5Ø4A
T81.5Ø5A
T81.5Ø6A
T81.5Ø7A
T81.5Ø8A
T81.5Ø9A
T81.51ØA
T81.511A
T81.512A
T81.513A
T81.514A
T81.515A
T81.516A
T81.517A
T81.518A
T81.519A
T81.52ØA
T81.521A
T81.522A
T81.523A
T81.524A
T81.525A
T81.526A
T81.527A
T81.528A
T81.529A
T81.53ØA
T81.531A
T81.532A
T81.533A
T81.534A
T81.535A
T81.536A
T81.537A
T81.538A
T81.539A
T81.59ØA
T81.591A
T81.592A
T81.593A
T81.594A
T81.595A
T81.596A
T81.597A
T81.598A
T81.599A
T81.6ØXA
T81.61XA
T81.69XA

HAC 02: Air Embolism

Secondary diagnosis not POA:

T8Ø.ØXXA

HAC 03: Blood Incompatibility

Secondary diagnosis not POA:

T8Ø.3ØXA
T8Ø.31ØA
T8Ø.311A
T8Ø.319A
T8Ø.39XA

HAC 04: Stage III and IV Pressure Ulcers

Secondary diagnosis not POA:

L89.ØØ3
L89.ØØ4
L89.Ø13
L89.Ø14
L89.Ø23
L89.Ø24
L89.1Ø3
L89.1Ø4
L89.113
L89.114
L89.123
L89.124
L89.133
L89.134
L89.143
L89.144
L89.153
L89.154
L89.2Ø3
L89.2Ø4
L89.213
L89.214
L89.223
L89.224
L89.3Ø3
L89.3Ø4
L89.313
L89.314
L89.323
L89.324
L89.43
L89.44
L89.5Ø3
L89.5Ø4
L89.513
L89.514
L89.523
L89.524
L89.6Ø3
L89.6Ø4
L89.613
L89.614
L89.623
L89.624
L89.813
L89.814
L89.893
L89.894
L89.93
L89.94

HAC 05: Falls and Trauma

Secondary diagnosis not POA:

M99.1Ø
M99.11
M99.18
SØ2.ØXXA
SØ2.ØXXB
SØ2.1Ø1A
SØ2.1Ø1B
SØ2.1Ø2A
SØ2.1Ø2B
SØ2.1Ø9A
SØ2.1Ø9B
SØ2.11ØA
SØ2.11ØB
SØ2.111A
SØ2.111B
SØ2.112A
SØ2.112B
SØ2.113A
SØ2.113B
SØ2.118A
SØ2.118B
SØ2.119A
SØ2.119B
SØ2.11AA
SØ2.11AB
SØ2.11BA
SØ2.11BB
SØ2.11CA
SØ2.11CB
SØ2.11DA
SØ2.11DB
SØ2.11EA
SØ2.11EB
SØ2.11FA
SØ2.11FB
SØ2.11GA
SØ2.11GB
SØ2.11HA
SØ2.11HB
SØ2.19XA
SØ2.19XB
SØ2.2XXB
SØ2.3ØXA
SØ2.3ØXB
SØ2.31XA
SØ2.31XB
SØ2.32XA
SØ2.32XB
SØ2.4ØØA
SØ2.4ØØB
SØ2.4Ø1A
SØ2.4Ø1B
SØ2.4Ø2A
SØ2.4Ø2B
SØ2.4ØAA
SØ2.4ØAB
SØ2.4ØBA
SØ2.4ØBB
SØ2.4ØCA
SØ2.4ØCB
SØ2.4ØDA
SØ2.4ØDB
SØ2.4ØEA
SØ2.4ØEB
SØ2.4ØFA
SØ2.4ØFB
SØ2.411A
SØ2.411B
SØ2.412A
SØ2.412B
SØ2.413A
SØ2.413B
SØ2.42XA
SØ2.42XB
SØ2.6ØØA
SØ2.6ØØB
SØ2.6Ø1A
SØ2.6Ø1B
SØ2.6Ø2A
SØ2.6Ø2B
SØ2.6Ø9A
SØ2.6Ø9B
SØ2.61ØA
SØ2.61ØB
SØ2.611A
SØ2.611B
SØ2.612A
SØ2.612B
SØ2.62ØA
SØ2.62ØB
SØ2.621A
SØ2.621B
SØ2.622A
SØ2.622B
SØ2.63ØA
SØ2.63ØB
SØ2.631A
SØ2.631B
SØ2.632A
SØ2.632B
SØ2.64ØA
SØ2.64ØB
SØ2.641A
SØ2.641B
SØ2.642A
SØ2.642B
SØ2.65ØA
SØ2.65ØB
SØ2.651A
SØ2.651B
SØ2.652A
SØ2.652B
SØ2.66XA
SØ2.66XB
SØ2.67ØA
SØ2.67ØB
SØ2.671A
SØ2.671B
SØ2.672A
SØ2.672B
SØ2.69XA
SØ2.69XB
SØ2.8ØXA
SØ2.8ØXB
SØ2.81XA
SØ2.81XB
SØ2.82XA
SØ2.82XB
SØ2.91XA
SØ2.91XB
SØ2.92XA
SØ2.92XB
SØ6.ØX1A
SØ6.ØX9A
SØ6.1X1A
SØ6.1X2A
SØ6.1X3A
SØ6.1X4A
SØ6.1X5A
SØ6.1X6A
SØ6.1X7A
SØ6.1X8A
SØ6.1X9A
SØ6.2X1A
SØ6.2X2A
SØ6.2X3A
SØ6.2X4A
SØ6.2X5A
SØ6.2X6A
SØ6.2X7A
SØ6.2X8A
SØ6.2X9A
SØ6.3Ø1A
SØ6.3Ø2A
SØ6.3Ø3A
SØ6.3Ø4A
SØ6.3Ø5A
SØ6.3Ø6A
SØ6.3Ø7A
SØ6.3Ø8A
SØ6.3Ø9A
SØ6.31ØA
SØ6.311A
SØ6.312A
SØ6.313A
SØ6.314A
SØ6.315A
SØ6.316A
SØ6.317A
SØ6.318A
SØ6.319A
SØ6.32ØA
SØ6.321A
SØ6.322A
SØ6.323A
SØ6.324A
SØ6.325A
SØ6.326A
SØ6.327A
SØ6.328A
SØ6.329A
SØ6.33ØA
SØ6.331A
SØ6.332A
SØ6.333A
SØ6.334A
SØ6.335A
SØ6.336A
SØ6.337A
SØ6.338A
SØ6.339A
SØ6.34ØA
SØ6.341A
SØ6.342A
SØ6.343A
SØ6.344A
SØ6.345A
SØ6.346A
SØ6.347A
SØ6.348A
SØ6.349A
SØ6.35ØA
SØ6.351A
SØ6.352A
SØ6.353A
SØ6.354A
SØ6.355A
SØ6.356A
SØ6.357A
SØ6.358A
SØ6.359A
SØ6.36ØA
SØ6.361A
SØ6.362A
SØ6.363A
SØ6.364A
SØ6.365A
SØ6.366A
SØ6.367A
SØ6.368A
SØ6.369A

HAC 05: Falls and Trauma (continued)

SØ6.37ØA
SØ6.371A
SØ6.372A
SØ6.373A
SØ6.374A
SØ6.375A
SØ6.376A
SØ6.377A
SØ6.378A
SØ6.379A
SØ6.38ØA
SØ6.381A
SØ6.382A
SØ6.383A
SØ6.384A
SØ6.385A
SØ6.386A
SØ6.387A
SØ6.388A
SØ6.389A
SØ6.4XØA
SØ6.4X1A
SØ6.4X2A
SØ6.4X3A
SØ6.4X4A
SØ6.4X5A
SØ6.4X6A
SØ6.4X7A
SØ6.4X8A
SØ6.4X9A
SØ6.5XØA
SØ6.5X1A
SØ6.5X2A
SØ6.5X3A
SØ6.5X4A
SØ6.5X5A
SØ6.5X6A
SØ6.5X7A
SØ6.5X8A
SØ6.5X9A
SØ6.6XØA
SØ6.6X1A
SØ6.6X2A
SØ6.6X3A
SØ6.6X4A
SØ6.6X5A
SØ6.6X6A
SØ6.6X7A
SØ6.6X8A
SØ6.6X9A
SØ6.811A
SØ6.812A
SØ6.813A
SØ6.814A
SØ6.815A
SØ6.816A
SØ6.817A
SØ6.818A
SØ6.819A
SØ6.821A
SØ6.822A
SØ6.823A
SØ6.824A
SØ6.825A
SØ6.826A
SØ6.827A
SØ6.828A
SØ6.829A
SØ6.891A
SØ6.892A
SØ6.893A
SØ6.894A
SØ6.895A
SØ6.896A
SØ6.897A
SØ6.898A
SØ6.899A
SØ6.9X1A
SØ6.9X2A
SØ6.9X3A
SØ6.9X4A
SØ6.9X5A
SØ6.9X6A
SØ6.9X7A
SØ6.9X8A
SØ6.9X9A
SØ7.ØXXA
SØ7.1XXA
SØ7.8XXA
SØ7.9XXA
S12.ØØØA
S12.ØØØB
S12.ØØ1A
S12.ØØ1B
S12.Ø1XA
S12.Ø1XB
S12.Ø2XA
S12.Ø2XB
S12.Ø3ØA
S12.Ø3ØB
S12.Ø31A
S12.Ø31B
S12.Ø4ØA
S12.Ø4ØB
S12.Ø41A
S12.Ø41B
S12.Ø9ØA
S12.Ø9ØB
S12.Ø91A
S12.Ø91B
S12.1ØØA
S12.1ØØB
S12.1Ø1A
S12.1Ø1B
S12.11ØA
S12.11ØB
S12.111A
S12.111B
S12.112A
S12.112B
S12.12ØA
S12.12ØB
S12.121A
S12.121B
S12.13ØA
S12.13ØB
S12.131A
S12.131B
S12.14XA
S12.14XB
S12.15ØA
S12.15ØB
S12.151A
S12.151B
S12.19ØA
S12.19ØB
S12.191A
S12.191B
S12.2ØØA
S12.2ØØB
S12.2Ø1A
S12.2Ø1B
S12.23ØA
S12.23ØB
S12.231A
S12.231B
S12.24XA
S12.24XB
S12.25ØA
S12.25ØB
S12.251A
S12.251B
S12.29ØA
S12.29ØB
S12.291A
S12.291B
S12.3ØØA
S12.3ØØB
S12.3Ø1A
S12.3Ø1B
S12.33ØA
S12.33ØB
S12.331A
S12.331B
S12.34XA
S12.34XB
S12.35ØA
S12.35ØB
S12.351A
S12.351B
S12.39ØA
S12.39ØB
S12.391A
S12.391B
S12.4ØØA
S12.4ØØB
S12.4Ø1A
S12.4Ø1B
S12.43ØA
S12.43ØB
S12.431A
S12.431B
S12.44XA
S12.44XB
S12.45ØA
S12.45ØB
S12.451A
S12.451B
S12.49ØA
S12.49ØB
S12.491A
S12.491B
S12.5ØØA
S12.5ØØB
S12.5Ø1A
S12.5Ø1B
S12.53ØA
S12.53ØB
S12.531A
S12.531B
S12.54XA
S12.54XB
S12.55ØA
S12.55ØB
S12.551A
S12.551B
S12.59ØA
S12.59ØB
S12.591A
S12.591B
S12.6ØØA
S12.6ØØB
S12.6Ø1A
S12.6Ø1B
S12.63ØA
S12.63ØB
S12.631A
S12.631B
S12.64XA
S12.64XB
S12.65ØA
S12.65ØB
S12.651A
S12.651B
S12.69ØA
S12.69ØB
S12.691A
S12.691B
S12.8XXA
S12.9XXA
S13.ØXXA
S13.1ØØA
S13.1Ø1A
S13.11ØA
S13.111A
S13.12ØA
S13.121A
S13.13ØA
S13.131A
S13.14ØA
S13.141A
S13.15ØA
S13.151A
S13.16ØA
S13.161A
S13.17ØA
S13.171A
S13.18ØA
S13.181A
S13.2ØXA
S13.29XA
S14.1Ø1A
S14.1Ø2A
S14.1Ø3A
S14.1Ø4A
S14.1Ø5A
S14.1Ø6A
S14.1Ø7A
S14.111A
S14.112A
S14.113A
S14.114A
S14.115A
S14.116A
S14.117A
S14.121A
S14.122A
S14.123A
S14.124A
S14.125A
S14.126A
S14.127A
S14.131A
S14.132A
S14.133A
S14.134A
S14.135A
S14.136A
S14.137A
S14.151A
S14.152A
S14.153A
S14.154A
S14.155A
S14.156A
S14.157A
S17.ØXXA
S17.8XXA
S17.9XXA
S22.ØØØA
S22.ØØØB
S22.ØØ1A
S22.ØØ1B
S22.ØØ2A
S22.ØØ2B
S22.ØØ8A
S22.ØØ8B
S22.ØØ9A
S22.ØØ9B
S22.Ø1ØA
S22.Ø1ØB
S22.Ø11A
S22.Ø11B
S22.Ø12A
S22.Ø12B
S22.Ø18A
S22.Ø18B
S22.Ø19A
S22.Ø19B
S22.Ø2ØA
S22.Ø2ØB
S22.Ø21A
S22.Ø21B
S22.Ø22A
S22.Ø22B
S22.Ø28A
S22.Ø28B
S22.Ø29A
S22.Ø29B
S22.Ø3ØA
S22.Ø3ØB
S22.Ø31A
S22.Ø31B
S22.Ø32A
S22.Ø32B
S22.Ø38A
S22.Ø38B
S22.Ø39A
S22.Ø39B
S22.Ø4ØA
S22.Ø4ØB
S22.Ø41A
S22.Ø41B
S22.Ø42A
S22.Ø42B
S22.Ø48A
S22.Ø48B
S22.Ø49A
S22.Ø49B
S22.Ø5ØA
S22.Ø5ØB
S22.Ø51A
S22.Ø51B
S22.Ø52A
S22.Ø52B
S22.Ø58A
S22.Ø58B
S22.Ø59A
S22.Ø59B
S22.Ø6ØA
S22.Ø6ØB
S22.Ø61A
S22.Ø61B
S22.Ø62A
S22.Ø62B
S22.Ø68A
S22.Ø68B
S22.Ø69A
S22.Ø69B
S22.Ø7ØA
S22.Ø7ØB
S22.Ø71A
S22.Ø71B
S22.Ø72A
S22.Ø72B
S22.Ø78A
S22.Ø78B
S22.Ø79A
S22.Ø79B
S22.Ø8ØA
S22.Ø8ØB
S22.Ø81A
S22.Ø81B
S22.Ø82A
S22.Ø82B
S22.Ø88A
S22.Ø88B
S22.Ø89A
S22.Ø89B
S22.2ØXA
S22.2ØXB
S22.21XA
S22.21XB
S22.22XA
S22.22XB
S22.23XA
S22.23XB
S22.24XA
S22.24XB
S22.31XA
S22.31XB
S22.32XA
S22.32XB
S22.39XA
S22.39XB
S22.41XA
S22.41XB
S22.42XA
S22.42XB
S22.43XA
S22.43XB
S22.49XA
S22.49XB
S22.5XXA
S22.5XXB
S22.9XXA
S22.9XXB
S24.1Ø1A
S24.1Ø2A
S24.1Ø3A
S24.1Ø4A
S24.111A
S24.112A
S24.113A
S24.114A
S24.131A
S24.132A
S24.133A
S24.134A
S24.151A
S24.152A
S24.153A
S24.154A
S32.ØØØA
S32.ØØØB
S32.ØØ1A
S32.ØØ1B
S32.ØØ2A
S32.ØØ2B
S32.ØØ8A
S32.ØØ8B
S32.ØØ9A
S32.ØØ9B
S32.Ø1ØA
S32.Ø1ØB
S32.Ø11A
S32.Ø11B
S32.Ø12A
S32.Ø12B
S32.Ø18A
S32.Ø18B
S32.Ø19A
S32.Ø19B
S32.Ø2ØA
S32.Ø2ØB
S32.Ø21A
S32.Ø21B
S32.Ø22A
S32.Ø22B
S32.Ø28A
S32.Ø28B
S32.Ø29A
S32.Ø29B
S32.Ø3ØA

HAC 05: Falls and Trauma (continued)

S32.Ø3ØB
S32.Ø31A
S32.Ø31B
S32.Ø32A
S32.Ø32B
S32.Ø38A
S32.Ø38B
S32.Ø39A
S32.Ø39B
S32.Ø4ØA
S32.Ø4ØB
S32.Ø41A
S32.Ø41B
S32.Ø42A
S32.Ø42B
S32.Ø48A
S32.Ø48B
S32.Ø49A
S32.Ø49B
S32.Ø5ØA
S32.Ø5ØB
S32.Ø51A
S32.Ø51B
S32.Ø52A
S32.Ø52B
S32.Ø58A
S32.Ø58B
S32.Ø59A
S32.Ø59B
S32.1ØXA
S32.1ØXB
S32.11ØA
S32.11ØB
S32.111A
S32.111B
S32.112A
S32.112B
S32.119A
S32.119B
S32.12ØA
S32.12ØB
S32.121A
S32.121B
S32.122A
S32.122B
S32.129A
S32.129B
S32.13ØA
S32.13ØB
S32.131A
S32.131B
S32.132A
S32.132B
S32.139A
S32.139B
S32.14XA
S32.14XB
S32.15XA
S32.15XB
S32.16XA
S32.16XB
S32.17XA
S32.17XB
S32.19XA
S32.19XB
S32.2XXA
S32.2XXB
S32.3Ø1A
S32.3Ø1B
S32.3Ø2A
S32.3Ø2B
S32.3Ø9A
S32.3Ø9B
S32.311A
S32.311B
S32.312A
S32.312B
S32.313A
S32.313B
S32.314A
S32.314B
S32.315A
S32.315B
S32.316A
S32.316B
S32.391A
S32.391B
S32.392A
S32.392B
S32.399A
S32.399B
S32.4Ø1A
S32.4Ø1B
S32.4Ø2A
S32.4Ø2B
S32.4Ø9A
S32.4Ø9B
S32.411A
S32.411B
S32.412A
S32.412B
S32.413A
S32.413B
S32.414A
S32.414B
S32.415A
S32.415B
S32.416A
S32.416B
S32.421A
S32.421B
S32.422A
S32.422B
S32.423A
S32.423B
S32.424A
S32.424B
S32.425A
S32.425B
S32.426A
S32.426B
S32.431A
S32.431B
S32.432A
S32.432B
S32.433A
S32.433B
S32.434A
S32.434B
S32.435A
S32.435B
S32.436A
S32.436B
S32.441A
S32.441B
S32.442A
S32.442B
S32.443A
S32.443B
S32.444A
S32.444B
S32.445A
S32.445B
S32.446A
S32.446B
S32.451A
S32.451B
S32.452A
S32.452B
S32.453A
S32.453B
S32.454A
S32.454B
S32.455A
S32.455B
S32.456A
S32.456B
S32.461A
S32.461B
S32.462A
S32.462B
S32.463A
S32.463B
S32.464A
S32.464B
S32.465A
S32.465B
S32.466A
S32.466B
S32.471A
S32.471B
S32.472A
S32.472B
S32.473A
S32.473B
S32.474A
S32.474B
S32.475A
S32.475B
S32.476A
S32.476B
S32.481A
S32.481B
S32.482A
S32.482B
S32.483A
S32.483B
S32.484A
S32.484B
S32.485A
S32.485B
S32.486A
S32.486B
S32.491A
S32.491B
S32.492A
S32.492B
S32.499A
S32.499B
S32.5Ø1A
S32.5Ø1B
S32.5Ø2A
S32.5Ø2B
S32.5Ø9A
S32.5Ø9B
S32.511A
S32.511B
S32.512A
S32.512B
S32.519A
S32.519B
S32.591A
S32.591B
S32.592A
S32.592B
S32.599A
S32.599B
S32.6Ø1A
S32.6Ø1B
S32.6Ø2A
S32.6Ø2B
S32.6Ø9A
S32.6Ø9B
S32.611A
S32.611B
S32.612A
S32.612B
S32.613A
S32.613B
S32.614A
S32.614B
S32.615A
S32.615B
S32.616A
S32.616B
S32.691A
S32.691B
S32.692A
S32.692B
S32.699A
S32.699B
S32.81ØA
S32.81ØB
S32.811A
S32.811B
S32.82XA
S32.82XB
S32.89XA
S32.89XB
S32.9XXA
S32.9XXB
S34.1Ø1A
S34.1Ø2A
S34.1Ø3A
S34.1Ø4A
S34.1Ø5A
S34.1Ø9A
S34.111A
S34.112A
S34.113A
S34.114A
S34.115A
S34.119A
S34.121A
S34.122A
S34.123A
S34.124A
S34.125A
S34.129A
S34.131A
S34.132A
S34.139A
S34.3XXA
S42.ØØ1B
S42.ØØ2B
S42.ØØ9B
S42.Ø11B
S42.Ø12B
S42.Ø13B
S42.Ø14B
S42.Ø15B
S42.Ø16B
S42.Ø17B
S42.Ø18B
S42.Ø19B
S42.Ø21B
S42.Ø22B
S42.Ø23B
S42.Ø24B
S42.Ø25B
S42.Ø26B
S42.Ø31B
S42.Ø32B
S42.Ø33B
S42.Ø34B
S42.Ø35B
S42.Ø36B
S42.1Ø1B
S42.1Ø2B
S42.1Ø9B
S42.111B
S42.112B
S42.113B
S42.114B
S42.115B
S42.116B
S42.121B
S42.122B
S42.123B
S42.124B
S42.125B
S42.126B
S42.131B
S42.132B
S42.133B
S42.134B
S42.135B
S42.136B
S42.141B
S42.142B
S42.143B
S42.144B
S42.145B
S42.146B
S42.151B
S42.152B
S42.153B
S42.154B
S42.155B
S42.156B
S42.191B
S42.192B
S42.199B
S42.2Ø1A
S42.2Ø1B
S42.2Ø2A
S42.2Ø2B
S42.2Ø9A
S42.2Ø9B
S42.211A
S42.211B
S42.212A
S42.212B
S42.213A
S42.213B
S42.214A
S42.214B
S42.215A
S42.215B
S42.216A
S42.216B
S42.221A
S42.221B
S42.222A
S42.222B
S42.223A
S42.223B
S42.224A
S42.224B
S42.225A
S42.225B
S42.226A
S42.226B
S42.231A
S42.231B
S42.232A
S42.232B
S42.239A
S42.239B
S42.241A
S42.241B
S42.242A
S42.242B
S42.249A
S42.249B
S42.251A
S42.251B
S42.252A
S42.252B
S42.253A
S42.253B
S42.254A
S42.254B
S42.255A
S42.255B
S42.256A
S42.256B
S42.261A
S42.261B
S42.262A
S42.262B
S42.263A
S42.263B
S42.264A
S42.264B
S42.265A
S42.265B
S42.266A
S42.266B
S42.271A
S42.272A
S42.279A
S42.291A
S42.291B
S42.292A
S42.292B
S42.293A
S42.293B
S42.294A
S42.294B
S42.295A
S42.295B
S42.296A
S42.296B
S42.3Ø1A
S42.3Ø1B
S42.3Ø2A
S42.3Ø2B
S42.3Ø9A
S42.3Ø9B
S42.311A
S42.312A
S42.319A
S42.321A
S42.321B
S42.322A
S42.322B
S42.323A
S42.323B
S42.324A
S42.324B
S42.325A
S42.325B
S42.326A
S42.326B
S42.331A
S42.331B
S42.332A
S42.332B
S42.333A
S42.333B
S42.334A
S42.334B
S42.335A
S42.335B
S42.336A
S42.336B
S42.341A
S42.341B
S42.342A
S42.342B
S42.343A
S42.343B
S42.344A

HAC 05: Falls and Trauma (continued)

S42.344B
S42.345A
S42.345B
S42.346A
S42.346B
S42.351A
S42.351B
S42.352A
S42.352B
S42.353A
S42.353B
S42.354A
S42.354B
S42.355A
S42.355B
S42.356A
S42.356B
S42.361A
S42.361B
S42.362A
S42.362B
S42.363A
S42.363B
S42.364A
S42.364B
S42.365A
S42.365B
S42.366A
S42.366B
S42.391A
S42.391B
S42.392A
S42.392B
S42.399A
S42.399B
S42.4Ø1A
S42.4Ø1B
S42.4Ø2A
S42.4Ø2B
S42.4Ø9A
S42.4Ø9B
S42.411A
S42.411B
S42.412A
S42.412B
S42.413A
S42.413B
S42.414A
S42.414B
S42.415A
S42.415B
S42.416A
S42.416B
S42.421A
S42.421B
S42.422A
S42.422B
S42.423A
S42.423B
S42.424A
S42.424B
S42.425A
S42.425B
S42.426A
S42.426B
S42.431A
S42.431B
S42.432A
S42.432B
S42.433A
S42.433B
S42.434A
S42.434B
S42.435A
S42.435B
S42.436A
S42.436B
S42.441A
S42.441B
S42.442A
S42.442B
S42.443A
S42.443B
S42.444A
S42.444B
S42.445A
S42.445B
S42.446A
S42.446B
S42.447A
S42.447B
S42.448A
S42.448B
S42.449A
S42.449B
S42.451A
S42.451B
S42.452A
S42.452B
S42.453A
S42.453B
S42.454A
S42.454B
S42.455A
S42.455B
S42.456A
S42.456B
S42.461A
S42.461B
S42.462A
S42.462B
S42.463A
S42.463B
S42.464A
S42.464B
S42.465A
S42.465B
S42.466A
S42.466B
S42.471A
S42.471B
S42.472A
S42.472B
S42.473A
S42.473B
S42.474A
S42.474B
S42.475A
S42.475B
S42.476A
S42.476B
S42.481A
S42.482A
S42.489A
S42.491A
S42.491B
S42.492A
S42.492B
S42.493A
S42.493B
S42.494A
S42.494B
S42.495A
S42.495B
S42.496A
S42.496B
S42.9ØXA
S42.9ØXB
S42.91XA
S42.91XB
S42.92XA
S42.92XB
S43.2Ø1A
S43.2Ø2A
S43.2Ø3A
S43.2Ø4A
S43.2Ø5A
S43.2Ø6A
S43.211A
S43.212A
S43.213A
S43.214A
S43.215A
S43.216A
S43.221A
S43.222A
S43.223A
S43.224A
S43.225A
S43.226A
S49.ØØ1A
S49.ØØ2A
S49.ØØ9A
S49.Ø11A
S49.Ø12A
S49.Ø19A
S49.Ø21A
S49.Ø22A
S49.Ø29A
S49.Ø31A
S49.Ø32A
S49.Ø39A
S49.Ø41A
S49.Ø42A
S49.Ø49A
S49.Ø91A
S49.Ø92A
S49.Ø99A
S49.1Ø1A
S49.1Ø2A
S49.1Ø9A
S49.111A
S49.112A
S49.119A
S49.121A
S49.122A
S49.129A
S49.131A
S49.132A
S49.139A
S49.141A
S49.142A
S49.149A
S49.191A
S49.192A
S49.199A
S52.ØØ1B
S52.ØØ1C
S52.ØØ2B
S52.ØØ2C
S52.ØØ9B
S52.ØØ9C
S52.Ø11A
S52.Ø12A
S52.Ø19A
S52.Ø21B
S52.Ø21C
S52.Ø22B
S52.Ø22C
S52.Ø23B
S52.Ø23C
S52.Ø24B
S52.Ø24C
S52.Ø25B
S52.Ø25C
S52.Ø26B
S52.Ø26C
S52.Ø31B
S52.Ø31C
S52.Ø32B
S52.Ø32C
S52.Ø33B
S52.Ø33C
S52.Ø34B
S52.Ø34C
S52.Ø35B
S52.Ø35C
S52.Ø36B
S52.Ø36C
S52.Ø41B
S52.Ø41C
S52.Ø42B
S52.Ø42C
S52.Ø43B
S52.Ø43C
S52.Ø44B
S52.Ø44C
S52.Ø45B
S52.Ø45C
S52.Ø46B
S52.Ø46C
S52.Ø91B
S52.Ø91C
S52.Ø92B
S52.Ø92C
S52.Ø99B
S52.Ø99C
S52.1Ø1B
S52.1Ø1C
S52.1Ø2B
S52.1Ø2C
S52.1Ø9B
S52.1Ø9C
S52.111A
S52.112A
S52.119A
S52.121B
S52.121C
S52.122B
S52.122C
S52.123B
S52.123C
S52.124B
S52.124C
S52.125B
S52.125C
S52.126B
S52.126C
S52.131B
S52.131C
S52.132B
S52.132C
S52.133B
S52.133C
S52.134B
S52.134C
S52.135B
S52.135C
S52.136B
S52.136C
S52.181B
S52.181C
S52.182B
S52.182C
S52.189B
S52.189C
S52.2Ø1A
S52.2Ø1B
S52.2Ø1C
S52.2Ø2A
S52.2Ø2B
S52.2Ø2C
S52.2Ø9A
S52.2Ø9B
S52.2Ø9C
S52.211A
S52.212A
S52.219A
S52.221A
S52.221B
S52.221C
S52.222A
S52.222B
S52.222C
S52.223A
S52.223B
S52.223C
S52.224A
S52.224B
S52.224C
S52.225A
S52.225B
S52.225C
S52.226A
S52.226B
S52.226C
S52.231A
S52.231B
S52.231C
S52.232A
S52.232B
S52.232C
S52.233A
S52.233B
S52.233C
S52.234A
S52.234B
S52.234C
S52.235A
S52.235B
S52.235C
S52.236A
S52.236B
S52.236C
S52.241A
S52.241B
S52.241C
S52.242A
S52.242B
S52.242C
S52.243A
S52.243B
S52.243C
S52.244A
S52.244B
S52.244C
S52.245A
S52.245B
S52.245C
S52.246A
S52.246B
S52.246C
S52.251A
S52.251B
S52.251C
S52.252A
S52.252B
S52.252C
S52.253A
S52.253B
S52.253C
S52.254A
S52.254B
S52.254C
S52.255A
S52.255B
S52.255C
S52.256A
S52.256B
S52.256C
S52.261A
S52.261B
S52.261C
S52.262A
S52.262B
S52.262C
S52.263A
S52.263B
S52.263C
S52.264A
S52.264B
S52.264C
S52.265A
S52.265B
S52.265C
S52.266A
S52.266B
S52.266C
S52.271B
S52.271C
S52.272B
S52.272C
S52.279B
S52.279C
S52.281A
S52.281B
S52.281C
S52.282A
S52.282B
S52.282C
S52.283A
S52.283B
S52.283C
S52.291A
S52.291B
S52.291C
S52.292A
S52.292B
S52.292C
S52.299A
S52.299B
S52.299C
S52.3Ø1A
S52.3Ø1B
S52.3Ø1C
S52.3Ø2A
S52.3Ø2B
S52.3Ø2C
S52.3Ø9A
S52.3Ø9B
S52.3Ø9C
S52.311A
S52.312A
S52.319A
S52.321A
S52.321B
S52.321C
S52.322A
S52.322B
S52.322C
S52.323A
S52.323B
S52.323C
S52.324A
S52.324B
S52.324C
S52.325A
S52.325B
S52.325C
S52.326A
S52.326B
S52.326C
S52.331A
S52.331B

HAC 05: Falls and Trauma (continued)

S52.331C
S52.332A
S52.332B
S52.332C
S52.333A
S52.333B
S52.333C
S52.334A
S52.334B
S52.334C
S52.335A
S52.335B
S52.335C
S52.336A
S52.336B
S52.336C
S52.341A
S52.341B
S52.341C
S52.342A
S52.342B
S52.342C
S52.343A
S52.343B
S52.343C
S52.344A
S52.344B
S52.344C
S52.345A
S52.345B
S52.345C
S52.346A
S52.346B
S52.346C
S52.351A
S52.351B
S52.351C
S52.352A
S52.352B
S52.352C
S52.353A
S52.353B
S52.353C
S52.354A
S52.354B
S52.354C
S52.355A
S52.355B
S52.355C
S52.356A
S52.356B
S52.356C
S52.361A
S52.361B
S52.361C
S52.362A
S52.362B
S52.362C
S52.363A
S52.363B
S52.363C
S52.364A
S52.364B
S52.364C
S52.365A
S52.365B
S52.365C
S52.366A
S52.366B
S52.366C
S52.371A
S52.371B
S52.371C
S52.372A
S52.372B
S52.372C
S52.379A
S52.379B
S52.379C
S52.381A
S52.381B
S52.381C
S52.382A
S52.382B
S52.382C
S52.389A
S52.389B
S52.389C
S52.391A
S52.391B
S52.391C
S52.392A
S52.392B
S52.392C
S52.399A
S52.399B
S52.399C
S52.5Ø1A
S52.5Ø1B
S52.5Ø1C
S52.5Ø2A
S52.5Ø2B
S52.5Ø2C
S52.5Ø9A
S52.5Ø9B
S52.5Ø9C
S52.511A
S52.511B
S52.511C
S52.512A
S52.512B
S52.512C
S52.513A
S52.513B
S52.513C
S52.514A
S52.514B
S52.514C
S52.515A
S52.515B
S52.515C
S52.516A
S52.516B
S52.516C
S52.521A
S52.522A
S52.529A
S52.531A
S52.531B
S52.531C
S52.532A
S52.532B
S52.532C
S52.539A
S52.539B
S52.539C
S52.541A
S52.541B
S52.541C
S52.542A
S52.542B
S52.542C
S52.549A
S52.549B
S52.549C
S52.551A
S52.551B
S52.551C
S52.552A
S52.552B
S52.552C
S52.559A
S52.559B
S52.559C
S52.561A
S52.561B
S52.561C
S52.562A
S52.562B
S52.562C
S52.569A
S52.569B
S52.569C
S52.571A
S52.571B
S52.571C
S52.572A
S52.572B
S52.572C
S52.579A
S52.579B
S52.579C
S52.591A
S52.591B
S52.591C
S52.592A
S52.592B
S52.592C
S52.599A
S52.599B
S52.599C
S52.6Ø1A
S52.6Ø1B
S52.6Ø1C
S52.6Ø2A
S52.6Ø2B
S52.6Ø2C
S52.6Ø9A
S52.6Ø9B
S52.6Ø9C
S52.611A
S52.611B
S52.611C
S52.612A
S52.612B
S52.612C
S52.613A
S52.613B
S52.613C
S52.614A
S52.614B
S52.614C
S52.615A
S52.615B
S52.615C
S52.616A
S52.616B
S52.616C
S52.621A
S52.622A
S52.629A
S52.691A
S52.691B
S52.691C
S52.692A
S52.692B
S52.692C
S52.699A
S52.699B
S52.699C
S52.9ØXA
S52.9ØXB
S52.9ØXC
S52.91XA
S52.91XB
S52.91XC
S52.92XA
S52.92XB
S52.92XC
S59.ØØ1A
S59.ØØ2A
S59.ØØ9A
S59.Ø11A
S59.Ø12A
S59.Ø19A
S59.Ø21A
S59.Ø22A
S59.Ø29A
S59.Ø31A
S59.Ø32A
S59.Ø39A
S59.Ø41A
S59.Ø42A
S59.Ø49A
S59.Ø91A
S59.Ø92A
S59.Ø99A
S59.2Ø1A
S59.2Ø2A
S59.2Ø9A
S59.211A
S59.212A
S59.219A
S59.221A
S59.222A
S59.229A
S59.231A
S59.232A
S59.239A
S59.241A
S59.242A
S59.249A
S59.291A
S59.292A
S59.299A
S62.ØØ1B
S62.ØØ2B
S62.ØØ9B
S62.Ø11B
S62.Ø12B
S62.Ø13B
S62.Ø14B
S62.Ø15B
S62.Ø16B
S62.Ø21B
S62.Ø22B
S62.Ø23B
S62.Ø24B
S62.Ø25B
S62.Ø26B
S62.Ø31B
S62.Ø32B
S62.Ø33B
S62.Ø34B
S62.Ø35B
S62.Ø36B
S62.1Ø1B
S62.1Ø2B
S62.1Ø9B
S62.111B
S62.112B
S62.113B
S62.114B
S62.115B
S62.116B
S62.121B
S62.122B
S62.123B
S62.124B
S62.125B
S62.126B
S62.131B
S62.132B
S62.133B
S62.134B
S62.135B
S62.136B
S62.141B
S62.142B
S62.143B
S62.144B
S62.145B
S62.146B
S62.151B
S62.152B
S62.153B
S62.154B
S62.155B
S62.156B
S62.161B
S62.162B
S62.163B
S62.164B
S62.165B
S62.166B
S62.171B
S62.172B
S62.173B
S62.174B
S62.175B
S62.176B
S62.181B
S62.182B
S62.183B
S62.184B
S62.185B
S62.186B
S62.2Ø1B
S62.2Ø2B
S62.2Ø9B
S62.211B
S62.212B
S62.213B
S62.221B
S62.222B
S62.223B
S62.224B
S62.225B
S62.226B
S62.231B
S62.232B
S62.233B
S62.234B
S62.235B
S62.236B
S62.241B
S62.242B
S62.243B
S62.244B
S62.245B
S62.246B
S62.251B
S62.252B
S62.253B
S62.254B
S62.255B
S62.256B
S62.291B
S62.292B
S62.299B
S62.3ØØB
S62.3Ø1B
S62.3Ø2B
S62.3Ø3B
S62.3Ø4B
S62.3Ø5B
S62.3Ø6B
S62.3Ø7B
S62.3Ø8B
S62.3Ø9B
S62.31ØB
S62.311B
S62.312B
S62.313B
S62.314B
S62.315B
S62.316B
S62.317B
S62.318B
S62.319B
S62.32ØB
S62.321B
S62.322B
S62.323B
S62.324B
S62.325B
S62.326B
S62.327B
S62.328B
S62.329B
S62.33ØB
S62.331B
S62.332B
S62.333B
S62.334B
S62.335B
S62.336B
S62.337B
S62.338B
S62.339B
S62.34ØB
S62.341B
S62.342B
S62.343B
S62.344B
S62.345B
S62.346B
S62.347B
S62.348B
S62.349B
S62.35ØB
S62.351B
S62.352B
S62.353B
S62.354B
S62.355B
S62.356B
S62.357B
S62.358B
S62.359B
S62.36ØB
S62.361B
S62.362B
S62.363B
S62.364B
S62.365B
S62.366B
S62.367B
S62.368B
S62.369B
S62.39ØB
S62.391B
S62.392B
S62.393B
S62.394B
S62.395B
S62.396B
S62.397B
S62.398B
S62.399B
S62.5Ø1B
S62.5Ø2B
S62.5Ø9B
S62.511B

HAC 05: Falls and Trauma (continued)

S62.512B
S62.513B
S62.514B
S62.515B
S62.516B
S62.521B
S62.522B
S62.523B
S62.524B
S62.525B
S62.526B
S62.600B
S62.601B
S62.602B
S62.603B
S62.604B
S62.605B
S62.606B
S62.607B
S62.608B
S62.609B
S62.610B
S62.611B
S62.612B
S62.613B
S62.614B
S62.615B
S62.616B
S62.617B
S62.618B
S62.619B
S62.620B
S62.621B
S62.622B
S62.623B
S62.624B
S62.625B
S62.626B
S62.627B
S62.628B
S62.629B
S62.630B
S62.631B
S62.632B
S62.633B
S62.634B
S62.635B
S62.636B
S62.637B
S62.638B
S62.639B
S62.640B
S62.641B
S62.642B
S62.643B
S62.644B
S62.645B
S62.646B
S62.647B
S62.648B
S62.649B
S62.650B
S62.651B
S62.652B
S62.653B
S62.654B
S62.655B
S62.656B
S62.657B
S62.658B
S62.659B
S62.660B
S62.661B
S62.662B
S62.663B
S62.664B
S62.665B
S62.666B
S62.667B
S62.668B
S62.669B
S62.90XB
S62.91XB
S62.92XB
S72.001A
S72.001B
S72.001C
S72.002A
S72.002B
S72.002C
S72.009A
S72.009B
S72.009C
S72.011A
S72.011B
S72.011C
S72.012A
S72.012B
S72.012C
S72.019A
S72.019B
S72.019C
S72.021A
S72.021B
S72.021C
S72.022A
S72.022B
S72.022C
S72.023A
S72.023B
S72.023C
S72.024A
S72.024B
S72.024C
S72.025A
S72.025B
S72.025C
S72.026A
S72.026B
S72.026C
S72.031A
S72.031B
S72.031C
S72.032A
S72.032B
S72.032C
S72.033A
S72.033B
S72.033C
S72.034A
S72.034B
S72.034C
S72.035A
S72.035B
S72.035C
S72.036A
S72.036B
S72.036C
S72.041A
S72.041B
S72.041C
S72.042A
S72.042B
S72.042C
S72.043A
S72.043B
S72.043C
S72.044A
S72.044B
S72.044C
S72.045A
S72.045B
S72.045C
S72.046A
S72.046B
S72.046C
S72.051A
S72.051B
S72.051C
S72.052A
S72.052B
S72.052C
S72.059A
S72.059B
S72.059C
S72.061A
S72.061B
S72.061C
S72.062A
S72.062B
S72.062C
S72.063A
S72.063B
S72.063C
S72.064A
S72.064B
S72.064C
S72.065A
S72.065B
S72.065C
S72.066A
S72.066B
S72.066C
S72.091A
S72.091B
S72.091C
S72.092A
S72.092B
S72.092C
S72.099A
S72.099B
S72.099C
S72.101A
S72.101B
S72.101C
S72.102A
S72.102B
S72.102C
S72.109A
S72.109B
S72.109C
S72.111A
S72.111B
S72.111C
S72.112A
S72.112B
S72.112C
S72.113A
S72.113B
S72.113C
S72.114A
S72.114B
S72.114C
S72.115A
S72.115B
S72.115C
S72.116A
S72.116B
S72.116C
S72.121A
S72.121B
S72.121C
S72.122A
S72.122B
S72.122C
S72.123A
S72.123B
S72.123C
S72.124A
S72.124B
S72.124C
S72.125A
S72.125B
S72.125C
S72.126A
S72.126B
S72.126C
S72.131A
S72.131B
S72.131C
S72.132A
S72.132B
S72.132C
S72.133A
S72.133B
S72.133C
S72.134A
S72.134B
S72.134C
S72.135A
S72.135B
S72.135C
S72.136A
S72.136B
S72.136C
S72.141A
S72.141B
S72.141C
S72.142A
S72.142B
S72.142C
S72.143A
S72.143B
S72.143C
S72.144A
S72.144B
S72.144C
S72.145A
S72.145B
S72.145C
S72.146A
S72.146B
S72.146C
S72.21XA
S72.21XB
S72.21XC
S72.22XA
S72.22XB
S72.22XC
S72.23XA
S72.23XB
S72.23XC
S72.24XA
S72.24XB
S72.24XC
S72.25XA
S72.25XB
S72.25XC
S72.26XA
S72.26XB
S72.26XC
S72.301A
S72.301B
S72.301C
S72.302A
S72.302B
S72.302C
S72.309A
S72.309B
S72.309C
S72.321A
S72.321B
S72.321C
S72.322A
S72.322B
S72.322C
S72.323A
S72.323B
S72.323C
S72.324A
S72.324B
S72.324C
S72.325A
S72.325B
S72.325C
S72.326A
S72.326B
S72.326C
S72.331A
S72.331B
S72.331C
S72.332A
S72.332B
S72.332C
S72.333A
S72.333B
S72.333C
S72.334A
S72.334B
S72.334C
S72.335A
S72.335B
S72.335C
S72.336A
S72.336B
S72.336C
S72.341A
S72.341B
S72.341C
S72.342A
S72.342B
S72.342C
S72.343A
S72.343B
S72.343C
S72.344A
S72.344B
S72.344C
S72.345A
S72.345B
S72.345C
S72.346A
S72.346B
S72.346C
S72.351A
S72.351B
S72.351C
S72.352A
S72.352B
S72.352C
S72.353A
S72.353B
S72.353C
S72.354A
S72.354B
S72.354C
S72.355A
S72.355B
S72.355C
S72.356A
S72.356B
S72.356C
S72.361A
S72.361B
S72.361C
S72.362A
S72.362B
S72.362C
S72.363A
S72.363B
S72.363C
S72.364A
S72.364B
S72.364C
S72.365A
S72.365B
S72.365C
S72.366A
S72.366B
S72.366C
S72.391A
S72.391B
S72.391C
S72.392A
S72.392B
S72.392C
S72.399A
S72.399B
S72.399C
S72.401A
S72.401B
S72.401C
S72.402A
S72.402B
S72.402C
S72.409A
S72.409B
S72.409C
S72.411A
S72.411B
S72.411C
S72.412A
S72.412B
S72.412C
S72.413A
S72.413B
S72.413C
S72.414A
S72.414B
S72.414C
S72.415A
S72.415B
S72.415C
S72.416A
S72.416B
S72.416C
S72.421A
S72.421B
S72.421C
S72.422A
S72.422B
S72.422C
S72.423A
S72.423B
S72.423C
S72.424A
S72.424B
S72.424C
S72.425A
S72.425B
S72.425C
S72.426A
S72.426B
S72.426C
S72.431A
S72.431B
S72.431C
S72.432A
S72.432B
S72.432C
S72.433A
S72.433B
S72.433C
S72.434A

HAC 05: Falls and Trauma (continued)

S72.434B
S72.434C
S72.435A
S72.435B
S72.435C
S72.436A
S72.436B
S72.436C
S72.441A
S72.441B
S72.441C
S72.442A
S72.442B
S72.442C
S72.443A
S72.443B
S72.443C
S72.444A
S72.444B
S72.444C
S72.445A
S72.445B
S72.445C
S72.446A
S72.446B
S72.446C
S72.451A
S72.451B
S72.451C
S72.452A
S72.452B
S72.452C
S72.453A
S72.453B
S72.453C
S72.454A
S72.454B
S72.454C
S72.455A
S72.455B
S72.455C
S72.456A
S72.456B
S72.456C
S72.461A
S72.461B
S72.461C
S72.462A
S72.462B
S72.462C
S72.463A
S72.463B
S72.463C
S72.464A
S72.464B
S72.464C
S72.465A
S72.465B
S72.465C
S72.466A
S72.466B
S72.466C
S72.471A
S72.472A
S72.479A
S72.491A
S72.491B
S72.491C
S72.492A
S72.492B
S72.492C
S72.499A
S72.499B
S72.499C
S72.8X1A
S72.8X1B
S72.8X1C
S72.8X2A
S72.8X2B
S72.8X2C
S72.8X9A
S72.8X9B
S72.8X9C
S72.9ØXA
S72.9ØXB
S72.9ØXC
S72.91XA
S72.91XB
S72.91XC
S72.92XA
S72.92XB
S72.92XC
S73.ØØ1A
S73.ØØ2A
S73.ØØ3A
S73.ØØ4A
S73.ØØ5A
S73.ØØ6A
S73.Ø11A
S73.Ø12A
S73.Ø13A
S73.Ø14A
S73.Ø15A
S73.Ø16A
S73.Ø21A
S73.Ø22A
S73.Ø23A
S73.Ø24A
S73.Ø25A
S73.Ø26A
S73.Ø31A
S73.Ø32A
S73.Ø33A
S73.Ø34A
S73.Ø35A
S73.Ø36A
S73.Ø41A
S73.Ø42A
S73.Ø43A
S73.Ø44A
S73.Ø45A
S73.Ø46A
S77.ØØXA
S77.Ø1XA
S77.Ø2XA
S77.1ØXA
S77.11XA
S77.12XA
S79.ØØ1A
S79.ØØ2A
S79.ØØ9A
S79.Ø11A
S79.Ø12A
S79.Ø19A
S79.Ø91A
S79.Ø92A
S79.Ø99A
S79.1Ø1A
S79.1Ø2A
S79.1Ø9A
S79.111A
S79.112A
S79.119A
S79.121A
S79.122A
S79.129A
S79.131A
S79.132A
S79.139A
S79.141A
S79.142A
S79.149A
S79.191A
S79.192A
S79.199A
S82.ØØ1A
S82.ØØ1B
S82.ØØ1C
S82.ØØ2A
S82.ØØ2B
S82.ØØ2C
S82.ØØ9A
S82.ØØ9B
S82.ØØ9C
S82.Ø11A
S82.Ø11B
S82.Ø11C
S82.Ø12A
S82.Ø12B
S82.Ø12C
S82.Ø13A
S82.Ø13B
S82.Ø13C
S82.Ø14A
S82.Ø14B
S82.Ø14C
S82.Ø15A
S82.Ø15B
S82.Ø15C
S82.Ø16A
S82.Ø16B
S82.Ø16C
S82.Ø21A
S82.Ø21B
S82.Ø21C
S82.Ø22A
S82.Ø22B
S82.Ø22C
S82.Ø23A
S82.Ø23B
S82.Ø23C
S82.Ø24A
S82.Ø24B
S82.Ø24C
S82.Ø25A
S82.Ø25B
S82.Ø25C
S82.Ø26A
S82.Ø26B
S82.Ø26C
S82.Ø31A
S82.Ø31B
S82.Ø31C
S82.Ø32A
S82.Ø32B
S82.Ø32C
S82.Ø33A
S82.Ø33B
S82.Ø33C
S82.Ø34A
S82.Ø34B
S82.Ø34C
S82.Ø35A
S82.Ø35B
S82.Ø35C
S82.Ø36A
S82.Ø36B
S82.Ø36C
S82.Ø41A
S82.Ø41B
S82.Ø41C
S82.Ø42A
S82.Ø42B
S82.Ø42C
S82.Ø43A
S82.Ø43B
S82.Ø43C
S82.Ø44A
S82.Ø44B
S82.Ø44C
S82.Ø45A
S82.Ø45B
S82.Ø45C
S82.Ø46A
S82.Ø46B
S82.Ø46C
S82.Ø91A
S82.Ø91B
S82.Ø91C
S82.Ø92A
S82.Ø92B
S82.Ø92C
S82.Ø99A
S82.Ø99B
S82.Ø99C
S82.1Ø1A
S82.1Ø1B
S82.1Ø1C
S82.1Ø2A
S82.1Ø2B
S82.1Ø2C
S82.1Ø9A
S82.1Ø9B
S82.1Ø9C
S82.111A
S82.111B
S82.111C
S82.112A
S82.112B
S82.112C
S82.113A
S82.113B
S82.113C
S82.114A
S82.114B
S82.114C
S82.115A
S82.115B
S82.115C
S82.116A
S82.116B
S82.116C
S82.121A
S82.121B
S82.121C
S82.122A
S82.122B
S82.122C
S82.123A
S82.123B
S82.123C
S82.124A
S82.124B
S82.124C
S82.125A
S82.125B
S82.125C
S82.126A
S82.126B
S82.126C
S82.131A
S82.131B
S82.131C
S82.132A
S82.132B
S82.132C
S82.133A
S82.133B
S82.133C
S82.134A
S82.134B
S82.134C
S82.135A
S82.135B
S82.135C
S82.136A
S82.136B
S82.136C
S82.141A
S82.141B
S82.141C
S82.142A
S82.142B
S82.142C
S82.143A
S82.143B
S82.143C
S82.144A
S82.144B
S82.144C
S82.145A
S82.145B
S82.145C
S82.146A
S82.146B
S82.146C
S82.151A
S82.151B
S82.151C
S82.152A
S82.152B
S82.152C
S82.153A
S82.153B
S82.153C
S82.154A
S82.154B
S82.154C
S82.155A
S82.155B
S82.155C
S82.156A
S82.156B
S82.156C
S82.161A
S82.162A
S82.169A
S82.191A
S82.191B
S82.191C
S82.192A
S82.192B
S82.192C
S82.199A
S82.199B
S82.199C
S82.2Ø1A
S82.2Ø1B
S82.2Ø1C
S82.2Ø2A
S82.2Ø2B
S82.2Ø2C
S82.2Ø9A
S82.2Ø9B
S82.2Ø9C
S82.221A
S82.221B
S82.221C
S82.222A
S82.222B
S82.222C
S82.223A
S82.223B
S82.223C
S82.224A
S82.224B
S82.224C
S82.225A
S82.225B
S82.225C
S82.226A
S82.226B
S82.226C
S82.231A
S82.231B
S82.231C
S82.232A
S82.232B
S82.232C
S82.233A
S82.233B
S82.233C
S82.234A
S82.234B
S82.234C
S82.235A
S82.235B
S82.235C
S82.236A
S82.236B
S82.236C
S82.241A
S82.241B
S82.241C
S82.242A
S82.242B
S82.242C
S82.243A
S82.243B
S82.243C
S82.244A
S82.244B
S82.244C
S82.245A
S82.245B
S82.245C
S82.246A
S82.246B
S82.246C
S82.251A
S82.251B
S82.251C
S82.252A
S82.252B
S82.252C
S82.253A
S82.253B
S82.253C
S82.254A
S82.254B
S82.254C
S82.255A
S82.255B
S82.255C
S82.256A
S82.256B
S82.256C
S82.261A
S82.261B
S82.261C
S82.262A
S82.262B
S82.262C
S82.263A
S82.263B
S82.263C
S82.264A
S82.264B
S82.264C
S82.265A
S82.265B
S82.265C
S82.266A
S82.266B

HAC 05: Falls and Trauma (continued)

S82.266C
S82.291A
S82.291B
S82.291C
S82.292A
S82.292B
S82.292C
S82.299A
S82.299B
S82.299C
S82.3Ø1B
S82.3Ø1C
S82.3Ø2B
S82.3Ø2C
S82.3Ø9B
S82.3Ø9C
S82.311A
S82.312A
S82.319A
S82.391B
S82.391C
S82.392B
S82.392C
S82.399B
S82.399C
S82.4Ø1B
S82.4Ø1C
S82.4Ø2B
S82.4Ø2C
S82.4Ø9B
S82.4Ø9C
S82.421B
S82.421C
S82.422B
S82.422C
S82.423B
S82.423C
S82.424B
S82.424C
S82.425B
S82.425C
S82.426B
S82.426C
S82.431B
S82.431C
S82.432B
S82.432C
S82.433B
S82.433C
S82.434B
S82.434C
S82.435B
S82.435C
S82.436B
S82.436C
S82.441B
S82.441C
S82.442B
S82.442C
S82.443B
S82.443C
S82.444B
S82.444C
S82.445B
S82.445C
S82.446B
S82.446C
S82.451B
S82.451C
S82.452B
S82.452C
S82.453B
S82.453C
S82.454B
S82.454C
S82.455B
S82.455C
S82.456B
S82.456C
S82.461B
S82.461C
S82.462B
S82.462C
S82.463B
S82.463C
S82.464B
S82.464C
S82.465B
S82.465C
S82.466B
S82.466C
S82.491B
S82.491C
S82.492B
S82.492C
S82.499B
S82.499C
S82.51XB
S82.51XC
S82.52XB
S82.52XC
S82.53XB
S82.53XC
S82.54XB
S82.54XC
S82.55XB
S82.55XC
S82.56XB
S82.56XC
S82.61XB
S82.61XC
S82.62XB
S82.62XC
S82.63XB
S82.63XC
S82.64XB
S82.64XC
S82.65XB
S82.65XC
S82.66XB
S82.66XC
S82.831B
S82.831C
S82.832B
S82.832C
S82.839B
S82.839C
S82.841B
S82.841C
S82.842B
S82.842C
S82.843B
S82.843C
S82.844B
S82.844C
S82.845B
S82.845C
S82.846B
S82.846C
S82.851B
S82.851C
S82.852B
S82.852C
S82.853B
S82.853C
S82.854B
S82.854C
S82.855B
S82.855C
S82.856B
S82.856C
S82.861B
S82.861C
S82.862B
S82.862C
S82.863B
S82.863C
S82.864B
S82.864C
S82.865B
S82.865C
S82.866B
S82.866C
S82.871B
S82.871C
S82.872B
S82.872C
S82.873B
S82.873C
S82.874B
S82.874C
S82.875B
S82.875C
S82.876B
S82.876C
S82.891B
S82.891C
S82.892B
S82.892C
S82.899B
S82.899C
S82.9ØXB
S82.9ØXC
S82.91XB
S82.91XC
S82.92XB
S82.92XC
S89.ØØ1A
S89.ØØ2A
S89.ØØ9A
S89.Ø11A
S89.Ø12A
S89.Ø19A
S89.Ø21A
S89.Ø22A
S89.Ø29A
S89.Ø31A
S89.Ø32A
S89.Ø39A
S89.Ø41A
S89.Ø42A
S89.Ø49A
S89.Ø91A
S89.Ø92A
S89.Ø99A
S92.ØØ1B
S92.ØØ2B
S92.ØØ9B
S92.Ø11B
S92.Ø12B
S92.Ø13B
S92.Ø14B
S92.Ø15B
S92.Ø16B
S92.Ø21B
S92.Ø22B
S92.Ø23B
S92.Ø24B
S92.Ø25B
S92.Ø26B
S92.Ø31B
S92.Ø32B
S92.Ø33B
S92.Ø34B
S92.Ø35B
S92.Ø36B
S92.Ø41B
S92.Ø42B
S92.Ø43B
S92.Ø44B
S92.Ø45B
S92.Ø46B
S92.Ø51B
S92.Ø52B
S92.Ø53B
S92.Ø54B
S92.Ø55B
S92.Ø56B
S92.Ø61B
S92.Ø62B
S92.Ø63B
S92.Ø64B
S92.Ø65B
S92.Ø66B
S92.1Ø1B
S92.1Ø2B
S92.1Ø9B
S92.111B
S92.112B
S92.113B
S92.114B
S92.115B
S92.116B
S92.121B
S92.122B
S92.123B
S92.124B
S92.125B
S92.126B
S92.131B
S92.132B
S92.133B
S92.134B
S92.135B
S92.136B
S92.141B
S92.142B
S92.143B
S92.144B
S92.145B
S92.146B
S92.151B
S92.152B
S92.153B
S92.154B
S92.155B
S92.156B
S92.191B
S92.192B
S92.199B
S92.2Ø1B
S92.2Ø2B
S92.2Ø9B
S92.211B
S92.212B
S92.213B
S92.214B
S92.215B
S92.216B
S92.221B
S92.222B
S92.223B
S92.224B
S92.225B
S92.226B
S92.231B
S92.232B
S92.233B
S92.234B
S92.235B
S92.236B
S92.241B
S92.242B
S92.243B
S92.244B
S92.245B
S92.246B
S92.251B
S92.252B
S92.253B
S92.254B
S92.255B
S92.256B
S92.3Ø1B
S92.3Ø2B
S92.3Ø9B
S92.311B
S92.312B
S92.313B
S92.314B
S92.315B
S92.316B
S92.321B
S92.322B
S92.323B
S92.324B
S92.325B
S92.326B
S92.331B
S92.332B
S92.333B
S92.334B
S92.335B
S92.336B
S92.341B
S92.342B
S92.343B
S92.344B
S92.345B
S92.346B
S92.351B
S92.352B
S92.353B
S92.354B
S92.355B
S92.356B
S92.811B
S92.812B
S92.819B
S92.9Ø1B
S92.9Ø2B
S92.9Ø9B
T2Ø.3ØXA
T2Ø.311A
T2Ø.312A
T2Ø.319A
T2Ø.32XA
T2Ø.33XA
T2Ø.34XA
T2Ø.35XA
T2Ø.36XA
T2Ø.37XA
T2Ø.39XA
T2Ø.7ØXA
T2Ø.711A
T2Ø.712A
T2Ø.719A
T2Ø.72XA
T2Ø.73XA
T2Ø.74XA
T2Ø.75XA
T2Ø.76XA
T2Ø.77XA
T2Ø.79XA
T21.3ØXA
T21.31XA
T21.32XA
T21.33XA
T21.34XA
T21.35XA
T21.36XA
T21.37XA
T21.39XA
T21.7ØXA
T21.71XA
T21.72XA
T21.73XA
T21.74XA
T21.75XA
T21.76XA
T21.77XA
T21.79XA
T22.3ØXA
T22.311A
T22.312A
T22.319A
T22.321A
T22.322A
T22.329A
T22.331A
T22.332A
T22.339A
T22.341A
T22.342A
T22.349A
T22.351A
T22.352A
T22.359A
T22.361A
T22.362A
T22.369A
T22.391A
T22.392A
T22.399A
T22.7ØXA
T22.711A
T22.712A
T22.719A
T22.721A
T22.722A
T22.729A
T22.731A
T22.732A
T22.739A
T22.741A
T22.742A
T22.749A
T22.751A
T22.752A
T22.759A
T22.761A
T22.762A
T22.769A
T22.791A
T22.792A
T22.799A
T23.3Ø1A
T23.3Ø2A
T23.3Ø9A
T23.311A
T23.312A
T23.319A
T23.321A
T23.322A
T23.329A
T23.331A
T23.332A
T23.339A
T23.341A
T23.342A
T23.349A
T23.351A
T23.352A
T23.359A

HAC 05: Falls and Trauma (continued)

T23.361A
T23.362A
T23.369A
T23.371A
T23.372A
T23.379A
T23.391A
T23.392A
T23.399A
T23.701A
T23.702A
T23.709A
T23.711A
T23.712A
T23.719A
T23.721A
T23.722A
T23.729A
T23.731A
T23.732A
T23.739A
T23.741A
T23.742A
T23.749A
T23.751A
T23.752A
T23.759A
T23.761A
T23.762A
T23.769A
T23.771A
T23.772A
T23.779A
T23.791A
T23.792A
T23.799A
T24.301A
T24.302A
T24.309A
T24.311A
T24.312A
T24.319A
T24.321A
T24.322A
T24.329A
T24.331A
T24.332A
T24.339A
T24.391A
T24.392A
T24.399A
T24.701A
T24.702A
T24.709A
T24.711A
T24.712A
T24.719A
T24.721A
T24.722A
T24.729A
T24.731A
T24.732A
T24.739A
T24.791A
T24.792A
T24.799A
T25.311A
T25.312A
T25.319A
T25.321A
T25.322A
T25.329A
T25.331A
T25.332A
T25.339A
T25.391A
T25.392A
T25.399A
T25.711A
T25.712A
T25.719A
T25.721A
T25.722A
T25.729A
T25.731A
T25.732A
T25.739A
T25.791A
T25.792A
T25.799A
T26.20XA
T26.21XA
T26.22XA
T26.70XA
T26.71XA
T26.72XA
T27.0XXA
T27.1XXA
T27.2XXA
T27.3XXA
T27.4XXA
T27.5XXA
T27.6XXA
T27.7XXA
T28.1XXA
T28.2XXA
T28.6XXA
T28.7XXA
T31.10
T31.11
T31.20
T31.21
T31.22
T31.30
T31.31
T31.32
T31.33
T31.40
T31.41
T31.42
T31.43
T31.44
T31.50
T31.51
T31.52
T31.53
T31.54
T31.55
T31.60
T31.61
T31.62
T31.63
T31.64
T31.65
T31.66
T31.70
T31.71
T31.72
T31.73
T31.74
T31.75
T31.76
T31.77
T31.80
T31.81
T31.82
T31.83
T31.84
T31.85
T31.86
T31.87
T31.88
T31.90
T31.91
T31.92
T31.93
T31.94
T31.95
T31.96
T31.97
T31.98
T31.99
T32.10
T32.11
T32.20
T32.21
T32.22
T32.30
T32.31
T32.32
T32.33
T32.40
T32.41
T32.42
T32.43
T32.44
T32.50
T32.51
T32.52
T32.53
T32.54
T32.55
T32.60
T32.61
T32.62
T32.63
T32.64
T32.65
T32.66
T32.70
T32.71
T32.72
T32.73
T32.74
T32.75
T32.76
T32.77
T32.80
T32.81
T32.82
T32.83
T32.84
T32.85
T32.86
T32.87
T32.88
T32.90
T32.91
T32.92
T32.93
T32.94
T32.95
T32.96
T32.97
T32.98
T32.99
T33.011A
T33.012A
T33.019A
T33.02XA
T33.09XA
T33.1XXA
T33.2XXA
T33.3XXA
T33.40XA
T33.41XA
T33.42XA
T33.511A
T33.512A
T33.519A
T33.521A
T33.522A
T33.529A
T33.531A
T33.532A
T33.539A
T33.60XA
T33.61XA
T33.62XA
T33.70XA
T33.71XA
T33.72XA
T33.811A
T33.812A
T33.819A
T33.821A
T33.822A
T33.829A
T33.831A
T33.832A
T33.839A
T33.90XA
T33.99XA
T34.011A
T34.012A
T34.019A
T34.02XA
T34.09XA
T34.1XXA
T34.2XXA
T34.3XXA
T34.40XA
T34.41XA
T34.42XA
T34.511A
T34.512A
T34.519A
T34.521A
T34.522A
T34.529A
T34.531A
T34.532A
T34.539A
T34.60XA
T34.61XA
T34.62XA
T34.70XA
T34.71XA
T34.72XA
T34.811A
T34.812A
T34.819A
T34.821A
T34.822A
T34.829A
T34.831A
T34.832A
T34.839A
T34.90XA
T34.99XA
T67.0XXA
T69.021A
T69.022A
T69.029A
T70.3XXA
T71.111A
T71.112A
T71.113A
T71.114A
T71.121A
T71.122A
T71.123A
T71.124A
T71.131A
T71.132A
T71.133A
T71.134A
T71.141A
T71.143A
T71.144A
T71.151A
T71.152A
T71.153A
T71.154A
T71.161A
T71.162A
T71.163A
T71.164A
T71.191A
T71.192A
T71.193A
T71.194A
T71.20XA
T71.21XA
T71.29XA
T71.9XXA
T75.1XXA

HAC 06: Catheter Associated Urinary Tract Infection (UTI)

Secondary diagnosis not POA:

T83.511A
T83.518A

With or Without

Secondary diagnosis (also not POA) of:

B37.41
B37.49
N10
N11.9
N12
N13.6
N15.1
N28.84
N28.85
N28.86
N30.00
N30.01
N34.0
N39.0

HAC 07: Vascular Catheter Associated Infection

Secondary diagnosis not POA:

T80.211A
T80.212A
T80.218A
T80.219A

HAC 08: Surgical Site Infection of Mediastinitis Following Coronary Bypass Graft (CABG) Procedures

Secondary diagnosis not POA:

J98.51
J98.59

AND

Any of the following procedures:

0210083	Bypass Coronary Artery, One Artery from Coronary Artery with Zooplastic Tissue, Open Approach
0210088	Bypass Coronary Artery, One Artery from Right Internal Mammary with Zooplastic Tissue, Open Approach
0210089	Bypass Coronary Artery, One Artery from Left Internal Mammary with Zooplastic Tissue, Open Approach
021008C	Bypass Coronary Artery, One Artery from Thoracic Artery with Zooplastic Tissue, Open Approach
021008F	Bypass Coronary Artery, One Artery from Abdominal Artery with Zooplastic Tissue, Open Approach
021008W	Bypass Coronary Artery, One Artery from Aorta with Zooplastic Tissue, Open Approach
0210093	Bypass Coronary Artery, One Artery from Coronary Artery with Autologous Venous Tissue, Open Approach
0210098	Bypass Coronary Artery, One Artery from Right Internal Mammary with Autologous Venous Tissue, Open Approach
0210099	Bypass Coronary Artery, One Artery from Left Internal Mammary with Autologous Venous Tissue, Open Approach
021009C	Bypass Coronary Artery, One Artery from Thoracic Artery with Autologous Venous Tissue, Open Approach
021009F	Bypass Coronary Artery, One Artery from Abdominal Artery with Autologous Venous Tissue, Open Approach
021009W	Bypass Coronary Artery, One Artery from Aorta with Autologous Venous Tissue, Open Approach
02100A3	Bypass Coronary Artery, One Artery from Coronary Artery with Autologous Arterial Tissue, Open Approach
02100A8	Bypass Coronary Artery, One Artery from Right Internal Mammary with Autologous Arterial Tissue, Open Approach
02100A9	Bypass Coronary Artery, One Artery from Left Internal Mammary with Autologous Arterial Tissue, Open Approach
02100AC	Bypass Coronary Artery, One Artery from Thoracic Artery with Autologous Arterial Tissue, Open Approach
02100AF	Bypass Coronary Artery, One Artery from Abdominal Artery with Autologous Arterial Tissue, Open Approach
02100AW	Bypass Coronary Artery, One Artery from Aorta with Autologous Arterial Tissue, Open Approach
02100J3	Bypass Coronary Artery, One Artery from Coronary Artery with Synthetic Substitute, Open Approach
02100J8	Bypass Coronary Artery, One Artery from Right Internal Mammary with Synthetic Substitute, Open Approach
02100J9	Bypass Coronary Artery, One Artery from Left Internal Mammary with Synthetic Substitute, Open Approach
02100JC	Bypass Coronary Artery, One Artery from Thoracic Artery with Synthetic Substitute, Open Approach
02100JF	Bypass Coronary Artery, One Artery from Abdominal Artery with Synthetic Substitute, Open Approach
02100JW	Bypass Coronary Artery, One Artery from Aorta with Synthetic Substitute, Open Approach
02100K3	Bypass Coronary Artery, One Artery from Coronary Artery with Nonautologous Tissue Substitute, Open Approach
02100K8	Bypass Coronary Artery, One Artery from Right Internal Mammary with Nonautologous Tissue Substitute, Open Approach
02100K9	Bypass Coronary Artery, One Artery from Left Internal Mammary with Nonautologous Tissue Substitute, Open Approach
02100KC	Bypass Coronary Artery, One Artery from Thoracic Artery with Nonautologous Tissue Substitute, Open Approach
02100KF	Bypass Coronary Artery, One Artery from Abdominal Artery with Nonautologous Tissue Substitute, Open Approach
02100KW	Bypass Coronary Artery, One Artery from Aorta with Nonautologous Tissue Substitute, Open Approach
02100Z3	Bypass Coronary Artery, One Artery from Coronary Artery, Open Approach
02100Z8	Bypass Coronary Artery, One Artery from Right Internal Mammary, Open Approach
02100Z9	Bypass Coronary Artery, One Artery from Left Internal Mammary, Open Approach
02100ZC	Bypass Coronary Artery, One Artery from Thoracic Artery, Open Approach
02100ZF	Bypass Coronary Artery, One Artery from Abdominal Artery, Open Approach
0210483	Bypass Coronary Artery, One Artery from Coronary Artery with Zooplastic Tissue, Percutaneous Endoscopic Approach
0210488	Bypass Coronary Artery, One Artery from Right Internal Mammary with Zooplastic Tissue, Percutaneous Endoscopic Approach
0210489	Bypass Coronary Artery, One Artery from Left Internal Mammary with Zooplastic Tissue, Percutaneous Endoscopic Approach
021048C	Bypass Coronary Artery, One Artery from Thoracic Artery with Zooplastic Tissue, Percutaneous Endoscopic Approach
021048F	Bypass Coronary Artery, One Artery from Abdominal Artery with Zooplastic Tissue, Percutaneous Endoscopic Approach
021048W	Bypass Coronary Artery, One Artery from Aorta with Zooplastic Tissue, Percutaneous Endoscopic Approach
0210493	Bypass Coronary Artery, One Artery from Coronary Artery with Autologous Venous Tissue, Percutaneous Endoscopic Approach
0210498	Bypass Coronary Artery, One Artery from Right Internal Mammary with Autologous Venous Tissue, Percutaneous Endoscopic Approach
0210499	Bypass Coronary Artery, One Artery from Left Internal Mammary with Autologous Venous Tissue, Percutaneous Endoscopic Approach
021049C	Bypass Coronary Artery, One Artery from Thoracic Artery with Autologous Venous Tissue, Percutaneous Endoscopic Approach
021049F	Bypass Coronary Artery, One Artery from Abdominal Artery with Autologous Venous Tissue, Percutaneous Endoscopic Approach
021049W	Bypass Coronary Artery, One Artery from Aorta with Autologous Venous Tissue, Percutaneous Endoscopic Approach
02104A3	Bypass Coronary Artery, One Artery from Coronary Artery with Autologous Arterial Tissue, Percutaneous Endoscopic Approach
02104A8	Bypass Coronary Artery, One Artery from Right Internal Mammary with Autologous Arterial Tissue, Percutaneous Endoscopic Approach
02104A9	Bypass Coronary Artery, One Artery from Left Internal Mammary with Autologous Arterial Tissue, Percutaneous Endoscopic Approach
02104AC	Bypass Coronary Artery, One Artery from Thoracic Artery with Autologous Arterial Tissue, Percutaneous Endoscopic Approach
02104AF	Bypass Coronary Artery, One Artery from Abdominal Artery with Autologous Arterial Tissue, Percutaneous Endoscopic Approach
02104AW	Bypass Coronary Artery, One Artery from Aorta with Autologous Arterial Tissue, Percutaneous Endoscopic Approach
02104J3	Bypass Coronary Artery, One Artery from Coronary Artery with Synthetic Substitute, Percutaneous Endoscopic Approach
02104J8	Bypass Coronary Artery, One Artery from Right Internal Mammary with Synthetic Substitute, Percutaneous Endoscopic Approach
02104J9	Bypass Coronary Artery, One Artery from Left Internal Mammary with Synthetic Substitute, Percutaneous Endoscopic Approach
02104JC	Bypass Coronary Artery, One Artery from Thoracic Artery with Synthetic Substitute, Percutaneous Endoscopic Approach
02104JF	Bypass Coronary Artery, One Artery from Abdominal Artery with Synthetic Substitute, Percutaneous Endoscopic Approach
02104JW	Bypass Coronary Artery, One Artery from Aorta with Synthetic Substitute, Percutaneous Endoscopic Approach
02104K3	Bypass Coronary Artery, One Artery from Coronary Artery with Nonautologous Tissue Substitute, Percutaneous Endoscopic Approach
02104K8	Bypass Coronary Artery, One Artery from Right Internal Mammary with Nonautologous Tissue Substitute, Percutaneous Endoscopic Approach
02104K9	Bypass Coronary Artery, One Artery from Left Internal Mammary with Nonautologous Tissue Substitute, Percutaneous Endoscopic Approach
02104KC	Bypass Coronary Artery, One Artery from Thoracic Artery with Nonautologous Tissue Substitute, Percutaneous Endoscopic Approach

HAC 08: Surgical Artery Infection of Mediastinitis Following Coronary Bypass Graft (CABG) Procedures (continued)

Ø21Ø4KF Bypass Coronary Artery, One Artery from Abdominal Artery with Nonautologous Tissue Substitute, Percutaneous Endoscopic Approach
Ø21Ø4KW Bypass Coronary Artery, One Artery from Aorta with Nonautologous Tissue Substitute, Percutaneous Endoscopic Approach
Ø21Ø4Z3 Bypass Coronary Artery, One Artery from Coronary Artery, Percutaneous Endoscopic Approach
Ø21Ø4Z8 Bypass Coronary Artery, One Artery from Right Internal Mammary, Percutaneous Endoscopic Approach
Ø21Ø4Z9 Bypass Coronary Artery, One Artery from Left Internal Mammary, Percutaneous Endoscopic Approach
Ø21Ø4ZC Bypass Coronary Artery, One Artery from Thoracic Artery, Percutaneous Endoscopic Approach
Ø21Ø4ZF Bypass Coronary Artery, One Artery from Abdominal Artery, Percutaneous Endoscopic Approach
Ø211Ø83 Bypass Coronary Artery, Two Arteries from Coronary Artery with Zooplastic Tissue, Open Approach
Ø211Ø88 Bypass Coronary Artery, Two Arteries from Right Internal Mammary with Zooplastic Tissue, Open Approach
Ø211Ø89 Bypass Coronary Artery, Two Arteries from Left Internal Mammary with Zooplastic Tissue, Open Approach
Ø211Ø8C Bypass Coronary Artery, Two Arteries from Thoracic Artery with Zooplastic Tissue, Open Approach
Ø211Ø8F Bypass Coronary Artery, Two Arteries from Abdominal Artery with Zooplastic Tissue, Open Approach
Ø211Ø8W Bypass Coronary Artery, Two Arteries from Aorta with Zooplastic Tissue, Open Approach
Ø211Ø93 Bypass Coronary Artery, Two Arteries from Coronary Artery with Autologous Venous Tissue, Open Approach
Ø211Ø98 Bypass Coronary Artery, Two Arteries from Right Internal Mammary with Autologous Venous Tissue, Open Approach
Ø211Ø99 Bypass Coronary Artery, Two Arteries from Left Internal Mammary with Autologous Venous Tissue, Open Approach
Ø211Ø9C Bypass Coronary Artery, Two Arteries from Thoracic Artery with Autologous Venous Tissue, Open Approach
Ø211Ø9F Bypass Coronary Artery, Two Arteries from Abdominal Artery with Autologous Venous Tissue, Open Approach
Ø211Ø9W Bypass Coronary Artery, Two Arteries from Aorta with Autologous Venous Tissue, Open Approach
Ø211ØA3 Bypass Coronary Artery, Two Arteries from Coronary Artery with Autologous Arterial Tissue, Open Approach
Ø211ØA8 Bypass Coronary Artery, Two Arteries from Right Internal Mammary with Autologous Arterial Tissue, Open Approach
Ø211ØA9 Bypass Coronary Artery, Two Arteries from Left Internal Mammary with Autologous Arterial Tissue, Open Approach
Ø211ØAC Bypass Coronary Artery, Two Arteries from Thoracic Artery with Autologous Arterial Tissue, Open Approach
Ø211ØAF Bypass Coronary Artery, Two Arteries from Abdominal Artery with Autologous Arterial Tissue, Open Approach
Ø211ØAW Bypass Coronary Artery, Two Arteries from Aorta with Autologous Arterial Tissue, Open Approach
Ø211ØJ3 Bypass Coronary Artery, Two Arteries from Coronary Artery with Synthetic Substitute, Open Approach
Ø211ØJ8 Bypass Coronary Artery, Two Arteries from Right Internal Mammary with Synthetic Substitute, Open Approach
Ø211ØJ9 Bypass Coronary Artery, Two Arteries from Left Internal Mammary with Synthetic Substitute, Open Approach
Ø211ØJC Bypass Coronary Artery, Two Arteries from Thoracic Artery with Synthetic Substitute, Open Approach
Ø211ØJF Bypass Coronary Artery, Two Arteries from Abdominal Artery with Synthetic Substitute, Open Approach
Ø211ØJW Bypass Coronary Artery, Two Arteries from Aorta with Synthetic Substitute, Open Approach
Ø211ØK3 Bypass Coronary Artery, Two Arteries from Coronary Artery with Nonautologous Tissue Substitute, Open Approach
Ø211ØK8 Bypass Coronary Artery, Two Arteries from Right Internal Mammary with Nonautologous Tissue Substitute, Open Approach
Ø211ØK9 Bypass Coronary Artery, Two Arteries from Left Internal Mammary with Nonautologous Tissue Substitute, Open Approach
Ø211ØKC Bypass Coronary Artery, Two Arteries from Thoracic Artery with Nonautologous Tissue Substitute, Open Approach
Ø211ØKF Bypass Coronary Artery, Two Arteries from Abdominal Artery with Nonautologous Tissue Substitute, Open Approach
Ø211ØKW Bypass Coronary Artery, Two Arteries from Aorta with Nonautologous Tissue Substitute, Open Approach
Ø211ØZ3 Bypass Coronary Artery, Two Arteries from Coronary Artery, Open Approach
Ø211ØZ8 Bypass Coronary Artery, Two Arteries from Right Internal Mammary, Open Approach
Ø211ØZ9 Bypass Coronary Artery, Two Arteries from Left Internal Mammary, Open Approach
Ø211ØZC Bypass Coronary Artery, Two Arteries from Thoracic Artery, Open Approach
Ø211ØZF Bypass Coronary Artery, Two Arteries from Abdominal Artery, Open Approach
Ø211483 Bypass Coronary Artery, Two Arteries from Coronary Artery with Zooplastic Tissue, Percutaneous Endoscopic Approach
Ø211488 Bypass Coronary Artery, Two Arteries from Right Internal Mammary with Zooplastic Tissue, Percutaneous Endoscopic Approach
Ø211489 Bypass Coronary Artery, Two Arteries from Left Internal Mammary with Zooplastic Tissue, Percutaneous Endoscopic Approach
Ø21148C Bypass Coronary Artery, Two Arteries from Thoracic Artery with Zooplastic Tissue, Percutaneous Endoscopic Approach
Ø21148F Bypass Coronary Artery, Two Arteries from Abdominal Artery with Zooplastic Tissue, Percutaneous Endoscopic Approach
Ø21148W Bypass Coronary Artery, Two Arteries from Aorta with Zooplastic Tissue, Percutaneous Endoscopic Approach
Ø211493 Bypass Coronary Artery, Two Arteries from Coronary Artery with Autologous Venous Tissue, Percutaneous Endoscopic Approach
Ø211498 Bypass Coronary Artery, Two Arteries from Right Internal Mammary with Autologous Venous Tissue, Percutaneous Endoscopic Approach
Ø211499 Bypass Coronary Artery, Two Arteries from Left Internal Mammary with Autologous Venous Tissue, Percutaneous Endoscopic Approach
Ø21149C Bypass Coronary Artery, Two Arteries from Thoracic Artery with Autologous Venous Tissue, Percutaneous Endoscopic Approach
Ø21149F Bypass Coronary Artery, Two Arteries from Abdominal Artery with Autologous Venous Tissue, Percutaneous Endoscopic Approach
Ø21149W Bypass Coronary Artery, Two Arteries from Aorta with Autologous Venous Tissue, Percutaneous Endoscopic Approach
Ø2114A3 Bypass Coronary Artery, Two Arteries from Coronary Artery with Autologous Arterial Tissue, Percutaneous Endoscopic Approach
Ø2114A8 Bypass Coronary Artery, Two Arteries from Right Internal Mammary with Autologous Arterial Tissue, Percutaneous Endoscopic Approach
Ø2114A9 Bypass Coronary Artery, Two Arteries from Left Internal Mammary with Autologous Arterial Tissue, Percutaneous Endoscopic Approach
Ø2114AC Bypass Coronary Artery, Two Arteries from Thoracic Artery with Autologous Arterial Tissue, Percutaneous Endoscopic Approach
Ø2114AF Bypass Coronary Artery, Two Arteries from Abdominal Artery with Autologous Arterial Tissue, Percutaneous Endoscopic Approach
Ø2114AW Bypass Coronary Artery, Two Arteries from Aorta with Autologous Arterial Tissue, Percutaneous Endoscopic Approach
Ø2114J3 Bypass Coronary Artery, Two Arteries from Coronary Artery with Synthetic Substitute, Percutaneous Endoscopic Approach
Ø2114J8 Bypass Coronary Artery, Two Arteries from Right Internal Mammary with Synthetic Substitute, Percutaneous Endoscopic Approach
Ø2114J9 Bypass Coronary Artery, Two Arteries from Left Internal Mammary with Synthetic Substitute, Percutaneous Endoscopic Approach
Ø2114JC Bypass Coronary Artery, Two Arteries from Thoracic Artery with Synthetic Substitute, Percutaneous Endoscopic Approach

HAC 08: Surgical Site Infection of Mediastinitis Following Coronary Bypass Graft (CABG) Procedures (continued)

Ø2114JF Bypass Coronary Artery, Two Arteries from Abdominal Artery with Synthetic Substitute, Percutaneous Endoscopic Approach
Ø2114JW Bypass Coronary Artery, Two Arteries from Aorta with Synthetic Substitute, Percutaneous Endoscopic Approach
Ø2114K3 Bypass Coronary Artery, Two Arteries from Coronary Artery with Nonautologous Tissue Substitute, Percutaneous Endoscopic Approach
Ø2114K8 Bypass Coronary Artery, Two Arteries from Right Internal Mammary with Nonautologous Tissue Substitute, Percutaneous Endoscopic Approach
Ø2114K9 Bypass Coronary Artery, Two Arteries from Left Internal Mammary with Nonautologous Tissue Substitute, Percutaneous Endoscopic Approach
Ø2114KC Bypass Coronary Artery, Two Arteries from Thoracic Artery with Nonautologous Tissue Substitute, Percutaneous Endoscopic Approach
Ø2114KF Bypass Coronary Artery, Two Arteries from Abdominal Artery with Nonautologous Tissue Substitute, Percutaneous Endoscopic Approach
Ø2114KW Bypass Coronary Artery, Two Arteries from Aorta with Nonautologous Tissue Substitute, Percutaneous Endoscopic Approach
Ø2114Z3 Bypass Coronary Artery, Two Arteries from Coronary Artery, Percutaneous Endoscopic Approach
Ø2114Z8 Bypass Coronary Artery, Two Arteries from Right Internal Mammary, Percutaneous Endoscopic Approach
Ø2114Z9 Bypass Coronary Artery, Two Arteries from Left Internal Mammary, Percutaneous Endoscopic Approach
Ø2114ZC Bypass Coronary Artery, Two Arteries from Thoracic Artery, Percutaneous Endoscopic Approach
Ø2114ZF Bypass Coronary Artery, Two Arteries from Abdominal Artery, Percutaneous Endoscopic Approach
Ø212Ø83 Bypass Coronary Artery, Three Arteries from Coronary Artery with Zooplastic Tissue, Open Approach
Ø212Ø88 Bypass Coronary Artery, Three Arteries from Right Internal Mammary with Zooplastic Tissue, Open Approach
Ø212Ø89 Bypass Coronary Artery, Three Arteries from Left Internal Mammary with Zooplastic Tissue, Open Approach
Ø212Ø8C Bypass Coronary Artery, Three Arteries from Thoracic Artery with Zooplastic Tissue, Open Approach
Ø212Ø8F Bypass Coronary Artery, Three Arteries from Abdominal Artery with Zooplastic Tissue, Open Approach
Ø212Ø8W Bypass Coronary Artery, Three Arteries from Aorta with Zooplastic Tissue, Open Approach
Ø212Ø93 Bypass Coronary Artery, Three Arteries from Coronary Artery with Autologous Venous Tissue, Open Approach
Ø212Ø98 Bypass Coronary Artery, Three Arteries from Right Internal Mammary with Autologous Venous Tissue, Open Approach
Ø212Ø99 Bypass Coronary Artery, Three Arteries from Left Internal Mammary with Autologous Venous Tissue, Open Approach
Ø212Ø9C Bypass Coronary Artery, Three Arteries from Thoracic Artery with Autologous Venous Tissue, Open Approach
Ø212Ø9F Bypass Coronary Artery, Three Arteries from Abdominal Artery with Autologous Venous Tissue, Open Approach
Ø212Ø9W Bypass Coronary Artery, Three Arteries from Aorta with Autologous Venous Tissue, Open Approach
Ø212ØA3 Bypass Coronary Artery, Three Arteries from Coronary Artery with Autologous Arterial Tissue, Open Approach
Ø212ØA8 Bypass Coronary Artery, Three Arteries from Right Internal Mammary with Autologous Arterial Tissue, Open Approach
Ø212ØA9 Bypass Coronary Artery, Three Arteries from Left Internal Mammary with Autologous Arterial Tissue, Open Approach
Ø212ØAC Bypass Coronary Artery, Three Arteries from Thoracic Artery with Autologous Arterial Tissue, Open Approach
Ø212ØAF Bypass Coronary Artery, Three Arteries from Abdominal Artery with Autologous Arterial Tissue, Open Approach
Ø212ØAW Bypass Coronary Artery, Three Arteries from Aorta with Autologous Arterial Tissue, Open Approach
Ø212ØJ3 Bypass Coronary Artery, Three Arteries from Coronary Artery with Synthetic Substitute, Open Approach
Ø212ØJ8 Bypass Coronary Artery, Three Arteries from Right Internal Mammary with Synthetic Substitute, Open Approach
Ø212ØJ9 Bypass Coronary Artery, Three Arteries from Left Internal Mammary with Synthetic Substitute, Open Approach
Ø212ØJC Bypass Coronary Artery, Three Arteries from Thoracic Artery with Synthetic Substitute, Open Approach
Ø212ØJF Bypass Coronary Artery, Three Arteries from Abdominal Artery with Synthetic Substitute, Open Approach
Ø212ØJW Bypass Coronary Artery, Three Arteries from Aorta with Synthetic Substitute, Open Approach
Ø212ØK3 Bypass Coronary Artery, Three Arteries from Coronary Artery with Nonautologous Tissue Substitute, Open Approach
Ø212ØK8 Bypass Coronary Artery, Three Arteries from Right Internal Mammary with Nonautologous Tissue Substitute, Open Approach
Ø212ØK9 Bypass Coronary Artery, Three Arteries from Left Internal Mammary with Nonautologous Tissue Substitute, Open Approach
Ø212ØKC Bypass Coronary Artery, Three Arteries from Thoracic Artery with Nonautologous Tissue Substitute, Open Approach
Ø212ØKF Bypass Coronary Artery, Three Arteries from Abdominal Artery with Nonautologous Tissue Substitute, Open Approach
Ø212ØKW Bypass Coronary Artery, Three Arteries from Aorta with Nonautologous Tissue Substitute, Open Approach
Ø212ØZ3 Bypass Coronary Artery, Three Arteries from Coronary Artery, Open Approach
Ø212ØZ8 Bypass Coronary Artery, Three Arteries from Right Internal Mammary, Open Approach
Ø212ØZ9 Bypass Coronary Artery, Three Arteries from Left Internal Mammary, Open Approach
Ø212ØZC Bypass Coronary Artery, Three Arteries from Thoracic Artery, Open Approach
Ø212ØZF Bypass Coronary Artery, Three Arteries from Abdominal Artery, Open Approach
Ø212483 Bypass Coronary Artery, Three Arteries from Coronary Artery with Zooplastic Tissue, Percutaneous Endoscopic Approach
Ø212488 Bypass Coronary Artery, Three Arteries from Right Internal Mammary with Zooplastic Tissue, Percutaneous Endoscopic Approach
Ø212489 Bypass Coronary Artery, Three Arteries from Left Internal Mammary with Zooplastic Tissue, Percutaneous Endoscopic Approach
Ø21248C Bypass Coronary Artery, Three Arteries from Thoracic Artery with Zooplastic Tissue, Percutaneous Endoscopic Approach
Ø21248F Bypass Coronary Artery, Three Arteries from Abdominal Artery with Zooplastic Tissue, Percutaneous Endoscopic Approach
Ø21248W Bypass Coronary Artery, Three Arteries from Aorta with Zooplastic Tissue, Percutaneous Endoscopic Approach
Ø212493 Bypass Coronary Artery, Three Arteries from Coronary Artery with Autologous Venous Tissue, Percutaneous Endoscopic Approach
Ø212498 Bypass Coronary Artery, Three Arteries from Right Internal Mammary with Autologous Venous Tissue, Percutaneous Endoscopic Approach
Ø212499 Bypass Coronary Artery, Three Arteries from Left Internal Mammary with Autologous Venous Tissue, Percutaneous Endoscopic Approach
Ø21249C Bypass Coronary Artery, Three Arteries from Thoracic Artery with Autologous Venous Tissue, Percutaneous Endoscopic Approach
Ø21249F Bypass Coronary Artery, Three Arteries from Abdominal Artery with Autologous Venous Tissue, Percutaneous Endoscopic Approach
Ø21249W Bypass Coronary Artery, Three Arteries from Aorta with Autologous Venous Tissue, Percutaneous Endoscopic Approach
Ø2124A3 Bypass Coronary Artery, Three Arteries from Coronary Artery with Autologous Arterial Tissue, Percutaneous Endoscopic Approach
Ø2124A8 Bypass Coronary Artery, Three Arteries from Right Internal Mammary with Autologous Arterial Tissue, Percutaneous Endoscopic Approach
Ø2124A9 Bypass Coronary Artery, Three Arteries from Left Internal Mammary with Autologous Arterial Tissue, Percutaneous Endoscopic Approach
Ø2124AC Bypass Coronary Artery, Three Arteries from Thoracic Artery with Autologous Arterial Tissue, Percutaneous Endoscopic Approach

HAC 08: Surgical Site Infection of Mediastinitis Following Coronary Bypass Graft (CABG) Procedures (continued)

Ø2124AF Bypass Coronary Artery, Three Arteries from Abdominal Artery with Autologous Arterial Tissue, Percutaneous Endoscopic Approach
Ø2124AW Bypass Coronary Artery, Three Arteries from Aorta with Autologous Arterial Tissue, Percutaneous Endoscopic Approach
Ø2124J3 Bypass Coronary Artery, Three Arteries from Coronary Artery with Synthetic Substitute, Percutaneous Endoscopic Approach
Ø2124J8 Bypass Coronary Artery, Three Arteries from Right Internal Mammary with Synthetic Substitute, Percutaneous Endoscopic Approach
Ø2124J9 Bypass Coronary Artery, Three Arteries from Left Internal Mammary with Synthetic Substitute, Percutaneous Endoscopic Approach
Ø2124JC Bypass Coronary Artery, Three Arteries from Thoracic Artery with Synthetic Substitute, Percutaneous Endoscopic Approach
Ø2124JF Bypass Coronary Artery, Three Arteries from Abdominal Artery with Synthetic Substitute, Percutaneous Endoscopic Approach
Ø2124JW Bypass Coronary Artery, Three Arteries from Aorta with Synthetic Substitute, Percutaneous Endoscopic Approach
Ø2124K3 Bypass Coronary Artery, Three Arteries from Coronary Artery with Nonautologous Tissue Substitute, Percutaneous Endoscopic Approach
Ø2124K8 Bypass Coronary Artery, Three Arteries from Right Internal Mammary with Nonautologous Tissue Substitute, Percutaneous Endoscopic Approach
Ø2124K9 Bypass Coronary Artery, Three Arteries from Left Internal Mammary with Nonautologous Tissue Substitute, Percutaneous Endoscopic Approach
Ø2124KC Bypass Coronary Artery, Three Arteries from Thoracic Artery with Nonautologous Tissue Substitute, Percutaneous Endoscopic Approach
Ø2124KF Bypass Coronary Artery, Three Arteries from Abdominal Artery with Nonautologous Tissue Substitute, Percutaneous Endoscopic Approach
Ø2124KW Bypass Coronary Artery, Three Arteries from Aorta with Nonautologous Tissue Substitute, Percutaneous Endoscopic Approach
Ø2124Z3 Bypass Coronary Artery, Three Arteries from Coronary Artery, Percutaneous Endoscopic Approach
Ø2124Z8 Bypass Coronary Artery, Three Arteries from Right Internal Mammary, Percutaneous Endoscopic Approach
Ø2124Z9 Bypass Coronary Artery, Three Arteries from Left Internal Mammary, Percutaneous Endoscopic Approach
Ø2124ZC Bypass Coronary Artery, Three Arteries from Thoracic Artery, Percutaneous Endoscopic Approach
Ø2124ZF Bypass Coronary Artery, Three Arteries from Abdominal Artery, Percutaneous Endoscopic Approach
Ø213Ø83 Bypass Coronary Artery, Four or More Arteries from Coronary Artery with Zooplastic Tissue, Open Approach
Ø213Ø88 Bypass Coronary Artery, Four or More Arteries from Right Internal Mammary with Zooplastic Tissue, Open Approach
Ø213Ø89 Bypass Coronary Artery, Four or More Arteries from Left Internal Mammary with Zooplastic Tissue, Open Approach
Ø213Ø8C Bypass Coronary Artery, Four or More Arteries from Thoracic Artery with Zooplastic Tissue, Open Approach
Ø213Ø8F Bypass Coronary Artery, Four or More Arteries from Abdominal Artery with Zooplastic Tissue, Open Approach
Ø213Ø8W Bypass Coronary Artery, Four or More Arteries from Aorta with Zooplastic Tissue, Open Approach
Ø213Ø93 Bypass Coronary Artery, Four or More Arteries from Coronary Artery with Autologous Venous Tissue, Open Approach
Ø213Ø98 Bypass Coronary Artery, Four or More Arteries from Right Internal Mammary with Autologous Venous Tissue, Open Approach
Ø213Ø99 Bypass Coronary Artery, Four or More Arteries from Left Internal Mammary with Autologous Venous Tissue, Open Approach
Ø213Ø9C Bypass Coronary Artery, Four or More Arteries from Thoracic Artery with Autologous Venous Tissue, Open Approach
Ø213Ø9F Bypass Coronary Artery, Four or More Arteries from Abdominal Artery with Autologous Venous Tissue, Open Approach
Ø213Ø9W Bypass Coronary Artery, Four or More Arteries from Aorta with Autologous Venous Tissue, Open Approach
Ø213ØA3 Bypass Coronary Artery, Four or More Arteries from Coronary Artery with Autologous Arterial Tissue, Open Approach
Ø213ØA8 Bypass Coronary Artery, Four or More Arteries from Right Internal Mammary with Autologous Arterial Tissue, Open Approach
Ø213ØA9 Bypass Coronary Artery, Four or More Arteries from Left Internal Mammary with Autologous Arterial Tissue, Open Approach
Ø213ØAC Bypass Coronary Artery, Four or More Arteries from Thoracic Artery with Autologous Arterial Tissue, Open Approach
Ø213ØAF Bypass Coronary Artery, Four or More Arteries from Abdominal Artery with Autologous Arterial Tissue, Open Approach
Ø213ØAW Bypass Coronary Artery, Four or More Arteries from Aorta with Autologous Arterial Tissue, Open Approach
Ø213ØJ3 Bypass Coronary Artery, Four or More Arteries from Coronary Artery with Synthetic Substitute, Open Approach
Ø213ØJ8 Bypass Coronary Artery, Four or More Arteries from Right Internal Mammary with Synthetic Substitute, Open Approach
Ø213ØJ9 Bypass Coronary Artery, Four or More Arteries from Left Internal Mammary with Synthetic Substitute, Open Approach
Ø213ØJC Bypass Coronary Artery, Four or More Arteries from Thoracic Artery with Synthetic Substitute, Open Approach
Ø213ØJF Bypass Coronary Artery, Four or More Arteries from Abdominal Artery with Synthetic Substitute, Open Approach
Ø213ØJW Bypass Coronary Artery, Four or More Arteries from Aorta with Synthetic Substitute, Open Approach
Ø213ØK3 Bypass Coronary Artery, Four or More Arteries from Coronary Artery with Nonautologous Tissue Substitute, Open Approach
Ø213ØK8 Bypass Coronary Artery, Four or More Arteries from Right Internal Mammary with Nonautologous Tissue Substitute, Open Approach
Ø213ØK9 Bypass Coronary Artery, Four or More Arteries from Left Internal Mammary with Nonautologous Tissue Substitute, Open Approach
Ø213ØKC Bypass Coronary Artery, Four or More Arteries from Thoracic Artery with Nonautologous Tissue Substitute, Open Approach
Ø213ØKF Bypass Coronary Artery, Four or More Arteries from Abdominal Artery with Nonautologous Tissue Substitute, Open Approach
Ø213ØKW Bypass Coronary Artery, Four or More Arteries from Aorta with Nonautologous Tissue Substitute, Open Approach
Ø213ØZ3 Bypass Coronary Artery, Four or More Arteries from Coronary Artery, Open Approach
Ø213ØZ8 Bypass Coronary Artery, Four or More Arteries from Right Internal Mammary, Open Approach
Ø213ØZ9 Bypass Coronary Artery, Four or More Arteries from Left Internal Mammary, Open Approach
Ø213ØZC Bypass Coronary Artery, Four or More Arteries from Thoracic Artery, Open Approach
Ø213ØZF Bypass Coronary Artery, Four or More Arteries from Abdominal Artery, Open Approach
Ø213483 Bypass Coronary Artery, Four or More Arteries from Coronary Artery with Zooplastic Tissue, Percutaneous Endoscopic Approach
Ø213488 Bypass Coronary Artery, Four or More Arteries from Right Internal Mammary with Zooplastic Tissue, Percutaneous Endoscopic Approach
Ø213489 Bypass Coronary Artery, Four or More Arteries from Left Internal Mammary with Zooplastic Tissue, Percutaneous Endoscopic Approach
Ø21348C Bypass Coronary Artery, Four or More Arteries from Thoracic Artery with Zooplastic Tissue, Percutaneous Endoscopic Approach
Ø21348F Bypass Coronary Artery, Four or More Arteries from Abdominal Artery with Zooplastic Tissue, Percutaneous Endoscopic Approach
Ø21348W Bypass Coronary Artery, Four or More Arteries from Aorta with Zooplastic Tissue, Percutaneous Endoscopic Approach
Ø213493 Bypass Coronary Artery, Four or More Arteries from Coronary Artery with Autologous Venous Tissue, Percutaneous Endoscopic Approach
Ø213498 Bypass Coronary Artery, Four or More Arteries from Right Internal Mammary with Autologous Venous Tissue, Percutaneous Endoscopic Approach

HAC 08: Surgical Site Infection of Mediastinitis Following Coronary Bypass Graft (CABG) Procedures (continued)

Ø213499 Bypass Coronary Artery, Four or More Arteries from Left Internal Mammary with Autologous Venous Tissue, Percutaneous Endoscopic Approach
Ø21349C Bypass Coronary Artery, Four or More Arteries from Thoracic Artery with Autologous Venous Tissue, Percutaneous Endoscopic Approach
Ø21349F Bypass Coronary Artery, Four or More Arteries from Abdominal Artery with Autologous Venous Tissue, Percutaneous Endoscopic Approach
Ø21349W Bypass Coronary Artery, Four or More Arteries from Aorta with Autologous Venous Tissue, Percutaneous Endoscopic Approach
Ø2134A3 Bypass Coronary Artery, Four or More Arteries from Coronary Artery with Autologous Arterial Tissue, Percutaneous Endoscopic Approach
Ø2134A8 Bypass Coronary Artery, Four or More Arteries from Right Internal Mammary with Autologous Arterial Tissue, Percutaneous Endoscopic Approach
Ø2134A9 Bypass Coronary Artery, Four or More Arteries from Left Internal Mammary with Autologous Arterial Tissue, Percutaneous Endoscopic Approach
Ø2134AC Bypass Coronary Artery, Four or More Arteries from Thoracic Artery with Autologous Arterial Tissue, Percutaneous Endoscopic Approach
Ø2134AF Bypass Coronary Artery, Four or More Arteries from Abdominal Artery with Autologous Arterial Tissue, Percutaneous Endoscopic Approach
Ø2134AW Bypass Coronary Artery, Four or More Arteries from Aorta with Autologous Arterial Tissue, Percutaneous Endoscopic Approach
Ø2134J3 Bypass Coronary Artery, Four or More Arteries from Coronary Artery with Synthetic Substitute, Percutaneous Endoscopic Approach
Ø2134J8 Bypass Coronary Artery, Four or More Arteries from Right Internal Mammary with Synthetic Substitute, Percutaneous Endoscopic Approach
Ø2134J9 Bypass Coronary Artery, Four or More Arteries from Left Internal Mammary with Synthetic Substitute, Percutaneous Endoscopic Approach
Ø2134JC Bypass Coronary Artery, Four or More Arteries from Thoracic Artery with Synthetic Substitute, Percutaneous Endoscopic Approach
Ø2134JF Bypass Coronary Artery, Four or More Arteries from Abdominal Artery with Synthetic Substitute, Percutaneous Endoscopic Approach
Ø2134JW Bypass Coronary Artery, Four or More Arteries from Aorta with Synthetic Substitute, Percutaneous Endoscopic Approach
Ø2134K3 Bypass Coronary Artery, Four or More Arteries from Coronary Artery with Nonautologous Tissue Substitute, Percutaneous Endoscopic Approach
Ø2134K8 Bypass Coronary Artery, Four or More Arteries from Right Internal Mammary with Nonautologous Tissue Substitute, Percutaneous Endoscopic Approach
Ø2134K9 Bypass Coronary Artery, Four or More Arteries from Left Internal Mammary with Nonautologous Tissue Substitute, Percutaneous Endoscopic Approach
Ø2134KC Bypass Coronary Artery, Four or More Arteries from Thoracic Artery with Nonautologous Tissue Substitute, Percutaneous Endoscopic Approach
Ø2134KF Bypass Coronary Artery, Four or More Arteries from Abdominal Artery with Nonautologous Tissue Substitute, Percutaneous Endoscopic Approach
Ø2134KW Bypass Coronary Artery, Four or More Arteries from Aorta with Nonautologous Tissue Substitute, Percutaneous Endoscopic Approach
Ø2134Z3 Bypass Coronary Artery, Four or More Arteries from Coronary Artery, Percutaneous Endoscopic Approach
Ø2134Z8 Bypass Coronary Artery, Four or More Arteries from Right Internal Mammary, Percutaneous Endoscopic Approach
Ø2134Z9 Bypass Coronary Artery, Four or More Arteries from Left Internal Mammary, Percutaneous Endoscopic Approach
Ø2134ZC Bypass Coronary Artery, Four or More Arteries from Thoracic Artery, Percutaneous Endoscopic Approach
Ø2134ZF Bypass Coronary Artery, Four or More Arteries from Abdominal Artery, Percutaneous Endoscopic Approach

HAC 09: Manifestations of Poor Glycemic Control

Secondary diagnosis not POA:

EØ8.ØØ
EØ8.Ø1
EØ8.1Ø
EØ9.ØØ
EØ9.Ø1
EØ9.1Ø
E1Ø.1Ø
E11.ØØ
E11.Ø1
E13.ØØ
E13.Ø1
E13.1Ø
E15

HAC 10: Deep Vein Thrombosis (DVT) or Pulmonary Embolism (PE) with Total Knee or Hip Replacement

Secondary diagnosis not POA:

I26.Ø2
I26.Ø9
I26.92
I26.99
I82.4Ø1
I82.4Ø2
I82.4Ø3
I82.4Ø9
I82.411
I82.412
I82.413
I82.419
I82.421
I82.422
I82.423
I82.429
I82.431
I82.432
I82.433
I82.439
I82.441
I82.442
I82.443
I82.449
I82.491
I82.492
I82.493
I82.499
I82.4Y1
I82.4Y2
I82.4Y3
I82.4Y9
I82.4Z1
I82.4Z2
I82.4Z3
I82.4Z9

AND

Any of the following procedures:

ØSR9Ø19 Replacement of Right Hip Joint with Metal Synthetic Substitute, Cemented, Open Approach
ØSR9Ø1A Replacement of Right Hip Joint with Metal Synthetic Substitute, Uncemented, Open Approach
ØSR9Ø1Z Replacement of Right Hip Joint with Metal Synthetic Substitute, Open Approach
ØSR9Ø29 Replacement of Right Hip Joint with Metal on Polyethylene Synthetic Substitute, Cemented, Open Approach
ØSR9Ø2A Replacement of Right Hip Joint with Metal on Polyethylene Synthetic Substitute, Uncemented, Open Approach
ØSR9Ø2Z Replacement of Right Hip Joint with Metal on Polyethylene Synthetic Substitute, Open Approach
ØSR9Ø39 Replacement of Right Hip Joint with Ceramic Synthetic Substitute, Cemented, Open Approach
ØSR9Ø3A Replacement of Right Hip Joint with Ceramic Synthetic Substitute, Uncemented, Open Approach
ØSR9Ø3Z Replacement of Right Hip Joint with Ceramic Synthetic Substitute, Open Approach
ØSR9Ø49 Replacement of Right Hip Joint with Ceramic on Polyethylene Synthetic Substitute, Cemented, Open Approach
ØSR9Ø4A Replacement of Right Hip Joint with Ceramic on Polyethylene Synthetic Substitute, Uncemented, Open Approach
ØSR9Ø4Z Replacement of Right Hip Joint with Ceramic on Polyethylene Synthetic Substitute, Open Approach
ØSR9Ø69 Replacement of Right Hip Joint with Oxidized Zirconium on Polyethylene Synthetic Substitute, Cemented, Open Approach
ØSR9Ø6A Replacement of Right Hip Joint with Oxidized Zirconium on Polyethylene Synthetic Substitute, Uncemented, Open Approach
ØSR9Ø6Z Replacement of Right Hip Joint with Oxidized Zirconium on Polyethylene Synthetic Substitute, Open Approach
ØSR9Ø7Z Replacement of Right Hip Joint with Autologous Tissue Substitute, Open Approach
ØSR9ØJ9 Replacement of Right Hip Joint with Synthetic Substitute, Cemented, Open Approach
ØSR9ØJA Replacement of Right Hip Joint with Synthetic Substitute, Uncemented, Open Approach
ØSR9ØJZ Replacement of Right Hip Joint with Synthetic Substitute, Open Approach

HAC 10: Deep Vein Thrombosis (DVT) or Pulmonary Embolism (PE) with Total Knee or Hip Replacement (continued)

ØSR9ØKZ Replacement of Right Hip Joint with Nonautologous Tissue Substitute, Open Approach
ØSRAØØ9 Replacement of Right Hip Joint, Acetabular Surface with Polyethylene Synthetic Substitute, Cemented, Open Approach
ØSRAØØA Replacement of Right Hip Joint, Acetabular Surface with Polyethylene Synthetic Substitute, Uncemented, Open Approach
ØSRAØØZ Replacement of Right Hip Joint, Acetabular Surface with Polyethylene Synthetic Substitute, Open Approach
ØSRAØ19 Replacement of Right Hip Joint, Acetabular Surface with Metal Synthetic Substitute, Cemented, Open Approach
ØSRAØ1A Replacement of Right Hip Joint, Acetabular Surface with Metal Synthetic Substitute, Uncemented, Open Approach
ØSRAØ1Z Replacement of Right Hip Joint, Acetabular Surface with Metal Synthetic Substitute, Open Approach
ØSRAØ39 Replacement of Right Hip Joint, Acetabular Surface with Ceramic Synthetic Substitute, Cemented, Open Approach
ØSRAØ3A Replacement of Right Hip Joint, Acetabular Surface with Ceramic Synthetic Substitute, Uncemented, Open Approach
ØSRAØ3Z Replacement of Right Hip Joint, Acetabular Surface with Ceramic Synthetic Substitute, Open Approach
ØSRAØ7Z Replacement of Right Hip Joint, Acetabular Surface with Autologous Tissue Substitute, Open Approach
ØSRAØJ9 Replacement of Right Hip Joint, Acetabular Surface with Synthetic Substitute, Cemented, Open Approach
ØSRAØJA Replacement of Right Hip Joint, Acetabular Surface with Synthetic Substitute, Uncemented, Open Approach
ØSRAØJZ Replacement of Right Hip Joint, Acetabular Surface with Synthetic Substitute, Open Approach
ØSRAØKZ Replacement of Right Hip Joint, Acetabular Surface with Nonautologous Tissue Substitute, Open Approach
ØSRBØ19 Replacement of Left Hip Joint with Metal Synthetic Substitute, Cemented, Open Approach
ØSRBØ1A Replacement of Left Hip Joint with Metal Synthetic Substitute, Uncemented, Open Approach
ØSRBØ1Z Replacement of Left Hip Joint with Metal Synthetic Substitute, Open Approach
ØSRBØ29 Replacement of Left Hip Joint with Metal on Polyethylene Synthetic Substitute, Cemented, Open Approach
ØSRBØ2A Replacement of Left Hip Joint with Metal on Polyethylene Synthetic Substitute, Uncemented, Open Approach
ØSRBØ2Z Replacement of Left Hip Joint with Metal on Polyethylene Synthetic Substitute, Open Approach
ØSRBØ39 Replacement of Left Hip Joint with Ceramic Synthetic Substitute, Cemented, Open Approach
ØSRBØ3A Replacement of Left Hip Joint with Ceramic Synthetic Substitute, Uncemented, Open Approach
ØSRBØ3Z Replacement of Left Hip Joint with Ceramic Synthetic Substitute, Open Approach
ØSRBØ49 Replacement of Left Hip Joint with Ceramic on Polyethylene Synthetic Substitute, Cemented, Open Approach
ØSRBØ4A Replacement of Left Hip Joint with Ceramic on Polyethylene Synthetic Substitute, Uncemented, Open Approach
ØSRBØ4Z Replacement of Left Hip Joint with Ceramic on Polyethylene Synthetic Substitute, Open Approach
ØSRBØ69 Replacement of Left Hip Joint with Oxidized Zirconium on Polyethylene Synthetic Substitute, Cemented, Open Approach
ØSRBØ6A Replacement of Left Hip Joint with Oxidized Zirconium on Polyethylene Synthetic Substitute, Uncemented, Open Approach
ØSRBØ6Z Replacement of Left Hip Joint with Oxidized Zirconium on Polyethylene Synthetic Substitute, Open Approach
ØSRBØ7Z Replacement of Left Hip Joint with Autologous Tissue Substitute, Open Approach
ØSRBØJ9 Replacement of Left Hip Joint with Synthetic Substitute, Cemented, Open Approach
ØSRBØJA Replacement of Left Hip Joint with Synthetic Substitute, Uncemented, Open Approach
ØSRBØJZ Replacement of Left Hip Joint with Synthetic Substitute, Open Approach
ØSRBØKZ Replacement of Left Hip Joint with Nonautologous Tissue Substitute, Open Approach
ØSRCØ69 Replacement of Right Knee Joint with Oxidized Zirconium on Polyethylene Synthetic Substitute, Cemented, Open Approach
ØSRCØ6A Replacement of Right Knee Joint with Oxidized Zirconium on Polyethylene Synthetic Substitute, Uncemented, Open Approach
ØSRCØ6Z Replacement of Right Knee Joint with Oxidized Zirconium on Polyethylene Synthetic Substitute, Open Approach
ØSRCØ7Z Replacement of Right Knee Joint with Autologous Tissue Substitute, Open Approach
ØSRCØJ9 Replacement of Right Knee Joint with Synthetic Substitute, Cemented, Open Approach
ØSRCØJA Replacement of Right Knee Joint with Synthetic Substitute, Uncemented, Open Approach
ØSRCØJZ Replacement of Right Knee Joint with Synthetic Substitute, Open Approach
ØSRCØKZ Replacement of Right Knee Joint with Nonautologous Tissue Substitute, Open Approach
ØSRDØ69 Replacement of Left Knee Joint with Oxidized Zirconium on Polyethylene Synthetic Substitute, Cemented, Open Approach
ØSRDØ6A Replacement of Left Knee Joint with Oxidized Zirconium on Polyethylene Synthetic Substitute, Uncemented, Open Approach
ØSRDØ6Z Replacement of Left Knee Joint with Oxidized Zirconium on Polyethylene Synthetic Substitute, Open Approach
ØSRDØ7Z Replacement of Left Knee Joint with Autologous Tissue Substitute, Open Approach
ØSRDØJ9 Replacement of Left Knee Joint with Synthetic Substitute, Cemented, Open Approach
ØSRDØJA Replacement of Left Knee Joint with Synthetic Substitute, Uncemented, Open Approach
ØSRDØJZ Replacement of Left Knee Joint with Synthetic Substitute, Open Approach
ØSRDØKZ Replacement of Left Knee Joint with Nonautologous Tissue Substitute, Open Approach
ØSREØØ9 Replacement of Left Hip Joint, Acetabular Surface with Polyethylene Synthetic Substitute, Cemented, Open Approach
ØSREØØA Replacement of Left Hip Joint, Acetabular Surface with Polyethylene Synthetic Substitute, Uncemented, Open Approach
ØSREØØZ Replacement of Left Hip Joint, Acetabular Surface with Polyethylene Synthetic Substitute, Open Approach
ØSREØ19 Replacement of Left Hip Joint, Acetabular Surface with Metal Synthetic Substitute, Cemented, Open Approach
ØSREØ1A Replacement of Left Hip Joint, Acetabular Surface with Metal Synthetic Substitute, Uncemented, Open Approach
ØSREØ1Z Replacement of Left Hip Joint, Acetabular Surface with Metal Synthetic Substitute, Open Approach
ØSREØ39 Replacement of Left Hip Joint, Acetabular Surface with Ceramic Synthetic Substitute, Cemented, Open Approach
ØSREØ3A Replacement of Left Hip Joint, Acetabular Surface with Ceramic Synthetic Substitute, Uncemented, Open Approach
ØSREØ3Z Replacement of Left Hip Joint, Acetabular Surface with Ceramic Synthetic Substitute, Open Approach
ØSREØ7Z Replacement of Left Hip Joint, Acetabular Surface with Autologous Tissue Substitute, Open Approach
ØSREØJ9 Replacement of Left Hip Joint, Acetabular Surface with Synthetic Substitute, Cemented, Open Approach
ØSREØJA Replacement of Left Hip Joint, Acetabular Surface with Synthetic Substitute, Uncemented, Open Approach
ØSREØJZ Replacement of Left Hip Joint, Acetabular Surface with Synthetic Substitute, Open Approach
ØSREØKZ Replacement of Left Hip Joint, Acetabular Surface with Nonautologous Tissue Substitute, Open Approach
ØSRRØ19 Replacement of Right Hip Joint, Femoral Surface with Metal Synthetic Substitute, Cemented, Open Approach
ØSRRØ1A Replacement of Right Hip Joint, Femoral Surface with Metal Synthetic Substitute, Uncemented, Open Approach
ØSRRØ1Z Replacement of Right Hip Joint, Femoral Surface with Metal Synthetic Substitute, Open Approach

HAC 10: Deep Vein Thrombosis (DVT) or Pulmonary Embolism (PE) with Total Knee or Hip Replacement (continued)

ØSRRØ39 Replacement of Right Hip Joint, Femoral Surface with Ceramic Synthetic Substitute, Cemented, Open Approach
ØSRRØ3A Replacement of Right Hip Joint, Femoral Surface with Ceramic Synthetic Substitute, Uncemented, Open Approach
ØSRRØ3Z Replacement of Right Hip Joint, Femoral Surface with Ceramic Synthetic Substitute, Open Approach
ØSRRØ7Z Replacement of Right Hip Joint, Femoral Surface with Autologous Tissue Substitute, Open Approach
ØSRRØJ9 Replacement of Right Hip Joint, Femoral Surface with Synthetic Substitute, Cemented, Open Approach
ØSRRØJA Replacement of Right Hip Joint, Femoral Surface with Synthetic Substitute, Uncemented, Open Approach
ØSRRØJZ Replacement of Right Hip Joint, Femoral Surface with Synthetic Substitute, Open Approach
ØSRRØKZ Replacement of Right Hip Joint, Femoral Surface with Nonautologous Tissue Substitute, Open Approach
ØSRSØ19 Replacement of Left Hip Joint, Femoral Surface with Metal Synthetic Substitute, Cemented, Open Approach
ØSRSØ1A Replacement of Left Hip Joint, Femoral Surface with Metal Synthetic Substitute, Uncemented, Open Approach
ØSRSØ1Z Replacement of Left Hip Joint, Femoral Surface with Metal Synthetic Substitute, Open Approach
ØSRSØ39 Replacement of Left Hip Joint, Femoral Surface with Ceramic Synthetic Substitute, Cemented, Open Approach
ØSRSØ3A Replacement of Left Hip Joint, Femoral Surface with Ceramic Synthetic Substitute, Uncemented, Open Approach
ØSRSØ3Z Replacement of Left Hip Joint, Femoral Surface with Ceramic Synthetic Substitute, Open Approach
ØSRSØ7Z Replacement of Left Hip Joint, Femoral Surface with Autologous Tissue Substitute, Open Approach
ØSRSØJ9 Replacement of Left Hip Joint, Femoral Surface with Synthetic Substitute, Cemented, Open Approach
ØSRSØJA Replacement of Left Hip Joint, Femoral Surface with Synthetic Substitute, Uncemented, Open Approach
ØSRSØJZ Replacement of Left Hip Joint, Femoral Surface with Synthetic Substitute, Open Approach
ØSRSØKZ Replacement of Left Hip Joint, Femoral Surface with Nonautologous Tissue Substitute, Open Approach
ØSRTØ7Z Replacement of Right Knee Joint, Femoral Surface with Autologous Tissue Substitute, Open Approach
ØSRTØJ9 Replacement of Right Knee Joint, Femoral Surface with Synthetic Substitute, Cemented, Open Approach
ØSRTØJA Replacement of Right Knee Joint, Femoral Surface with Synthetic Substitute, Uncemented, Open Approach
ØSRTØJZ Replacement of Right Knee Joint, Femoral Surface with Synthetic Substitute, Open Approach
ØSRTØKZ Replacement of Right Knee Joint, Femoral Surface with Nonautologous Tissue Substitute, Open Approach
ØSRUØ7Z Replacement of Left Knee Joint, Femoral Surface with Autologous Tissue Substitute, Open Approach
ØSRUØJ9 Replacement of Left Knee Joint, Femoral Surface with Synthetic Substitute, Cemented, Open Approach
ØSRUØJA Replacement of Left Knee Joint, Femoral Surface with Synthetic Substitute, Uncemented, Open Approach
ØSRUØJZ Replacement of Left Knee Joint, Femoral Surface with Synthetic Substitute, Open Approach
ØSRUØKZ Replacement of Left Knee Joint, Femoral Surface with Nonautologous Tissue Substitute, Open Approach
ØSRVØ7Z Replacement of Right Knee Joint, Tibial Surface with Autologous Tissue Substitute, Open Approach
ØSRVØJ9 Replacement of Right Knee Joint, Tibial Surface with Synthetic Substitute, Cemented, Open Approach
ØSRVØJA Replacement of Right Knee Joint, Tibial Surface with Synthetic Substitute, Uncemented, Open Approach
ØSRVØJZ Replacement of Right Knee Joint, Tibial Surface with Synthetic Substitute, Open Approach
ØSRVØKZ Replacement of Right Knee Joint, Tibial Surface with Nonautologous Tissue Substitute, Open Approach
ØSRWØ7Z Replacement of Left Knee Joint, Tibial Surface with Autologous Tissue Substitute, Open Approach
ØSRWØJ9 Replacement of Left Knee Joint, Tibial Surface with Synthetic Substitute, Cemented, Open Approach
ØSRWØJA Replacement of Left Knee Joint, Tibial Surface with Synthetic Substitute, Uncemented, Open Approach
ØSRWØJZ Replacement of Left Knee Joint, Tibial Surface with Synthetic Substitute, Open Approach
ØSRWØKZ Replacement of Left Knee Joint, Tibial Surface with Nonautologous Tissue Substitute, Open Approach
ØSU9ØBZ Supplement Right Hip Joint with Resurfacing Device, Open Approach
ØSUAØBZ Supplement Right Hip Joint, Acetabular Surface with Resurfacing Device, Open Approach
ØSUBØBZ Supplement Left Hip Joint with Resurfacing Device, Open Approach
ØSUEØBZ Supplement Left Hip Joint, Acetabular Surface with Resurfacing Device, Open Approach
ØSURØBZ Supplement Right Hip Joint, Femoral Surface with Resurfacing Device, Open Approach
ØSUSØBZ Supplement Left Hip Joint, Femoral Surface with Resurfacing Device, Open Approach

HAC 11: Surgical Site Infection Following Bariatric Surgery

Principal diagnosis of:
E66.Ø1

AND

Secondary diagnosis not POA:
K68.11
K95.Ø1
K95.81
T81.4XXA

AND

Any of the following procedures:

ØD16Ø79 Bypass Stomach to Duodenum with Autologous Tissue Substitute, Open Approach
ØD16Ø7A Bypass Stomach to Jejunum with Autologous Tissue Substitute, Open Approach
ØD16Ø7B Bypass Stomach to Ileum with Autologous Tissue Substitute, Open Approach
ØD16Ø7L Bypass Stomach to Transverse Colon with Autologous Tissue Substitute, Open Approach
ØD16ØJ9 Bypass Stomach to Duodenum with Synthetic Substitute, Open Approach
ØD16ØJA Bypass Stomach to Jejunum with Synthetic Substitute, Open Approach
ØD16ØJB Bypass Stomach to Ileum with Synthetic Substitute, Open Approach
ØD16ØJL Bypass Stomach to Transverse Colon with Synthetic Substitute, Open Approach
ØD16ØK9 Bypass Stomach to Duodenum with Nonautologous Tissue Substitute, Open Approach
ØD16ØKA Bypass Stomach to Jejunum with Nonautologous Tissue Substitute, Open Approach
ØD16ØKB Bypass Stomach to Ileum with Nonautologous Tissue Substitute, Open Approach
ØD16ØKL Bypass Stomach to Transverse Colon with Nonautologous Tissue Substitute, Open Approach
ØD16ØZ9 Bypass Stomach to Duodenum, Open Approach
ØD16ØZA Bypass Stomach to Jejunum, Open Approach
ØD16ØZB Bypass Stomach to Ileum, Open Approach
ØD16ØZL Bypass Stomach to Transverse Colon, Open Approach
ØD16479 Bypass Stomach to Duodenum with Autologous Tissue Substitute, Percutaneous Endoscopic Approach
ØD1647A Bypass Stomach to Jejunum with Autologous Tissue Substitute, Percutaneous Endoscopic Approach
ØD1647B Bypass Stomach to Ileum with Autologous Tissue Substitute, Percutaneous Endoscopic Approach
ØD1647L Bypass Stomach to Transverse Colon with Autologous Tissue Substitute, Percutaneous Endoscopic Approach
ØD164J9 Bypass Stomach to Duodenum with Synthetic Substitute, Percutaneous Endoscopic Approach
ØD164JA Bypass Stomach to Jejunum with Synthetic Substitute, Percutaneous Endoscopic Approach
ØD164JB Bypass Stomach to Ileum with Synthetic Substitute, Percutaneous Endoscopic Approach
ØD164JL Bypass Stomach to Transverse Colon with Synthetic Substitute, Percutaneous Endoscopic Approach
ØD164K9 Bypass Stomach to Duodenum with Nonautologous Tissue Substitute, Percutaneous Endoscopic Approach
ØD164KA Bypass Stomach to Jejunum with Nonautologous Tissue Substitute, Percutaneous Endoscopic Approach
ØD164KB Bypass Stomach to Ileum with Nonautologous Tissue Substitute, Percutaneous Endoscopic Approach

HAC 11: Surgical Site Infection Following Bariatric Surgery (continued)

ØD164KL Bypass Stomach to Transverse Colon with Nonautologous Tissue Substitute, Percutaneous Endoscopic Approach
ØD164Z9 Bypass Stomach to Duodenum, Percutaneous Endoscopic Approach
ØD164ZA Bypass Stomach to Jejunum, Percutaneous Endoscopic Approach
ØD164ZB Bypass Stomach to Ileum, Percutaneous Endoscopic Approach
ØD164ZL Bypass Stomach to Transverse Colon, Percutaneous Endoscopic Approach
ØD16879 Bypass Stomach to Duodenum with Autologous Tissue Substitute, Via Natural or Artificial Opening Endoscopic
ØD1687A Bypass Stomach to Jejunum with Autologous Tissue Substitute, Via Natural or Artificial Opening Endoscopic
ØD1687B Bypass Stomach to Ileum with Autologous Tissue Substitute, Via Natural or Artificial Opening Endoscopic
ØD1687L Bypass Stomach to Transverse Colon with Autologous Tissue Substitute, Via Natural or Artificial Opening Endoscopic
ØD168J9 Bypass Stomach to Duodenum with Synthetic Substitute, Via Natural or Artificial Opening Endoscopic
ØD168JA Bypass Stomach to Jejunum with Synthetic Substitute, Via Natural or Artificial Opening Endoscopic
ØD168JB Bypass Stomach to Ileum with Synthetic Substitute, Via Natural or Artificial Opening Endoscopic
ØD168JL Bypass Stomach to Transverse Colon with Synthetic Substitute, Via Natural or Artificial Opening Endoscopic
ØD168K9 Bypass Stomach to Duodenum with Nonautologous Tissue Substitute, Via Natural or Artificial Opening Endoscopic
ØD168KA Bypass Stomach to Jejunum with Nonautologous Tissue Substitute, Via Natural or Artificial Opening Endoscopic
ØD168KB Bypass Stomach to Ileum with Nonautologous Tissue Substitute, Via Natural or Artificial Opening Endoscopic
ØD168KL Bypass Stomach to Transverse Colon with Nonautologous Tissue Substitute, Via Natural or Artificial Opening Endoscopic
ØD168Z9 Bypass Stomach to Duodenum, Via Natural or Artificial Opening Endoscopic
ØD168ZA Bypass Stomach to Jejunum, Via Natural or Artificial Opening Endoscopic
ØD168ZB Bypass Stomach to Ileum, Via Natural or Artificial Opening Endoscopic
ØD168ZL Bypass Stomach to Transverse Colon, Via Natural or Artificial Opening Endoscopic
ØDV64CZ Restriction of Stomach with Extraluminal Device, Percutaneous Endoscopic Approach

HAC 12: Surgical Site Infection Following Certain Orthopedic Procedures of the Spine, Shoulder, and Elbow

Secondary diagnosis not POA:

K68.11
T81.4XXA
T84.6ØXA
T84.61ØA
T84.611A
T84.612A
T84.613A
T84.614A
T84.615A
T84.619A
T84.63XA
T84.69XA
T84.7XXA

AND

Any of the following procedures:

ØRGØØ7Ø Fusion of Occipital-cervical Joint with Autologous Tissue Substitute, Anterior Approach, Anterior Column, Open Approach
ØRGØØ71 Fusion of Occipital-cervical Joint with Autologous Tissue Substitute, Posterior Approach, Posterior Column, Open Approach
ØRGØØ7J Fusion of Occipital-cervical Joint with Autologous Tissue Substitute, Posterior Approach, Anterior Column, Open Approach
ØRGØØAØ Fusion of Occipital-cervical Joint with Interbody Fusion Device, Anterior Approach, Anterior Column, Open Approach
ØRGØØAJ Fusion of Occipital-cervical Joint with Interbody Fusion Device, Posterior Approach, Anterior Column, Open Approach
ØRGØØJØ Fusion of Occipital-cervical Joint with Synthetic Substitute, Anterior Approach, Anterior Column, Open Approach
ØRGØØJ1 Fusion of Occipital-cervical Joint with Synthetic Substitute, Posterior Approach, Posterior Column, Open Approach
ØRGØØJJ Fusion of Occipital-cervical Joint with Synthetic Substitute, Posterior Approach, Anterior Column, Open Approach
ØRGØØKØ Fusion of Occipital-cervical Joint with Nonautologous Tissue Substitute, Anterior Approach, Anterior Column, Open Approach
ØRGØØK1 Fusion of Occipital-cervical Joint with Nonautologous Tissue Substitute, Posterior Approach, Posterior Column, Open Approach
ØRGØØKJ Fusion of Occipital-cervical Joint with Nonautologous Tissue Substitute, Posterior Approach, Anterior Column, Open Approach
ØRGØ37Ø Fusion of Occipital-cervical Joint with Autologous Tissue Substitute, Anterior Approach, Anterior Column, Percutaneous Approach
ØRGØ371 Fusion of Occipital-cervical Joint with Autologous Tissue Substitute, Posterior Approach, Posterior Column, Percutaneous Approach
ØRGØ37J Fusion of Occipital-cervical Joint with Autologous Tissue Substitute, Posterior Approach, Anterior Column, Percutaneous Approach
ØRGØ3AØ Fusion of Occipital-cervical Joint with Interbody Fusion Device, Anterior Approach, Anterior Column, Percutaneous Approach
ØRGØ3AJ Fusion of Occipital-cervical Joint with Interbody Fusion Device, Posterior Approach, Anterior Column, Percutaneous Approach
ØRGØ3JØ Fusion of Occipital-cervical Joint with Synthetic Substitute, Anterior Approach, Anterior Column, Percutaneous Approach
ØRGØ3J1 Fusion of Occipital-cervical Joint with Synthetic Substitute, Posterior Approach, Posterior Column, Percutaneous Approach
ØRGØ3JJ Fusion of Occipital-cervical Joint with Synthetic Substitute, Posterior Approach, Anterior Column, Percutaneous Approach
ØRGØ3KØ Fusion of Occipital-cervical Joint with Nonautologous Tissue Substitute, Anterior Approach, Anterior Column, Percutaneous Approach
ØRGØ3K1 Fusion of Occipital-cervical Joint with Nonautologous Tissue Substitute, Posterior Approach, Posterior Column, Percutaneous Approach
ØRGØ3KJ Fusion of Occipital-cervical Joint with Nonautologous Tissue Substitute, Posterior Approach, Anterior Column, Percutaneous Approach
ØRGØ47Ø Fusion of Occipital-cervical Joint with Autologous Tissue Substitute, Anterior Approach, Anterior Column, Percutaneous Endoscopic Approach
ØRGØ471 Fusion of Occipital-cervical Joint with Autologous Tissue Substitute, Posterior Approach, Posterior Column, Percutaneous Endoscopic Approach
ØRGØ47J Fusion of Occipital-cervical Joint with Autologous Tissue Substitute, Posterior Approach, Anterior Column, Percutaneous Endoscopic Approach
ØRGØ4AØ Fusion of Occipital-cervical Joint with Interbody Fusion Device, Anterior Approach, Anterior Column, Percutaneous Endoscopic Approach
ØRGØ4AJ Fusion of Occipital-cervical Joint with Interbody Fusion Device, Posterior Approach, Anterior Column, Percutaneous Endoscopic Approach
ØRGØ4JØ Fusion of Occipital-cervical Joint with Synthetic Substitute, Anterior Approach, Anterior Column, Percutaneous Endoscopic Approach
ØRGØ4J1 Fusion of Occipital-cervical Joint with Synthetic Substitute, Posterior Approach, Posterior Column, Percutaneous Endoscopic Approach
ØRGØ4JJ Fusion of Occipital-cervical Joint with Synthetic Substitute, Posterior Approach, Anterior Column, Percutaneous Endoscopic Approach
ØRGØ4KØ Fusion of Occipital-cervical Joint with Nonautologous Tissue Substitute, Anterior Approach, Anterior Column, Percutaneous Endoscopic Approach
ØRGØ4K1 Fusion of Occipital-cervical Joint with Nonautologous Tissue Substitute, Posterior Approach, Posterior Column, Percutaneous Endoscopic Approach
ØRGØ4KJ Fusion of Occipital-cervical Joint with Nonautologous Tissue Substitute, Posterior Approach, Anterior Column, Percutaneous Endoscopic Approach
ØRG1Ø7Ø Fusion of Cervical Vertebral Joint with Autologous Tissue Substitute, Anterior Approach, Anterior Column, Open Approach
ØRG1Ø71 Fusion of Cervical Vertebral Joint with Autologous Tissue Substitute, Posterior Approach, Posterior Column, Open Approach
ØRG1Ø7J Fusion of Cervical Vertebral Joint with Autologous Tissue Substitute, Posterior Approach, Anterior Column, Open Approach

HAC 12: Surgical Site Infection Following Certain Orthopedic Procedures of the Spine, Shoulder, and Elbow (continued)

ØRG10AØ Fusion of Cervical Vertebral Joint with Interbody Fusion Device, Anterior Approach, Anterior Column, Open Approach
ØRG10AJ Fusion of Cervical Vertebral Joint with Interbody Fusion Device, Posterior Approach, Anterior Column, Open Approach
ØRG10JØ Fusion of Cervical Vertebral Joint with Synthetic Substitute, Anterior Approach, Anterior Column, Open Approach
ØRG10J1 Fusion of Cervical Vertebral Joint with Synthetic Substitute, Posterior Approach, Posterior Column, Open Approach
ØRG10JJ Fusion of Cervical Vertebral Joint with Synthetic Substitute, Posterior Approach, Anterior Column, Open Approach
ØRG10KØ Fusion of Cervical Vertebral Joint with Nonautologous Tissue Substitute, Anterior Approach, Anterior Column, Open Approach
ØRG10K1 Fusion of Cervical Vertebral Joint with Nonautologous Tissue Substitute, Posterior Approach, Posterior Column, Open Approach
ØRG10KJ Fusion of Cervical Vertebral Joint with Nonautologous Tissue Substitute, Posterior Approach, Anterior Column, Open Approach
ØRG137Ø Fusion of Cervical Vertebral Joint with Autologous Tissue Substitute, Anterior Approach, Anterior Column, Percutaneous Approach
ØRG1371 Fusion of Cervical Vertebral Joint with Autologous Tissue Substitute, Posterior Approach, Posterior Column, Percutaneous Approach
ØRG137J Fusion of Cervical Vertebral Joint with Autologous Tissue Substitute, Posterior Approach, Anterior Column, Percutaneous Approach
ØRG13AØ Fusion of Cervical Vertebral Joint with Interbody Fusion Device, Anterior Approach, Anterior Column, Percutaneous Approach
ØRG13AJ Fusion of Cervical Vertebral Joint with Interbody Fusion Device, Posterior Approach, Anterior Column, Percutaneous Approach
ØRG13JØ Fusion of Cervical Vertebral Joint with Synthetic Substitute, Anterior Approach, Anterior Column, Percutaneous Approach
ØRG13J1 Fusion of Cervical Vertebral Joint with Synthetic Substitute, Posterior Approach, Posterior Column, Percutaneous Approach
ØRG13JJ Fusion of Cervical Vertebral Joint with Synthetic Substitute, Posterior Approach, Anterior Column, Percutaneous Approach
ØRG13KØ Fusion of Cervical Vertebral Joint with Nonautologous Tissue Substitute, Anterior Approach, Anterior Column, Percutaneous Approach
ØRG13K1 Fusion of Cervical Vertebral Joint with Nonautologous Tissue Substitute, Posterior Approach, Posterior Column, Percutaneous Approach
ØRG13KJ Fusion of Cervical Vertebral Joint with Nonautologous Tissue Substitute, Posterior Approach, Anterior Column, Percutaneous Approach
ØRG147Ø Fusion of Cervical Vertebral Joint with Autologous Tissue Substitute, Anterior Approach, Anterior Column, Percutaneous Endoscopic Approach
ØRG1471 Fusion of Cervical Vertebral Joint with Autologous Tissue Substitute, Posterior Approach, Posterior Column, Percutaneous Endoscopic Approach
ØRG147J Fusion of Cervical Vertebral Joint with Autologous Tissue Substitute, Posterior Approach, Anterior Column, Percutaneous Endoscopic Approach
ØRG14AØ Fusion of Cervical Vertebral Joint with Interbody Fusion Device, Anterior Approach, Anterior Column, Percutaneous Endoscopic Approach
ØRG14AJ Fusion of Cervical Vertebral Joint with Interbody Fusion Device, Posterior Approach, Anterior Column, Percutaneous Endoscopic Approach
ØRG14JØ Fusion of Cervical Vertebral Joint with Synthetic Substitute, Anterior Approach, Anterior Column, Percutaneous Endoscopic Approach
ØRG14J1 Fusion of Cervical Vertebral Joint with Synthetic Substitute, Posterior Approach, Posterior Column, Percutaneous Endoscopic Approach
ØRG14JJ Fusion of Cervical Vertebral Joint with Synthetic Substitute, Posterior Approach, Anterior Column, Percutaneous Endoscopic Approach
ØRG14KØ Fusion of Cervical Vertebral Joint with Nonautologous Tissue Substitute, Anterior Approach, Anterior Column, Percutaneous Endoscopic Approach
ØRG14K1 Fusion of Cervical Vertebral Joint with Nonautologous Tissue Substitute, Posterior Approach, Posterior Column, Percutaneous Endoscopic Approach
ØRG14KJ Fusion of Cervical Vertebral Joint with Nonautologous Tissue Substitute, Posterior Approach, Anterior Column, Percutaneous Endoscopic Approach
ØRG207Ø Fusion of 2 or more Cervical Vertebral Joints with Autologous Tissue Substitute, Anterior Approach, Anterior Column, Open Approach
ØRG2071 Fusion of 2 or more Cervical Vertebral Joints with Autologous Tissue Substitute, Posterior Approach, Posterior Column, Open Approach
ØRG207J Fusion of 2 or more Cervical Vertebral Joints with Autologous Tissue Substitute, Posterior Approach, Anterior Column, Open Approach
ØRG20AØ Fusion of 2 or more Cervical Vertebral Joints with Interbody Fusion Device, Anterior Approach, Anterior Column, Open Approach
ØRG20AJ Fusion of 2 or more Cervical Vertebral Joints with Interbody Fusion Device, Posterior Approach, Anterior Column, Open Approach
ØRG20JØ Fusion of 2 or more Cervical Vertebral Joints with Synthetic Substitute, Anterior Approach, Anterior Column, Open Approach
ØRG20J1 Fusion of 2 or more Cervical Vertebral Joints with Synthetic Substitute, Posterior Approach, Posterior Column, Open Approach
ØRG20JJ Fusion of 2 or more Cervical Vertebral Joints with Synthetic Substitute, Posterior Approach, Anterior Column, Open Approach
ØRG20KØ Fusion of 2 or more Cervical Vertebral Joints with Nonautologous Tissue Substitute, Anterior Approach, Anterior Column, Open Approach
ØRG20K1 Fusion of 2 or more Cervical Vertebral Joints with Nonautologous Tissue Substitute, Posterior Approach, Posterior Column, Open Approach
ØRG20KJ Fusion of 2 or more Cervical Vertebral Joints with Nonautologous Tissue Substitute, Posterior Approach, Anterior Column, Open Approach
ØRG237Ø Fusion of 2 or more Cervical Vertebral Joints with Autologous Tissue Substitute, Anterior Approach, Anterior Column, Percutaneous Approach
ØRG2371 Fusion of 2 or more Cervical Vertebral Joints with Autologous Tissue Substitute, Posterior Approach, Posterior Column, Percutaneous Approach
ØRG237J Fusion of 2 or more Cervical Vertebral Joints with Autologous Tissue Substitute, Posterior Approach, Anterior Column, Percutaneous Approach
ØRG23AØ Fusion of 2 or more Cervical Vertebral Joints with Interbody Fusion Device, Anterior Approach, Anterior Column, Percutaneous Approach
ØRG23AJ Fusion of 2 or more Cervical Vertebral Joints with Interbody Fusion Device, Posterior Approach, Anterior Column, Percutaneous Approach
ØRG23JØ Fusion of 2 or more Cervical Vertebral Joints with Synthetic Substitute, Anterior Approach, Anterior Column, Percutaneous Approach
ØRG23J1 Fusion of 2 or more Cervical Vertebral Joints with Synthetic Substitute, Posterior Approach, Posterior Column, Percutaneous Approach
ØRG23JJ Fusion of 2 or more Cervical Vertebral Joints with Synthetic Substitute, Posterior Approach, Anterior Column, Percutaneous Approach
ØRG23KØ Fusion of 2 or more Cervical Vertebral Joints with Nonautologous Tissue Substitute, Anterior Approach, Anterior Column, Percutaneous Approach
ØRG23K1 Fusion of 2 or more Cervical Vertebral Joints with Nonautologous Tissue Substitute, Posterior Approach, Posterior Column, Percutaneous Approach
ØRG23KJ Fusion of 2 or more Cervical Vertebral Joints with Nonautologous Tissue Substitute, Posterior Approach, Anterior Column, Percutaneous Approach
ØRG247Ø Fusion of 2 or more Cervical Vertebral Joints with Autologous Tissue Substitute, Anterior Approach, Anterior Column, Percutaneous Endoscopic Approach
ØRG2471 Fusion of 2 or more Cervical Vertebral Joints with Autologous Tissue Substitute, Posterior Approach, Posterior Column, Percutaneous Endoscopic Approach

HAC 12: Surgical Site Infection Following Certain Orthopedic Procedures of the Spine, Shoulder, and Elbow (continued)

ØRG247J Fusion of 2 or more Cervical Vertebral Joints with Autologous Tissue Substitute, Posterior Approach, Anterior Column, Percutaneous Endoscopic Approach
ØRG24AØ Fusion of 2 or more Cervical Vertebral Joints with Interbody Fusion Device, Anterior Approach, Anterior Column, Percutaneous Endoscopic Approach
ØRG24AJ Fusion of 2 or more Cervical Vertebral Joints with Interbody Fusion Device, Posterior Approach, Anterior Column, Percutaneous Endoscopic Approach
ØRG24JØ Fusion of 2 or more Cervical Vertebral Joints with Synthetic Substitute, Anterior Approach, Anterior Column, Percutaneous Endoscopic Approach
ØRG24J1 Fusion of 2 or more Cervical Vertebral Joints with Synthetic Substitute, Posterior Approach, Posterior Column, Percutaneous Endoscopic Approach
ØRG24JJ Fusion of 2 or more Cervical Vertebral Joints with Synthetic Substitute, Posterior Approach, Anterior Column, Percutaneous Endoscopic Approach
ØRG24KØ Fusion of 2 or more Cervical Vertebral Joints with Nonautologous Tissue Substitute, Anterior Approach, Anterior Column, Percutaneous Endoscopic Approach
ØRG24K1 Fusion of 2 or more Cervical Vertebral Joints with Nonautologous Tissue Substitute, Posterior Approach, Posterior Column, Percutaneous Endoscopic Approach
ØRG24KJ Fusion of 2 or more Cervical Vertebral Joints with Nonautologous Tissue Substitute, Posterior Approach, Anterior Column, Percutaneous Endoscopic Approach
ØRG4Ø7Ø Fusion of Cervicothoracic Vertebral Joint with Autologous Tissue Substitute, Anterior Approach, Anterior Column, Open Approach
ØRG4Ø71 Fusion of Cervicothoracic Vertebral Joint with Autologous Tissue Substitute, Posterior Approach, Posterior Column, Open Approach
ØRG4Ø7J Fusion of Cervicothoracic Vertebral Joint with Autologous Tissue Substitute, Posterior Approach, Anterior Column, Open Approach
ØRG4ØAØ Fusion of Cervicothoracic Vertebral Joint with Interbody Fusion Device, Anterior Approach, Anterior Column, Open Approach
ØRG4ØAJ Fusion of Cervicothoracic Vertebral Joint with Interbody Fusion Device, Posterior Approach, Anterior Column, Open Approach
ØRG4ØJØ Fusion of Cervicothoracic Vertebral Joint with Synthetic Substitute, Anterior Approach, Anterior Column, Open Approach
ØRG4ØJ1 Fusion of Cervicothoracic Vertebral Joint with Synthetic Substitute, Posterior Approach, Posterior Column, Open Approach
ØRG4ØJJ Fusion of Cervicothoracic Vertebral Joint with Synthetic Substitute, Posterior Approach, Anterior Column, Open Approach
ØRG4ØKØ Fusion of Cervicothoracic Vertebral Joint with Nonautologous Tissue Substitute, Anterior Approach, Anterior Column, Open Approach
ØRG4ØK1 Fusion of Cervicothoracic Vertebral Joint with Nonautologous Tissue Substitute, Posterior Approach, Posterior Column, Open Approach
ØRG4ØKJ Fusion of Cervicothoracic Vertebral Joint with Nonautologous Tissue Substitute, Posterior Approach, Anterior Column, Open Approach
ØRG437Ø Fusion of Cervicothoracic Vertebral Joint with Autologous Tissue Substitute, Anterior Approach, Anterior Column, Percutaneous Approach
ØRG4371 Fusion of Cervicothoracic Vertebral Joint with Autologous Tissue Substitute, Posterior Approach, Posterior Column, Percutaneous Approach
ØRG437J Fusion of Cervicothoracic Vertebral Joint with Autologous Tissue Substitute, Posterior Approach, Anterior Column, Percutaneous Approach
ØRG43AØ Fusion of Cervicothoracic Vertebral Joint with Interbody Fusion Device, Anterior Approach, Anterior Column, Percutaneous Approach
ØRG43AJ Fusion of Cervicothoracic Vertebral Joint with Interbody Fusion Device, Posterior Approach, Anterior Column, Percutaneous Approach
ØRG43JØ Fusion of Cervicothoracic Vertebral Joint with Synthetic Substitute, Anterior Approach, Anterior Column, Percutaneous Approach
ØRG43J1 Fusion of Cervicothoracic Vertebral Joint with Synthetic Substitute, Posterior Approach, Posterior Column, Percutaneous Approach
ØRG43JJ Fusion of Cervicothoracic Vertebral Joint with Synthetic Substitute, Posterior Approach, Anterior Column, Percutaneous Approach
ØRG43KØ Fusion of Cervicothoracic Vertebral Joint with Nonautologous Tissue Substitute, Anterior Approach, Anterior Column, Percutaneous Approach
ØRG43K1 Fusion of Cervicothoracic Vertebral Joint with Nonautologous Tissue Substitute, Posterior Approach, Posterior Column, Percutaneous Approach
ØRG43KJ Fusion of Cervicothoracic Vertebral Joint with Nonautologous Tissue Substitute, Posterior Approach, Anterior Column, Percutaneous Approach
ØRG447Ø Fusion of Cervicothoracic Vertebral Joint with Autologous Tissue Substitute, Anterior Approach, Anterior Column, Percutaneous Endoscopic Approach
ØRG4471 Fusion of Cervicothoracic Vertebral Joint with Autologous Tissue Substitute, Posterior Approach, Posterior Column, Percutaneous Endoscopic Approach
ØRG447J Fusion of Cervicothoracic Vertebral Joint with Autologous Tissue Substitute, Posterior Approach, Anterior Column, Percutaneous Endoscopic Approach
ØRG44AØ Fusion of Cervicothoracic Vertebral Joint with Interbody Fusion Device, Anterior Approach, Anterior Column, Percutaneous Endoscopic Approach
ØRG44AJ Fusion of Cervicothoracic Vertebral Joint with Interbody Fusion Device, Posterior Approach, Anterior Column, Percutaneous Endoscopic Approach
ØRG44JØ Fusion of Cervicothoracic Vertebral Joint with Synthetic Substitute, Anterior Approach, Anterior Column, Percutaneous Endoscopic Approach
ØRG44J1 Fusion of Cervicothoracic Vertebral Joint with Synthetic Substitute, Posterior Approach, Posterior Column, Percutaneous Endoscopic Approach
ØRG44JJ Fusion of Cervicothoracic Vertebral Joint with Synthetic Substitute, Posterior Approach, Anterior Column, Percutaneous Endoscopic Approach
ØRG44KØ Fusion of Cervicothoracic Vertebral Joint with Nonautologous Tissue Substitute, Anterior Approach, Anterior Column, Percutaneous Endoscopic Approach
ØRG44K1 Fusion of Cervicothoracic Vertebral Joint with Nonautologous Tissue Substitute, Posterior Approach, Posterior Column, Percutaneous Endoscopic Approach
ØRG44KJ Fusion of Cervicothoracic Vertebral Joint with Nonautologous Tissue Substitute, Posterior Approach, Anterior Column, Percutaneous Endoscopic Approach
ØRG6Ø7Ø Fusion of Thoracic Vertebral Joint with Autologous Tissue Substitute, Anterior Approach, Anterior Column, Open Approach
ØRG6Ø71 Fusion of Thoracic Vertebral Joint with Autologous Tissue Substitute, Posterior Approach, Posterior Column, Open Approach
ØRG6Ø7J Fusion of Thoracic Vertebral Joint with Autologous Tissue Substitute, Posterior Approach, Anterior Column, Open Approach
ØRG6ØAØ Fusion of Thoracic Vertebral Joint with Interbody Fusion Device, Anterior Approach, Anterior Column, Open Approach
ØRG6ØAJ Fusion of Thoracic Vertebral Joint with Interbody Fusion Device, Posterior Approach, Anterior Column, Open Approach
ØRG6ØJØ Fusion of Thoracic Vertebral Joint with Synthetic Substitute, Anterior Approach, Anterior Column, Open Approach
ØRG6ØJ1 Fusion of Thoracic Vertebral Joint with Synthetic Substitute, Posterior Approach, Posterior Column, Open Approach
ØRG6ØJJ Fusion of Thoracic Vertebral Joint with Synthetic Substitute, Posterior Approach, Anterior Column, Open Approach
ØRG6ØKØ Fusion of Thoracic Vertebral Joint with Nonautologous Tissue Substitute, Anterior Approach, Anterior Column, Open Approach
ØRG6ØK1 Fusion of Thoracic Vertebral Joint with Nonautologous Tissue Substitute, Posterior Approach, Posterior Column, Open Approach
ØRG6ØKJ Fusion of Thoracic Vertebral Joint with Nonautologous Tissue Substitute, Posterior Approach, Anterior Column, Open Approach
ØRG637Ø Fusion of Thoracic Vertebral Joint with Autologous Tissue Substitute, Anterior Approach, Anterior Column, Percutaneous Approach
ØRG6371 Fusion of Thoracic Vertebral Joint with Autologous Tissue Substitute, Posterior Approach, Posterior Column, Percutaneous Approach

HAC 12: Surgical Site Infection Following Certain Orthopedic Procedures of the Spine, Shoulder, and Elbow (continued)

ØRG637J Fusion of Thoracic Vertebral Joint with Autologous Tissue Substitute, Posterior Approach, Anterior Column, Percutaneous Approach
ØRG63AØ Fusion of Thoracic Vertebral Joint with Interbody Fusion Device, Anterior Approach, Anterior Column, Percutaneous Approach
ØRG63AJ Fusion of Thoracic Vertebral Joint with Interbody Fusion Device, Posterior Approach, Anterior Column, Percutaneous Approach
ØRG63JØ Fusion of Thoracic Vertebral Joint with Synthetic Substitute, Anterior Approach, Anterior Column, Percutaneous Approach
ØRG63J1 Fusion of Thoracic Vertebral Joint with Synthetic Substitute, Posterior Approach, Posterior Column, Percutaneous Approach
ØRG63JJ Fusion of Thoracic Vertebral Joint with Synthetic Substitute, Posterior Approach, Anterior Column, Percutaneous Approach
ØRG63KØ Fusion of Thoracic Vertebral Joint with Nonautologous Tissue Substitute, Anterior Approach, Anterior Column, Percutaneous Approach
ØRG63K1 Fusion of Thoracic Vertebral Joint with Nonautologous Tissue Substitute, Posterior Approach, Posterior Column, Percutaneous Approach
ØRG63KJ Fusion of Thoracic Vertebral Joint with Nonautologous Tissue Substitute, Posterior Approach, Anterior Column, Percutaneous Approach
ØRG647Ø Fusion of Thoracic Vertebral Joint with Autologous Tissue Substitute, Anterior Approach, Anterior Column, Percutaneous Endoscopic Approach
ØRG6471 Fusion of Thoracic Vertebral Joint with Autologous Tissue Substitute, Posterior Approach, Posterior Column, Percutaneous Endoscopic Approach
ØRG647J Fusion of Thoracic Vertebral Joint with Autologous Tissue Substitute, Posterior Approach, Anterior Column, Percutaneous Endoscopic Approach
ØRG64AØ Fusion of Thoracic Vertebral Joint with Interbody Fusion Device, Anterior Approach, Anterior Column, Percutaneous Endoscopic Approach
ØRG64AJ Fusion of Thoracic Vertebral Joint with Interbody Fusion Device, Posterior Approach, Anterior Column, Percutaneous Endoscopic Approach
ØRG64JØ Fusion of Thoracic Vertebral Joint with Synthetic Substitute, Anterior Approach, Anterior Column, Percutaneous Endoscopic Approach
ØRG64J1 Fusion of Thoracic Vertebral Joint with Synthetic Substitute, Posterior Approach, Posterior Column, Percutaneous Endoscopic Approach
ØRG64JJ Fusion of Thoracic Vertebral Joint with Synthetic Substitute, Posterior Approach, Anterior Column, Percutaneous Endoscopic Approach
ØRG64KØ Fusion of Thoracic Vertebral Joint with Nonautologous Tissue Substitute, Anterior Approach, Anterior Column, Percutaneous Endoscopic Approach
ØRG64K1 Fusion of Thoracic Vertebral Joint with Nonautologous Tissue Substitute, Posterior Approach, Posterior Column, Percutaneous Endoscopic Approach
ØRG64KJ Fusion of Thoracic Vertebral Joint with Nonautologous Tissue Substitute, Posterior Approach, Anterior Column, Percutaneous Endoscopic Approach
ØRG7Ø7Ø Fusion of 2 to 7 Thoracic Vertebral Joints with Autologous Tissue Substitute, Anterior Approach, Anterior Column, Open Approach
ØRG7Ø71 Fusion of 2 to 7 Thoracic Vertebral Joints with Autologous Tissue Substitute, Posterior Approach, Posterior Column, Open Approach
ØRG7Ø7J Fusion of 2 to 7 Thoracic Vertebral Joints with Autologous Tissue Substitute, Posterior Approach, Anterior Column, Open Approach
ØRG7ØAØ Fusion of 2 to 7 Thoracic Vertebral Joints with Interbody Fusion Device, Anterior Approach, Anterior Column, Open Approach
ØRG7ØAJ Fusion of 2 to 7 Thoracic Vertebral Joints with Interbody Fusion Device, Posterior Approach, Anterior Column, Open Approach
ØRG7ØJØ Fusion of 2 to 7 Thoracic Vertebral Joints with Synthetic Substitute, Anterior Approach, Anterior Column, Open Approach
ØRG7ØJ1 Fusion of 2 to 7 Thoracic Vertebral Joints with Synthetic Substitute, Posterior Approach, Posterior Column, Open Approach
ØRG7ØJJ Fusion of 2 to 7 Thoracic Vertebral Joints with Synthetic Substitute, Posterior Approach, Anterior Column, Open Approach
ØRG7ØKØ Fusion of 2 to 7 Thoracic Vertebral Joints with Nonautologous Tissue Substitute, Anterior Approach, Anterior Column, Open Approach
ØRG7ØK1 Fusion of 2 to 7 Thoracic Vertebral Joints with Nonautologous Tissue Substitute, Posterior Approach, Posterior Column, Open Approach
ØRG7ØKJ Fusion of 2 to 7 Thoracic Vertebral Joints with Nonautologous Tissue Substitute, Posterior Approach, Anterior Column, Open Approach
ØRG737Ø Fusion of 2 to 7 Thoracic Vertebral Joints with Autologous Tissue Substitute, Anterior Approach, Anterior Column, Percutaneous Approach
ØRG7371 Fusion of 2 to 7 Thoracic Vertebral Joints with Autologous Tissue Substitute, Posterior Approach, Posterior Column, Percutaneous Approach
ØRG737J Fusion of 2 to 7 Thoracic Vertebral Joints with Autologous Tissue Substitute, Posterior Approach, Anterior Column, Percutaneous Approach
ØRG73AØ Fusion of 2 to 7 Thoracic Vertebral Joints with Interbody Fusion Device, Anterior Approach, Anterior Column, Percutaneous Approach
ØRG73AJ Fusion of 2 to 7 Thoracic Vertebral Joints with Interbody Fusion Device, Posterior Approach, Anterior Column, Percutaneous Approach
ØRG73JØ Fusion of 2 to 7 Thoracic Vertebral Joints with Synthetic Substitute, Anterior Approach, Anterior Column, Percutaneous Approach
ØRG73J1 Fusion of 2 to 7 Thoracic Vertebral Joints with Synthetic Substitute, Posterior Approach, Posterior Column, Percutaneous Approach
ØRG73JJ Fusion of 2 to 7 Thoracic Vertebral Joints with Synthetic Substitute, Posterior Approach, Anterior Column, Percutaneous Approach
ØRG73KØ Fusion of 2 to 7 Thoracic Vertebral Joints with Nonautologous Tissue Substitute, Anterior Approach, Anterior Column, Percutaneous Approach
ØRG73K1 Fusion of 2 to 7 Thoracic Vertebral Joints with Nonautologous Tissue Substitute, Posterior Approach, Posterior Column, Percutaneous Approach
ØRG73KJ Fusion of 2 to 7 Thoracic Vertebral Joints with Nonautologous Tissue Substitute, Posterior Approach, Anterior Column, Percutaneous Approach
ØRG747Ø Fusion of 2 to 7 Thoracic Vertebral Joints with Autologous Tissue Substitute, Anterior Approach, Anterior Column, Percutaneous Endoscopic Approach
ØRG7471 Fusion of 2 to 7 Thoracic Vertebral Joints with Autologous Tissue Substitute, Posterior Approach, Posterior Column, Percutaneous Endoscopic Approach
ØRG747J Fusion of 2 to 7 Thoracic Vertebral Joints with Autologous Tissue Substitute, Posterior Approach, Anterior Column, Percutaneous Endoscopic Approach
ØRG74AØ Fusion of 2 to 7 Thoracic Vertebral Joints with Interbody Fusion Device, Anterior Approach, Anterior Column, Percutaneous Endoscopic Approach
ØRG74AJ Fusion of 2 to 7 Thoracic Vertebral Joints with Interbody Fusion Device, Posterior Approach, Anterior Column, Percutaneous Endoscopic Approach
ØRG74JØ Fusion of 2 to 7 Thoracic Vertebral Joints with Synthetic Substitute, Anterior Approach, Anterior Column, Percutaneous Endoscopic Approach
ØRG74J1 Fusion of 2 to 7 Thoracic Vertebral Joints with Synthetic Substitute, Posterior Approach, Posterior Column, Percutaneous Endoscopic Approach
ØRG74JJ Fusion of 2 to 7 Thoracic Vertebral Joints with Synthetic Substitute, Posterior Approach, Anterior Column, Percutaneous Endoscopic Approach
ØRG74KØ Fusion of 2 to 7 Thoracic Vertebral Joints with Nonautologous Tissue Substitute, Anterior Approach, Anterior Column, Percutaneous Endoscopic Approach
ØRG74K1 Fusion of 2 to 7 Thoracic Vertebral Joints with Nonautologous Tissue Substitute, Posterior Approach, Posterior Column, Percutaneous Endoscopic Approach
ØRG74KJ Fusion of 2 to 7 Thoracic Vertebral Joints with Nonautologous Tissue Substitute, Posterior Approach, Anterior Column, Percutaneous Endoscopic Approach
ØRG8Ø7Ø Fusion of 8 or More Thoracic Vertebral Joints with Autologous Tissue Substitute, Anterior Approach, Anterior Column, Open Approach
ØRG8Ø71 Fusion of 8 or More Thoracic Vertebral Joints with Autologous Tissue Substitute, Posterior Approach, Posterior Column, Open Approach
ØRG8Ø7J Fusion of 8 or More Thoracic Vertebral Joints with Autologous Tissue Substitute, Posterior Approach, Anterior Column, Open Approach

HAC 12: Surgical Site Infection Following Certain Orthopedic Procedures of the Spine, Shoulder, and Elbow (continued)

ØRG8ØAØ Fusion of 8 or More Thoracic Vertebral Joints with Interbody Fusion Device, Anterior Approach, Anterior Column, Open Approach
ØRG8ØAJ Fusion of 8 or More Thoracic Vertebral Joints with Interbody Fusion Device, Posterior Approach, Anterior Column, Open Approach
ØRG8ØJØ Fusion of 8 or More Thoracic Vertebral Joints with Synthetic Substitute, Anterior Approach, Anterior Column, Open Approach
ØRG8ØJ1 Fusion of 8 or More Thoracic Vertebral Joints with Synthetic Substitute, Posterior Approach, Posterior Column, Open Approach
ØRG8ØJJ Fusion of 8 or More Thoracic Vertebral Joints with Synthetic Substitute, Posterior Approach, Anterior Column, Open Approach
ØRG8ØKØ Fusion of 8 or More Thoracic Vertebral Joints with Nonautologous Tissue Substitute, Anterior Approach, Anterior Column, Open Approach
ØRG8ØK1 Fusion of 8 or More Thoracic Vertebral Joints with Nonautologous Tissue Substitute, Posterior Approach, Posterior Column, Open Approach
ØRG8ØKJ Fusion of 8 or More Thoracic Vertebral Joints with Nonautologous Tissue Substitute, Posterior Approach, Anterior Column, Open Approach
ØRG837Ø Fusion of 8 or More Thoracic Vertebral Joints with Autologous Tissue Substitute, Anterior Approach, Anterior Column, Percutaneous Approach
ØRG8371 Fusion of 8 or More Thoracic Vertebral Joints with Autologous Tissue Substitute, Posterior Approach, Posterior Column, Percutaneous Approach
ØRG837J Fusion of 8 or More Thoracic Vertebral Joints with Autologous Tissue Substitute, Posterior Approach, Anterior Column, Percutaneous Approach
ØRG83AØ Fusion of 8 or More Thoracic Vertebral Joints with Interbody Fusion Device, Anterior Approach, Anterior Column, Percutaneous Approach
ØRG83AJ Fusion of 8 or More Thoracic Vertebral Joints with Interbody Fusion Device, Posterior Approach, Anterior Column, Percutaneous Approach
ØRG83JØ Fusion of 8 or More Thoracic Vertebral Joints with Synthetic Substitute, Anterior Approach, Anterior Column, Percutaneous Approach
ØRG83J1 Fusion of 8 or More Thoracic Vertebral Joints with Synthetic Substitute, Posterior Approach, Posterior Column, Percutaneous Approach
ØRG83JJ Fusion of 8 or More Thoracic Vertebral Joints with Synthetic Substitute, Posterior Approach, Anterior Column, Percutaneous Approach
ØRG83KØ Fusion of 8 or More Thoracic Vertebral Joints with Nonautologous Tissue Substitute, Anterior Approach, Anterior Column, Percutaneous Approach
ØRG83K1 Fusion of 8 or More Thoracic Vertebral Joints with Nonautologous Tissue Substitute, Posterior Approach, Posterior Column, Percutaneous Approach
ØRG83KJ Fusion of 8 or More Thoracic Vertebral Joints with Nonautologous Tissue Substitute, Posterior Approach, Anterior Column, Percutaneous Approach
ØRG847Ø Fusion of 8 or More Thoracic Vertebral Joints with Autologous Tissue Substitute, Anterior Approach, Anterior Column, Percutaneous Endoscopic Approach
ØRG8471 Fusion of 8 or More Thoracic Vertebral Joints with Autologous Tissue Substitute, Posterior Approach, Posterior Column, Percutaneous Endoscopic Approach
ØRG847J Fusion of 8 or More Thoracic Vertebral Joints with Autologous Tissue Substitute, Posterior Approach, Anterior Column, Percutaneous Endoscopic Approach
ØRG84AØ Fusion of 8 or More Thoracic Vertebral Joints with Interbody Fusion Device, Anterior Approach, Anterior Column, Percutaneous Endoscopic Approach
ØRG84AJ Fusion of 8 or More Thoracic Vertebral Joints with Interbody Fusion Device, Posterior Approach, Anterior Column, Percutaneous Endoscopic Approach
ØRG84JØ Fusion of 8 or More Thoracic Vertebral Joints with Synthetic Substitute, Anterior Approach, Anterior Column, Percutaneous Endoscopic Approach
ØRG84J1 Fusion of 8 or More Thoracic Vertebral Joints with Synthetic Substitute, Posterior Approach, Posterior Column, Percutaneous Endoscopic Approach
ØRG84JJ Fusion of 8 or More Thoracic Vertebral Joints with Synthetic Substitute, Posterior Approach, Anterior Column, Percutaneous Endoscopic Approach
ØRG84KØ Fusion of 8 or More Thoracic Vertebral Joints with Nonautologous Tissue Substitute, Anterior Approach, Anterior Column, Percutaneous Endoscopic Approach
ØRG84K1 Fusion of 8 or More Thoracic Vertebral Joints with Nonautologous Tissue Substitute, Posterior Approach, Posterior Column, Percutaneous Endoscopic Approach
ØRG84KJ Fusion of 8 or More Thoracic Vertebral Joints with Nonautologous Tissue Substitute, Posterior Approach, Anterior Column, Percutaneous Endoscopic Approach
ØRGAØ7Ø Fusion of Thoracolumbar Vertebral Joint with Autologous Tissue Substitute, Anterior Approach, Anterior Column, Open Approach
ØRGAØ71 Fusion of Thoracolumbar Vertebral Joint with Autologous Tissue Substitute, Posterior Approach, Posterior Column, Open Approach
ØRGAØ7J Fusion of Thoracolumbar Vertebral Joint with Autologous Tissue Substitute, Posterior Approach, Anterior Column, Open Approach
ØRGAØAØ Fusion of Thoracolumbar Vertebral Joint with Interbody Fusion Device, Anterior Approach, Anterior Column, Open Approach
ØRGAØAJ Fusion of Thoracolumbar Vertebral Joint with Interbody Fusion Device, Posterior Approach, Anterior Column, Open Approach
ØRGAØJØ Fusion of Thoracolumbar Vertebral Joint with Synthetic Substitute, Anterior Approach, Anterior Column, Open Approach
ØRGAØJ1 Fusion of Thoracolumbar Vertebral Joint with Synthetic Substitute, Posterior Approach, Posterior Column, Open Approach
ØRGAØJJ Fusion of Thoracolumbar Vertebral Joint with Synthetic Substitute, Posterior Approach, Anterior Column, Open Approach
ØRGAØKØ Fusion of Thoracolumbar Vertebral Joint with Nonautologous Tissue Substitute, Anterior Approach, Anterior Column, Open Approach
ØRGAØK1 Fusion of Thoracolumbar Vertebral Joint with Nonautologous Tissue Substitute, Posterior Approach, Posterior Column, Open Approach
ØRGAØKJ Fusion of Thoracolumbar Vertebral Joint with Nonautologous Tissue Substitute, Posterior Approach, Anterior Column, Open Approach
ØRGA37Ø Fusion of Thoracolumbar Vertebral Joint with Autologous Tissue Substitute, Anterior Approach, Anterior Column, Percutaneous Approach
ØRGA371 Fusion of Thoracolumbar Vertebral Joint with Autologous Tissue Substitute, Posterior Approach, Posterior Column, Percutaneous Approach
ØRGA37J Fusion of Thoracolumbar Vertebral Joint with Autologous Tissue Substitute, Posterior Approach, Anterior Column, Percutaneous Approach
ØRGA3AØ Fusion of Thoracolumbar Vertebral Joint with Interbody Fusion Device, Anterior Approach, Anterior Column, Percutaneous Approach
ØRGA3AJ Fusion of Thoracolumbar Vertebral Joint with Interbody Fusion Device, Posterior Approach, Anterior Column, Percutaneous Approach
ØRGA3JØ Fusion of Thoracolumbar Vertebral Joint with Synthetic Substitute, Anterior Approach, Anterior Column, Percutaneous Approach
ØRGA3J1 Fusion of Thoracolumbar Vertebral Joint with Synthetic Substitute, Posterior Approach, Posterior Column, Percutaneous Approach
ØRGA3JJ Fusion of Thoracolumbar Vertebral Joint with Synthetic Substitute, Posterior Approach, Anterior Column, Percutaneous Approach
ØRGA3KØ Fusion of Thoracolumbar Vertebral Joint with Nonautologous Tissue Substitute, Anterior Approach, Anterior Column, Percutaneous Approach
ØRGA3K1 Fusion of Thoracolumbar Vertebral Joint with Nonautologous Tissue Substitute, Posterior Approach, Posterior Column, Percutaneous Approach
ØRGA3KJ Fusion of Thoracolumbar Vertebral Joint with Nonautologous Tissue Substitute, Posterior Approach, Anterior Column, Percutaneous Approach
ØRGA47Ø Fusion of Thoracolumbar Vertebral Joint with Autologous Tissue Substitute, Anterior Approach, Anterior Column, Percutaneous Endoscopic Approach

HAC 12: Surgical Site Infection Following Certain Orthopedic Procedures of the Spine, Shoulder, and Elbow (continued)

ØRGA471 Fusion of Thoracolumbar Vertebral Joint with Autologous Tissue Substitute, Posterior Approach, Posterior Column, Percutaneous Endoscopic Approach
ØRGA47J Fusion of Thoracolumbar Vertebral Joint with Autologous Tissue Substitute, Posterior Approach, Anterior Column, Percutaneous Endoscopic Approach
ØRGA4AØ Fusion of Thoracolumbar Vertebral Joint with Interbody Fusion Device, Anterior Approach, Anterior Column, Percutaneous Endoscopic Approach
ØRGA4AJ Fusion of Thoracolumbar Vertebral Joint with Interbody Fusion Device, Posterior Approach, Anterior Column, Percutaneous Endoscopic Approach
ØRGA4JØ Fusion of Thoracolumbar Vertebral Joint with Synthetic Substitute, Anterior Approach, Anterior Column, Percutaneous Endoscopic Approach
ØRGA4J1 Fusion of Thoracolumbar Vertebral Joint with Synthetic Substitute, Posterior Approach, Posterior Column, Percutaneous Endoscopic Approach
ØRGA4JJ Fusion of Thoracolumbar Vertebral Joint with Synthetic Substitute, Posterior Approach, Anterior Column, Percutaneous Endoscopic Approach
ØRGA4KØ Fusion of Thoracolumbar Vertebral Joint with Nonautologous Tissue Substitute, Anterior Approach, Anterior Column, Percutaneous Endoscopic Approach
ØRGA4K1 Fusion of Thoracolumbar Vertebral Joint with Nonautologous Tissue Substitute, Posterior Approach, Posterior Column, Percutaneous Endoscopic Approach
ØRGA4KJ Fusion of Thoracolumbar Vertebral Joint with Nonautologous Tissue Substitute, Posterior Approach, Anterior Column, Percutaneous Endoscopic Approach
ØRGEØ4Z Fusion of Right Sternoclavicular Joint with Internal Fixation Device, Open Approach
ØRGEØ7Z Fusion of Right Sternoclavicular Joint with Autologous Tissue Substitute, Open Approach
ØRGEØJZ Fusion of Right Sternoclavicular Joint with Synthetic Substitute, Open Approach
ØRGEØKZ Fusion of Right Sternoclavicular Joint with Nonautologous Tissue Substitute, Open Approach
ØRGE34Z Fusion of Right Sternoclavicular Joint with Internal Fixation Device, Percutaneous Approach
ØRGE37Z Fusion of Right Sternoclavicular Joint with Autologous Tissue Substitute, Percutaneous Approach
ØRGE3JZ Fusion of Right Sternoclavicular Joint with Synthetic Substitute, Percutaneous Approach
ØRGE3KZ Fusion of Right Sternoclavicular Joint with Nonautologous Tissue Substitute, Percutaneous Approach
ØRGE44Z Fusion of Right Sternoclavicular Joint with Internal Fixation Device, Percutaneous Endoscopic Approach
ØRGE47Z Fusion of Right Sternoclavicular Joint with Autologous Tissue Substitute, Percutaneous Endoscopic Approach
ØRGE4JZ Fusion of Right Sternoclavicular Joint with Synthetic Substitute, Percutaneous Endoscopic Approach
ØRGE4KZ Fusion of Right Sternoclavicular Joint with Nonautologous Tissue Substitute, Percutaneous Endoscopic Approach
ØRGFØ4Z Fusion of Left Sternoclavicular Joint with Internal Fixation Device, Open Approach
ØRGFØ7Z Fusion of Left Sternoclavicular Joint with Autologous Tissue Substitute, Open Approach
ØRGFØJZ Fusion of Left Sternoclavicular Joint with Synthetic Substitute, Open Approach
ØRGFØKZ Fusion of Left Sternoclavicular Joint with Nonautologous Tissue Substitute, Open Approach
ØRGF34Z Fusion of Left Sternoclavicular Joint with Internal Fixation Device, Percutaneous Approach
ØRGF37Z Fusion of Left Sternoclavicular Joint with Autologous Tissue Substitute, Percutaneous Approach
ØRGF3JZ Fusion of Left Sternoclavicular Joint with Synthetic Substitute, Percutaneous Approach
ØRGF3KZ Fusion of Left Sternoclavicular Joint with Nonautologous Tissue Substitute, Percutaneous Approach
ØRGF44Z Fusion of Left Sternoclavicular Joint with Internal Fixation Device, Percutaneous Endoscopic Approach
ØRGF47Z Fusion of Left Sternoclavicular Joint with Autologous Tissue Substitute, Percutaneous Endoscopic Approach
ØRGF4JZ Fusion of Left Sternoclavicular Joint with Synthetic Substitute, Percutaneous Endoscopic Approach
ØRGF4KZ Fusion of Left Sternoclavicular Joint with Nonautologous Tissue Substitute, Percutaneous Endoscopic Approach
ØRGGØ4Z Fusion of Right Acromioclavicular Joint with Internal Fixation Device, Open Approach
ØRGGØ7Z Fusion of Right Acromioclavicular Joint with Autologous Tissue Substitute, Open Approach
ØRGGØJZ Fusion of Right Acromioclavicular Joint with Synthetic Substitute, Open Approach
ØRGGØKZ Fusion of Right Acromioclavicular Joint with Nonautologous Tissue Substitute, Open Approach
ØRGG34Z Fusion of Right Acromioclavicular Joint with Internal Fixation Device, Percutaneous Approach
ØRGG37Z Fusion of Right Acromioclavicular Joint with Autologous Tissue Substitute, Percutaneous Approach
ØRGG3JZ Fusion of Right Acromioclavicular Joint with Synthetic Substitute, Percutaneous Approach
ØRGG3KZ Fusion of Right Acromioclavicular Joint with Nonautologous Tissue Substitute, Percutaneous Approach
ØRGG44Z Fusion of Right Acromioclavicular Joint with Internal Fixation Device, Percutaneous Endoscopic Approach
ØRGG47Z Fusion of Right Acromioclavicular Joint with Autologous Tissue Substitute, Percutaneous Endoscopic Approach
ØRGG4JZ Fusion of Right Acromioclavicular Joint with Synthetic Substitute, Percutaneous Endoscopic Approach
ØRGG4KZ Fusion of Right Acromioclavicular Joint with Nonautologous Tissue Substitute, Percutaneous Endoscopic Approach
ØRGHØ4Z Fusion of Left Acromioclavicular Joint with Internal Fixation Device, Open Approach
ØRGHØ7Z Fusion of Left Acromioclavicular Joint with Autologous Tissue Substitute, Open Approach
ØRGHØJZ Fusion of Left Acromioclavicular Joint with Synthetic Substitute, Open Approach
ØRGHØKZ Fusion of Left Acromioclavicular Joint with Nonautologous Tissue Substitute, Open Approach
ØRGH34Z Fusion of Left Acromioclavicular Joint with Internal Fixation Device, Percutaneous Approach
ØRGH37Z Fusion of Left Acromioclavicular Joint with Autologous Tissue Substitute, Percutaneous Approach
ØRGH3JZ Fusion of Left Acromioclavicular Joint with Synthetic Substitute, Percutaneous Approach
ØRGH3KZ Fusion of Left Acromioclavicular Joint with Nonautologous Tissue Substitute, Percutaneous Approach
ØRGH44Z Fusion of Left Acromioclavicular Joint with Internal Fixation Device, Percutaneous Endoscopic Approach
ØRGH47Z Fusion of Left Acromioclavicular Joint with Autologous Tissue Substitute, Percutaneous Endoscopic Approach
ØRGH4JZ Fusion of Left Acromioclavicular Joint with Synthetic Substitute, Percutaneous Endoscopic Approach
ØRGH4KZ Fusion of Left Acromioclavicular Joint with Nonautologous Tissue Substitute, Percutaneous Endoscopic Approach
ØRGJØ4Z Fusion of Right Shoulder Joint with Internal Fixation Device, Open Approach
ØRGJØ7Z Fusion of Right Shoulder Joint with Autologous Tissue Substitute, Open Approach
ØRGJØJZ Fusion of Right Shoulder Joint with Synthetic Substitute, Open Approach
ØRGJØKZ Fusion of Right Shoulder Joint with Nonautologous Tissue Substitute, Open Approach
ØRGJ34Z Fusion of Right Shoulder Joint with Internal Fixation Device, Percutaneous Approach
ØRGJ37Z Fusion of Right Shoulder Joint with Autologous Tissue Substitute, Percutaneous Approach
ØRGJ3JZ Fusion of Right Shoulder Joint with Synthetic Substitute, Percutaneous Approach
ØRGJ3KZ Fusion of Right Shoulder Joint with Nonautologous Tissue Substitute, Percutaneous Approach
ØRGJ44Z Fusion of Right Shoulder Joint with Internal Fixation Device, Percutaneous Endoscopic Approach
ØRGJ47Z Fusion of Right Shoulder Joint with Autologous Tissue Substitute, Percutaneous Endoscopic Approach
ØRGJ4JZ Fusion of Right Shoulder Joint with Synthetic Substitute, Percutaneous Endoscopic Approach
ØRGJ4KZ Fusion of Right Shoulder Joint with Nonautologous Tissue Substitute, Percutaneous Endoscopic Approach
ØRGKØ4Z Fusion of Left Shoulder Joint with Internal Fixation Device, Open Approach
ØRGKØ7Z Fusion of Left Shoulder Joint with Autologous Tissue Substitute, Open Approach
ØRGKØJZ Fusion of Left Shoulder Joint with Synthetic Substitute, Open Approach

HAC 12: Surgical Site Infection Following Certain Orthopedic Procedures of the Spine, Shoulder, and Elbow (continued)

ØRGKØKZ Fusion of Left Shoulder Joint with Nonautologous Tissue Substitute, Open Approach
ØRGK34Z Fusion of Left Shoulder Joint with Internal Fixation Device, Percutaneous Approach
ØRGK37Z Fusion of Left Shoulder Joint with Autologous Tissue Substitute, Percutaneous Approach
ØRGK3JZ Fusion of Left Shoulder Joint with Synthetic Substitute, Percutaneous Approach
ØRGK3KZ Fusion of Left Shoulder Joint with Nonautologous Tissue Substitute, Percutaneous Approach
ØRGK44Z Fusion of Left Shoulder Joint with Internal Fixation Device, Percutaneous Endoscopic Approach
ØRGK47Z Fusion of Left Shoulder Joint with Autologous Tissue Substitute, Percutaneous Endoscopic Approach
ØRGK4JZ Fusion of Left Shoulder Joint with Synthetic Substitute, Percutaneous Endoscopic Approach
ØRGK4KZ Fusion of Left Shoulder Joint with Nonautologous Tissue Substitute, Percutaneous Endoscopic Approach
ØRGLØ4Z Fusion of Right Elbow Joint with Internal Fixation Device, Open Approach
ØRGLØ5Z Fusion of Right Elbow Joint with External Fixation Device, Open Approach
ØRGLØ7Z Fusion of Right Elbow Joint with Autologous Tissue Substitute, Open Approach
ØRGLØJZ Fusion of Right Elbow Joint with Synthetic Substitute, Open Approach
ØRGLØKZ Fusion of Right Elbow Joint with Nonautologous Tissue Substitute, Open Approach
ØRGL34Z Fusion of Right Elbow Joint with Internal Fixation Device, Percutaneous Approach
ØRGL35Z Fusion of Right Elbow Joint with External Fixation Device, Percutaneous Approach
ØRGL37Z Fusion of Right Elbow Joint with Autologous Tissue Substitute, Percutaneous Approach
ØRGL3JZ Fusion of Right Elbow Joint with Synthetic Substitute, Percutaneous Approach
ØRGL3KZ Fusion of Right Elbow Joint with Nonautologous Tissue Substitute, Percutaneous Approach
ØRGL44Z Fusion of Right Elbow Joint with Internal Fixation Device, Percutaneous Endoscopic Approach
ØRGL45Z Fusion of Right Elbow Joint with External Fixation Device, Percutaneous Endoscopic Approach
ØRGL47Z Fusion of Right Elbow Joint with Autologous Tissue Substitute, Percutaneous Endoscopic Approach
ØRGL4JZ Fusion of Right Elbow Joint with Synthetic Substitute, Percutaneous Endoscopic Approach
ØRGL4KZ Fusion of Right Elbow Joint with Nonautologous Tissue Substitute, Percutaneous Endoscopic Approach
ØRGMØ4Z Fusion of Left Elbow Joint with Internal Fixation Device, Open Approach
ØRGMØ5Z Fusion of Left Elbow Joint with External Fixation Device, Open Approach
ØRGMØ7Z Fusion of Left Elbow Joint with Autologous Tissue Substitute, Open Approach
ØRGMØJZ Fusion of Left Elbow Joint with Synthetic Substitute, Open Approach
ØRGMØKZ Fusion of Left Elbow Joint with Nonautologous Tissue Substitute, Open Approach
ØRGM34Z Fusion of Left Elbow Joint with Internal Fixation Device, Percutaneous Approach
ØRGM35Z Fusion of Left Elbow Joint with External Fixation Device, Percutaneous Approach
ØRGM37Z Fusion of Left Elbow Joint with Autologous Tissue Substitute, Percutaneous Approach
ØRGM3JZ Fusion of Left Elbow Joint with Synthetic Substitute, Percutaneous Approach
ØRGM3KZ Fusion of Left Elbow Joint with Nonautologous Tissue Substitute, Percutaneous Approach
ØRGM44Z Fusion of Left Elbow Joint with Internal Fixation Device, Percutaneous Endoscopic Approach
ØRGM45Z Fusion of Left Elbow Joint with External Fixation Device, Percutaneous Endoscopic Approach
ØRGM47Z Fusion of Left Elbow Joint with Autologous Tissue Substitute, Percutaneous Endoscopic Approach
ØRGM4JZ Fusion of Left Elbow Joint with Synthetic Substitute, Percutaneous Endoscopic Approach
ØRGM4KZ Fusion of Left Elbow Joint with Nonautologous Tissue Substitute, Percutaneous Endoscopic Approach
ØRQEØZZ Repair Right Sternoclavicular Joint, Open Approach
ØRQE3ZZ Repair Right Sternoclavicular Joint, Percutaneous Approach
ØRQE4ZZ Repair Right Sternoclavicular Joint, Percutaneous Endoscopic Approach
ØRQEXZZ Repair Right Sternoclavicular Joint, External Approach
ØRQFØZZ Repair Left Sternoclavicular Joint, Open Approach
ØRQF3ZZ Repair Left Sternoclavicular Joint, Percutaneous Approach
ØRQF4ZZ Repair Left Sternoclavicular Joint, Percutaneous Endoscopic Approach
ØRQFXZZ Repair Left Sternoclavicular Joint, External Approach
ØRQGØZZ Repair Right Acromioclavicular Joint, Open Approach
ØRQG3ZZ Repair Right Acromioclavicular Joint, Percutaneous Approach
ØRQG4ZZ Repair Right Acromioclavicular Joint, Percutaneous Endoscopic Approach
ØRQGXZZ Repair Right Acromioclavicular Joint, External Approach
ØRQHØZZ Repair Left Acromioclavicular Joint, Open Approach
ØRQH3ZZ Repair Left Acromioclavicular Joint, Percutaneous Approach
ØRQH4ZZ Repair Left Acromioclavicular Joint, Percutaneous Endoscopic Approach
ØRQHXZZ Repair Left Acromioclavicular Joint, External Approach
ØRQJØZZ Repair Right Shoulder Joint, Open Approach
ØRQJ3ZZ Repair Right Shoulder Joint, Percutaneous Approach
ØRQJ4ZZ Repair Right Shoulder Joint, Percutaneous Endoscopic Approach
ØRQJXZZ Repair Right Shoulder Joint, External Approach
ØRQKØZZ Repair Left Shoulder Joint, Open Approach
ØRQK3ZZ Repair Left Shoulder Joint, Percutaneous Approach
ØRQK4ZZ Repair Left Shoulder Joint, Percutaneous Endoscopic Approach
ØRQKXZZ Repair Left Shoulder Joint, External Approach
ØRQLØZZ Repair Right Elbow Joint, Open Approach
ØRQL3ZZ Repair Right Elbow Joint, Percutaneous Approach
ØRQL4ZZ Repair Right Elbow Joint, Percutaneous Endoscopic Approach
ØRQLXZZ Repair Right Elbow Joint, External Approach
ØRQMØZZ Repair Left Elbow Joint, Open Approach
ØRQM3ZZ Repair Left Elbow Joint, Percutaneous Approach
ØRQM4ZZ Repair Left Elbow Joint, Percutaneous Endoscopic Approach
ØRQMXZZ Repair Left Elbow Joint, External Approach
ØRUEØ7Z Supplement Right Sternoclavicular Joint with Autologous Tissue Substitute, Open Approach
ØRUEØJZ Supplement Right Sternoclavicular Joint with Synthetic Substitute, Open Approach
ØRUEØKZ Supplement Right Sternoclavicular Joint with Nonautologous Tissue Substitute, Open Approach
ØRUE37Z Supplement Right Sternoclavicular Joint with Autologous Tissue Substitute, Percutaneous Approach
ØRUE3JZ Supplement Right Sternoclavicular Joint with Synthetic Substitute, Percutaneous Approach
ØRUE3KZ Supplement Right Sternoclavicular Joint with Nonautologous Tissue Substitute, Percutaneous Approach
ØRUE47Z Supplement Right Sternoclavicular Joint with Autologous Tissue Substitute, Percutaneous Endoscopic Approach
ØRUE4JZ Supplement Right Sternoclavicular Joint with Synthetic Substitute, Percutaneous Endoscopic Approach
ØRUE4KZ Supplement Right Sternoclavicular Joint with Nonautologous Tissue Substitute, Percutaneous Endoscopic Approach
ØRUFØ7Z Supplement Left Sternoclavicular Joint with Autologous Tissue Substitute, Open Approach
ØRUFØJZ Supplement Left Sternoclavicular Joint with Synthetic Substitute, Open Approach
ØRUFØKZ Supplement Left Sternoclavicular Joint with Nonautologous Tissue Substitute, Open Approach
ØRUF37Z Supplement Left Sternoclavicular Joint with Autologous Tissue Substitute, Percutaneous Approach
ØRUF3JZ Supplement Left Sternoclavicular Joint with Synthetic Substitute, Percutaneous Approach
ØRUF3KZ Supplement Left Sternoclavicular Joint with Nonautologous Tissue Substitute, Percutaneous Approach
ØRUF47Z Supplement Left Sternoclavicular Joint with Autologous Tissue Substitute, Percutaneous Endoscopic Approach
ØRUF4JZ Supplement Left Sternoclavicular Joint with Synthetic Substitute, Percutaneous Endoscopic Approach

Appendix J: Hospital Acquired Conditions

HAC 12: Surgical Site Infection Following Certain Orthopedic Procedures of the Spine, Shoulder, and Elbow (continued)

ØRUF4KZ Supplement Left Sternoclavicular Joint with Nonautologous Tissue Substitute, Percutaneous Endoscopic Approach
ØRUGØ7Z Supplement Right Acromioclavicular Joint with Autologous Tissue Substitute, Open Approach
ØRUGØJZ Supplement Right Acromioclavicular Joint with Synthetic Substitute, Open Approach
ØRUGØKZ Supplement Right Acromioclavicular Joint with Nonautologous Tissue Substitute, Open Approach
ØRUG37Z Supplement Right Acromioclavicular Joint with Autologous Tissue Substitute, Percutaneous Approach
ØRUG3JZ Supplement Right Acromioclavicular Joint with Synthetic Substitute, Percutaneous Approach
ØRUG3KZ Supplement Right Acromioclavicular Joint with Nonautologous Tissue Substitute, Percutaneous Approach
ØRUG47Z Supplement Right Acromioclavicular Joint with Autologous Tissue Substitute, Percutaneous Endoscopic Approach
ØRUG4JZ Supplement Right Acromioclavicular Joint with Synthetic Substitute, Percutaneous Endoscopic Approach
ØRUG4KZ Supplement Right Acromioclavicular Joint with Nonautologous Tissue Substitute, Percutaneous Endoscopic Approach
ØRUHØ7Z Supplement Left Acromioclavicular Joint with Autologous Tissue Substitute, Open Approach
ØRUHØJZ Supplement Left Acromioclavicular Joint with Synthetic Substitute, Open Approach
ØRUHØKZ Supplement Left Acromioclavicular Joint with Nonautologous Tissue Substitute, Open Approach
ØRUH37Z Supplement Left Acromioclavicular Joint with Autologous Tissue Substitute, Percutaneous Approach
ØRUH3JZ Supplement Left Acromioclavicular Joint with Synthetic Substitute, Percutaneous Approach
ØRUH3KZ Supplement Left Acromioclavicular Joint with Nonautologous Tissue Substitute, Percutaneous Approach
ØRUH47Z Supplement Left Acromioclavicular Joint with Autologous Tissue Substitute, Percutaneous Endoscopic Approach
ØRUH4JZ Supplement Left Acromioclavicular Joint with Synthetic Substitute, Percutaneous Endoscopic Approach
ØRUH4KZ Supplement Left Acromioclavicular Joint with Nonautologous Tissue Substitute, Percutaneous Endoscopic Approach
ØRUJØ7Z Supplement Right Shoulder Joint with Autologous Tissue Substitute, Open Approach
ØRUJØJZ Supplement Right Shoulder Joint with Synthetic Substitute, Open Approach
ØRUJØKZ Supplement Right Shoulder Joint with Nonautologous Tissue Substitute, Open Approach
ØRUJ37Z Supplement Right Shoulder Joint with Autologous Tissue Substitute, Percutaneous Approach
ØRUJ3JZ Supplement Right Shoulder Joint with Synthetic Substitute, Percutaneous Approach
ØRUJ3KZ Supplement Right Shoulder Joint with Nonautologous Tissue Substitute, Percutaneous Approach
ØRUJ47Z Supplement Right Shoulder Joint with Autologous Tissue Substitute, Percutaneous Endoscopic Approach
ØRUJ4JZ Supplement Right Shoulder Joint with Synthetic Substitute, Percutaneous Endoscopic Approach
ØRUJ4KZ Supplement Right Shoulder Joint with Nonautologous Tissue Substitute, Percutaneous Endoscopic Approach
ØRUKØ7Z Supplement Left Shoulder Joint with Autologous Tissue Substitute, Open Approach
ØRUKØJZ Supplement Left Shoulder Joint with Synthetic Substitute, Open Approach
ØRUKØKZ Supplement Left Shoulder Joint with Nonautologous Tissue Substitute, Open Approach
ØRUK37Z Supplement Left Shoulder Joint with Autologous Tissue Substitute, Percutaneous Approach
ØRUK3JZ Supplement Left Shoulder Joint with Synthetic Substitute, Percutaneous Approach
ØRUK3KZ Supplement Left Shoulder Joint with Nonautologous Tissue Substitute, Percutaneous Approach
ØRUK47Z Supplement Left Shoulder Joint with Autologous Tissue Substitute, Percutaneous Endoscopic Approach
ØRUK4JZ Supplement Left Shoulder Joint with Synthetic Substitute, Percutaneous Endoscopic Approach
ØRUK4KZ Supplement Left Shoulder Joint with Nonautologous Tissue Substitute, Percutaneous Endoscopic Approach
ØRULØ7Z Supplement Right Elbow Joint with Autologous Tissue Substitute, Open Approach
ØRULØJZ Supplement Right Elbow Joint with Synthetic Substitute, Open Approach
ØRULØKZ Supplement Right Elbow Joint with Nonautologous Tissue Substitute, Open Approach
ØRUL37Z Supplement Right Elbow Joint with Autologous Tissue Substitute, Percutaneous Approach
ØRUL3JZ Supplement Right Elbow Joint with Synthetic Substitute, Percutaneous Approach
ØRUL3KZ Supplement Right Elbow Joint with Nonautologous Tissue Substitute, Percutaneous Approach
ØRUL47Z Supplement Right Elbow Joint with Autologous Tissue Substitute, Percutaneous Endoscopic Approach
ØRUL4JZ Supplement Right Elbow Joint with Synthetic Substitute, Percutaneous Endoscopic Approach
ØRUL4KZ Supplement Right Elbow Joint with Nonautologous Tissue Substitute, Percutaneous Endoscopic Approach
ØRUMØ7Z Supplement Left Elbow Joint with Autologous Tissue Substitute, Open Approach
ØRUMØJZ Supplement Left Elbow Joint with Synthetic Substitute, Open Approach
ØRUMØKZ Supplement Left Elbow Joint with Nonautologous Tissue Substitute, Open Approach
ØRUM37Z Supplement Left Elbow Joint with Autologous Tissue Substitute, Percutaneous Approach
ØRUM3JZ Supplement Left Elbow Joint with Synthetic Substitute, Percutaneous Approach
ØRUM3KZ Supplement Left Elbow Joint with Nonautologous Tissue Substitute, Percutaneous Approach
ØRUM47Z Supplement Left Elbow Joint with Autologous Tissue Substitute, Percutaneous Endoscopic Approach
ØRUM4JZ Supplement Left Elbow Joint with Synthetic Substitute, Percutaneous Endoscopic Approach
ØRUM4KZ Supplement Left Elbow Joint with Nonautologous Tissue Substitute, Percutaneous Endoscopic Approach
ØSGØØ7Ø Fusion of Lumbar Vertebral Joint with Autologous Tissue Substitute, Anterior Approach, Anterior Column, Open Approach
ØSGØØ71 Fusion of Lumbar Vertebral Joint with Autologous Tissue Substitute, Posterior Approach, Posterior Column, Open Approach
ØSGØØ7J Fusion of Lumbar Vertebral Joint with Autologous Tissue Substitute, Posterior Approach, Anterior Column, Open Approach
ØSGØØAØ Fusion of Lumbar Vertebral Joint with Interbody Fusion Device, Anterior Approach, Anterior Column, Open Approach
ØSGØØAJ Fusion of Lumbar Vertebral Joint with Interbody Fusion Device, Posterior Approach, Anterior Column, Open Approach
ØSGØØJØ Fusion of Lumbar Vertebral Joint with Synthetic Substitute, Anterior Approach, Anterior Column, Open Approach
ØSGØØJ1 Fusion of Lumbar Vertebral Joint with Synthetic Substitute, Posterior Approach, Posterior Column, Open Approach
ØSGØØJJ Fusion of Lumbar Vertebral Joint with Synthetic Substitute, Posterior Approach, Anterior Column, Open Approach
ØSGØØKØ Fusion of Lumbar Vertebral Joint with Nonautologous Tissue Substitute, Anterior Approach, Anterior Column, Open Approach
ØSGØØK1 Fusion of Lumbar Vertebral Joint with Nonautologous Tissue Substitute, Posterior Approach, Posterior Column, Open Approach
ØSGØØKJ Fusion of Lumbar Vertebral Joint with Nonautologous Tissue Substitute, Posterior Approach, Anterior Column, Open Approach
ØSGØ37Ø Fusion of Lumbar Vertebral Joint with Autologous Tissue Substitute, Anterior Approach, Anterior Column, Percutaneous Approach
ØSGØ371 Fusion of Lumbar Vertebral Joint with Autologous Tissue Substitute, Posterior Approach, Posterior Column, Percutaneous Approach
ØSGØ37J Fusion of Lumbar Vertebral Joint with Autologous Tissue Substitute, Posterior Approach, Anterior Column, Percutaneous Approach
ØSGØ3AØ Fusion of Lumbar Vertebral Joint with Interbody Fusion Device, Anterior Approach, Anterior Column, Percutaneous Approach

HAC 12: Surgical Site Infection Following Certain Orthopedic Procedures of the Spine, Shoulder, and Elbow (continued)

ØSGØ3AJ Fusion of Lumbar Vertebral Joint with Interbody Fusion Device, Posterior Approach, Anterior Column, Percutaneous Approach
ØSGØ3JØ Fusion of Lumbar Vertebral Joint with Synthetic Substitute, Anterior Approach, Anterior Column, Percutaneous Approach
ØSGØ3J1 Fusion of Lumbar Vertebral Joint with Synthetic Substitute, Posterior Approach, Posterior Column, Percutaneous Approach
ØSGØ3JJ Fusion of Lumbar Vertebral Joint with Synthetic Substitute, Posterior Approach, Anterior Column, Percutaneous Approach
ØSGØ3KØ Fusion of Lumbar Vertebral Joint with Nonautologous Tissue Substitute, Anterior Approach, Anterior Column, Percutaneous Approach
ØSGØ3K1 Fusion of Lumbar Vertebral Joint with Nonautologous Tissue Substitute, Posterior Approach, Posterior Column, Percutaneous Approach
ØSGØ3KJ Fusion of Lumbar Vertebral Joint with Nonautologous Tissue Substitute, Posterior Approach, Anterior Column, Percutaneous Approach
ØSGØ47Ø Fusion of Lumbar Vertebral Joint with Autologous Tissue Substitute, Anterior Approach, Anterior Column, Percutaneous Endoscopic Approach
ØSGØ471 Fusion of Lumbar Vertebral Joint with Autologous Tissue Substitute, Posterior Approach, Posterior Column, Percutaneous Endoscopic Approach
ØSGØ47J Fusion of Lumbar Vertebral Joint with Autologous Tissue Substitute, Posterior Approach, Anterior Column, Percutaneous Endoscopic Approach
ØSGØ4AØ Fusion of Lumbar Vertebral Joint with Interbody Fusion Device, Anterior Approach, Anterior Column, Percutaneous Endoscopic Approach
ØSGØ4AJ Fusion of Lumbar Vertebral Joint with Interbody Fusion Device, Posterior Approach, Anterior Column, Percutaneous Endoscopic Approach
ØSGØ4JØ Fusion of Lumbar Vertebral Joint with Synthetic Substitute, Anterior Approach, Anterior Column, Percutaneous Endoscopic Approach
ØSGØ4J1 Fusion of Lumbar Vertebral Joint with Synthetic Substitute, Posterior Approach, Posterior Column, Percutaneous Endoscopic Approach
ØSGØ4JJ Fusion of Lumbar Vertebral Joint with Synthetic Substitute, Posterior Approach, Anterior Column, Percutaneous Endoscopic Approach
ØSGØ4KØ Fusion of Lumbar Vertebral Joint with Nonautologous Tissue Substitute, Anterior Approach, Anterior Column, Percutaneous Endoscopic Approach
ØSGØ4K1 Fusion of Lumbar Vertebral Joint with Nonautologous Tissue Substitute, Posterior Approach, Posterior Column, Percutaneous Endoscopic Approach
ØSGØ4KJ Fusion of Lumbar Vertebral Joint with Nonautologous Tissue Substitute, Posterior Approach, Anterior Column, Percutaneous Endoscopic Approach
ØSG1Ø7Ø Fusion of 2 or More Lumbar Vertebral Joints with Autologous Tissue Substitute, Anterior Approach, Anterior Column, Open Approach
ØSG1Ø71 Fusion of 2 or More Lumbar Vertebral Joints with Autologous Tissue Substitute, Posterior Approach, Posterior Column, Open Approach
ØSG1Ø7J Fusion of 2 or More Lumbar Vertebral Joints with Autologous Tissue Substitute, Posterior Approach, Anterior Column, Open Approach
ØSG1ØAØ Fusion of 2 or More Lumbar Vertebral Joints with Interbody Fusion Device, Anterior Approach, Anterior Column, Open Approach
ØSG1ØAJ Fusion of 2 or More Lumbar Vertebral Joints with Interbody Fusion Device, Posterior Approach, Anterior Column, Open Approach
ØSG1ØJØ Fusion of 2 or More Lumbar Vertebral Joints with Synthetic Substitute, Anterior Approach, Anterior Column, Open Approach
ØSG1ØJ1 Fusion of 2 or More Lumbar Vertebral Joints with Synthetic Substitute, Posterior Approach, Posterior Column, Open Approach
ØSG1ØJJ Fusion of 2 or More Lumbar Vertebral Joints with Synthetic Substitute, Posterior Approach, Anterior Column, Open Approach
ØSG1ØKØ Fusion of 2 or More Lumbar Vertebral Joints with Nonautologous Tissue Substitute, Anterior Approach, Anterior Column, Open Approach
ØSG1ØK1 Fusion of 2 or More Lumbar Vertebral Joints with Nonautologous Tissue Substitute, Posterior Approach, Posterior Column, Open Approach
ØSG1ØKJ Fusion of 2 or More Lumbar Vertebral Joints with Nonautologous Tissue Substitute, Posterior Approach, Anterior Column, Open Approach
ØSG137Ø Fusion of 2 or More Lumbar Vertebral Joints with Autologous Tissue Substitute, Anterior Approach, Anterior Column, Percutaneous Approach
ØSG1371 Fusion of 2 or More Lumbar Vertebral Joints with Autologous Tissue Substitute, Posterior Approach, Posterior Column, Percutaneous Approach
ØSG137J Fusion of 2 or More Lumbar Vertebral Joints with Autologous Tissue Substitute, Posterior Approach, Anterior Column, Percutaneous Approach
ØSG13AØ Fusion of 2 or More Lumbar Vertebral Joints with Interbody Fusion Device, Anterior Approach, Anterior Column, Percutaneous Approach
ØSG13AJ Fusion of 2 or More Lumbar Vertebral Joints with Interbody Fusion Device, Posterior Approach, Anterior Column, Percutaneous Approach
ØSG13JØ Fusion of 2 or More Lumbar Vertebral Joints with Synthetic Substitute, Anterior Approach, Anterior Column, Percutaneous Approach
ØSG13J1 Fusion of 2 or More Lumbar Vertebral Joints with Synthetic Substitute, Posterior Approach, Posterior Column, Percutaneous Approach
ØSG13JJ Fusion of 2 or More Lumbar Vertebral Joints with Synthetic Substitute, Posterior Approach, Anterior Column, Percutaneous Approach
ØSG13KØ Fusion of 2 or More Lumbar Vertebral Joints with Nonautologous Tissue Substitute, Anterior Approach, Anterior Column, Percutaneous Approach
ØSG13K1 Fusion of 2 or More Lumbar Vertebral Joints with Nonautologous Tissue Substitute, Posterior Approach, Posterior Column, Percutaneous Approach
ØSG13KJ Fusion of 2 or More Lumbar Vertebral Joints with Nonautologous Tissue Substitute, Posterior Approach, Anterior Column, Percutaneous Approach
ØSG147Ø Fusion of 2 or More Lumbar Vertebral Joints with Autologous Tissue Substitute, Anterior Approach, Anterior Column, Percutaneous Endoscopic Approach
ØSG1471 Fusion of 2 or More Lumbar Vertebral Joints with Autologous Tissue Substitute, Posterior Approach, Posterior Column, Percutaneous Endoscopic Approach
ØSG147J Fusion of 2 or More Lumbar Vertebral Joints with Autologous Tissue Substitute, Posterior Approach, Anterior Column, Percutaneous Endoscopic Approach
ØSG14AØ Fusion of 2 or More Lumbar Vertebral Joints with Interbody Fusion Device, Anterior Approach, Anterior Column, Percutaneous Endoscopic Approach
ØSG14AJ Fusion of 2 or More Lumbar Vertebral Joints with Interbody Fusion Device, Posterior Approach, Anterior Column, Percutaneous Endoscopic Approach
ØSG14JØ Fusion of 2 or More Lumbar Vertebral Joints with Synthetic Substitute, Anterior Approach, Anterior Column, Percutaneous Endoscopic Approach
ØSG14J1 Fusion of 2 or More Lumbar Vertebral Joints with Synthetic Substitute, Posterior Approach, Posterior Column, Percutaneous Endoscopic Approach
ØSG14JJ Fusion of 2 or More Lumbar Vertebral Joints with Synthetic Substitute, Posterior Approach, Anterior Column, Percutaneous Endoscopic Approach
ØSG14KØ Fusion of 2 or More Lumbar Vertebral Joints with Nonautologous Tissue Substitute, Anterior Approach, Anterior Column, Percutaneous Endoscopic Approach
ØSG14K1 Fusion of 2 or More Lumbar Vertebral Joints with Nonautologous Tissue Substitute, Posterior Approach, Posterior Column, Percutaneous Endoscopic Approach
ØSG14KJ Fusion of 2 or More Lumbar Vertebral Joints with Nonautologous Tissue Substitute, Posterior Approach, Anterior Column, Percutaneous Endoscopic Approach
ØSG3Ø7Ø Fusion of Lumbosacral Joint with Autologous Tissue Substitute, Anterior Approach, Anterior Column, Open Approach
ØSG3Ø71 Fusion of Lumbosacral Joint with Autologous Tissue Substitute, Posterior Approach, Posterior Column, Open Approach

HAC 12: Surgical Site Infection Following Certain Orthopedic Procedures of the Spine, Shoulder, and Elbow (continued)

ØSG3Ø7J Fusion of Lumbosacral Joint with Autologous Tissue Substitute, Posterior Approach, Anterior Column, Open Approach
ØSG3ØAØ Fusion of Lumbosacral Joint with Interbody Fusion Device, Anterior Approach, Anterior Column, Open Approach
ØSG3ØAJ Fusion of Lumbosacral Joint with Interbody Fusion Device, Posterior Approach, Anterior Column, Open Approach
ØSG3ØJØ Fusion of Lumbosacral Joint with Synthetic Substitute, Anterior Approach, Anterior Column, Open Approach
ØSG3ØJ1 Fusion of Lumbosacral Joint with Synthetic Substitute, Posterior Approach, Posterior Column, Open Approach
ØSG3ØJJ Fusion of Lumbosacral Joint with Synthetic Substitute, Posterior Approach, Anterior Column, Open Approach
ØSG3ØKØ Fusion of Lumbosacral Joint with Nonautologous Tissue Substitute, Anterior Approach, Anterior Column, Open Approach
ØSG3ØK1 Fusion of Lumbosacral Joint with Nonautologous Tissue Substitute, Posterior Approach, Posterior Column, Open Approach
ØSG3ØKJ Fusion of Lumbosacral Joint with Nonautologous Tissue Substitute, Posterior Approach, Anterior Column, Open Approach
ØSG337Ø Fusion of Lumbosacral Joint with Autologous Tissue Substitute, Anterior Approach, Anterior Column, Percutaneous Approach
ØSG3371 Fusion of Lumbosacral Joint with Autologous Tissue Substitute, Posterior Approach, Posterior Column, Percutaneous Approach
ØSG337J Fusion of Lumbosacral Joint with Autologous Tissue Substitute, Posterior Approach, Anterior Column, Percutaneous Approach
ØSG33AØ Fusion of Lumbosacral Joint with Interbody Fusion Device, Anterior Approach, Anterior Column, Percutaneous Approach
ØSG33AJ Fusion of Lumbosacral Joint with Interbody Fusion Device, Posterior Approach, Anterior Column, Percutaneous Approach
ØSG33JØ Fusion of Lumbosacral Joint with Synthetic Substitute, Anterior Approach, Anterior Column, Percutaneous Approach
ØSG33J1 Fusion of Lumbosacral Joint with Synthetic Substitute, Posterior Approach, Posterior Column, Percutaneous Approach
ØSG33JJ Fusion of Lumbosacral Joint with Synthetic Substitute, Posterior Approach, Anterior Column, Percutaneous Approach
ØSG33KØ Fusion of Lumbosacral Joint with Nonautologous Tissue Substitute, Anterior Approach, Anterior Column, Percutaneous Approach
ØSG33K1 Fusion of Lumbosacral Joint with Nonautologous Tissue Substitute, Posterior Approach, Posterior Column, Percutaneous Approach
ØSG33KJ Fusion of Lumbosacral Joint with Nonautologous Tissue Substitute, Posterior Approach, Anterior Column, Percutaneous Approach
ØSG347Ø Fusion of Lumbosacral Joint with Autologous Tissue Substitute, Anterior Approach, Anterior Column, Percutaneous Endoscopic Approach
ØSG3471 Fusion of Lumbosacral Joint with Autologous Tissue Substitute, Posterior Approach, Posterior Column, Percutaneous Endoscopic Approach
ØSG347J Fusion of Lumbosacral Joint with Autologous Tissue Substitute, Posterior Approach, Anterior Column, Percutaneous Endoscopic Approach
ØSG34AØ Fusion of Lumbosacral Joint with Interbody Fusion Device, Anterior Approach, Anterior Column, Percutaneous Endoscopic Approach
ØSG34AJ Fusion of Lumbosacral Joint with Interbody Fusion Device, Posterior Approach, Anterior Column, Percutaneous Endoscopic Approach
ØSG34JØ Fusion of Lumbosacral Joint with Synthetic Substitute, Anterior Approach, Anterior Column, Percutaneous Endoscopic Approach
ØSG34J1 Fusion of Lumbosacral Joint with Synthetic Substitute, Posterior Approach, Posterior Column, Percutaneous Endoscopic Approach
ØSG34JJ Fusion of Lumbosacral Joint with Synthetic Substitute, Posterior Approach, Anterior Column, Percutaneous Endoscopic Approach
ØSG34KØ Fusion of Lumbosacral Joint with Nonautologous Tissue Substitute, Anterior Approach, Anterior Column, Percutaneous Endoscopic Approach
ØSG34K1 Fusion of Lumbosacral Joint with Nonautologous Tissue Substitute, Posterior Approach, Posterior Column, Percutaneous Endoscopic Approach
ØSG34KJ Fusion of Lumbosacral Joint with Nonautologous Tissue Substitute, Posterior Approach, Anterior Column, Percutaneous Endoscopic Approach
ØSG7Ø4Z Fusion of Right Sacroiliac Joint with Internal Fixation Device, Open Approach
ØSG7Ø7Z Fusion of Right Sacroiliac Joint with Autologous Tissue Substitute, Open Approach
ØSG7ØJZ Fusion of Right Sacroiliac Joint with Synthetic Substitute, Open Approach
ØSG7ØKZ Fusion of Right Sacroiliac Joint with Nonautologous Tissue Substitute, Open Approach
ØSG734Z Fusion of Right Sacroiliac Joint with Internal Fixation Device, Percutaneous Approach
ØSG737Z Fusion of Right Sacroiliac Joint with Autologous Tissue Substitute, Percutaneous Approach
ØSG73JZ Fusion of Right Sacroiliac Joint with Synthetic Substitute, Percutaneous Approach
ØSG73KZ Fusion of Right Sacroiliac Joint with Nonautologous Tissue Substitute, Percutaneous Approach
ØSG744Z Fusion of Right Sacroiliac Joint with Internal Fixation Device, Percutaneous Endoscopic Approach
ØSG747Z Fusion of Right Sacroiliac Joint with Autologous Tissue Substitute, Percutaneous Endoscopic Approach
ØSG74JZ Fusion of Right Sacroiliac Joint with Synthetic Substitute, Percutaneous Endoscopic Approach
ØSG74KZ Fusion of Right Sacroiliac Joint with Nonautologous Tissue Substitute, Percutaneous Endoscopic Approach
ØSG8Ø4Z Fusion of Left Sacroiliac Joint with Internal Fixation Device, Open Approach
ØSG8Ø7Z Fusion of Left Sacroiliac Joint with Autologous Tissue Substitute, Open Approach
ØSG8ØJZ Fusion of Left Sacroiliac Joint with Synthetic Substitute, Open Approach
ØSG8ØKZ Fusion of Left Sacroiliac Joint with Nonautologous Tissue Substitute, Open Approach
ØSG834Z Fusion of Left Sacroiliac Joint with Internal Fixation Device, Percutaneous Approach
ØSG837Z Fusion of Left Sacroiliac Joint with Autologous Tissue Substitute, Percutaneous Approach
ØSG83JZ Fusion of Left Sacroiliac Joint with Synthetic Substitute, Percutaneous Approach
ØSG83KZ Fusion of Left Sacroiliac Joint with Nonautologous Tissue Substitute, Percutaneous Approach
ØSG844Z Fusion of Left Sacroiliac Joint with Internal Fixation Device, Percutaneous Endoscopic Approach
ØSG847Z Fusion of Left Sacroiliac Joint with Autologous Tissue Substitute, Percutaneous Endoscopic Approach
ØSG84JZ Fusion of Left Sacroiliac Joint with Synthetic Substitute, Percutaneous Endoscopic Approach
ØSG84KZ Fusion of Left Sacroiliac Joint with Nonautologous Tissue Substitute, Percutaneous Endoscopic Approach
XRGØØF3 Fusion of Occipital-cervical Joint using Radiolucent Porous Interbody Fusion Device, Open Approach, New Technology Group 3
XRG1Ø92 Fusion of Cervical Vertebral Joint using Nanotextured Surface Interbody Fusion Device, Open Approach, New Technology Group 2
XRG1ØF3 Fusion of Cervical Vertebral Joint using Radiolucent Porous Interbody Fusion Device, Open Approach, New Technology Group 3
XRG2Ø92 Fusion of 2 or more Cervical Vertebral Joints using Nanotextured Surface Interbody Fusion Device, Open Approach, New Technology Group 2
XRG2ØF3 Fusion of 2 or more Cervical Vertebral Joints using Radiolucent Porous Interbody Fusion Device, Open Approach, New Technology Group 3
XRG4Ø92 Fusion of Cervicothoracic Vertebral Joint using Nanotextured Surface Interbody Fusion Device, Open Approach, New Technology Group 2
XRG4ØF3 Fusion of Cervicothoracic Vertebral Joint using Radiolucent Porous Interbody Fusion Device, Open Approach, New Technology Group 3

HAC 12: Surgical Site Infection Following Certain Orthopedic Procedures of the Spine, Shoulder, and Elbow (continued)

XRG6Ø92 Fusion of Thoracic Vertebral Joint using Nanotextured Surface Interbody Fusion Device, Open Approach, New Technology Group 2
XRG6ØF3 Fusion of Thoracic Vertebral Joint using Radiolucent Porous Interbody Fusion Device, Open Approach, New Technology Group 3
XRG7Ø92 Fusion of 2 to 7 Thoracic Vertebral Joints using Nanotextured Surface Interbody Fusion Device, Open Approach, New Technology Group 2
XRG7ØF3 Fusion of 2 to 7 Thoracic Vertebral Joints using Radiolucent Porous Interbody Fusion Device, Open Approach, New Technology Group 3
XRG8Ø92 Fusion of 8 or more Thoracic Vertebral Joints using Nanotextured Surface Interbody Fusion Device, Open Approach, New Technology Group 2
XRG8ØF3 Fusion of 8 or more Thoracic Vertebral Joints using Radiolucent Porous Interbody Fusion Device, Open Approach, New Technology Group 3
XRGAØ92 Fusion of Thoracolumbar Vertebral Joint using Nanotextured Surface Interbody Fusion Device, Open Approach, New Technology Group 2
XRGAØF3 Fusion of Thoracolumbar Vertebral Joint using Radiolucent Porous Interbody Fusion Device, Open Approach, New Technology Group 3
XRGBØ92 Fusion of Lumbar Vertebral Joint using Nanotextured Surface Interbody Fusion Device, Open Approach, New Technology Group 2
XRGBØF3 Fusion of Lumbar Vertebral Joint using Radiolucent Porous Interbody Fusion Device, Open Approach, New Technology Group 3
XRGCØ92 Fusion of 2 or more Lumbar Vertebral Joints using Nanotextured Surface Interbody Fusion Device, Open Approach, New Technology Group 2
XRGCØF3 Fusion of 2 or more Lumbar Vertebral Joints using Radiolucent Porous Interbody Fusion Device, Open Approach, New Technology Group 3
XRGDØ92 Fusion of Lumbosacral Joint using Nanotextured Surface Interbody Fusion Device, Open Approach, New Technology Group 2
XRGDØF3 Fusion of Lumbosacral Joint using Radiolucent Porous Interbody Fusion Device, Open Approach, New Technology Group 3

HAC 13: Surgical Site Infection (SSI) Following Cardiac Implantable Electronic Device (CIED) Procedures

Secondary diagnosis not POA:

K68.11
T81.4XXA
T82.6XXA
T82.7XXA

AND

Any of the following procedures:

Ø2H43JZ Insertion of Pacemaker Lead into Coronary Vein, Percutaneous Approach
Ø2H43KZ Insertion of Defibrillator Lead into Coronary Vein, Percutaneous Approach
Ø2H43MZ Insertion of Cardiac Lead into Coronary Vein, Percutaneous Approach
Ø2H63JZ Insertion of Pacemaker Lead into Right Atrium, Percutaneous Approach
Ø2H63MZ Insertion of Cardiac Lead into Right Atrium, Percutaneous Approach
Ø2H73JZ Insertion of Pacemaker Lead into Left Atrium, Percutaneous Approach
Ø2H73MZ Insertion of Cardiac Lead into Left Atrium, Percutaneous Approach
Ø2HK3JZ Insertion of Pacemaker Lead into Right Ventricle, Percutaneous Approach
Ø2HL3JZ Insertion of Pacemaker Lead into Left Ventricle, Percutaneous Approach
Ø2HNØJZ Insertion of Pacemaker Lead into Pericardium, Open Approach
Ø2HNØMZ Insertion of Cardiac Lead into Pericardium, Open Approach
Ø2HN3JZ Insertion of Pacemaker Lead into Pericardium, Percutaneous Approach
Ø2HN3MZ Insertion of Cardiac Lead into Pericardium, Percutaneous Approach
Ø2HN4JZ Insertion of Pacemaker Lead into Pericardium, Percutaneous Endoscopic Approach
Ø2HN4MZ Insertion of Cardiac Lead into Pericardium, Percutaneous Endoscopic Approach
Ø2PAØMZ Removal of Cardiac Lead from Heart, Open Approach
Ø2PA3MZ Removal of Cardiac Lead from Heart, Percutaneous Approach
Ø2PA4MZ Removal of Cardiac Lead from Heart, Percutaneous Endoscopic Approach
Ø2PAXMZ Removal of Cardiac Lead from Heart, External Approach
Ø2WAØMZ Revision of Cardiac Lead in Heart, Open Approach
Ø2WA3MZ Revision of Cardiac Lead in Heart, Percutaneous Approach
Ø2WA4MZ Revision of Cardiac Lead in Heart, Percutaneous Endoscopic Approach
ØJH6Ø4Z Insertion of Pacemaker, Single Chamber into Chest Subcutaneous Tissue and Fascia, Open Approach
ØJH6Ø5Z Insertion of Pacemaker, Single Chamber Rate Responsive into Chest Subcutaneous Tissue and Fascia, Open Approach
ØJH6Ø6Z Insertion of Pacemaker, Dual Chamber into Chest Subcutaneous Tissue and Fascia, Open Approach
ØJH6Ø7Z Insertion of Cardiac Resynchronization Pacemaker Pulse Generator into Chest Subcutaneous Tissue and Fascia, Open Approach
ØJH6Ø8Z Insertion of Defibrillator Generator into Chest Subcutaneous Tissue and Fascia, Open Approach
ØJH6Ø9Z Insertion of Cardiac Resynchronization Defibrillator Pulse Generator into Chest Subcutaneous Tissue and Fascia, Open Approach
ØJH6ØPZ Insertion of Cardiac Rhythm Related Device into Chest Subcutaneous Tissue and Fascia, Open Approach
ØJH634Z Insertion of Pacemaker, Single Chamber into Chest Subcutaneous Tissue and Fascia, Percutaneous Approach
ØJH635Z Insertion of Pacemaker, Single Chamber Rate Responsive into Chest Subcutaneous Tissue and Fascia, Percutaneous Approach
ØJH636Z Insertion of Pacemaker, Dual Chamber into Chest Subcutaneous Tissue and Fascia, Percutaneous Approach
ØJH637Z Insertion of Cardiac Resynchronization Pacemaker Pulse Generator into Chest Subcutaneous Tissue and Fascia, Percutaneous Approach
ØJH638Z Insertion of Defibrillator Generator into Chest Subcutaneous Tissue and Fascia, Percutaneous Approach
ØJH639Z Insertion of Cardiac Resynchronization Defibrillator Pulse Generator into Chest Subcutaneous Tissue and Fascia, Percutaneous Approach
ØJH63PZ Insertion of Cardiac Rhythm Related Device into Chest Subcutaneous Tissue and Fascia, Percutaneous Approach
ØJH8Ø4Z Insertion of Pacemaker, Single Chamber into Abdomen Subcutaneous Tissue and Fascia, Open Approach
ØJH8Ø5Z Insertion of Pacemaker, Single Chamber Rate Responsive into Abdomen Subcutaneous Tissue and Fascia, Open Approach
ØJH8Ø6Z Insertion of Pacemaker, Dual Chamber into Abdomen Subcutaneous Tissue and Fascia, Open Approach
ØJH8Ø7Z Insertion of Cardiac Resynchronization Pacemaker Pulse Generator into Abdomen Subcutaneous Tissue and Fascia, Open Approach
ØJH8Ø8Z Insertion of Defibrillator Generator into Abdomen Subcutaneous Tissue and Fascia, Open Approach
ØJH8Ø9Z Insertion of Cardiac Resynchronization Defibrillator Pulse Generator into Abdomen Subcutaneous Tissue and Fascia, Open Approach
ØJH8ØPZ Insertion of Cardiac Rhythm Related Device into Abdomen Subcutaneous Tissue and Fascia, Open Approach
ØJH834Z Insertion of Pacemaker, Single Chamber into Abdomen Subcutaneous Tissue and Fascia, Percutaneous Approach
ØJH835Z Insertion of Pacemaker, Single Chamber Rate Responsive into Abdomen Subcutaneous Tissue and Fascia, Percutaneous Approach
ØJH836Z Insertion of Pacemaker, Dual Chamber into Abdomen Subcutaneous Tissue and Fascia, Percutaneous Approach
ØJH837Z Insertion of Cardiac Resynchronization Pacemaker Pulse Generator into Abdomen Subcutaneous Tissue and Fascia, Percutaneous Approach
ØJH838Z Insertion of Defibrillator Generator into Abdomen Subcutaneous Tissue and Fascia, Percutaneous Approach
ØJH839Z Insertion of Cardiac Resynchronization Defibrillator Pulse Generator into Abdomen Subcutaneous Tissue and Fascia, Percutaneous Approach
ØJH83PZ Insertion of Cardiac Rhythm Related Device into Abdomen Subcutaneous Tissue and Fascia, Percutaneous Approach
ØJPTØPZ Removal of Cardiac Rhythm Related Device from Trunk Subcutaneous Tissue and Fascia, Open Approach
ØJPT3PZ Removal of Cardiac Rhythm Related Device from Trunk Subcutaneous Tissue and Fascia, Percutaneous Approach
ØJWTØPZ Revision of Cardiac Rhythm Related Device in Trunk Subcutaneous Tissue and Fascia, Open Approach
ØJWT3PZ Revision of Cardiac Rhythm Related Device in Trunk Subcutaneous Tissue and Fascia, Percutaneous Approach

HAC 14: Iatrogenic Pneumothorax with Venous Catheterization

Secondary diagnosis not POA:

J95.811

AND

Any of the following procedures:

- Ø2H633Z Insertion of Infusion Device into Right Atrium, Percutaneous Approach
- Ø2HK33Z Insertion of Infusion Device into Right Ventricle, Percutaneous Approach
- Ø2HS33Z Insertion of Infusion Device into Right Pulmonary Vein, Percutaneous Approach
- Ø2HS43Z Insertion of Infusion Device into Right Pulmonary Vein, Percutaneous Endoscopic Approach
- Ø2HT33Z Insertion of Infusion Device into Left Pulmonary Vein, Percutaneous Approach
- Ø2HT43Z Insertion of Infusion Device into Left Pulmonary Vein, Percutaneous Endoscopic Approach
- Ø2HV33Z Insertion of Infusion Device into Superior Vena Cava, Percutaneous Approach
- Ø2HV43Z Insertion of Infusion Device into Superior Vena Cava, Percutaneous Endoscopic Approach
- Ø5HØ33Z Insertion of Infusion Device into Azygos Vein, Percutaneous Approach
- Ø5HØ43Z Insertion of Infusion Device into Azygos Vein, Percutaneous Endoscopic Approach
- Ø5H133Z Insertion of Infusion Device into Hemiazygos Vein, Percutaneous Approach
- Ø5H143Z Insertion of Infusion Device into Hemiazygos Vein, Percutaneous Endoscopic Approach
- Ø5H333Z Insertion of Infusion Device into Right Innominate Vein, Percutaneous Approach
- Ø5H343Z Insertion of Infusion Device into Right Innominate Vein, Percutaneous Endoscopic Approach
- Ø5H433Z Insertion of Infusion Device into Left Innominate Vein, Percutaneous Approach
- Ø5H443Z Insertion of Infusion Device into Left Innominate Vein, Percutaneous Endoscopic Approach
- Ø5H533Z Insertion of Infusion Device into Right Subclavian Vein, Percutaneous Approach
- Ø5H543Z Insertion of Infusion Device into Right Subclavian Vein, Percutaneous Endoscopic Approach
- Ø5H633Z Insertion of Infusion Device into Left Subclavian Vein, Percutaneous Approach
- Ø5H643Z Insertion of Infusion Device into Left Subclavian Vein, Percutaneous Endoscopic Approach
- Ø5HM33Z Insertion of Infusion Device into Right Internal Jugular Vein, Percutaneous Approach
- Ø5HN33Z Insertion of Infusion Device into Left Internal Jugular Vein, Percutaneous Approach
- Ø5HP33Z Insertion of Infusion Device into Right External Jugular Vein, Percutaneous Approach
- Ø5HQ33Z Insertion of Infusion Device into Left External Jugular Vein, Percutaneous Approach
- ØJH63XZ Insertion of Vascular Access Device into Chest Subcutaneous Tissue and Fascia, Percutaneous Approach

Appendix K: Coding Exercises and Answers

Using the ICD-10-PCS tables construct the code that accurately represents the procedure performed.

Medical Surgical Section

Procedure	Code
1. Excision of malignant melanoma from skin of right ear	
2. Laparoscopy with excision of endometrial implant from left ovary	
3. Percutaneous needle core biopsy of right kidney	
4. EGD with gastric biopsy	
5. Open endarterectomy of left common carotid artery	
6. Excision of basal cell carcinoma of lower lip	
7. Open excision of tail of pancreas	
8. Percutaneous biopsy of right gastrocnemius muscle	
9. Sigmoidoscopy with sigmoid polypectomy	
10. Open excision of lesion from right Achilles tendon	
11. Open resection of cecum	
12. Total excision of pituitary gland, open	
13. Explantation of left failed kidney, open	
14. Open left axillary total lymphadenectomy	
15. Laparoscopic-assisted vaginal hysterectomy	
16. Right total mastectomy, open	
17. Open resection of papillary muscle	
18. Total retropubic prostatectomy, open	
19. Laparoscopic cholecystectomy	
20. Endoscopic bilateral total maxillary sinusectomy	
21. Amputation at right elbow level	
22. Right below-knee amputation, proximal tibia/fibula	
23. Fifth ray carpometacarpal joint amputation, left hand	
24. Right leg and hip amputation through ischium	
25. DIP joint amputation of right thumb	
26. Right wrist joint amputation	
27. Trans-metatarsal amputation of foot at left big toe	
28. Mid-shaft amputation, right humerus	
29. Left fourth toe amputation, mid-proximal phalanx	
30. Right above-knee amputation, distal femur	
31. Cryotherapy of wart on left hand	
32. Percutaneous radiofrequency ablation of right vocal cord lesion	
33. Left heart catheterization with laser destruction of arrhythmogenic focus, A-V node	
34. Cautery of nosebleed	
35. Transurethral endoscopic laser ablation of prostate	
36. Percutaneous cautery of oozing varicose vein, left calf	

Procedure	Code
37. Laparoscopy with destruction of endometriosis, bilateral ovaries	
38. Laser coagulation of right retinal vessel hemorrhage, percutaneous	
39. Thoracoscopic pleurodesis, left side	
40. Percutaneous insertion of Greenfield IVC filter	
41. Forceps total mouth extraction, upper and lower teeth	
42. Removal of left thumbnail	
43. Extraction of right intraocular lens without replacement, percutaneous	
44. Laparoscopy with needle aspiration of ova for in vitro fertilization	
45. Nonexcisional debridement of skin ulcer, right foot	
46. Open stripping of abdominal fascia, right side	
47. Hysteroscopy with D&C, diagnostic	
48. Liposuction for medical purposes, left upper arm	
49. Removal of tattered right ear drum fragments with tweezers	
50. Microincisional phlebectomy of spider veins, right lower leg	
51. Routine Foley catheter placement	
52. Incision and drainage of external anal abscess	
53. Percutaneous drainage of ascites	
54. Laparoscopy with left ovarian cystotomy and drainage	
55. Laparotomy and drain placement for liver abscess, right lobe	
56. Right knee arthrotomy with drain placement	
57. Thoracentesis of left pleural effusion	
58. Phlebotomy of left median cubital vein for polycythemia vera	
59. Percutaneous chest tube placement for right pneumothorax	
60. Endoscopic drainage of left ethmoid sinus	
61. External ventricular CSF drainage catheter placement via burr hole	
62. Removal of foreign body, right cornea	
63. Percutaneous mechanical thrombectomy, left brachial artery	
64. Esophagogastroscopy with removal of bezoar from stomach	
65. Foreign body removal, skin of left thumb	
66. Transurethral cystoscopy with removal of bladder stone	
67. Forceps removal of foreign body in right nostril	
68. Laparoscopy with excision of old suture from mesentery	
69. Incision and removal of right lacrimal duct stone	
70. Nonincisional removal of intraluminal foreign body from vagina	
71. Right common carotid endarterectomy, open	
72. Open excision of retained sliver, subcutaneous tissue of left foot	
73. Extracorporeal shockwave lithotripsy (ESWL), bilateral ureters	

Procedure	Code
74. Endoscopic retrograde cholangiopancreatography (ERCP) with lithotripsy of common bile duct stone	
75. Thoracotomy with crushing of pericardial calcifications	
76. Transurethral cystoscopy with fragmentation of bladder calculus	
77. Hysteroscopy with intraluminal lithotripsy of left fallopian tube calcification	
78. Division of right foot tendon, percutaneous	
79. Left heart catheterization with division of bundle of HIS	
80. Open osteotomy of capitate, left hand	
81. EGD with esophagotomy of esophagogastric junction	
82. Sacral rhizotomy for pain control, percutaneous	
83. Laparotomy with exploration and adhesiolysis of right ureter	
84. Incision of scar contracture, right elbow	
85. Frenulotomy for treatment of tongue-tie syndrome	
86. Right shoulder arthroscopy with coracoacromial ligament release	
87. Mitral valvulotomy for release of fused leaflets, open approach	
88. Percutaneous left Achilles tendon release	
89. Laparoscopy with lysis of peritoneal adhesions	
90. Manual rupture of right shoulder joint adhesions under general anesthesia	
91. Open posterior tarsal tunnel release	
92. Laparoscopy with freeing of left ovary and fallopian tube	
93. Liver transplant with donor matched liver	
94. Orthotopic heart transplant using porcine heart	
95. Right lung transplant, open, using organ donor match	
96. Transplant of large intestine, organ donor match	
97. Left kidney/pancreas organ bank transplant	
98. Replantation of avulsed scalp	
99. Reattachment of severed right ear	
100. Reattachment of traumatic left gastrocnemius avulsion, open	
101. Closed replantation of three avulsed teeth, lower jaw	
102. Reattachment of severed left hand	
103. Right open palmaris longus tendon transfer	
104. Endoscopic radial to median nerve transfer	
105. Fasciocutaneous flap closure of left thigh, open	
106. Transfer left index finger to left thumb position, open	
107. Percutaneous fascia transfer to fill defect, right neck	
108. Trigeminal to facial nerve transfer, percutaneous endoscopic	
109. Endoscopic left leg flexor hallucis longus tendon transfer	
110. Right scalp advancement flap to right temple	
111. Bilateral TRAM pedicle flap reconstruction status post mastectomy, muscle only, open	
112. Skin transfer flap closure of complex open wound, left lower back	
113. Open fracture reduction, right tibia	
114. Laparoscopy with gastropexy for malrotation	
115. Left knee arthroscopy with reposition of anterior cruciate ligament	
116. Open transposition of ulnar nerve	
117. Closed reduction with percutaneous internal fixation of right femoral neck fracture	
118. Trans-vaginal intraluminal cervical cerclage	
119. Cervical cerclage using Shirodkar technique	
120. Thoracotomy with banding of left pulmonary artery using extraluminal device	
121. Restriction of thoracic duct with intraluminal stent, percutaneous	
122. Craniotomy with clipping of cerebral aneurysm	
123. Nonincisional, transnasal placement of restrictive stent in right lacrimal duct	
124. Catheter-based temporary restriction of blood flow in abdominal aorta for treatment of cerebral ischemia	
125. Percutaneous ligation of esophageal vein	
126. Percutaneous embolization of left internal carotid-cavernous fistula	
127. Laparoscopy with bilateral occlusion of fallopian tubes using Hulka extraluminal clips	
128. Open suture ligation of failed AV graft, left brachial artery	
129. Percutaneous embolization of vascular supply, intracranial meningioma	
130. Percutaneous embolization of right uterine artery, using coils	
131. Open occlusion of left atrial appendage, using extraluminal pressure clips	
132. Percutaneous suture exclusion of left atrial appendage, via femoral artery access	
133. ERCP with balloon dilation of common bile duct	
134. PTCA of two coronary arteries, LAD with stent placement, RCA with no stent	
135. Cystoscopy with intraluminal dilation of bladder neck stricture	
136. Open dilation of old anastomosis, left femoral artery	
137. Dilation of upper esophageal stricture, direct visualization, with Bougie sound	
138. PTA of right brachial artery stenosis	
139. Transnasal dilation and stent placement in right lacrimal duct	
140. Hysteroscopy with balloon dilation of bilateral fallopian tubes	
141. Tracheoscopy with intraluminal dilation of tracheal stenosis	
142. Cystoscopy with dilation of left ureteral stricture, with stent placement	
143. Open gastric bypass with Roux-en-Y limb to jejunum	
144. Right temporal artery to intracranial artery bypass using Gore-Tex graft, open	

Procedure	Code
145. Tracheostomy formation with tracheostomy tube placement, percutaneous	
146. PICVA (percutaneous in situ coronary venous arterialization) of single coronary artery	
147. Open left femoral-popliteal artery bypass using cadaver vein graft	
148. Shunting of intrathecal cerebrospinal fluid to peritoneal cavity using synthetic shunt	
149. Colostomy formation, open, transverse colon to abdominal wall	
150. Open urinary diversion, left ureter, using ileal conduit to skin	
151. CABG of LAD using left internal mammary artery, open off-bypass	
152. Open pleuroperitoneal shunt, right pleural cavity, using synthetic device	
153. Percutaneous placement of ventriculoperitoneal shunt for treatment of hydrocephalus	
154. End-of-life replacement of spinal neurostimulator generator, multiple array, in lower abdomen	
155. Percutaneous insertion of spinal neurostimulator lead, lumbar spinal cord	
156. Percutaneous replacement of broken pacemaker lead in left atrium	
157. Open placement of dual chamber pacemaker generator in chest wall	
158. Percutaneous placement of venous central line in right internal jugular, with tip in superior vena cava	
159. Open insertion of multiple channel cochlear implant, left ear	
160. Percutaneous placement of Swan-Ganz catheter in pulmonary trunk	
161. Bronchoscopy with insertion of Low Dose, Pd-103 brachytherapy seeds, right main bronchus	
162. Open insertion of interspinous process device into lumbar vertebral joint	
163. Open placement of bone growth stimulator, left femoral shaft	
164. Cystoscopy with placement of brachytherapy seeds in prostate gland	
165. Percutaneous insertion of Greenfield IVC filter	
166. Full-thickness skin graft to right lower arm, autograft (do not code graft harvest for this exercise)	
167. Excision of necrosed left femoral head with bone bank bone graft to fill the defect, open	
168. Penetrating keratoplasty of right cornea with donor matched cornea, percutaneous approach	
169. Bilateral mastectomy with concomitant saline breast implants, open	
170. Excision of abdominal aorta with Gore-Tex graft replacement, open	
171. Total right knee arthroplasty with insertion of total knee prosthesis	
172. Bilateral mastectomy with free TRAM flap reconstruction	
173. Tenonectomy with graft to right ankle using cadaver graft, open	

Procedure	Code
174. Mitral valve replacement using porcine valve, open	
175. Percutaneous phacoemulsification of right eye cataract with prosthetic lens insertion	
176. Transcatheter replacement of pulmonary valve using of bovine jugular vein valve	
177. Total left hip replacement using ceramic on ceramic prosthesis, without bone cement	
178. Aortic valve annuloplasty using ring, open	
179. Laparoscopic repair of left inguinal hernia with marlex plug	
180. Autograft nerve graft to right median nerve, percutaneous endoscopic (do not code graft harvest for this exercise)	
181. Exchange of liner in femoral component of previous left hip replacement, open approach	
182. Anterior colporrhaphy with polypropylene mesh reinforcement, open approach	
183. Implantation of CorCap cardiac support device, open approach	
184. Abdominal wall herniorrhaphy, open, using synthetic mesh	
185. Tendon graft to strengthen injured left shoulder using autograft, open (do not code graft harvest for this exercise)	
186. Onlay lamellar keratoplasty of left cornea using autograft, external approach	
187. Resurfacing procedure on right femoral head, open approach	
188. Exchange of drainage tube from right hip joint	
189. Tracheostomy tube exchange	
190. Change chest tube for left pneumothorax	
191. Exchange of cerebral ventriculostomy drainage tube	
192. Foley urinary catheter exchange	
193. Open removal of lumbar sympathetic neurostimulator lead	
194. Nonincisional removal of Swan-Ganz catheter from right pulmonary artery	
195. Laparotomy with removal of pancreatic drain	
196. Extubation, endotracheal tube	
197. Nonincisional PEG tube removal	
198. Transvaginal removal of brachytherapy seeds	
199. Transvaginal removal of extraluminal cervical cerclage	
200. Incision with removal of K-wire fixation, right first metatarsal	
201. Cystoscopy with retrieval of left ureteral stent	
202. Removal of nasogastric drainage tube for decompression	
203. Removal of external fixator, left radial fracture	
204. Trimming and reanastomosis of stenosed femorofemoral synthetic bypass graft, open	
205. Open revision of right hip replacement, with readjustment of prosthesis	
206. Adjustment of position, pacemaker lead in left ventricle, percutaneous	
207. External repositioning of Foley catheter to bladder	
208. Taking out loose screw and putting larger screw in fracture repair plate, left tibia	

Procedure	Code
209. Revision of totally implantable VAD port placement in chest wall, causing patient discomfort, open	
210. Thoracotomy with exploration of right pleural cavity	
211. Diagnostic laryngoscopy	
212. Exploratory arthrotomy of left knee	
213. Colposcopy with diagnostic hysteroscopy	
214. Digital rectal exam	
215. Diagnostic arthroscopy of right shoulder	
216. Endoscopy of maxillary sinus	
217. Laparotomy with palpation of liver	
218. Transurethral diagnostic cystoscopy	
219. Colonoscopy, discontinued at sigmoid colon	
220. Percutaneous mapping of basal ganglia	
221. Heart catheterization with cardiac mapping	
222. Intraoperative whole brain mapping via craniotomy	
223. Mapping of left cerebral hemisphere, percutaneous endoscopic	
224. Intraoperative cardiac mapping during open heart surgery	
225. Hysteroscopy with cautery of post-hysterectomy oozing and evacuation of clot	
226. Open exploration and ligation of post-op arterial bleeder, left forearm	
227. Control of post-operative retroperitoneal bleeding via laparotomy	
228. Reopening of thoracotomy site with drainage and control of post-op hemopericardium	
229. Arthroscopy with drainage of hemarthrosis at previous operative site, right knee	
230. Radiocarpal fusion of left hand with internal fixation, open	
231. Posterior spinal fusion at L1-L3 level with BAK cage interbody fusion device, open	
232. Intercarpal fusion of right hand with bone bank bone graft, open	
233. Sacrococcygeal fusion with bone graft from same operative site, open	
234. Interphalangeal fusion of left great toe, percutaneous pin fixation	
235. Suture repair of left radial nerve laceration	
236. Laparotomy with suture repair of blunt force duodenal laceration	
237. Perineoplasty with repair of old obstetric laceration, open	
238. Suture repair of right biceps tendon (upper arm) laceration, open	
239. Closure of abdominal wall stab wound	
240. Cosmetic face lift, open, no other information available	
241. Bilateral breast augmentation with silicone implants, open	
242. Cosmetic rhinoplasty with septal reduction and tip elevation using local tissue graft, open	
243. Abdominoplasty (tummy tuck), open	
244. Liposuction of bilateral thighs	
245. Creation of penis in female patient using tissue bank donor graft	

Procedure	Code
246. Creation of vagina in male patient using synthetic material	
247. Laparoscopic vertical (sleeve) gastrectomy	
248. Left uterine artery embolization with intraluminal biosphere injection	

Obstetrics

Procedure	Code
1. Abortion by dilation and evacuation following laminaria insertion	
2. Manually assisted spontaneous abortion	
3. Abortion by abortifacient insertion	
4. Bimanual pregnancy examination	
5. Extraperitoneal C-section, low transverse incision	
6. Fetal spinal tap, percutaneous	
7. Fetal kidney transplant, laparoscopic	
8. Open in utero repair of congenital diaphragmatic hernia	
9. Laparoscopy with total excision of tubal pregnancy	
10. Transvaginal removal of fetal monitoring electrode	

Placement

Procedure	Code
1. Placement of packing material, right ear	
2. Mechanical traction of entire left leg	
3. Removal of splint, right shoulder	
4. Placement of neck brace	
5. Change of vaginal packing	
6. Packing of wound, chest wall	
7. Sterile dressing placement to left groin region	
8. Removal of packing material from pharynx	
9. Placement of intermittent pneumatic compression device, covering entire right arm	
10. Exchange of pressure dressing to left thigh	

Administration

Procedure	Code
1. Peritoneal dialysis via indwelling catheter	
2. Transvaginal artificial insemination	
3. Infusion of total parenteral nutrition via central venous catheter	
4. Esophagogastroscopy with Botox injection into esophageal sphincter	
5. Percutaneous irrigation of knee joint	
6. Systemic infusion of recombinant tissue plasminogen activator (r-tPA) via peripheral venous catheter	
7. Transfusion of antihemophilic factor, (nonautologous) via arterial central line	
8. Transabdominal in vitro fertilization, implantation of donor ovum	
9. Autologous bone marrow transplant via central venous line	
10. Implantation of anti-microbial envelope with cardiac defibrillator placement, open	

Procedure	Code
11. Sclerotherapy of brachial plexus lesion, alcohol injection	
12. Percutaneous peripheral vein injection, glucarpidase	
13. Introduction of anti-infective envelope into subcutaneous tissue, open	

Measurement and Monitoring

Procedure	Code
1. Cardiac stress test, single measurement	
2. EGD with biliary flow measurement	
3. Right and left heart cardiac catheterization with bilateral sampling and pressure measurements	
4. Temperature monitoring, rectal	
5. Peripheral venous pulse, external, single measurement	
6. Holter monitoring	
7. Respiratory rate, external, single measurement	
8. Fetal heart rate monitoring, transvaginal	
9. Visual mobility test, single measurement	
10. Left ventricular cardiac output monitoring from pulmonary artery wedge (Swan-Ganz) catheter	
11. Olfactory acuity test, single measurement	

Extracorporeal or Systemic Assistance and Performance

Procedure	Code
1. Intermittent mechanical ventilation, 16 hours	
2. Liver dialysis, single encounter	
3. Cardiac countershock with successful conversion to sinus rhythm	
4. IPPB (intermittent positive pressure breathing) for mobilization of secretions, 22 hours	
5. Renal dialysis, 12 hours	
6. IABP (intra-aortic balloon pump) continuous	
7. Intra-operative cardiac pacing, continuous	
8. ECMO (extracorporeal membrane oxygenation), central	
9. Controlled mechanical ventilation (CMV), 45 hours	
10. Pulsatile compression boot with intermittent inflation	

Extracorporeal or Systemic Therapies

Procedure	Code
1. Donor thrombocytapheresis, single encounter	
2. Bili-lite phototherapy, series treatment	
3. Whole body hypothermia, single treatment	
4. Circulatory phototherapy, single encounter	
5. Shock wave therapy of plantar fascia, single treatment	
6. Antigen-free air conditioning, series treatment	
7. TMS (transcranial magnetic stimulation), series treatment	
8. Therapeutic ultrasound of peripheral vessels, single treatment	
9. Plasmapheresis, series treatment	
10. Extracorporeal electromagnetic stimulation (EMS) for urinary incontinence, single treatment	

Osteopathic

Procedure	Code
1. Isotonic muscle energy treatment of right leg	
2. Low velocity-high amplitude osteopathic treatment of head	
3. Lymphatic pump osteopathic treatment of left axilla	
4. Indirect osteopathic treatment of sacrum	
5. Articulatory osteopathic treatment of cervical region	

Other Procedures

Procedure	Code
1. Near infrared spectroscopy of leg vessels	
2. CT computer assisted sinus surgery	
3. Suture removal, abdominal wall	
4. Isolation after infectious disease exposure	
5. Robotic assisted open prostatectomy	
6. In vitro fertilization	

Chiropractic

Procedure	Code
1. Chiropractic treatment of lumbar region using long lever specific contact	
2. Chiropractic manipulation of abdominal region, indirect visceral	
3. Chiropractic extra-articular treatment of hip region	
4. Chiropractic treatment of sacrum using long and short lever specific contact	
5. Mechanically-assisted chiropractic manipulation of head	

Imaging

Procedure	Code
1. Noncontrast CT of abdomen and pelvis	
2. Intravascular ultrasound, left subclavian artery	
3. Fluoroscopic guidance for insertion of central venous catheter in SVC, low osmolar contrast	
4. Chest x-ray, AP/PA and lateral views	

Procedure	Code
5. Endoluminal ultrasound of gallbladder and bile ducts	
6. MRI of thyroid gland, contrast unspecified	
7. Esophageal videofluoroscopy study with oral barium contrast	
8. Portable x-ray study of right radius/ulna shaft, standard series	
9. Routine fetal ultrasound, second trimester twin gestation	
10. CT scan of bilateral lungs, high osmolar contrast with densitometry	
11. Fluoroscopic guidance for percutaneous transluminal angioplasty (PTA) of left common femoral artery, low osmolar contrast	

Nuclear Medicine

Procedure	Code
1. Tomo scan of right and left heart, unspecified radiopharmaceutical, qualitative gated rest	
2. Technetium pentetate assay of kidneys, ureters, and bladder	
3. Uniplanar scan of spine using technetium oxidronate, with first-pass study	
4. Thallous chloride tomographic scan of bilateral breasts	
5. PET scan of myocardium using rubidium	
6. Gallium citrate scan of head and neck, single plane imaging	
7. Xenon gas nonimaging probe of brain	
8. Upper GI scan, radiopharmaceutical unspecified, for gastric emptying	
9. Carbon 11 PET scan of brain with quantification	
10. Iodinated albumin nuclear medicine assay, blood plasma volume study	

Radiation Therapy

Procedure	Code
1. Plaque radiation of left eye, single port	
2. 8 MeV photon beam radiation to brain	
3. IORT of colon, 3 ports	
4. HDR brachytherapy of prostate using palladium-103	
5. Electron radiation treatment of right breast, with custom device	
6. Hyperthermia oncology treatment of pelvic region	
7. Contact radiation of tongue	
8. Heavy particle radiation treatment of pancreas, four risk sites	
9. LDR brachytherapy to spinal cord using iodine	
10. Whole body Phosphorus 32 administration with risk to hematopoetic system	

Physical Rehabilitation and Diagnostic Audiology

Procedure	Code
1. Bekesy assessment using audiometer	
2. Individual fitting of left eye prosthesis	
3. Physical therapy for range of motion and mobility, patient right hip, no special equipment	
4. Bedside swallow assessment using assessment kit	
5. Caregiver training in airway clearance techniques	
6. Application of short arm cast in rehabilitation setting	
7. Verbal assessment of patient's pain level	
8. Caregiver training in communication skills using manual communication board	
9. Group musculoskeletal balance training exercises, whole body, no special equipment	
10. Individual therapy for auditory processing using tape recorder	

Mental Health

Procedure	Code
1. Cognitive-behavioral psychotherapy, individual	
2. Narcosynthesis	
3. Light therapy	
4. ECT (electroconvulsive therapy), unilateral, multiple seizure	
5. Crisis intervention	
6. Neuropsychological testing	
7. Hypnosis	
8. Developmental testing	
9. Vocational counseling	
10. Family psychotherapy	

Substance Abuse Treatment

Procedure	Code
1. Naltrexone treatment for drug dependency	
2. Substance abuse treatment family counseling	
3. Medication monitoring of patient on methadone maintenance	
4. Individual interpersonal psychotherapy for drug abuse	
5. Patient in for alcohol detoxification treatment	
6. Group motivational counseling	
7. Individual 12-step psychotherapy for substance abuse	
8. Post-test infectious disease counseling for IV drug abuser	
9. Psychodynamic psychotherapy for drug dependent patient	
10. Group cognitive-behavioral counseling for substance abuse	

New Technology

Procedure	Code
1. Infusion of ceftazidime via peripheral venous catheter	

Answers to Coding Exercises

Medical Surgical Section

Procedure	Code
1. Excision of malignant melanoma from skin of right ear	ØHB2XZZ
2. Laparoscopy with excision of endometrial implant from left ovary	ØUB14ZZ
3. Percutaneous needle core biopsy of right kidney	ØTBØ3ZX
4. EGD with gastric biopsy	ØDB68ZX
5. Open endarterectomy of left common carotid artery	Ø3CJØZZ
6. Excision of basal cell carcinoma of lower lip	ØCB1XZZ
7. Open excision of tail of pancreas	ØFBGØZZ
8. Percutaneous biopsy of right gastrocnemius muscle	ØKBS3ZX
9. Sigmoidoscopy with sigmoid polypectomy	ØDBN8ZZ
10. Open excision of lesion from right Achilles tendon	ØLBNØZZ
11. Open resection of cecum	ØDTHØZZ
12. Total excision of pituitary gland, open	ØGTØØZZ
13. Explantation of left failed kidney, open	ØTT1ØZZ
14. Open left axillary total lymphadenectomy	Ø7T6ØZZ (RESECTION is coded for cutting out a chain of lymph nodes.)
15. Laparoscopic-assisted vaginal hysterectomy	ØUT9FZZ
16. Right total mastectomy, open	ØHTTØZZ
17. Open resection of papillary muscle	Ø2TDØZZ (The papillary muscle refers to the heart and is found in the *Heart and Great Vessels* body system.)
18. Total retropubic prostatectomy, open	ØVTØØZZ
19. Laparoscopic cholecystectomy	ØFT44ZZ
20. Endoscopic bilateral total maxillary sinusectomy	Ø9TQ8ZZ, Ø9TR8ZZ
21. Amputation at right elbow level	ØX6BØZZ
22. Right below-knee amputation, proximal tibia/fibula	ØY6HØZ1 (The qualifier *High* here means the portion of the tib/fib closest to the knee.)
23. Fifth ray carpometacarpal joint amputation, left hand	ØX6KØZ8 (A *complete* ray amputation is through the carpometacarpal joint.)
24. Right leg and hip amputation through ischium	ØY62ØZZ (The *Hindquarter* body part includes amputation along any part of the hip bone.)
25. DIP joint amputation of right thumb	ØX6LØZ3 (The qualifier *low* here means through the distal interphalangeal joint.)
26. Right wrist joint amputation	ØX6JØZØ (Amputation at the wrist joint is actually complete amputation of the hand.)
27. Trans-metatarsal amputation of foot at left big toe	ØY6NØZ9 (A *partial* amputation is through the shaft of the metatarsal bone.)
28. Mid-shaft amputation, right humerus	ØX68ØZ2
29. Left fourth toe amputation, mid-proximal phalanx	ØY6WØZ1 (The qualifier *High* here means anywhere along the proximal phalanx.)
30. Right above-knee amputation, distal femur	ØY6CØZ3
31. Cryotherapy of wart on left hand	ØH5GXZZ
32. Percutaneous radiofrequency ablation of right vocal cord lesion	ØC5T3ZZ
33. Left heart catheterization with laser destruction of arrhythmogenic focus, A-V node	Ø2583ZZ
34. Cautery of nosebleed	Ø95KXZZ
35. Transurethral endoscopic laser ablation of prostate	ØV5Ø8ZZ
36. Percutaneous cautery of oozing varicose vein, left calf	Ø65Y3ZZ
37. Laparoscopy with destruction of endometriosis, bilateral ovaries	ØU524ZZ
38. Laser coagulation of right retinal vessel hemorrhage, percutaneous	Ø85G3ZZ (The *Retinal Vessel* body-part values are in the *Eye* body system.)
39. Thoracoscopic pleurodesis, left side	ØB5P4ZZ
40. Percutaneous insertion of Greenfield IVC filter	Ø6HØ3DZ
41. Forceps total mouth extraction, upper and lower teeth	ØCDWXZ2, ØCDXXZ2
42. Removal of left thumbnail	ØHDQXZZ (No separate body-part value is given for thumbnail, so this is coded to *Fingernail*.)
43. Extraction of right intraocular lens without replacement, percutaneous	Ø8DJ3ZZ
44. Laparoscopy with needle aspiration of ova for in vitro fertilization	ØUDN4ZZ
45. Nonexcisional debridement of skin ulcer, right foot	ØHDMXZZ
46. Open stripping of abdominal fascia, right side	ØJD8ØZZ
47. Hysteroscopy with D&C, diagnostic	ØUDB8ZX
48. Liposuction for medical purposes, left upper arm	ØJDF3ZZ (The *Percutaneous* approach is inherent in the liposuction technique.)
49. Removal of tattered right ear drum fragments with tweezers	Ø9D77ZZ
50. Microincisional phlebectomy of spider veins, right lower leg	Ø6DY3ZZ
51. Routine Foley catheter placement	ØT9B7ØZ
52. Incision and drainage of external anal abscess	ØD9QXZZ
53. Percutaneous drainage of ascites	ØW9G3ZZ (This is drainage of the cavity and not the peritoneal membrane itself.)
54. Laparoscopy with left ovarian cystotomy and drainage	ØU914ZZ
55. Laparotomy and drain placement for liver abscess, right lobe	ØF91ØØZ
56. Right knee arthrotomy with drain placement	ØS9CØØZ
57. Thoracentesis of left pleural effusion	ØW9B3ZZ (This is drainage of the pleural cavity)
58. Phlebotomy of left median cubital vein for polycythemia vera	Ø59C3ZZ (The median cubital vein is a branch of the basilic vein)

Procedure	Code
59. Percutaneous chest tube placement for right pneumothorax	ØW993ØZ
60. Endoscopic drainage of left ethmoid sinus	Ø99V4ZZ
61. External ventricular CSF drainage catheter placement via burr hole	ØØ963ØZ
62. Removal of foreign body, right cornea	Ø8C8XZZ
63. Percutaneous mechanical thrombectomy, left brachial artery	Ø3C83ZZ
64. Esophagogastroscopy with removal of bezoar from stomach	ØDC68ZZ
65. Foreign body removal, skin of left thumb	ØHCGXZZ (There is no specific value for thumb skin, so the procedure is coded to *Hand*.)
66. Transurethral cystoscopy with removal of bladder stone	ØTCB8ZZ
67. Forceps removal of foreign body in right nostril	Ø9CKXZZ (Nostril is coded to the *Nasal mucosa and soft tissue* body-part value.)
68. Laparoscopy with excision of old suture from mesentery	ØDCV4ZZ
69. Incision and removal of right lacrimal duct stone	Ø8CXØZZ
70. Nonincisional removal of intraluminal foreign body from vagina	ØUCG7ZZ (The approach *External* is also a possibility. It is assumed here that since the patient went to the doctor to have the object removed, that it was not in the vaginal orifice.)
71. Right common carotid endarterectomy, open	Ø3CHØZZ
72. Open excision of retained sliver, subcutaneous tissue of left foot	ØJCRØZZ
73. Extracorporeal shockwave lithotripsy (ESWL), bilateral ureters	ØTF6XZZ, ØTF7XZZ (The *Bilateral Ureter* body-part value is not available for the root operation FRAGMENTATION, so the procedures are coded separately.)
74. Endoscopic retrograde cholangiopancreatography (ERCP) with lithotripsy of common bile duct stone	ØFF98ZZ (ERCP is performed through the mouth to the biliary system via the duodenum, so the approach value is *Via Natural or Artificial Opening Endoscopic*.)
75. Thoracotomy with crushing of pericardial calcifications	Ø2FNØZZ
76. Transurethral cystoscopy with fragmentation of bladder calculus	ØTFB8ZZ
77. Hysteroscopy with intraluminal lithotripsy of left fallopian tube calcification	ØUF68ZZ
78. Division of right foot tendon, percutaneous	ØL8V3ZZ
79. Left heart catheterization with division of bundle of HIS	Ø2883ZZ
80. Open osteotomy of capitate, left hand	ØP8NØZZ (The capitate is one of the carpal bones of the hand.)
81. EGD with esophagotomy of esophagogastric junction	ØD948ZZ
82. Sacral rhizotomy for pain control, percutaneous	Ø18R3ZZ
83. Laparotomy with exploration and adhesiolysis of right ureter	ØTN6ØZZ

Procedure	Code
84. Incision of scar contracture, right elbow	ØHNDXZZ (The skin of the elbow region is coded to *Lower Arm*.)
85. Frenulotomy for treatment of tongue-tie syndrome	ØCN7XZZ (The frenulum is coded to the body-part value *Tongue*.)
86. Right shoulder arthroscopy with coracoacromial ligament release	ØMN14ZZ
87. Mitral valvulotomy for release of fused leaflets, open approach	Ø2NGØZZ
88. Percutaneous left Achilles tendon release	ØLNP3ZZ
89. Laparoscopy with lysis of peritoneal adhesions	ØDNW4ZZ
90. Manual rupture of right shoulder joint adhesions under general anesthesia	ØRNJXZZ
91. Open posterior tarsal tunnel release	Ø1NGØZZ (The nerve released in the posterior tarsal tunnel is the tibial nerve.)
92. Laparoscopy with freeing of left ovary and fallopian tube	ØUN14ZZ, ØUN64ZZ
93. Liver transplant with donor matched liver	ØFYØØZØ
94. Orthotopic heart transplant using porcine heart	Ø2YAØZ2 (The donor heart comes from an animal [pig], so the qualifier value is *Zooplastic*.)
95. Right lung transplant, open, using organ donor match	ØBYKØZØ
96. Transplant of large intestine, organ donor match	ØDYEØZØ
97. Left kidney/pancreas organ bank transplant	ØFYGØZØ, ØTY1ØZØ
98. Replantation of avulsed scalp	ØHMØXZZ
99. Reattachment of severed right ear	Ø9MØXZZ
100. Reattachment of traumatic left gastrocnemius avulsion, open	ØKMTØZZ
101. Closed replantation of three avulsed teeth, lower jaw	ØCMXXZ1
102. Reattachment of severed left hand	ØXMKØZZ
103. Right open palmaris longus tendon transfer	ØLX5ØZZ
104. Endoscopic radial to median nerve transfer	Ø1X64Z5
105. Fasciocutaneous flap closure of left thigh, open	ØJXMØZC (The qualifier identifies the body layers in addition to fascia included in the procedure.)
106. Transfer left index finger to left thumb position, open	ØXXPØZM
107. Percutaneous fascia transfer to fill defect, right neck	ØJX43ZZ
108. Trigeminal to facial nerve transfer, percutaneous endoscopic	ØØXK4ZM
109. Endoscopic left leg flexor hallucis longus tendon transfer	ØLXP4ZZ
110. Right scalp advancement flap to right temple	ØHXØXZZ
111. Bilateral TRAM pedicle flap reconstruction status post mastectomy, muscle only, open	ØKXKØZ6, ØKXLØZ6 (The transverse rectus abdominus muscle (TRAM) flap is coded for each flap developed.)
112. Skin transfer flap closure of complex open wound, left lower back	ØHX6XZZ
113. Open fracture reduction, right tibia	ØQSGØZZ
114. Laparoscopy with gastropexy for malrotation	ØDS64ZZ
115. Left knee arthroscopy with reposition of anterior cruciate ligament	ØMSP4ZZ

Procedure	Code
116. Open transposition of ulnar nerve	Ø1S4ØZZ
117. Closed reduction with percutaneous internal fixation of right femoral neck fracture	ØQS634Z
118. Trans-vaginal intraluminal cervical cerclage	ØUVC7DZ
119. Cervical cerclage using Shirodkar technique	ØUVC7ZZ
120. Thoracotomy with banding of left pulmonary artery using extraluminal device	Ø2VRØCZ
121. Restriction of thoracic duct with intraluminal stent, percutaneous	Ø7VK3DZ
122. Craniotomy with clipping of cerebral aneurysm	Ø3VGØCZ (The clip is placed lengthwise on the outside wall of the widened portion of the vessel.)
123. Nonincisional, transnasal placement of restrictive stent in right lacrimal duct	Ø8VX7DZ
124. Catheter-based temporary restriction of blood flow in abdominal aorta for treatment of cerebral ischemia	Ø4VØ3DJ
125. Percutaneous ligation of esophageal vein	Ø6L33ZZ
126. Percutaneous embolization of left internal carotid-cavernous fistula	Ø3LL3DZ
127. Laparoscopy with bilateral occlusion of fallopian tubes using Hulka extraluminal clips	ØUL74CZ
128. Open suture ligation of failed AV graft, left brachial artery	Ø3L8ØZZ
129. Percutaneous embolization of vascular supply, intracranial meningioma	Ø3LG3DZ
130. Percutaneous embolization of right uterine artery, using coils	Ø4LE3DT
131. Open occlusion of left atrial appendage, using extraluminal pressure clips	Ø2L7ØCK
132. Percutaneous suture exclusion of left atrial appendage, via femoral artery access	Ø2L73ZK
133. ERCP with balloon dilation of common bile duct	ØF798ZZ
134. PTCA of two coronary arteries, LAD with stent placement, RCA with no stent	Ø27Ø3DZ, Ø27Ø3ZZ (A separate procedure is coded for each artery dilated, since the device value differs for each artery.)
135. Cystoscopy with intraluminal dilation of bladder neck stricture	ØT7C8ZZ
136. Open dilation of old anastomosis, left femoral artery	Ø47LØZZ
137. Dilation of upper esophageal stricture, direct visualization, with Bougie sound	ØD717ZZ
138. PTA of right brachial artery stenosis	Ø3773ZZ
139. Transnasal dilation and stent placement in right lacrimal duct	Ø87X7DZ
140. Hysteroscopy with balloon dilation of bilateral fallopian tubes	ØU778ZZ
141. Tracheoscopy with intraluminal dilation of tracheal stenosis	ØB718ZZ
142. Cystoscopy with dilation of left ureteral stricture, with stent placement	ØT778DZ
143. Open gastric bypass with Roux-en-Y limb to jejunum	ØD16ØZA
144. Right temporal artery to intracranial artery bypass using Gore-Tex graft, open	Ø31SØJG
145. Tracheostomy formation with tracheostomy tube placement, percutaneous	ØB113F4
146. PICVA (percutaneous in situ coronary venous arterialization) of single coronary artery	Ø21Ø3D4

Procedure	Code
147. Open left femoral-popliteal artery bypass using cadaver vein graft	Ø41LØKL
148. Shunting of intrathecal cerebrospinal fluid to peritoneal cavity using synthetic shunt	ØØ16ØJ6
149. Colostomy formation, open, transverse colon to abdominal wall	ØD1LØZ4
150. Open urinary diversion, left ureter, using ileal conduit to skin	ØT17ØZC
151. CABG of LAD using left internal mammary artery, open off-bypass	Ø21ØØZ9
152. Open pleuroperitoneal shunt, right pleural cavity, using synthetic device	ØW19ØJG
153. Percutaneous placement of ventriculoperitoneal shunt for treatment of hydrocephalus	ØØ163J6
154. End-of-life replacement of spinal neurostimulator generator, multiple array, in lower abdomen	ØJH8ØDZ (Taking out of the old generator is coded separately to the root operation *Removal*)
155. Percutaneous insertion of spinal neurostimulator lead, lumbar spinal cord	ØØHV3MZ
156. Percutaneous replacement of broken pacemaker lead in left atrium	Ø2H73JZ (Taking out the broken pacemaker lead is coded separately to the root operation *Removal*.)
157. Open placement of dual chamber pacemaker generator in chest wall	ØJH6Ø6Z
158. Percutaneous placement of venous central line in right internal jugular, with tip in superior vena cava	Ø2HV33Z
159. Open insertion of multiple channel cochlear implant, left ear	Ø9HEØ6Z
160. Percutaneous placement of Swan-Ganz catheter in pulmonary trunk	Ø2HP32Z (The Swan-Ganz catheter is coded to the device value *Monitoring Device* because it monitors pulmonary artery output.)
161. Bronchoscopy with insertion of Low Dose Pd-103 brachytherapy seeds, right main bronchus	ØBHØ81Z, DB11BB2
162. Open insertion of interspinous process device into lumbar vertebral joint	ØSHØØBZ
163. Open placement of bone growth stimulator, left femoral shaft	ØQHYØMZ
164. Cystoscopy with placement of brachytherapy seeds in prostate gland	ØVHØ81Z
165. Percutaneous insertion of Greenfield IVC filter	Ø6HØ3DZ
166. Full-thickness skin graft to right lower arm, autograft (do not code graft harvest for this exercise)	ØHRDX73
167. Excision of necrosed left femoral head with bone bank bone graft to fill the defect, open	ØQR7ØKZ
168. Penetrating keratoplasty of right cornea with donor matched cornea, percutaneous approach	Ø8R83KZ
169. Bilateral mastectomy with concomitant saline breast implants, open	ØHRVØJZ
170. Excision of abdominal aorta with Gore-Tex graft replacement, open	Ø4RØØJZ
171. Total right knee arthroplasty with insertion of total knee prosthesis	ØSRCØJZ
172. Bilateral mastectomy with free TRAM flap reconstruction	ØHRVØ76
173. Tenonectomy with graft to right ankle using cadaver graft, open	ØLRSØKZ

Procedure	Code
174. Mitral valve replacement using porcine valve, open	Ø2RGØ8Z
175. Percutaneous phacoemulsification of right eye cataract with prosthetic lens insertion	Ø8RJ3JZ
176. Transcatheter replacement of pulmonary valve using of bovine jugular vein valve	Ø2RH38Z
177. Total left hip replacement using ceramic on ceramic prosthesis, without bone cement	ØSRBØ3A
178. Aortic valve annuloplasty using ring, open	Ø2UFØJZ
179. Laparoscopic repair of left inguinal hernia with marlex plug	ØYU64JZ
180. Autograft nerve graft to right median nerve, percutaneous endoscopic (do not code graft harvest for this exercise)	Ø1U547Z
181. Exchange of liner in femoral component of previous left hip replacement, open approach	ØSUSØ9Z (Taking out of the old liner is coded separately to the root operation *Removal*)
182. Anterior colporrhaphy with polypropylene mesh reinforcement, open approach	ØJUCØJZ
183. Implantation of CorCap cardiac support device, open approach	Ø2UAØJZ
184. Abdominal wall herniorrhaphy, open, using synthetic mesh	ØWUFØJZ
185. Tendon graft to strengthen injured left shoulder using autograft, open (do not code graft harvest for this exercise)	ØLU2Ø7Z
186. Onlay lamellar keratoplasty of left cornea using autograft, external approach	Ø8U9X7Z
187. Resurfacing procedure on right femoral head, open approach	ØSURØBZ
188. Exchange of drainage tube from right hip joint	ØS2YXØZ
189. Tracheostomy tube exchange	ØB21XFZ
190. Change chest tube for left pneumothorax	ØW2BXØZ
191. Exchange of cerebral ventriculostomy drainage tube	ØØ2ØXØZ
192. Foley urinary catheter exchange	ØT2BXØZ (This is coded to *Drainage Device* because urine is being drained.)
193. Open removal of lumbar sympathetic neurostimulator lead	Ø1PYØMZ
194. Nonincisional removal of Swan-Ganz catheter from right pulmonary artery	Ø2PYX2Z
195. Laparotomy with removal of pancreatic drain	ØFPGØØZ
196. Extubation, endotracheal tube	ØBP1XDZ
197. Nonincisional PEG tube removal	ØDP6XUZ
198. Transvaginal removal of brachytherapy seeds	ØUPH71Z
199. Transvaginal removal of extraluminal cervical cerclage	ØUPD7CZ
200. Incision with removal of K-wire fixation, right first metatarsal	ØQPNØ4Z
201. Cystoscopy with retrieval of left ureteral stent	ØTP98DZ
202. Removal of nasogastric drainage tube for decompression	ØDP6XØZ
203. Removal of external fixator, left radial fracture	ØPPJX5Z
204. Trimming and reanastomosis of stenosed femorofemoral synthetic bypass graft, open	Ø4WYØJZ
205. Open revision of right hip replacement, with readjustment of prosthesis	ØSW9ØJZ
206. Adjustment of position, pacemaker lead in left ventricle, percutaneous	Ø2WA3MZ
207. External repositioning of Foley catheter to bladder	ØTWBXØZ

Procedure	Code
208. Taking out loose screw and putting larger screw in fracture repair plate, left tibia	ØQWHØ4Z
209. Revision of totally implantable VAD port placement in chest wall, causing patient discomfort, open	ØJWTØWZ
210. Thoracotomy with exploration of right pleural cavity	ØWJ9ØZZ
211. Diagnostic laryngoscopy	ØCJS8ZZ
212. Exploratory arthrotomy of left knee	ØSJDØZZ
213. Colposcopy with diagnostic hysteroscopy	ØUJD8ZZ
214. Digital rectal exam	ØDJD7ZZ
215. Diagnostic arthroscopy of right shoulder	ØRJJ4ZZ
216. Endoscopy of maxillary sinus	Ø9JY4ZZ
217. Laparotomy with palpation of liver	ØFJØØZZ
218. Transurethral diagnostic cystoscopy	ØTJB8ZZ
219. Colonoscopy, discontinued at sigmoid colon	ØDJD8ZZ
220. Percutaneous mapping of basal ganglia	ØØK83ZZ
221. Heart catheterization with cardiac mapping	Ø2K83ZZ
222. Intraoperative whole brain mapping via craniotomy	ØØKØØZZ
223. Mapping of left cerebral hemisphere, percutaneous endoscopic	ØØK74ZZ
224. Intraoperative cardiac mapping during open heart surgery	Ø2K8ØZZ
225. Hysteroscopy with cautery of post-hysterectomy oozing and evacuation of clot	ØW3R8ZZ
226. Open exploration and ligation of post-op arterial bleeder, left forearm	ØX3FØZZ
227. Control of post-operative retroperitoneal bleeding via laparotomy	ØW3HØZZ
228. Reopening of thoracotomy site with drainage and control of post-op hemopericardium	ØW3DØZZ
229. Arthroscopy with drainage of hemarthrosis at previous operative site, right knee	ØY3F4ZZ
230. Radiocarpal fusion of left hand with internal fixation, open	ØRGPØ4Z
231. Posterior spinal fusion at L1-L3 level with BAK cage interbody fusion device, open	ØSG1ØAJ
232. Intercarpal fusion of right hand with bone bank bone graft, open	ØRGQØKZ
233. Sacrococcygeal fusion with bone graft from same operative site, open	ØSG5Ø7Z
234. Interphalangeal fusion of left great toe, percutaneous pin fixation	ØSGQ34Z
235. Suture repair of left radial nerve laceration	Ø1Q6ØZZ (The approach value is *Open*, though the surgical exposure may have been created by the wound itself.)
236. Laparotomy with suture repair of blunt force duodenal laceration	ØDQ9ØZZ
237. Perineoplasty with repair of old obstetric laceration, open	ØWQNØZZ
238. Suture repair of right biceps tendon (upper arm) laceration, open	ØLQ3ØZZ
239. Closure of abdominal wall stab wound	ØWQFØZZ
240. Cosmetic face lift, open, no other information available	ØWØ2ØZZ
241. Bilateral breast augmentation with silicone implants, open	ØHØVØJZ
242. Cosmetic rhinoplasty with septal reduction and tip elevation using local tissue graft, open	Ø9ØKØ7Z
243. Abdominoplasty (tummy tuck), open	ØWØFØZZ

Procedure	Code
244. Liposuction of bilateral thighs	ØJØL3ZZ, ØJØM3ZZ
245. Creation of penis in female patient using tissue bank donor graft	ØW4NØK1
246. Creation of vagina in male patient using synthetic material	ØW4MØJØ
247. Laparoscopic vertical (sleeve) gastrectomy	ØDB64Z3
248. Left uterine artery embolization with intraluminal biosphere injection	Ø4LF3DU

Obstetrics

Procedure	Code
1. Abortion by dilation and evacuation following laminaria insertion	1ØAØ7ZW
2. Manually assisted spontaneous abortion	1ØEØXZZ (Since the pregnancy was not artificially terminated, this is coded to *Delivery* because it captures the procedure objective. The fact that it was an abortion will be identified in the diagnosis code.)
3. Abortion by abortifacient insertion	1ØAØ7ZX
4. Bimanual pregnancy examination	1ØJØ7ZZ
5. Extraperitoneal C-section, low transverse incision	1ØDØØZ2
6. Fetal spinal tap, percutaneous	1Ø9Ø3ZA
7. Fetal kidney transplant, laparoscopic	1ØYØ4ZS
8. Open in utero repair of congenital diaphragmatic hernia	1ØQØØZK (Diaphragm is classified to the *Respiratory* body system in the *Medical and Surgical* section.)
9. Laparoscopy with total excision of tubal pregnancy	1ØT24ZZ
10. Transvaginal removal of fetal monitoring electrode	1ØPØ73Z

Placement

Procedure	Code
1. Placement of packing material, right ear	2Y42X5Z
2. Mechanical traction of entire left leg	2W6MXØZ
3. Removal of splint, right shoulder	2W5AX1Z
4. Placement of neck brace	2W32X3Z
5. Change of vaginal packing	2YØ4X5Z
6. Packing of wound, chest wall	2W44X5Z
7. Sterile dressing placement to left groin region	2W27X4Z
8. Removal of packing material from pharynx	2Y5ØX5Z
9. Placement of intermittent pneumatic compression device, covering entire right arm	2W18X7Z
10. Exchange of pressure dressing to left thigh	2WØPX6Z

Administration

Procedure	Code
1. Peritoneal dialysis via indwelling catheter	3E1M39Z
2. Transvaginal artificial insemination	3EØP7LZ
3. Infusion of total parenteral nutrition via central venous catheter	3EØ436Z
4. Esophagogastroscopy with Botox injection into esophageal sphincter	3EØG8GC (Botulinum toxin is a paralyzing agent with temporary effects; it does not sclerose or destroy the nerve.)
5. Percutaneous irrigation of knee joint	3E1U38Z
6. Systemic infusion of recombinant tissue plasminogen activator (r-tPA) via peripheral venous catheter	3EØ3317
7. Transfusion of antihemophilic factor, (nonautologous) via arterial central line	3Ø263V1
8. Transabdominal in vitro fertilization, implantation of donor ovum	3EØP3Q1
9. Autologous bone marrow transplant via central venous line	3Ø243GØ
10. Implantation of anti-microbial envelope with cardiac defibrillator placement, open	3EØ1Ø2A
11. Sclerotherapy of brachial plexus lesion, alcohol injection	3EØT3TZ
12. Percutaneous peripheral vein injection, glucarpidase	3EØ33GQ
13. Introduction of anti-infective envelope into subcutaneous tissue, open	3EØ1Ø2A

Measurement and Monitoring

Procedure	Code
1. Cardiac stress test, single measurement	4AØ2XM4
2. EGD with biliary flow measurement	4AØC85Z
3. Right and left heart cardiac catheterization with bilateral sampling and pressure measurements	4AØ23N8
4. Temperature monitoring, rectal	4A1Z7KZ
5. Peripheral venous pulse, external, single measurement	4AØ4XJ1
6. Holter monitoring	4A12X45
7. Respiratory rate, external, single measurement	4AØ9XCZ
8. Fetal heart rate monitoring, transvaginal	4A1H7CZ
9. Visual mobility test, single measurement	4AØ7X7Z
10. Left ventricular cardiac output monitoring from pulmonary artery wedge (Swan-Ganz) catheter	4A1239Z
11. Olfactory acuity test, single measurement	4AØ8XØZ

Extracorporeal or Systemic Assistance and Performance

Procedure	Code
1. Intermittent mechanical ventilation, 16 hours	5A1935Z
2. Liver dialysis, single encounter	5A1C00Z
3. Cardiac countershock with successful conversion to sinus rhythm	5A2204Z
4. IPPB (intermittent positive pressure breathing) for mobilization of secretions, 22 hours	5A09358
5. Renal dialysis, 12 hours	5A1D80Z
6. IABP (intra-aortic balloon pump) continuous	5A02210
7. Intra-operative cardiac pacing, continuous	5A1223Z
8. ECMO (extracorporeal membrane oxygenation), central	5A1522F
9. Controlled mechanical ventilation (CMV), 45 hours	5A1945Z
10. Pulsatile compression boot with intermittent inflation	5A02115 (This is coded to the function value *Cardiac Output*, because the purpose of such compression devices is to return blood to the heart faster.)

Extracorporeal or Systemic Therapies

Procedure	Code
1. Donor thrombocytapheresis, single encounter	6A550Z2
2. Bili-lite phototherapy, series treatment	6A601ZZ
3. Whole body hypothermia, single treatment	6A4Z0ZZ
4. Circulatory phototherapy, single encounter	6A650ZZ
5. Shock wave therapy of plantar fascia, single treatment	6A930ZZ
6. Antigen-free air conditioning, series treatment	6A0Z1ZZ
7. TMS (transcranial magnetic stimulation), series treatment	6A221ZZ
8. Therapeutic ultrasound of peripheral vessels, single treatment	6A750Z6
9. Plasmapheresis, series treatment	6A551Z3
10. Extracorporeal electromagnetic stimulation (EMS) for urinary incontinence, single treatment	6A210ZZ

Osteopathic

Procedure	Code
1. Isotonic muscle energy treatment of right leg	7W06X8Z
2. Low velocity-high amplitude osteopathic treatment of head	7W00X5Z
3. Lymphatic pump osteopathic treatment of left axilla	7W07X6Z
4. Indirect osteopathic treatment of sacrum	7W04X4Z
5. Articulatory osteopathic treatment of cervical region	7W01X0Z

Other Procedures

Procedure	Code
1. Near infrared spectroscopy of leg vessels	8E023DZ
2. CT computer assisted sinus surgery	8E09XBG (The primary procedure is coded separately.)
3. Suture removal, abdominal wall	8E0WXY8
4. Isolation after infectious disease exposure	8E0ZXY6
5. Robotic assisted open prostatectomy	8E0W0CZ (The primary procedure is coded separately.)
6. In vitro fertilization	8E0ZXY1

Chiropractic

Procedure	Code
1. Chiropractic treatment of lumbar region using long lever specific contact	9WB3XGZ
2. Chiropractic manipulation of abdominal region, indirect visceral	9WB9XCZ
3. Chiropractic extra-articular treatment of hip region	9WB6XDZ
4. Chiropractic treatment of sacrum using long and short lever specific contact	9WB4XJZ
5. Mechanically-assisted chiropractic manipulation of head	9WB0XKZ

Imaging

Procedure	Code
1. Noncontrast CT of abdomen and pelvis	BW21ZZZ
2. Intravascular ultrasound, left subclavian artery	B342ZZ3
3. Fluoroscopic guidance for insertion of central venous catheter in SVC, low osmolar contrast	B5181ZA
4. Chest x-ray, AP/PA and lateral views	BW03ZZZ
5. Endoluminal ultrasound of gallbladder and bile ducts	BF43ZZZ
6. MRI of thyroid gland, contrast unspecified	BG34YZZ
7. Esophageal videofluoroscopy study with oral barium contrast	BD11YZZ
8. Portable x-ray study of right radius/ulna shaft, standard series	BP0JZZZ
9. Routine fetal ultrasound, second trimester twin gestation	BY4DZZZ
10. CT scan of bilateral lungs, high osmolar contrast with densitometry	BB240ZZ
11. Fluoroscopic guidance for percutaneous transluminal angioplasty (PTA) of left common femoral artery, low osmolar contrast	B41G1ZZ

Nuclear Medicine

Procedure	Code
1. Tomo scan of right and left heart, unspecified radiopharmaceutical, qualitative gated rest	C226YZZ
2. Technetium pentetate assay of kidneys, ureters, and bladder	CT631ZZ
3. Uniplanar scan of spine using technetium oxidronate, with first-pass study	CP151ZZ
4. Thallous chloride tomographic scan of bilateral breasts	CH22SZZ
5. PET scan of myocardium using rubidium	C23GQZZ
6. Gallium citrate scan of head and neck, single plane imaging	CW1BLZZ
7. Xenon gas nonimaging probe of brain	CØ5ØVZZ
8. Upper GI scan, radiopharmaceutical unspecified, for gastric emptying	CD15YZZ
9. Carbon 11 PET scan of brain with quantification	CØ3ØBZZ
10. Iodinated albumin nuclear medicine assay, blood plasma volume study	C763HZZ

Radiation Therapy

Procedure	Code
1. Plaque radiation of left eye, single port	D8YØFZZ
2. 8 MeV photon beam radiation to brain	DØØ11ZZ
3. IORT of colon, 3 ports	DDY5CZZ
4. HDR brachytherapy of prostate using palladium-103	DV1Ø9BZ
5. Electron radiation treatment of right breast, with custom device	DMØ13ZZ
6. Hyperthermia oncology treatment of pelvic region	DWY68ZZ
7. Contact radiation of tongue	D9Y57ZZ
8. Heavy particle radiation treatment of pancreas, four risk sites	DFØ34ZZ
9. LDR brachytherapy to spinal cord using iodine	DØ16B9Z
10. Whole body Phosphorus 32 administration with risk to hematopoetic system	DWY5GFZ

Physical Rehabilitation and Diagnostic Audiology

Procedure	Code
1. Bekesy assessment using audiometer	F13Z31Z
2. Individual fitting of left eye prosthesis	FØDZ8UZ
3. Physical therapy for range of motion and mobility, patient right hip, no special equipment	FØ7LØZZ
4. Bedside swallow assessment using assessment kit	FØØZHYZ
5. Caregiver training in airway clearance techniques	FØFZ8ZZ
6. Application of short arm cast in rehabilitation setting	FØDZ7EZ (Inhibitory cast is listed in the equipment reference table under E, *Orthosis*.)
7. Verbal assessment of patient's pain level	FØ2ZFZZ
8. Caregiver training in communication skills using manual communication board	FØFZJMZ (Manual communication board is listed in the equipment reference table under M, *Augmentative/Alternative Communication*.)
9. Group musculoskeletal balance training exercises, whole body, no special equipment	FØ7M6ZZ (Balance training is included in the motor treatment reference table under *Therapeutic Exercise*.)
10. Individual therapy for auditory processing using tape recorder	FØ9Z2KZ (Tape recorder is listed in the equipment reference table under *Audiovisual Equipment*.)

Mental Health

Procedure	Code
1. Cognitive-behavioral psychotherapy, individual	GZ58ZZZ
2. Narcosynthesis	GZGZZZZ
3. Light therapy	GZJZZZZ
4. ECT (electroconvulsive therapy), unilateral, multiple seizure	GZB1ZZZ
5. Crisis intervention	GZ2ZZZZ
6. Neuropsychological testing	GZ13ZZZ
7. Hypnosis	GZFZZZZ
8. Developmental testing	GZ1ØZZZ
9. Vocational counseling	GZ61ZZZ
10. Family psychotherapy	GZ72ZZZ

Substance Abuse Treatment

Procedure	Code
1. Naltrexone treatment for drug dependency	HZ94ZZZ
2. Substance abuse treatment family counseling	HZ63ZZZ
3. Medication monitoring of patient on methadone maintenance	HZ81ZZZ
4. Individual interpersonal psychotherapy for drug abuse	HZ54ZZZ
5. Patient in for alcohol detoxification treatment	HZ2ZZZZ
6. Group motivational counseling	HZ47ZZZ
7. Individual 12-step psychotherapy for substance abuse	HZ53ZZZ
8. Post-test infectious disease counseling for IV drug abuser	HZ3CZZZ
9. Psychodynamic psychotherapy for drug dependent patient	HZ5CZZZ
10. Group cognitive-behavioral counseling for substance abuse	HZ42ZZZ

New Technology

Procedure	Code
1. Infusion of ceftazidime via peripheral venous catheter	XWØ3321

Appendix L: Procedure Combination Tables

The tables below were developed to help simplify the relationship between ICD-10-PCS coding and MS-DRG assignment. The Centers for Medicare & Medicaid Services (CMS) has identified in the MS-DRG v35 Definitions Manual certain procedure combinations that must occur in order to assign a specific MS-DRG. There are many factors influencing MS-DRG assignment, including principal and secondary diagnoses, MCC or CC use, sex of the patient, and discharge status. These tables should be used only as a guide.

DRG ØØ1-ØØ2 Heart Transplant or Implant of Heart Assist System

Heart Transplant

Replacement of Right and Left Ventricle Ø2RKØJZ and Ø2RLØJZ

Insertion With Removal of Heart Assist System

Type of Heart Assist System	Code as appropriate Insertion by approach	Code also as appropriate Removal of Heart Assist System by approach
Biventricular External	Ø2HA[Ø,3,4]RS	Ø2PA[Ø,3,4]RZ
External	Ø2HA[Ø,4]RZ	Ø2PA[Ø,3,4]RZ

Revision With Removal of Heart Assist System

Type of Heart Assist System	Code as appropriate Revision by approach	Code also as appropriate Removal of Heart Assist System by approach
Implantable	Ø2WA[Ø,3,4]QZ	Ø2PA[Ø,3,4]RZ
External	Ø2WA[Ø,3,4]RZ	Ø2PA[Ø,3,4]RZ

DRG ØØ8 Simultaneous Pancreas/Kidney Transplant

Transplanted Body Part Laterality	Code Transplant as appropriate by tissue type			Code also Pancreas Transplant as appropriate by tissue type		
	Allogeneic	Syngeneic	Zooplastic	Allogeneic	Syngeneic	Zooplastic
Kidney, Right	ØTYØØZØ	ØTYØØZ1	ØTYØØZ2	ØFYGØZØ	ØFYGØZ1	ØFYGØZ2
Kidney, Left	ØTY1ØZØ	ØTY1ØZ1	ØTY1ØZ2	ØFYGØZØ	ØFYGØZ1	ØFYGØZ2

DRG Ø23-Ø27 Craniotomy

Site of Neurostimulator Lead	Code as appropriate Insertion of Lead by approach	Code also as appropriate Insertion of Device by type and subcutaneous site						
		Neuro-stimulator Generator	Stimulator Multiple Array Code as appropriate by approach			Stimulator Multiple Array, Rechargeable Code as appropriate by approach		
		Skull	Chest	Back	Abdomen	Chest	Back	Abdomen
Brain	ØØHØ[Ø,3,4]MZ	ØNHØØNZ	ØJH6[Ø,3]DZ	ØJH7[Ø,3]DZ	ØJH8[Ø,3]DZ	ØJH6[Ø,3]EZ	ØJH7[Ø,3]EZ	ØJH8[Ø,3]EZ
Cerebral Ventricle	ØØH6[Ø,3,4]MZ	ØNHØØNZ	ØJH6[Ø,3]DZ	ØJH7[Ø,3]DZ	ØJH8[Ø,3]DZ	ØJH6[Ø,3]EZ	ØJH7[Ø,3]EZ	ØJH8[Ø,3]EZ

DRG Ø28-Ø3Ø Spinal Procedures

Generator Type	Insertion of Generator by Site			Code also as appropriate Insertion of Neurostimulator Lead by approach	
	Chest	Abdomen	Back	Spinal Canal	Spinal Cord
Single Array	ØJH6[Ø,3]BZ	ØJH8[Ø,3]BZ	ØJH7[Ø,3]BZ	ØØHU[Ø,3,4]MZ	ØØHV[Ø,3,4]MZ
Single Array, Rechargeable	ØJH6[Ø,3]CZ	ØJH8[Ø,3]CZ	ØJH7[Ø,3]CZ	ØØHU[Ø,3,4]MZ	ØØHV[Ø,3,4]MZ
Multiple Array	ØJH6[Ø,3]DZ	ØJH8[Ø,3]DZ	ØJH7[Ø,3]DZ	ØØHU[Ø,3,4]MZ	ØØHV[Ø,3,4]MZ
Multiple Array, Rechargable	ØJH6[Ø,3]EZ	—	ØJH7[Ø,3]EZ	ØØHU[Ø,3,4]MZ	ØØHV[Ø,3,4]MZ
Multiple Array, Rechargable	—	ØJH8[Ø,3]EZ	—	ØØHU[Ø,3,4]MZ	ØØHVØMZ
Multiple Array, Rechargable	—	ØJH8ØEZ	—	—	ØØHV[3,4]MZ

DRG Ø4Ø-Ø42 Peripheral and Cranial Nerve and Other Nervous System Procedures

Insertion of Neurostimulator Lead With Device

Site of Neurostimulator Lead	Code as appropriate Insertion by approach	Code also as appropriate Insertion of Device by type and subcutaneous site					
		Stimulator Single Array Code as appropriate by approach			Stimulator Single Array, Rechargeable Code as appropriate by approach		
		Chest	Back	Abdomen	Chest	Back	Abdomen
Cranial Nerve	ØØHE[Ø,3,4]MZ	ØJH6[Ø,3]BZ	ØJH7[Ø,3]BZ	ØJH8[Ø,3]BZ	ØJH6[Ø,3]CZ	ØJH7[Ø,3]CZ	ØJH8[Ø,3]CZ
Peripheral Nerve	Ø1HY[Ø,3,4]MZ	ØJH6[Ø,3]BZ	ØJH7[Ø,3]BZ	ØJH8[Ø,3]BZ	ØJH6[Ø,3]CZ	ØJH7[Ø,3]CZ	ØJH8[Ø,3]CZ
Stomach	ØDH6[Ø,3,4]MZ	ØJH6[Ø,3]BZ	ØJH7[Ø,3]BZ	ØJH8[Ø,3]BZ	ØJH6[Ø,3]CZ	ØJH7[Ø,3]CZ	ØJH8[Ø,3]CZ
Azygos vein	Ø5HØ[Ø,3,4]MZ	ØJH6[Ø,3]BZ	ØJH7[Ø,S]BZ	ØJH8[Ø,3]BZ	ØJH6[Ø,3]CZ	ØJH7[Ø,S]CZ	ØJH8[Ø,3]CZ
Innominate Vein, Right	Ø5H3[Ø,3,4]MZ	ØJH6[Ø,3]BZ	ØJH7[Ø,S]BZ	ØJH8[Ø,3]BZ	ØJH6[Ø,3]CZ	ØJH7[Ø,S]CZ	ØJH8[Ø,3]CZ
Innominate Vein, Left	Ø5H4[Ø,3,4]MZ	ØJH6[Ø,3]BZ	ØJH7[Ø,S]BZ	ØJH8[Ø,3]BZ	ØJH6[Ø,3]CZ	ØJH7[Ø,S]CZ	ØJH8[Ø,3]CZ
		Stimulator Multiple Array Code as appropriate by approach			Stimulator Multiple Array, Rechargeable Code as appropriate by approach		
		Chest	Back	Abdomen	Chest	Back	Abdomen
Cranial Nerve	ØØHE[Ø,3,4]MZ	ØJH6[Ø,3]DZ	ØJH7[Ø,3]DZ	ØJH8[Ø,3]DZ	ØJH6[Ø,3]EZ	ØJH7[Ø,3]EZ	ØJH8[Ø,3]EZ
Peripheral Nerve	Ø1HY[Ø,3,4]MZ	ØJH6[Ø,3]DZ	ØJH7[Ø,3]DZ	ØJH8[Ø,3]DZ	ØJH6[Ø,3]EZ	ØJH7[Ø,3]EZ	ØJH8[Ø,3]EZ
Stomach	ØDH6[Ø,3,4]MZ	ØJH6[Ø,3]DZ	ØJH7[Ø,3]DZ	ØJH8[Ø,3]DZ	ØJH6[Ø,3]EZ	ØJH7[Ø,3]EZ	ØJH8[Ø,3]EZ
Azygos vein	Ø5HØ[Ø,3,4]MZ	ØJH6[Ø,3]DZ	ØJH7[Ø,S]DZ	ØJH8[Ø,3]DZ	ØJH6[Ø,3]EZ	ØJH7[Ø,S]EZ	ØJH8[Ø,3]EZ
Innominate Vein, Right	Ø5H3[Ø,3,4]MZ	ØJH6[Ø,3]DZ	ØJH7[Ø,S]DZ	ØJH8[Ø,3]DZ	ØJH6[Ø,3]EZ	ØJH7[Ø,S]EZ	ØJH8[Ø,3]EZ
Innominate Vein, Left	Ø5H4[Ø,3,4]MZ	ØJH6[Ø,3]DZ	ØJH7[Ø,S]DZ	ØJH8[Ø,3]DZ	ØJH6[Ø,3]EZ	ØJH7[Ø,S]EZ	ØJH8[Ø,3]EZ

DRG 222-227 Cardiac Defibrillator Implant

Insertion of Generator With Insertion of Lead(s) into Coronary Vein, Atrium or Ventricle

Generator Type	Insertion of Generator by Site		Code also as appropriate Insertion of Leads by site				
	Chest	Abdomen	Coronary Vein	Atrium		Ventricle	
				Right	Left	Right	Left
Defibrillator	ØJH6[Ø,3]8Z	ØJH8[Ø,3]8Z	Ø2H4[Ø,4]KZ	Ø2H6[Ø,3,4]KZ	Ø2H7[Ø,3,4]KZ	Ø2HK[Ø,3,4]KZ	Ø2HL[Ø,3,4]KZ
Cardiac Resynch Defibrillator Pulse Generator	ØJH6[Ø,3]9Z	ØJH8[Ø,3]9Z	Ø2H4[Ø,3,4]KZ or Ø2H43[J,M]Z	Ø2H6[Ø,3,4]KZ	Ø2H7[Ø,3,4]KZ	Ø2HK[Ø,3,4]KZ	Ø2HL[Ø,3,4]KZ
Contractility Modulation Device	ØJH6[Ø,3]AZ	ØJH8[Ø,3]AZ	—	—	—	—	Ø2HL[Ø,3,4]MZ

Insertion of Generator with Insertion of Lead(s) into Pericardium

Generator Type	Insertion of Generator by Site		Code also as appropriate Insertion of Leads by Type		
	Chest	Abdomen	Pericardium		
			Pacemaker	Defibrillator	Cardiac
Defibrillator	ØJH6[Ø,3]8Z	ØJH8[Ø,3]8Z	Ø2HN[Ø,3,4]JZ	Ø2HN[Ø,3,4]KZ	Ø2HN[Ø,3,4]MZ
Cardiac Resynch Defibrillator Pulse Generator	ØJH6[Ø,3]9Z	ØJH8[Ø,3]9Z	Ø2HN[Ø,3,4]JZ	Ø2HN[Ø,3,4]KZ	Ø2HN[Ø,3,4]MZ

DRG 326-328 Stomach, Esophageal and Duodenal Procedures

Site	Resection by Open Approach	Code also as appropriate Resection of Pancreas by Open Approach
Duodenum	ØDT9ØZZ	ØFTGØZZ

DRG 344-346 Minor Small and Large Bowel Procedures

Site	Repair by Open Approach	Code also as appropriate Repair by external approach of Abdominal Wall Stoma
Small Intestine	ØDQ8ØZZ	ØWQFXZ2
Duodenum	ØDQ9ØZZ	ØWQFXZ2
Jejunum	ØDQAØZZ	ØWQFXZ2
Ileum	ØDQBØZZ	ØWQFXZ2
Large Intestine	ØDQEØZZ	ØWQFXZ2
Large Intestine, Right	ØDQFØZZ	ØWQFXZ2
Large Intestine, Left	ØDQGØZZ	ØWQFXZ2
Cecum	ØDQHØZZ	ØWQFXZ2
Ascending Colon	ØDQKØZZ	ØWQFXZ2
Transverse Colon	ØDQLØZZ	ØWQFXZ2
Descending Colon	ØDQMØZZ	ØWQFXZ2
Sigmoid Colon	ØDQNØZZ	ØWQFXZ2

DRG 456-458 Spinal Fusion Except Cervical with Spinal Curvature/Malignancy/Infection or Extensive Fusions

Fusion of Thoracic and Lumbar Vertebra, Anterior Column

2 to 7 Thoracic Vertebra		Code also 2 or more Lumbar Vertebra	
ØRG[Ø,3,4][7,A,J,K,Z]Ø	XRG7ØF3	ØSG1[Ø,3,4][7,A,J,K,Z]Ø	XRGCØF3

Fusion of Thoracic and Lumbar Vertebra, Posterior Column

2 to 7 Thoracic Vertebra			Code also 2 or more Lumbar Vertebra		
Posterior Approach	Anterior Approach	New Technology	Posterior Approach	Anterior Approach	New Technology
ØRG7[Ø,3,4][7,J,K,Z]1	ØRG7[Ø,3,4][7,A,J,K,Z]J	XRG7Ø92 XRG7ØF3	ØSG1[Ø,3,4][7,J,K,Z]1	ØSG1[Ø,3,4][7,A,J,K,Z]J	XRGCØ92 XRGCØF3

DRG 466-468 Revision of Hip or Knee Replacement

Open Removal of Hip Joint Spacer, Liner, or Resurfacing Device With Supplement of Liner

Body Part	Removal Spacer/Liner/Resurfacing Device	Code also as appropriate Supplement of Body Part by Site		
		Joint	Acetabular Surface	Femoral Surface
Hip, RT	ØSP9Ø[8,9,B]Z	ØSU9Ø9Z	ØSUAØ9Z	ØSURØ9Z
Hip, LT	ØSPBØ[8,9,B]Z	ØSUBØ9Z	ØSUEØ9Z	ØSUSØ9Z

Open Removal of Hip Joint Spacer, Liner, Resurfacing Device, or Synthetic Substitute With Replacement

Body Part	Removal Spacer/Liner/Resurfacing Device/Synthetic Substitute	Code also as appropriate Replacement of Body Part by Device Type						
		Polyethylene	Metal	Metal on Poly	Ceramic	Ceramic on Poly	Oxidized Zirc on Poly	Synth Subst
Hip, RT	ØSP9Ø[8,9,B,J]Z	—	ØSR9Ø1[9,A,Z]	ØSR9Ø2[9,A,Z]	ØSR9Ø3[9,A,Z]	ØSR9Ø4[9,A,Z]	ØSR9Ø6[9,A,Z]	ØSR9ØJ[9,A,Z]
Hip, LT	ØSPBØ[8,9,B,J]Z	—	ØSRBØ1[9,A,Z]	ØSRBØ2[9,A,Z]	ØSRBØ3[9,A,Z]	ØSRBØ4[9,A,Z]	ØSRBØ6[9,A,Z]	ØSRBØJ[9,A,Z]
Acetabular Surface, RT	ØSP9Ø[8,9,B,J]Z	ØSRAØØ[9,A,Z]	ØSRAØ1[9,A,Z]	—	ØSRAØ3[9,A,Z]	—	—	ØSRAØJ[9,A,Z]
Acetabular Surface, LT	ØSPBØ[8,9,B,J]Z	ØSREØØ[9,A,Z]	ØSREØ1[9,A,Z]	—	ØSREØ3[9,A,Z]	—	—	ØSREØJ[9,A,Z]
Femoral Surface, RT	ØSP9Ø[8,9,B,J]Z	—	ØSRRØ1[9,A,Z]	—	ØSRRØ3[9,A,Z]	—	—	ØSRRØJ[9,A,Z]
Femoral Surface, LT	ØSPBØ[8,9,B,J]Z	—	ØSRSØ1[9,A,Z]	—	ØSRSØ3[9,A,Z]	—	—	ØSRSØJ[9,A,Z]

DRG 466-468 Revision of Hip or Knee Replacement *(Continued)*

Percutaneous Endoscopic Removal of Hip Joint Spacer or Synthetic Substitute With Supplement of Liner

Body Part	Removal Spacer/Synthetic Substitute	Code also as appropriate Supplement of Body Part by Site		
		Joint	Acetabular Surface	Femoral Surface
Hip, RT	ØSP94[8,J]Z	ØSU9Ø9Z	ØSUAØ9Z	ØSURØ9Z
Hip, LT	ØSPB4[8,J]Z	ØSUBØ9Z	ØSUEØ9Z	ØSUSØ9Z

Percutaneous Endoscopic Removal of Hip Joint Spacer or Synthetic Substitute With Replacement

Body Part	Removal Spacer/Synthetic Substitute	Code also as appropriate Replacement of Body Part by Device Type					
		Polyethylene	Metal	Metal on Poly	Ceramic	Ceramic on Poly	Synth Subst
Hip, RT	ØSP94[8,J]Z	—	ØSR9Ø1[9,A,Z]	ØSR9Ø2[9,A,Z]	ØSR9Ø3[9,A,Z]	ØSR9Ø4[9,A,Z]	ØSR9ØJ[9,A,Z]
Hip, LT	ØSPB4[8,J]Z	—	ØSRBØ1[9,A,Z]	ØSRBØ2[9,A,Z]	ØSRBØ3[9,A,Z]	ØSRBØ4[9,A,Z]	ØSRBØJ[9,A,Z]
Acetabular Surface, RT	ØSP94[8,J]Z	ØSRAØØ[9,A,Z]	ØSRAØ1[9,A,Z]	—	ØSRAØ3[9,A,Z]	—	ØSRAØJ[9,A,Z]
Acetabular Surface, LT	ØSPB4[8,J]Z	ØSREØØ[9,A,Z]	ØSREØ1[9,A,Z]	—	ØSREØ3[9,A,Z]	—	ØSREØJ[9,A,Z]
Femoral Surface, RT	ØSP94[8,J]Z	—	ØSRRØ1[9,A,Z]	—	ØSRRØ3[9,A,Z]	—	ØSRRØJ[9,A,Z]
Femoral Surface, LT	ØSPB4[8,J]Z	—	ØSRSØ1[9,A,Z]	—	ØSRSØ3[9,A,Z]	—	ØSRSØJ[9,A,Z]

Removal of Hip Joint Surface With Hip Joint Replacement

Body Part	Removal of Spacer/Liner/Resurfacing Device/Synthetic Substitute	Code also as appropriate Replacement of Hip Joint				
		Metal	Metal on Poly	Ceramic	Ceramic on Poly	Synth Subst
Acetabular Surface, RT	ØSPA[Ø,4]JZ	ØSR9Ø1[9,A,Z]	ØSR9Ø2[9,A,Z]	ØSR9Ø3[9,A,Z]	ØSR9Ø4[9,A,Z]	ØSR9ØJ[9,A,Z]
Acetabular Surface, LT	ØSPE[Ø,4]JZ	ØSRBØ1[9,A,Z]	ØSRBØ2[9,A,Z]	ØSRBØ3[9,A,Z]	ØSRBØ4[9,A,Z]	ØSRBØJ[9,A,Z]
Femoral Surface, RT	ØSPR[Ø,4]JZ	ØSR9Ø1[9,A,Z]	ØSR9Ø2[9,A,Z]	ØSR9Ø3[9,A,Z]	ØSR9Ø4[9,A,Z]	ØSR9ØJ[9,A,Z]
Femoral Surface, LT	ØSPS[Ø,4]JZ	ØSRBØ1[9,A,Z]	ØSRBØ2[9,A,Z]	ØSRBØ3[9,A,Z]	ØSRBØ4[9,A,Z]	ØSRBØJ[9,A,Z]

Removal of Hip Joint Surface with Replacement with New Joint Acetabular Surface

Body Part	Removal of Spacer/Liner/Resurfacing Device/Synthetic Substitute	Code also as appropriate Replacement of Acetabular Surface			
		Polyethylene	Metal	Ceramic	Synth Subst
Acetabular Surface, RT	ØSPA[Ø,4]JZ	ØSRAØØ[9,A,Z]	ØSRAØ1[9,A,Z]	ØSRAØ3[9,A,Z]	ØSRAØJ[9,A,Z]
Acetabular Surface, LT	ØSPE[Ø,4]JZ	ØSREØØ[9,A,Z]	ØSREØ1[9,A,Z]	ØSREØ3[9,A,Z]	ØSREØJ[9,A,Z]
Femoral Surface, RT	ØSPR[Ø,4]JZ	ØSRAØØ[9,A,Z]	ØSRAØ1[9,A,Z]	ØSRAØ3[9,A,Z]	ØSRAØJ[9,A,Z]
Femoral Surface, LT	ØSPS[Ø,4]JZ	ØSREØØ[9,A,Z]	ØSREØ1[9,A,Z]	ØSREØ3[9,A,Z]	ØSREØJ[9,A,Z]

Removal of Hip Joint Surface With Replacement with New Joint Femoral Surface

Body Part	Removal of Spacer/Liner/Resurfacing Device/Synthetic Substitute	Code also as appropriate Replacement of Femoral Surface		
		Metal	Ceramic	Synth Subst
Acetabular Surface, RT	ØSPA[Ø,4]JZ	ØSRRØ1[9,A,Z]	ØSRRØ3[9,A,Z]	ØSRRØJ[9,A,Z]
Acetabular Surface, LT	ØSPE[Ø,4]JZ	ØSRSØ1[9,A,Z]	ØSRSØ3[9,A,Z]	ØSRSØJ[9,A,Z]
Femoral Surface, RT	ØSPR[Ø,4]JZ	ØSRRØ1[9,A,Z]	ØSRRØ3[9,A,Z]	ØSRRØJ[9,A,Z]
Femoral Surface, LT	ØSPS[Ø,4]JZ	ØSRSØ1[9,A,Z]	ØSRSØ3[9,A,Z]	ØSRSØJ[9,A,Z]

Percutaneous Endoscopic Removal of Hip Joint Surface With Supplement of Liner

Body Part	Removal of Spacer/Liner/Resurfacing Device/Synthetic Substitute	Code also as appropriate Body Part by Site		
		Joint	Acetabular Surface	Femoral Surface
Acetabular Surface, RT	ØSPA4JZ	ØSU9Ø9Z	ØSUAØ9Z	ØSURØ9Z
Acetabular Surface, LT	ØSPE4JZ	ØSUBØ9Z	ØSUEØ9Z	ØSUSØ9Z
Femoral Surface, RT	ØSPR4JZ	ØSU9Ø9Z	ØSUAØ9Z	ØSURØ9Z
Femoral Surface, LT	ØSPS4JZ	ØSUBØ9Z	ØSUEØ9Z	ØSUSØ9Z

DRG 466-468 Revision of Hip or Knee Replacement *(Continued)*

Removal of Knee Joint, Liner, With Replacement

Body Part	Removal of Liner	Code also as appropriate Replacement of Body Part				
		Joint	Oxidized Zirc on Poly	Unicondylar	Femoral Surface	Tibial Surface
Knee, RT	ØSPCØ9Z	ØSRCØJ[9,A,Z]	ØSRCØ6[9,A,Z]	ØSRCØL[9,A,Z]	ØSRTØJ[9,A,Z]	ØSRVØJ[9,A,Z]
Knee, LT	ØSPDØ9Z	ØSRDØJ[9,A,Z]	ØSRDØ6[9,A,Z]	ØSRDØL[9,A,Z]	ØSRUØJ[9,A,Z]	ØSRWØJ[9,A,Z]

Removal of Knee Joint, Spacer, With Replacement

Body Part	Removal of Spacer	Code also as appropriate Replacement of Body Part			
		Joint	Oxidized Zirc on Poly	Femoral Surface	Tibial Surface
Knee, RT	ØSPC[Ø,3,4]8Z	ØSRCØJ[9,A,Z]	ØSRCØ6[9,A,Z]	ØSRTØJ[9,A,Z]	ØSRVØJ[9,A,Z]
Knee, LT	ØSPD[Ø,3,4]8Z	ØSRDØJ[9,A,Z]	ØSRDØ6[9,A,Z]	ØSRUØJ[9,A,Z]	ØSRWØJ[9,A,Z]

Removal of Knee Joint, Synthetic Substitute, With Replacement

Body Part	Removal of Synthetic Substitute	Code also as appropriate Replacement of Body Part				
		Joint	Oxidized Zirc on Poly	Unicondylar	Femoral Surface	Tibial Surface
Knee, RT	ØSPC[Ø,4]JZ	ØSRCØJ[9,A,Z]	ØSRCØ6[9,A,Z]	ØSRCØL[9,A,Z]	ØSRTØJ[9,A,Z]	ØSRVØJ[9,A,Z]
Knee, LT	ØSPD[Ø,4]JZ	ØSRDØJ[9,A,Z]	ØSRDØ6[9,A,Z]	ØSRDØL[9,A,Z]	ØSRUØJ[9,A,Z]	ØSRWØJ[9,A,Z]

Open Removal of Knee Joint, Patellar Surface, With Replacement

Body Part	Removal of Patellar Surface	Code also as appropriate Replacement of Body Part			
		Joint	Oxidized Zirc on Poly	Femoral Surface	Tibial Surface
Knee, RT	ØSPCØJC	ØSRCØJ[9,A,Z]	ØSRCØ6[9,A,Z]	ØSRTØJ[9,A,Z]	ØSRVØJ[9,A,Z]
Knee, LT	ØSPDØJC	ØSRDØJ[9,A,Z]	ØSRDØ6[9,A,Z]	ØSRUØJ[9,A,Z]	ØSRWØJ[9,A,Z]

Percutaneous Endoscopic Removal of Knee Joint, Patellar Surface, With Replacement

Body Part	Removal of Patellar Surface	Code also as appropriate Replacement of Body Part	
		Joint	Oxidized Zirc on Poly
Knee, RT	ØSPC4JC	ØSRCØJ[9,A,Z]	ØSRCØ6[9,A,Z]
Knee, LT	ØSPD4JC	ØSRDØJ[9,A,Z]	ØSRDØ6[9,A,Z]

Removal of Knee Joint, Synthetic Substitute, With Replacement

Body Part	Removal of Synthetic Sustitute	Code also as appropriate Replacement of Body Part			
		Joint	Oxidized Zirc on Poly	Femoral Surface	Tibial Surface
Femoral Surface, RT	ØSPT[Ø,4]JZ	ØSRCØJ[9,A,Z]	ØSRCØ6[9,A,Z]	ØSRTØJ[9,A,Z]	ØSRVØJ[9,A,Z]
Femoral Surface, LT	ØSPU[Ø,4]JZ	ØSRDØJ[9,A,Z]	ØSRDØ6[9,A,Z]	ØSRUØJ[9,A,Z]	ØSRWØJ[9,A,Z]
Tibial Surface, RT	ØSPV[Ø,4]JZ	ØSRCØJ[9,A,Z]	ØSRCØ6[9,A,Z]	ØSRTØJ[9,A,Z]	ØSRVØJ[9,A,Z]
Tibial Surface, LT	ØSPW[Ø,4]JZ	ØSRDØJ[9,A,Z]	ØSRDØ6[9,A,Z]	ØSRUØJ[9,A,Z]	ØSRWØJ[9,A,Z]

DRG 485-489 Knee Procedures

Joint	Removal of Liner by open approach	Code also as appropriate Supplement of Tibial Surface by Site
Knee, RT	ØSPCØ9Z	ØSUVØ9Z
Knee, LT	ØSPDØ9Z	ØSUWØ9Z

DRG 515-517 Other Musculoskeletal System and Connective Tissue Procedures

Site	Reposition of Vertebra by percutaneous approach	Code also as appropriate Supplement With Synthetic Substitute by Percutaneous Approach at site of Repositioned Vertebra
Cervical	ØPS33ZZ	ØPU33JZ
Coccyx	ØQSS3ZZ	ØQUS3JZ
Lumbar	ØQSØ3ZZ	ØQUØ3JZ
Sacrum	ØQS13ZZ	ØQU13JZ
Thoracic	ØPS43ZZ	ØPU43JZ

DRG 518-52Ø Back and Neck Procedures, Except Spinal Fusion, or Disc Devices/Neurostimulators

Generator Type	Insertion of Generator by Site			Code also as appropriate Insertion Neurostimulator Lead by approach and Site	
	Chest	Abdomen	Back	Spinal Canal	Spinal Cord
Single Array	ØJH6[Ø,3]BZ	ØJH8[Ø,3]BZ	ØJH7[Ø,3]BZ	ØØHU[Ø,3,4]MZ	ØØHV[Ø,3,4]MZ
Single Array, Rechargeable	ØJH6[Ø,3]CZ	ØJH8[Ø,3]CZ	ØJH7[Ø,3]CZ	ØØHU[Ø,3,4]MZ	ØØHV[Ø,3,4]MZ
Multiple Array	ØJH6[Ø,3]DZ	ØJH8[Ø,3]DZ	ØJH7[Ø,3]DZ	ØØHU[Ø,3,4]MZ	ØØHV[Ø,3,4]MZ
Multiple Array, Rechargable	ØJH6[Ø,3]EZ	—	ØJH7[Ø,3]EZ	ØØHU[Ø,3,4]MZ	ØØHV[Ø,3,4]MZ
Multiple Array, Rechargable	—	ØJH8[Ø,3]EZ	—	ØØHU[Ø,3,4]MZ	ØØHVØMZ
Multiple Array, Rechargable	—	ØJH8ØEZ	—	—	ØØHV[3,4]MZ

DRG 582-583 Mastectomy for Malignancy

Site	Resection by Open approach	Code also as appropriate Resection of Lymph Nodes by Open approach by site			Code also as appropriate Resection of Thorax Muscle by Open approach	
		Axillary	Internal Mammary	Thorax	Right	Left
Breast, Right	ØHTTØZZ	Ø7T5ØZZ	Ø7T8ØZZ	Ø7T7ØZZ	ØKTHØZZ	—
Breast, Left	ØHTUØZZ	Ø7T6ØZZ	Ø7T9ØZZ	Ø7T7ØZZ	—	ØKTJØZZ
Breast, Bilateral	ØHTVØZZ	Ø7T5ØZZ and Ø7T6ØZZ	Ø7T8ØZZ and Ø7T9ØZZ	Ø7T7ØZZ	ØKTHØZZ	ØKTJØZZ

DRG 584-585 Breast Biopsy, Local Excision and Other Breast procedures

Resection of Breast With Resection of Lymph Nodes and Thorax Muscle

Site	Resection by Open approach	Code also as appropriate Resection of Lymph Nodes by Open approach by site			Code also as appropriate Resection of Thorax Muscle by Open approach	
		Axillary	Internal Mammary	Thorax	Right	Left
Breast, Right	ØHTTØZZ	Ø7T5ØZZ	Ø7T8ØZZ	Ø7T7ØZZ	ØKTHØZZ	—
Breast, Left	ØHTUØZZ	Ø7T6ØZZ	Ø7T9ØZZ	Ø7T7ØZZ	—	ØKTJØZZ
Breast, Bilateral	ØHTVØZZ	Ø7T5ØZZ and Ø7T6ØZZ	Ø7T8ØZZ and Ø7T9ØZZ	Ø7T7ØZZ	ØKTHØZZ	ØKTJØZZ

Replacement of Breast Tissue

Site	Replacement by Percutaneous approach with Autologous Tissue	Code also as appropriate Extraction of Subcutaneous Tissue by Percutaneous approach					
		Abdomen	Back	Buttock	Chest	Leg, Upper, Right	Leg, Upper, Left
Breast, Right	ØHRT37Z	ØJD83ZZ	ØJD73ZZ	ØJD93ZZ	ØJD63ZZ	ØJDL3ZZ	ØJDM3ZZ
Breast, Left	ØHRU37Z	ØJD83ZZ	ØJD73ZZ	ØJD93ZZ	ØJD63ZZ	ØJDL3ZZ	ØJDM3ZZ
Breast, Bilateral	ØHRV37Z	ØJD83ZZ	ØJD73ZZ	ØJD93ZZ	ØJD63ZZ	ØJDL3ZZ	ØJDM3ZZ

DRG 628-630 Other Endocrine, Nutritional and Metabolic Procedures

Open Removal of Hip Joint Spacer, Liner, Resurfacing Device, or Synthetic Substitute With Replacement

Body Part	Removal Spacer/ Liner/Resurfacing Device/Synthetic Substitute	Code also as appropriate Replacement of Body Part by Device Type					
		Polyethylene	Metal	Metal on Poly	Ceramic	Ceramic on Poly	Synth Subst
Hip, RT	ØSP9Ø[8,9,B,J]Z	—	ØSR9Ø1[9,A,Z]	ØSR9Ø2[9,A,Z]	ØSR9Ø3[9,A,Z]	ØSR9Ø4[9,A,Z]	ØSR9ØJ[9,A,Z]
Hip, LT	ØSPBØ[8,9,B,J]Z	—	ØSRBØ1[9,A,Z]	ØSRBØ2[9,A,Z]	ØSRBØ3[9,A,Z]	ØSRBØ4[9,A,Z]	ØSRBØJ[9,A,Z]
Acetabular Surface, RT	ØSP9Ø[8,9,B,J]Z	ØSRAØØ[9,A,Z]	ØSRAØ1[9,A,Z]	—	ØSRAØ3[9,A,Z]	—	ØSRAØJ[9,A,Z]
Acetabular Surface, LT	ØSPBØ[8,9,B,J]Z	ØSREØØ[9,A,Z]	ØSREØ1[9,A,Z]	—	ØSREØ3[9,A,Z]	—	ØSREØJ[9,A,Z]
Femoral Surface, RT	ØSP9Ø[8,9,B,J]Z	—	ØSRRØ1[9,A,Z]	—	ØSRRØ3[9,A,Z]	—	ØSRRØJ[9,A,Z]
Femoral Surface, LT	ØSPBØ[8,9,B,J]Z	—	ØSRSØ1[9,A,Z]	—	ØSRSØ3[9,A,Z]	—	ØSRSØJ[9,A,Z]

Open Removal of Hip Joint Spacer, Liner, or Resurfacing Device With Supplement of Liner

Body Part	Removal Spacer/Liner/ Resurfacing Device	Code also as appropriate Supplement of Body Part		
		Joint	Acetabular Surface	Femoral Surface
Hip, RT	ØSP9Ø[8,9,B]Z	ØSU9Ø9Z	ØSUAØ9Z	ØSURØ9Z
Hip, LT	ØSPBØ[8,9,B]Z	ØSUBØ9Z	ØSUEØ9Z	ØSUSØ9Z

Percutaneous Endoscopic Removal of Hip Joint Spacer or Synthetic Substitute With Replacement

Body Part	Removal Spacer/Synthetic Substitute	Code also as appropriate Replacement of Body Part by Device Type					
		Polyethylene	Metal	Metal on Poly	Ceramic	Ceramic on Poly	Synth Subst
Hip, RT	ØSP94[8,J]Z	—	ØSR9Ø1[9,A,Z]	ØSR9Ø2[9,A,Z]	ØSR9Ø3[9,A,Z]	ØSR9Ø4[9,A,Z]	ØSR9ØJ[9,A,Z]
Hip, LT	ØSPB4[8,J]Z	—	ØSRBØ1[9,A,Z]	ØSRBØ2[9,A,Z]	ØSRBØ3[9,A,Z]	ØSRBØ4[9,A,Z]	ØSRBØJ[9,A,Z]
Acetabular Surface, RT	ØSP94[8,J]Z	ØSRAØØ[9,A,Z]	ØSRAØ1[9,A,Z]	—	ØSRAØ3[9,A,Z]	—	ØSRAØJ[9,A,Z]
Acetabular Surface, LT	ØSPB4[8,J]Z	ØSREØØ[9,A,Z]	ØSREØ1[9,A,Z]	—	ØSREØ3[9,A,Z]	—	ØSREØJ[9,A,Z]
Femoral Surface, RT	ØSP94[8,J]Z	—	ØSRRØ1[9,A,Z]	—	ØSRRØ3[9,A,Z]	—	ØSRRØJ[9,A,Z]
Femoral Surface, LT	ØSPB4[8,J]Z	—	ØSRSØ1[9,A,Z]	—	ØSRSØ3[9,A,Z]	—	ØSRSØJ[9,A,Z]

Percutaneous Endoscopic Removal of Hip Joint Spacer or Synthetic Substitute With Supplement of Liner

Body Part	Removal Spacer/Synthetic Substitute	Code also as appropriate Supplement of Body Part by Site		
		Joint	Acetabular Surface	Femoral Surface
Hip, RT	ØSP94[8,J]Z	ØSU9Ø9Z	ØSUAØ9Z	ØSURØ9Z
Hip, LT	ØSPB4[8,J]Z	ØSUBØ9Z	ØSUEØ9Z	ØSUSØ9Z

Removal of Hip Joint Surface with Replacement with New Joint Acetabular Surface

Body Part	Removal of Spacer/ Liner/Resurfacing Device/Synthetic Substitute	Code also as appropriate Replacement of Acetabular Surface			
		Polyethylene	Metal	Ceramic	Synth Subst
Acetabular Surface, RT	ØSPA[Ø,4]JZ	ØSRAØØ[9,A,Z]	ØSRAØ1[9,A,Z]	ØSRAØ3[9,A,Z]	ØSRAØJ[9,A,Z]
Acetabular Surface, LT	ØSPE[Ø,4]JZ	ØSREØØ[9,A,Z]	ØSREØ1[9,A,Z]	ØSREØ3[9,A,Z]	ØSREØJ[9,A,Z]
Femoral Surface, RT	ØSPR[Ø,4]JZ	ØSRAØØ[9,A,Z]	ØSRAØ1[9,A,Z]	ØSRAØ3[9,A,Z]	ØSRAØJ[9,A,Z]
Femoral Surface, LT	ØSPS[Ø,4]JZ	ØSREØØ[9,A,Z]	ØSREØ1[9,A,Z]	ØSREØ3[9,A,Z]	ØSREØJ[9,A,Z]

DRG 628-630 Other Endocrine, Nutritional and Metabolic Procedures *(Continued)*

Removal of Hip Joint Surface With Replacement with New Joint Femoral Surface

Body Part	Removal of Spacer/ Liner/Resurfacing Device/Synthetic Substitute	Code also as appropriate Replacement of Femoral Surface		
		Metal	Ceramic	Synth Subst
Acetabular Surface, RT	ØSPA[Ø,4]JZ	ØSRRØ1[9,A,Z]	ØSRRØ3[9,A,Z]	ØSRRØJ[9,A,Z]
Acetabular Surface, LT	ØSPE[Ø,4]JZ	ØSRSØ1[9,A,Z]	ØSRSØ3[9,A,Z]	ØSRSØJ[9,A,Z]
Femoral Surface, RT	ØSPR[Ø,4]JZ	ØSRRØ1[9,A,Z]	ØSRRØ3[9,A,Z]	ØSRRØJ[9,A,Z]
Femoral Surface, LT	ØSPS[Ø,4]JZ	ØSRSØ1[9,A,Z]	ØSRSØ3[9,A,Z]	ØSRSØJ[9,A,Z]

Percutaneous Endoscopic Removal of Hip Joint Surface With Supplement of Liner

Body Part	Removal of Spacer/ Liner/Resurfacing Device/Synthetic Substitute	Code also as appropriate Body Part by Site		
		Joint	Acetabular Surface	Femoral Surface
Acetabular Surface, RT	ØSPA4JZ	ØSU9Ø9Z	ØSUAØ9Z	ØSURØ9Z
Acetabular Surface, LT	ØSPE4JZ	ØSUBØ9Z	ØSUEØ9Z	ØSUSØ9Z
Femoral Surface, RT	ØSPR4JZ	ØSU9Ø9Z	ØSUAØ9Z	ØSURØ9Z
Femoral Surface, LT	ØSPS4JZ	ØSUBØ9Z	ØSUEØ9Z	ØSUSØ9Z

Removal of Knee Joint, Liner, With Replacement

Body Part	Removal of Liner	Code also as appropriate Replacement of Body Part			
		Joint	Unicondylar	Femoral Surface	Tibial Surface
Knee, RT	ØSPCØ9Z	ØSRCØJ[9,A,Z]	ØSRCØL[9,A,Z]	ØSRTØJ[9,A,Z]	ØSRVØJ[9,A,Z]
Knee, LT	ØSPDØ9Z	ØSRDØJ[9,A,Z]	ØSRDØL[9,A,Z]	ØSRUØJ[9,A,Z]	ØSRWØJ[9,A,Z]

Removal of Knee Joint, Patellar Surface, With Replacement

Body Part	Removal of Patellar Surface	Code also as appropriate Replacement of Body Part	
		Femoral Surface	Tibial Surface
Knee, RT	ØSPC[Ø,4]JC	ØSRTØJ[9,A]	ØSRVØJ[9,A]
Knee, LT	ØSPD[Ø,4]JC	ØSRUØJ[9,A]	ØSRWØJ[9,A,Z]

Removal of Knee Joint, Synthetic Substitute, With Replacement

Body Part	Removal of Synthetic Sustitute	Code also as appropriate Replacement of Body Part	
		Femoral Surface	Tibial Surface
Knee, RT	ØSPC[Ø,4]JZ	ØSRTØJ[9,A]	ØSRVØJ[9,A]
Knee, LT	ØSPD[Ø,4]JZ	ØSRUØJ[9,A]	ØSRWØJ[9,A,Z]
Femoral Surface, RT	ØSPT[Ø,4]JZ	ØSRTØJ[9,A]	ØSRVØJ[9,A]
Femoral Surface, LT	ØSPU[Ø,4]JZ	ØSRUØJ[9,A]	ØSRWØJ[9,A,Z]
Tibial Surface, RT	ØSPV[Ø,4]JZ	ØSRTØJ[9,A]	ØSRVØJ[9,A]
Tibial Surface, LT	ØSPW[Ø,4]JZ	ØSRUØJ[9,A]	ØSRWØJ[9,A,Z]

DRG 662-664 Minor Bladder Procedure

Repair of Bladder	Code also as appropriate Repair of Abdominal Wall	
	with Stoma	without Stoma
ØTQB[Ø,3,4]ZZ	ØWQFXZ2	ØWQFXZZ

DRG 665-667 Prostatectomy

Site	Resection by approach				Code also as appropriate Resection of Seminal Vesicles, Bilateral by approach	
	Open	Percutaneous Endoscopic	Via Natural or Artificial Opening	Via Natural or Artificial Opening Endoscopic	Open	Percutaneous Endoscopic
Prostate	ØVTØØZZ	ØVTØ4ZZ	ØVTØ7ZZ	ØVTØ8ZZ	ØVT3ØZZ	ØVT34ZZ

DRG 7Ø7-7Ø8 Major Male Pelvic Procedures

Site	Resection by approach				Code also as appropriate Resection of Seminal Vesicles, Bilateral by approach	
	Open	Percutaneous Endoscopic	Via Natural or Artificial Opening	Via Natural or Artificial Opening Endoscopic	Open	Percutaneous Endoscopic
Prostate	ØVTØØZZ	ØVTØ4ZZ	ØVTØ7ZZ	ØVTØ8ZZ	ØVT3ØZZ	ØVT34ZZ

DRG 734-735 Pelvic Evisceration, Radical Hysterectomy and Radical Vulvectomy

Pelvic Evisceration

Resection by Site						
Bladder	Cervix	Fallopian Tubes, Bilateral	Ovaries, Bilateral	Urethra	Uterus	Vagina
ØTTBØZZ	ØUTCØZZ	ØUT7ØZZ	ØUT2ØZZ	ØTTDØZZ	ØUT9ØZZ	ØUTGØZZ

Radical Hysterectomy

Approach	Resection by Site		
	Cervix	Uterus	Uterine Support Structure
Vaginal	ØUTC[7,8]ZZ	ØUT9[7,8]ZZ	ØUT4[7,8]ZZ
Abdominal, Endoscopic	ØUTC4ZZ	ØUT9[4,F]ZZ	ØUT44ZZ
Abdominal, Open	ØUTCØZZ	ØUT9ØZZ	ØUT4ØZZ

Radical Vulvectomy

Resection by Site	Code also as appropriate Excision of Inguinal Lymph Nodes by Approach	
Vulva	Right	Left
ØUTM[Ø,X]ZZ	Ø7BH[Ø,4]ZZ	Ø7BJ[Ø,4]ZZ

Non-OR procedure combinations

Note: The following table identifies procedure combinations that are considered Non-OR even though one or more procedures of the combination are considered valid DRG OR procedures

Dilation With Removal of Intraluminal Device - Via Natural or Artificial Opening

Code as appropriate Dilation by Site					Code also as appropriate Removal of Intraluminal Device by Site	
Hepatic Duct, Right	Hepatic Duct, Left	Cystic Duct	Common Bile Duct	Pancreatic Duct	Hepatobiliary Duct	Pancreatic Duct
ØF75[7,8]DZ	ØF76[7,8]DZ	ØF78[7,8]DZ	ØF79[7,8]DZ	ØF7D[7,8]DZ	ØFPB[7,8]DZ	ØFPD[7,8]DZ

Insertion With Removal of Intraluminal Device

Code as appropriate Insertion of Intraluminal Device into Hepatobiliary Duct	Code also as appropriate Removal of Intraluminal Device by Approach and Site			
	Via Natural or Artificial Opening		External	
	Hepatobiliary Duct	Pancreatic Duct	Hepatobiliary Duct	Pancreatic Duct
ØFHB[7,8]DZ	ØFPB[7,8]DZ	ØFPD[7,8]DZ	—	—
ØFHB7DZ	—	—	ØFPBXDZ	ØFPDXDZ

Notes

Notes